Editor

JOHN MARQUIS CONVERSE, M.D.

Lawrence D. Bell Professor of Plastic Surgery,
New York University School of Medicine

Assistant Editor

JOSEPH G. McCARTHY, M.D.

Associate Professor of Surgery (Plastic Surgery),
New York University School of Medicine

Editor, section on The Hand

J. WILLIAM LITTLER, M.D.

Chief of Plastic and Reconstructive Surgery,
The Roosevelt Hospital, New York City

SECOND EDITION

RECONSTRUCTIVE PLASTIC SURGERY

*Principles and Procedures
in Correction, Reconstruction
and Transplantation*

VOLUME ONE
GENERAL PRINCIPLES

W. B. SAUNDERS COMPANY

Philadelphia   London   Toronto   Mexico City   Rio de Janeiro   Sydney   Tokyo

W. B. Saunders Company: West Washington Square
Philadelphia, PA 19105

1 St. Anne's Road
Eastbourne, East Sussex BN21 3UN, England

1 Goldthorne Avenue
Toronto, Ontario M8Z 5T9, Canada

Complete Set	0-7216-2691-2
Volume 1	0-7216-2680-7
Volume 2	0-7216-2681-5
Volume 3	0-7216-2682-3
Volume 4	0-7216-2683-1
Volume 5	0-7216-2684-X
Volume 6	0-7216-2685-8
Volume 7	0-7216-2686-6

Reconstructive Plastic Surgery

Last digit is the print number: 9   8

CONTRIBUTORS

JEROME E. ADAMSON, M.D.

Professor of Surgery (Plastic Surgery), Eastern Virginia Medical School. Director, Department of Plastic and Reconstructive Surgery, Medical Center Hospitals, Inc., Norfolk, Virginia. Consultant, Plastic and Hand Surgery, U.S. Public Health Hospital, Norfolk, Virginia; Veterans Administration Hospital, Hampton, Virginia; and U.S. Naval Hospitals, Portsmouth, Virginia, and Bethesda, Maryland.

HANS ANDERL, M.D.

Surgeon in Chief, University Hospital for Plastic and Reconstructive Surgery, Innsbruck, Austria.

STEPHAN ARIYAN, M.D.

Assistant Professor of Surgery, Section of Plastic and Reconstructive Surgery, Yale University School of Medicine, New Haven. Consultant, Veterans Administration Hospital, West Haven, Connecticut.

VINKO ARNERI, M.D.

Professor of Plastic Surgery and Specialist in General Surgery, Military Medical Academy, Belgrade. Director, Klinika za Plasticku Hirurgiju, V.M.A., Belgrade, Yugoslavia.

FRANKLIN L. ASHLEY, M.D.

Adjunct Professor of Surgery, Division of Plastic Surgery, UCLA Center for the Health Sciences, Los Angeles. Attending Physician, St. John's Hospital, Santa Monica, California.

SHERRELL J. ASTON, M.D.

Assistant Professor of Surgery (Plastic Surgery), New York University School of Medicine. Assistant Attending Surgeon, Institute of Reconstructive Plastic Surgery, New York University Medical Center. Chief, Plastic Surgery Service, Veterans Administration Hospital, New York; Associate Attending Surgeon, Manhattan Eye, Ear and Throat Hospital, New York.

FRITZ H. BACH, M.D.

Professor, Medical Genetics, and Director, Immunobiology Research Center, University of Wisconsin Medical School, Madison, Wisconsin.

VAHRAM Y. BAKAMJIAN, M.D.

Assistant Research Professor of Surgery, State University of New York at Buffalo; Clinical Associate Professor of Plastic Surgery, The University of Rochester School of Medicine and Dentistry; Clinical Associate Professor of Surgery, Stanford University.

Associate Chief, Department of Head and Neck Surgery, Roswell Park Memorial Institute, Buffalo, New York.

DONALD L. BALLANTYNE, JR., Ph.D.

Professor of Experimental Surgery, New York University School of Medicine. Chief of Microsurgical Research Laboratories, Institute of Reconstructive Plastic Surgery, New York University Medical Center, New York.

FRITZ E. BARTON, M.D.

Clinical Instructor in Surgery (Plastic Surgery), University of Texas Southwestern Medical School, Dallas. Assistant Attending Surgeon (Plastic Surgery), Baylor University Medical Center, Dallas; Associate Attending Surgeon (Plastic Surgery), Gaston Episcopal Hospital, Dallas, Texas.

ROBERT W. BEASLEY, M.D.

Professor of Surgery (Plastic Surgery), New York University School of Medicine. Director of Hand Surgery Service, Institute of Reconstructive Plastic Surgery, New York University Medical Center; Consultant, Department of Plastic Surgery, Manhattan Eye, Ear and Throat Hospital; Visiting Surgeon and Director, Hand Surgery Service, Bellevue Hospital, New York.

RICHARD J. BELLUCCI, M.D.

Professor and Chairman, Department of Otolaryngology, New York Medical College. Surgeon Director and Chairman, Department of Otolaryngology, Manhattan Eye, Ear and Throat Hospital; Attending Otolaryngologist, Flower Fifth Avenue Hospital, Metropolitan Hospital, St. Luke's Hospital, and New York Hospital, New York.

TRUMAN G. BLOCKER, JR., M.D.

Professor of Surgery (Plastic and Maxillofacial Surgery) and President Emeritus, The University of Texas Medical Branch, Galveston, Texas.

PHILIP C. BONANNO, M.D.

Clinical Associate Professor of Surgery (Plastic Surgery), New York University School of Medicine. Assistant Attending Surgeon, Institute of Reconstructive Plastic Surgery, New York University Medical Center, and Veterans Administration Hospital; Assistant Visiting Surgeon, Bellevue Hospital; Attending Surgeon, United Hospital and Northern Westchester Hospital, New York.

RAYMOND O. BRAUER, M.D.

Associate Clinical Professor of Plastic Surgery, Baylor University College of Medicine; Clinical Associate Professor of Surgery, M.D. Anderson Hospital. Active Staff, Hermann Hospital, St. Luke's Hospital, Memorial Hospital, and Methodist Hospital; Chief of Plastic Surgery, St. Joseph's Hospital and Park Plaza Hospital, Houston, Texas.

BURT BRENT, M.D.

Assistant Clinical Professor and Research Advisor in Plastic Surgery, Stanford University School of Medicine. Surgeon, Stanford University Medical Center and Affiliated Hospitals, Stanford, California.

EARL Z. BROWNE, JR., M.D.

Assistant Professor, Division of Plastic Surgery, University of Utah College of Medicine. Surgeon, University Medical Center, Salt Lake City, Utah.

JOHN C. BULL, JR., M.D.

Active Staff, Phoenix Baptist Hospital, Good Samaritan Hospital, Saint Joseph's Hospital, and John C. Lincoln Hospital, Phoenix, Arizona.

PETER M. CALAMEL, M.B., B.D.S., F.R.C.S.(C)

Associate Chief, Department of Head and Neck Surgery, Roswell Park Memorial Institute, Buffalo, New York.

ROSS M. CAMPBELL, M.D.

Formerly Associate Professor of Clinical Surgery (Plastic Surgery), New York University School of Medicine, and Attending Surgeon in Plastic Surgery, Institute of Reconstructive Plastic Surgery, New York University Medical Center, New York.

BRADFORD CANNON, M.D.

Clinical Professor of Surgery (Emeritus), Harvard Medical School. Senior Consulting Staff, Massachusetts General Hospital, Boston, Massachusetts.

PHILLIP R. CASSON, M.B., F.R.C.S.

Associate Professor of Surgery (Plastic Surgery), New York University School of Medicine. Attending Surgeon, Institute of Reconstructive Plastic Surgery, New York University Medical Center; Bellevue Hospital; Manhattan Eye, Ear and Throat Hospital, and Veterans Administration Hospital, New York.

ROBERT A. CHASE, M.D.

Emile Holman Professor of Surgery and Professor of Anatomy, Stanford University School of Medicine, Stanford, California.

PETER J. COCCARO, D.D.S.

Research Professor of Clinical Surgery (Orthodontics), New York University Medical Center. Associate Professor of Clinical Orthodontics, New York University College of Dentistry. Director of Craniofacial Research, Center for Craniofacial Anomalies, Institute of Reconstructive Plastic Surgery, New York University Medical Center, New York.

CLAUDE C. COLEMAN, JR., M.D.

Associate Clinical Professor of Plastic Surgery, Medical College of Virginia School of Medicine. Director, Head and Neck Surgery, Richmond Memorial Hospital; Chief, Plastic Surgery, Henrico Doctors Hospital, Richmond, Virginia.

JOHN MARQUIS CONVERSE, M.D.

Lawrence D. Bell Professor of Plastic Surgery, New York University School of Medicine; Director, Institute of Reconstructive Plastic Surgery, New York University Medical Center; Director of Plastic Surgery Service, Bellevue Hospital; Consultant in Plastic Surgery, Manhattan Eye, Ear and Throat Hospital and Veterans Administration Hospital, New York.

JOHN D. CONSTABLE, M.D.

Assistant Clinical Professor of Surgery, Harvard Medical School. Visiting Surgeon, Massachusetts General Hospital, Boston, Massachusetts.

STEPHEN G. E. COOLEY, M.D.

Clinical Instructor, Department of Surgery and Department of Orthopedic Surgery and Rehabilitation, University of Miami School of Medicine. Attending Surgeon, Variety Children's Hospital; Staff Surgeon, Victoria Hospital, Miami, Florida.

BARD COSMAN, M.D.

Associate Professor of Clinical Surgery, Columbia University College of Physicians and Surgeons. Associate Attending Surgeon, Presbyterian Hospital, New York; Attending Plastic Surgeon, St. Elizabeth's Division of St. Clare's Hospital and Medical Center, New York; Consultant Plastic Surgeon, Blythedale Hospital for Children, Valhalla, New York.

GEORGE F. CRIKELAIR, M.D.

Professor of Clinical Surgery, Columbia University College of Physicians and Surgeons. Director, Plastic Surgery Service, Columbia-Presbyterian Medical Center. Attending Surgeon, Presbyterian Hospital and St. Elizabeth's Division of St. Clare's Hospital and Medical Center, New York; Attending Surgeon, Valley Hospital, Ridgewood, New Jersey.

DAVID A. CROCKFORD, M.A., M.B., F.R.C.S.

Clinical Lecturer in Plastic Surgery, University of Newcastle-upon-Tyne. Consultant Plastic Surgeon, Royal Victoria Infirmary, Newcastle-upon-Tyne, England.

THOMAS D. CRONIN, M.D.

Clinical Professor of Plastic Surgery, Baylor University College of Medicine. Director, Plastic Surgery Residency Program, St. Joseph's Hospital; Chief, Plastic Surgery, St. Luke's Episcopal Hospital and Texas Children's Hospital; Chief Emeritus, Plastic Surgery, Hermann Hospital; Emeritus Staff, Methodist Hospital; Active Staff, Twelve Oaks and Park Plaza Hospitals, Houston, Texas.

DOUGLAS S. DAHL, M.D.

Assistant Professor of Surgery, University of Utah College of Medicine. Active Staff, University Medical Center, Salt Lake City, Utah.

JOSÉ DELGADO, M.D.

Clinical Associate Professor of Surgery (Plastic Surgery), New York University School of Medicine. Associate Attending Surgeon, Institute of Reconstructive Plastic Surgery, New York University Medical Center, Bellevue Hospital, and Manhattan Eye, Ear and Throat Hospital, New York.

WALLACE M. DENNISON, M.D., F.R.C.S.(Ed.), F.R.C.S.(Glasg.)

Formerly Barclay Lecturer in Surgery of Childhood, University of Glasgow; Senior Surgeon and Chairman of the Division of Surgery, Royal Hospital for Sick Children and Surgical Paediatric Unit, Stobhill Hospital, Glasgow; Paediatric Surgeon, Royal Maternity Hospital, Glasgow, Scotland.

CHARLES J. DEVINE, JR., M.D.

Professor and Chairman, Department of Urology, Eastern Virginia Medical School. Chief, Department of Urology, Medical Center Hospitals, Inc. and DePaul Hospital; Active Staff, Children's Hospital of the King's Daughters, General Hospital of Virginia Beach, Bayside Hospital, and Chesapeake General Hospital, Norfolk, Virginia.

PATRICK C. DEVINE, M.D.

Professor, Department of Urology, Eastern Virginia Medical School. Director, Urology Residency Program, Medical Center Hospitals, Inc. and DePaul Hospital; Active Staff, Children's Hospital of the King's Daughters, Norfolk, Virginia; Consultant, U.S. Naval Hospital, Portsmouth, and Veterans Administration Center, Hampton, Virginia.

REED O. DINGMAN, M.D., D.D.S., D.Sc.

Professor Emeritus of Surgery (Plastic Surgery), University of Michigan School of Medicine. Active Staff, University of Michigan Medical Center and St. Joseph Mercy Hospital, Ann Arbor, Michigan.

MARIO DOBRKOVSKY, M.D.

Plastic Surgeon, Shriners Burns Institute, Galveston, Texas.

MILTON T. EDGERTON, JR., M.D.

Professor and Chairman, Department of Plastic Surgery, University of Virginia School of Medicine. Plastic Surgeon in Chief, University of Virginia Medical Center, Charlottesville; Consultant Plastic Surgeon, Clinical Center (Cancer Division) of The National Institutes of Health, Bethesda, Maryland; Plastic Surgeon, Veterans Administration Hospital, Salem, Virginia.

RAY E. ELLIOTT, JR., M.D.

Associate Clinical Professor of Plastic Surgery and Orthopedic Surgery (Hand), Albany Medical College. Attending Plastic Surgeon, Albany Medical Center Hospital, Albany Memorial Hospital, Albany Veterans Administration Hospital, Cohoes Memorial Hospital, and Child's Hospital, Albany, New York.

MIROSLAV FÁRA, M.D., D.Sc.

Professor of Plastic Surgery, Charles University. Deputy Chief of The Clinic of Plastic Surgery, Prague, Czechoslovakia.

BERNARD F. FETTER, M.D.

Professor of Pathology, Duke University Medical Center, Durham, North Carolina.

ADRIAN E. FLATT, M.D., M.Chir., F.R.C.S.

Professor of Orthopaedic Surgery, University of Iowa College of Medicine. Director, Division of Hand Surgery, University Hospitals, Iowa City, Iowa.

BROMLEY S. FREEMAN, M.D.

Clinical Professor of Plastic Surgery, Baylor University College of Medicine; Clinical Associate in Plastic Surgery, The University of Texas Medical School at Houston. Attending Plastic Surgeon, Methodist Hospital, St. Luke's Hospital, Heights Hospital, St. Joseph's Hospital, Memorial Baptist Hospital, Veterans Administration Hospital, Ben Taub General Hospital, and Hermann Hospital; Consultant in Plastic Surgery, Texas Children's Hospital and Diagnostic Center Hospital, Houston, Texas.

LEONARD T. FURLOW, M.D.

Clinical Associate Professor of Plastic Surgery, University of Florida School of Medicine. Attending Plastic Surgeon, Alachua General Hospital and North Florida Regional Hospital; Consultant in Plastic Surgery, Veterans Administration Hospital, Gainesville, Florida.

JOHN C. GAISFORD, M.D.

Chief, Division of Surgery, Western Pennsylvania Hospital, Pittsburgh, Pennsylvania.

WILLIAM S. GARRETT, JR., M.D.

Clinical Assistant Professor of Surgery (Plastic Surgery), University of Pittsburgh School of Medicine. Active Staff, Presbyterian-University Hospital and Children's Hospital of Pittsburgh, Pennsylvania.

NICHOLAS G. GEORGIADE, M.D., D.D.S.

Professor and Chairman, Division of Plastic, Maxillofacial and Oral Surgery, Duke University Medical Center. Attending Plastic Surgeon, Duke University Medical Center, Watts Hospital, and Lincoln Hospital; Consultant in Plastic, Maxillofacial and Oral Surgery, Veterans Administration Hospital, Durham, North Carolina.

RALPH GER, M.D.

Professor of Surgery and Professor of Anatomy, Albert Einstein College of Medicine. Director of Surgery, Hospital of the Albert Einstein College of Medicine, Bronx, New York.

THOMAS GIBSON, M.B., D.Sc., F.R.C.S.

Senior Lecturer in Tissue Transplantation, University of Glasgow; Visiting Professor in BioEngineering, University of Strathclyde. Regional Director, Glasgow and West of Scotland Regional Plastic and Oral Surgery Unit, Canniesburn Hospital, Glasgow, Scotland.

WILLIAM C. GRABB, M.D.

Professor of Surgery (Plastic Surgery), and Chief, Section of Plastic Surgery, University of Michigan Medical School. Staff Surgeon, University of Michigan Hospital, St. Joseph Mercy Hospital, and Veterans Administration Hospital, Ann Arbor, Michigan.

CARL V. GRANGER, M.D.

Professor and Chairman, Department of Physical and Rehabilitation Medicine, Tufts University School of Medicine. Physiatrist-in-Chief (Specialist in Physical Medicine and Rehabilitation), Rehabilitation Institute, New England Medical Center Hospital, Boston, Massachusetts.

CARY L. GUY, M.D.

Clinical Associate Professor of Surgery (Plastic Surgery), New York University School of Medicine. Associate Attending Surgeon, Institute of Reconstructive Plastic Surgery, New York University Medical Center; Assistant Visiting Surgeon, Bellevue Hospital; Attending Plastic Surgeon, Manhattan Eye, Ear and Throat Hospital, New York.

DWIGHT C. HANNA, III, M.D.

Chief, Department of Plastic and Reconstructive Surgery, Western Pennsylvania Hospital, Pittsburgh, Pennsylvania.

JOSEPH W. HAYHURST, M.D.

Clinical Assistant Professor of Plastic Surgery, University of Oklahoma College of Medicine. Director of the Microsurgery Unit, Presbyterian Hospital, Oklahoma City, Oklahoma.

VINCENT R. HENTZ, M.D.

Clinical Assistant Professor of Surgery, Stanford University School of Medicine. Chief of Hand Clinic, Stanford University Hospital, Stanford; Assistant Chief, Plastic Surgery Section, Veterans Administration Hospital, Palo Alto, California.

JAMES H. HERNDON, M.D.

Assistant Clinical Professor of Surgery (Orthopedic), Michigan State University College of Human Medicine. Orthopedic Surgeon, Blodgett Memorial Medical Center and Mary Free Bed Hospital and Rehabilitation Center; Consultant Orthopedic Surgeon, Butterworth Hospital, Grand Rapids, Michigan.

V. MICHAEL HOGAN, M.D.

Associate Professor of Clinical Surgery (Plastic Surgery), New York University School of Medicine; Assistant Clinical Professor of Dentistry, New York University College of Dentistry. Chief, Cleft Palate Clinic, Institute of Reconstructive Plastic Surgery, New York University Medical Center; Associate Attending Surgeon, University Hospital and Bellevue Hospital; Attending Surgeon, Manhattan Eye, Ear and Throat Hospital, New York.

HERBERT HÖHLER, M.D.

Chief of the Department of Plastic and Reconstructive Surgery, St. Markus Krankenhaus, Frankfurt am Main, Germany.

CHARLES E. HORTON, M.D.

Professor and Chairman, Department of Plastic Surgery, Eastern Virginia Medical School. Chief of Plastic Surgery, Medical Center Hospitals, Inc.; Consultant, DePaul Hospital and Children's Hospital of the King's Daughters, Norfolk, Virginia.

JOHN T. HUESTON, M.S.(Melb.), F.R.C.S., F.R.A.C.S.

Lecturer in Plastic Surgery, University of Melbourne. Consultant Plastic Surgeon, The Royal Melbourne Hospital, Melbourne, Australia.

RICHARD P. JOBE, M.D.

Clinical Associate Professor of Surgery, Stanford University School of Medicine. Surgical Staff, Stanford University Hospital; El Camino Hospital; Veterans Administration Hospital, Palo Alto; and Valley Medical Center, San Jose, California.

DAVID M. C. JU, M.D.

Associate Clinical Professor of Surgery, Columbia University College of Physicians and Surgeons. Associate Attending Surgeon, Presbyterian Hospital, New York.

HENRY K. KAWAMOTO, JR., M.D., D.D.S.

Assistant Clinical Professor, Division of Plastic Surgery, UCLA Center for the Health Sciences, Los Angeles. Attending Plastic Surgeon, Saint John's Hospital and Health Center and Santa Monica Hospital Medical Center, Santa Monica, California.

JOHN J. KEYSER, M.D.

Assistant Attending Surgeon in Plastic, Reconstructive and Hand Surgery, The Roosevelt Hospital, New York.

DAVID M. KNIZE, M.D.

Assistant Clinical Professor in Plastic Surgery, University of Colorado School of Medicine. Attending Plastic Surgeon, Colorado General Hospital, Denver General Hospital, Veterans Administration Hospital, Swedish-Porter Medical Center, Presbyterian Hospital and Children's Hospital, Denver, Colorado.

NORMAN J. KNORR, M.D.

Professor of Psychiatry, Professor of Plastic Surgery, and Associate Dean, University of Virginia School of Medicine. Director, Psychiatric Liaison Consultation Service, University of Virginia Medical Center, Charlottesville; Consultant, Eastern State Hospital, Williamsburg, Virginia.

THOMAS J. KRIZEK, M.D.

Professor of Surgery (Plastic Surgery), Yale University School of Medicine. Chief, Section of Plastic and Reconstructive Surgery, Yale–New Haven Medical Center, New Haven, Connecticut.

SERGE KRUPP, M.D.

Surgeon in Chief, Division of Plastic Surgery, Clinic for Plastic and Reconstructive Surgery, University of Basel, Switzerland.

DUANE L. LARSON, M.D.

Professor of Surgery and Director of the University Burn Unit, The University of Texas Medical Branch. Chief of Staff and Chief Surgeon, Shriners Burns Institute, Galveston, Texas.

RALPH A. LATHAM, B.D.S., Ph.D.

Professor of Paediatric Dentistry, University of Western Ontario, London, Ontario, Canada.

STEPHEN R. LEWIS, M.D.

Professor of Surgery and Chief, Division of Plastic Surgery, The University of Texas Medical Branch. Consultant, St. Mary's Infirmary and Galveston County Memorial Hospital, Galveston, Texas.

J. WILLIAM LITTLER, M.D.

Clinical Professor of Surgery, Columbia University College of Physicians and Surgeons. Attending Surgeon, The Roosevelt Hospital, New York.

J. J. LONGACRE, M.D., Ph.D.†

Late Associate Clinical Professor of Surgery (Plastic Surgery), University of Cincinnati College of Medicine. Attending Plastic Surgeon, Cincinnati General Hospital and Children's Hospital; Director of Plastic Surgery Department, Christ Hospital; Director of Cleft Palate and Craniofacial Clinics, Children's Hospital, Cincinnati, Ohio.

JOHN B. LYNCH, M.D.

Professor and Chairman, Department of Plastic Surgery, Vanderbilt University School of Medicine. Chief of Plastic Surgery, Vanderbilt University Hospital and Nashville Metropolitan General Hospital; Attending Plastic Surgeon, Veterans Administration Hospital, Nashville, Tennessee.

SEAMUS LYNCH, M.D.

Clinical Associate Professor of Anesthesiology, Cornell University Medical College. Director, Department of Anesthesiology, Manhattan Eye, Ear and Throat Hospital; Attending Anesthesiologist, New York Hospital, New York.

JOSEPH G. McCARTHY, M.D.

Associate Professor of Surgery (Plastic Surgery), New York University School of Medicine. Associate Director, Institute of Reconstructive Plastic Surgery, New York University Medical Center. Attending Surgeon, University Hospital, Bellevue Hospital, Manhattan Eye, Ear and Throat Hospital, and Veterans Administration Hospital, New York.

ROBERT M. McCORMACK, M.D.

Professor of Plastic Surgery, Chairman, Division of Plastic Surgery, and Vice-Chairman of Department of Surgery, University of Rochester School of Medicine and Dentistry. Chief Surgeon in Plastic Surgery, Strong Memorial Hospital, Rochester, New York.

JOHN B. McCRAW, M.D.

Associate Clinical Professor of Plastic Surgery, Eastern Virginia Medical School. Attending Surgeon, Medical Center Hospitals, Inc., Norfolk, Virginia; Consultant to Public Health and U.S. Naval Hospitals, Portsmouth, Virginia, and Bethesda, Maryland.

IAN A. McGREGOR, Ch.M., F.R.C.S., F.R.C.S.(Glasg.)

Honorary Clinical Lecturer in Plastic Surgery, University of Glasgow. Consultant Plastic Surgeon, Regional Plastic Surgery Unit, Canniesburn Hospital, and Royal Infirmary and Western Infirmary, Glasgow, Scotland.

---

†Deceased.

FRANCES COOKE MACGREGOR, M.A.

Clinical Associate Professor of Surgery (Sociology), New York University School of Medicine. Sociologist, Institute of Reconstructive Plastic Surgery, New York University Medical Center, New York.

W. BRANDON MACOMBER, M.D.

Professor of Plastic and Reconstructive Surgery, Albany Medical College. Chief of Plastic Surgery, Albany Medical Center Hospital, St. Peter's Hospital, Child's Hospital, Memorial Hospital, and Veterans Administration Hospital, Albany, New York.

FRED M. MASSEY, M.D.

Chief, Gynecologic Oncology, Wilford Hall U.S.A.F. Medical Center, Lackland Air Force Base, Texas.

FRANK W. MASTERS, M.D.

Professor of Surgery, University of Kansas Medical Center. Professor and Chief, Section of Plastic Surgery, Vice Chairman, Department of Surgery, and Associate Dean for Clinical Affairs, University of Kansas Medical Center; Active Staff, St. Luke's Hospital and Veterans Administration Hospital, Kansas City, Missouri.

LESLEY MATHIESON, L.C.S.T.

Senior Speech Therapist, The Middlesex Hospital, London, England.

EUGENE MEYER, M.D.

Professor of Psychiatry and Professor of Medicine, The Johns Hopkins University School of Medicine. Psychiatrist, Physician-in-Charge, OPD-Psychosomatic Clinic, The Johns Hopkins Hospital; Consultant, Sinai Hospital, Baltimore City Hospitals, and Sheppard and Enoch Pratt Hospital, Baltimore, Maryland.

HANNO MILLESI, M.D.

Professor of Plastic Surgery, University of Vienna. Chief of Plastic Surgery Unit, First Surgical University Clinic, Vienna, Austria.

DANIEL C. MORELLO, M.D.

Clinical Instructor in Surgery (Plastic Surgery), New York University School of Medicine. Associate Attending Surgeon, United Hospital, Port Chester; Assistant Attending Surgeon, Manhattan Eye, Ear and Throat Hospital, Northern Westchester Hospital, St. Agnes Hospital, and White Plains Hospital, New York.

HUGHLETT L. MORRIS, Ph.D.

Professor, Department of Otolaryngology and Maxillofacial Surgery and Department of Speech Pathology and Audiology, The University of Iowa, Iowa City, Iowa.

IAN R. MUNRO, F.R.C.S.(C.)

Assistant Professor of Surgery, University of Toronto. Staff Plastic Surgeon, Hospital for Sick Children and Sunnybrook Hospital, Toronto, Canada.

ROSS H. MUSGRAVE, M.D.

Clinical Professor of Surgery (Plastic Surgery), University of Pittsburgh. Active Staff, Presbyterian-University Hospital and Children's Hospital, Pittsburgh, Pennsylvania.

JOHN CLARKE MUSTARDÉ, M.B., Ch.B., D.O.M.S., F.R.C.S., F.R.C.S.(Glasg.)

Clinical Lecturer in Plastic Surgery, University of Glasgow. Consultant Plastic Surgeon, West of Scotland Plastic Surgery Unit, Canniesburn Hospital, Glasgow; Royal Hospital for Sick Children, Glasgow; Ballochmyle Hospital, Ayrshire; and Seafield Sick Children's Hospital, Ayr, Scotland.

ZVI NEUMAN, M.D.†

Professor of Plastic and Maxillofacial Surgery, Hebrew University Hadassah Medical School. Chief, Department of Plastic and Maxillofacial Surgery, Hadassah University Hospital, Jerusalem, Israel.

B. M. O'BRIEN, M.S., F.R.C.S., F.R.A.C.S.

Director of Microsurgery Unit and Assistant Plastic Surgeon, St. Vincent's Hospital, Melbourne, Australia.

F. X. PALETTA, M.D.

Professor of Clinical Surgery and Director of Plastic Surgery, St. Louis University School of Medicine. Director of Cleft Palate Clinic, Cardinal Glennon Hospital for Children; Consultant in Plastic Surgery, Cochran's Veterans Hospital, St. Louis City Hospital, St. Mary's Hospital, and Missouri Pacific Hospital, St. Louis, Missouri.

ERLE E. PEACOCK, M.D.

Department of Surgery, University of Arizona College of Medicine, Tucson.

LYNDON A. PEER, M.D.

Formerly Clinical Professor of Plastic and Reconstructive Surgery, Seton Hall Medical and Dental College, Newark, and Director of Plastic Surgery and of Research, St. Barnabas Medical Center, Livingston, New Jersey.

KENNETH L. PICKRELL, M.D.

Professor of Plastic and Reconstructive Surgery, Duke University Medical Center. Consultant Plastic Surgeon, Veterans Administration Hospitals, Durham and Fayetteville, and Memorial Hospital, Greensboro, North Carolina.

IVO PITANGUY, M.D.

Professor of Plastic and Reconstructive Surgery, Catholic University of Rio de Janeiro. Chief, Plastic Reconstructive Unit, Santa Casa do Rio de Janeiro General Hospital, Rio de Janeiro, Brazil.

JOAN M. PLATT, M.D.

Clinical Associate, University of Connecticut Health Center, Farmington. Courtesy Staff with Assignment, Hartford Hospital, Hartford; Associate in Plastic Surgery, Newington Children's Hospital, Newington, Connecticut.

GEORGE L. POPKIN, M.D.

Professor of Clinical Dermatology, New York University School of Medicine. Attending in Dermatology, Skin and Cancer Unit, New York University Medical Center, New York.

PETER RANDALL, M.D.

Professor of Plastic Surgery, University of Pennsylvania School of Medicine. Chief of Plastic Surgery, Children's Hospital of Philadelphia and Lankenau Hospital; Associate Chief of Plastic Surgery, Hospital of the University of Pennsylvania, Philadelphia, Pennsylvania.

†Deceased.

FELIX T. RAPAPORT, M.D.

Professor of Surgery and Director, Transplantation and Immunology Division, New York University School of Medicine. Director of Research, Institute of Reconstructive Plastic Surgery, New York University Medical Center. Associate Attending Surgeon, University Hospital; Visiting Surgeon, Bellevue Hospital; Consultant, Veterans Administration Hospital, New York.

THOMAS D. REES, M.D.

Clinical Professor of Surgery (Plastic Surgery), New York University School of Medicine. Attending Surgeon, Institute of Reconstructive Plastic Surgery, New York University Medical Center. Visiting Surgeon, Bellevue Hospital; Chairman, Department of Plastic Surgery, Manhattan Eye, Ear and Throat Hospital, New York.

PERRY ROBINS, M.D.

Associate Professor of Clinical Dermatology, New York University School of Medicine. Attending Physician, University Hospital, Bellevue Hospital, and Veterans Administration Hospital, New York.

DAVID W. ROBINSON, M.D.

Professor of Surgery and Director, Gene and Barbara Burnett Burn Center, University of Kansas Medical Center. Active Staff, University of Kansas Medical Center, St. Luke's Hospital, and Veterans Administration Hospital, Kansas City, Missouri.

BLAIR O. ROGERS, M.D.

Associate Professor of Clinical Surgery (Plastic Surgery), New York University School of Medicine. Attending Surgeon, Institute of Reconstructive Plastic Surgery, New York University Medical Center. Attending Surgeon, Department of Plastic Surgery, Manhattan Eye, Ear and Throat Hospital, New York.

R. B. ROSS, D.D.S., F.R.C.S.(C.)

Assistant Professor of Dentistry, University of Toronto. Chief of Dentistry, The Hospital for Sick Children, Toronto, Canada.

BURGOS T. SAYOC, M.D.

Doctor of Medicine and Surgery, University of the Philippines. Surgeon-Director, Sayoc Eye, Ear, Nose and Throat Clinic and Hospital, Quezon City, Philippines.

MARTIN F. SCHWARTZ, Ph.D.

Research Associate Professor of Surgery (Speech Pathology), New York University School of Medicine. Speech Pathologist, Institute of Reconstructive Plastic Surgery, New York University Medical Center, New York.

WILLIAM W. SHAW, M.D.

Instructor in Surgery (Plastic Surgery), New York University School of Medicine. Assistant Attending Surgeon, Institute of Reconstructive Plastic Surgery, New York University Medical Center. Chief, Plastic Surgery, Bellevue Hospital, New York.

ALAN R. SHONS, M.D., Ph.D.

Assistant Professor of Surgery, University of Minnesota School of Medicine. Chief, Division of Plastic Surgery, University of Minnesota Hospital; Active Staff, St. Paul Ramsey Hospital and Veterans Administration Hospital, Minneapolis, Minnesota.

BYRON SMITH, M.D.

Clinical Professor of Ophthalmology, New York Medical College. Consultant in Oculoplastic Surgery, Manhattan Eye, Ear and Throat Hospital and The New York Eye-Ear Infirmary, New York.

JAMES W. SMITH, M.D.

Associate Professor of Clinical Surgery (Plastic Surgery), Cornell University Medical College. Associate Attending Surgeon (Plastic Surgery), New York Hospital; Attending Plastic Surgeon, Veterans Administration Hospital, Bronx; Assistant Attending Surgeon (Plastic Surgery), Arthur C. Logan Hospital and Knickerbocker Hospital, New York.

CLIFFORD C. SNYDER, M.D.

Professor and Chairman, Division of Plastic Surgery, University of Utah College of Medicine. Chief, Surgical Services, Veterans Administration Hospital; Chief, Plastic Surgery Service, Shriners Hospital for Crippled Children, Salt Lake City, Utah.

REUVEN K. SNYDERMAN, M.D.

Clinical Professor of Surgery (Plastic Surgery), College of Medicine and Dentistry of New Jersey, Rutgers Medical School. Chief, Section of Plastic and Reconstructive Surgery, Rariton Valley Hospital, Greenbrook; Attending Physician, Department of Surgery, Division of Plastic and Reconstructive Surgery, Princeton Medical Center, Princeton, New Jersey.

DUANE C. SPRIESTERSBACH, Ph.D.

Professor of Speech Pathology, University of Iowa, Iowa City, Iowa.

RICHARD BOIES STARK, M.D.

Professor of Clinical Surgery, Columbia University College of Physicians and Surgeons. Attending Surgeon in Charge of Plastic Surgery, St. Luke's Hospital, New York.

CHESTER A. SWINYARD, M.D., Ph.D.

Professor of Rehabilitation Medicine, New York University School of Medicine. Attending Physician, Institute of Rehabilitation Medicine, New York University Medical Center. Associate Attending Physician, Bellevue Hospital, New York.

RADFORD C. TANZER, M.D.

Clinical Professor of Plastic Surgery Emeritus, Dartmouth Medical School, Hanover, New Hampshire. Consultant in Plastic Surgery, Veterans Administration Hospital, White River Junction, Vermont.

JAMES S. THOMPSON, M.D.

Attending Hand Surgeon, Memorial Mission Hospital and St. Joseph's Hospital, Asheville, North Carolina.

NOEL THOMPSON, M.S., F.R.C.S.

Clinical Tutor and Specialist Examiner in Plastic Surgery, University of London. Consultant Plastic Surgeon, The Middlesex Hospital, London, and the Plastic Surgery Centre, Mount Vernon Hospital, Northwood, Middlesex, England.

AUGUSTUS J. VALAURI, D.D.S.

Professor of Surgery (Maxillofacial Prosthetics), New York University School of Medicine; Clinical Associate Professor of Removable Prosthodontics, New York University College of Dentistry. Chief of the Maxillofacial Prosthetics Service, Institute of Reconstructive Plastic Surgery, New York University Medical Center; Acting Chief of Dental Service, Manhattan Eye, Ear and Throat Hospital; Attending Staff, Bellevue Hospital; Consultant, Veterans Administration Hospital, New York.

MARK K. H. WANG, M.D.

Clinical Professor of Plastic Surgery, Albany Medical College. Attending Plastic Surgeon, Albany Medical Center Hospital, St. Peter's Hospital, Child's Hospital, Memorial Hospital, and Veterans Administration Hospital, Albany, New York.

R. C. A. WEATHERLEY-WHITE, M.D.

Associate Clinical Professor of Surgery (Plastic Surgery), University of Colorado Medical School. Director, Plastic Surgery Division, Denver General Hospital; Coordinator, Cleft Palate Clinic, Children's Hospital, Denver, Colorado.

MENACHEM RON WEXLER, M.D.

Associate Professor of Plastic Surgery, Hebrew University Hadassah Medical School. Chief Surgeon, Department of Plastic and Maxillofacial Surgery, Hadassah University Hospital, Jerusalem, Israel.

DONALD WOOD-SMITH, M.B., F.R.C.S.E.

Associate Professor of Surgery (Plastic Surgery), New York University School of Medicine. Surgeon Director, Department of Plastic Surgery, Manhattan Eye, Ear and Throat Hospital; Attending Surgeon, Institute of Reconstructive Plastic Surgery, New York University Medical Center; Visiting Surgeon in Plastic Surgery, Bellevue Hospital; Attending Surgeon, Veterans Administration Hospital; Consultant, New York Eye and Ear Infirmary, New York.

PREFACE
to the Second Edition

The first edition of *Reconstructive Plastic Surgery*, widely distributed throughout the world, was considered by many to be the standard reference for plastic surgeons. A second edition is long overdue. There were a number of factors in the delay: an upsurge of activity at the Institute of Reconstructive Plastic Surgery; fulfillment of a promise made to V. H. Kazanjian to write a third edition of our book *The Surgical Treatment of Facial Injuries*, published in 1974; and the rapid advances in plastic surgical concepts and techniques since 1964. Constant revision has been required to keep the contents of the chapters up to date.

Not since World War II has plastic surgery gained so much prestige or have so many advances been made as in the last decade: evolution of new concepts in flap surgery based on expanding knowledge of skin circulation; increased understanding of the biology of wound healing and tissue transplantation; reduction in burn morbidity and mortality; reconstruction of the face by complex craniofacial osteotomies; introduction of the microscope into vascular and nerve repair, enabling the free transfer of composite tissue and the replantation of severed parts; new concepts in the treatment of acute injuries and deformities of the upper extremity; and refinements in surgery of the aging face. This edition incorporates these and other advances, which have been built on a foundation of surgical principles established in the past.

The titles of the one hundred chapters that make up this work constitute a listing of subjects that encompass and define the scope of plastic surgery. A perusal of the table of contents shows that *Reconstructive Plastic Surgery* covers many subjects that have been considered the appanage or special endowment of allied specialties. The word "allied" is particularly applicable to a philosophy that implies teamwork, a collaboration of specialists. An ecumenical approach benefits both patient and surgeon. The plastic surgeon can learn from his colleagues in the clinical fields and from research workers in basic sciences, thus enlarging the body of knowledge of the specialty.

Since my early training I have witnessed the fragmentation of general surgery and the rise of new surgical specialties and of subspecialties. Forecasting "Surgery in the twenty-first century," J. Englebert Dunphy wrote, "Surgical care will be delivered exclusively by specialists and at varying levels of primary to tertiary care. Specialization will be even greater than at present so that the old-fashioned general surgeon of the past will disappear. Very difficult or complicated operations within the established specialties will be performed by superspecialists" (Surgery, *75*:332, 1974).

But how to coordinate the activities of the superspecialists? The answer is the orchestral concept. The virtuosi play their individual instruments, but the orchestra conductor ensures harmony and the success of the concert—a word that originally meant an understanding or harmony between a number of persons. No single plastic surgeon can be an expert in all areas of the specialty. The solution, therefore, is the team. The resident in training thus benefits from the teaching of each expert within the group of specialists.

It is difficult to unite all aspects of plastic surgery under one roof. A multiple hospital organization offers the resident exposure to the greatest variety of clinical problems and those of allied specialties. Such an arrangement exists at the New York University Medical Center, which includes the Institute of Reconstructive Plastic Surgery in the University Hospital, Bellevue Hospital Medical Center, the New York Veterans Hospital, and a teaching affiliation with the Department of Plastic Surgery at the Manhattan Eye, Ear and Throat Hospital.

In the Preface to the first edition I gave tribute to the many coauthors who contributed to its success. My gratitude and indebtedness is again expressed to those who revised their chapters and to the new authors who introduced new ideas and techniques. Together we were able to rejuvenate a text which, after being reprinted a number of times, is widely read 13 years after its publication.

Dr. J. William Littler, master of hand surgery, has edited the section on surgery of the upper extremity. He has left his imprint and injected his own philosophy of diagnosis and treatment throughout the section.

Dr. Joseph G. McCarthy, Associate Director of the Institute, has given talent, time and energy to make possible the completion of this extensive revision and has made many original suggestions which have enhanced its usefulness.

We can confidently predict the progressive growth of our specialty, a specialty with unlimited possibilities engendered by the fertile imagination of the plastic surgeon, whose ideal combines a vision of the desirable with an appreciation of the attainable.

JOHN MARQUIS CONVERSE, M.D.

ACKNOWLEDGMENTS

To all of my associates in the Institute of Reconstructive Plastic Surgery I owe a debt of gratitude, for together we have achieved a level of expertise which none of us could have reached individually: Sherrell J. Aston, M.D.; Daniel C. Baker, M.D.; Robert W. Beasley, M.D.; Robert W. Bernard, M.D.; Philip C. Bonanno, M.D.; Ross M. Campbell, M.D.; Phillip R. Casson, F.R.C.S.; José Delgado, M.D.; Cary L. Guy, M.D.; V. Michael Hogan, M.D.; Joseph G. McCarthy, M.D.; Daniel C. Morello, M.D.; Thomas D. Rees, M.D.; Blair O. Rogers, M.D.; William W. Shaw, M.D.; and Donald Wood-Smith, F.R.C.S.E.

There are many others whose collaboration during each day's work must be mentioned here. I have had a long and fruitful association with Byron Smith in the treatment of orbital deformities. Felix T. Rapaport, director of research and president-elect of the Transplantation Society, has been a close associate and friend since the initiation of transplantation research many years ago. Donald L. Ballantyne now heads an experimental and clinical laboratory for microsurgery. Our dental colleagues Peter J. Coccaro, director of craniofacial research, and Augustus J. Valauri, chief of maxillofacial prosthetics, have provided indispensable help in the treatment of patients with craniofacial and maxillofacial deformities.

To all members of the multidisciplinary team at the New York University Medical Center and in particular to radiologist Melvin Becker and neurosurgeons Joseph M. Ransohoff and Fred Epstein I express warm thanks for unstinting and talented collaboration. Frances Cooke Macgregor has worked with me since the beginning of my career on the psychological and sociological problems associated with facial deformities. Her books and articles have earned her a special status as an authority on this important aspect of our specialty.

Now turning to the task of preparing this second edition, my debt to my coeditors and to the contributing writers has been mentioned in the Preface. Over two hundred personal communications were received from authoritative sources, illuminating and clarifying particular points. Each of these communications has been duly acknowledged in the text.

A number of our residents have assisted in the arduous task of reading proof. Thanks are expressed to Doctors Daniel C. Baker, Fritz E. Barton, Henry Kawamoto, David M. Knize, Hissam Maiwandi, Daniel C. Morello, Gerald H. Pitman, Robert E. Reber and William W. Shaw.

Pauline Porowski, R.N., again demonstrated her devotion and ability to maintain order in an abundance of manuscripts, galley proof, page proof, drawings and photographs, as well as to locate missing references. Typing and retyping manuscripts is an often thankless task; appreciation is expressed to Caren Crane, Joan Hercke, Janette Swords, Marjorie Bent, Patricia Anderson and Winifred Bridgman.

Two talented people with very special skills have been associated with me ever since I started working in New York soon after World War II. Miss Daisy Stilwell, pupil of Max Brödel, in addition to her unquestioned talent, has acquired through the years a knowledge of plastic surgery which has enabled her to edit the numerous illustrations. Mr. Don Allen is an outstanding professional in medical photography.

Deep-felt appreciation is expressed to Mr. Henry Steeger, President, and the Trustees of the Society for the Facially Disfigured, who established and are supporting the Institute, to Mr. DeWitt Wallace for his continued backing, to Mr. Charles Wohlstetter for making possible the establishment of the Center for Craniofacial Anomalies, and to the foundations and individuals who have helped in so many ways. Mr. Robert E. Bochat, executive director of the Society for the Facially Disfigured and my administrative assistant, has been the indispensable link between the diverse activities of our Institute.

From a small clinic built on a roof at the Manhattan Eye, Ear and Throat Hospital in 1955 grew the concept of a full-scale Institute of Reconstructive Plastic Surgery at the New York University Medical Center. Dr. Ivan L. Bennett, Jr., Dean and Provost, Dr. Frank Cole Spencer, George David Stewart Professor of Surgery, Dr. Howard A. Rusk and many other colleagues are thanked for providing, at the New York University Medical Center, the environment for the development of the Institute and its programs.

Our publishers the W. B. Saunders Company and particularly editors Ruth Hope and RoseMarie Sorrentino, illustration coordinator Kathleen Collier and production manager Herbert J. Powell, Jr. deserve the gratitude of all who have participated in the task of assembling the body of knowledge to be found in these seven volumes.

Each volume, as in the first edition, has been kept to a size that is easy to handle. Each also contains the index to the entire book for the convenience of the reader. Placing each of the illustrations in proximity to the relevant text has been a problem that required careful planning in many chapters. It could not be entirely resolved despite painstaking care. The reader will be indulgent when he realizes that special attention has been given to this task.

A special word of appreciation is extended to the Williams & Wilkins Company for graciously allowing reproduction of numerous illustrations that originally appeared in *The Surgical Treatment of Facial Injuries* (herein cited briefly as "Kazanjian and Converse").

Finally it must be recognized that in spite of the effort that has been devoted to the matter, errors may remain, and in particular accurate acknowledgment of historical priorities may have eluded both authors and editors.

J. M. C.

PREFACE
to the First Edition

This treatise is the result of the concerted efforts of my coauthors; to them I express my indebtedness and my gratitude.

The work attempts to assemble present-day knowledge concerning the rapidly growing field of reconstructive plastic surgery. Each author was asked to treat the subject assigned to him in the manner he felt most suitable. Because of limitations in the already lengthy text, many distinguished plastic surgeons who have made important contributions to the specialty could not be included as coauthors. They will find, however, that their work has been referred to repeatedly in the various chapters.

My friend Dr. J. William Littler, master of hand surgery, added immeasurably to the value of the work by editing, illustrating and contributing to the section devoted to surgery of the hand and upper extremity.

Special care has been taken to ensure uniformity of the terminology throughout the text, which is the terminology generally employed in the specialty journals of the English speaking world. An effort was made to clarify and simplify the language and apply simple terms in the place of the pedantic terms often favored by the medical profession. English has become the international language of medicine. May this simplification of the text make it more understandable throughout the world.

The text has been divided into seven parts: 1, General Principles; 2, The Head and Neck; 3, The Hand and Upper Extremity; 4, The Lower Extremity; 5, The Trunk; 6, The Genitourinary System and Anorectal Malformations; and 7, Tissue Transplantation and Burn Shock.

For the convenience of the reader, the text has been published in five volumes. Ernest Hemingway once stated that no book should be so large that it could not be read in bed, and it is hoped that the reader will find these volumes easier to handle than the originally projected two large volumes.

The opening chapters deal with the basic principles of plastic surgery. The philosophy of plastic surgery cannot be taught in a textbook, however, but only through the guidance of a master surgeon in the clinical management of the patient. There is never a day that I do not give silent tribute to my own teachers, Kazanjian and Gillies, and feel privileged to attempt to teach others as they have taught me.

Specialization in surgery was a consequence of the development of abdominal surgery. Prior to his entry into the abdominal cavity, the surgeon's activity was largely confined to what was often referred to as "external pathology," in contra-distinction to "internal pathology" considered to be amenable to medical care only. Specialization was necessary when the surgeon's activities became too diversified as new fields of surgical endeavor were developed.

Recognition of plastic surgery by the medical profession, now an accomplished fact, was slow. Saving life and restoring function have been the mission of the physician; the concept of surgery for the improvement of facial appearance, of corrective or cosmetic surgery, was more difficult to accept. Changing concepts have resulted from the reclamation of severly injured individuals by workers in the various aspects of rehabilitation; from the often dramatic results obtained through reconstructive surgery, particularly in victims of war; from the recognition of the importance of the teachings of psychiatry and of the need for corrective surgery for the mental well-being of the patient.

The sheer ever-increasing numbers of individuals who are the victims of accidents, who suffer disability and disfigurement from the resection of tissue for the eradication of tumors, or as a result of a destructive disease such as leprosy, or who are born with a congenital malformation have created a demand for highly skilled professional care.

Disfigurements of the body and, in particular, because of its special social significance, disfigurement of the face, have deep psychologic repercussions. Perhaps in no field of medicine is the careful psychologic evaluation and handling of the patient more necessary than in plastic surgery. The finality of the surgical result may not be accepted by the patient, who must be led progressively to the realization that his remaining physical handicap must not preclude his return to active social participation. If success in plastic surgery, as Gillies has stated, is a matter of balance between beauty and blood supply, success in the psychologic handling of the patient is a matter of balance between hope and truth — hope: the patient expects total correction of his deformity and the solution of all his associated problems; truth: an improvement, small or large, can be achieved but may not meet the patient's expectations of total recovery. These aspects are discussed in Chapters 15 and 16.

Volumes 2 and 3 of the text deal with the corrective and reconstructive surgery of deformities of the head and neck, including cleft lip and palate, a frequent congenital deformity.

Volume 4 covers the reconstructive surgery of the hand and extremities. The face and hands have many aspects in common from the viewpoint of the plastic surgeon. They are exposed areas of the body; their shape and movements characterize the individual; they participate in communication and social interaction. The face and hands are activated by a finely differentiated musculature; the fine movements of the digits are reminiscent of the delicate shades of expression produced by the facial musculature of expression. Surgery of the hand requires a thorough understanding of the anatomic, physiologic and functional aspects of hand disabilities.

Plastic surgery of various deformities of the trunk, including the breast, of the genitourinary system, of anorectal malformations, and recent advances in transplantation are described in Volume 5 of the text.

The plastic surgeon, that daily transplanter, must consider himself akin to the transplantation biologist. Transplantation biology is at the forefront of the phenomenal advances in surgery of recent years. Transplantation of tissues and replacement of structures and organs, physiologically worn out, resected for disease or amputated in accidents, will be one of the major tasks of the surgeon of the future. The plastic surgeon, because of his experience in transplantation in his clinical practice, his ability to perform delicate and intricate techniques, is admirably suited by temperament and training to play a leading role in the development of transplantation surgery. The teaching of transplantation biology should become an integral part of the teaching of the plastic surgery resident.

Preoccupied by the details of surgical technique, the plastic surgeon may find himself devoting the major portion of his vital energy to activities in the operating room. Progress is made through the application of a sum of knowledge to the resolution of a particular problem and time must be allowed for the necessary observations and conclusions. A rationing of activities, an efficient distribution of effort are best achieved if the surgeon has a well organized hospital service. This requires the attribution of a sufficient number of hospital beds, operating rooms and research facilities. Good quality patient care goes hand in hand with resident teaching and research activities.

Emphasis must be laid upon the need for the interdisciplinary approach to many of the complex clinical problems of plastic surgery. Collaboration with members of the allied surgical specialties, of medicine, dentistry, speech pathology, psychiatry and the social sciences is often required to achieve the physical and psychosocial rehabilitation of the patient.

Because of the diversity of plastic surgery in its various clinical applications, the future plastic surgeon should receive the broadest possible preliminary training in surgery and the surgical specialties. A trained surgeon prior to his residency in plastic surgery, he will soon begin to see the solution to the various clinical problems through the eyes of a plastic surgeon; he will learn to make the diagnosis of the deformity and to visualize repair in terms of fit and form; where to make his incisions; how to design a flap; when to graft to ensure maximum survival. He has become a plastic surgeon because he is thinking as a plastic surgeon and is now capable of applying the principles of plastic surgery to any area of the body.

JOHN MARQUIS CONVERSE, M.D.

CONTENTS

VOLUME 1

Part One. General Principles

CHAPTER 1
INTRODUCTION TO PLASTIC SURGERY 3

John Marquis Converse

CHAPTER 2
THE PHYSICAL PROPERTIES OF SKIN 69

Thomas Gibson

CHAPTER 3
REPAIR AND REGENERATION 78

Erle E. Peacock

CHAPTER 4
CONGENITAL MALFORMATIONS: GENERAL CONSIDERATIONS 104

Chester A. Swinyard

CHAPTER 5
TRANSPLANTATION BIOLOGY 126

Alan R. Shons, John Marquis Converse and Felix T. Rapaport

GENETICS OF TRANSPLANTATION 139

Fritz H. Bach

CHAPTER 6
TRANSPLANTATION OF SKIN: GRAFTS AND FLAPS 152

John Marquis Converse, Joseph G. McCarthy,
Raymond O. Brauer and Donald L. Ballantyne

Dᴇʀᴍᴀʟ Oᴠᴇʀɢʀᴀғᴛɪɴɢ 183

Noel Thompson

Rᴇɪɴɴᴇʀᴠᴀᴛɪᴏɴ ᴏғ Sᴋɪɴ Tʀᴀɴsᴘʟᴀɴᴛs....................... 226

Joan M. Platt

Tʀᴀɴsᴘʟᴀɴᴛᴀᴛɪᴏɴ ᴏғ Hᴀɪʀ-Bᴇᴀʀɪɴɢ Sᴄᴀʟᴘ 229

Jerome E. Adamson

CHAPTER 7
TRANSPLANTATION OF DERMIS 240

Noel Thompson

CHAPTER 8
TRANSPLANTATION OF FAT 251

Lyndon A. Peer

CHAPTER 9
TRANSPLANTATION OF FASCIA 262

Reuven K. Snyderman

CHAPTER 10
TRANSPLANTATION OF TENDON 266

D. A. Crockford

CHAPTER 11
TRANSPLANTATION OF SKELETAL MUSCLE 293

Noel Thompson

CHAPTER 12
TRANSPLANTATION OF CARTILAGE 301

Thomas Gibson

CHAPTER 13
TRANSPLANTATION OF BONE 313

J. J. Longacre, John Marquis Converse and David M. Knize

CHAPTER 14
**PRINCIPLES AND TECHNIQUES OF
MICROVASCULAR SURGERY** 340

B. M. O'Brien and J. W. Hayhurst

CHAPTER 15
INORGANIC IMPLANTS 392
Thomas D. Rees, Richard P. Jobe and Donald L. Ballantyne, Jr.

CHAPTER 16
SCARS AND KELOIDS 413
George F. Crikelair, David M. C. Ju and Bard Cosman

CHAPTER 17
SURGICAL AND CHEMICAL PLANING OF THE SKIN 442
Ross M. Campbell

CHAPTER 18
THERMAL BURNS 464
John B. Lynch and Truman G. Blocker, Jr.

ELECTRICAL BURNS 512
John Marquis Converse and Donald Wood-Smith

CHAPTER 19
COLD INJURY 516
David M. Knize

CHAPTER 20
RADIATION EFFECTS: BIOLOGICAL AND SURGICAL CONSIDERATIONS 531
Stephan Ariyan and Thomas J. Krizek

CHAPTER 21
PSYCHIATRIC ASPECTS OF PLASTIC SURGERY 549
Eugene Meyer and Norman J. Knorr

CHAPTER 22
A SOCIAL SCIENCE APPROACH TO THE STUDY OF FACIAL DEFORMITIES AND PLASTIC SURGERY 565
Frances Cooke Macgregor

CHAPTER 23
THE ROLE OF THE ANESTHESIOLOGIST IN PLASTIC SURGERY 585
Seamus Lynch

VOLUME 2

Part Two. The Head and Neck

CHAPTER 24

**THE CLINICAL MANAGEMENT OF FACIAL INJURIES
AND FRACTURES OF THE FACIAL BONES** 599

Reed O. Dingman and John Marquis Converse

CHAPTER 25

ORBITAL AND NASO-ORBITAL FRACTURES 748

John Marquis Converse, Byron Smith and Donald Wood-Smith

CHAPTER 26

FACIAL INJURIES IN CHILDREN 794

John Marquis Converse and Reed O. Dingman

CHAPTER 27

**DEFORMITIES OF THE FOREHEAD, SCALP
AND CALVARIUM** 822

J. J. Longacre and John Marquis Converse

CHAPTER 28

**DEFORMITIES OF THE EYELIDS AND ADNEXA,
ORBIT AND THE ZYGOMA**

*John Marquis Converse, Byron Smith, Mark K. H. Wang,
W. Brandon Macomber, John Clarke Mustardé, Burgos T. Sayoc,
Ray A. Elliott, Jr., Augustus J. Valauri, Serge Krupp and
Donald Wood-Smith*

THE EYELIDS AND THEIR ADNEXA 858

SURGICAL CORRECTION OF THE ORIENTAL EYELID 947

DEFORMITIES OF THE EYEBROW 956

THE ORBIT 962

DEFECTS OF THE LACRIMAL SYSTEM 980

MALUNITED FRACTURES OF THE ORBIT 989

CHAPTER 29

**CORRECTIVE AND RECONSTRUCTIVE SURGERY OF
THE NOSE** 1040

CORRECTIVE RHINOPLASTY 1040

John Marquis Converse

CONGENITAL CHOANAL ATRESIA 1163

John Marquis Converse, Donald Wood-Smith and William W. Shaw

CONGENITAL TUMORS OF THE NOSE 1169

Mark K. H. Wang and W. Brandon Macomber

CONGENITAL ANOMALIES OF THE NOSE............................ 1178

Mark K. H. Wang

RHINOPHYMA.. 1185

Bromley S. Freeman

MALIGNANT TUMORS OF THE NOSE 1192

John Marquis Converse and Phillip R. Casson

DEFORMITIES OF THE SKIN OF THE NOSE 1195

John Marquis Converse

DEFORMITIES OF THE LINING OF THE NOSE...................... 1199

John Marquis Converse

FULL-THICKNESS LOSS OF NASAL TISSUE....................... 1209

John Marquis Converse

VOLUME 3

CHAPTER 30
DEFORMITIES OF THE JAWS 1288

*John Marquis Converse, Henry K. Kawamoto, Jr.,
Donald Wood-Smith, Peter J. Coccaro and Joseph G. McCarthy*

CHAPTER 31
DISTURBANCES OF THE TEMPOROMANDIBULAR JOINT....... 1521

Nicholas G. Georgiade

CHAPTER 32
DEFORMITIES OF THE LIPS AND CHEEKS 1540

*John Marquis Converse, Donald Wood-Smith, W. Brandon Macomber
and Mark K. H. Wang*

CHAPTER 33
FACIAL BURNS 1595

*John Marquis Converse, Joseph G. McCarthy, Mario Dobrkovsky
and Duane L. Larson*

CHAPTER 34
DEFORMITIES OF THE CERVICAL REGION 1643

Thomas D. Cronin

CHAPTER 35
DEFORMITIES OF THE AURICLE.................................... 1671

Congenital Deformities 1671
Radford C. Tanzer

Congenital Auricular Malformation: Indications,
Contraindications and Timing of Middle Ear Surgery:
An Otologist's Viewpoint.. 1719
Richard J. Bellucci

Acquired Deformities.. 1724
John Marquis Converse and Burt Brent

CHAPTER 36
FACIAL PALSY 1774
Bromley S. Freeman

Autogenous Muscle Grafts in the Reconstruction of the
Paralyzed Face.. 1841
Noel Thompson

Reconstruction of the Face Through Cross-Face
Nerve Transplantation in Facial Paralysis......................... 1848
Hans Anderl

CHAPTER 37
ESTHETIC SURGERY FOR THE AGING FACE............................ 1868
Cary L. Guy, John Marquis Converse and Daniel C. Morello

VOLUME 4

CHAPTER 38
CLEFT LIP AND PALATE: INTRODUCTION............................ 1930
*John Marquis Converse, V. Michael Hogan and
Joseph G. McCarthy*

CHAPTER 39
EMBRYOLOGY OF CLEFT LIP AND PALATE 1941
Richard B. Stark

CHAPTER 40
**THE ANATOMY OF THE FACIAL SKELETON IN CLEFT
LIP AND PALATE** 1950
R. A. Latham

CHAPTER 41
THE MUSCULATURE OF CLEFT LIP AND PALATE................. 1966
Miroslav Fára

CHAPTER 42
FACIAL GROWTH IN CLEFT LIP AND PALATE........................ 1989
R. B. Ross

CHAPTER 43
THE UNILATERAL CLEFT LIP 2016
Ross H. Musgrave and William S. Garrett, Jr.

CHAPTER 44
THE BILATERAL CLEFT LIP WITH BILATERAL CLEFT
OF THE PRIMARY PALATE 2048
Thomas D. Cronin

CHAPTER 45
CLEFT PALATE 2090
Richard B. Stark

SUBMUCOUS CLEFT PALATE 2104
Miroslav Fára and R. C. A. Weatherley-White

CHAPTER 46
RARE CRANIOFACIAL CLEFTS.. 2116
Henry K. Kawamoto, Jr., Mark K. H. Wang and W. Brandon Macomber

CHAPTER 47
SECONDARY DEFORMITIES OF CLEFT LIP, CLEFT LIP
AND NOSE, AND CLEFT PALATE... 2165
John Marquis Converse, V. Michael Hogan and Fritz E. Barton

CHAPTER 48
BONE GRAFTING IN THE CLEFT PALATE PATIENT 2205
John Marquis Converse and David M. Knize

CHAPTER 49
ORTHODONTICS IN CLEFT LIP AND PALATE CHILDREN 2213
Peter J. Coccaro and Augustus J. Valauri

CHAPTER 50
THE ROBIN ANOMALAD: MICROGNATHIA AND
GLOSSOPTOSIS WITH AIRWAY OBSTRUCTION 2235
Peter Randall

CHAPTER 51
SPEECH PROBLEMS OF PATIENTS WITH CLEFT LIP
AND PALATE.. 2246
Duane C. Spriestersbach and Hughlett L. Morris

CHAPTER 52
VELOPHARYNGEAL INCOMPETENCE.................................... 2268
V. Michael Hogan and Martin F. Schwartz

CLEFT PALATE PROSTHETICS 2283
Augustus J. Valauri

CHAPTER 53
**EMBRYOLOGY OF THE FACE AND INTRODUCTION TO
CRANIOFACIAL ANOMALIES** 2296
Blair O. Rogers

CHAPTER 54
CRANIOFACIAL MICROSOMIA...................................... 2359
*John Marquis Converse, Joseph G. McCarthy, Donald Wood-Smith
and Peter J. Coccaro*

CHAPTER 55
MANDIBULOFACIAL DYSOSTOSIS 2401
Blair O. Rogers

CHAPTER 56
PRINCIPLES OF CRANIOFACIAL SURGERY 2427
*John Marquis Converse, Joseph G. McCarthy, Donald Wood-Smith
and Peter J. Coccaro*

RESHAPING THE CRANIAL VAULT................................... 2492
Ian R. Munro

VOLUME 5

CHAPTER 57
**GENERAL PRINCIPLES IN THE SURGICAL TREATMENT
OF PATIENTS WITH HEAD AND NECK CANCER** 2509
Milton T. Edgerton, Jr., and John C. Bull, Jr.

CHAPTER 58
**SURGICAL TREATMENT OF DISEASE OF THE
SALIVARY GLANDS**.. 2521
David W. Robinson and Frank W. Masters

CHAPTER 59
TUMORS OF THE JAW 2547
Nicholas G. Georgiade and Bernard F. Fetter

CHAPTER 60
MALIGNANT TUMORS OF THE MAXILLA 2574
Franklin L. Ashley, Philip C. Bonanno and Phillip R. Casson

CHAPTER 61
OROMANDIBULAR TUMORS: RECONSTRUCTIVE ASPECTS 2589
John C. Gaisford and Dwight C. Hanna, III

CHAPTER 62
RECONSTRUCTION FOLLOWING EXCISION OF INTRAORAL AND MANDIBULAR TUMORS 2642
Ian A. McGregor

CHAPTER 63
OROPHARYNGEO-ESOPHAGEAL RECONSTRUCTIVE SURGERY 2697
Vahram Y. Bakamjian and Peter M. Calamel

CHAPTER 64
TUMORS INVOLVING THE CRANIOFACIAL SKELETON 2757
Claude C. Coleman, Jr.

CHAPTER 65
TUMORS OF THE SKIN 2776
A DERMATOLOGIST'S VIEWPOINT 2776
George L. Popkin
A PLASTIC SURGEON'S VIEWPOINT 2817
F. X. Paletta
MALIGNANT MELANOMA 2841
Phillip R. Casson
SUPERFICIAL FORMS OF SKIN CANCER 2853
F. X. Paletta
CHEMOSURGERY 2880
Phillip R. Casson and Perry Robins

CHAPTER 66
CONGENITAL CYSTS AND TUMORS OF THE NECK 2902
Raymond O. Brauer

CHAPTER 67
MAXILLOFACIAL PROSTHETICS 2917
Augustus J. Valauri

VOLUME 6

Part Three. The Hand and Upper Extremity
Edited by J. William Littler, M.D.

CHAPTER 68
SURGERY OF THE HAND: INTRODUCTION 2953
J. William Littler

CHAPTER 69
SURGICAL ANATOMY OF THE HAND 2957
Robert A. Chase

CHAPTER 70
EXAMINATION OF THE HAND 2964
J. William Littler, James H. Herndon and James S. Thompson

THE NAILS 2976
J. J. Keyser

ELECTRODIAGNOSTIC EXAMINATION 2981
Carl V. Granger

CHAPTER 71
DRESSINGS AND SPLINTS 2991
James S. Thompson and J. William Littler

CHAPTER 72
PRINCIPLES OF MANAGING ACUTE HAND INJURIES 3000
Robert W. Beasley

CHAPTER 73
**PRINCIPLES OF RECONSTRUCTIVE SURGERY
OF THE HAND** 3103
J. William Littler

CHAPTER 74
**CONSERVATION OF USABLE STRUCTURES
IN INJURED HANDS** 3154
Robert A. Chase

CHAPTER 75
THE DIGITAL EXTENSOR-FLEXOR SYSTEM 3166
J. William Littler

CHAPTER 76
REPAIR OF PERIPHERAL NERVES 3215
William C. Grabb and J. W. Smith

NERVE GRAFTING 3227
Hanno Millesi

CHAPTER 77
REPLANTATION SURGERY 3243
B. M. O'Brien

CHAPTER 78
**RESTORATION OF POWER AND STABILITY IN THE
PARTIALLY PARALYZED HAND** 3266
J. William Littler

CHAPTER 79
**THE SURGICAL MANAGEMENT OF CONGENITAL
HAND ANOMALIES** 3306
Vincent R. Hentz and J. William Littler

CHAPTER 80
RECONSTRUCTION OF THE THUMB IN TRAUMATIC LOSS ... 3350
J. William Littler

CHAPTER 81
THE BURNED UPPER EXTREMITY 3368

BURNS OF THE HAND 3368
Erle E. Peacock, Jr.

THE IMMEDIATE MANAGEMENT OF BURNS OF THE DORSAL
HAND SURFACE (EMPHASIS ON EARLY TANGENTIAL EXCISION) 3381
Menachem Ron Wexler and Zvi Neuman

BURNS OF THE AXILLA AND ELBOW 3391
Robert W. Beasley

CHAPTER 82
DUPUYTREN'S CONTRACTURE 3403
John T. Hueston

CHAPTER 83
NERVE AND TENDON ENTRAPMENT SYNDROMES 3428

THE CARPAL TUNNEL SYNDROME 3428
Radford C. Tanzer

ULNAR TUNNEL SYNDROME 3437
J. William Littler

STENOSING DIGITAL TENDOVAGINITIS 3440
J. William Littler

DEQUERVAIN'S DISEASE (STENOSING TENDOVAGINITIS) 3443
J. William Littler

CHAPTER 84
TUMORS OF THE HAND AND FOREARM 3449
Stephen G. E. Cooley

CHAPTER 85
THE ARTHRITIC HAND 3507
Adrian E. Flatt

VOLUME 7

Part Four. The Lower Extremity

CHAPTER 86
**RECONSTRUCTIVE SURGERY OF THE
LOWER EXTREMITY** 3521
*Bradford Cannon, John D. Constable, Leonard T. Furlow,
Joseph W. Hayhurst, Joseph G. McCarthy and John B. McCraw*

CLOSURE OF DEFECTS OF THE LOWER EXTREMITY
BY MUSCLE FLAPS 3549
Ralph Ger

CLOSURE OF DEFECTS OF THE LOWER EXTREMITY
BY MYOCUTANEOUS FLAPS 3560
John B. McCraw

CHAPTER 87
LYMPHEDEMA 3567
Stephen R. Lewis

Part Five. The Trunk

CHAPTER 88
CHEST WALL RECONSTRUCTION 3609
Sherrell J. Aston and Kenneth L. Pickrell

CHAPTER 89
PLASTIC SURGERY OF THE BREAST 3661
Thomas D. Rees

RECONSTRUCTION OF THE FEMALE BREAST AFTER
RADICAL MASTECTOMY 3710
Herbert Höhler

CHAPTER 90
**RECONSTRUCTIVE SURGERY OF THE
ABDOMINAL WALL**.. 3727
Sherrell J. Aston and Kenneth L. Pickrell

Spina Bifida.. 3749
John C. Mustardé and Wallace M. Dennison

CHAPTER 91
THE PRESSURE SORE 3763
Ross M. Campbell and José P. Delgado

CHAPTER 92
**DERMOLIPECTOMY OF THE ABDOMINAL WALL, THIGHS,
BUTTOCKS AND UPPER EXTREMITY** 3800
Ivo Pitanguy

Part Six. The Genitourinary System

CHAPTER 93
EMBRYOLOGY OF THE GENITOURINARY SYSTEM 3827
Clifford C. Snyder, Douglas S. Dahl and Earl Z. Browne, Jr.

CHAPTER 94
**HYPOSPADIAS: SOME HISTORICAL ASPECTS AND THE
EVOLUTION OF TECHNIQUES OF TREATMENT** 3835
Donald Wood-Smith

CHAPTER 95
HYPOSPADIAS 3845
Charles E. Horton and Charles J. Devine, Jr.

CHAPTER 96
EPISPADIAS AND EXSTROPHY OF THE BLADDER 3862
Clifford C. Snyder and Earl Z. Browne, Jr.

CHAPTER 97
STRICTURES OF THE MALE URETHRA 3883
Patrick C. Devine and Charles E. Horton

Peyronie's Disease 3895
Charles E. Horton and Charles J. Devine, Jr.

CHAPTER 98
RECONSTRUCTION OF THE MALE GENITALIA 3902
Vinko Arneri

CHAPTER 99

ABNORMALITIES OF THE EXTERNAL FEMALE GENITALIA... 3922
Richard Boies Stark

VAGINAL RECONSTRUCTION FOLLOWING ABLATIVE SURGERY
BY GRACILIS MYOCUTANEOUS FLAPS 3926
John B. McCraw and Fred M. Massey

CHAPTER 100

INTERSEX PROBLEMS AND HERMAPHRODITISM 3930
Clifford C. Snyder and Earl Z. Browne, Jr.

EPILOGUE 3970

INDEX i

Part One

GENERAL
PRINCIPLES

CHAPTER 1

INTRODUCTION TO PLASTIC SURGERY

JOHN MARQUIS CONVERSE, M.D.

What is Plastic Surgery? Plastic surgery is a specialized branch of surgery concerned with deformities and defects of the integument and the underlying musculoskeletal framework.

The origins of the art of plastic surgery, rooted in ancient history, are related to the relief of facial deformity, in particular to reconstruction of the amputated nose, and thus the restoration of the individual, the person. A person: the noun person is derived from the Latin "persona," which signified the mask that actors wore and then, by metonymy, the role played by the actor, the personage he represented in the play (persona dramatis). The word has gradually become synonymous, in general, with personality, with the idea of individuality, the individual.

We have taken for granted that each human face is different, that no human face has ever been reduplicated among the millions that surround us and the billions that have preceded us. Not even a facial feature has ever been reproduced. The uniqueness of the individual, which extends to the subcellular level, is the clue to the diversity of the facial features of man, his facial expression with its infinite variants, the timbre of his voice, his posture, his movements, and the entire mysterious psychosomatic complex that constitutes the personality of a human being.

It was only many centuries later, in the nineteenth century, that the principles and techniques of plastic surgery were applied to other areas of the body. Surgery of the hand was developed only in the present century.

Because of the special nature of plastic surgery, it is largely concerned with form, as is implied in the term "plastic." Functional aspects of plastic surgery are also important: for example, reestablishing the continuity of the mandible to permit mastication, restoring the function of the hand, or making possible the healing of a compound fracture of the tibia by providing adequate soft tissue coverage over the fractured bone.

A paramount quality required for plastic surgery is a sense of form, an esthetic judgment, and an ability to visualize the end result. Webster in his foreword to the textbook by Gillies and Millard, *The Principles and Art of Plastic Surgery* (1957), quotes from Aristotle's "On the Parts of Animals": "Art, indeed, consists in the conception of the result to be produced before its realization in the material." Perhaps this quality is the most essential requisite for a plastic surgeon; it is the quality that distinguishes the artist from the technician.

The term "plastique" was used by Desavit in 1798. "Plastic surgery" was part of the title of Zeis's book, *Handbuch der plastischen Chirurgie,* in 1838. Von Graefe was the first to employ the term "plastic" in his monograph entitled *Rhinoplastik* published in Berlin in 1818. In most countries, the term "plastic surgery" designates the specialty.

3

Until the end of the nineteenth century, plastic surgery was essentially reconstructive. With the perfection of techniques, the correction of minor defects that are congenital in nature or secondary to aging came to be practiced. Thus corrective or *esthetic* surgery in contradistinction to *reconstructive* surgery provided another challenge for the plastic surgeon. Although no clear distinction between the two types of plastic surgery is required, there being an esthetic aspect in reconstructive surgery and often a reconstructive aspect in esthetic surgery, the terms *reconstructive* and *esthetic* are convenient only to differentiate between the surgery of major and minor defects.

Gillies often mentioned a definition which I recall. He defined reconstructive surgery as an attempt to restore the individual to the normal; esthetic surgery, he stated, attempts to surpass the normal. The relief of facial disfigurement, the restoration of function, the closure of defects—these are easily understood goals and imperative surgical procedures. But what is the "normal"? Esthetic concepts have changed from century to century, from decade to decade, and from culture to culture.

A review of the progressive development of plastic surgery helps one to understand the present status of the specialty—thus the following brief account of the history of plastic surgery. Additional historical data are included in many chapters of this text.

THE AGES OF PLASTIC SURGERY

In an address to the Royal College of Physicians Winston Churchill remarked, "The longer you look back, the further you can look forward." Similarly, the thoughts, struggles, and efforts of those who have preceded us form the foundations of the present-day practice of plastic surgery. Plastic surgery is one of the oldest forms of surgery. Its often told history will not be reviewed in detail in this textbook. The reader is referred to the works listed in the bibliography at the end of the chapter.

Although ancient man practiced trephination of the skull, specialized surgery appears to have been practiced by the Babylonians during the time of Hammurabi (circa 1950 B.C.) when the operation for cataract was performed as a legitimate surgical procedure.

In India, Sushruta, the Hippocrates of the sixth or seventh century before Christ (Rogers, 1967), described operations for the reconstruction of the nose and the earlobes in the Sushruta samita (translated by Bhishagratna, 1916). Amputation of the nose was a common practice to punish criminals and the inhabitants of conquered cities. The operation was performed by members of a caste of potters known as the Koomas (see Chapter 29, p. 1209). Knowledge of these operations probably filtered through the Persians, the Greeks, the Arabs, the Nestorian Christian communities in India, Persia, and Iraq and through Jewish scholars to Rome (Gnudi and Webster, 1950).

Celsus (25 B.C. to 50 A.D.) used advancement flaps (Fig. 1–1, *A* to *C*). It is not clear whether the flaps were raised prior to advancement, as was done in the nineteenth century under the name of "flaps according to the French method" or "gliding flaps" ("lambeaux par glissement"). He was probably the originator of the island flap with a subcutaneous pedicle (Fig. 1–1, *D, E*.).

Galen (130 to 200 A.D.) did not concern himself with plastic surgery techniques. Progress in surgical techniques during the period of the Roman Empire was epitomized by Paulus Aegineta (625 to 690 A.D.), thought to have been a major link between the medical learning of the Hindu and Arab schools and the increasing number of Western scholars during his lifetime. He may be considered one of the originators of plastic surgery as we know it today (Rogers, 1974). He described

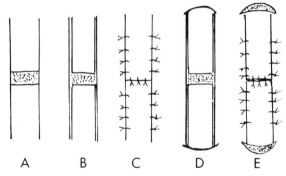

FIGURE 1–1. Operation for cure of a mutilation (of nose, lips, or ears), as performed by Celsus (25 B.C.–50 A.D.) *A*, Quadrilateral incisions for the excision of the mutilation. *B*, Skin and underlying tissue raised as flaps on opposite sides of the excised area. *C*, Flaps drawn together and sutured to cover the area. *D*, Semilunar incisions to relieve tension. *E*, Relaxed flaps drawn together, leaving two lunate raw areas to heal by secondary intention. (From Spencer, W. G.: Celsus: De medicina; with an English translation. Vol. 3. Cambridge, Mass., Harvard University Press, 1938. Redrawn from B. O. Rogers, in Wood-Smith, D., and Porowski, P. C.: Nursing Care of the Plastic Surgery Patient. St. Louis, Mo., C. V. Mosby Company, 1967.)

procedures varying from the treatment of nasal and jaw fractures to operations for hypospadias. With the death of Paulus Aegineta, the enrichment of medical and surgical knowledge provided by the Greco-Roman period came to an end.

The rise of Islam enhanced the prestige of Arabic medicine. It has been suggested that contacts between the Arabs, the invaders of Sicily, and the local practitioners, such as members of the Branca family, led to the transmission of the art of reconstructive rhinoplasty as practiced in ancient India. Occidental medicine thus is indebted to Arabic medicine. Arabian scholars in the 8th century A.D. provided Arabic translations of the work of the famed Indian practitioner Sushruta, which were subsequently translated into Latin (Gnudi and Webster, 1950).

The Renaissance

The period of the Renaissance or rebirth of civilization which marked the transition from the Middle Ages emerged in Italy in the fourteenth century, reaching its height during the fifteenth and sixteenth centuries. The cultural enrichment spread throughout Europe, often intermingling with older interests and forces and flourishing in different lands.

During the first half of the fifteenth century, plastic surgery came to be practiced in Sicily by members of the Branca family. Sicily was a center of Arabic, Greek, and Occidental learning during the earlier centuries, and it is thought that the elder Branca used the method of repair described by Sushruta. Antonio Branca, the son, abandoned the ancient Indian method and was probably the first to use a flap from the arm to repair mutilated lips and ears.

During the sixteenth century the Vianeo family practiced the art of plastic surgery in the region of Calabria in the southwestern part of the Italian peninsula. A number of other practitioners appeared to have repaired mutilated noses. Symonds' observations (1935) on the increase of violence during the period from 1530 to 1600 are of particular interest: "Compared with the middle ages, compared with the Renaissance, this period is distinguished by extraordinary ferocity of temper and by an almost unparalleled facility of blood shed."

Remarks of Paré. The need for reconstructive operations during the sixteenth century due to the frequent duels and clashes of armed men appears to have coincided with an increased interest in this branch of surgery. The renowned surgeon Ambroise Paré warned, however, of the extreme difficulty and discomfort of the operation for the repair of a mutilated nose:

We have testimony of this from a gentleman named the Cadet of St. Thoan, who, having lost his nose and having long worn one of silver, became angry at the remark that there was never a lack of laughing matter when he was present. And having heard that there was in Italy a master re-maker of lost noses, he went to find him, and he made a new one for him in the way described above as an infinite number of people have since seen him, not without the great marvelling of those who had known him before with a silver nose. Such a thing is not impossible; nevertheless it seems to me very difficult and burdensome to the patient, both because of the trouble of keeping the head down with the arm for so long a time, and because of the pain of the incisions made in healthy parts, cutting and lifting away the part of the flesh of the arm to form the nose; in addition, this flesh is not of the same quality nor similar to that of the nose, and even when agglutinated and reformed it can never be of the same shape and color as that which was former in the place of the lost nose, likewise the openings of the nostrils can never be as they were originally."

Paré apparently shared the common misunderstanding concerning the arm flap technique of nose repair, as he named the biceps muscle as the donor site and specified 40 days as the period requisite for union.

Paré's negative attitude was all the more surprising as he expressed the horror of his contemporaries for facial mutilations in his book published in 1575:

Having arrived in the town. I entered a stable and there I found four soldiers who were dead and three who were leaning against the wall, their faces completely disfigured and they could not see nor could they hear or speak and their clothes were still smoking from the gun powder that had burnt them. As I was looking at them with pity, an old soldier approached me and asked me if there was any way by which I could cure them: I answered that there was no way. Suddenly he approached each one of them and cut his throat, gently and without anger. Seeing this cruel action I told him that he was a bad man to have done this. He answered that he prayed God that if he should be so afflicted there would be someone who would render him the same service rather than allow him to languish miserably.

Work of Tagliacozzi. It would appear that Paré never came to know the work of the man who was to lay the cornerstone of modern plastic surgery, Gaspare Tagliacozzi of Bologna. The work of Tagliacozzi, particularly in nose reconstruction, was renowned throughout Europe. His treatise "De Curtorum Chirurgia per Insitionem," published in 1597, summarizes his life's work. In describing the technique of preparing the arm flap for transplantation to reconstruct the nose, he specified the delayed flap and in Chapter 10, "The proper age of the flap when we make the implanting," he stated, "It is not well to implant the flap in its age of infancy because then it is not strong enough, it has suffered the violence of the first operation, and is subject to inflammation or hemorrhage. Nor is its youth the proper time as it is then still not firm enough and is subject to various evils. Nor yet should one await its old age, for by then it has become too wrinkled, blanched, pallid and juiceless." But "when it has reached the age of manhood and has entirely hardened, and now begins to be turned, strong enough and fortified to sustain the force of the operation, it is necessary to take the flap, and to join it with the missing parts in the new union of grafting, for it cannot be done better or more safely. Thus it will satisfy the hopes of ourselves and of the patient abundantly. Between the taking up of the flap and the insertion (about fourteen days) the patient is not limited as to diet and may go about freely" (Gnudi and Webster, 1950).

The Seventeenth and Eighteenth Centuries: The Decline

Tagliacozzi's technique was probably little practiced during the seventeenth and eighteenth centuries. The decline of plastic surgery after the death of Tagliacozzi parallels the decline of surgery, which was languishing throughout all of Europe, particularly in Italy. The errors which Tagliacozzi had combated so vigorously augmented the misconception and fears that stifled its acceptance. Finally the whole subject, including Tagliacozzi's name, became the object of ridicule from the pens of the wits of the polite society of the eighteenth century.

The greatest hindrance to the acceptance and use of plastic surgical operations came from a misconception that reparative tissue could be taken from a slave or person other than the patient and that under such circumstances, a kind of mystic sympathy existed between the new nose and the person from whom it had been taken, causing the nose to die when the original donor died.

The encyclopedist or "philosophes," a group of scientific determinists (Diderot published the first volume of the "encyclopédie" in 1751), had great influence during the eighteenth century. One of the encyclopedists, Voltaire, wrote a satirical poem concerning the "sympathetic" slave, the donor tissue having been taken from a slave's buttocks. Ironically, the age of enlightenment was not an age of enlightenment for plastic surgery. Although it has been stated that the Faculty of Medicine of Paris interdicted face repairing during the eighteenth century, there appears to be no truth to the statement. What did happen was that a thesis, "Whether defective noses can be remade from the arm," was rejected by the Faculty. The jokes about "nose and face repairing" during this period, although more cruel, were not unlike the jokes made during the period of development of esthetic surgery in our era.

Second Rebirth

A Report from India. In October, 1794, a letter was written to Mr. Urban, the editor of the Gentleman's Magazine published in London. The letter stated that a friend in India had communicated to the author the following report on a hitherto unknown operation which had long been practiced successfully in those parts. The letter concerned an incident that had occurred in the Third Mysore War waged by the British East Indian forces against Sultan Tippoo.

Cowasjee, a bullock-driver with the English army in the war of 1792, was made a prisoner by Tippoo, who cut off his nose, and one of his hands. In this state, he joined the Bombay army near Seringapatam, and is now a pensioner of the Honorable East India Company. For about twelve months, he was wholly without a nose; when he had a new one put on, by a Mahratta surgeon.... This operation is not uncommon in India, and has been practiced from time immemorial.

Two of the medical gentlemen, Mr. Thomas Cruso, and Mr. James Findlay, of Bombay, have seen it performed as follows: a thin plate of wax is fitted to the stump of the nose, so as to make a nose of good appearance; it is then flattened, and laid on the forehead. A line is drawn round the wax, which is then of no further use; and the operator then dissects off as much skin as it covered, leaving undivided a small slip between the eyes. This slip preserves the circulation, till an union has taken place between the new and old parts.

The cicatrix of the stump of the nose is next pared off; and, immediately behind this raw part, an incision is made through the skin, which passes round both alae, and goes along the upper lip. The skin is now brought down from the forehead; and, being twisted half round, its edge is inserted into this incision; so that a nose is formed with a double hold, above, and with its alae and septum below, fixed in the incision.

A little Terra Japonica is softened with water, and, being spread on slips of cloth, five or six of these are placed over each other, to secure the joining. No other dressing than this cement is used for four days; it is then removed, and cloths, dipped in *ghee* (a kind of butter), are supplied. The connecting slip of skin is divided about the twenty-fifth day, when a little more dissecting is necessary to improve the appearance of the new nose.

For five or six days after the operation, the patient is made to lie on his back; and on the tenth day, bits of soft cloth are put into the nostrils to keep them sufficiently open. This operation is always successful. The artifical nose is secure, and looks nearly as well as the natural one; nor is the scar on the forehead very observable, after a length of time.

Chance played a part, as it often does. Joseph Carpue, who at the time was 30 years old, read the story of Cowasjee and there rose before his eyes the images of all those hapless souls whose faces had been shattered. If such an operation were possible in India, he reasoned, it should also be possible in Europe. He began seeking more detailed reports of the operation. He questioned all the army men and civil servants who returned to London from India, in the hope that they might be able to give him some information. Altogether, he devoted nearly 20 years to investigating this matter. Carpue even located Lieutenant-Colonel Ward, who had been commander of the unit to which Cowasjee belonged and who had witnessed the operation. Cowasjee had fallen into Tippoo's hands along with four other Indian soliders. All five had had their noses and hands cut off and had been sent back to the English troops as terrifying examples. They were a ghastly sight. Leaves had been bound over the stumps of their wrists to stop the bleeding, but the horrible vestiges of their noses had not even been bandaged.

Another chance encounter occurred when Ward noticed a scar on the bridge of a peddler's nose and inquired what it was from. The peddler admitted that his original nose had been cut off by the headman of his home village in punishment for adultery. He pointed out another scar on his forehead and described how an artist had shaped a new nose out of the skin of his forehead for him. This operation was often performed, he said, because the punishment of cutting off a nose was so common. Ward then sent for the practitioner who lived some 400 miles away. The man came to Poohnah, where he performed the operation described in the Gentleman's Magazine in 1794.

Carpue located physicians who had witnessed the operation. Barry, who had worked for the East India Company, informed him that the operation had taken 1½ hours and that it had been performed with an old razor which had to be repeatedly honed in the course of the

operation. Carpue obtained another report that indicated that the art of nose operations in India was widely practiced by the Koomas, a caste of brickmakers (or potters) in Hindustan. At the beginning of the operation the patient was given betel and arrack. During the operation he had to lie flat on the floor with both hands at the side, and despite the intense pain, the man would unfailingly lie without stirring.

The practice of cutting off noses was common in India to punish thieves, adulterers, and prisoners of war. Only 24 years before the story published in the Gentleman's Magazine, Protwinarajan, the king of Ghorka, captured the city of Kirtipor in Ceylon in 1770. The King ordered a census taken by cutting off the noses and lips of all the inhabitants, even the smallest children. The population figure was then to be determined by a count of cut-off noses. Kirtipor was afterwards renamed Naskatapoor, meaning the city of severed noses.

Carpue's Experience. Carpue hesitated to perform the operation until September, 1814. A man came to call on him who wore a black patch over his face. He said, "I heard in Gibraltar that you can restore lost noses, and that you are the only man who knows the method. I have come here to beg your aid." The stranger removed the patch. In place of the nose was a gaping red hole. The patient told the following story:

In 1801 I entered the Egyptian army as a fledgling officer. There I suffered an attack of jaundice, and the army doctors prescribed mercury. From this you will probably assume that in truth I suffered from a syphilitic disease. I know that syphilis also destroys noses. But I can prove by the testimony of my doctors that I never had any such disease. The mercury which was administered to me in Egypt, then in Malta, then in Ireland, and finally here in London, poisoned me and in the end resulted in the loss of my nose.

Carpue pointed out to the patient that the English climate differed in some essential features from the climate in India. The new nose might drop off from freezing or become purulent.

Early in October, 1814, Carpue decided to risk the operation. Carpue first made a test to determine whether healing would occur or whether the mercury poisoning had undermined the soundness of the apparently healthy parts of the face. Carpue took a scalpel and made several incisions close to the root of the nose; within a few days the incisions were already beginning to heal. On October 23, the operation took place. Carpue formed the model of the nose out of wax in accordance with the descriptions of the Indian procedure. He then flattened the model, laid it on the patient's forehead, and drew a line around it with red paint. Then he had the patient lie on his back on the operating table, his head supported by a pillow. The patient refused to be held, although Carpue warned him that the operation would be unusually painful.

Carpue drew lines with the red paint around the stub of the nose, where he would have to make incisions in order to insert the edges of the new nasal skin. The patient did not stir as the knife cut the outlines of the flap on the forehead and freed the skin from the frontal bone. By the end of 9 minutes, according to the friend who had accompanied the patient, Carpue was placing the lowest part of the new nose into the incision above the upper lip and suturing it ligature by ligature while the blood continued to run from the forehead across the patient's face. After having sutured the two sides of the nose, he cut out the nostril openings and inserted lint to keep them open. Carpue endeavored to bring the edges of the wound on the forehead as much into contact as possible. The patient opened his mouth and said, "It was no child's play—extremely painful—but there was no use complaining." The officer with the watch came up to the foot of the bed and announced 37 minutes. Then he shook hands heartily with Carpue.

The nose had been covered with a dressing, and the sick room was kept at a torrid temperature in order to simulate the temperature of India. On the third day Carpue removed the dressing in the presence of his assistants and the officer who kept time during the operation. When the dressing was removed, the officer exclaimed, "My God, there is a nose."

Carpue's second patient was Captain Latham, whose nose was mutilated in the Battle of Albusera in Spain on May 16, 1810, during the Napoleonic Wars; the operation was performed 5 years later.

Rapid Adoption of Rhinoplasty. Von Graefe, who became Professor of Surgery at the University of Berlin, interrupting his academic career to assume the responsibilities of Surgeon General of the Prussian Army at the end of the Napoleonic Wars (1813 to 1815), reported three cases of reconstructive rhinoplasty in 1818 in which he had employed the Tagliacotian, the Indian, and a modification of the original Tagliacotian procedure, consisting of the immediate application of the flap to the nose without a period of delay; he also short-ened to 6 days, when possible, the period during which the arm was attached to the head. Other than Carpue's report (1816), Von Graefe's *Rhinoplastik* (1818) was the first treatise on plastic surgery after Tagliacozzi (1597), and his work stimulated the development of plastic surgery throughout Europe and the United States.

The recognition of the historical contribution of Tagliacozzi was epitomized by Delpech in his two volumes (1823–1828): "Nothing is more exact than his observations, nothing more wise than his precepts. . . . Tagliacozzi's method was a stroke of genius which can become extremely fruitful in skilled hands. . . ." Delpech wrote not only about his rhinoplastic operations but also on reconstruction of the lips, urethroplasty, and other plastic surgical procedures.

Dieffenbach, a younger contemporary of von Graefe, was instrumental in enlarging the scope of plastic surgery. His clinical work was monumental in its variety, inventiveness, and breadth of scope. Among his numerous publications, the best known is his *Die operative Chirurgie*, published in 1845 and 1848 in two volumes. John Staige Davis (1941) stated that his "methods and principles have not been improved upon and are still constantly employed."

During the first half of the nineteenth century Labat (1834) and Blandin (1836) wrote the first treatises on plastic surgery in France.

Serre in 1842 published his "Traité sur l'art de restaurer les déformités de la face" (treatise on the art of repairing deformities of the face). Serre was the chief exponent of the sliding (advancement) flap technique, the so-called French method, an adaptation of the technique of Celsus.

The names of two great surgeons of the nineteenth century cannot be omitted: Dupuytren, particularly for his operations for Dupuytren's contracture and his classification of burns according to their depth, and von Langenbeck, who succeeded Dieffenbach, for his contributions to cleft palate and jaw surgery.

During the remainder of the nineteenth century, hundreds of papers appeared on the subject of plastic surgery and either surgical treatises devoted entirely to plastic surgery (Zeis's *Handbuch der plastischen Chirurgie*, published in 1838; Jobert's* *Traite de*

---

*Jobert was often referred to as "Jobert (de Lamballe)" after the custom of the time of designating the man by the city from which he originated.

Chirurgie Plastique, published in 1849) or substantive portions of surgical treatises, such as the works of Roux in 1854 and Verneuil in 1877, were published.

A book which also included plastic surgery in its title was published in 1842 by von Ammon and Baumgarten and was translated into French and Italian. In England, Liston devoted a considerable discussion to various plastic surgical procedures in his textbooks published in 1831 and 1837. In France the textbooks of Velpeau (1839) and Malgaigne (1849) also contained sections on plastic surgery. A number of Italian surgeons were performing plastic surgical operations. Sabbatini published a book in 1838 describing the history of plastic surgery. The American edition of *Velpeau's Operative Surgery* published in 1851 included, in the first volume under the section "Anaplasty or Autoplasty," a concluding American appendix which described a variety of reconstructive procedures by Pancoast and Mutter of Philadelphia as well as by Mott, Post, and Buck of New York. The publications of Blasius (1839–1843) and a number of other surgeons give an excellent picture of the great advances made during the first half of the nineteenth century. One of the outstanding works published in Russia in 1869 was the *Manual of Operative Surgery* by Szymanowski.

The Birth of Skin Grafting

Although Bünger, a colleague of von Graefe, had applied a skin graft from the thigh to the nose in 1823, Baronio (1804) had performed experimental skin grafts on sheep, and later Warren (1840) in Boston had transplanted a full-thickness skin graft to the ala of the nose, the full clinical import of skin grafting was recognized only near the last quarter of the century.

An event took place shortly before the Franco-Prussian War which was to add to the armamentarium of the plastic surgeon: the development of the skin graft. In 1869 Reverdin reported the hastening of the healing of granulating wounds by what he called "epidermic" grafts. On December 8, 1869, before the Imperial Society of Surgery of Paris, Reverdin showed a patient on whom he had applied, on a granulating surface, a segment of skin excised from the superficial portion of the integument approximately 2 by 3 mm in size. Reverdin was an intern working in the service of Guyon. In the discussion that followed, Guyon

stated, "A single experiment is not conclusive . . . . The question of the future of the epidermic graft is today before you. . . . Dr. Reverdin has, on my advice, presented this patient to draw attention to this new method and to receive the recognition which it merits." Claude Bernard, in person, presented Reverdin's work before the Academy of Sciences.

The technique of skin grafting was further developed when Ollier in 1872 described the clinical application of a dermoepidermic graft 4 by 8 cm in size; Thiersch (1874) advocated the use of larger sheets of dermoepidermic grafts to cover wounds and emphasized the importance of the dermal component. The grafts were thin split-thickness skin grafts often referred to in the English and German literature as "Thiersch" grafts; credit should be given to Ollier and the grafts designated as "Ollier-Thiersch" grafts. Lawson (1870), Lefort (1872), and Wolfe (1876) described the use of a full-thickness graft for the treatment of eyelid ectropion; Krause (1893) perfected the technique.

The nineteenth century literature was compiled and classified by Nélaton and Ombrédanne in two books published in 1904 and 1907, and the first American textbook, *Plastic Surgery—Its Principles and Practice,* by Staige Davis, was published in 1919.

It is significant that the early development of plastic surgery appears to have been closely linked to the development of reconstruction of the nose; a parallel is found during the twentieth century when corrective rhinoplasty preceded the development of esthetic surgery (see Chapters 29 and 37).

The Twentieth Century

The Period of Growth (1914 to 1939). World War I (1914 to 1918), often referred to as the Great War, appears to have been the crucial starting point for the development of the concept of plastic surgery which we know today. One may consider that World War II marks the beginning of the period of healthy adolescence; the period of 25 years extending from 1914 to 1939 then represents the period of growth.

Tactical maneuvering rapidly became limited during the first World War as the war of movement ceased and the conflict became stabilized on the western front. Casualties mounted to appalling figures, and trench warfare was responsible for ever-increasing numbers of max-illofacial wounds.

The influx of patients with gunshot wounds of the face into the military hospitals during World War I required the organization of specialized centers. Few surgeons knew how to cope with the problem. It was realized that the makeshift methods employed in the past were inadequate and that these patients would require specialized care. A number of treatment centers were established by the French Army, one of which was headed by an outstanding reconstructive surgeon, Morestin. Morestin was a native of the Carribean island of Martinique and was of part Negro extraction. Well known prior to World War I for his work in the application of the Z-plasty technique to linear contractures and for developing techniques of cartilage grafting, Morestin conducted an active service at the Val-de-Grâce Military Hospital in Paris. Morestin was one of the first surgeons to show that the skin and subcutaneous tissue could be widely undermined without being subject to necrosis (Converse, 1968).

Morestin died prematurely, a victim of the great influenza epidemic of 1917–1918, and left a void in French plastic surgery. The concept of adapting dental techniques to the treatment of gunshot wounds of the face was foreign to Morestin, who disdained the services of the dental surgeon and claimed, "I can do everything with my scalpel." He rendered an incommensurable service by unwittingly being responsible for Sir Harold Gillies' interest in plastic surgery.

Gillies was an otolaryngologist attached to a British general hospital at Rouen, France. A friend of his, an American dentist named Roberts, having returned from a trip to Paris where he had seen Morestin operate, urged Gillies to go to Paris. Gillies told me that he watched Morestin repair a large facial defect by means of a large undelayed cervicothoracic flap. Gillies was inspired by what he saw and with the help of Sir William Arbuthnot Lane, his army consultant, a unit was established at the Aldershot Military Hospital. This measure was taken as part of the preparation being made for the Somme offensive (Clarkson, 1966). It is interesting that there appears to have been no further contact between Gillies and Morestin until Morestin's death; Morestin even closed the door of his operating room to Gillies.

A center was subsequently established at the Queen Mary Hospital, Sidcup, Kent. Here Gillies, assisted by Kilner, developed a vast treatment center for British and allied military casualties. Many allied medical officers came to Sidcup to learn plastic surgery; among these were Ferris Smith from the United States, Waldron and Risdon from Canada, and Newland and Pickerill from Australia and New Zealand. Gillies was fortunate to have as an associate a dental officer, Kelsey Fry, who applied dental techniques to the many maxillofacial reconstructive problems the surgeons were trying to solve.

Paralleling the development at Sidcup, another center situated not far from the front lines was actively functioning at Etaples, near Boulogne, under the direction of Varaztad H. Kazanjian. Kazanjian, a dental surgeon on the faculty of the Harvard Dental School, had volunteered to serve in the First Harvard Unit attached to the British Expeditionary Force. Kazanjian applied his knowledge of prosthetic dentistry to the early treatment of gunshot wounds of the face. He perfected methods of fixation of jaw fragments and of the utilization of prosthetic devices prior to the late primary closure of facial wounds. Gillies told me of the remarkable condition of those patients received by him at Sidcup who had been treated by Kazanjian at Etaples before their evacuation to England.

Kazanjian's participation in the Harvard Unit was the result of a chance encounter in Boston; he was invited to join as the dental surgeon of the unit and accepted. In 1920 he returned to the United States, entered Harvard Medical School, and continued his unusual career to become one of the world's leading plastic surgeons. Kazanjian was an immigrant to the United States at the age of 16, and his is truly one of the great success stories. His enthusiasm and interest never flagged, as I can personally attest, from the many long evenings we spent together writing our first book (Kazanjian and Converse, 1949).

There was American participation in World War I prior to the offical entry of the United States in 1917. Volunteers such as Kazanjian, Waldron, and Ferris Smith have already been mentioned. Others served with the American Ambulance Hospital in Neuilly, a Paris suburb. A hospital was installed in a school, symbolically called the Lycée Pasteur, through donations given by supporters of the American Hospital of Paris. Blake, a surgeon at St. Luke's Hospital in New York, had moved to Paris and did much surgery on the war wounded, including bone grafting for loss of bone in the mandible. Two American dental surgeons who had practiced for years in Paris—Davenport and Hayes—did outstanding work in the fixation of jaw fragments in wounded French soldiers at the American Hospital.

At the outbreak of World War I there was no recognized specialty of plastic surgery in the United States. Most general surgeons practiced reconstructive surgery and a few showed interest in this type of work. There were a considerable number of oral surgeons, such as Brophy, Gilmer, Cryer, Marshall, G. V. I. Brown, and Chalmers J. Lyons who, as a result of their dental training, took a special interest in surgical diseases of the mouth and jaws, particularly cleft lip and palate.

When the United States entered the War in 1917, Surgeon General Gorgas organized, under the Division of Surgery, certain sections in the Surgeon General's office, among them a section on head surgery which included subsections of ophthalmology, otolaryngology, brain surgery, and oral and plastic surgery. Vilray P. Blair of Saint Louis headed the last-named section and chose Robert H. Ivy as his assistant. Blair was well known for his work and had written a book, *Surgery and Diseases of the Mouth and Jaws* (1912). As early as 1907 Blair had attempted the surgical correction of mandibular prognathism in collaboration with Edward H. Angle, the orthodontist who is often considered the father of the American school of orthodontics. Blair conceived the idea of setting up teams, each consisting of a general surgeon and a dental surgeon who could pool their respective talents. Officers assigned to these teams were sent to special short courses of instruction in several medical and dental schools. A revised edition of Blair's textbook was prepared and distributed to Army hospitals. A number of officers were sent for short periods of observation and training at British and French hospital centers. Attempts were made to concentrate on patients with face and jaw injuries at Base Hospital 115, Vichy.

In the United States three centers were established where most of the patients with face and jaw injuries were sent on arrival from overseas. These were General Hospital No. 11 at Cape May, New Jersey; General Hospital No. 2, Fort McKinley, Maryland; and Walter Reed General Hospital, Washington, D.C. Later, two other centers were established at Columbus Barracks, Ohio, and Jefferson Barracks, Missouri (Ivy, 1948). By the end of the war, names such as Gillies in England, Morestin in France, Lexer, Ganzer, and Lindemann in Germany, Esser and Pichler in Austria, and Burian in Czechoslovakia became widely known, these men being characterized as specialists in plastic surgery or in jaw and face surgery.

One can consider, therefore, that World War I was the beginning of the era during which plastic surgery became a surgical specialty. After the war, national and international congresses began to include in their scientific programs papers concerned with the methods of treatment of the victims of the war and demonstrating new surgical possibilities. This was the period when one saw the facially mutilated. Ernest Hemingway (1964), recalling the clients of a particular Parisian café, wrote: "There were other people too who lived in the quarter and came to Lilas, and some of them wore Croix de Guerre ribbons in their lapels and others also had the yellow and green of the Médaille Militaire, and I watched how well they were overcoming the handicap of the loss of limbs, and saw the quality of their artificial eyes and the degree of skill with which their faces had been reconstructed. There was always an almost iridescent shiny cast about the considerably reconstructed face, rather like that of a well packed ski run and we respected these clients. . . ." There were many others whose faces contained gaping holes, who had no lower jaws; these were the veterans whose faces could not be reconstructed. They formed an organization of mutual aid, "Les Gueules Cassées" ("the broken faces"). In view of the vast number of casualties, the rehabilitation task did not end with the war but continued for a number of years until as many as possible of the mutilated veterans were rehabilitated.

A number of publications appeared at this time. Important books were written by Staige Davis (1919) and Gillies (1920), and the contributions of surgeons and dentists during the war were described in a publication, "La Revue Maxillo-faciale," which appeared in 1919 and 1920. Ivy (1918, 1923) summarized the new knowledge in plastic surgery acquired during the war. A 1921 paper by Blair, "Reconstructive surgery of the face," illustrates the high degree of proficiency achieved in the rehabilitation of the war disfigured. Other important publications during this period included those of Velter (1917), Steinschneider (1917), Lexer (1919, 1920), Delagenière (1921), and Mauclaire (1922).

Gillies has told me that, following the closure of the Queen's Hospital in Sidcup, Kilner and he wondered how they were going to be able to specialize in the field of plastic surgery. When one thinks of the rapid development of plastic surgery during the past 25 years, it is difficult to realize that there was so little demand in civilian life for the services of the plastic surgeon in the early 1920's. The increase in birth defects, automobile and industrial accidents, ablative cancer surgery, and burns; the rapid rise in requests for esthetic surgery; and the competitive industrial society are some of the causes for the increased demands for plastic surgery.

With the advent of peace and a period of relative prosperity, there appeared a new branch of plastic surgery which was designated as "esthetic" or "cosmetic." Joseph, an orthopedic surgeon in Berlin, who is justly regarded as the founder of modern corrective rhinoplasty, was at the apogee of his career; he gave courses which were attended by two pioneers of modern corrective rhinoplasty in the United States, Aufricht and Safian. In France, Passot, Noel, and others were performing surgical procedures for the correction of the aging face.

A considerable emphasis was given to the teaching of plastic surgery during this period by the organization of international courses by Lemaitre, an associate professor at the Faculty of Medicine of Paris and chief of an otolaryngologic service in a Paris hospital. Lemaitre had been in charge of a large maxillofacial center at Vichy during the war and had met a number of Allied officers, notably Blair and Ivy. In 1925 he organized an international clinic in his service at the Hôpital Saint-Louis, which was conducted on a yearly basis until 1928. Gillies also held a series of operative demonstrations, and in the following years Eastman Sheehan, Ferris Smith, Kilner, and Joseph conducted courses which were well attended. There being no other way of learning plastic surgery at this time, a number of surgeons from various parts of Europe and from the United States received their training at these courses. Among these the most illustrious was Sanvenero-Rosselli of Milan, the president of the Fourth International Congress of Plastic Surgery held in Rome in October, 1967 (Figs. 1–2 and 1–3).

An important contribution to the literature of plastic surgery in the 1920's was Ferris Smith's *Reconstructive Surgery,* which appeared in 1928. Ferris Smith, who had acquired a reputation as a distinguished oto-

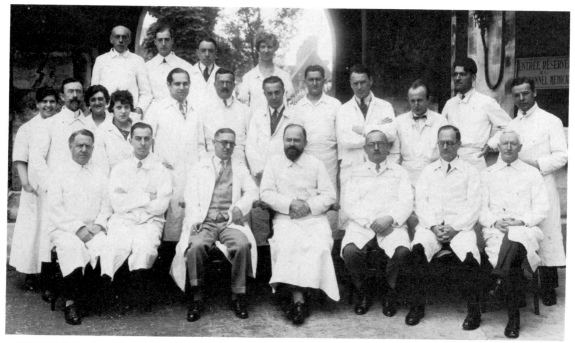

FIGURE 1–2. A photograph taken at the Hospital Saint-Louis in Paris in 1927 following the International Clinic. From left to right (seated): Myron Metzenbaum (Cleveland), Gustavo Sanvenero-Rosselli (Milan), Ferris Smith (Grand Rapids), Fernand Lemaitre, Paris; the next two are unidentified; extreme right: W. T. Coughlin (New York). Standing behind M. Metzenbaum: M. Roy (Quebec). (From Converse J. M.: Plastic surgery: The 20th century: The period of growth (1914–1939). Surg. Clin. North Am., *47*:261, 1967.)

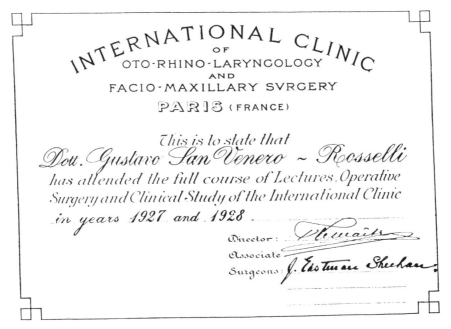

FIGURE 1–3. Diploma given to Dr. G. Sanvenero-Rosselli following his attendance at the International Clinic held in Paris in 1927 and 1928. The document is signed by Fernand Lemaitre and J. Eastman Sheehan. (From Converse, J. M.: Plastic surgery: The 20th century. The period of growth (1914–1939). *Surg. Clin. North Am.*, *47:*261, 1967.)

laryngologist, was particularly interested in the technique of repeated partial excision and the use of local flaps on the face. Many considered him one of the finest technicians of his day. Even in those days he had an appreciation of atraumatic technique, and, above all, he placed emphasis on detail.

In the 1920's and 1930's three personalities—John Staige Davis, Vilray Papin Blair, and Harold Delf Gillies—helped to shape the present concepts of plastic surgery as it is practiced in the English-speaking world.

Staige Davis was probably the first outstanding surgeon to devote his entire practice to plastic surgery. When there was little recognition for plastic surgery, Davis, working alone and with little encouragement from his own medical school, made many important contributions over the years—contributions that remain significant even today. His textbook *Plastic Surgery*, published in 1919, was the first book of its kind in the English language. This textbook provided the reader with an extensive review of the literature, a critical appraisal by the author of the methods described, and a voluminous description of his own experience.

A significant surgical contribution by Staige Davis was "the small deep skin graft," often referred to, particularly in foreign countries, as the Davis graft*. Halsted had devised the technique, but to Davis belongs the merit of its diffusion in the surgical world. Prior to the development of modern methods of skin grafting, the small deep graft was invaluable in resurfacing granulating areas. Many of Davis' papers remain classics even today. Among these are his papers concerning the theory and practical applications of the Z-plasty (1931), which he often referred to as the "Z-incision." He stressed the value of partial excision of scars (1929), a technique that was to be widely used. His studies on the vascularization of skin grafts in 1925 and the delay of skin flaps in 1933 (German, Finesilver, and Davis) remain valid today and have been repeatedly confirmed by later workers.

Blair and Gillies had a profound influence on the development of plastic surgery, not only in English-speaking countries but also throughout the world at large. Their influence was exerted not only in scientific aspects but also in helping to shape plastic surgery into its present organizational lines.

Each of these men contributed outstandingly to the field of skin transplantation. Gillies de-

---

*The "small deep skin graft" is usually referred to as a "pinch graft."

veloped the tube flap, coincidentally with Fila-tov (1917), and showed many applications of the new technique in his book *Plastic Surgery of the Face* (1920). Blair defined the process of delay in nontubulated flaps in his paper, "The delayed transfer of long pedicled flaps in plastic surgery," published in 1921.

The development of the technique of split-thickness skin grafting and the paper on the subject by Blair and his pupil Barrett Brown (1929) constitute a landmark in the history of skin grafting. The thicker split-thickness graft gave a more durable type of repair with less shrinkage and wrinkling than the thin Thiersch graft generally used by surgeons for covering raw surfaces and granulating wounds, or the small, deep, so-called "pinch" grafts which resulted in even more contraction and scarring.

To facilitate removal of the split-thickness skin graft, Blair developed a special skin grafting knife and the Blair suction box, which, connected with a negative pressure apparatus, facilitated traction of the skin and flattening of the donor area during the cutting of the graft. In numerous articles written in subsequent years, the St. Louis group emphasized the value of early grafting in skin defects resulting from burns and other types of injuries, and the principle that the best dressing for a wound with loss of skin was a skin graft. *Skin Grafting* by Brown and McDowell (1939) rendered a great service to patients and surgeons during World War II. Converse (1942) emphasized the importance of early skin grafting in war wounds.

The Development of the Dermatome. Skin grafting was greatly facilitated by the development of the dermatome by Earl C. Padgett and George F. Hood, the latter a mechanical engineer. Padgett described the three-quarter thickness skin graft, with qualities comparable to those of a full-thickness graft, in 1939. Webster (1956), in a beautifully written and sensitive eulogy of Vilray Blair, recounted an incident that took place during his period of observation at Blair's clinic in the fall of 1927. "One day, while scrubbing for an operation, dressed in his white shirt and trousers, and all white sneakers, with a gauze swathe tied about his face and head, he walked away from the sink and paced up and down, scrubbing his hands and humming to himself. Suddenly he whirled about and burst out in his high reedy voice: 'Webster, did you ever see 'em split leather with a machine?'" It was undoubtedly his interest in an invention of this kind that stimu-

lated Padgett to produce the dermatome ten years later. Padgett had been trained by Blair.

The idea of calibration, one of the chief advantages of the dermatome, was not a new one. Finochietto, an Argentine surgeon, had devised a calibrated knife as early as 1920. Humby, while serving as a house surgeon at the Great Ormond Street Hospital for Sick Children in London, added a roller to the Blair knife which permitted calibration of the graft. The Padgett dermatome, by providing a relatively easy mechanical means for the removal of split-thickness grafts, placed the technique of skin grafting into the hands of all surgeons. I can recall, during my period of training, a group of general surgeons at the Massachusetts General Hospital gathering around Kazanjian to watch him cut a large split-thickness graft free hand. In those days skin grafting was a specialized technique of the plastic surgeon; today it should be a routine procedure in the hands of all surgeons. The service rendered by the dermatome in making possible the frequent use of split-thickness grafting during World War II was immeasurable in terms of saving many lives and limbs.

The development of split-thickness grafting was essentially an American contribution. When I arrived in England to work with Gillies in August, 1940, the first Padgett dermatomes had just been received. In Gillies' hands, skin grafting was still an exceptional procedure in reconstructive surgery of the face, and local or distant skin flaps were more commonly employed. Skin grafting was mostly of the thin Thiersch graft variety, or of the relatively small full-thickness type, known in England as Wolfe grafts. Gillies, in the course of his characteristically humorous and very instructive teaching clinics, would ask us how we would repair a certain defect. Then he would turn to me and say: "If you tell me you are going to use a graft I will send you back to America!" Of course, in many cases he was right, for certainly his was a great school for learning the art of utilization of local tissue. Archibald H. McIndoe, his pupil, was the first British surgeon to utilize split-thickness skin grafting on a large scale for the early and also the definitive repair of burns. Skin grafting was not extensively used in either France or Germany. A visit to a number of German plastic surgery centers a few weeks after the end of World War II showed a predilection for skin flap repair; the dermatome was not known in these countries on the European continent.

Aside from their many scientific contributions, too numerous to be included in this short historical review, Blair and Gillies were instrumental in establishing the specialty of plastic surgery on a solid footing.

Blair can justly be considered the father of the American Board of Plastic Surgery, which was established in 1937 (Fig. 1–4). In 1936, in an editorial entitled "Surgery, Specialty Surgery, and 'Plastic Surgery,'" Blair had intimated the need for a Plastic Surgery Board.

It is difficult for a young plastic surgeon to realize the flimsy status of plastic surgery 40 years ago. That status is well exemplified by a personal experience. At the end of World War I, my family moved to Paris where my father was sent by the United States Public Health Service to supervise the health status (preventive medicine) of the returning American Expeditionary Force, and a few years later my father joined the staff of the American Hospital in Paris. After graduating from medical school in Paris and being trained in general surgery, I decided to become a plastic surgeon. On my way to Boston, I spent a few days in New York. My father had corresponded with a former fellow resident, now a general practitioner, who was kind enough to invite me to dinner. At coffee time he turned to me and said, "Now young man, what are you going to do?" When I told him I intended to be trained as a plastic surgeon he fell silent, and I could guess the workings of his mind: "How disappointing it must be for my old friend George to have a son who wants to become a plastic surgeon!"

Again, to quote Webster: "At that time the public generally considered plastic surgeons as 'face lifters' and 'nose whittlers.' To be sure, a few surgeons throughout the country were known for their capabilities in the special fields of plastic surgery. There were also those who were close to the border of being ethical, if not unethical, in their practice, and some were definitely below that level. Blair felt that those slightly below the ethical line could be raised if given proper recognition, and those with special abilities should be recognized and their qualities brought to bear for the good of the specialty of plastic surgery."

Staige Davis in Baltimore, Ivy and Warren B. Davis in Philadelphia, Kazanjian in Boston, Blair, Brown, Byars, and their associates in St. Louis, Pierce in San Francisco, Peer in New-

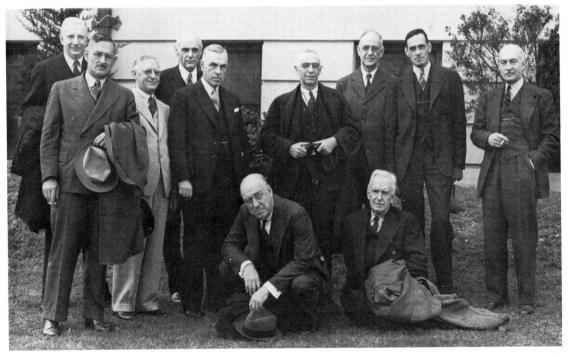

FIGURE 1–4. The first annual meeting of the American Board of Plastic Surgery held in Galveston, Texas, February 2, 1938. From left to right standing: William S. Kiskadden, George Warren Pierce, Ferris Smith, William E. Ladd, Fulton Risdon, Robert H. Ivy, John Staige Davis, Harold L. D. Kirkham, and Jerome P. Webster. Seated: George M. Dorrance and Vilray Papin Blair. (From Converse, J. M.: Plastic surgery: The 20th century. The period of growth (1914–1939). Surg. Clin. North Am., *47*:261, 1967.)

ark, Ferris Smith in Grand Rapids, Webster, Eastman Sheehan, Maliniac, and John M. Wheeler and Wendell L. Hughes, the latter two ophthalmic plastic surgeons in New York, were well known and respected. Safian and Aufricht in New York were perfecting the techniques of corrective rhinoplasty. Many surgeons were practicing corrective rhinoplasty after having taken courses in Europe either with Joseph in Berlin in the 1920's, or in other centers such as Vienna, where such courses were also available.

Opportunities for learning plastic surgery were few in the 1930's. Preceptorships were not numerous, and there were few well-organized plastic surgery services in the hospitals. One of the first active hospital services in the United States was that organized by Eastman Sheehan at the Postgraduate Hospital, the predecessor to our own Institute of Reconstructive Plastic Surgery at the New York University Medical Center. Sheehan trained Straatsma, Milton Adams, Peer, and Barsky. Sheehan was a brilliant technician who had a predilection for operating upon members of the European nobility and was not averse to publicity. He wrote a number of books and did much work on the wounded of the armies of General Franco during the Spanish Civil War.

By an unusual set of circumstances, Sheehan was responsible for the establishment of the Nuffield Professorship of Plastic Surgery at Oxford University. Through personal friendship with Lord and Lady Nuffield (he had sutured the thyroid incision following an operation by Lahey upon Lady Nuffield—with goat hair!), he was offered the Nuffield chair of Plastic Surgery. Because Sheehan had been classified as a Fascist following his activities in Spain, Lord Nuffield was obliged to intervene with Prime Minister Churchill in order to obtain a visa permitting him to enter England. The Council of Oxford University, however, disapproved of his appointment, and T. Pomfret Kilner was appointed the first (and unfortunately last) Nuffield Professor of Plastic Surgery.

Before the establishment of approved residencies and with the exception of the few available preceptorships, the only method of learning was observation, and there were well trodden paths to St. Louis, Baltimore, New York, Boston, and London. One of the most active and well-organized hospital services was that of Burian in Prague. I had the privilege of spending two weeks with Burian in 1938 in his new hospital service, which had been established with the aid of the Rockefeller Foundation.

A residency in maxillofacial surgery was established by Ivy in Philadelphia. Another residency was started at King's County Hospital in Brooklyn by Coakley. For a number of years Ivy's residents spent an additional year in Coakley's service. Webster established his residency program in New York on January 1, 1939, the first resident being the late Milton Dupertuis. Webster's residency program graduated a whole generation of plastic surgeons, many of whom are today leaders in the field.

A curious phenomen was the publication in 1939 of a book, *Surgery of Injury and Plastic Repair*, by Fomon. Not a plastic surgeon but a medical writer, Fomon had proposed to Kazanjian that he write a book for him. When Kazanjian declined the offer, Fomon made a similar proposition to Eastman Sheehan, who accepted. Some disagreement occurred subsequently, and Fomon published a book under his own name. Although deficient in many ways, the deficiencies reflecting the author's inexperience, the book rendered a service by collecting the known techniques, some of which were well illustrated, and assembling a vast and accurate bibliography.

In Great Britian, prior to World War II, plastic surgery was a monopoly in the hands of Gillies, McIndoe, Mowlem, all from New Zealand, and Kilner, an Englishman. McIndoe, who had been trained in surgery at the Mayo Clinic, was consultant to the Royal Air Force, and Kilner was in charge of plastic surgery at the Ministry of Pensions. These surgeons were active in a number of London hospitals.

A Swedish surgeon, Ragnell, was trained in England by Gillies, returning to Stockholm in the 1930's, where he later headed a service established at the Karolinska Institute. This was the beginning of the Swedish school of plastic surgery.

Léon Dufourmentel, an otolaryngologist, son-in-law of Sébileau, who was professor of otolaryngology at the University of Paris during World War I and during the immediate postwar period, unfortunately was not appointed head of one of the Paris hospital services and was obliged to restrict his activities to private practice. This fact, in addition to the untimely death of Morestin, was responsible for a long period of stagnation in the development of reconstructive plastic surgery in France. Plastic surgery became commonly known as "chirurgie esthetique," and it was not until after World War II that a new and dynamic generation of plastic surgeons arose. This generation has reached surgical maturity and is making notable contributions to our surgical specialty.

Victor Veau, a pediatric surgeon (Converse, 1962), started making his surgical contributions to the treatment of cleft lip and palate in the early 1920's and doing his outstanding research in the embryology of cleft lip in the 1930's. Lexer, a general surgeon (May, 1962) in Germany, summarized his own work in reconstructive surgery in his treatise *Die gesamte Wiederherstellungschirurgie,* published in 1931.

The period between the two wars also saw the birth of the oldest plastic surgery society, the American Association of Oral and Plastic Surgeons, which was established in 1921. The name of the society was changed to American Association of Plastic Surgeons in 1941. Annual meetings were held; these were small, intimate gatherings until World War II. The meetings comprised operating room sessions at which members gathered around their host and watched him operate. Under the leadership of Maliniac, Aufricht, Palmer, and Peer, another society, the American Society of Plastic and Reconstructive Surgeons, was established in 1931. The proceedings of the Society were published in a European publication, *Revue de Chirurgie Plastique,* until 1940, after which the Society published its own proceedings.

A picturesque individualist between the two World Wars was Esser, a Dutch surgeon who had volunteered to work with the Austrian army during World War I. Esser did much of his work in Vienna during the war and made a number of notable contributions, such as the application of the rotation flap to the repair of facial defects, the artery island flap which he termed the "biologic flap," and the important contribution of the "epithelial" or skin graft inlay technique.

Following the war, Esser appears to have led the life of a wandering surgeon. For a long period of time he was established in Munich and then in Monte Carlo. In the late 1930's he conceived the grandiose plan of establishing a world center for plastic surgery. For this purpose he requested an audience with Benito Mussolini. In the Palazzo Venezia, Mussolini had his desk at the end of an enormous room, and the visitor walked the long distance under the steady gaze of the head of the Fascist state. It is said that Esser picked up a chair and sat down next to Il Duce, much to the lat-

ter's amazement. He then requested an island in "Mare Nostrum" (Mussolini's Imperial Roman term for the Mediterranean Sea) in which to establish the world center for plastic surgery! The advent of World War II put an end to this grandiose plan.

The first issue of the *Revue de Chirurgie Plastique* was published in 1931 under the editorship of Coelst (Fig. 1–5). Coelst was a practitioner in Brussels, Belgium, who does not appear to have had any official university or hospital appointments. Through his personal initiative and efforts, he assembled a series of papers of good quality for the period. At the suggestion of Esser, the name of the publication was later changed to *Revue de Chirurgie Structive* (Fig. 1–6). Esser pointed out, quite correctly, that "plastic" was a poor term which did not define the speciality, and that the term "structive," derived from the Latin *structo* (I build), was more appropriate. Coelst brought together an international editorial board of high quality which included many well-known names (see Fig. 1–6). The papers were published in whatever language was preferred by the author and summarized in English, German, and French. By contrast with this early effort, the American journal *Plastic and Reconstructive Surgery* and the *British Journal of Plastic Surgery* commenced publication only after World War II.

In 1931 the first congress of the French Society of Reparative and Esthetic Surgery was held in Paris. This group published in book form the papers read at the congress, edited by Claoué and Dartigues. Participants in the congress and authors of the papers published in the *Revue* comprised, in addition to the few full-time practicing plastic surgeons, general surgeons, otolaryngologists, ophthalmologists, oral and dental surgeons, and orthodontists who were involved either full or part time in the various aspects of plastic surgery.

Of major interest in the history of this period was the establishment in 1936 of a European Society of Structive Surgery, which held its first congress in Brussels in that year (Fig. 1–7). Eminent personalities in the field such as Gillies, Esser, and Kilner participated. The second congress was held in the following year in London, and the third in Milan in 1938. At the time of the Milan congress there appeared the first issue of a new international review entitled *Plastica Chirurgica*, edited by Sanvenero-Rosselli, who established a teaching course for the training of plastic surgeons in

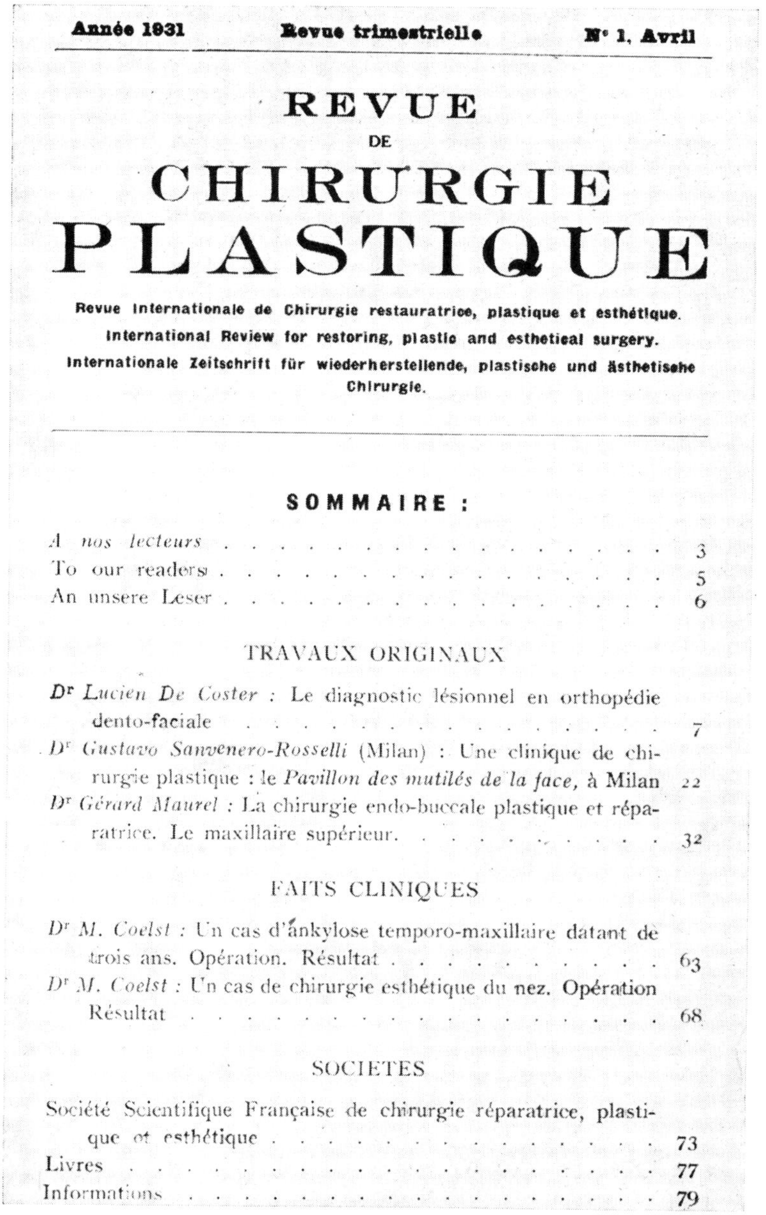

Année 1931   Revue trimestrielle   N° 1, Avril

REVUE
DE
CHIRURGIE
PLASTIQUE

Revue internationale de Chirurgie restauratrice, plastique et esthétique.
International Review for restoring, plastic and esthetical surgery.
Internationale Zeitschrift für wiederherstellende, plastische und ästhetische Chirurgie.

SOMMAIRE :

A nos lecteurs 3
To our readers 5
An unsere Leser 6

TRAVAUX ORIGINAUX

Dʳ *Lucien De Coster* : Le diagnostic lésionnel en orthopédie
    dento-faciale 7
Dʳ *Gustavo Sanvenero-Rosselli* (Milan) : Une clinique de chi-
    rurgie plastique : le *Pavillon des mutilés de la face*, à Milan 22
Dʳ *Gérard Maurel* : La chirurgie endo-buccale plastique et répa-
    ratrice. Le maxillaire supérieur. 32

FAITS CLINIQUES

Dʳ *M. Coelst* : Un cas d'ankylose temporo-maxillaire datant de
    trois ans. Opération. Résultat 63
Dʳ *M. Coelst* : Un cas de chirurgie esthétique du nez. Opération
    Résultat 68

SOCIETES

Société Scientifique Française de chirurgie réparatrice, plasti-
    que et esthétique 73
Livres 77
Informations 79

FIGURE 1–5. Title page of the first issue of the Revue de Chirurgie Plastique. (From Converse, J. M.: Plastic surgery: The 20th century. The period of growth (1914–1939). Surg. Clin. North Am., *47*:261, 1967.)

Italy. The publication of subsequent issues was interrupted by the advent of World War II. These international congresses of the European Society of Structive Surgery represented the high point of development of plastic surgery prior to World War II. The contributions to the congresses were of high quality and represented milestones of progress toward recognition, not only by the public at large but also by the academic world, of the existence of this new branch of surgery.

Throughout the period between the wars looms the towering figure of Sterling Bunnell. Bunnell, along with other great pioneers — Alan Kanavel, Sumner L. Koch, Hugh Auchincloss, Condict W. Cutler, in the United States; Frederick Wood-Jones, the anatomist, in Great Britain; and Marc Iselin, in France — originated the anatomical and physiologic concepts of reconstructive hand surgery. This type of reconstructive plastic surgery reached its fruition during World War II after the establishment of specialized hand centers under the consultantship of Bunnell.

6ᵉ Année.   Nᵒˢ 3 et 4, Décembre 1936.

REVUE
DE
CHIRURGIE
STRUCTIVE

(Ancienne Revue de Chirurgie Plastique)

Revue Internationale de Chirurgie restauratrice et plastique
International Review for restoring, and plastic Surgery.
Internationale Zeitschrift für wiederherstellende
und plastische Chirurgie.

Directeur-Fondateur : Dr **M. COELST** (Bruxelles)

FIGURE 1-6. Title page of the first issue of the Revue de Chirurgie Structive. (From Converse, J. M.: Plastic surgery: The 20th century. The period of growth (1914–1936). Surg. Clin. North Am., *47*:261, 1967.)

Collaborateurs : MM. les Professeurs et Docteurs :
Albee, F.-H. *(New-York)* — Anopol, G. *(New-York)* — Aubert *(Marseille)* — Bames, H.-O. *(Los Angeles)* — Bettman, A.-G. *(Portland)* — Boisson, R. *(Bruxelles)* — Bourguet, J. *(Paris)* — Burian, F. *(Prague)* — Claoué, Ch. *(Paris)* — Corachan, M. *(Barcelona)* — Dantlo, R. *(Moyeuvre)* — Dantrelle *(Paris)* — Darcissac, M. *(Paris)* — Dartigues *(Paris)* — Decoster, L. *(Bruxelles)* — Deselaers, A. *(Barcelona)* — Dieulafé *(Toulouse)* — Dobrzaniecki, W. *(Lwow)* — Dufourmentel, L. *(Paris)* — Eastman-Sheehan *(New-York)* — Esser, J.-F.-S. *(Monaco)* — Ferrari, R.-C. *(Buenos-Aires)* — Ferris Smith *(Grand Rapids)* — Fruhwald *(Wien)* — Gumpert, M. *(New-York)* — Halle, M. *(Berlin)* — Hofer, Otto *(Wien)* — Horno Alcorta *(Zaragoza)* — Ivanissevich, O. *(Buenos-Aires)* — Ivy, R.-H. *(Philadelphia)* — Jiano, J. *(Bucarest)* — Joseph, J. *(Berlin)* † — Karfik *(Prague)* — Kilner, T.-P. *(London)* — Kubertova, E. *(Prague)* — Lapierre, V. *(Lyon)* — Larroudé, C. *(Lisboa)* — Lexer *(München)* — Lumière, A. *(Lyon)* — Lyons, Hunt *(New-York)* — Madureira, A. *(Lisboa)* — Maliniak, J.-W. *(New-York)* — Manna, A. *(Roma)* — Marchal *(Anvers)* — Maurel, Gérard *(Paris)* — Michalek-Grodzki *(Warszawa)* — O' Connor, C.-B. *(San-Francisco)* — Passot, R. *(Paris)* † — Péri, M. *(Alger)* — Pierre-Robin *(Paris)* — Pohl, L. *(Wien)* — Pont, A. *(Lyon)* — Portmann, G. *(Bordeaux)* — Prevot *(Marseille)* — Raul *(Thionville)* — Rebello-Neto *(Sao Paulo)* — Réthi *(Budapest)* — Rocher *(Bordeaux)* — Roy, J.-N. *(Montréal)* — Sanvenero-Rosselli *(Milano)* — Sargnon *(Lyon)* — Schultz, J.-H. *(Berlin)* — Sercer, A. *(Zagreb)* — Simon, Paul-W. *(Berlin)* — Straith, C.-L. *(Detroit)* — Stephan Wahl *(New-York)* — Ulrich *(Paris)* — Wallet *(Paris)* — Warren Pierce, G. *(San Franscisco)* — Wodak, E. *(Prague)* — Gerald Brown O'Connor M. D. *San Francisco)*.

Rédaction : **Centre de Chirurgie Structive**
3, Boulevard du Centenaire
Administration : **17, Rue de la Longue-Haie, Bruxelles**

Abonnement pour quatre numéros :
Belgique. 20 belgas ; Etranger, 25 ou 30 belgas selon les conventions postales.

Plastic surgery has long passed the stage when it was more or less confined to the correction of nasal deformities or earlier, during World War I, to maxillofacial surgery. The pioneers of plastic surgery were actually individualists who operated within the framework of their own specialized fields — dental surgeons, otolaryngologists, ophthalmologists, orthopedic surgeons, and others. Many had little or no training in general surgery.

World War II and the Growth to Maturity. Since World War II the scope of plastic surgery has changed. During this conflict it was necessary to treat a great many complicated fractures, to replace lost structures, to treat

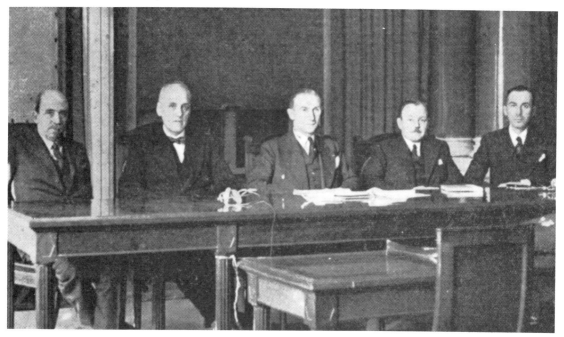

FIGURE 1–7. Officers of the First European Congress of Structive Surgery held in Brussels in October, 1936. From left to right: Sir Harold Gillies, J. F. S. Esser, M. Coelst, T. Pomfret Kilner, and G. Sanvenero-Rosselli. (From Converse, J. M.: Plastic surgery: The 20th century. The period of growth (1914–1939). Surg. Clin. North Am., *47*:261, 1967.)

paraplegic pressure sores, frostbite, and burns, and to prepare soft tissues for orthopedic surgery and the repair of peripheral nerves. Impetus was given to the development of surgery of the hand and the treatment of burns, as well as research in tissue transplantation. In this way, reconstructive plastic surgery, as it is now known, came into being.

As its scope increased over the years, the training of plastic surgeons had to be extended. The additional training entails extensive experience in the basic disciplines, primarily those of general surgery. Only when equipped with the knowledge of general principles common to all fields of surgery can the surgeon be admitted to specialized training in plastic surgery. He should not work in isolation but should be in close contact with all other fields of surgery and medicine, from which he draws benefits and, in return, to which he contributes his specialized knowledge.

World War II saw considerable development in plastic surgery. Because of the fear of massive civilian casualties resulting from air raids, special centers were established in strategic locations in Great Britain for the treatment of both civilian and military casualties under the direction of the Emergency Medical Service. Gillies was the leader in insisting on adequate facilities for the treatment of all patients requiring plastic surgery, military or civilian, including those with severe burns. From the beginning of the war it became obvious that tank warfare would cause numerous burns. During the Battle of Britain the pilots of fighter aircraft were ordered to land their planes in flame in order that they could be repaired and returned to intercept German bombers. As a result many of the Royal Air Force pilots were severely burned.

The Plastic Surgery and Jaw Centers in Great Britain became teaching centers for surgeons of the Western Allies, and considerable progress resulted during this period. Similar units were organized in the United States in a certain number of Army and Navy General Hospitals. Hand surgery centers were also established and generally associated with Plastic Surgery Centers under the guidance of Bunnell.

Plastic surgery gained much stature among the medical profession and the public at large as a result of the accomplishments of plastic surgeons during World War II. Since World War II plastic surgeons have contributed much, not only to the clinical field of plastic and reconstructive surgery but also to research, especially in the field of transplantation (see Chapter 5).

Plastic surgery today offers a wide field for research in transplantation, implantation, genetics, growth and development, speech pathology, and the newer fields of microsurgery and craniofacial surgery pioneered by plastic surgeons.

THE SCOPE OF PLASTIC SURGERY

Verdan stated in his opening speech on the occasion of the tenth anniversary of the foundation of the Swiss Society of Plastic and Reconstructive Surgery in 1974:

It is true that plastic surgery is a specialty that is difficult to define and that all the other surgical specialties with the exception of pediatric surgery have a regional character which is anatomically defined. The plastic surgeon extends his surgical activities not only to the skin and its adnexa but also to certain subjacent tissues in locations as diverse as the face and hands, the neck and abdominal wall, the extremities and the genitourinary apparatus, the breasts and scalp. To the term plastic surgery is added the adjective "reconstructive" which implies an extension of the plastic surgeon's activities to the most diverse reconstructive procedures such as vascular and microvascular surgery, peripheral nerve surgery, transplantation of muscles and tendons and arthroplasties thus overlapping the specialty of orthopedic surgery.

With the development of craniofacial surgery by Tessier and his associates (1967), the plastic surgeon finds himself invading the interior of the cranium, the private domain of the neurosurgeon. Thus, as Vilain (1965) has stated, the plastic surgeon is probably the last of the general surgeons. Unfortunately the general public often envisions plastic surgery as esthetic surgery, essentially the correction of relatively minor defects and the repair of the manifestations of the ravages of aging. The increased popularity of plastic surgery has not lessened this misconception.

It is interesting that the development of the modern era of plastic surgery dating from World War I originated from the activities of surgeons of disparate specialties. Morestin and Blair were general surgeons; Ivy and Kazanjian were originally dental surgeons; Gillies was an otolaryngologist, to name only a few who were the pioneers of the modern era. It is therefore understandable that practitioners of other surgical specialities lay claim to certain plastic surgical procedures which fall into the domain of their specialty. It is just as reasonable that the plastic surgeon abstain from performing operations for which he has not been trained as for the specialists in allied specialties to engage in plastic surgery procedures for which they are not qualified. In many cases plastic surgery is competently performed in specialized areas of oral surgery, otolaryngology, ophthalmology and orthopedic surgery.

J. William Littler, who acquired extensive experience in hand surgery during World War II under the overall guidance of Sterling Bunnell, played a decisive role in bringing hand surgery into the field of plastic surgery in the United States. Littler, the editor of the hand section of this text, decided to become a plastic surgeon. His influence has been preponderant, and he has trained innumerable plastic surgeons in this special field of surgery.

Prior to World War II, Burian in Prague had established one of the world's best plastic surgery services; in 1948 Burian was appointed Professor and Chairman of the Department of Plastic Surgery at Charles University. However, the fragmentation of plastic surgery occurred early on the European continent probably because of the emphasis on maxillofacial surgery needed for the large number of facial gunshot wounds inflicted upon the thousands of survivors of World War I.

In Vienna von Eiselsberg, the general surgeon and professor of surgery at the Allgemeines Krankenhaus, sought a close and intimate collaboration with Pichler, a dentist and physician, as early as 1903. Pichler, the son of a dentist, was sent to Chicago by his father to study under Black at the Northwestern University. After his return to Vienna he started to practice dentistry and worked closely with Eiselsberg. Eiselsberg applied for a maxillofacial unit to furnish Pichler with a position. In 1915, the Austrian Imperial Reserve Hospital No. 17 was organized, and Foramitti and Esser from Holland were among its experienced surgeons, capable of performing plastic surgery. In 1917 the outpatient department was also opened to civilians, but the beneficial work of the unit was terminated at the end of the war. It was Eiselsberg who made every effort to preserve the facilities. He succeeded by applying to the university and the government by stating that "the unit would not only be most beneficial for so many patients and the teaching of students, but also to attract foreign physicians and patients."

Thus it was the personal efforts of a general

surgeon that led to the foundation of one of the schools of maxillofacial surgery in Austria.

Wilflingseder, who trained under Gillies, became the head of a division of plastic surgery at the University Hospital in Innsbruck in 1957. In 1966 a chair of Plastic and Reconstructive Surgery was founded for Wilflingseder, and a Department of Plastic Surgery was placed under his direction.

In Germany, departments of maxillofacial surgery originated in the military hospitals for the facially disfigured early in the 1920's. These were headed by Axhausen in Berlin, Rosenthal in Leipzig, and Lindemann in Düsseldorf. These three men became the founders of German face and jaw surgery and were later joined by the much younger Wassmund. The pupils of these men, especially Schuchardt and Schmid, led the transition from maxillofacial to plastic surgery.

In Hamburg the Nordwestdeutschen Kieferklinik was established after World War II, when Schuchardt was asked to come to Hamburg, and he transferred 200 wounded soliders from a hospital in Schleswig-Holstein, the province north of Hamburg. Schuchardt had managed to bring these soldiers out of an area occupied by the Russians.

These separate origins explain why there are two disparate German societies of plastic surgeons. The Vereinigung Deutscher Plastischer Chirurgen strives to have plastic surgery considered as a specialty in its own right; the older, dental-oriented group clings to a regional specialty concept (Kiefer und Gesichtschirurgie: jaw and face surgery). There is also the Society of Plastic and Reconstructive Surgery, which developed as a section, later a branch, of the Deutsche Gesellschaft für Chirurgie. Its membership is open to all doctors who are interested in plastic surgery.

In France, surgeons trained in Great Britain and the United States after World War II rapidly established the French School under the leadership of Claude Dufourmentel (the son of Léon Dufourmentel) and Morel-Fatio; they were followed by surgeons in Switzerland and other countries of Europe and throughout the world. Marino and Malbec provided leadership for the specialty in South America.

Ten years after the end of World War II, in 1955, the International Association of Plastic Surgeons was organized under the aegis of Tord Skoog and held its first International Congress in Stockholm.

The presently thriving specialty of plastic surgery in Australia began under the leadership of Rank and Wakefield after they had acquired additional training in England and experience during World War II. Penn, who had served as chief of a hospital for the wounded requiring plastic surgery during World War II, was the founder of the specialty in South Africa. As a specialist in dermatology and urology, Ohmori, the founder of the Japanese Society of Plastic and Reconstructive Surgery, treated patients with scar contractures from burns at the Tokyo Metropolitan Police Hospital. While attending a course on dermatology at Harvard Medical School in 1952, Ohmori spent most of his time watching Bradford Cannon performing plastic surgical operations at the Massachusetts General Hospital. He acquired further knowledge in England and Scotland, the United States and Australia. A training program was started in 1958 at Tokyo University Hospital and the Tokyo Metropolitan Police Hospital.

Plastic Surgery as a Specialty: Its Future

During the early part of the nineteenth century prior to the discovery of general anesthesia and prior to the surgeon's entry into the abdominal cavity, the surgeon was mostly concerned with what was referred to as "external pathology." This explains the large number of reconstructive plastic surgical operations performed during this period.

Specialization came much later, especially during the present century with increasing impetus. Even the "general" surgeon is becoming a specialist in many respects. Let us read the words of a Professor of Surgery, Francis Moore (quoted by Edgerton, 1974): "Are we to go along with the concept that those who operate on the face, the neck, the head, the lip, the eye, the hand, and the breast are the *only* persons who should do any of those operations?" A plastic surgeon's answer is: "Of course, the answer is 'no,' but in the case of many *particular* operations in those regions, if the plastic surgeon can do these operations not only *better,* but also more *safely* and more efficiently *without increasing the medical cost,* then those operations probably should be done by a plastic surgeon whenever one is available. We must deliver reconstruction not only better, but also more efficiently" (Edgerton, 1974).

The principles of plastic surgical techniques are special, and the conceptual application of these principles requires indoctrination. Once indoctrinated, the plastic surgeon can apply these concepts in any area of the body if he has had basic training in "general" surgery. During his surgical training he must seek training in as many areas of surgical endeavor as possible.

Postresidency fellowships in various countries and continuing education symposia such as those organized by the Educational Foundation of the American Society of Plastic and Reconstructive Surgeons are available to those who require additional training. The education of the plastic surgeon, as for all members of the medical profession, is a continuing obligation during his entire professional career.

Whether in a university setting or in large-city private practice, the answer to complete, efficient coverage of all phases of plastic surgery is the team approach. After a broad training in general surgery with periods of training in the surgical specialties and in plastic surgery, each plastic surgeon of the team subspecializes in his area of preference. The team should include not only plastic surgeons but also members of allied specialties in the field of medicine and dentistry. Thus the various talents are centralized for the benefit of the patient. The multidisciplinary approach has been brought to the foreground in the treatment of craniofacial malformations. Various surgical, medical, and dental specialists and representatives of the basic sciences are members of the team. It is the interdisciplinary interchange that makes for surgical progress and provides for the optimal care of the patient.

In smaller cities and towns the plastic surgeon will find himself called upon to solve problems which the general surgeon or other specialists will find necessary to refer to him. He will cover the broad field of plastic surgery, seek collaboration with other specialists, and refer to the large centers those patients he feels he is not equipped to treat.

Esthetic surgery is here to stay as a legitimate subspecialty of plastic surgery. Because of the psychological component in the patient's motivation in this type of corrective surgery (see Chapters 21 and 22), the indications for surgery should be carefully evaluated. The psychological and, often, vocational gains resulting from esthetic surgery, whether large or small, often have a considerable impact on the patient's life style. It is appreciation by the lay public of the results obtained that has led to increasing demands for this type of surgery.

Tagliacozzi wrote, "We reconstruct and complete parts which nature had given but which were destroyed by fate, and we do so not so much for the enjoyment of the eye as for psychic comfort to the afflicted."

Tagliacozzi was damned, exhumed, and buried in unconsecrated ground because of his reconstructive nasal operations, which were against nature and illegal. Only in our time have the problems and purpose of plastic surgery been valued theologically. Pope Pius XII declared on October 14, 1958:

"If we consider physical beauty in its Christian light and if we respect the conditions set by our moral teachings, then esthetic surgery is not in contradiction to the will of God, in that it restores the perfection of that greatest work of creation, man" (Wilflingseder, 1975).

FACE TO FACE WITH DEFORMITY

The plastic surgeon must first make an accurate evaluation of the deformity, of the degree of displacement of the tissues, of the extent of the defect, and of the functional disability. Is the deformity apparent or real? What is the extent of the true defect? Having made his appraisal, he must then consider various methods of treatment in relation to the type of deformity, the age of the patient, and the patient's mental attitude toward the surgery. The methods to be employed are also considered: a simple and rapid technique may give an adequate result; a more intricate type of repair may give a better permanent result. Which is the best suited to the particular patient? A primary defect may be satisfactorily repaired, but the result may be obtained at the expense of a secondary defect which is a more serious deformity than the original one.

Certainly, detailed plastic surgery and a superior final result are possible only in the patient who is willing to give the highest degree of cooperation. The demands of the patient stimulate the surgeon toward progress. In the developing countries the patient may be satisfied with a type of result that would not satisfy the patient who lives in a country where competition for employment and social status requires that he achieve the best result possible in appearance and function. Careful diagnosis for the restoration of function is of particular importance in hand surgery.

Planning Repair

In planning the repair, the surgeon must choose from many methods of treatment: shifting of local tissue; transplantation of tissue from a distance; skin flaps; grafts of skin, dermis, fat, fascia, tendon, or muscle; the restoration of the skeletal framework by bone or cartilage; suture or grafting of nerves; the transposition or grafting of muscles. He must consider the advisability of the use of inorganic implants in certain favorable sites.

The unhurried, deliberate, judicious approach to the problem at hand is the key to success in plastic surgery. Only if the true extent of the deformity is fully appreciated can an adequate plan of treatment be established. It is true that in some types of cases the "wait and see" approach can be employed with impunity. The motto may be: "Let's get in and see!" A retracted, scarred area is excised, the true defect becomes evident after retraction of the surrounding soft tissues, and the defect is covered with skin grafts. With this approach the surgeon would find himself in trouble had he planned a skin flap from a distant area, for the flap would not fit the defect unless careful measurements had been made prior to surgery.

The Apparent Versus the True Defect

In many cases the defect is evident. In a deformity of the mandible, the change in the occlusal relationships of the teeth provides a satisfactory guide to the size of the defect. A retracted, everted lower eyelid may be compared to the contralateral lower eyelid and an accurate estimate of the required amount of skin readily obtained; a missing ala may be compared to its unaffected twin and the size of the composite graft to repair the nasal defect readily evaluated.

A method of actually mapping the extent of the true defect and comparing it with the apparent defect is illustrated in Figure 1–8. Measurements are made from landmarks such as the acromion and the styloid process, and in this manner the size of the area to be covered by grafts or a flap can be evaluated with a certain degree of precision. When the defect is bilateral, as in an extensive contracture of the cervical area resulting from burns (Fig. 1–9, A), fixed points at the mental symphysis and the sternal notch permit one to obtain a fairly accurate evaluation of the amount of missing skin by measuring the distance between these two points in another individual of approximately the same size and comparing this distance with that between similar points in the patient.

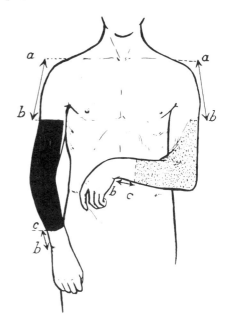

FIGURE 1–8. The true defect versus the apparent defect. Drawing illustrating a severe burn contracture of the left upper extremity. Because of the contracture, the apparent defect is smaller than the true defect plotted on the right upper extremity. Fixed points, such as the acromion and the styloid process of the ulna, are employed to obtain the distances a-b and c-d which, when transferred to the unaffected extremity, permit estimation of the upper and lower limits of the true defect.

The apparent defect is often the result of the loss of tissue followed by the contraction and contracture of the adjacent parts (Fig. 1–9, B). The apparent defect may also be a relative one: the chin may appear deviated to one side because of a deviation of the nose; the nose may appear too prominent in the profile because of lack of development of the mental symphysis. In establishing the diagnosis of a facial deformity, it is essential to place the face according to the Frankfort horizontal and the midsagittal plane (see Fig. 1–11). In this position many facial discrepancies become evident.

Aids in Planning

There is no substitute for the careful clinical examination of the patient. In deformities of the face, photographs taken in standardized positions according to the Frankfort horizontal and the midsagittal plane of the face are of assistance in establishing a diagnosis and a plan

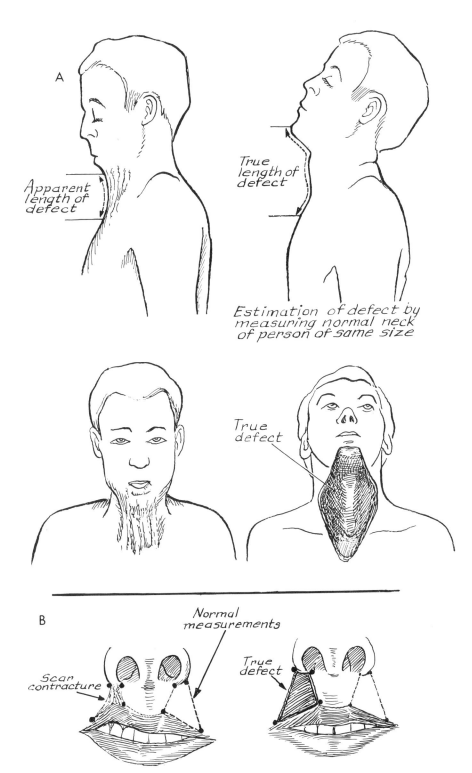

FIGURE 1–9. True versus apparent defect. *A,* In bilateral involvement, as in neck contractures, a measurement between two fixed points (mental symphysis and sternal notch) in an unaffected individual of the same size gives the length of the true defect. *B,* Upper lip scar and contracture. The apparent defect is smaller because of the resulting contracture of the adjacent parts. (From Kazanjian and Converse.)

of treatment. Serial photographs are indispensable for following progress. Facial casts aid in planning contour restoration or other changes in form but are usually not required in the average case. Bony deformities require a careful roentgenographic examination; cephalometric roentgenograms are of invaluable assistance in planning changes in the form of the skeletal framework of the face.

The team approach is essential for progress. Many problems in plastic surgery require consultation with specialists in other fields. The collaboration of dental specialists is essential in the treatment of such problems as jaw fractures, cleft lip and palate, and other craniofacial malformations and in reconstruction following excisional surgery for malignant disease. Postoperative physiotherapy, guided by the surgeon, is an important part of hand rehabilitation.

There are certain intangible qualities which make for excellence in plastic surgery; a sense of proportion and contour, esthetic judgment, and attention to minute detail may spell the difference between success and failure. The part-time plastic surgeon may not have these qualities. The everyday preoccupation with problems which require solution makes for excellence.

Not the least of the aspects of treatment is the psychological support provided by the surgeon and his team; psychiatric treatment is obligatory in some cases. The psychological make-up of the patient often influences the technique or repair; simple methods may be required in problem cases.

A characteristic of plastic surgery is its diversity, both in the problems to be solved and in the methods available to solve the problems. "There are more ways than one to skin a cat": there is the simple and effective way, and there is also the complicated way. The beginner will often choose the most devious route when he is blind to the most obviously simple. One of the most important aspects of residency training is to impart the importance, after a diagnosis of the deformity has been made, of considering in turn all possible methods of treatment, weighing the alternatives, and choosing the most suitable.

Regional Entities of the Face and Neck

In reconstructive procedures in the face, for example, in skin grafting for burn contractures,

it is important to observe the confines of the regional entity of the face (Fig. 1–10). The first of these is the forehead, extending from the eyebrows to the hairline. The regional entity of the forehead should be preserved when a large forehead flap is employed in reconstructing the cheek; for example, a one-piece split-thickness skin graft will provide a satisfactory esthetic result. Other regional entities are the orbital region, the nasal region, the region of the lips, limited laterally by the nasolabial folds and secondary lines of expression situated laterally to the angle of the mouth, and the labiomental fold. The region of the cheek is subdivided into two entities, an anterior, which is soft, pliable and mobile, and a posterior, extending over the parotid-masseteric region, which is relatively firm and less mobile.

Interpretation of the Deformity

The deformity may be minor to an impartial observer. To the patient, however, the deformity may assume a magnitude out of all proportion to reality. One of the main purposes of plastic surgery is to restore the mental health of the patient, thus permitting a return to active social participation. The psychological

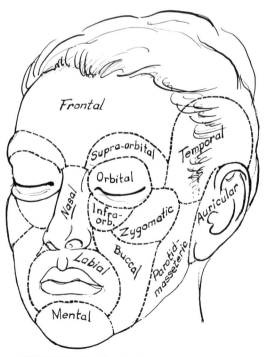

FIGURE 1–10.   Regional entities of the face.

trauma suffered by the patient may be related to the injury and the circumstances of the accident or may be due to comments of relatives or friends. One of the distressing aspects of this type of surgery is that the successful repair of even major traumatic deformities is not necessarily followed by a cure. Deep seated psychological disturbances may persist.

In major deformities, physical diagnosis is more obvious, but in many serious disfigurements, despite the significant progress made in surgery, the appreciable improvement achieved does not always restore the physical appearance of the patient. The severity of the psychological disturbance is not necessarily related to the severity of the deformity, nor is it directly proportional to the degree of improvement accomplished by surgery. Cultural aspects complicate this picture. A classic example is the scar resulting from the Heidelberg duels, considered an emblem of an individual's manliness rather than a disfigurement. Severe facial disfigurement is one of the worst physical and psychosocial handicaps (see Chapters 21 and 22).

In civilized man the face alone remains unclothed and exposed. An injury resulting in distortion of the features thus sets the unfortunate individual apart in a highly organized society where a premium is placed upon beauty and facial symmetry. Because disfigurement of the face becomes a serious social handicap, the surgical treatment of facial injuries is of special significance, as it serves to restore the inner feelings of happiness and well-being in addition to the outer appearance and function.

The need for the rehabilitation of the facially disfigured is well recognized in the present era. Around 1950 a change took place in regard to the treatment of patients requiring massive resection for head and neck cancer. The disease-oriented surgeon proceeded, in the past, with the necessary mutilating surgery following the philosophy that all means are good to preserve life, irrespective of the esthetic and functional consequences to the patient. This philosophy no longer prevails: the patient demands more than the preservation of life. The quality of life is important to the patient as is the quantity of life which the wide resection of hard and soft tissues is able to achieve. While the anticipation that radical extirpative surgery gives the best chance for a cure is reassuring to the surgeon, the expectation that satisfactory reconstruction is feasible is also comforting to the patient.

Body Image

The body image is a basic component of our self concept and our feeling of personal identity. It includes both the mental picture we have of our physical characteristics and our attitudes toward these characteristics. It stems from both conscious and unconscious sources (Macgregor, 1974*a, b*).

The body image develops slowly and undergoes many changes in the course of growth and development. The perception of one's physical characteristics begins to take shape probably around the age of 6 months of life when the infant explores and discovers his body. Later, as he begins to play with other children, he gradually develops a vague idea of what his body can or cannot do. This is the beginning of the body concept. As time goes on, the attitudes of others play a major role in the image he has of his body and its parts.

A patient can incur a deformity or undergo correction of the deformity, but his reactions may well depend on the reactions of others, which may in turn bring about a change in his *body concept*. Some people incorporate defects or corrections in the body image, while others retain a distorted image. By using preoperative photographs of the patient or a mirror to determine how the patient views himself, it is often possible to learn to what extent the patient's perception of himself is realistic or unrealistic.

Aids in Diagnosis

The diagnosis of a defect and the distinction between the true defect and the apparent defect has been discussed earlier in the chapter. The plastic surgeon is confronted with difficult decisions and diagnoses in facial deformities and abnormalities. In addition to the clinical examination, clinical photographs and a summary knowledge of artistic anatomy are of invaluable assistance.

ANTHROPOMETRIC POINTS OF THE FACE

Physical anthropologists employ methods of measurement which permit determination of significant likenesses and differences between individuals and races. These standardized measurements are useful when attempting to restore the structure and contour of the deformed face. Among the commonly employed anthropometric points (Fig. 1–11) are: *trichion,* an imprecise landmark, the midpoint at the hairline on the forehead; *nasion,* the most anterior point of the midline of the frontonasal suture; *subnasale,* the point beneath the nasal spine where the nasal columella merges with the upper lip in the mid-sagittal plane; *pogonion,* the most anterior point on the contour of the chin; *menton,* the lowest point on the symphyseal outline; and *gnathion,* the point obtained by bisecting the facial and mandibular planes. The mid-sagittal line, a vertical line passing through these points, divides the face into halves. *Tragion* is the notch immediately above the tragus of the ear; *orbitale* is the lowest point on the infraorbital margin; the Frankfort horizontal passes through these points.

Measurements of facial dimensions are taken according to three planes: vertical (facial length), frontal (facial width), and sagittal (facial depth). Facial width is obtained by measuring the distance between the most prominent points on the zygomatic bones. Facial depth is determined by measuring the distance from the external auditory canal to various points such as nasion, subnasale, and gnathion. The distance between pogonion and gonion, the tip of the angle of the jaw, determines the length of the body of the mandible; the distance from the nasion to the tip of the nose equals the length of the nose.

Horizontal lines passing through trichion, nasion, subnasale, and menton divide the physiognomic face into thirds, theoretically of equal height; in practice, however, each third of the face differs in size from the others.

Some Principles of Artistic Anatomy

Beauty has no universal criteria and varies from culture to culture and from century to century (Fig. 1–12). Burkhardt (1929) cites the work of Firenzuola (1802) on female beauty written in the 16th century: "The nose, which chiefly determines the value of the profile, must recede gently and uniformly in the direction of the eyes; where the cartilage ceases there may be a slight elevation, but not so marked so as to make the nose aquiline, which is not pleasing in women...." As delicacies of details, he mentions a dimple in the upper lip, a certain fullness of the lower lip, and a tempting smile in the left corner of the mouth. Such a description would infer that the smile of "La Gioconda" (the Mona Lisa) is not necessarily one of mystery but rather a habit induced by what was considered the style of the period. Large hips and a robust body were much admired as recently as the Victorian age; crease lines around the neck were called the "necklace of Venus" (Fig. 1–13).

Contemporary standards of beauty are epitomized in advertisements showing young,

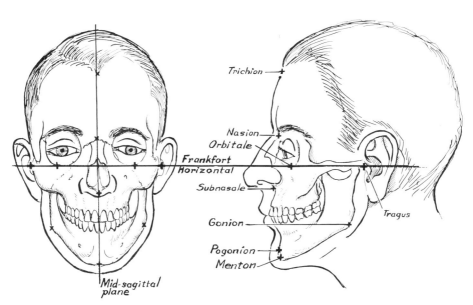

FIGURE 1–11.   Anthropometric points of the face. *A,* Frontal view. Note Frankfort horizontal line and mid-sagittal plane. *B,* Lateral view showing the anthropometric points of the face.

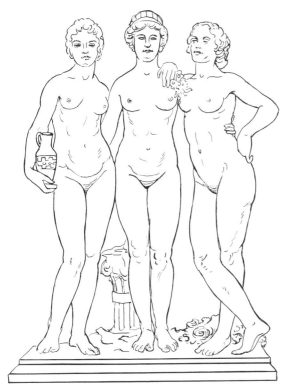

FIGURE 1–12. The three graces, a statue by Paul Richer, representing three different types: the female of antiquity (left), the Renaissance woman (center), and modern woman (right). It appears that the same model (circa 1914) posed for all three studies.

the human form as are the artists who specialize in portraits or nudes.

Leonardo de Vinci sketched and measured many faces and figures to determine geometrically what he called "the divine proportions." Many of his measurements and divisions remain the basic tools in art school for teaching life classes in drawing. Figure 1–15 is a penline copy of a well known crayon sketch by Leonardo in which he appears to have analyzed the shape and relationships of the various features of the face. No descriptive accompanying notes explain his geometric lines. The following illustration (Fig. 1–16, *A*) is also a tracing of a sketch by Leonardo. A translation of his notes reads as follows: "Proportions of the head. From the eyebrow to the junction of the lip with the chin, and from there to the posterior angle of the jaw, and from there to the upper edge of the ear near the temple, there is a perfect square, the side of which measures half a head, and the hollow of the cheek bone is halfway between the tip of the nose and the back portion of the jaw." Figure 1–16, *B* shows distortion of the square in Apert's syndrome.

If one takes the same Leonardo sketch and superimposes the ear (Fig. 1–17), his following note is understood. "From the edge of the orbit to the ear, there is the same distance as the length of the ear, in other words one-third

slender-bodied models with perfectly proportioned facial features. Beauty basically reflects an assemblage of esthetic properties which commands approbation in the specific culture.

Today people are turning to plastic surgeons in increasing numbers to give them these valued features, to correct minor defects, and to repair the ravages of age. It is their hope that such surgery will improve their life style in a highly competitive society which places considerable emphasis on youth and accepted standards of beauty.

Figure 1–14 illustrates in tracings from pre- and postoperative photographs how far nature may stray from ideals of beauty, and the results of the surgeon's attempt to correct nature's mistakes.

Proportions of Human Form. In making his corrections, the surgeon tries to reform the affected body or face to an acceptable cultural standard. In doing so, he must also be as well acquainted with the accepted proportions of

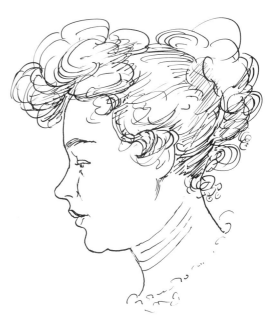

FIGURE 1–13. The necklace of Venus.

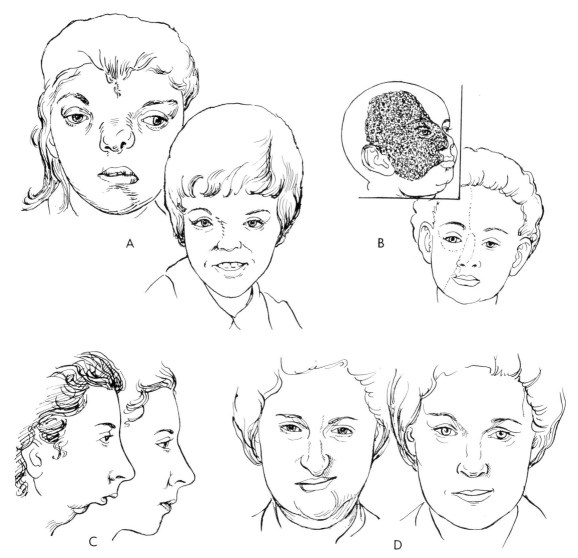

FIGURE 1–14. Examples of nature's mistakes and surgical correction (tracings from pre- and postoperative photographs). *A*, Orbital hypertelorism. *B*, Hairy nevus. *C*, Micrognathia. *D*, Mandibular asymmetry.

of the head." It would then apparently follow that the distance from the hairline to the chin is three ears long and also three noses long. He wrote, "The distances from the chin to the nose and from the hairline to the eyebrows are equal, each of them to the height of the ear and to one-third of the face."

Other proportions of the face taught in art schools today are still credited to Leonardo. For example, the distance between the eyes is equal to the width of one eye (Fig. 1–18, *A*). It is also pointed out that, in the ideal Caucasian form, the nostrils should not flare more laterally than a line dropped vertically from the medial canthus (Fig. 1–18, *B*–line "f"). The mouth should extend laterally to a line dropped from the medial margin of the limbus (Fig. 1–18–line "e"). Beyond this point the mouth is too large. Figure 1–18, *C* is a tracing from a photograph of a patient with orbital hypertelorism, showing the wide deviation from normal measurements. The eyes are two lengths apart, and lines "e" and "f" are no longer vertical.

In considering the face in relation to the body, one should remember that the face from chin to hairline is the same length as the hand, and the nose is the same length as that of the

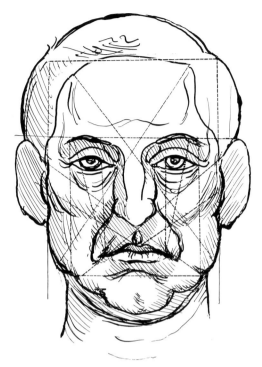

FIGURE 1-15. Tracing of a sketch by Leonardo da Vinci. An analysis of the relationships of the various facial structures.

thumb (Fig. 1–19, *A*). The eyes are situated in the exact center of the head, between the top of the skull and the chin (Fig. 1–19, *B*). The patient shown in Figure 1–20, *A* has, if the mouth were closed, eyes placed three-fifths of the distance down from the top of the head to the chin. His appearance suggests mental deficiency. This impression is corrected in the sketch (Fig. 1–20, *B*) by placing a normal-sized cranium above the same features and closing the mouth so that the chin is shorter and the teeth are in occlusion. Figure 1–21 shows a patient with the eyes set too high in the face.

Eyebrows should always lift as they follow the rim of the orbit laterally, to give a youthful appearance (Fig. 1–22, *A*). The brow should never follow the same curvature as the two lines just below it—the line of the contour of the globe and the line of the upper rim of the orbital cavity. The repetition of three lines of the same curvature is not artistic and gives an uninteresting appearance (Fig. 1–22, *B*). An older, more serious appearance is characteristic of individuals with brows slanting downward as they progress laterally (Fig. 1–22, *C*).

On straightforward vision, the rim of the upper eyelid should touch the edge of the

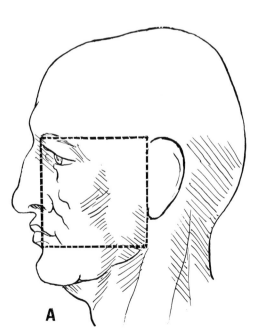

A

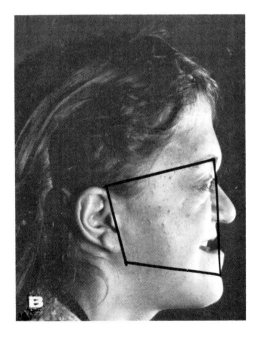

FIGURE 1-16. *A*, The square in the face described by Leonardo (after Leonardo). *B*, Distortion of the square in Apert's syndrome (acrocephalosyndactyly).

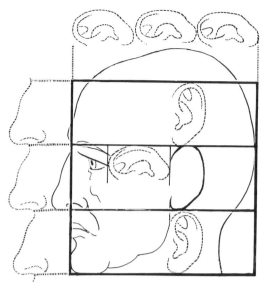

FIGURE 1-17. Leonardo's measurements of the face superimposed on a tracing of a sketch by him.

lower lid was considered to be a sign of psychoneurosis or psychosis. It is doubtful whether many psychiatrists would agree with Brödel's observation. Certainly this would not hold true with elderly people.

George Bridgman, long considered the finest instructor of life drawing in America, at the Art Students League in New York City, evolved a system of simplifying and blocking masses of human figures into geometric shapes and giving them increased definition. Constructive anatomy was an integral part of the course. Bridgman saw four distinct forms in the face: (1) the square or rectangular forehead; (2) the flat cheekbone area; (3) the triangular form of the lower jaw; and (4) an erect cylindrical form on which are placed the base of the nose and the mouth (Fig. 1–24, *A–C*). Bridgman (1973) saw the nose as a wedge (Fig. 1–24, *D*), with its root in the forehead and its base in the upper lip. While Bridgman's knowledge of the substructures of the nose leaves something to be desired, he was able to simplify the nose in his drawings. He described two wedges meeting on the bridge of the nose (Fig. 1–24, *E–G*) and tapering toward the forehead and the bulbous tip, and remarked that the bulb rises from the middle of the upper

pupil; the lower lid touches the limbus (Fig. 1–23, *A*). It was pointed out by Max Brödel, the father of medical art in America, that the white of the eye showing between the limbus and the

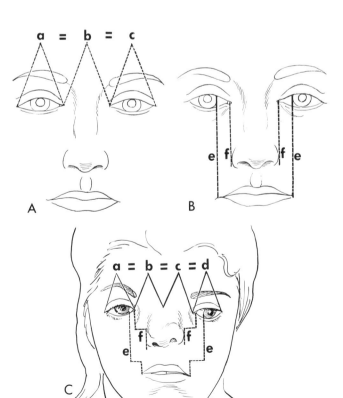

FIGURE 1-18. Proportions of the face. *A,* Ideal relationships of the eyes and the interorbital space. *B,* Ideal relationships of the nostrils, the corners of the mouth, and the eyes. *C,* Tracing from a photograph of a patient with orbital hypertelorism, showing the distorted relationships.

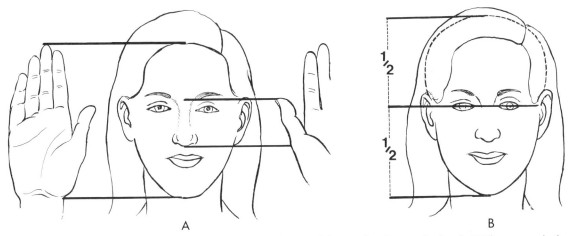

FIGURE 1–19. *A,* The hand has the same length as the face, and the nose is as long as the thumb. *B,* The eyes are in the exact middle of the head.

lip (septum), expands into a bulbous tip, flows over the sides, and flares out to form the wings of the nostrils.

Artists of the past have taught that the upper lip is composed of three muscles and the lower lip of two muscles. They taught that the preliminary sketch should be diagrammed to show these divisions (Fig. 1–25) and thereby facilitate production of the finished product (Fig. 1–26) by giving the student a simple understanding of the subtle lip form. Figure 1–26 is a drawing of the lips diagrammed in Figure 1–25: *A,* lips of a young man; *B,* lips of a young woman; *C,* lips of a young girl.

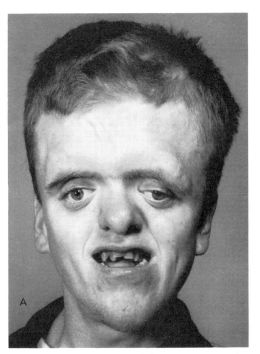
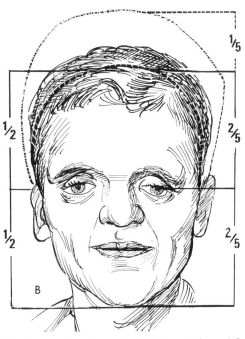

FIGURE 1–20. A knowledge of the correct proportions of the face can be of a great value in analyzing a deformity. *A,* Photograph of patient with acrocephalosyndactyly (Apert's syndrome). *B,* The tracing of the photograph (dotted) demonstrates the increase in size of the cranial vault.

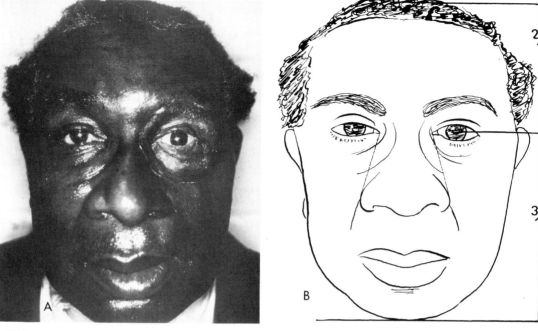

FIGURE 1–21. *A*, Patient with an unusually low cranial vault. Note also the position of the nostrils in relation to the medial canthi. (The patient happens to have a left orbital prosthesis.) *B*, Drawing shows the high position of the eyes.

Most artists have difficulty in drawing the ear because of a lack of understanding of the anatomy (Fig. 1–27, *A*). It appears to be a complex structure because of the intricate con-

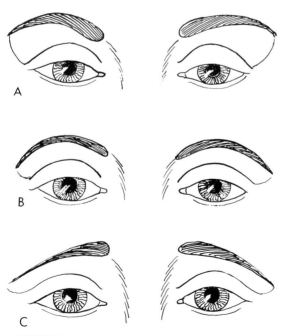

FIGURE 1–22. *A*, Preferred placement of the eyebrow. *B, C*, Less attractive position of the eyebrow.

volutions. Simplification of the structure into an elongated "C" for the helix, a "Y" for the superior and inferior crura, the triangular fossa, and the concha, and a "U" for the lobule (Fig. 1–27, *B*) renders it understandable (Fig. 1–27, *C*). Any surgeon planning reconstruction of the ear should first practice drawing it or modeling it in clay.

The length of the body in relation to the head varies according to the artist. Leonardo claimed the head to be one-eighth the length of the body, the leg from the crest of the ilium to the base of the heel one-half the length of the body, and the distance from the fingertip to the center of the chin one-half the length of the body. At that time Leonardo was interested in the Platonian theory of the geometric representation of the universe as discussed in the book of Fra Luca Pacciola (circa 1445–1514), with whom Leonardo collaborated. According to the position in which one places the human body, the body may be enclosed within a square because of the equal dimensions of the arm-span and the body height when they are perpendicular to each other, in a circle when the limbs are more or less in abduction, and in a pentagon (the Pythagorean symbol of a microcosm). Leonardo's plates to this effect expressed an esthetic rule rather than an anthropologic fact, and he later abandoned that

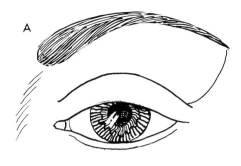

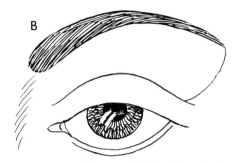

FIGURE 1–23. *A,* The upper lid should touch the pupil on forward gaze. The lower lid should touch the limbus. *B,* The sclera of the eye should not show between the limbus and the lower lid ("scleral show").

concept. Richer (1920) of the Ecole des Beaux Arts in Paris taught that the body length equaled 7½ heads (Fig. 1–28). Richer further divided the body into masses for study and analysis, as shown in Figure 1–29.

Figure 1–29, *E* is a copy of a diagram by Lanteri of the Ecole des Beaux Arts, which shows his view of the circumscribed forms or masses of the face. It should be noted that both Lanteri and Bridgman see the infraorbital area as part of the flat zygomatic area, not as a separate mass, as the cosmetic surgeon would see it. Leonardo paid considerable attention to the infraorbital area in many drawings (see Figure 1–15), emphasizing the area in older faces and in his own self-portrait.

PHOTOGRAPHY

Photography is essential for diagnostic purposes, as a record of the progress made in multiple-stage operations and as a "before" and "after" record of the surgical result. Photographs are also important medicolegal records.

Gillies, at the First International Congress of Plastic Surgery in Stockholm in his speech at the Congress banquet, said facetiously, "I have been asked to speak about the important advances in plastic surgery. I think the most important advance is photography!"

In facial surgery the photograph serves as a means of determining how the patient views himself and thus of learning to what extent the patient's perception of himself is realistic or unrealistic. In the severely disfigured patient, total rehabilitation often cannot be achieved; the comparison of the preoperative and postoperative photographs will help the patient to perceive the improvement achieved. "Did I really look like that?" is his frequent comment.

Consistency in Medical Photography: Standards for Comparison.   Any surgeon attending a convention or congress will notice the frequent absence of any type of standard of comparison between preoperative and postoperative photographs of patients; the position, the lighting, and the exposure vary. Often the preoperative photograph shows the patient in the position and under the lighting and exposure which show the deformity at its worst; the postoperative view may be taken at an angle, with flat lighting, and with the most favorable photographic exposure. The surgeon does not mean to be dishonest, but he is. The same observation applies to publications. When the surgeon takes his own photographs with a direct flash attachment, he is bound to obtain differences in exposure, and he is also dependent upon the developer of the pictures.

A professional photographer is always desirable but is not always available. Some advice from Mr. Don Allen, the photographer of the Institute of Reconstructive Plastic Surgery since 1947, is pertinent.

The Role of the Medical Photographer.   The medical photographer must ask himself the following questions: What is the purpose of the photographs? How do they differ from ordinary photography? The photographer must be closely associated with the field of medicine, usually through a hospital affiliation. Most of his work is governed by a strict set of rules. Photographers outside the medical field remark that they are nearly totally bound up by confining limitations; this is true. The main confining limitation is *consistency.* Consistency is the constant challenge.

A medical photograph must be an accurate, pictorial (visual) record relative to a certain

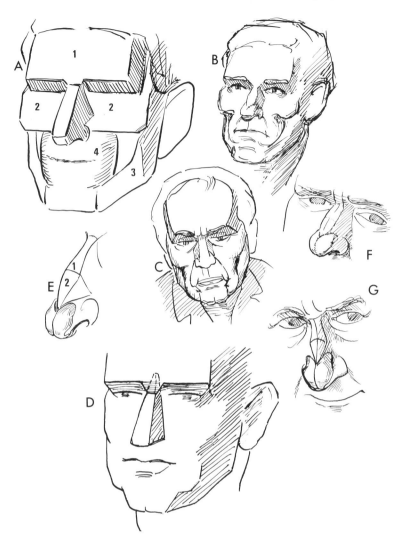

FIGURE 1–24. *A, B, C,* Geometric shapes in the face. *D,* The nose seen as a wedge inserting into the forehead. *E,* Two wedges shown meeting at the bridge of the nose. *F, G,* Variations in the nasal wedges.

condition. It may stand alone as a single photograph tied to a single date, or as part of a continuing, comparable record of the progress achieved by staged surgical procedures over an indeterminate period. To ensure its reliability the photograph must be consistent in quality, position, and accuracy.

Color transparencies serve a dual purpose, since good black and white photographs can be made through internegatives. There are many good color processing laboratories available throughout the world to give anyone fast, quality service. Color transparencies are also useful in illustrating lectures.

Vast amounts of visual records would be lost if it were not for the color-loaded, single lens reflex camera in the hands of either the doctor, nurse, or technician. When the original color photograph or its black and white reproduction is not of top quality, more than likely the culprit is the lighting. Most of the camera units incorporate a single-source strobe light, which is almost always mounted close to the lens axis, a feature which tends to produce a photograph without the contour details obtained by adequate lighting. This is an unavoidable characteristic, but the fact that the unit will produce consistently good color and exposure makes the unit most valuable.

The four major factors relating to these goals are the studio, the camera, the patient, and the lighting.

The *studio* should be large enough to make use of a focal length lens angle long enough to yield no distortion and to permit photographing patients full length. Appropriate

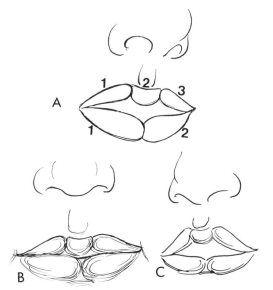

FIGURE 1-25. Diagram showing how to draw the lips. The prolabial and two lateral segments above; two segments below.

eye level markers—or fixed points to aid the patient in holding a given position—should be available. This requires a secure and comfortable chair of the correct height that can easily be moved.

The *camera* should be of the single-lens, reflex type with interchangeable lenses, and good optics, capable of strobe-synchronization. The single-lens reflex helps to achieve a correct camera angle.

The *patient* should be photographed in a comfortable atmosphere, without make-up, distracting clothes, interfering hair, or jewelry. Long hair should be cleared from the face.

The *lighting* is usually achieved by employing a set of at least three studio-type strobe light heads equipped with modeling lights. Strict lighting rules produce constant results. One must remember that the camera does not lie, but the lighting can and will unless careful attention is given at all times.

The patient's face should be placed in a position in accord with the horizontal (Frankfort) and mid-sagittal planes of the face (see Fig. 1-11).

Illustrations. There are several basic views to demonstrate proper alignment, correct and consistent lighting, and relative magnification: full-face view (Fig. 1-30), submental views (2) (Fig. 1-31), matching three-quarter anterior views (2) (Fig. 1-32), and matching left and right profile views (Fig. 1-33).

The production of each patient photograph

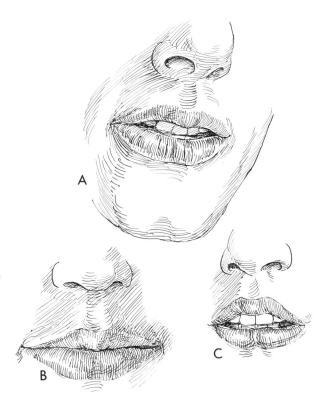

FIGURE 1-26. Drawings of the lips from the diagram in Figure 1-25.

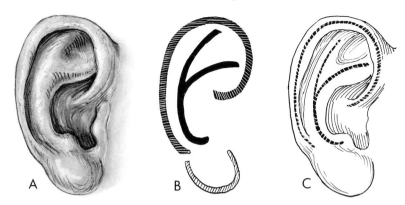

FIGURE 1–27.   Simplifying the ear into an elongated "C" for the helix, a "Y" for the superior and inferior crura, the triangular fossa, and the concha, and a "U" for the lobule.

must be guided by (1) proper positioning of the patient; (2) proper camera angle approach; (3) controlled lighting; (4) consistent photographic technique; and (5) proper laboratory finishing.

The photographic laboratory offers the final control. Magnification and alignment must be maintained at this, the final stage.

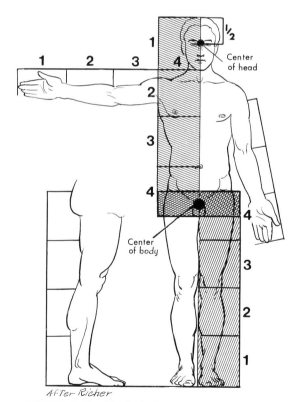

FIGURE 1–28.   The body is 7½ to 8 heads high. The distance from fingertips to chin is 4 heads in men, less in women because of the narrower shoulders. (Adapted from Richer, P.: Morphologie de la Femme. Plon-Nourrit et Cie, 1920.)

The Black and White Print Versus the Color Transparency.   If the photographs are taken under the conditions described above, a transparency is as accurate a document as a black and white print. The print has the advantage, however, that it can be more easily examined and placed on the wall of the operating room, where, because of its larger size, it can be readily and more accurately examined.

THE PLASTIC SURGEON AND THE INTEGUMENT

Although the plastic surgeon is concerned with the repair of the skeletal framework, muscles, tendons, nerves, and vessels, he must, in order to ensure a successful result, obtain adequate cutaneous covering of his underlying surgical procedures. He must, therefore, be an expert in the management of soft tissue wounds, whether operative or traumatic in origin.

Elasticity, Extensibility, and Resiliency of the Skin

The plastic surgeon's tasks in repair and reconstruction involve both soft and hard tissue. The tissue that occupies the majority of his operating time is the integument, the skin (see Anatomy of the Skin in Chapter 6). The skin is elastic, extensible, and resilient; these characteristics vary from birth to old age.

Lines of Tension.   Skin possesses a degree of elasticity owing to the presence of elastic

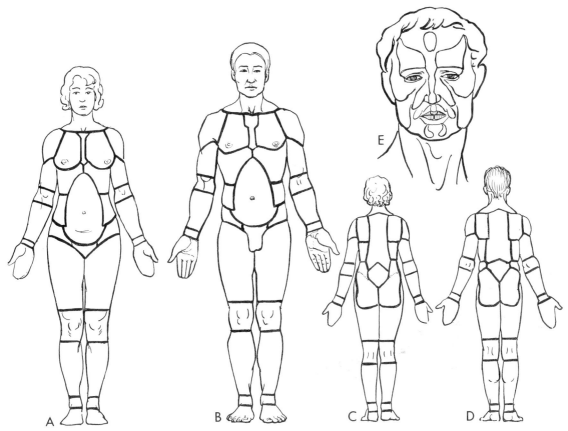

FIGURE 1–29. *A, B, C, D,* Divisions of the body surface for the purpose of artistic analysis (after Richer). *E,* Masses of the face (after Lanteri).

fibers in the dermis. Elastic fibers are disposed in bundles with the collagen fibers, many of them looped spirally around collagen fibers, and are distributed through the dermis, becoming finer toward the surface of the dermis (see Chapter 2). The elasticity maintains the skin in a state of constant tension. This is demonstrated by the gaping of wounds following incision, and also by the immediate contraction of skin grafts as they are removed from the donor site; the thicker the skin graft, the greater the amount of elastic tissue and associated contraction. The elasticity and extensibility of the skin facilitates the shifting of skin flaps. Degeneration of the elastic tissue in the skin of the aged is a contributing factor in the relaxation of the skin of the face and the formation of excess skin folds, which serve as a source of skin for flap repair.

The collagen and elastic fiber bundles of the skin are arranged along "lines of tension." The existence of lines of tension in the skin was first noted by Dupuytren (1832) in describing wounds of the skin made by penetrating instruments. He reported the case of a cobbler who committed suicide by stabbing himself with an awl; the awl was pointed at the tip and round in section, but the wounds in the cobbler's skin were linear in outline, as though made by the blade of a knife.

Langer (1861) found that, following puncture of the skin in various parts of the body, the puncture holes had a tendency to open in a direction corresponding to the normal tension of the skin. Langer considered that human skin was less extensible in the direction of the lines of tension than across them. He attributed this fact to the structure of skin, which he described as consisting of a network of rhomboid meshes permitting greater tension in the direction of the shorter diameter. When placed under tension, the fibers straighten and the meshes are stretched; the fibers themselves are stretched when tension is continued.

Langer's concept was not corroborated by practical experience, as Langer's lines were

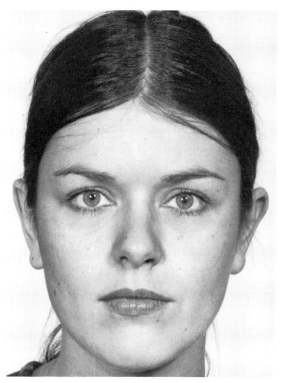

FIGURE 1-30. Full-face photograph. The face is oriented according to the Frankfort horizontal and mid-sagittal planes (see Fig. 1–11, *A*).

found to run across natural creases and flexion lines. Practical experience has shown that wounds heal better and scars are less conspicuous when incisions are made within, or parallel to, natural flexion lines or lines of facial expression. Cox (1941), working under the direction of Wood-Jones, made sections of tissue removed from a wound incised parallel to a flexion line. Sections of skin made in two planes, one exactly at right angles and another exactly parallel to the long axis of a wound, indicated a striking difference in structure according to the plane of the section. Sections taken at right angles to the long axis of the wound showed a marked preponderance of connective tissue and elastic fibers cut transversely; sections parallel to the long axis of the wound showed that the majority of fibers extended longitudinally.

Gibson (1967) has shown that, when skin is stretched, collagen and elastic fibers become aligned in the direction of the stretch (see Chapter 2). This condition exists in the lines of expression or creases of flexion. Wounds within or parallel to these lines are less subject to tension from the activity of the underlying musculature which has produced the lines of tension.

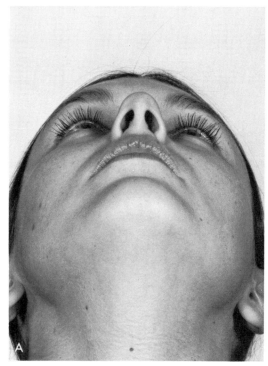 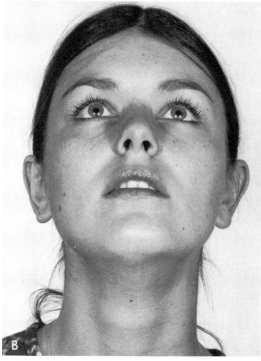

FIGURE 1-31. Submental views. *A*, Base of the nasal pyramid. *B*, Submental view showing the base of the nasal pyramid, the dorsum of the face, and the general facial configuration.

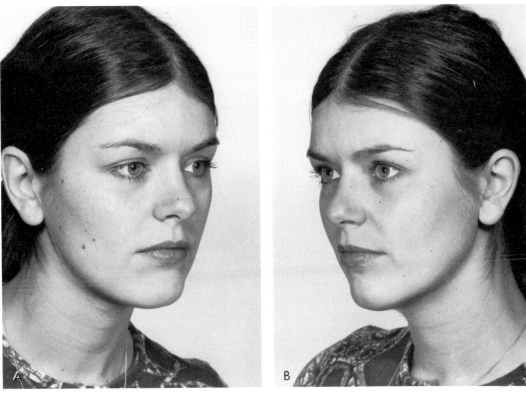

FIGURE 1–32. Three-quarter anterior views of the face.

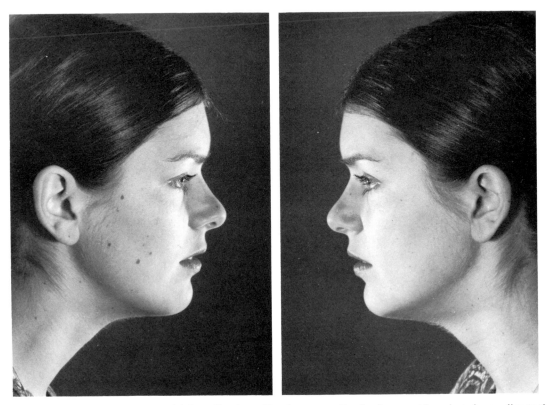

FIGURE 1–33. Matching right and left profile views. For the true profile, the face must be oriented according to the Frankfort horizontal, as illustrated in Figure 1–11, *B*.

The Lines of Minimal Tension. In a cutaneous defect, maximal contraction results in a scar (contracture) whose long axis crosses the lines of minimal tension at right angles. The lines of minimal tension are the result of adaptation to function, the skin being constantly pulled and stretched by the underlying muscle and joint. The connective tissue, collagen, and elastic fibers are arranged in bundles which are perpendicular to the underlying muscles. A scar parallel to the lines is not subject to the intermittent pull of the subjacent muscles—thus the term "lines of minimal tension" (Converse, 1964), indicating that a scar placed within a line of minimal tension or parallel to it will be submitted to minimal tension during the period of healing. Gibson (see Chapter 2) refers to these lines as "lines of maximal tension," indicating thereby that the bundles of connective tissue, collagen, and elastic fibers are submitted to a longitudinal maximum tension within or parallel to the line of tension. Borges (1974) prefers the term "relaxed skin tension lines" in describing these lines.

In an ordinary section of human skin, the collagen fibers of the dermis appear to be arranged haphazardly. If the skin is held in a stretch position during fixation, a proportion of the fibers will be found oriented along the lines of stretch.

In the head and neck, the lines of minimal tension (Fig. 1–34) are the response to adaptation to two different types of functional mechanisms. The first type is represented by the *lines of habitual expression in the face,* such as the lines in the forehead, the eyelids, the nasolabial folds, and other lines of expression around the mouth. The second type, the *lines of skin relaxation* (such as the horizontal circular lines in the neck), results from movements of flexion and extension. Lines of relaxation, of flexion and extension, are formed in the various areas of the body—the trunk, the limbs, the hands and feet.

A scar which traverses the lines of minimal tension of the skin at right angles is subjected to constant changes in tension as the result of the activity of the underlying musculature; hypertrophy of the scar develops. Only a slightly visible scar results when incisions in the neck are made within a skin fold or crease, or are parallel to the fold. Considerable width can be excised on either side of an incision parallel to or in the skin folds without materially increasing tension when the wound is closed, for the skin around the folds is loose and redundant.

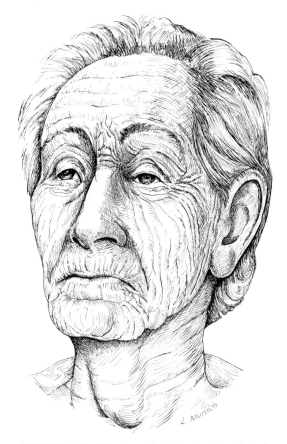

FIGURE 1–34. The lines of minimal tension of the face and neck.

Lines of Expression. Lines of expression are produced by repeated and habitual contraction of the underlying muscles of facial expression. In some regions a number of muscles act in unison. The nasolabial fold, for example, represents the area of junction between the skin of the lip, which is tightly bound to the underlying orbicularis oris muscle, and the more loosely bound skin of the cheek over the buccal fat pad. The nasolabial fold is also formed by muscular contraction of the zygomaticus, quadratus labii superioris, and caninus muscles, and in part by the risorius and buccinator muscles.

The supraorbital wrinkle lines and the transverse lines of the forehead are caused by the contraction of the frontalis muscle, which is inserted into the skin of the lower forehead. In the upper eyelids, many fine perpendicular strands of fibers of the levator aponeurosis terminate in the dermis of the skin and in the tarsus to form the tarsal fold. Similar insertions in the lower lid create the fine horizontal lines of the lower lid, which are accentuated by the contraction of the orbicularis oculi muscle. The sphincter action of the orbicularis oculi muscle is altered by its origin and insertion at two fixed points, the canthal tendon at the medial canthus and the lateral canthal tendon and raphé at the lateral canthus. Contraction of the lateral portion of the muscle produces lines; wrinkles are at right angles to the action of the muscle. In the upper portion of the dorsum of the nose, the corrugator supercilii and orbicularis ocul muscles act somewhat antagonistically to the frontalis to form the almost vertical lines observed during the act of frowning.

The oblique lines on the side of the nose are the consequence of the action of the angular head of the quadratus labii superioris and the procerus muscles. The vertical lines in the lower part of the nose are caused by the contraction of the transverse portion of the nasalis muscle. Crease lines develop radially from the oral fissure. At the angles of the mouth, however, the combined action of the quadratus labii superioris and other muscles in this region causes the lines to blend with those of the nasolabial fold. The formation of the lines on the lateral aspect of the chin results from the action of the triangularis, quadratus labii inferioris, and mentalis muscles.

The transverse lines across the neck separate folds of excess skin, permitting extension of the neck. Near the chest the horizontal neck lines assume a more oblique direction.

Every individual possesses lines of expression that become more apparent when the muscles contract. Wrinkles are less evident in young individuals; however, in old age skin creases and wrinkles are more numerous because the skin, through degenerative changes, has lost its elasticity and becomes redundant. Because the skin is less elastic and also redundant, it is incapable of assuming its smooth appearance at the termination of muscular contraction.

Choice of the Site of Incision. The size and direction of an elective incision should always be chosen in relation to the lines of minimal tension. For example, when planning an incision in the thorax for the removal of costal cartilage, flexion of the thorax shows the position of the skin folds, and the incision is placed in this position. When the incision thus placed does not provide the best exposure of the underlying structures, it is lengthened. Because of the better quality of scar obtained, the longer incision will still be less visible than a

shorter incision placed at right angles to the skin fold; in children, incisions in this area have a notable tendency to hypertrophy. No amount of care in suturing or in the approximation of wound edges will help if the scar is in a position unfavorable to minimal scarring, i.e., at right angles or oblique to the lines of minimal tension.

Although the lines of expression and flexion creases generally coincide with the lines of minimal tension and are the best guide to the placing of incisions, there are exceptions. On the hand, for example, wrinkles produced by hyperextending the thumb and flexing the metacarpal joint of the index finger do not represent the lines of minimal tension (Fig. 1–35). Another exception is the submental fold. An incision made within this fold often heals in an inverted manner, resulting in a bulging of the adjacent tissue; an incision made along the posterior aspect of the inferior border of the mental symphysis is preferable.

Certain areas are particularly unfavorable and tend to heal in a hypertrophic manner (see Chapter 16) following wounds and surgical incisions. The most notable of these areas are the shoulder and the presternal area, which

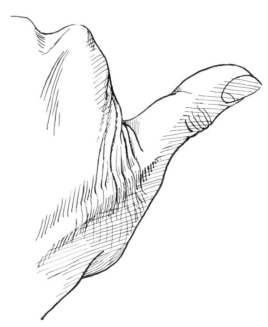

FIGURE 1–35. The wrinkles produced by hyperextending the thumb and flexing the metacarpal joint of the index finger do not represent the lines of minimal tension.

involves exceptional skin tension, especially in the woman with pendulous breasts. Man, originally a quadriped, became a biped; in the erect position the upper extremities hang loosely, and the skin of the shoulder is thus placed under tension. Only in the elderly do anteroposterior folds appear in this area as the skin loses its elasticity and becomes lax.

The Influence of Age. During infancy and the major part of childhood, the skin has its maximum elasticity; it is also padded by a type of adipose tissue, familiarly termed "baby fat," which maintains the skin at its maximum distention. As the aging process takes place, the skin loses much of its elasticity, and the subcutaneous fat changes in character and quantity; the skin folds and wrinkles increase with the progressive relaxation of the skin (see Chapter 37).

The greater elasticity and extensibility of the skin in infants and young children make possible the use of large rotation and advancement flaps to cover defects. The aged patient with relaxed skin has a similar advantage, making possible types of reconstructive procedures which would not provide satisfactory results in young adults.

One of the few compensations of old age is the inconspicuous scar, the result of the relaxation of the skin.

TIMING OF REPAIR

In the treatment of congenital deformities, a number of problems are posed. A major problem is the age at which surgical treatment should be administered. Some deformities must be remedied within a few days after birth, and a number of surgeons have made it their practice to repair a cleft lip in the newborn baby before the mother and child leave the hospital; many other surgeons prefer to wait until the child is 3 or 4 months old before performing the corrective surgery, feeling that the increase in the size of the structures will allow for more accurate repair and that the child is also more physiologically equipped to withstand surgical trauma. Other elective procedures are best postponed until the infant is at least 1 year old, as the morbidity at this age is decreased; a postponement until the child is 5 years old may be advisable if cooperation of the patient is required. In congenital hypopla-

sia of the auricle or microtia, it is usually preferable to reconstruct a new auricle prior to school age in order to avoid psychologic trauma, although the construction of the auricle is easier when the child is older because of the greater availability of costal cartilage and the larger area of available skin in the auricular area.

In developmental malformations, it has been the practice in the past to wait until completion of growth before undertaking reconstructive surgery. This philosophy has been the practice in craniofacial malformations, for example, although postponement of surgery often resulted in progressive accentuation of the malformation. Should these malformations be surgically corrected prior to the achievement of growth? Such a problem is also posed in the treatment of the patient with a cleft lip and/or palate; it has been felt by some that surgery interfered with growth and that postponement of operation was desirable in order to permit growth to progress unimpeded. A change of attitude in recent years has lead to a more selective approach to the timing of reconstructive surgery during the growth and development of the patient.

In craniofacial malformations, such as craniofacial dysostosis (Crouzon), acrocephalosyndactyly (Apert), or hemifacial microsomia, it is preferable to wait until the eruption of a sufficient number of permanent teeth (age 9 or 10 years) to provide sufficient anchorage for orthodontic or other types of appliances for intermaxillary fixation.

The type of plastic surgery that is practiced in cancer differs from the definitive type of surgery done for the repair of congenital malformations or deformities following trauma. Preoccupation with the eradication of malignant disease predominates in the plan of treatment.

In the treatment of oromandibular cancer, if primary reconstruction is not performed after resection of the soft tissues of the lips, cheeks, floor of the mouth, and mandible, constant drooling is present and retention of food is difficult. Unable to feed himself, having to be fed through a tube, the patient has a repulsive appearance to onlookers and even to himself. Outwardly alive, he is inwardly dead (see Chapters 57 to 67).

In other types of cases—after resection of the nose, for example—primary reconstructive surgery is not indicated. A secondary procedure to reconstruct the nose after an interval of a few months is preferable (see Chapter 29).

CHOICE OF THE METHOD OF REPAIR

cessful matching of the skin results in a conspicuous "patch."

Consideration of the Age and Sex of the Patient

The quality of the repair depends upon the surgeon's operative skill and judgment in selecting the operative procedure. Sound clinical judgment in the choice of the method of repair is one of the difficult aspects in the teaching of plastic surgery. The student of plastic surgery peruses books and publications which contain the description, both textual and illustrative, of many operative procedures. Certain procedures are an excellent choice for the patient in the older age group, in whom the relaxed, aging tissues provide an ample supply of tissue to permit closure of the donor site with minimal tension and a relatively inconspicuous scar. Secondary deformities caused by the transfer of regional flaps to repair the defects are also of relatively lesser import in the aged patient, whose main problem may be solely functional. A similar technique may be totally inapplicable in the younger patient.

The method of repair is also influenced by the sex of the patient. For example, flaps may be transferred from the chest in male patients, a procedure which may not be cosmetically acceptable to the female patient.

Camouflage versus Osteotomy

Facial appearance may be improved by a type of camouflage exemplified by the procedure employed in malunited fracture of the zygoma. By this procedure contour is restored by an onlay bone graft in preference to attempting to reposition the zygoma, a more difficult surgical task in some cases.

Color and Texture Match

When transferring skin to the face, a satisfactory match in color, thickness, and texture is important, for the skin of the transplant must harmonize with the surrounding tissue. The choice of tissue borrowed from another area of the body to repair a defect of the soft tissue of the face requires careful consideration. The texture and color of the skin of the face and neck differ from those of other areas. Unsuc-

The Barter Principle

When skin is borrowed from one area of the face to repair another, the secondary deformity may be discernible, but the procedure is often desirable because a closer match of tissue is obtained than when a flap is transferred from a distant area. The principle simplifies reconstruction and avoids conspicuous disparity in the color and texture of the skin. In this process of "robbing Peter to pay Paul," the price paid is at the discretion of the surgeon. It seems obvious that good clinical judgment reduces the cost of the barter to a minimum.

One example of the principle of barter is the use of a forehead flap for subtotal reconstruction of the nose. The forehead tissue is employed for this procedure because the best results in terms of color and texture match are obtained by the use of forehead skin. A major portion of the flap is replaced in its original site after detaching the pedicle, leaving a portion of the flap to form the reconstructed nose. A secondary defect remains on the forehead. This defect is repaired by the most suitable skin available in order to minimize the secondary deformity. Full-thickness skin removed from the supraclavicular or retroauricular areas offers a suitable color match. The supraclavicular defect can usually be closed primarily, and the defect behind the ear is repaired by a split-thickness skin graft from the thigh or abdomen, which, although darker than the surrounding skin, is camouflaged behind the ear. This is a good barter; by contrast, a split-thickness graft placed upon the forehead represents an unsatisfactory repair of the secondary defect.

The Principle of Shifting the Defect

This principle is applied in the transfer of a defect from an area which is either less conspicuous or less important from a functional point of view. For example, a defect may require a flap of tissue from the adjacent skin in order to provide the thickness of both skin and underlying subcutaneous tissue. The procedure is accomplished by closing the primary defect with an adjacent rotation or transposition flap; the secondary defect is then repaired quite satisfactorily by a skin graft or another local flap. For example, when a flap is raised from the preauricular area and is shifted forward to repair a zygomatic defect, skin of suitable color and texture is used in addition to the subcutaneous tissue removed with the flap from over the parotid-masseter fascia. The secondary defect can be repaired by a full-thickness retroauricular graft; the vascularization of the graft is assured, and the esthetic result is excellent. The deficiency in the subcutaneous tissue is less obvious in the preauricular area, a less conspicuous portion of the face than the zygomatic area.

Other examples of the principle of shifting the defect are the closure of a median forehead defect by two rotation flaps and the use of skin grafts to repair the secondary defects produced by the mobilization of the rotation flaps; the restoration of an alar defect by shifting the remaining nasal tissue downward to form the new alar border and reconstructing the resulting full-thickness defect of the side of the nose by flaps; and the reconstruction of a median defect of the lower lip by shifting the remaining lateral portion of the lower lip to the midline and repairing the laterally situated secondary defect by means of an Estlander flap from the upper lip.

Reasons for Postponing the Operation

Temporary or even indefinite postponement of reconstructive or esthetic surgery may occasionally be necessary for reasons which include infection, insufficient lapse of time after healing of the primary wound, and psychological factors. Varying periods of time, depending upon the vascularity of the region, should be permitted to elapse after the healing of the original wound before reconstruction is initiated. Latent infection disappears during this period, and gradual softening of scar tissue occurs by reestablishment of the hemic and lymphatic circulation.

The passage of time softens and smooths scars, skin grafts, and flaps, permitting the repaired tissues to adapt themselves to the underlying structures. The surgeon must allow sufficient time to elapse to permit revascularization and softening of scar before proceeding to a later stage in reconstruction.

The initial tendency to hypertrophic scarring diminishes with the passage of time; this is particularly true in deformities due to burns. Reconstructive procedures are more successful after the tendency to hypertrophic scarring has disappeared. The disruption of the immunologic machinery of a severely burned patient may necessitate postponement of reconstruction for six months to one year (see Chapter 33).

After other types of traumatic injuries, at least four to six months should elapse before undertaking the secondary repair of scars, skin grafts and flaps, and bone and cartilage grafts. Secondary corrective operations on the nose should be postponed for at least six months.

PLASTIC SURGICAL TECHNIQUE

The modern plastic surgeon has at his disposal an armamentarium including special needle-holders capable of holding small, fine-honed needles, delicate forceps, hooks, hemostatic forceps, and many other instruments which are used manually or driven mechanically or by a turbine. The basic principles of plastic surgery technique have been admirably reviewed in the English language by McGregor (1975) and Grabb and Smith (1973).

The making of incisions at right angles to the skin, careful hemostasis with fine-tipped hemostats which grasp only the blood vessel itself with as little surrounding tissue as possible, gentleness in handling the tissues to avoid devitalization: these are points of technique that are well known but cannot be overstressed. Hematoma is the most frequent cause of failure in plastic surgical operations. The use of precise electrocoagulation, with fine-tipped instruments grasping the bleeding vessel, is an efficient and rapid method of obtaining hemostasis. The use of small, flat, perforated suction tubes attached to a suction apparatus has reduced the incidence of hematoma and infection when they are placed under widely undermined areas and skin flaps.

Suturing

Various techniques were used in the period of Ambroise Paré (1575). Figures 1–36 and 1–37 are redrawn from Paré's works. Figure 1–36 represents the "twisted suture" (la suture entortillée); a straight needle penetrated both edges of the wound and suture material was twisted in a figure-of-eight fashion around the ends of the needle. This technique was employed until the discovery of anesthesia in the

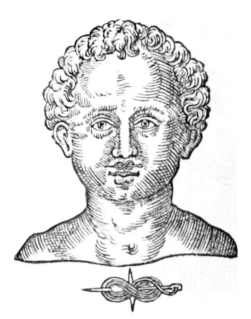

needle to encircle a larger amount of tissue at the periphery of the wound than in the depth of the wound; inversion is also obtained by placing the sutures superficially in the skin.

Subcuticular (subdermal) buried sutures are placed on the undersurface of the cutis (dermis) with the knot downward beneath the dermis; these are useful approximating sutures if tension is present and a widened scar is feared (Fig. 1–42). Special sutures such as vertical mattress sutures (Fig. 1–43) are also useful to evert the wound edges and maintain the skin coapted to the underlying fascial layer.

The *mattress suture,* either horizontal or vertical, *with a dermal component* (Fig. 1–44), the suture being placed through the undersurface of the dermis, is useful at the scalp-skin junction if there is tension. The dermal component avoids suture marks in the skin. The suture also gives excellent approximation of the edge of a skin flap to the edge of the recipient site; the dermal component is placed through the dermis of the flap. The suture assists in joining a thicker wound edge to a thinner

nineteenth century and was used in early cleft lip repairs. Another technique shown by Paré approximates the wound edges by means of sutures passed through cloth glued to the skin surface (la suture agglutinée) (Fig. 1–37). These methods of suturing wounds were still being used until the first part of the nineteenth century. Approximation of the wound edges, or reinforcement of the sutured wound, was revived by the introduction of porous paper-tape Steri-strips (Fig. 1–38).

Precise approximation of skin edges without undue tension ensures primary healing with minimum scarring. The *everting interrupted suture* is the most frequently employed type of suture in plastic surgery (Fig. 1–39). The needle penetrates the skin close to the incision line, diverging from the edge of the wound in order to encircle a larger amount of tissue in the lower depths of the skin than at the periphery. In this manner the suture everts as well as approximates (Fig. 1–40).

The *inverting suture* is required in approximating the skin in the construction of a tube flap or in the establishment of a skin fold in the upper lid by inverting the skin edge toward the upper edge of the tarsus (Fig. 1–41). Inversion is obtained by changing the pathway of the

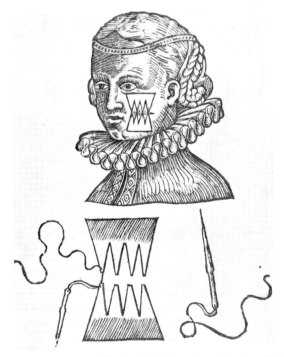

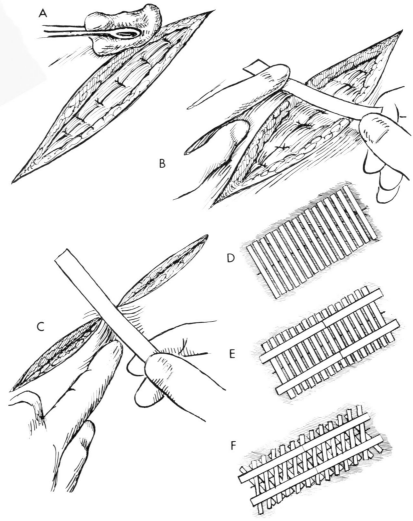

FIGURE 1–38. The Steri-tape technique of skin closure. *A,* Deep layers of wound have been sutured. Skin surface around periphery of wound is cleansed with grease solvent. *B, C,* First strip is applied and center of the wound approximated. *D, E, F,* Completion of adhesive strip closure.

wound edge and equalizing the level of the epithelial layers (Fig. 1–44).

In some areas, as satisfactory an approximation can be obtained by the use of a carefully inserted *continuous running suture* as by interrupted sutures (Fig. 1–45).

Subcutaneous sutures are also employed to obtain layer by layer closure in deep wounds, to eliminate dead space under a flap, and to assist in relieving tension in an advancement flap. The *removable continuous subcuticular suture* (Fig. 1–46) is of particular value in children, whose skin is normally under greater tension than that of the adult and in whom suture marks are apt to occur. Each suture should penetrate the undersurface of the

dermis 1 or 2 mm from the wound edge in order to obtain slight eversion and good approximation. The continuous subcuticular suture may be left in place for a longer period, thus ensuring the maturation of collagen in the wound without danger of suture marks. A precaution must be taken in using a subcuticular suture; the suture must be looped through the skin at intervals, depending on the length of the wound and the area of the body in which it is located. If this precaution is not taken, the suture may resist removal. One solution, in this eventuality, is to leave the suture subcutaneously. Nylon is well tolerated. The protruding ends of the suture are buried by the procedure illustrated in Figure 1–47. Stainless

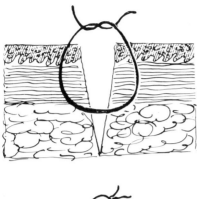

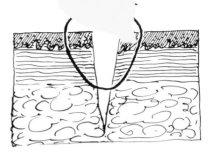

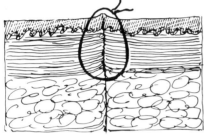

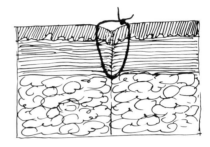

FIGURE 1–39. Correct manner of placing a suture to produce eversion. Needle should be placed to form a wider loop deep in the tissue to obtain eversion.

FIGURE 1–41. Placing suture to produce inversion. Inversion of wound edges is produced when loop is wider superficially than it is deep in the tissues.

steel wire has also proved satisfactory as a removable continuous subcuticular suture.

Variations in Technique in Wound Suturing. It may be advisable to leave a base of scar tissue and suture the wound edges over the base

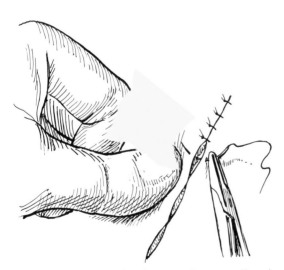

FIGURE 1–40. Placing interrupted sutures. Eversion can often be obtained by slight thumb pressure, by lightly applied fine tooth forceps or by means of a skin hook.

after excising the superficial portion of a depressed scar (Fig. 1–48). An ingenious technique to diminish tension on skin is that advocated by Millard (1970) (Fig. 1–49). A flap of subcutaneous fat may also be advanced from beneath one wound edge to bolster up a thinner opposing wound edge.

"Depuckering" the Pucker. When the two sides of an elliptical wound are of equal length, the wound may be closed without a resulting pucker at one end. If the two sides are unequal or if the ellipse has a wide curvature, a pucker or "dog-ear" is inevitable. The problem then is to "depucker" without unduly extending the length of the wound. The technique shown in Figure 1–50 has given the best results.

Pressure Dressings

A pressure dressing eliminates dead space, prevents hematoma formation, and immobilizes skin-grafted areas. A compressive dressing also encourages venous return, enhancing circulation in the area which it covers. Circulation is also promoted by elevation of the operated part. The need for a compressive dressing varies according to the type of opera-

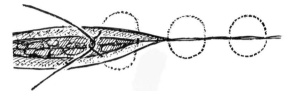

FIGURE 1–42. Interrupted subcuticular mattress sutures.

tion and the area in which the operation is performed. In most skin grafting procedures, the compressive dressing may be the most important part of the operation, ensuring as it does the close coaptation of the graft to the recipient site. Skin grafting may be done without a compressive dressing in certain selected cases in which careful observation ensures that the graft remains in contact with the recipient bed (see Chapter 6). Compressive dressings are not necessary in certain types of procedures in which only the integument is involved, and may be dispensed with if they are uncomfortable to the patient. The open method of treatment (Wallace, 1949) may be preferable in the treatment of burns or of abraded areas, as the absence of a dressing appears to favor epithelization. A pressure dressing may also be unnecessary when the wound has been closed without undermining the edges of the wound.

Suction tubes have replaced pressure dressings in areas where they are difficult to apply, e.g., the cervical area following the elevation of skin flaps for a neck dissection. Hematoma is probably the most frequent complication in plastic surgery.

Infections in Plastic Surgery

It is an undeniable fact that two factors have been responsible for progress in plastic surgery: the advent of antibiotics, and progress in the techniques of anesthesia and postoperative support of the patient.

Prior to the discovery of sulfanilamide, penicillin, and other antibiotics, the plastic surgeon lived under a Sword of Damocles: infection, that threatened to ruin the result of a carefully planned operation.

In general, plastic surgical procedures in the region of the head and neck are relatively immune from infection because of the rich vascular supply of the head and neck. However, if there is possible contamination by oral bacteria

and if craniofacial operations are undertaken in which the risk of meningeal infection is high, antibiotic prophylaxis should be considered. If antibiotics are administered, they should be given for 24 hours preoperatively.

Staphylococcus aureus is the most common offending pathogen in recent surveys of plastic surgery units (Converse and McCarthy, 1972; Morrison, Lister and Holmes, 1972). In view of this fact, an antistaphylococcal agent is indicated, either for antibiotic prophylaxis or for treatment of established infections.

Absolute indications for antibiotic prophylaxis are: traumatic wounds that are heavily contaminated; wounds in which debridement or cleansing are not possible; thermal burns; operative sites associated with heavy contamination or established infection; operations in which inorganic implants are inserted; operations in patients prone to infections (impoverished blood supply, carrier state, undernutrition, changes in host defense mechanisms, and remote preexisting infection).

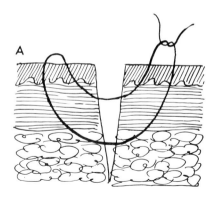

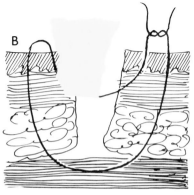

FIGURE 1–43. Vertical mattress suture. *A,* Usual type of mattress suture for approximating and everting wound edges. *B,* "Tacking" type of vertical mattress suture, extending into deep fascia to obliterate dead space under wound.

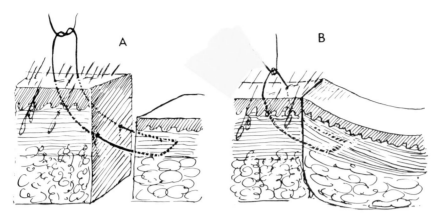

FIGURE 1–44. Horizontal mattress suture with an intradermal component. *A, B,* Eversion of thinner skin to obtain adequate approximation with thicker scalp tissue.

The two major causes of postoperative infection remain: rough handling of tissues, resulting in devitalized tissue in the wound, and hematoma, a natural culture medium.

A survey studying the role of preoperative antibiotics in plastic surgery was conducted by Krizek, Ross, and Robson (1975). Questionnaires were distributed to plastic surgeons, and 1025 responded. According to Krizek and his coworkers, who have quoted Ellis (1969), the availability of antibiotics has "neither eliminated surgical infection as a threat nor even reduced the incidence of infection in most cases." Plastic surgeons who practiced prior to the advent of antibiotics (personal communications from Aufricht, Kazanjian and Straatsma) have told me that in simple rhinoplastic operations, osteitis along the lines of osteotomy and abscess formation were occasional complications. Would craniofacial surgery be feasible without antibiotics? Or bone grafting through the intraoral approach?

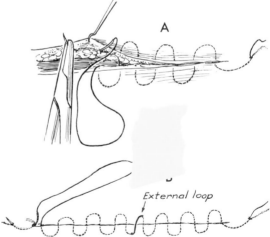

FIGURE 1–46. Continuous subcuticular pull-out suture. *A,* The suture has been placed through the epidermal surface and is introduced into the wound through the dermis. A hook everts the wound edge, permitting the needle to penetrate the undersurface of the dermis. The suture is looped to and fro. *B,* The subcuticular sutures are being completed and the needle is penetrating the dermis and is being brought out through the epidermis. Note that the suture is brought out through the skin halfway across the wound (or more often in longer wounds) to facilitate its eventual removal. Failure to take this precaution may result in breakage of the suture when an attempt is made to remove it.

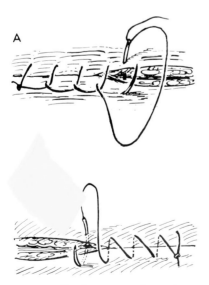

FIGURE 1–45. Continuous running suture and lock stitch. *A,* Continuous locking suture. *B,* Continuous non-locking suture.

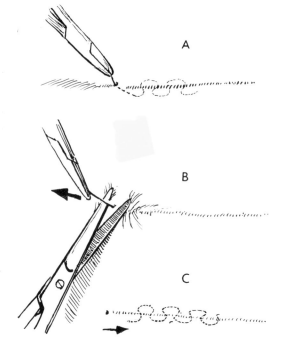

FIGURE 1–47. What to do if a subcuticular suture cannot be removed or a portion of it ruptures during removal. *A,* The protruding end is grasped with a hemostat. *B,* Traction is exerted by the hemostat, and pressure is applied on the skin by the blades of scissors. *C,* The end of the suture retracts under the skin. Nylon is usually well tolerated when left permanently.

Transplantation

"To transplant" (from the Latin verb *transplantare*) designates the removal of a colony of living cells from a donor area and its transfer to a recipient site where it is capable of propagating a lineage of living cells. The term is employed for the transfer of tissues or an organ from one part of the body to another, or from one individual to another. The term "graft" (from the French *greffe*) is essentially synonymous with the term "transplant."

Various terms have become accepted to define the modes of transplantation: "autograft" designates a graft transferred from one area to another in the same individual; "allograft" ("homograft") defines a graft transplanted between individuals of the same species; "xenograft" ("heterograft") indicates the transplantation of tissue between individuals of different species.

The term "isograft" is usually employed to designate an allograft between highly inbred (genetically pure) strains of animals. "Syngenesiotransplantation" is the grafting of tissue, not between two individuals of ordinary genetic diversity, as in the homograft, but between individuals of close genetic relationship. "Brephoplasty" (May, 1934) indicates the grafting of embryonic tissues.

"Replantation" designates the surgical pro-

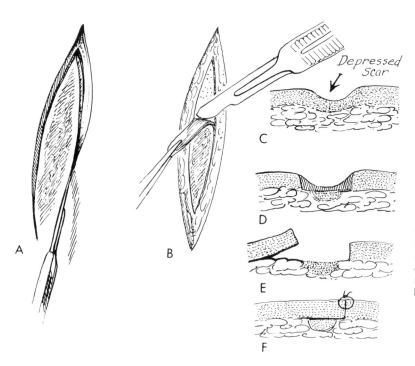

FIGURE 1–48. Partial excision of the scar. *A, B,* In a depressed scar it may be advisable to leave a base of scar tissue and suture the wound edges over the base, excising the superficial portion of the scar. *C,* Sectional view illustrating the depressed scar. *D,* Cross-lined area illustrates the excised portion of the scar. *E,* The undermining of one side of the wound. *F,* The wound edge has been advanced over the scar and sutured to the contralateral side.

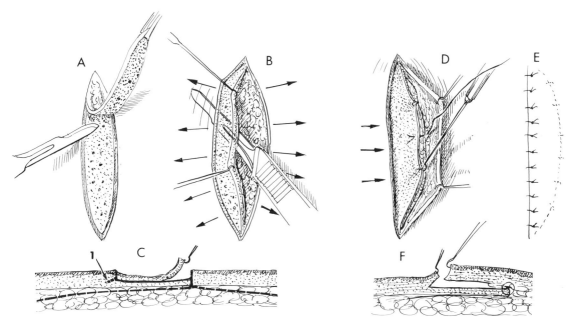

FIGURE 1–49. Another use of scar tissue after split-thickness excision of scar to diminish tension on sutured wound. *A*, Partial excision of scar. *B*, Remaining scar tissue is undermined. *C*, Split-thickness excision of scar. Note short incision (1) made to receive advancement flap. *D*, Flap of dermal scar is advanced and sutured subcutaneously into undermined area on opposite side of scar. The purpose of this technique is to release tension from sutured wound. (After Millard, D. R.: Scar repair by double-vested principle. Plast. Reconstr. Surg., *45*:616, 1970.)

cedure whereby tissue or a structure is replaced into its original site.

The term "implantation" is employed in this text to designate the insertion into the tissues

of a foreign, relatively inert material referred to as an "inorganic implant" (see Chapter 15).

Two methods of skin transplantation are available, mediate and immediate. In *mediate*

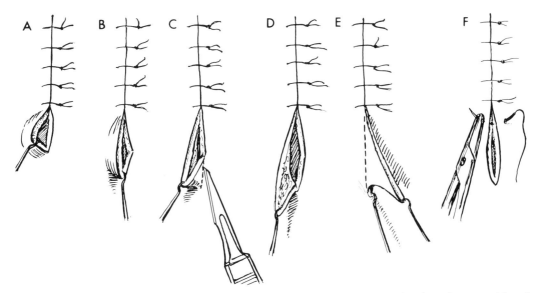

FIGURE 1–50. "Depuckering" the pucker (or removal of a dog-ear). *A*, The excessive tissue is retracted by a hook. *B*, A hook is placed at the end of the incision. *C*, The hook retracts the tissue laterally, and a sharp, pointed blade (#11) makes an incision in direct prolongation of the sutured wound. *D*, The resultant flap is retracted. *E*, The flap of excess tissue is overlapped over the proposed line of suture. Note the hook exerting traction at the end of the incision line. The dotted lines indicate the line of incision for the removal of the excess tissue. *F*, The remainder of the wound is sutured.

transplantation of skin, the survival of the transplant is ensured by a pedicle to which it remains attached until vessels have grown into the flap from the recipient site, thus the term "skin flap" (see Chapter 6).

In *immediate* transplantation of skin, a portion of skin is completely detached from its vascular connections, and revascularization of the transplant is accomplished by vascular connections and ingrowth of vessels from the host site; this type of free transplant is known as a "skin graft" (see Chapter 6). The development of microvascular surgery has permitted the immediate transfer of a skin flap, the *microvascular free flap* (see Chapter 14).

Transplantation of other tissues, such as dermis (Chapter 7), fat (Chapter 8), fascia (Chapter 9), tendon (Chapter 10), muscle (Chapter 11), cartilage (Chapter 12), bone (Chapter 13), and nerve (Chapter 76), is discussed in individual chapters.

There are specific indications for the use of inorganic implants as useful adjuncts to other surgical procedures (Chapter 15).

The Raw Area, the Straight Line, and Wound Tension: Three Enemies of the Plastic Surgeon

The first enemy is a wound devoid of integument. The wound contracts; the result is an uncontrollable contracture with deformity and functional impairment. If it cannot contract, the wound may progress toward an indolent ulcer. Skin covering should always be provided by direct approximation, the transplantation of a skin graft, or the transfer of a flap. In the reconstruction of a full-thickness defect of the cheek or the nose, for example, a lining as well as a surface covering should be provided.

The straight line not situated within, or parallel to, a line of minimal tension is the second enemy of the plastic surgeon since contraction along the straight line causes distortion and contracture and results in hypertrophy of the resulting scar. The straight line must be interrupted by a Z-plasty or W-plasty in order to distribute the contractile forces in more than one direction. This principle is the basis of techniques developed to avoid retraction of straight scars that run at variance with the lines of minimal tension. The Z-plasty is the plastic surgeon's best friend, and the W-plasty, rapidly increasing in popularity, is the plastic surgeon's second best friend. The

straight line, when situated in a favorable site and when the wound edges are sutured meticulously and with precision, is not an enemy: the resulting hairline scar will be inconspicuous (see Chapter 16).

Wound tension should be avoided at all costs. Undermining the wound edges is helpful but usually gives only partial relief of tension. Disruption of wounds, cross-hatching stitch marks, widening of scars, and necrosis of flaps are the consequences of excessive wound tension. Skin grafts or skin flaps are required when direct approximation of the wound edges cannot be achieved without tension.

THE Z-PLASTY

One of the most widely employed techniques in plastic surgery is the Z-plasty, characterized by the transposition of two triangularly shaped flaps (Fig. 1–51). The Z-plasty serves three purposes: (1) lengthening of a linear scar con-

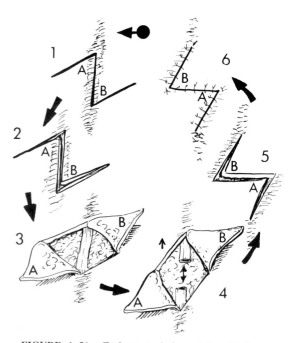

FIGURE 1–51. Z-plasty technique (after McGregor). *1*, Design. Central limb designed along scar. Both limbs are equal in length. Angles A and B are 60°. *2, 3*, Flaps are incised and raised. *4*, Release of deeper portion of scar. *5*, Transposition of triangular flaps. *6*, Wounds are approximated. Note lengthening and new direction of scar.

tracture; (2) dispersal of the scar, thus breaking up the straight scar; and (3) realigning the scar within the lines of minimal tension. Elongation and interruption of the straight line and release of linear scar contracture prevent its recurrence.

Development of the Z-plasty. Borges (1974) has researched the origin and development of the Z-plasty. The first procedures consisted of a single transposition flap, hardly what we could call a true Z-plasty. Such procedures were described by Fricke (1829), Horner (1837), and Denonvilliers (1854). These procedures involved the transposition of a flap from the temporal area or from the cheek to correct ectropion of the upper or lower eyelid. Mc-Curdy published a number of articles on what he called the "Z-plastic method" between 1898 and 1924. Although his first Z-plasty procedures were not true Z-plasties, he is credited with the current popularization of the Z-plasty technique. Berger in 1904 was the first to describe a true Z-plasty.

The first description of multiple Z-plasties was written by Morestin in 1914. The flaps were incised and allowed to shift in place without undermining. According to Woolf and Broadbent (1972), the geometric principles involved in the Z-plasty were first described by Limberg in 1929. Limberg's classic book (1946) contains a description of the many applications of the Z-plasty technique. Davis and Kitlowski (1939) reviewed their experience with the use of the Z-plasty, and Davis reviewed the practical applications of the principle in 1946. McGregor (1957) also discussed the theoretical basis of the Z-plasty. The books

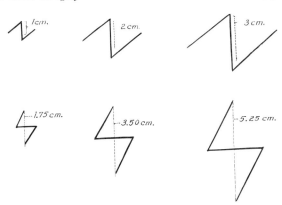

FIGURE 1–53. The greater gain in length with a Z-plasty as the length of the central limb is increased (angles remain constant.) Lower row shows theoretical linear increase. (After Grabb, W. C., and Smith, J. E.: Plastic Surgery—A Concise Guide to Clinical Practice. 2nd Ed. Boston, Little, Brown and Company, 1973.)

of Kazanjian and Converse (1959, 1974) and of Grabb and Smith (1968, 1973) have also discussed this technique in considerable detail. Borges (1973) published a book, the subject matter of which is entirely devoted to the Z- and W-plasties.

Technique of the Z-plasty. In the classic Z-plasty the two triangular flaps of skin and subcutaneous tissue of equal size are delimited by the three incisions of equal length cut at a 60° angle (see Fig. 1–51); the line of contracture is thus broken and also lengthened (Fig. 1–52). The length of the central limb and the angles of the Z determine the size of the flaps. The longer the central limb, the more lengthening is obtained, all the limbs being of the same length (Fig. 1–53). If the incisions outlining the Z-plasty are not of the same length, puckering of the flaps will result (Fig. 1–54). (See exceptions under Variations in the Z-plasty Technique.)

In addition to its lengthening effect, the value of the Z-plasty lies in the redistribution of tension and dispersal of the scar (Fig. 1–55).

Staige Davis had noted (1931) that release of scar contracture by means of the Z-plasty technique resulted in an improvement in the quality of the scar tissue, the tissue becoming softer and better appearing. He reaffirmed this observation in subsequent papers (Davis and Kitlowski, 1939; Davis, 1946).

A modification of collagen structure has been demonstrated in the scarred area following a Z-plasty procedure (Longacre and asso-

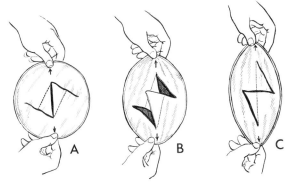

FIGURE 1–52. Elongation obtained by the Z-plasty (after Limberg).

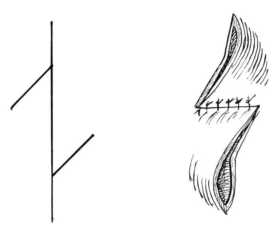

FIGURE 1–54. Puckering of the flaps results when the central member and limbs of the Z-plasty are of unequal length.

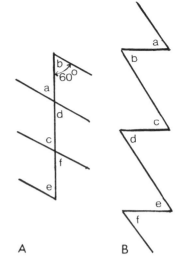

FIGURE 1–56. Multiple Z-plasty technique (after Davis and Kitlowski, 1939). *A,* Design. *B,* Final appearance following transposition of flaps. The technique is preferred to a single large Z-plasty in the revision of long, linear scars.

ciates, 1966). Both depressed scars and hypertrophic scars often become inconspicuous following excision and the breaking up of the linear contracture by one or multiple Z-plasties.

A Z-plasty in the middle of a long scar breaks the continuity and elongates the scar. Multiple Z-plasties (Fig. 1–56) have been employed successfully in long, linear, contracted scars.

Amount of Elongation According to the Z-flap Design. Much has been written about the degree of elongation obtained by varying the angles of the segments of the Z-plasty. While the geometric calculations appear accurate on paper, there are too many unpredictable factors in the patient to make them reliable. Theoretical considerations, while they are demonstrable on a piece of rubber sheeting or chamois skin, where the tension is equally distributed, are useless from a clinical point of

view. Skin tension varies because of the presence of scar tissue which is unequally distributed, and is not the same on both sides of the contracture. In the usual clinical situation when one needs to elongate an area because of distortion of landmarks or web formation (frequently following burns), one uses the most useful Z-plasty angle, which is 60 degrees. Greater elongation can be obtained by the use of wide flaps (see The Four-Flap Z-plasty).

The Use of the Z-plasty to Realign the Scar within the Lines of Minimal Tension. The Z-plasty (or W-plasty, see p. 60) should not be used if the scar does not cross a line of minimal tension. Resection by elliptical incision (fusiform excision) is indicated.

It takes courage deliberately to increase the length of a clean linear scar, even though it is unsatisfactory because it crosses the lines of minimal tension. No amount of care in meticulously suturing the wound will help if the scar is in an unfavorable position.

The application of the Z-plasty principle for the realignment of a scar crossing a line of minimal tension is most useful but requires careful consideration. The angles of the Z-flaps vary according to the obliquity of the scar in relation to the lines of minimal tension and may be considerably less than 60°. The more oblique the scar, the more acute the angle of

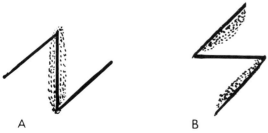

FIGURE 1–55. Dispersal of scar follows tranposition of the flaps in a Z-plasty (stippled area represents scar tissue).

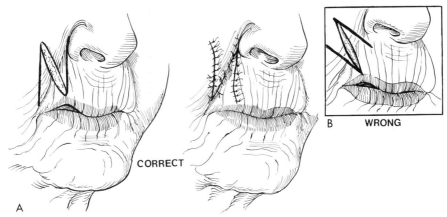

FIGURE 1-57. The angles of the Z-flaps vary according to the obliquity of the scar and its relation to the line of minimal tension; the more oblique the scar, the more acute the angle of the Z-flaps. *A*, Note that the scar is traversing the nasolabial fold obliquely. The flaps have been designed. The angles are less than 60 degrees. *B*, Flaps have been transposed. The Z was designed so that the ends of the limbs fall into the nasolabial fold. *Insert*, wrong design of the Z-plasty: the limbs of the Z cross the lines of minimal tension (After Borges, A. F., and Alexander, J. E.: Relaxed skin tension lines, Z-plasties on scars and fusiform excision of lesions. Br. J. Plast. Surg., *15*:242, 1962.)

the Z-flaps. This concept is illustrated in Figure 1–57; in the realignment of a scar crossing the nasolabial fold, the angles of the Z-flaps may be more acute. It is necessary to design the Z so that the end of the limbs falls into the nasolabial fold.

The closer the scar is directed toward a right angle crossing of the lines of minimal tension, the more the angles of the Z-plasty limbs approach 60°.

In the design of any Z-plasty, the limbs should follow the lines of minimal tension (Fig. 1–58, *A*). Thus, after transposition, the limbs follow the lines of minimal tension. Should the design be made in the opposite direction, the Z would cross the lines of minimal tension (Fig. 1–58, *B*).

Figure 1–59, *B* illustrates the advantage of two small Z-plasties over one large Z-plasty

(Fig. 1–59, *A*) in breaking up the scar into smaller components separated by normal tissue. Figure 1–59, *C* illustrates a Z-plasty whose central limb is placed in the middle of a long scar; as stated earlier, an improvement is

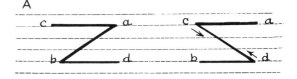

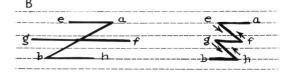

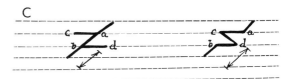

FIGURE 1-59. *A*, Inadequacy of a single large Z-plasty. The direction of the scar (central limb) is reversed, but its direction is not improved in relation to the lines of minimal tension and its length is not broken up into smaller scars. *B*, If one designs two or more Z-plasties, the long scar is divided into smaller, less contractile segments. *C*, A Z-plasty in the middle of a long scar interrupts the longitudinal contraction of the scar and elongates it (after Borges and Alexander).

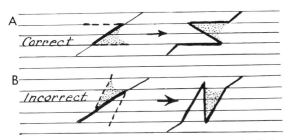

FIGURE 1-58. In the design of a Z-plasty, the limbs should follow the lines of minimal tension. *A*, Correct design. *B*, Incorrect design: the limbs of the Z would cross the lines of minimal tension (after Borges and Alexander).

achieved by the lengthening, relaxation, and interruption of the longitudinal tension.

Variations in the Z-plasty Technique

UNEQUAL TRIANGLES. Triangles of an unequal size are indicated in the Z-plasty when the skin on one side of the central segment is loose and the other side requires more elongation, particularly in burn patients when the resection of the scar tissue on that side is not indicated (Fig. 1–60). This is an application of the "half-Z" procedure, which consists of a flap which is fitted into an incision made in the opposing wound edge and is a technique for lengthening the short side (Fig. 1–61). One incision is made almost at right angles to the border of the defect on the short side, while the other forms a more acute triangular flap on the long side. The width of the base of the triangle determines the amount of lengthening of the short side, into which it is inserted. This technique can be employed only when the tis-

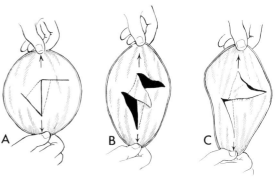

FIGURE 1–61. Half-Z technique. *A*, Arrows indicate direction of elongation; Z-incision is indicated. *B*, Preparation of Z-flaps. *C*, Elongation obtained by Z-plasty technique (after Limberg, 1946.) The insertion of the triangular flap into the horizontal incision elongates the right bank (in drawing) more than the left bank.

sues are soft and pliable. The length of the limbs of the Z-plasty may also vary when the irregular scar requires lengthening and relaxation (Fig. 1–62). The S-plasty (Fig. 1–63) is employed in cervical contractures, as the tips of the flaps are less susceptible to necrosis than those with the acute angle of the classic Z-plasty. It is especially indicated when the involved area includes healed, burned skin or skin graft (Converse, 1964).

DOUBLE OPPOSING Z-PLASTIES. Double opposing Z-plasties (Fig. 1–64) are particularly effective in breaking up a line of contracture when the anatomical position of the contracture does not permit the use of large flaps, such as in the medial canthal region for the correction of epicanthal folds (Converse and Smith, 1966). Double opposing Z-plasties are also useful in diminishing the size of the Z-flaps when the vascularization of the flaps is precarious, such as is frequent in burn contractures. Double opposing Z-plasties with small flaps are as effective in contracture release as the single Z-plasty with larger flaps. Opposing Z-plasties may also be placed at each end of a linear scar for the purpose of elongating a retractile scar (Converse, 1964).

THE FOUR-FLAP Z-PLASTY. The four-flap Z-plasty was described in Limberg's book in 1946 (Fig. 1–65). It has been utilized to achieve a maximum gain in length with the ease of the classic 60° angle flaps and without the difficulty of transfer of flaps with a wider angle.

The technique consists of outlining wide angle flaps, each flap then being divided into

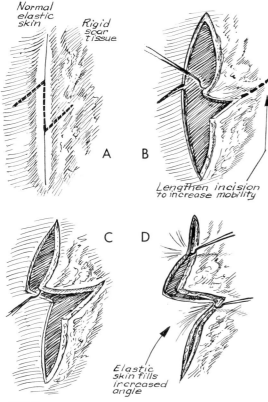

FIGURE 1–60. Z-plasty with flaps of unequal size. *A*, Scarred area in which one bank consists of thin, elastic skin, whereas the other bank contains thick, rigid, scarred skin. *B*, Central scar has been excised. Z-flap on scarred bank has been elongated to provide greater mobility. *C*, *D*, Transposition of flaps.

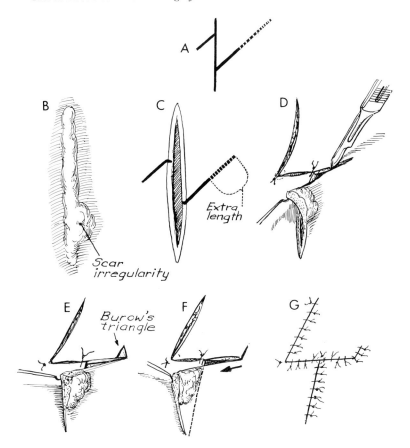

FIGURE 1–62. Z-plasty with unequal triangles. *A*, Z-plasty. *B*, Scar tissue. *C*, Main portion of scar is excised through elliptical incisions. Z-flaps (*A* to *D*) are outlined. *D*, Flaps are being transposed. Additional scar tissue excision is required as indicated. *E*, In order to avoid a pucker, a small Burow's triangle is excised as indicated in *E*. Flap containing scar tissue is advanced. *F*, Scar tissue is excised. *G*, Completion of Z-plasty with unequal triangles.

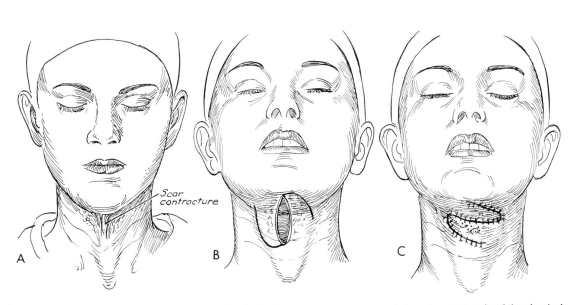

FIGURE 1–63. S-plasty. Rounded ends of flap in S-plasty ensure better survival than the acute ends of the classical Z-plasty. The S-plasty is useful when the skin surrounding the scar contracture is scarred from a healed thermal burn. *A*, Scar contracture of neck. *B*, S-plasty. *C*, S-plasty has been completed.

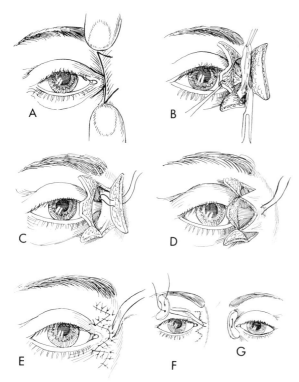

FIGURE 1–64. Double opposing Z-plasties. Two Z-plasties done in opposing directions constitute an excellent technique for relaxing tension and releasing contracture of a linear scar. This technique is of particular usefulness in areas where only small flaps may be designed, such as the nasoorbital valley in which an epicanthal fold may result from a scar in the vicinity of the medial canthus. Limited amount of tissue in the confined nasoorbital valley limits the size of the Z-flaps. Double opposing Z-plasties with small flaps are as effective as a single Z-plasty with large flaps. *A*, Design of opposing Z-plasties. *B*, Flaps are raised, and deep scar tissue is excised. *C*, Transosseous wires (see Chapter 28) have been placed through the bony skeleton of the nose for fixation of the canthal buttons (see *F* and *G*). *D*, Flaps have been transposed. *E*, Double opposing Z-plastics completed. *F*, *G*, Canthal buttons maintained by through-and-through wiring assure coaptation of the flaps to the underlying skeleton and prevent hematoma formation (see also Chapter 28).

two separate flaps, thus converting the usual two-flap Z-plasty into a four-flap Z-plasty.

A modification was introduced by Iselin (1962). His "plastie en Z rectifiés" was used to correct a contracture of the thumb web.

Iselin's technique has been employed by Woolf and Broadbent (1972) for a contracted web space in the hand (Fig. 1–66), for axillary contractures following burns (Fig. 1–67), and for minor cases of syndactyly. Furnas (1965) has studied the four-flap Z-plasty in considerable detail (Fig. 1–68) and has suggested a

number of applications of the technique (stenosis of external auditory canal, of a tracheal stoma, of the urethral meatus, of a colostomy and end-to-side vessel anastomosis).

THE W-PLASTY

The W-plasty (Borges, 1959) consists of the imbrication of triangles of skin on each side of the excised scar.

A surgical technique resembling the W-plasty was described by Ombrédanne in 1937 and was employed by him for the correction of a congenital constricting band of the lower extremity (Fig. 1–69).

Hazrati (1952) has described a compound right angle Z-plasty. Borges (1973) has pointed out that this technique might well represent the missing link between the multiple Z-plasties and the W-plasty technique (Fig. 1–70).

In order to produce triangles of equal size, a metal pattern can be employed (Fig. 1–71). A large hemostat bends the soft metal band into a series of 60° angles. The size of the triangle is determined by the width of the limb of the particular hemostat.

The pattern is painted with surgical ink and applied to one side of the scar; a similar procedure is repeated on the opposite side of the

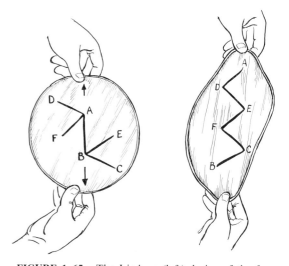

FIGURE 1–65. The Limberg (left) design of the four-flap Z-plasty. The technique consists of outlining wide angle flaps, which are then divided into separate flaps converting the usual two flap Z-plasty into a four-flap design (right). Elongation obtained after transfer of the four flaps.

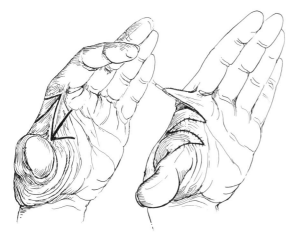

FIGURE 1-66. Application of the four-flap technique for a contracted web space in the hand. (Left) design of the four-flap Z-plasty. (Right) After transfer of the flaps (after Woolf and Broadbent.)

scar. The metal pattern is not essential, as the design can be easily made freehand by the operator.

At the end of the scar, the triangles are smaller and the length of the limbs of the W are tapered (Fig. 1–72, *A*). With a sharp pointed scalpel, the limbs of the W-plasty are incised on each side alternatively. In this fashion the tissues are firmer and easier to incise than if one entire edge is prepared before incising the opposing edge. After each triangle is outlined, the tip of the triangle on the contralateral side should be placed at the midpoint of the base of the opposing triangle (Fig. 1–72, *B*).

Each triangular flap is approximately 5 mm in length and has an angle of approximately 55° in vertical or almost vertical scars (scars that cross the lines of minimal tension at right angles). As the inclination of a scar in relation

to the minimal tension lines becomes more acute, the angles of each triangular flap become more obtuse (Fig. 1–72, *B*). Borges (1971) advocates gradually increasing the angles until they reach 90°, when the scar traverses the line of minimal tension at an angle of more than 60°.

A continuous subcuticular suture of 4–0 monofilament nylon should be employed to approximate the angles. The subcuticular suture should be placed halfway between the apex and the base of each triangle in order to avoid buckling of the flaps. Additional approximation is obtained with interrupted 6–0 nylon sutures.

Indications and Contraindications of Z- and W-Plasties. The Z-plasty and W-plasty techniques have two common denominators: they break up the straight linear scar into smaller components, and they improve the direction of the scar in relation to the lines of minimal tension.

The Z-plasty has the advantage that it elongates a contractile scar, changes the direction of the scar, when correctly done, and places it more nearly parallel to the lines of minimal tension. The Z-plasty also has the advantage of utilizing all of the available skin, as it is possible in some cases to perform the Z-plasty without excising the scar, if tissue is scarce. The change that takes place in the character and quality of the scar when tension is relaxed was mentioned earlier in the chapter. The Z-plasty elongates the linear scar, thereby relaxing tension; it also permits readjustment of displaced tissue.

Rarely are two cicatricial deformities exactly alike; each case must be studied carefully on its own merits and the various methods of repair weighed from every standpoint in relation to that particular scar.

The Z-plasty is preferable to the W-plasty

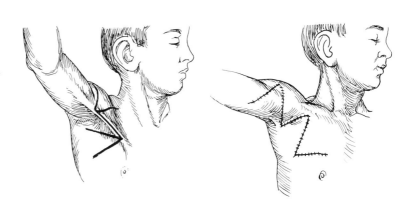

FIGURE 1-67. Application of the four-flap technique for the correction of an axillary contracture following a thermal burn. (Left) Design of the four-flap Z-plasty. (Right) Correction obtained after transfer of the flaps.

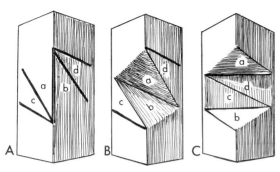

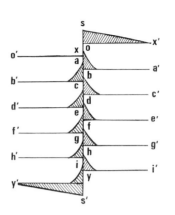

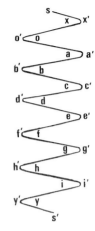

FIGURE 1–68. Four-flap Z-plasty, showing three interlocking tetrahedrons. *A*, Flaps in initial position (a=b= 45° tip angle, c=d=30° tip angle. *B*, Transposition of a and b demonstrates first tetrahedron. *C*, Additional transposition demonstrates third tetrahedron (after Furnas).

FIGURE 1–70. The compound right angle Z-plasty (after Hazrati). (Left) Design of the compound right angle Z-plasty. (Right) After transfer of the flaps (after Borges).

in areas where there is either too much skin tension or too little skin tension. Other areas on the face permit the use of the W-plasty (forehead, temporal skin, and the skin of the cheeks and chin). A horizontal scar extending across the lower lip or chin can be repaired by a W-plasty.

The main disadvantage of the Z-plasty, when improperly designed and/or placed, is that it elongates the scar excessively and enlarges the area it occupies. However, the Z-plasty nearly always improves the condition for which it is applied. The longer segments of the Z-plasty are another disadvantage over the W-plasty. It is possible to counteract this danger by Z-plasties with smaller limbs, such as the double opposing Z-plasty, and by multiple Z-plasties. In oblique scars traversing the

lines of minimal tension at an angle of less than 30°, a Z-plasty procedure is preferable to a W-plasty. When the scar is almost parallel to the lines of minimal tension, the entire scar or the major portion of the scar should be excised by elliptical incisions parallel to the lines of minimal tension.

The W-plasty also has the advantage of having smaller triangular limbs, which break up the scar into smaller components and relieve the bowstring effect.

When the W-plasty is employed, there is no displacement of anatomical landmarks, as there is no transposition of tissue. W-plasties are indicated on scars of the face that are per-

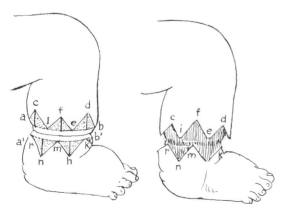

FIGURE 1–69. Ombrédanne's technique for the relief of a congenital constricting band of the lower extremity. (Left) Design of the flaps. (Right) After excision of the constricting band, the flaps are ready to be sutured (after Borges).

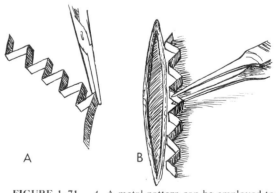

FIGURE 1–71. *A*, A metal pattern can be employed to assist in designing the W-plasty. A piece of metal is bent into a series of angles by means of a hemostat. *B*, One side of the metal pattern is painted with Bonney's blue by means of a cotton-tipped applicator. Pattern is then applied to skin, leaving an imprint.

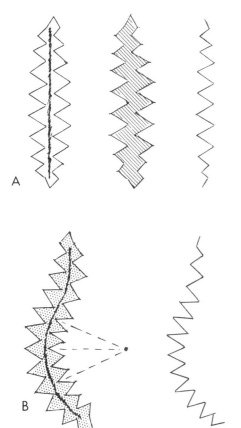

pendicular or nearly perpendicular to the lines of minimal tension. As stated earlier, they find their best application in scars that cross the lines of minimal tension on the forehead, cheeks, temporal area and chin. They also have the ability to restore the normal contour of the scarred cheek.

The W-plasty has the disadvantage of increasing rather than decreasing the tension in the area of the scar because of the necessary sacrifice of tissue. It should be reserved, therefore, for scars surrounded by plentiful tissue. When elongation of the linear scar is required, the Z-plasty is always preferable.

The W-plasty and the Z-plasty may have application in patients with multiple scars, or in different parts of the same scar.

If irregularities (and not hypertrophic scars) in the surface area persist following either a Z-plasty or a W-plasty, a single (or a repeated) dermabrasion done at a suitable time interval after the operation will improve the surface contour.

Excision, Z-plasty, and Skin Grafting in Wide Hypertrophic Scars. Wide hypertrophic scars require excision, Z-plasty, and skin grafting to cover the remaining defect. The thicker the skin graft, the better the result (Skoog, 1963). After an area of hypertrophic scarring has been dissected along the subcicatricial plane of loose connective tissue and resected, only a full-thickness or three-quarter thickness graft will minimize subsequent contraction, wrinkling, and possible recurrence of hypertrophic scarring (see also Chapter 16).

FIGURE 1–72. W-plasty. *A*, W-plasty for repair of a straight scar. Triangles become smaller at the end of the scar, and the length of the limbs of the flap is tapered to avoid puckering. *B*, On a curved scar, the angles of the inner aspect of the curve should be more acute than the angles of the outer aspect of the curve (after Borges).

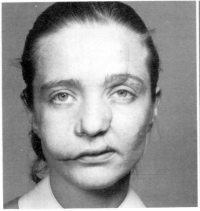
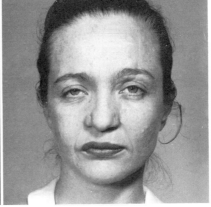

FIGURE 1–73. Z-plasty and W-plasty in scars resulting from massive partial avulsion of facial tissue. *A*, Massive partial avulsion of soft tissues of face. Flap sheared from facial skeleton extended from left side of forehead through left eyebrow and upper eyelid downward along lateral wall of nose, through upper lip on left side, through right angle of mouth backward to an area situated immediately in front of right auricle. Massive lymphatic obstruction resulting from scar caused long-term lymphedema. *B*, Final result obtained.

Z-plasty and W-plasty in Depressed Scars of Partially Avulsed Trapdoor Flaps. The patient whose photographs are shown in Figure 1–73, *A* suffered a massive partial avulsion of the soft tissues of the face when she was projected through the windshield of the automobile in which she was a right front seat passenger when it was involved in a head-on collision with another vehicle.

Lymphatic obstruction by the deeply penetrating scar resulted in long-term lymphedema of the soft tissues of the face, which accentuated the deep indentation produced by the scar. Interdigitation between edematous and normal tissue bordering the scar by Z-plasty and W-plasty, as well as excision of the scar, assists in promoting lymphatic vessel regrowth across the scar and progressive amelioration of the lymphedema (Fig. 1–73, *B*).

The same principles apply to the U-shaped scar which follows the healing of the trapdoor flaps. Excision of the scar, partial or total, combined with Z-plasty, W-plasty, and surgical abrasion, often results in an acceptable appearance (see Chapter 16).

REPEATED PARTIAL EXCISIONS
(Morestin, 1915; Davis, 1929; Smith, 1950)

Partial excision may be preferable in the eradication of pigmented nevi or of wide scars in which total excision and suture cannot be accomplished without tension. Multiple repeated partial excisions are indicated in areas surrounded by loose tissue. Serial excisions are done at suitable intervals, provided that sufficient loose tissue is available and that distortion of the eyelids, nose, or lips does not result; distortion must be avoided. Wide undermining of the surrounding skin is essential. The technique has its limitations, however, as excessive repeated excisions may cause contracture.

The technique of multiple partial excision has its best application in infants in whom the skin is more elastic than in the adult; closure of the resulting defect is thus facilitated. In the aged patient the looseness of the skin and the excess of skin also favors this technique.

REFERENCES

Ammon, F. A. von, and Baumgarten, M.: Die plastische Chirurgie nach ihren bisherigen Leistungen Kritisch dargestellt. Berlin, Reimer, 1842.

Artz, C. P., and Moncrief, J. A.: The Treatment of Burns. Philadelphia, W. B. Saunders Company, 1969.

Baronio, G.: Degli Innesti Animali, Stamperia e Fonderia del Genio, Milan, 1804.

Barsky, A. J., Kahn, S., and Simon, B. E.: Principles and Practice of Plastic Surgery. New York, Mc-Graw-Hill Book Company, 1964.

Berger, P.: Autoplastie par dédoublement de la palmure et échange des lambeaux. *In* Berger, P., and Banzet, S. (Eds.): Chirurgie Orthopédique. Paris, G. Steinheil. 1904, p. 180.

Bhishagratna, K. K.: An English translation of the Sushruta samhita based on original Sanskrit text. 3 Vols. Calcutta, Bose, 1916, p. 107.

Blair, V. P.: Surgery and Diseases of the Mouth and Jaws. St. Louis, Mo., C. V. Mosby Company, 1912.

Blair, V. P.: The delayed transfer of long pedicle flaps in plastic surgery. Surg. Gynecol. Obstet., *33*:261, 1921.

Blair, V. P.: Reconstruction surgery of the face. Surg. Gynecol. Obstet., *34*:701, 1922.

Blair, V. P., and Brown, J. B.: Use and uses of large split skin grafts of intermediate thickness. Surg. Gynecol. Obstet., *49*:82, 1929.

Blandin, P. F.: De l'autoplastie, ou restauration des parties du corps, qui ont été détruites, à la faveur, d'un emprunt fait à d'autres parties plus ou moins éloignées. Thesis, Urtubie, Paris, 1836.

Blasius, E.: Gaumennaht Staphylorraphie. *In* Handbuch der Chirurgie. Vol. 2. Halle, E. Anton, 1839–1843.

Bloch, B., and Hastings, G. W.: Plastics in Surgery. Springfield, Ill., Charles C Thomas, Publisher, 1967.

Borges, A. F.: Improvement of antitension-line scars by the W-plastic operation. Br. J. Plast. Surg., *12*:29, 1959.

Borges, A. F.: Historical review of the Z- and W-plasty revisions of linear scars. Int. Surg., *56*:182, 1971.

Borges, A. F.: Elective Incisions and Scar Revision. Boston, Little, Brown and Company, 1973.

Borges, A. F.: The five single Z-plastics. Va. Med. Monthly, *101*:618, 1974.

Borges, A. F., and Alexander, J. E.: Relaxed skin tension lines, Z-plasties on scars and fusiform excision of lesions. Br. J. Plast. Surg., *15*:242, 1962.

Borges, A. F., and Gibson, T.: The original Z-plasty. Br. J. of Surg., *22*:237, 1973.

Bridgman, G.: Complete Guide to Drawing from Life. New York, Sterling Publishing Company, 1973.

Brown, J. B., and McDowell, F.: Skin Grafting. Philadelphia, J. B. Lippincott Company, 1939.

Bünger, C.: Gelungener Versuch einer Nasenbildung aus einem völlig getrennten Hautstück aus dem Beine. J. Chir. Augenh. Berlin, 1823.

Burkhardt, J.: The Civilization of the Renaissance in Italy. New York, Harper and Brothers, 1929.

Bzoch, K. R.: Communicative Disorders Related to Cleft Lip and Palate. Boston, Little, Brown and Company, 1972.

Carpue, J. C.: An account of two successful operations for restoring a lost nose from the integuments of the forehead. London, Longman, 1816.

Clarkson, P.: Sir Harold Gillies. Br. Med. J., *2*:641, 1966.

Conley, J., and Dickinson, J. T.: Plastic and Reconstructive Surgery of the Face and Neck. New York, Grune & Stratton, 1972.

Converse, J. M.: Early skin grafting in war wounds of the extremities. Ann. Surg., *115*:321, 1942.

Converse, J. M.: Victor Veau (1871–1949). The contributions of a pioneer. Plast. Reconstr. Surg., *30*:225, 1962.

Converse, J. M.: Introduction to plastic surgery. *In* Converse, J. M. (Ed.): Reconstructive Plastic Surgery. 1st Ed. Ch. 1, p. 16, Fig. 1–17. Philadelphia, W. B. Saunders Company, 1964.

Converse, J. M.: The classic reprint: La réduction graduelle des difformités tégumentaires, by H. Morestin, M. D., Paris (Bull. et mém. Soc. chir. Paris, *41*:1233, 1915), Translated from the French. Plast. Reconstr. Surg., *42*:163, 1968.

Converse, J. M.: Kazanjian and Converse. Surgical Treatment of Facial Injuries. 3rd Ed. Baltimore, The Williams & Wilkins Company, 1974.

Converse, J. M., and McCarthy, J. G.: Infections in plastic surgery. Surg. Clin. North Am., *52*:1459, 1972.

Converse, J. M., and Smith, B.: Naso-orbital fractures and traumatic deformities of the medial canthus. Plast. Reconstr. Surg., *38*:147, 1966.

Cox, H. T.: The cleavage lines of skin. Br. J. Surg., *29*:234, 1941.

Davis, J. S.: Plastic surgery – Its principles and Practice, Philadelphia, P. Blakiston's Son & Company, 1919.

Davis, J. S.: Removal of wide scars and large disfigurements of the skin by gradual partial excision with closure. Ann. Surg., *90*:645, 1929.

Davis, J. S.: Relaxation of scar contractures by means of the Z-, or reversed Z-type incision; stressing use of scar infiltrated tissues. Ann. Surg., *94*:871, 1931.

Davis, J. S.: The story of plastic surgery. Ann. Surg., *113*:641, 1941.

Davis, J. S.: Present evaluation of the merits of the Z-plasty operation. Plast. Reconstr. Surg., *1*:26, 1946.

Davis, J. S., and Kitlowski, E. A.: The theory and practical use of the Z-incision for the relief of scar constriction. Ann. Surg., *109*:1001, 1939.

Davis, J. S., and Traut, H. F.: Origin and development of blood supply of whole thickness skin grafts. Ann. Surg., *82*:871, 1925.

Delagenière, H.: Greffes Ostéo-périostiques. J. Chir., *17*:305, 1921.

Delpech, J. M.: Chirurgie Clinique de Montpellier, ou Observations et Réflexions Tirées des Travaux de Chirurgie de cette Ecole. Paris, Gabon et Cie, 1823–1828.

Denecke, H. J., and Meyer, R.: Plastic Surgery of Head and Neck: Corrective and Reconstructive Rhinoplasty. Translated from the German by L. Oxtoby. New York, Springer-Verlag, 1967.

Denonvilliers, C. P.: Présentation de Malades. Bull. Soc. Chir. (Paris), *5*:35, 118, 1854.

Derganc, M.: Present Clinical Aspects of Burns: A Symposium. Maribor, Yugoslavia, Mariborski, 1968.

Desault, P. J.: Oeuvres Chirurgicales ou Exposé de la Doctrine et de la Plastique. Vol. 2. Paris, Megegnon, 1798.

Diderot, D.: Encyclopédie, ou Dictionnaire Raisonné des Sciences, des Arts et des Métiers, par une Société des gens de lettres. Vol. 1. Paris, 1751.

Dieffenbach, J. F.: Die operative Chirurgie. Leipzig, F. A. Brockhaus, 1845–1848.

Dingman, R. O., and Natvig, P.: Surgery of Facial Fractures. Philadelphia, W. B. Saunders Company, 1964.

Dolecek, R.: Metabolic Response of the Burned Organism. Springfield, Ill., Charles C Thomas, Publisher, 1969.

Donaghy, R. M. P., and Gazi Yasargil, M. (Eds.): Microvascular Surgery. St. Louis, Mo., C. V. Mosby Company, 1967.

Dunphy, J. E., and Van Winkle, H. W. (Eds.): Repair and Regeneration: The Scientific Basis for Surgical Practice. New York, McGraw-Hill Book Company, 1969.

Dupuytren, G.: Leçons orales de clinique chirurgicale, faites à l'Hôtel-Dieu de Paris. Paris, G. Baillière, 1832–1834.

Edgerton, M. T.: The role of plastic surgery in academic medicine. Presidential address. Plast. Reconstr. Surg., *54*:523, 1974.

Ellis, H.: The place of antibiotics in surgical practice. Ann. R. Coll. Surg., England, *45*:162, 1969.

Enlow, D. H.: The Human Face. New York, Harper & Row, 1968.

Epstein, E.: Skin Surgery. 3rd Ed. Springfield, Ill., Charles C Thomas, Publisher, 1970.

Filatov, V. P.: Plastie à tige ronde. Vestnik oftal., No. 5, 1917.

Finochietto, E.: Presentaçion de instrumentos. Prensa Med. Argent., *6*:356, 1920.

Firenzuola: Opere di Firenzuola, Milan, 1802.

Fomon, S.: Surgery of Injury and Plastic Repair. Baltimore, The Williams & Wilkins Company, 1939.

Fox, C. L. (Ed.): Annals of the New York Academy of Sciences. Early Treatment of Severe Burns. Vol. 150, Art. 3, October 3 to 5, 1966.

Fox, S. A.: Lid Surgery. Current Concepts. New York, Grune & Stratton, 1972.

Fricke, J. C. G.: Bildung neuer Augenlider (Blepharoplastik) nach Zerstörung und dadurch hervorgebrachter Auswartwendung derselben. Hamburg, Perthes & Basser, 1829.

Furnas, D. W.: The tetrahedral Z-plasty. Plast. Reconstr. Surg., *35*:291, 1965.

Furnas, D. W.: A Bedside Outline for the Treatment of Burns. Springfield, Ill., Charles C Thomas, Publisher, 1969.

Gaisford, J. C. (Ed.): Symposium on Cancer of the Head and Neck. Vol. 2. St. Louis, Mo., C. V. Mosby Company, 1969.

Gentleman's Magazine: A communication to the editor, Mr. Urban, signed B. L. and dated Oct. 9, 1794. Vol. 64, Part Two, pp. 891–892; engraved illustration between pp. 882 and 883. London, Nichols, 1794.

German, W., Finesilver, E. M., and Davis, J. S.: Establishment of circulation in tubed skin. Arch. Surg., *26*:27, 1933.

Gibson, H. L.: Medical Photography. Rochester, N.Y., Eastman Kodak Company, 1973.

Gibson, T.: Biochemical properties of skin. Surg. Clin. North Am., *47*:279, 1967.

Gillies, H. D.: Plastic Surgery of the Face. London, Oxford University Press, 1920.

Gillies, H. D., and Millard, D. R., Jr.: Principles and Art of Plastic Surgery. Boston, Little, Brown and Company, 1957.

Gnudi, M. T., and Webster, J. P.: The life and times of Gasparo Tagliacozzi. New York, Herbert Reichner, 1950.

Goldwyn, R. M.: The Unfavorable Result in Plastic Surgery: Avoidance and Treatment. Boston, Little, Brown and Company, 1972.

Grabb, W. C., and Smith, J. E.: Plastic Surgery – A Concise Guide to Clinical Practice. Boston, Little, Brown and Company, 1968. 2nd Ed., 1973.

Grabb, W. C., Rosenstein, S. W., and Bozach, K. R.: Cleft Lip and Palate: Surgical, Dental and Speech Aspects. Boston, Little, Brown and Company, 1971.

Graefe, C. F. von: Rhinoplastik; oder, Die kunst den verlust der Nase organisch zu ersetzen in ihren früheren Verhältnissen erforscht und durch neue Verfahrungsweisen zur höheren Vollkommenheit gefördert. Berlin, In der Realschulbuchhandlung, 1818.

Hazrati, E.: Compound right angle Z-plasty. Plast. Reconstr. Surg., *10*:133, 1952.

Hemingway, E.: A Moveable Feast. New York, Charles Schribner's & Sons, 1964, p. 82.

Hines, E., and Kent, J.: Surgical Treatment of Developmental Jaw Deformities. St. Louis, Mo., C. V. Mosby Company, 1972.

Holts, R., and Huber, H.: Early Treatment of Cleft Lip and Palate. Berne and Stuttgart, Hans Huber, 1964.

Horner, W. E.: Clinical Report on the Surgical Department of the Philadelphia Hospital, Blockley, for the Months of May, June, and July, 1837. Am. J. Med. Sci., *21*:99, 1837.

Horton, C. E.: Plastic and Reconstructive Surgery of the Genital Area. Boston, Little, Brown and Company, 1973.

Hueston, J. T. (Ed.): Transactions of the Fifth International Congress of Plastic and Reconstructive Surgery, Melbourne, February 22–26, 1971. Australia, Butterworth & Company, 1971.

Iselin, M.: La plastie en Z rectifiés. Ann. Chir. Plast., 7:295, 1962.

Ivy, R. H.: War injuries of the face and jaws (Internatl. Abstr. Surg.). Surg. Gynecol. Obstet., 27:101, 1918.

Ivy, R. H.: Plastic and reconstructive surgery of the face. Internatl. Abstr. Surg., 36:1, 1923.

Ivy, R. H.: War injuries of the face and jaws (Internatl. Abstr. Surg.). Surg. Gynecol. & Studies of the College of Physicians of Philadelphia, 16:42, 1948.

Jobert (de Lamballe), A. J.: Traité de Chirurgie Plastique. Paris, J. B. Baillière et fils, 1849.

Joseph, J.: Nasenplastik und sonstige Gesichtsplastik nebst einem Anhang uber Mammaplastik: Ein Atlas und Lehrbuch. Leipzig, Berlin, 1928.

Kazanjian, V. H., and Converse, J. M.: The Surgical Treatment of Facial Injuries. Baltimore, The Williams & Wilkins Company, 1949. 2nd Ed., 1959. 3rd Ed., 1974.

Krause, F.: Ueber die Transplantation grosser, ungestielter Hautlappen. Dtsch. Gesell. Chir. Vehandl., 22:46, 1893.

Krizek, T. J., Ross, N., and Robson, M. C.: The current use of prophylactic antibiotics in plastic and reconstructive surgery. Plast. Reconstr. Surg., 55:21, 1975.

Labat, L.: De la rhinoplastie, art de restaurer ou de refaire complètemente le nez. Thesis, Paris, 1834.

Langer, C.: Zur Anatomie und Physiologie der Haut. Sitzungsb. Acad. Wissensch., 45:223, 1861.

Lawson, G.: On the successful transplantation of portions of skin for the closure of large granulating surface. Lancet, 2:708, 1870.

LeFort, L.: Blépharoplastie par un lambeau complétement détaché due bras et reporté à la face. Insuccès. Bull. Soc. Chir. (Paris), *1*:39, 1872.

Lexer, E.: Die freien Transplantationen. Stuttgart, F. Enke, 1919–1924.

Lexer, E.: Die gesamte Wiederherstellungschirurgie. Leipzig, J. A. Barth, 1931.

Limberg, A. A.: Skin plastic with shifting triangular flaps. Translated from the Russian. Leningrad Tram. Institute, 8:62, 1929.

Limberg, A. A.: Matematicheskie Osnovuy Mestnoy Plastiki Na Poverchnosti Chelovecheskogo Tela, Medgiz, 1946.

Liston, R.: Practical Surgery. London, J & A Churchill, 1831–1837.

Longacre, J. J.: Cleft Palate Deformation. Springfield, Ill., Charles C Thomas, Publisher, 1970.

Longacre, J. J.: Scar Tissue, Its use and Abuse: The Surgical Correction of Deformation Due to Hypertrophic Scar and the Prevention of Its Formation. Springfield, Ill., Charles C Thomas, Publisher, 1972.

Longacre, J. J.: Rehabilitation of the Facially Disfigured. Springfield, Ill., Charles C Thomas, Publisher, 1973.

Longacre, J. J., Seghers, M. J., Berry, H. K., Wood, R. W., Munick, L. H., Johnson, H. A., and Chumekamsi, D.: L'ultrastructure du collagène et la relation avec la correction des cicatrices hypertrophiques. Ann. Chir. Plast., 9:111, 1966.

Lynch, J. B., and Lewis, S. R. (Eds.): Symposium on the Treatment of Burns. Vol. V. St. Louis, Mo., C. V. Mosby Company, 1973.

MacComb, W. S., and Fletcher, G. H.: Cancer of the Head and Neck. Baltimore, The Williams & Wilkins Company, 1967.

McCurdy, S. L.: Manual of Orthopedic Surgery. Pittsburgh, Nicholson Press, 1898.

McCurdy, S. L.: Plastic operations to elongate cicatricial contractions across joints. Cleveland Med. J., 3:123, 1904.

McCurdy, S. L.: Z-plastic surgery. Surg. Gynecol. Obstet., 16:209, 1913.

McCurdy, S. L.: Z-plastic surgery. Int. J. Surg., 30:389, 1917.

McCurdy, S. L.: Correction of burn scar deformity by the Z-plastic method. J. Bone Joint Surg., 6:683, 1924.

Macgregor, F. C.: Personal communication, 1974a.

Macgregor, F. C.: Transformation and Identity. The Face and Plastic Surgery. New York, Quadrangle, The New York Times Book Company, 1974b.

McGregor, I. A.: The theoretical basis of the Z-plasty. Br. J. Plast. Surg., 9:256, 1957.

McGregor, I. A.: Fundamental Techniques of Plastic Surgery and Their Surgical Applications. 6th Ed. Baltimore, The Williams and Wilkins Company, 1975.

Malgaigne, J. F.: Manuel de Médicine Opératoire. Paris, G. Baillière, 1849.

Maliniac, J. W.: Breast Deformities and Their Repair. Baltimore, Waverly Press, 1950. Reissued by Krieger Publishing Company, Huntington, N.Y., 1971.

Masters, F. W., and Lewis, J. R.: Symposium on Aesthetic Surgery of the Face, Eyelid, and Breast. Vol. IV. St. Louis, Mo., C. V. Mosby Company, 1972.

Mauclaire, P.: Les Greffes Chirurgicales. Vol. 1. Paris, G. Baillière, 1922.

May, H.: Erich Lexer, A biographical sketch. Plast. Reconstr. Surg., 29:141, 1962.

May, H.: Reconstructive and Reparative Surgery. 3rd Ed. Philadelphia, F. A. Davis Company, 1971.

May, R. M.: La greffe brephoplastique sous-cutanée de la thyroide chez le rat. Comptes rendus. Acad. Sci., 199:807, 1934.

Millard, D. R.: Scar repair by double-vested principle. Plast. Reconstr. Surg., 45:616, 1970.

Morestin, H.: De la correction des flexions permanentes des doigts consectives aux panaris et aux phlegmons de la paume de la main. Rev. Chir., 50:1, 1914.

Morestin, H.: La reduction graduelle des difformités tégumentaires. Bull. Mém. Soc. Chir. Paris, 41:1233, 1915.

Morrison, R. B., Lister, G. D., and Holmes, J. H.: Wound sepsis in a plastic surgery unit. Br. J. Plast. Surg., 25:435, 1972.

Mustardé, J. C.: Repair and Reconstruction in the Orbital Region. A Practical Guide. Baltimore, The Williams & Wilkins Company, 1966.

Mustardé, J. C.: Plastic Surgery in Infancy and Childhood. Edinburgh, E. & S. Livingstone, 1971.

Nélaton, C., and Ombrédann, L.: La Rhinoplastie. Paris, G. Steinheil, 1904.

Nélaton, C., and Ombrédanne, L.: Les Autoplasties. Paris, G. Steinheil, 1907

Ollier, L.: Greffes cutanée ou autoplastique. Bull. Acad. Méd., *1*:243, 1872.

Ombrédanne, L.: Maladie Amniotique. *In* Ombrédanne, L., and Mathieu, P. (Eds.): Traité de Chirurgie Orthopédique. Vol. 1. Masson et Cie, Paris, 1937, p. 44.

Padgett, E. C.: Skin grafting in severe burns. Am. J. Surg., *43*:626, 1939.

Paletta, F. X.: Pediatric Plastic Surgery. Vol. I, Trauma. St. Louis, Mo., C. V. Mosby Company, 1967.

Paparella, M. M., and Shumrick, D. A.: Otolaryngology. Vol. III, Head and Neck. Philadelphia, W. B. Saunders Company, 1973.

Paré, A.: Les oeuvres de M. Ambroise Paré conseiller et premier chirurgien du roy. Avec les figures et portraicts tant de l'anatomic que des instruments de chirugie, et de plusieurs monstres. Le tout divisé en vingt-six livres, comme il est contenu en la page suyvent. Paris, G. Buone, 1575.

Paton, D., and Goldberg, M. F.: Injuries of the Eye, the Lids, and the Orbit. Diagnosis and Management. Philadelphia, W. B. Saunders Company, 1968.

Peacock, E. E., Jr., and Van Winkle, W., Jr.: Surgery and Biology of Wound Repair. Philadelphia, W. B. Saunders Company, 1970.

Peet, E.: Reconstruction Absence of Ear. Edinburgh, E. & S. Livingston, 1971.

Rankow, R. M.: An Atlas of the Face, Mouth and Neck. Philadelphia, W. B. Saunders Company, 1968.

Rapaport, F. T., and Dausset, J.: Human Transplantation. New York, Grune & Stratton, 1968.

Rapaport, F. T., Balner, H., and Kountz, S. L.: Transplantation Today. New York, Grune & Stratton, 1973.

Rees, T. D., and Wood-Smith, D.: Cosmetic Facial Surgery. Philadelphia, W. B. Saunders Company, 1973.

Reverdin, J. L.: Greffes épidermiques; expérience faite dans le service de M. le docteur Guyon, à l'Hopital Necker, pendant 1869. Bull. Soc. Impériale Chir. Paris, Series 2, Vol. 10, published in 1870.

Richer, P.: Morphologie de la Femme. Plon-Nourrit et Cie, 1920.

Rogers, B. O.: The historical evolution of plastic and reconstructive surgery. *In* Wood-Smith, D., and Porowski, P. (Eds.): Nursing Care of the Plastic Surgery Patient. St. Louis, Mo., C. V. Mosby Company, 1967.

Rogers, B. O.: Personal communication, 1974.

Ross, R. B., and Johnston, M. C.: Cleft Lip and Palate. Baltimore, The Williams & Wilkins Company, 1972.

Roux, P. J.: Quarante années de practique chirurgicale. Vol. I, Chirurgie réparatrice. Paris, Masson et cie, 1854.

Rowe, N. L., and Killey, H. C.: Fractures of the Facial Skeleton. 2nd Ed. Baltimore, The Williams & Wilkins Company, 1968.

Sabbatini, P.: Cenno storico dell'origine e progressi della rinoplastica e cheiloplastica, seguita dalla descrizione di queste operazioni sopra un solo individuo. Bologna, Belle Arti, 1838.

Sanvenero-Rosselli, G., and Boggio-Robutti, G. (Eds.): Transactions of the Fourth International Congress of Plastic and Reconstructive Surgery, Rome, October, 1967. Amsterdam, Excerpta Medica Foundation, 1969.

Schultz, R. C.: Facial Injuries. Chicago, Year Book Medical Publishers, 1970.

Serre, M.: Traité sur l'art de restaurer les difformités de la face, selon la méthode par deplacement, ou méthode française. Montpellier, L. Castel, 1842.

Shearer, W. L.: Oral Surgery: Cleft Palate and Lip. St. Paul, Minn., North Central Publishing Company, 1967.

Skoog, T.: Surgical Treatment of Burns. A Clinical Report of 789 Cases. Stockholm, Almquist & Wiksell, 1963.

Smith, B., and Cherubini, T. D.: Oculoplastic Surgery. St. Louis, Mo., C. V. Mosby Company, 1970.

Smith, B., and Converse, J. M. (Eds.): Proceedings of the Second International Symposium on Plastic and Reconstructive Surgery of the Eye and Adnexa. St. Louis, Mo., C. V. Mosby Company, 1967.

Smith, F.: Nelson's Looseleaf Reconstructive Surgery. Springfield, Ill., Charles C Thomas, Publisher, 1928.

Smith, F.: Plastic and Reconstructive Surgery. Philadelphia, W. B. Saunders Company, 1950.

Spriestersbach, D. C.: Psychological Aspects of the "Cleft Palate Problem" Vol. I, Vol. II, by D. C. Spriestersbach, G. R. Powers, and associates. Iowa City, University of Iowa Press, 1973.

Stark, R. B.: Cleft Palate: A Multidiscipline Approach. New York, Harper & Row, 1968.

Steinschneider, E.: Beitrage zur Kieferschusstherapie. Berlin, Urban, 1917.

Sunderland, S.: Nerves and Nerve Injuries. Baltimore, The Williams & Wilkins Company, 1968.

Symonds, J. A.: The Renaissance in Italy. New York, Cerf (The Modern Library), 1935.

Szymanowski, J. von: Handbuch der operativen Chirurgie. Braunschweig, F. Vieweg u. Shon, 1870.

Tagliacozzi, G.: De Curtorum chirurgia per Insitionem. Venice, Gaspare Bindoni, 1597.

Tessier, P., Guiot, G., Rougerie, J., Delbet, J. P., and Pastoriza, J.: Osteotomies cranio-naso-orbital-faciales. Hypertelorisme. Ann. Chir. Plast., *12*:103, 1967.

Thiersch, C.: Ueber die feineren anatomischen Veränderungen bei Aufheilung von Haut auf Granulationen. Arch. Klin. Chir., *17*:318, 1874.

Thompson, R. V. S.: Primary Repair of Soft Tissue Injuries. Melbourne, Australia, University Press, 1969.

Turtz, A. I. (Ed.): Proceedings of the Centennial Symposium Manhattan Eye, Ear and Throat Hospital. Vol. I, Ophthalmology. St. Louis, Mo., C. V. Mosby Company, 1969.

Velpeau, A. A. L. M.: Nouveau Eléments de Médecine Opératoire. Paris, J. B. Baillière, 1839.

Velpeau, A. A. L. M.: New Elements of Operative Surgery. 3rd American Ed. from last Paris Ed. Translated by P. S. Tousend under the supervision of Valentine Mott. New York, Wood, 1951.

Velter, E.: Plaies pénétrantes du crane par projectiles de guerre. Paris, A. Maloine et Fils, 1917.

Verneuil, A.: Mémoires de Chirurgie. Paris, B. Masson, 1877–1888.

Vilain, R.: La chirurgie de la medecine, medecine de le chirurgie et chirurgie de la chirurgie. Concours Medical, *92*:44, 1965.

Voltaire, François Marie Arouet de: Oeuvres completes. Vol. 42, pp. 413–414. Paris, Imprimerie de la Societé littéraire-bibliographique, 1785. (Dictionnaire philosophique. Vol. 6.)

Wallace, A. B.: Treatment of burns; return to basic principles. Br. J. Plast. Surg., *1*:233, 1949.

Warkany, J.: Congenital Malformations: Notes and Comments. Chicago, Year Book Medical Publishers, 1971.

Warren, J. M.: Rhinoplastic Operations. With Some Remarks on the Autoplastic Methods Usually Adopted for the Restoration of Parts Lost by Accident or Disease. Boston, Clapp, 1840.

Webster, J. P.: In Memoriam, Vilray Papin Blair. Plast. Reconstr. Surg., *18*:83, 1956.

Wilflingseder, G.: Personal communication, 1975.

Wolfe, J. R.: A new method of performing plastic operations. Med. Times and Gazette, *1*:608, 1876.

Wolff, D., Bellucci, R. J., and Eggston, A. A.: Surgical and Microscopic Anatomy of the Temporal Bone. New York, Hafner Publishing Company, 1971.

Wood-Smith, D., and Porowski, P. C.: Nursing Care of the Plastic Surgery Patient. St. Louis, Mo., C. V. Mosby Company, 1967.

Woolf, R. M., and Broadbent, T. R.: The four-flap Z-plasty. Plast. Reconstr. Surg., *49*:48, 1972.

Yules, R. B.: Atlas for Surgical Repair of Cleft Lip, Cleft Palate and Noncleft Velopharyngeal Incompetence. Springfield, Ill., Charles C Thomas, Publisher, 1971.

Zeis, E.: Handbuch der plastischen Chirurgie (nebsteiner Vorrede von J. F. Dieffenbach). Berlin, Reimer, 1838.

CHAPTER 2

THE PHYSICAL PROPERTIES OF SKIN

Thomas Gibson, D.Sc., F.R.C.S.

Although the plastic surgeon operates upon and transplants most of the tissues of the body, both soft and hard tissues, the cutaneous envelope of the human body, an essential organ, is the most frequently dealt with.

A knowledge of the physical properties of the skin is therefore appropriate. The placing of incisions, the transposition of skin flaps, and the behavior of skin grafts are influenced by its special characteristics.

The most significant characteristic of the physical properties of skin is their extreme variability: the physical characteristics differ at the same site on different individuals; they differ at different sites on the same individual; they differ in different directions at the same site; and at any site they change remarkably with age. It is probably a truism that each piece of skin is uniquely constructed, and the uniqueness of its physical properties depends mainly on the twin fibrous networks of collagen and elastin, which constitute the bulk of the dermis, and the pattern of their interwoven architecture.

The collagen fibers in the dermis (Figs. 2–1 and 2–2) are extremely long structures compared to their diameter. In the relaxed state in young subjects they are markedly convoluted but become less so with age. They appear to be randomly oriented and intertwined one with another; yet, when skin is stretched in any direction, the convolutions straighten out. Furthermore, as the load increases, an increasing number of the fibers becomes aligned in the direction of the stretching force, until finally there is a structure of parallel fibers which is highly resistant to further extension (Fig. 2–3). This behavior underlies the typical stress-strain curve for skin (Fig. 2–4) and explains what every surgeon knows: a certain amount of skin may be excised at any site and the wound closed easily, but there is a point beyond which no amount of hauling on sutures will effect closure.

Each collagen fiber is made up of hundreds of finer fibrils, and each fibril is, in turn, made up of several triple helical spiraled collagen molecules twisted into "super coils." (See Chapter 3.) Collagen shows structure within structure within structure. The multiple spring-like molecules resist extension, and the aggregated fibrils form a cable of great strength and limited extension, which is readily capable of bending in any direction as the fiber network moves. Finally the network provides free mobility to follow a wide range of body movements, but with a built-in limit to the amount of extension possible.

The collagen fibers illustrated are those which make up most of the thickness of the dermis. As they approach the epidermis, the fibers become much finer. The fine sub-epidermal fibers probably act as a damping link to protect the epithelial cells from the more acute and coarse movements of the fiber network.

The elastic fibers of the dermis are much finer than the collagen fibers and unlike

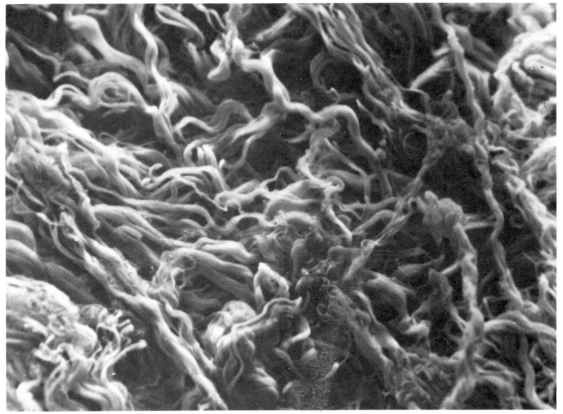

FIGURE 2–1. Scanning electron microscope (SEM) photograph of the collagen fibers of human dermis. (From Gibson, T., and Kenedi, R. M.: The structural components of the dermis. *In* Montagna, W., Bentley, J. P., and Dobson, R. L. (Eds.): The Dermis, 1970. Courtesy of Appleton-Century-Crofts, Publishing Division of Prentice-Hall, Inc., Englewood Cliffs, N.J.)

the latter have end to side junctions. Their function is to return the deformed collagen network to its relaxed condition. It is the elastic fibers which are in part responsible for the tension naturally occurring in skin.

Such a mobile microarchitecture requires a lubricant, and this is probably provided by the mucopolysaccharide ground substance and the tissue fluid lying around and between the fibers. It is noteworthy that each fibril in the fiber aggregate has a sheath of mucopolysaccharide which separates it from its fellows. Collagen does not exist in the body in a naked state; it is always associated with and covered by mucopolysaccharides.

Intertwined with the networks of collagen and elastin are three other networks: small blood vessels, nerve fibers, and lymphatics, respectively (Fig. 2–5). None of these structures contributes to the physical properties of skin, but their function may be interfered with when the fibrous networks through which they pass are deformed. Thus constriction of the

blood vessels will interfere with the blood supply and, if long continued, produce necrosis. Constriction of nerves causes pain, and interruption of the lymphatics results in edema.

The fibrous networks are transfixed in most parts of the body by a varying number of hairs (Fig. 2–6), which probably restrict the mobility of the dermis.

The varying physical properties of skin depend on the patterns of the fibrous weave of the dermis. For descriptive purposes these can be divided into three groups: (1) visco-elastic properties, (2) skin tension properties, and (3) skin extensibility.

THE VISCO-ELASTIC PROPERTIES OF SKIN

It is convenient to discuss these first since they are new concepts to most surgeons and yet are of considerable importance in studying the other physical properties of skin.

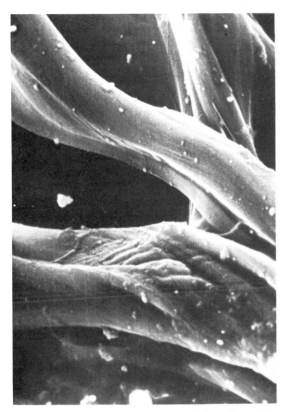

FIGURE 2–2. The smooth surface of the collagen fiber shown in a SEM study. (From Gibson, T., and Kenedi, R. M.: Factors affecting the mechanical characteristics of human skin. *In* Proceedings of the Centennial Symposium on Repair and Regeneration. New York, McGraw-Hill Book Company, 1968, p. 87.)

There are basically two visco-elastic properties: "creep" and "stress relaxation." Creep occurs when a piece of skin is stretched and the stretching force is kept constant; the skin will continue to extend, depending of course on the forces involved. Stress relaxation, the corollary of creep, occurs when a piece of skin is stretched for a given distance and that distance held constant; the force required to keep it stretched gradually decreases (Fig. 2–7).

It will be noted that time is required for creep and stress relaxation to occur. It is thus of paramount importance that any measurements made of the physical properties of skin and its behavior under stress are made during a standard time. Failure to appreciate this in previous studies has caused considerable confusion.

Creep, as a concept, is clinically important. It means that skin can be stretched by a significant, if small, amount. This can be of vital importance in such cases as the "just-too-small flap" or the "wound which just won't close." The usual technique is to place sharp, hooked retractors into the undersurface of the dermis on each side of the flap or wound and to pull them in opposite directions as hard as the surgeon and his assistant can, short of tearing the tissues. It has been found that if skin is "load cycled" (Fig. 2–8), the maximum extension is not usually obtained on the first loading. *It is therefore advisable when trying to stretch skin to repeat the extension three or four times.* One of the reasons for the visco-elasticity of skin is that, as the fibers in the dermis become aligned, tissue fluid and ground substance are progressively displaced from the network. The more fluid in the dermis, the greater the amount of creep obtainable, and the phenomenon is particularly evident and useful when handling flaps that have recently been delayed or moved.

Stress relaxation does not seem to have the same direct clinical relevance. It can, however, explain why the flap which appears to be sutured too tightly immediately postoperatively is often perfectly viable a few hours later.

SKIN TENSION

The naturally occurring tension in skin and skin extensibility are often confused and referred to loosely and inaccurately as "elasticity." They are certainly interrelated; skin will extend if increased tension is applied to it and, conversely, stretched skin is under increased tension. But they are distinct concepts and will be discussed separately.

Skin tension is of particular importance in wound healing. Clinical observation shows that it varies at different anatomical sites and in different directions at the same site. A sutured wound so oriented that the tension across it is maximum at that site is likely to produce a stretched hypertrophic scar. Plastic surgeons have learned to choose the direction of their incision wherever possible so that the tension across it is minimum and a fine linear scar is more probable. The concept of lines of tension is an old one, and for some time Langer's lines (Langer, 1861) were respected. However, Langer's lines are more a function of skin extensibility, and the only true lines of tension are the crease lines. Crease lines, whether caused by joint movement or the play of underlying muscles, are tension lines in the sense that the tension across them must be virtually

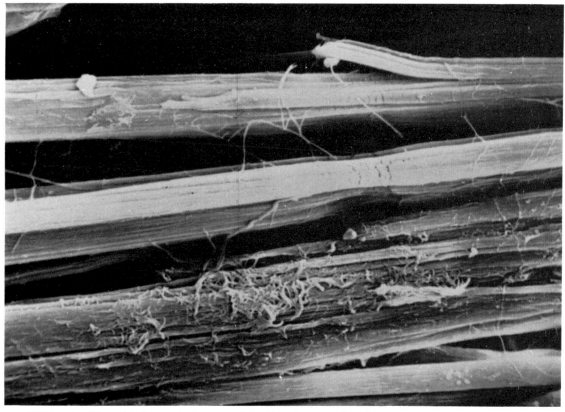

FIGURE 2-3. When skin is stretched, many of the fibers become aligned in a straight manner in the direction of stretch, thus imposing a limit on extensibility in that direction. (From Brown, I. A.: Structural and Mechanical Studies on Human Skin. Ph.D. Thesis, University of Strathclyde, Glasgow, 1971.)

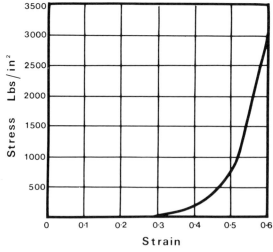

FIGURE 2-4. Typical stress-strain curve of human skin in tension. (From Gibson, T., and Kenedi, R. M.: The structural component of the dermis. *In* Montagna, W., Bentley, J. P., and Dobson, R. L. (Eds.): The Dermis, 1970. Courtesy of Appleton-Century-Crofts, Publishing Division of Prentice-Hall, Inc., Englewood Cliffs, N.J.)

nil; otherwise they would not have formed. The tension along a crease line is therefore higher than that across it. Sutured wounds which parallel creases are under the least possible tension at that site.

It would appear that there is a critical tension below which scars will not stretch but above which they will. Z-plasties around the head and neck often show a central limb which has stretched while the others have not, or vice versa.

Skin tension decreases with age, and the fine, almost undetectable scars which result in the lax skin of the elderly are well known; the same is true of the skin of the scrotum and the shaft of the penis. Conversely there are areas, such as the shoulder and presternum, where the tension existing in *all* directions seems to be greater than the critical value, and stretched, if not hypertrophic, scars are almost inevitable.

The tension naturally present in skin is presumably a function of the elastic fiber

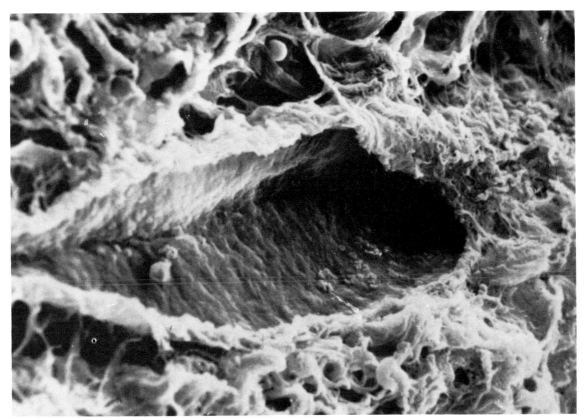

FIGURE 2–5. A small arteriole traversing the dermis. When the fiber network is deformed, the lumen may be obliterated, producing blanching and ultimately necrosis. (From Brown, I. A.: Structural and Mechanical Studies on Human Skin. Ph.D. Thesis, University of Strathclyde, Glasgow, 1971.)

network existing in a state of tension; collagen fibers have no power of retraction. In certain areas gravity must contribute significantly to skin tension. The shoulder girdle is rather like a coathanger supporting the skin of the chest and trunk, particularly in the female with the additional weight of the breasts. Such a condition may account for the high skin tension and stretched scars in the shoulder region.

Unfortunately it has not so far been possible to devise a technique which will measure tension in intact living skin, and absolute values to correlate with different kinds of scar remain unavailable.

The Effect of Increased Tension on Normal Skin

A certain degree of increased tension can persist in skin for long periods without stretching the skin or producing any obvious effects. The normal skin immediately adjacent to a flexion contracture due to burn scarring does not stretch and correct the defect in spite of recurrent tension. Furthermore, in serial excisions of nevi, it can be shown (Gibson and Kenedi, 1967) that the increased tension imposed on the skin by the elliptical excision will relax by only about 70 per cent after one year, and it is well known that overenthusiastic serial excisions can produce permanent deformity.

With higher tensions one of three phenomena may occur, depending on the force applied: stretching, rupture (striae formation), or blanching of the skin.

The skin *stretches* in such conditions as lymphedema and adiposity, and in the most severe cases a linear stretch of nine to ten times may occur. "Stretch" is probably not the correct term, since the skin maintains its thickness and indeed may be thicker than normal. This type of stretching depends on biological activity and growth and differs from the creep described above, which is purely physical in nature.

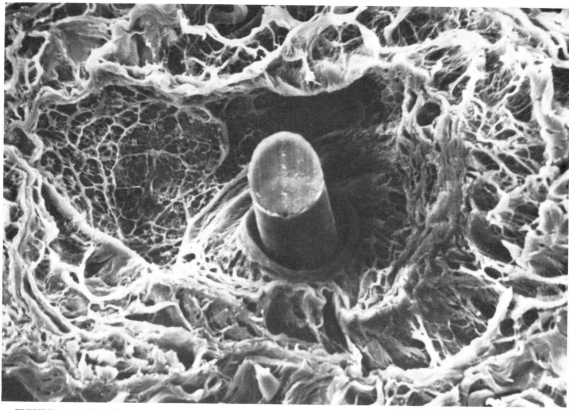

FIGURE 2–6. The fibrous networks are transfixed by hairs. A hair shaft surrounded by its follicle and by a sebaceous gland is shown attached to the main collagen network by fine fibrils. (From "A scanning electron microscope study of the effects of uniaxial tension on human skin" by Ian A. Brown. British Journal of Dermatology [1973] *89,* 383.)

Biological stretching of skin has no clinical value in plastic surgery, although if we knew more about the phenomenon and could harness it when necessary, it might theoretically obviate the need for skin grafts and flaps.

The dermis ruptures and striae form when an increasing load is applied at a faster rate than obtains in skin stretch. Striae are found in the skin of the pregnant abdomen, in the skin covering the rapidly increasing fat deposits in Cushing's disease, and even in skin over the expanding muscles of enthusiasts taking body-building exercises (Glashan, 1963; Strivens, 1963). They lie as a rule at right angles to Langer's lines which, as will be shown below, represent the direction of minimum extensibility. In other words, the fibers that stretch first and most are those oriented along Langer's lines, but whether they rupture or simply unravel from the weave has yet to be established. As Langer himself discovered, pregnancy imposes a different set of "lines" on a woman's abdominal skin than those shown in his original illustrations.

Blanching of the skin occurs when the fibrous network is deformed to such an extent that the lumina of the dermal blood vessels are obliterated and the blood flow is obstructed. If unrelieved, necrosis follows. Blanching may result from compression forces and can cause such lesions as decubitus ulcers. It is probably more familiar to the plastic surgeon as the result of a tension force when skin flaps are sutured into defects slightly too large or skin is advanced too far after wide undermining. It should be remembered that in the examples mentioned—flaps and undermined skin—the force required to produce blanching is usually much less than that required in uncut skin.

A zone of blanching across a flap can usually be relieved if the force is not too excessive, either by applying a stretching force and obtaining a modicum of creep, as described above, or by making a small incision just through the dermis in the center of and at right angles to the line of blanching. The latter maneuver divides the stretched, oriented fibers in the line of blanching and relaxes the collagen

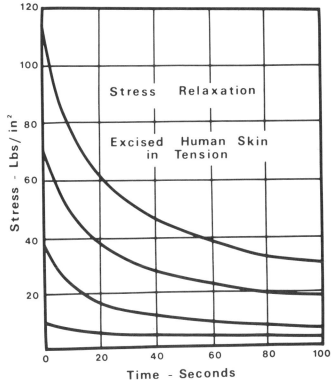

FIGURE 2–7. The stress relaxation which occurs in skin increases with the applied load. (From Gibson, T., and Kenedi, R. M.: The structural components of the dermis. *In* Montagna, W., Bentley, J. P., and Dobson, R. L. (Eds.): The Dermis, 1970. Courtesy of Appleton-Century-Crofts, Publishing Division of Prentice-Hall, Inc., Englewood Cliffs, N.J.)

network. It has been found experimentally that 60 per cent more force can be applied before blanching will recur in a band which divides to enclose the small incision (Kenedi, Gibson and Daly, 1965).

SKIN EXTENSIBILITY

Skin is extensible to allow for every possible body movement. Since none of our joints are universal, it follows that on most parts of the body skin will extend more in some directions than in others. Skin extensibility is greatest in infancy. As skin is repeatedly stretched and relaxed throughout life, the ability of the elastic tissue matrix to return skin from its extended state to its fully relaxed state is gradually lost, and skin extensibility is replaced by skin laxity, which fulfills the same role of permitting free body movement. It is skin extensibility and skin laxity which permit many plastic surgical procedures, particularly the complete closure of skin defects without the need for importing tissue from a distance.

Skin extensibility, unlike skin tension, can be readily measured in vivo, and the techniques vary from the approximation by the plastic surgeon of picking up a fold between finger and thumb to the use of highly sophisticated and precise instruments. The results of accurate measurement may differ in vitro and in vivo: when skin is extended, it contracts by a similar amount at right angles to the direction of extension. Should the ability to contract be limited in vivo, as circumferentially around a limb, extension along the limb is similarly influenced. Furthermore, in vivo skin is fixed to the underlying tissues to a varying degree, so that undermining will usually permit some further extension, although at the expense of the blood supply.

The Directional Variations in Skin Extensibility

Pinching up a fold of skin is good enough to ensure that two points can be approximated following skin excision or the rotation of a flap. It is inadequate at most sites, however, for detecting those directional differences in extensibility which may be of considerable clinical importance. The apparatus required for exact observations has been described elsewhere (Millington, Gibson, Evans and Barbenel, 1971). The varying extensions in different

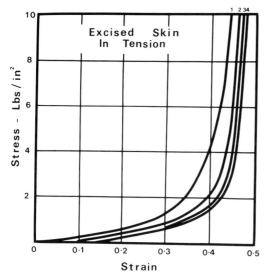

FIGURE 2–8. Repeated loading of skin shows varying curves until a stable state is attained in the region of curve 4. (From Gibson, T., and Kenedi, R. M.: The structural components of the dermis. *In* Montagna, W., Bentley, J. P., and Dobson, R. L. (Eds.): The Dermis, 1970. Courtesy of Appleton-Century-Crofts, Publishing Division of Prentice-Hall, Inc., Englewood Cliffs, N.J.)

directions for any given load can be recorded as ellipses in the manner shown in Figure 2–9, in which the various axes represent the extension obtained in that direction. When the extensibility ellipses are superimposed on Langer's lines, it is found that the axis of minimum extension corresponds almost exactly for the three areas examined: the anterior chest, abdomen, and front of thigh.

Although Langer's lines have often been referred to as lines of tension (they *may* in fact represent directions of maximum tension), Langer himself called them cleavage lines, and histologic examination will confirm that each little ellipse occurs by separation of parallel collagen fibers. Cox (1941) believed that this was the result of the collagen fibers being arranged parallel to Langer's lines around the body. However, the scanning electron microscope failed to confirm this concept. The explanation is that when a sharp, pointed, round-bodied instrument, as Langer used, is stabbed against the skin, the point first depresses the skin and increases the tension in all directions around the depression. The result is that the fibers first to be aligned will lie in the direction of minimum extensibility. When they are so aligned, resistance to further skin depression is greatly increased, and the point pierces the epidermis and splits the parallel fibers (Gibson, Stark and Kenedi, 1971).

Langer's lines are therefore lines of minimum extensibility; the two coincide almost exactly, and any minor discrepancies are well within the range of individual variation. The direction of maximum extensibility is at right angles to them. Thus if one were excising in the shape of an ellipse a skin tumor or a full-thickness skin graft, the greatest width would be obtained by placing the long axis of the ellipse along Langer's lines.

Langer (1862) in his studies with cadavers found that the tension along the cleavage line

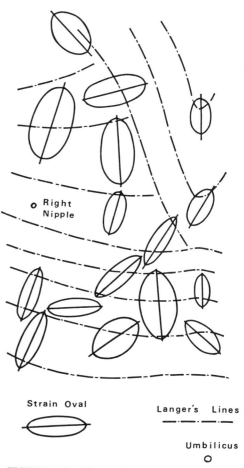

FIGURE 2–9. The ovals show graphically the varying extensibility of skin over the right side of the chest. Langer's lines are shown as background; there is good correlation between Langer's lines and the direction of minimum extensibility. (Average readings in a number of male subjects all under 30 years of age.) (From Gibson, T., and Kenedi, R. M.: The structural components of the dermis. *In* Montagna, W., Bentley, J. P., and Dobson, R. L. (Eds.): The Dermis, 1970. Courtesy of Appleton-Century-Crofts, Publishing Division of Prentice-Hall, Inc., Englewood Cliffs, N.J.)

was greater than that across it. A wound on the front of the thigh at right angles to the lines gaped much more than one parallel to them. That Langer's lines represent lines of maximum tension in the living, however, awaits the invention of a technique to measure skin tension on the intact body. Crease lines, which Langer himself stated coincided with his cleavage lines, are certainly lines of maximum tension,* as noted above, and this may well be true of all cleavage lines.

Langer also observed that the pattern of most of the cleavage lines was not innate but was imposed after birth, presumably because of increased joint movements. During the first year of life the pattern changed from that present in neonates to that which persisted into adult life. Even at this stage it was not necessarily permanent; pregnancy can change the direction of the cleavage lines on the abdominal skin, as presumably any long-continued period of increased tension may do.

---

*Maximal tension along the line, minimal tension upon the edges of a skin defect whose long axis is within, or parallel to, the line (see Chapter 1).

REFERENCES

Brown, I. A.: Structural and Mechanical Studies on Human Skin. Ph.D. Thesis, University of Strathclyde, Glasgow, 1971.

Brown, I. A.: A scanning electron microscope study of the effects of uniaxial tension on human skin. Br. J. Dermatol., *89*:383, 1973.

Cox, H. T.: The cleavage lines of the skin. Br. J. Surg., *29*:234, 1941.

Gibson, T., and Kenedi, R. M.: Biomechanical properties of skin. Surg. Clin. North Am., *47*:279, 1967.

Gibson, T., and Kenedi, R. M.: Factors affecting the mechanical characteristics of human skin. *In* Proceedings of the Centennial Symposium on Repair and Regeneration. New York, McGraw-Hill Book Company, 1968, p. 87.

Gibson, T., and Kenedi, R. M.: The structural components of the dermis. *In* Montagna, W., Bentley, J. P., and Dobson, R. L. (Eds.): The Dermis. New York, Appleton-Century-Crofts, 1970, p. 19.

Gibson, T., Stark, H., and Kenedi, R. M.: The significance of Langer's lines. *In* Hueston, J. T. (Ed.): Transactions of the Fifth International Congress of Plastic and Reconstructive Surgery. Australia, Butterworths, 1971, p. 1213.

Glashan, R. W.: Cutaneous striae. Br. Med. J., *1*:614, 1963.

Kenedi, R. M., Gibson, T., and Daly, C. H.: Bioengineering studies of the human skin. I. *In* Jackson, S. F., Harkness, R., Partridge, S., and Tristram, G. (Eds.): Structure and Function of Connective and Skeletal Tissues. London, Butterworths, 1965, p. 388.

Langer, K.: Zur Anatomie und Physiologie der Haut. I. Über die Spaltbarkeit der Cutis. S.-B. Akad. Wiss. Wien, *44*:19, 1861.

Langer, K.: Zur Anatomie und Physiologie der Haut. 2. Die Spannung der Cutis. S.-B. Akad. Wiss. Wien, *45*:133, 1862.

Millington, P. F., Gibson, T., Evans, J. H., and Barbenel, J. C.: Structural and mechanical aspects of connective tissue. *In* Kenedi, R. M. (Ed.): Advances in Bio-medical Engineering. London, Academic Press, 1971, p. 189.

Strivens, T.: Cutaneous striae. Br. Med. J., *1*:263, 1963.

CHAPTER 3

REPAIR AND REGENERATION

Erle E. Peacock, M.D.

In the practice of surgery, the rate of gain of tensile strength in a healing wound is the biological phenomenon of most concern to the patient and surgeon alike. Among the questions asked are: When can I get out of bed? When can I go back to work? When will the stitches come out? How long will the cast stay on? One can usually give the answers fairly accurately with only a superficial knowledge of the dynamics of collagen synthesis and collagen deposition in various areas of the body. The fact that no known biological alteration significantly accelerates the gain of tensile strength in a healing wound has made the study of wound healing unappealing to most surgeons at the present time. The repetitious duplication of investigative manipulations of wounds that increase the rate of gain in strength within a range which has only statistical significance has produced so many "false starts" that mild cynicism regarding the acceleration of healing in human patients is justified.

Actually, the search for a spot weld of human tissue is not within the realm of science fiction. Collagen, the major protein involved in providing tensile strength of an order required for normal use of a body part, is a crystalline protein which polymerizes and depolymerizes predictably under a wide range of physiologic conditions. Certainly there is ample collagen on each side of a fresh wound to provide strength if interaction of subunits across the wound could be established similar to that found in uninjured tissues. It has always seemed to the author that depolymerization and repolymerization reactions in already synthesized collagen are more likely to result in an extremely rapid gain in wound strength than methods which are dependent upon synthesis of new protein. The number of cells which must "be born," the length of time such cells require to "tool up" for efficient protein synthesis, and the relatively wasteful utilization of the first collagen synthesized are such complex biological phenomena that it seems almost ludicrous to search for a single catalyst or single biological manipulation to accelerate more than one, much less all, of the processes which contribute to wound healing.

The plastic surgeon has an entirely different view of wound healing. The time required to regain tensile strength is of little concern, while the qualitative end result is one of the most crucial factors in reconstructive surgery. In almost all of the chapters in these volumes, the techniques described are aimed at restoring a surface or an area in such a way that the end result of healing will result in the least possible interference with normal appearance and function. In some areas, such as the gliding surface of long tendons, this can be a most difficult task. The statement, "I dressed the wound, God healed it" (Ambroise Paré) simply does not produce predictably successful repairs of a lacerated flexor tendon or nerve, either in critical areas or under complicated conditions. Acceleration of healing in most reconstructive problems is not a major objective; the need to be able to control the manner in which the wound heals, however, is the single most critical factor in the search for excellence in reconstructive surgery. This chapter will briefly review the biological basis for much of what we currently do to assure minimal scar complications and will outline some of the differences which fundamental research in wound healing biology may make in restorative surgery in the years ahead.

The processes which most concern reconstructive surgeons are *contraction of a wound* and *synthesis of a scar*. Of course, *epithelization* is also important, but its importance lies more in the pathologic state (uncontrolled cell division) than in the normal resurfacing of a donor site or open wound. Unfortunately, however, surgeons often think of epithelization as being the same as regeneration of skin. It is extremely important to understand that skin is an organ—not a simple tissue, such as epithelium or fascia. Actually, skin is a very complex organ and like all compound organs, with the possible exception of liver, does not regenerate to any significant extent.

In the course of evolution, man lost the ability to regenerate compound organs and has only the relatively simple and often unsatisfactory substitute of healing to restore physical continuity. It is unfortunate, in some respects, that healing is rather uniformly regarded as being entirely beneficial. Of course, survival has been dependent upon even a crude method of restoring internal homeostasis after external injury; yet, the method by which restoration of integrity is accomplished may produce cosmetic and functional complications worse than the original wound. As an example, overhealing and its effect upon appearance is discussed in Chapter 16; the effect of overhealing on the function of internal organs, however, is not as clearly defined in most texts. It is not the lye burn of the esophagus or the toxic damage to the liver that is fatal to patients. It is the scar which forms during healing that results in serious dysphagia or fatal hepatic cirrhosis. Postoperative intestinal obstruction, stenosis of bile ducts, ureter, or urethra, and adhesions around tendons are not the direct effect of a surgical manipulation. Rather they are the consequences of the reparative process, in which wound contraction and fibrous protein synthesis were not controlled. Many possibilities for controlling healing are suggested by looking carefully at the various fundamental processes involved in the repair of human wounds.

EPITHELIZATION

The major function of epithelium is to act as a selective barrier between the body and its environment. The epithelial barrier in human beings prevents bacteria, toxic materials, and some radiation from gaining access to the internal milieu (of Claude Bernard). It also prevents or reduces the loss of fluid, electrolytes, and other substances from the underlying tissue. The barrier function is not absolute; toxic materials, when applied in appropriate solvents, can penetrate, and ionizing radiation can penetrate epithelium if the wavelength and energy are sufficient to do so. Nevertheless, epithelium acts as a primary defense against a hostile environment and is a major factor in maintaining internal homeostasis.

A piece of cellophane tape applied to the skin surface and then quickly detached will usually remove one layer of cells from the stratum corneum. The technique is called stripping, and, if the application is repeated in the same area, successive layers of cells will be removed (Pinkus, 1951). In this way it is possible to remove completely the stratum corneum; events that follow have been studied microscopically by taking small punch biopsies at repeated intervals. Such studies reveal that epithelial regeneration appears to be the result of mitosis of preexisting cells in the basal layer of the epidermis. Maximum increase in mitosis is noted 48 to 72 hours after injury (Sullivan and Epstein, 1963; Bullough, 1970). Some of the cells formed during mitosis migrate to the upper layers and without further division differentiate into keratinizing cells. Most of the cells in the basal layer enlarge after trauma, and the apparent effect of enlargement and mitosis is to squeeze some cells upward into the prickle cell layer of the epidermis. Because major regenerative activity occurs in the basal cell layer, the dermoepidermal junction is of considerable importance in the healing of epithelial wounds. In the normal state basal cells are firmly attached to the papillary layer, but following injury adhesion to the dermis is reduced; the cells migrate upward and are denuded more easily than in normal tissue. Thus, flattening of the rete pegs is one of the consequences of epithelial repair and has a great deal of significance in areas where healing has occurred entirely by epithelization.

For many years it was thought that specialized epithelial structures, such as the hair follicles and sebaceous glands, do not regenerate if they are totally destroyed. It has been demonstrated, however, that such appendages can regenerate by differentiation of migrated epidermal epithelium. Again, however, an area which has healed by epithelization alone and does not contain normal dermis and dermal structures is quite different from normal skin. Epithelium contains a large amount of water, and a body area covered only by epithelium has little resistance to mechanical disruption (Fig. 3–1). In addition, in the absence of rete pegs and epithelial appendages, vesicular formation and epithelial abrasions follow minimal trauma. Thus, biological forces which control all movement and division are seldom completely quiescent in an area where, in the absence of

dermis, epithelization was the only mechanism by which the wound healed.

Although mitosis does occur at the edge of a wound which is healing primarily by epithelization, cell dedifferentiation and movement are the primary biological phenomena responsible for the resurfacing of a denuded area (Gillman and Penn, 1956) (Figs. 3–2 and 3–3). At some stage during cell differentiation a point is reached at which the cell has no option but to continue performing a specialized function, and the cell will ultimately die completely clogged with keratin. Before that point, however, the cell can either differentiate to produce keratin or dedifferentiate to undergo mitosis or develop ameboid characteristics. Epithelization of a denuded area, of course, is accomplished by cells which are not sufficiently differentiated to undergo dedifferentiation to a motile form. Mobile cells develop ruffled membranes and begin to move in a direction where cell contact does not occur. The biological forces which are responsible for such movement are powerful and predictable and will continue for as long as the cell remains alive or until it meets a cell of similar type. Ruffled membranes are coated with a more adhesive surface than the rest of the cell, and when cells of similar type meet, adhesion occurs and the entire process reverts to a resting stage. The phenomenon is called *contact inhibition.*

In a wound in which it is not possible for contact inhibition to occur because the area is too large for resurfacing by epithelization alone or because any coverage is repeatedly traumatized, there is a continual stimulation to epithelial cellular dedifferentiation and ameboid motion. In addition, during long periods of stimulation to divide and become motile, some cells close to the wound margin can be shown to develop abnormal characteristics, including an acceleration of the mitosis rate.

The almost inevitable end result of continued attempts to resurface a wound by epithelization alone is epidermoid carcinoma. For all practical purposes, any wound in which re-epithelization is retarded long enough is in danger of malignant transformation. The mechanism by which this occurs has not been defined, but the factors which are responsible for dedifferentiation, ameboid motion, and, ultimately, an increased number of mitoses are some of the most powerful and predictable forces in human biology. That they ultimately become distorted or overpower normal control mechanisms is inexorable; the length of time required for such an unfortunate complication to

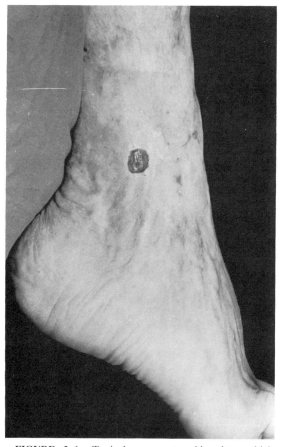

FIGURE 3–1. Typical recurrent ankle ulcer which healed only by epithelization and by some degree of fibrous protein synthesis.

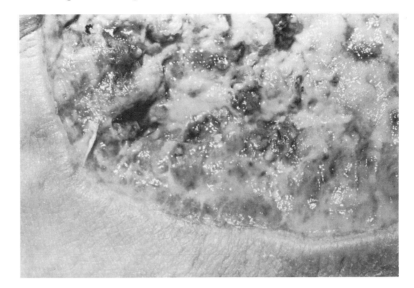

FIGURE 3–2. Radiation ulcer which cannot undergo wound contraction or fibrous protein synthesis because of damage to vital stem cells. Epithelization proceeds normally, as can be seen by the circumferential membrane extending in a central direction.

occur, however, may be quite variable. For example, when the original wound is the result of radiant energy, the length of time required for carcinoma to develop is directly proportional to the wavelength of the radiant energy. Thirty years may elapse before carcinoma (Marjolin's ulcer) develops in a scar resulting from thermal injury (radiation almost in the visible spectrum) (Fig. 3–4). However, injury caused by X-ray or gamma wave radiation (see Chapter 20) may produce a carcinoma in 12 to 24 months. Carcinoma developing in wounds caused by

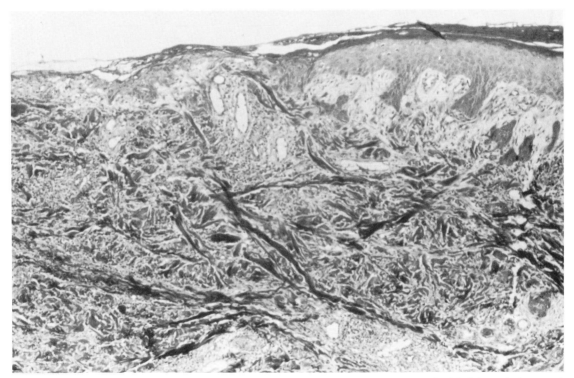

FIGURE 3–3. Microscopic appearance of advancing epithelial margin. The thickness of epithelial margin is approximately 20 cells at the base (right side of figure) but diminishes to one cell thickness at the leading edge (left side of figure). This suggests that cell movement rather than mitosis is the predominant biological mechanism involved.

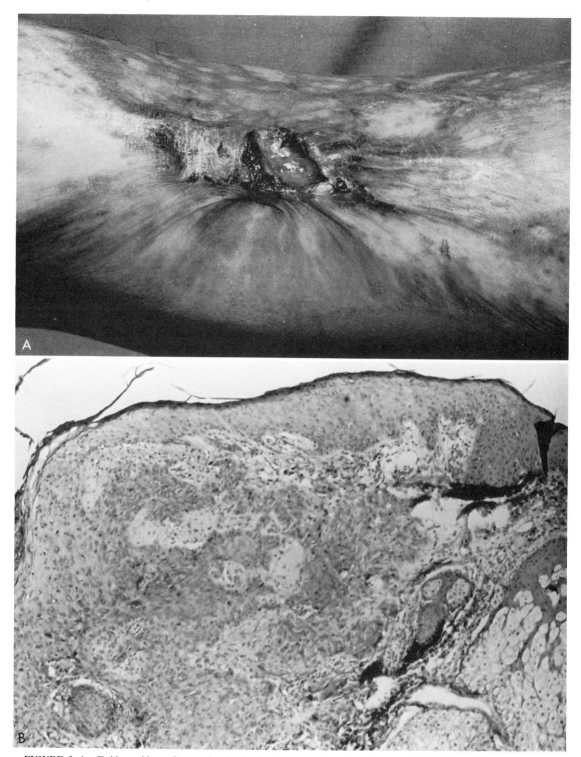

FIGURE 3–4. Epidermoid carcinoma developing in a 23 year old burn scar. *A*, Gross appearance. *B*, Microscopic appearance demonstrating piling up of excess epithelial cells rather than an edge of progressively diminishing thickness, as observed in the migrating cells in Figure 3.

mechanical injury or in chronic sinus tracts requires an even longer time interval to develop and is not as predictable as radiant energy–induced lesions.

At the moment, there is no known catalyst to accelerate the process of epithelization. It is known that cell movement occurs more rapidly against two surfaces than against a single one. Thus, a cover provided by an artificial material or a natural dressing, such as a scab, provides more than protection for delicate ameboid cells. The most important influence the surgeon can exert is to take reasonable measures to ensure that epithelization is not inhibited. Prevention of infection, protection from external trauma, and avoidance of chemical destruction from various drugs constitute sound wound treatment, as far as epithelization is concerned. Many substances have been studied for their epithelial stimulating powers; none has been found to increase ameboid motion or epithelial cellular division. Thus, the only reason for using a medicated gauze dressing is to assure that removal of the dressing will not cause stripping of the epithelial cells because of adherence to the dressing material. Actually, a scab is probably the best wound protection available. A scab must be cared for, however, as a dehydrated layer of crenated red blood cells is not a substantial covering and must be protected from external trauma (chemicals, mechanical force). The advancing edge of epithelial cells produces a collagenolytic enzyme which literally cuts through the interface between scab and dermis to prepare a "carpet" of fibrous tissue ahead of the advancing cells. The natural interaction between an overlying scab, the underlying dermis, and the advancing epithelial edge is one of the most complex and, teleologically speaking, superb biological phenomena in the body. It is probably not possible to improve on the natural effectiveness of these processes with current drugs, bandaging materials, or operative procedures.

CONTRACTION

It is important to distinguish between contraction and contracture. Contraction is an active biological process which is important in the closure of a wound in which loss of tissue has occurred. Contracture is the end result of such a wound and can be produced by the process of wound contraction or by fibrosis of tissue

which previously was elastic to some degree (Figs. 3–5 and 3–6). In large wounds characterized by loss of tissue, contraction is the most important process in healing (Fig. 3–7). Contracture, however, is the *bête noire* of the reconstructive surgeon, and one of the oldest axioms in plastic surgery is "recreate the wound before reconstructive surgery is started." Modern cell biology has uncovered many of the basic phenomena involved in the process of contraction, and some of these can be used to advantage by the reconstructive surgeon.

A review of recent work performed to identify specific processes in wound contraction may lead one to the conclusion that confusion still exists as to whether the contracting forces are located in the periphery or in the center of the wound. Actually, such confusion is probably due more to the study of different animal species and wound preparations than to the accumulation of conflicting data (Grillo and Gross, 1959). Animals which have a very mobile panniculus, such as the horse or rat, will respond to surgical manipulation of the contracting process differently than guinea pigs, rabbits, or human beings. A wound which is undergoing contraction in an animal with a

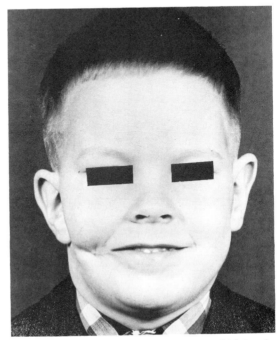

FIGURE 3–5. Example of a contracture which is relative in that the deep scar is apparent only when elasticity is required, as in the act of smiling. During repose no contracture is apparent.

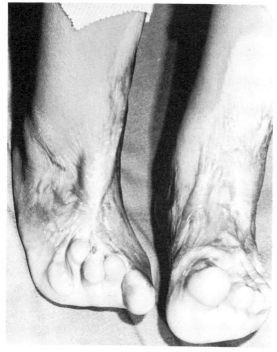

FIGURE 3-6. Typical "contracture" resulting from the process of *contraction* in a wound characterized by loss of tissue.

hypothesis that the main contractile elements are located in the dermal-subdermal interface at the margin of a contracting wound (Watts, Grillo, and Gross, 1958).

Wound contraction is a process mediated by living, healthy cells. Radiant energy, cell poisons, and death of the animal result in cessation of contraction (see Fig. 3-2).

A major advance in the understanding of wound contraction may have occurred with the discovery of a highly specialized form of fibroblast called a myofibroblast. A myofibroblast, as first described by Gabbiani, Ryan, and Majno (1971), is a typical fibroblast with a well-developed endocytoplasmic reticulum which also has many features of a smooth muscle cell. Such features include massive bundles of intracytoplasmic microfilaments,

movable panniculus will react in a different manner when an incision is made in the center of the granulation tissue than when a similar manipulation is performed in a wound which does not have a panniculus. Although there is not a single unifying hypothesis which explains all of the data at this time, most data can be explained by the work of Watts, Grillo, and Gross (1958), who identified the "picture frame area" just beneath the advancing skin margin as the area where the contractile process occurs. Phillips and Peacock (1964) felt the process originated in vertically oriented sites of locomotion and not in a horizontal ring of tissue which became smaller by excluding cells and reducing the circumference in a horizontal plane. Examination of the subdermal picture frame area has revealed the presence of large stellate cells which appear in greater number than elsewhere in the dermis. Subsequently, these cells have been shown to have ruffled membranes indicative of motile characteristics. Although other studies have indicated that some contractile forces originate in central granulation tissue, these experiments can be best explained as alterations in the panniculus which occur during contraction and do not, in the author's judgment, refute the earlier

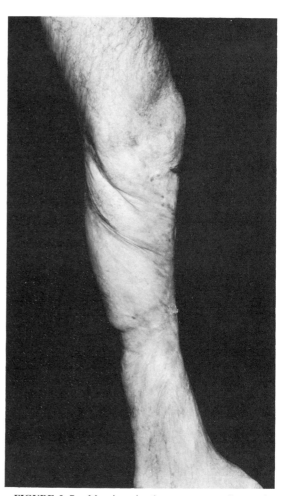

FIGURE 3-7. Massive circular movement of posterior unburned skin to close an anterior defect. As longitudinal movement is impossible in the center of the leg, circular movement occurs.

positive immunofluorescent labeling with human anti–smooth muscle serum, nuclear indentations indicative of contraction, and cell-to-stroma connections which would be necessary for cellular contraction to be imparted to whole tissue. Myofibroblasts are almost ubiquitous; they have been identified in virtually every type of tissue undergoing active contraction, including granulation tissue, tendon sheath, and palmar fascia in patients with Dupuytren's disease (Fig. 3–8). That wound contraction is almost entirely a cellular process and is not dependent on collagen synthesis was conclusively shown by the demonstration that wound contracture occurs normally in severely scorbutic animals. The contracture produced in a scorbutic animal is much less stable than that in a nonscorbutic one; only a small injury is required to release the contracture. The active process of moving the skin edges in a cen-

tripetal manner, however, is unchanged by preventing collagen synthesis.

A major advance in reconstructive surgery would be the ability to control wound contracture while at the same time permitting other aspects of wound healing to proceed uninhibited. One of the major functions of the reconstructive surgeon is to release contractures, and if it were possible to prevent contracture formation while epithelization or fibrous protein synthesis progressed in a normal fashion, the work of the reconstructive surgeon would be greatly simplified. Such a possibility is becoming increasingly more likely as the basic processes involved in wound contraction are elucidated. For example, whole granulation tissue preparations will contract when stimulated by histamine dihydrochloride, prostaglandins, or serotonin creatinine sulfate (5-hydroxytryptamine). Wound contraction can be inhibited in

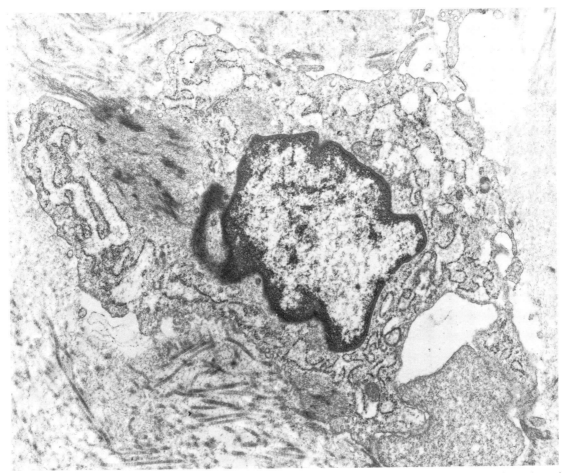

FIGURE 3–8. Typical myofibroblast. Note indented nuclear membrane, masses of contractile protein, and rough endocytoplasmic reticulum. Collagen fibrils are seen outside the cell membrane. This cell was found in the plantar fascia of a patient with chronic plantar contracture. × 24,000. (Courtesy of Dr. Edward Carlson, Department of Anatomy, College of Medicine, University of Arizona.)

living animals by topical application of a smooth muscle inhibitor, such as Trocinate (β-diethylaminoethyl diphenylthioacetate). At the moment, however, the available information can be used to advantage by plastic surgeons in the following ways.

Application of a split-thickness skin graft or skin flap on a contracting wound does not stop the contracting process. It may reduce the amount of contracture, but it certainly does not stop contraction. Thus, if wound contracture is to be avoided, a graft or flap must be placed very early, during the lag phase before contraction begins. Alternatively, the picture frame area must be excised and whatever contracture has occurred must be released before a graft or flap is applied. Otherwise, the graft and flap will become ruffled as the underlying wound bed contracts (Peacock and Van Winkle, 1970) (see Fig. 3–17, *A*).

It has been frequently stated that split-thickness skin grafts contract, whereas full-thickness grafts do not contract. However, it is the wound bed that contracts; grafts probably become reduced in size by extensive remodeling. Most split-thickness grafts are placed upon actively contracting wounds or wounds with granulation tissue, whereas full-thickness grafts are reserved for fresh surgical or traumatic wounds before secondary healing (including contraction) has commenced. Another process which is responsible for reduction in the size of split-thickness skin grafts which are not placed on contracting wounds is primary remodeling of the fibrous stroma of the transplanted dermis. This will be discussed later, but the point should now be made that the size of split-thickness skin grafts can be reduced by two entirely different mechanisms. One is contracture of the wound; this process produces a ruffled graft in a contracted area. The other process is internal remodeling of the graft itself. The latter phenomenon will produce a thin graft without pleats but will result in stretching of the surrounding skin to accommodate the smaller size of the graft. The basic processes involved in each are different, and prevention or correction of the end result also is different.

Cortisone will slightly retard wound contraction but will not prevent it completely. Small doses of cortisone have no effect on fibroblasts, and it is likely that larger doses primarily interfere with proliferation. Available data neither support nor defeat the hypothesis that the cells primarily involved in wound contracture are modified fibroblasts, as cells other than fibroblasts also respond in this manner to cortisone.

Finally, wound contraction is one of the few fundamental processes in wound healing that can be predicted. All the surgeon has to do is grasp the wound edges with forceps and pull them together. Whatever deformity is produced by such a maneuver (such as an ectropion, flexion of a joint, distortion of an eyebrow) will be identical to what will result from the biological process of wound contraction. The knowledge that skin does not regenerate but moves in a centripetal manner, as far as the redundant skin surrounding the wound will permit, makes it possible to predict the exact deformity which will be produced if contraction occurs. In areas where skin is redundant, an amazingly large defect can be closed by movement of the skin edges. In areas where there is little or no redundant skin (such as over the anterior tibia, the hand, face, or scalp of a young person), closure of the wound will either not completely occur or, even worse, will not occur without producing a deformity, because the skin is stretched in an area where function requires relative laxity.

STRUCTURE AND SYNTHESIS OF FIBROUS PROTEIN AND MATRIX

From both a functional and cosmetic standpoint, scar tissue is another *bête noire* of the reconstructive surgeon, and a large portion of his efforts are aimed at reducing the quantity and altering the quality of fibrous tissue. The major component of scar tissue is the fibrous protein, collagen. Refinements in electron microscopy and the development of biophysical and biochemical methods for studying protein structure at the molecular level have made it possible to study collagen intensively during the past two decades (Peacock, 1967a, b). As a result, we know almost as much about the molecular structure of collagen as we do about other important biological macromolecules, such as DNA. In addition, the dynamics of collagen synthesis and degradation have been measured in a number of species under varied conditions. The next several decades should be exciting if we are able to utilize this knowledge in controlling scar formation in human beings (Peacock, 1973).

The collagen molecule is one of the largest biological macromolecules. Frequently called tropocollagen and identified by being soluble in cold dilute salt solutions, it is approximately 3000 Å in length and 15 Å in width (Fig. 3–9). It consists of three coiled polypeptide chains, two of which are similar and are called alpha$_1$ chains; the other is slightly dissimilar and is called an alpha$_2$ chain. The primary structure carries an abundant sequence of amino acids in the form of a tripeptide, glycine-proline-hydroxyproline. Glycine is evenly distributed throughout the molecule, occurring as every third residue. The other amino acids, notably proline and hydroxyproline, glutamic and aspartic acids, lysine, hydroxylysine, and histidine, are not evenly distributed. Hydroxyproline and hydroxylysine are, for all practical purposes, found only in collagen and may be responsible for some of the unique physical properties which collagen fibrils impart to connective tissue.

The primary structure, as described above, is a linear polypeptide chain. The secondary structure is the basic tropocollagen molecule and consists of three chains of approximately equal length, each containing about 1000 amino acids, each of which is coiled in a left-handed helix. The chains are covalently cross-linked to form a dimer (beta form) or a trimer (gamma form). The tertiary structure is formed by twisting the three alpha chains into a right-handed "super" helix. This structure is stabilized by the formation of various cross links (hydrogen bonds, covalent bonds, and oppositely charged electrostatic groups) to form a rigid, rodlike molecule with a molecular weight of approximately 270,000. When tropocollagen is passed across the cell membrane, it has a polypeptide chain attached to the NH$_2$-terminal end that must be cleaved before intermolecular bonding occurs. Before cleavage of the terminal polypeptide, the collagen precursor is called procollagen (Schofield and Prockop, 1974). One of the functions which has been suggested for the NH$_2$-terminal peptide is that it facilitates correct association and alignment of the three chains and promotes proper formation of the triple helical structure. A critical en-

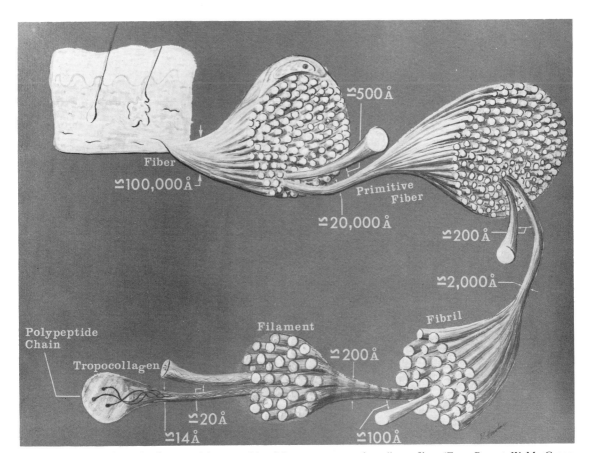

FIGURE 3–9. Schematic diagram of the assembly of the components of a collagen fiber. (From Bryant, W. M., Greenwell, J. E., and Weeks, P. M.: Alterations in collagen organization during dilatation of the cervix uteri. Surg. Gynecol. Obstet., *126*:27, 1968. Reproduced by permission of Surgery, Gynecology and Obstetrics.)

zyme in the formation of connective tissue, therefore, is procollagen peptidase, which separates the terminal peptide so that subsequent cross bonding can occur. Absence of this enzyme causes a pathologic condition known as dermatopraxia, which is characterized by extremely friable skin and other connective tissue disorders.

The quaternary structure is important in understanding the mechanism by which the physical properties of collagen are developed. It involves the aggregation of tropocollagen molecules into a stable biological unit of great mechanical strength. This is accomplished by formation of intermolecular cross links between adjacent molecules. Actually, there is a quarter-stagger overlay between molecules in such a way that a typical 640 Å repeating periodicity is seen in the ultrastructure band pattern. In addition, there is a small space between the head of one molecule and the tail of another in an adjacent chain. These spaces or holes may be important in the deposition of hydroxyapatite during the formation of bone and healing of fractures. By the formation of intermolecular cross links and the regular spacing of various subunits, a typical fibril is formed (see Fig. 3–9). The size of fibrils may be controlled by torsion on the helical molecular structure, which is necessary to bring potential cross linking sites into apposition and, to some extent, by interaction with mucopolysaccharides, which also utilize potential bonding sites.

Finally, factors as yet unidentified, control the physical weave of collagen fibrils and fibers to produce a connective tissue scar of varying proportions and physical characteristics. A diagram depicting the sequential stages of collagen arrangements is shown in Figure 3–9. As many factors enter into the final strength, elasticity, size, and shape of the scar; at present only some of them can be identified without knowing which ones are the most important in determining the physical and chemical characteristics of the collagen fiber. Nevertheless, the importance of the physical weave of the various subunits should not be underestimated. A nylon thread is relatively inelastic, yet a nylon stocking, as woven, is very elastic. Collagen fibrils in a long tendon are resistant to deforming forces, yet the same fibrils in the adventitia of the aorta easily accommodate pulsatile flow.

The synthesis of tropocollagen occurs in highly specialized cells called fibroblasts. It has been determined that fibroblasts are derived from specialized stem cells normally found along the adventitia of small blood vessels (Grillo, 1963). Apparently, each area of the body is independently endowed with fibroblasts, and when they are destroyed by radiation or other agents, the ability to synthesize collagen is removed. Some tissues, such as mature tendon, lack resident fibroblasts and are unable, therefore, to synthesize collagen. Other tissues, such as the loose areolar tissue found around long tendons, are especially well endowed with fibroblasts and are likely to produce heavy scar tissue when stimulated. The fibroblast is a stellate or spindle-shaped cell which can assume almost any shape, depending upon environmental influences. The most characteristic feature of an active fibroblast is an extensive, dilated, endoplasmic reticulum. The endoplasmic reticulum, or ergastoplasm, takes the form of long, intercommunicating cisternae which appear to be bounded by curved, double rows of polysomes attached to membranes. These structures are extremely important, as they are the sites of protein synthesis within the cell.

One critical reaction in the development of a collagen molecule is the hydroxylation of proline. There is evidence that hydroxylation occurs after a large polypeptide has been produced (Uitto and Prockop, 1974). It has been shown that molecular oxygen rather than water is the source of the oxygen atom in the hydroxyl group (Fujimoto and Tamiya, 1962). The entire hydroxylating system has been under intense study, and it has been determined that very precise cofactors, cosubstrates, and milieu conditions must exist for proline hydroxylation to occur. Cofactors such as iron, copper, alpha ketoglutarate, and ascorbic acid are needed. Essential enzymes, such as protocollagen hydroxylase and lysyl oxidase, can be assayed by measuring the utilization of some of these substances (Hutton, Tappel, and Udenfriend, 1967). Because there is urgent need for developing a method to control the synthesis of collagen selectively, a careful study of the cofactors, cosubstrates, and catalysts has been undertaken to find a way to inhibit collagen synthesis selectively without interfering with the synthesis of other important proteins, such as hemoglobin.

After the collagen molecule has been secreted through the Golgi apparatus into the extracellular milieu, rapid aggregation of molecules into young fibrils occurs. Aggregation occurs close to the cell membrane and results in formation of a collagen fibril, which becomes increasingly more insoluble as the compactness of the central molecules brings potential bonding sites together and inter- and intramolecular cross links are formed. Early in the cross-linking process, there are unfilled bonding sites which attract silver ions; thus young collagen is selectively stained by various silver stains and is frequently called reticulin.

The role of ground substance in fibril formation is not clearly understood but is probably related to the control of the size and possibly the orientation of fibrils and fibers (White, Shetlar, and Schilling, 1961). Unfortunately for the theorist, the actual sites by which glycoproteins combine with collagen molecules have been difficult to identify, and the exact manner in which these large molecules interact with collagen is not known. There seems to be a rough correlation, however, between the quantity and type of mucopolysaccharides present and some of the more important physical properties of mesenchymal tissues. Thus it seems likely that interaction between collagen and mucopolysaccharides is important in determining many of the physical characteristics which a scar imparts to healed tissue.

REMODELING OF COLLAGENOUS TISSUE

As every reconstructive surgeon knows, overhealing is a prominent feature of repair in most tissues. The callus of a healing fracture, keloids (Fig. 3–10), the hypertrophic appearance of scars (Fig. 3–11), and the unyielding adhe-

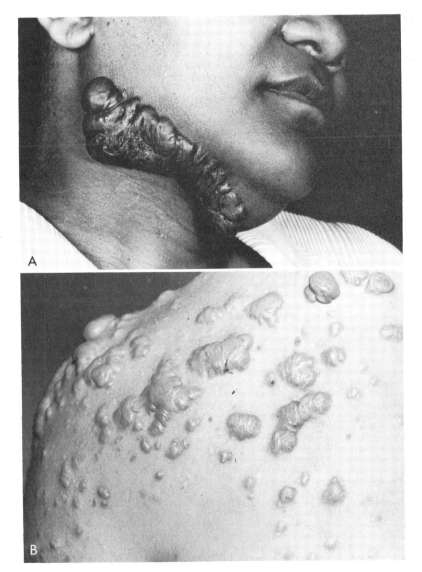

FIGURE 3–10. Overhealing of a type classified as keloid. Keloids following healing of a transverse cervical laceration (*A*) and acute acne on the shoulder (*B*). Note that the scars do not follow the outline of the original wound.

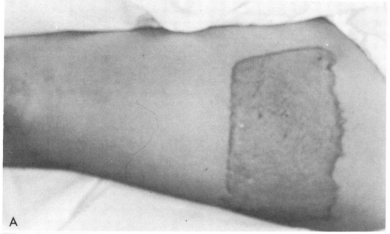

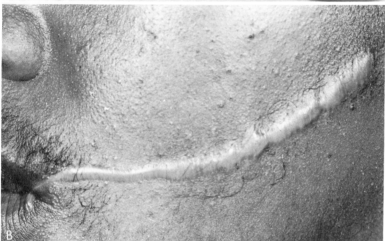

FIGURE 3–11. Overhealing of a type classified as hypertrophic scar. Note that the scar in the healed split-thickness skin donor site (*A*) and laceration of the cheek (*B*) follow the same general outline of the original wound.

FIGURE 3–12. Remodeling of scars. Both wounds are one year old. The difference in appearance is primarily due to the remodeling process. No evidence of hypertrophic scar was present three weeks after injury. The hypertrophic scar in the pectoral wound developed over a nine-month period, while normal scar development occurred in the tracheostomy incision.

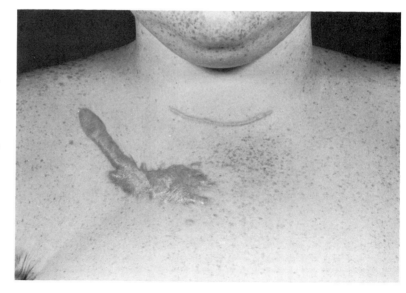

sions surrounding a repaired flexor tendon are but a few examples of excess scar formation. In addition, properties are imparted which are unwanted from the standpoint of recovering normal function and appearance (Figs. 3–12 and 3–13). It has also been appreciated that, in most people, there are natural mechanisms to reduce the effects of overhealing and, in some instances, produce a smaller scar or a scar with different physical characteristics than was originally synthesized. Such observations have meant, of course, that collagenolytic activity must be present in repaired tissue, even though actual identification and measurement of an enzyme capable of depolymerizing collagen are only recent events (Grillo and Gross, 1964). Identification of tissue collagenase (an enzyme attached to cells and not stored in tissue but manufactured for a specific purpose at a specific time) has made it possible to look at the healing wound as a balanced or unbalanced metabolic equation between collagen synthesis and collagen degradation. Tissue collagenase has been found in large amounts in human dermal scar tissue for as long as 30 years after a wound. It has also been found in hepatic cirrhosis and in the involuting gravid uterus. Actually, wherever connective tissue is undergoing involution, collagenolytic enzyme has been measured (Riley and Peacock, 1967).

Early investigations suggested that collagenolytic enzyme was produced almost entirely by epithelial cells (Grillo and Gross, 1964), but demonstrations of high collagenolytic enzyme activity in synovial and other mesenchymal tissue, which is devoid of epithelium, strongly suggest that connective tissue cells are also able to elaborate collagenolytic enzyme (Grillo and Gross, 1967). Unlike bacterial collagenase, which literally explodes the molecule, tissue collagenase neatly cleaves all three chains in the tropocollagen molecule at a point approximately two-fifths of the way along the main polypeptide chains. Ostensibly, the cleavage renders the molecule soluble, so that it can be carried away by the plasma circulation. Collagenolytic activity in tissue, hydroxyproline in polypeptides in circulating blood, and hydroxyproline excretion in the urine can be measured. The hypothesis that all three are the result of tissue collagen degradation with transport of the breakdown products to the kidneys where they are excreted is probably correct. There is, however, no positive evidence that the tissue, serum, and urine measurements are related to each other in this manner.

The relative timing of collagen synthesis and changes in the physical properties of a healing cutaneous wound are illustrated in Figure 3–14. Consideration of the scar in a clinically healed wound as a deposit of connective tissue, in or out of balance in terms of the ratio of collagen synthesis and deposition to collagenolytic activity, provides a theoretical explanation for many phenomena previously observed in cutaneous scars. The hypothesis also provides several avenues of approach to the control of scar formation.

As an example, one might consider three scars as variations in the equilibrium between collagen synthesis and degradation. These scars are a keloid, a relatively obscure cutan-

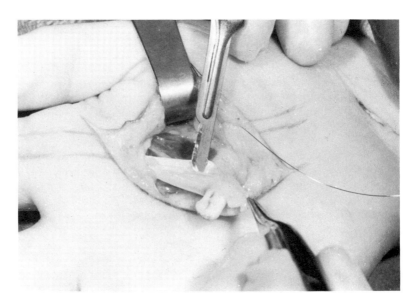

FIGURE 3–13. Scar tissue in the palm proximal to a finger injury. The newly synthesized collagen has remodeled around the distal end of a cut tendon to resemble normal tendon. This observation led pioneer hand surgeons to write and talk about "unsatisfied ends" and a tendon "sprouting filaments" which would attach to unmovable structures.

Comparison of Rate of New Collagen Deposition and Tensile Strength of Rat Skin Wounds

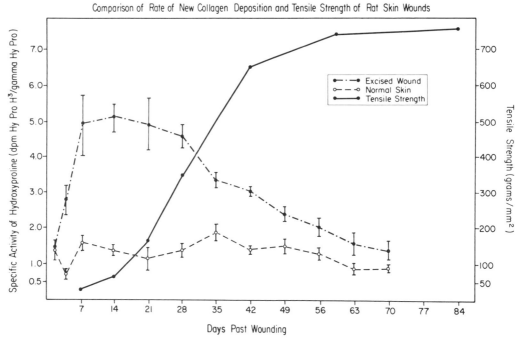

FIGURE 3–14. The relation of the rate of collagen synthesis to the gain of tensile strength of rat skin wounds. (From Madden, J. W., and Peacock, E. E., Jr.: Studies on the biology of collagen during wound healing. I. Rate of collagen synthesis and deposition in cutaneous wounds of the rat. Surgery, *64*:288, 1968. Tensile strength curve taken from Levenson, S. M., et al.: The healing of rat skin wounds. Ann. Surg. *161*:293, 1965.)

eous scar in a 42 day old wound, and a deteriorating scar in an ascorbic acid–deficient patient. While the scar in a normal 42 day old human cutaneous wound does not show any further increase or decrease in total collagen content, collagen synthesis, collagen deposition, and collagenolytic activity are greater than measured in unwounded skin. One must assume, therefore, that the rate of collagen synthesis and deposition and the rate of collagenolytic activity are in perfect equilibrium. If, through some genetic or other presently undefined factor collagenolytic activity becomes less than the rate of collagen synthesis and deposition, the scar would accrue more and more collagen until it developed the typical appearance of a keloid.

In keeping with the usual appearance of a keloid, the tendency would not appear for three to four weeks and would continue until mechanical or biological factors, such as blood supply, brought the synthetic and lytic factors into equilibrium. If collagen synthesis were partially or completely depressed by removing a cofactor, such as ascorbic acid, collagenolytic activity would exceed collagen synthesis, and a previously healed wound would grow weaker until the normal stress caused by skin elasticity and muscular activity produced dehiscence.

This is precisely what happens in scorbutic animals and people whose wounds had healed before the onset of scurvy. It is known that ascorbic acid is not needed to maintain the physical integrity of collagen under all circumstances. However, collagenous tissue in a state of dynamic equilibrium would obviously be altered dramatically by removing a cofactor needed for collagen synthesis. Between the extremes of dehiscence and keloid formation, other abnormalities could exist which would be explicable on the basis of unequal rates of collagen synthesis and destruction. Additional study of the factors which influence the rate of collagen synthesis and deposition and the rate of collagen destruction could be rewarding in understanding and controlling the deposition of scar following repair of a surface or deep injury.

FACTORS AFFECTING COLLAGEN METABOLISM

Several factors which influence collagen metabolism are under intensive study. The effect of cortisone on wound healing is probably more complex than present knowledge can explain. Cortisone inhibits but does not prevent synthesis of fibrous protein. In addition, there is some evidence that cortisone increases collagenolytic activity. The result is a delay in the gain of wound tensile strength without a complete interruption of scar formation. While other anabolic and catabolic hormones produce a mathematically significant effect in animals, the doses which have been utilized so far are much greater than those commonly used in the clinical practice of medicine.

Similarly, protein depletion, anemia, and the presence of a malignant neoplasm have a measurable effect on the gain of tensile strength in healing wounds in some species. In the case of protein depletion, however, deficiency of a single amino acid, methionine, appears more important than general protein depletion (Dunphy and Udupa, 1955); the effect of anemia, uremia, and other metabolic disturbances is not significant unless extremely harsh conditions are produced.

A wound is very much like a developing fetus in that it appears to have first call on the circulating building blocks present in the host. Relatively little protein is needed to produce a scar; an animal can be rather seriously protein-depleted and wound healing is unaffected. The most dramatic effect on wound healing produced by deficiency states is seen in ascorbic acid depletion; other nutritional deficiencies produce serious retardation of wound healing only under extreme conditions. Thus, the surgeon should usually look first at local factors to explain any abnormalities in wound healing. Systemic or general conditions seldom cause a significant delay or inhibition of the reparative phenomena.

CHANGES IN THE PHYSICAL PROPERTIES OF COLLAGEN

In addition to the possibilities for controlling collagen synthesis and deposition and collagenolytic activity after collagen has been synthesized, the physical properties of collagen can be controlled by manipulating intermediary metabolism. The most striking example of a defect in intermediate metabolism of collagen is lathyrism. Another more rare condition found primarily in cattle is dermatopraxia caused by a deficiency in the enzyme procollagen peptidase.

Lathyrism, described by Hippocrates, is a disease occasionally seen in human beings during times of famine. It is more frequently seen in animals who have eaten the common ground pea or the flowering sweet pea of the genus Lathyrus. The biochemical effect on connective tissues has been the same in all animals studied; the physiologic effect varies between species. Poultry with lathyrism usually succumb by rupture of a dissecting aneurysm of the aorta; young rats develop scoliosis and older rats develop massive abdominal hernias. Human beings develop hernias, scoliosis, and ruptured tendons (particularly at their bony insertion). In all species there is a noticeable decrease in the gain of tensile strength in healing wounds.

The cause of these deformities is interference with the cross-linking process during collagen maturation (Levene and Gross, 1959). The fact that supposedly mature tissues are also affected, but to a lesser extent, is further confirmation of the fact that all connective tissues are in a dynamic metabolic state. Any factor which affects newly synthesized collagen will ultimately have an effect on the physical properties of old fibrous tissue.

The active ingredient in sweet peas has been identified; it is a simple compound called β-aminopropionitrile or BAPN. Although many lathyrogenic agents have been identified, β-aminopropionitrile remains the most powerful one at this time (Levene, 1961). It is a monoamine oxidase inhibitor and primarily acts to prevent oxidative deamination of the E-amino group of lysine. This, in turn, prevents formation of aldehydes and thus prevents subsequent covalent cross linking. Lathyrogenic collagen shows a considerable increase in alpha chains and a decrease in beta and gamma chains. This finding is the major chemical difference between lathyritic and normal collagen; the physical difference is an enormous decrease in tensile strength of the fibrils and fibers.

Another agent which produces a similar physical effect is penicillamine (β,β-dimethylcysteine). The lathyrogenic effect of penicillamine was first noted in patients being treated for Wilson's disease. Penicillamine is a copper chelator, and it was first thought that the effect on connective tissue was due to chelation of trace metals (Nimni, Deshmukh, and Gerth, 1969). Later work has shown, however, that penicillamine reacts with formed aldehyde groups to block cross linking at a later stage than β-aminopropionitrile (which blocks formation of aldehyde groups). The end effect is the same, however, as cross links are inhibited and tensile strength is decreased (Nimni, Deshmukh, and Gerth, 1969).

Some recent evidence indicates that penicillamine also has a depolymerizing or uncoupling effect on previously formed cross links. If so, this is another distinct difference between the effect of penicillamine and that of β-aminopropionitrile. In contrast, β-aminopropionitrile acts solely on newly synthesized collagen by preventing the formation of aldehydes and subsequent cross links. It does not have any effect upon previously formed cross links.

In many respects, lathyrism is the only true collagen disease. Most of the conditions classified as collagen diseases are really the end result of poorly understood disease processes which have healed by the formation of copious amounts of collagenous tissue. In every such condition studied, the collagenous tissue is indistinguishable from normal collagen by ultrastructure, X-ray defraction, and amino acid analysis. Consequently, collagen should be considered as the ash or scar in these conditions rather than as a component of the fundamental disease process.

Penicillamine and β-aminopropionitrile have been investigated as agents which might control the physical properties of scar tissue in humans (Peacock and Madden, 1969). Both agents have been shown to interfere with cross linking in newly synthesized scar tissue; controlled studies have not been performed to measure the physiologic or biological benefits. Side reactions to these agents have not been completely investigated; such studies are underway and the next few years should make it possible to measure accurately the effect of induced, controlled lathyrism and to evaluate different agents and regimens which interfere with intermediate collagen metabolism without endangering general health.

In animals, the effect of controlled, induced lathyrism on the physical properties of adhesions around flexor tendons and the changes in periarticular collagen in immobilized joints strongly suggest that control of intermediate collagen metabolism may be a useful method for controlling the physical properties of human scar tissue. Although it seems doubtful at this time that β-aminopropionitrile or penicillamine will be the final drug of choice to interfere with cross linking, the principle of controlled, induced lathyrism appears to be a sound one, and a search must be made for ways to utilize

it in the safest possible manner (Peacock, 1973).

The first two attempts to produce controlled lathyrism in human beings were complicated by untoward signs and symptoms which apparently were the result of hypersensitivity or toxicity (Peacock and Madden, 1969). Recent experience with a highly purified product has eliminated the early complications of BAPN therapy; clinical trials of such therapy for urethral stenosis and joint surgery in the hand presently are going on under the supervision and control of the Food and Drug Administration. Because BAPN therapy of esophageal stenosis in dogs and joint stiffness in rats and dogs was successful, clinical trials of induced, controlled lathyrism in human patients must be conducted (Madden, Davis, Butler and Peacock, 1973).

CLINICAL APPLICATION OF BIOLOGICAL PRINCIPLES

The last few decades have witnessed the increasing influence on surgery of several basic science disciplines, such as bioengineering, biochemistry, and physiology. It seems likely that the next few decades will bring the results of recent advances in cellular and subcellular biology into the surgeon's armamentarium. Actually, present knowledge in fundamental biology is of considerable use to the biologically oriented surgeon in several ways. One important way is to provide a sound basis for much of what we do. By examining the biological basis for reconstructive surgical procedures, we can see why some have been successful while others, which were seemingly brilliant, have been disappointing. A knowledge of fundamental cellular and subcellular biology should make it possible to select procedures, choose sutures, understand reactions to injury, and anticipate disappointment much more accurately than we were able to do in the past. A few examples of the application of modern biology to problems in reconstructive surgery follow.

Skin

The biological basis for unsightly and restricting scars has been presented. A thorough understanding of the principles involved in the synthesis and deposition of collagen should make the surgeon less likely to use ionizing radiation to control the problem of hypertrophic scar formation. Knowledge that the dynamics of collagen synthesis and degradation change with time reinforces the importance of the temporal aspects of keloid and hypertrophic scar therapy. In addition, mechanical factors such as the effect of tension on collagen synthesis must be considered (see Chapter 2). An understanding of the lag period and the control of wound contraction provide an understanding of why the periphery of a wound is so important in the eventual appearance of a scar. In the surgical treatment of a keloid, partial excision, leaving a rim of scar tissue, provides a circumferential splint so that normal tissue tension or abnormal tissue movement will not add to the production of additional collagenous tissue. Conversely, if contraction of an open wound is to be stopped, the periphery of the wound must be excised or the process will continue, even if a skin graft or flap has been applied.

The selection and placement of sutures can be based on a sound biological principle by taking into consideration the relatively rapid and prolonged synthesis and deposition of collagen in scar tissue as compared to that in normal skin. When one adds to this the factor of accelerated collagenolytic activity during active remodeling of a scar, it is obvious why permanent subcuticular sutures in a fibrous protein structure such as dermis are necessary if widening of the scar is to be kept to a minimum. Absorbable sutures cannot maintain the physical integrity of the healing area for the period of time required for active remodeling. Although the clinical value of nonabsorbable subcuticular sutures has been questioned, the author prefers the use of nonabsorbable sutures in a predominantly fibrous protein structure (dermis) to maintain mechanical stability during the months required for collagen synthesis and collagenolysis to come into equilibrium before a stable scar is formed (Figs. 3–15 and 3–16).

The present knowledge concerning skin biology does not include a mechanism by which contraction of a skin graft might occur as a dynamic process. Modern studies of the contraction phenomenon have focused attention on the wound bed rather than on the graft and have made it possible to understand why previous misinterpretations of what actually occurred in a grafted wound undergoing contraction were so frequent. Realization that the contracting process is located in the periphery of the wound makes it possible to diagnose accurately whether a contracture is the result of a graft or flap having been placed upon an actively contracting wound (secondary contraction) or whether remodeling of the graft in response to other stimuli resulted in a contracture (primary contraction). Secondary treatment will be entirely different, of course, depending upon which basic process is involved (Fig. 3–17) (Madden, Morton, and Peacock, 1974).

The selection of a skin graft of proper thickness and the management of the donor site can also be placed on a sounder biological basis than was possible several decades ago. The basic biological premise is that skin is a complex organ which does not regenerate and that, when one transplants a skin graft, it is possible to determine precisely what the effect will be in both the recipient wound and the donor site. The key to such an analysis is realization that almost all the properties of skin (except those provided by keratin) are really properties of the dermis. Such important functions as regulation of temperature, secretion of glands, distribution of hair, skin elasticity, and reception of sensory stimuli all belong to the dermis. In addition, there are considerable, although less understood, inductive influences on the overlying epidermis which govern such important qualities as texture, pigmentation, and resistance to surface injury. Thus, one should think primarily in terms of how many of those qualities are needed in the recipient area, how many can be relinquished in the donor area, and what the cost will be in both sites should the transplant not survive (Fig. 3–18).

In the case of a 2-cm. diameter defect in the cheek of a youngster which has healed by contraction and epithelization with an unsightly scar and ectropion, all the major qualities of the skin are missing and all are needed for satisfactory restoration. It will be necessary, therefore, to take all the dermis from the recipient area; transplanting a split-thickness section of dermis would transfer only a portion of the desired qualities of normal skin to the recipient area. Fortunately, a full-thickness graft of this type can be removed without a major donor site problem.

In the patient with a 40 per cent burn, however, the qualities of dermis are not nearly as important, and the prime requisite is that the wound be healed by any mechanism before fatal complications occur. Rapid healing of the donor site, therefore, may mean the difference between life and death. Thus, a very thin graft is desirable. In the case of the full-thickness graft, wound conditions are optimal for vascu-

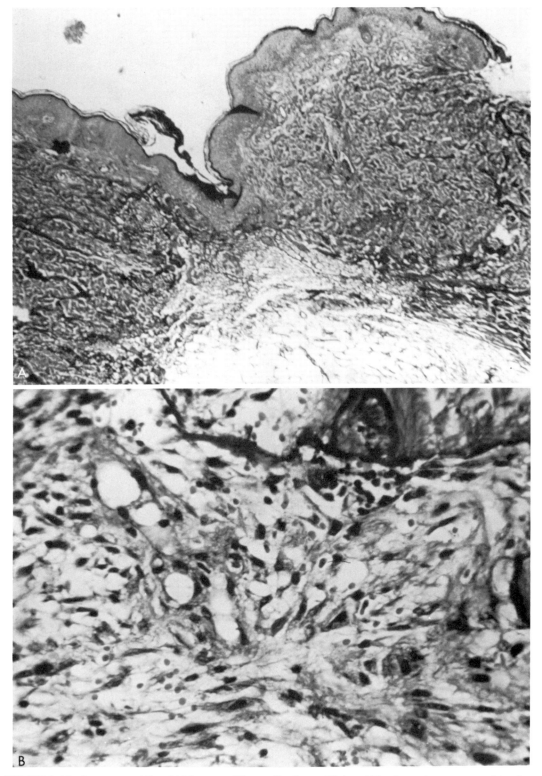

FIGURE 3–15. Low power (*A*) and high power (*B*) magnifications of 7 day old healing cutaneous wound in a human patient. Note that purposefully oriented large collagen fibers span the gap, and only a fine reticulum of newly synthesized collagen can be identified.

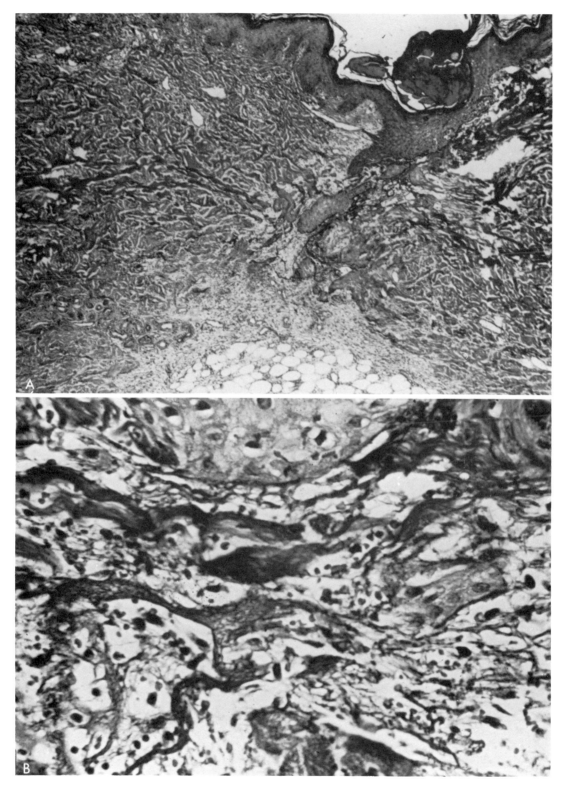

FIGURE 3–16. Low power (*A*) and high power (*B*) magnifications of 10 day old human cutaneous wound. Purposefully oriented fibrils are accruing additional collagen molecules and can be easily identified and correlated with a rapid gain in tensile strength.

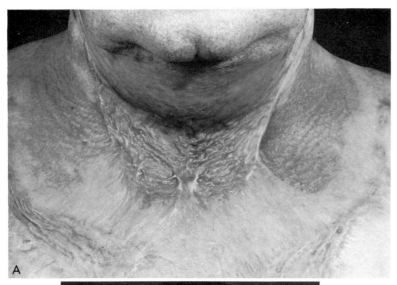

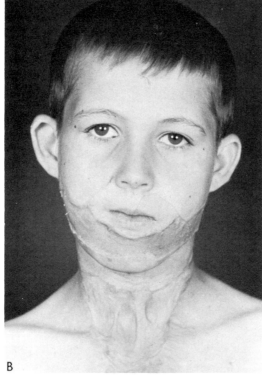

FIGURE 3–17. Two types of graft contracture resulting from entirely different biological processes. The wrinkled graft (*A*) is the result of wound contracture after the graft was transplanted. The thin, tight graft (*B*) on the chin has remodeled to a smaller dimension and has pulled cervical skin over the chin line.

larization, and the cost to the patient of failure of the graft to survive is not great as far as health is concerned. In the case of a patient with an extensive burn, recipient conditions are far from optimal, and the cost of failure of graft survival is extremely high.

Thus, from the standpoint of what is desirable in both the donor site and the recipient area and what will be the cost of failure in each

area, a split-thickness skin graft is unquestionably the best for one patient and a full-thickness graft is best for the other. Other situations may not be so clear-cut, but fundamental biological reasoning as illustrated by these two examples can be helpful in preventing mistakes, such as utilizing a full-thickness graft because of an erroneous assumption that split-thickness grafts contract or because some au-

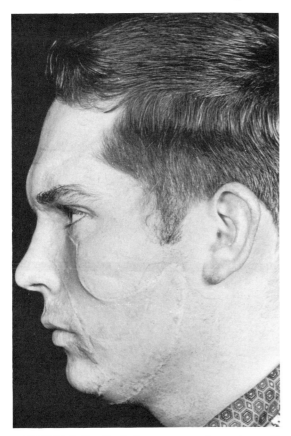

FIGURE 3-18. Typical appearance of a mature split-thickness skin graft on the face. Color, texture, thickness, and other differences are permanent, as only a portion of the skin was transplanted.

thority has recommended that a graft of a certain thickness be used in a particular area.

An area in which basic biological knowledge is badly needed involves the phenomenon of delay of a skin flap (see Chapter 6). Although there is considerable suggestive evidence that the fundamental process involved is release of various amines and kinins which cause the smooth muscle or pre- and postcapillary sphincters to utilize more effectively the normal dermal circulation, the older concept that tissues could be "taught to live with less oxygen" is one that has not yet been completely refuted (Skinner and Costen, 1968). It has seemed to this author that we have tended to put the cart a little in front of the horse by searching in an almost blind fashion for some test to determine when the circulation for a flap is ready for transfer. The possibility of finding a test for a biological phenomenon before the phenomenon has been identified or understood is doubtful.

Tendon

Fundamental biological research in the healing of long tendons has been helpful in directing further laboratory investigation and in altering the clinical approach to the repair of tendon lacerations (see Chapter 72). Highlights of this work include identification and emphasis of the "one wound" concept, which directs attention to secondary remodeling of a single scar or portion of a single scar rather than to control of synthesis and deposition of collagen in the wound. The factors which seem to be important in secondary scar remodeling are biological as well as mechanical in nature.

Mechanical factors include selection of sutures, approximation of tendon ends, and surgical manipulations involving the sheath or a substitute for the sheath. Biological factors include induction of scar tissue in the recipient area by transplanted tissue and the relatively segmental nature of tendon vascular patterns. The result has been concern about the type and amount of tissue which is moved with a graft, as well as the condition of the graft.

Such studies explain why a sheath formed by the usual wound reaction to implanted Silastic, a composite tissue graft of the entire sheath and internal flexor tendon mechanism, or biological control of inter- and intramolecular cross linking in tendon adhesions appear promising as methods of obtaining predictable tendon gliding function. Research during the immediate post World War II years was concerned primarily with refining mechanical techniques and investigating pharmacologic adjuvants. More biologically oriented investigations during recent years have shifted emphasis to the secondary remodeling of scar tissue as the fundamental process involved in developing gliding function and have opened a number of new approaches, such as utilization of the principle of controlled, induced lathyrism to influence the physical characteristics of restraining peritendinous adhesions (Fig. 3-19). The three major new approaches to tendon repair in the last decade — Silastic induction of tendon sheath, transplantation of composite tissue allografts to the flexor sheath, and biological control of the physical properties of tendon adhesions by induced lathyrism — have been based on rather fundamental studies in the biology of tendon healing.

Nerves

The basic biological processes involved in the healing of a peripheral nerve are, in many re-

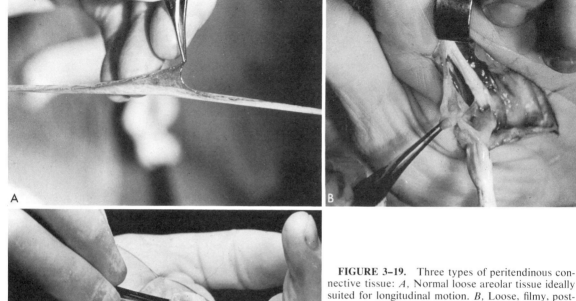

FIGURE 3–19. Three types of peritendinous connective tissue: *A*, Normal loose areolar tissue ideally suited for longitudinal motion. *B*, Loose, filmy, post-injury adhesions which have remodeled to permit excellent longitudinal motion. *C*, Dense, fibrous adhesions which have remodeled to resemble normal tendon and do not permit adequate longitudinal motion.

spects, quite the opposite from those involved in healing of a tendon. Whereas mature tendons do not contain cells capable of synthesizing collagen and are dependent upon extraneous connective tissue for development of tensile strength, peripheral nerves contain stem cells with the capability of differentiating into fibroblasts and are able to acquire all of the needed tensile strength without contributions from external tissues. In addition, great tensile strength is not required in reconstituted peripheral nerves; a reduction in the amount of scar tissue might actually enhance axoplasmic regeneration.

In the case of an injured or repaired tendon, therefore, satisfactory healing is virtually impossible following mechanical isolation. True progress in developing gliding function has resulted from concentration on secondary remodeling of scar tissue — not prevention of scar synthesis. In the case of peripheral nerves, however, although far less work has been done on the fundamental mechanism of healing, it appears that isolation of a nerve anastomosis may be highly desirable. In addition, anything

which could be done to decrease the amount of synthesized collagen is theoretically desirable from the standpoint of subsequent axoplasm regeneration (see Chapter 76).

Reduction in the number of sutures, surgical manipulation of nerve ends, and isolation of a nerve anastomosis appear to be sound principles in light of present biological information on nerve healing. The fact that a divided facial nerve left within the bony canal of the temporal bone, without any attempt to coapt the ends, regenerates much better than a laceration of the same nerve in connective tissue outside of the bony canal strongly supports the hypothesis that a reduction in fixative devices and isolation of the nerve ends are sound theoretical and practical principles of nerve repair.

Such reasoning probably does not support the microdissection of nerve ends to identify funicular patterns or the insertion of funicular sutures. It does support further search for methods of isolating a nerve anastomosis without producing constriction while axoplasm regeneration and internal healing are occurring. Working on the hypothesis that avoidance of any longitudinal tension was desirable from the standpoint of reduction of scar tissue and regeneration of axoplasm, Millesi, Meissl, and Berger (1972) performed a large number of interfascicular nerve grafts in the median and ulnar nerves of human patients (see Chapter 76). Lack of satisfactory controls and direct measurements, always the plague of human neurologic research, has prevented meaningful evaluation of results from interfascicular grafting.

Bone

Bone is one tissue in which continued search for a method to accelerate healing is clearly justified. In the case of other tissues, the time required for healing is not a serious deterrent to reconstructive surgery; the spot weld of a soft tissue wound is not a first priority problem in the minds of most investigators. In the case of bone, however, the need for a more rapid amalgamation of the various subunits following reduction of a fracture does have a high priority in the opinion of most clinicians and virtually all patients. Scanty biological data relating to the clinical problem have been of value primarily in treating delayed healing, not in accelerating normal healing. Such important discoveries as the importance of tissue oxygen tension, participation of cells in the endosteum rather than cells in the periosteum, and the effect of various types of bone grafts as inductors of bone formation have aided the clinician.

Unfortunately, however, most of the work on bone induction has been done in rabbits or other animals which have a very high propensity for bone induction in soft tissues. With the exception of a few tissues which have a high phosphatase activity (e.g., urinary bladder), human tissues cannot be induced to form bone so easily. There seems to be little doubt at the moment, however, that autogenous cancellous bone provides the best inductor of bone synthesis and is therefore the best material for bone grafts utilized primarily for the treatment of nonunion or threatened nonunion.

The precise biological effect of cancellous bone is not clear at this time. A bone induction principle has been rather crudely identified in animals, but the exact composition of such a principle has not been fully elucidated, although it does seem to be found primarily in the demineralized collagen matrix of dentin and ox bone (Urist, Dowell, Hay and Strates, 1968). Such discoveries have suggested that the E-amino groups of lysine and hydroxylysine in the collagen matrix are in some way essential to the calcification mechanism. In human bone, presumably, there is a local mechanism which either prevents utilization of these sites by a blocking agent or removes the blocking agent. Such a possibility may be closely related to phosphatase activity, and it has been suggested that phosphate rather than calcium is the key ion in a nucleation mechanism in bone (Glimcher, François, and Krane, 1965).

Many investigators still support the older concept, however, that calcium is the controlling ion in nucleation. It is interesting that calcification can proceed normally in collagens which have been deaminated, but the presence of carboxyl groups appears absolutely essential. Although a unifying hypothesis is not available, most workers have come to the conclusion that E-amino groups are not involved in calcification, but that blocking them with a bulky group, such as dinitrofluorobenzene, will inhibit calcification because of steric interference at the actual nucleation site. Such an explanation raises the question of whether the nucleation center resides in a monosaccharide or disaccharide attached to a hydroxylysine residue of collagen, and whether formation of a sugar phosphate at this point could readily be hindered by attaching a bulky group to the E-amino group of hydroxylysine.

At the moment, various theories of calcification suggest that a phosphate ion is transferred from a phosphate ester, possibly ATP, by a phosphokinase to a hexose in a strategic location on the collagen molecule. Alternatively, the hydroxyapatite crystal may be formed by a two-step hydrolytic reaction involving ATP-calcium complexes. This theory leaves unexplained, however, the close and specific association of hydroxyapatite with collagen fibrils. The phosphate ester and probably essential enzymes may be locally produced by osteoblasts and chondroblasts. Calcification is hindered or promoted by mucopolysaccharides, and, in fact, these substances may interact with the inorganic constitutents in different ways, according to the particular compartment being observed. Polyphosphates in tissue fluids also may inhibit calcification, and bone cells may produce phosphatases to neutralize them. It is likely that calcium binding to protein also must occur for nucleation to ensue. However, it is more likely that a particular steric configuration must exist between bound calcium and bound phosphate for a crystal lattice to form.

Subsequent crystal growth occurs in the same manner as similar crystal growth elsewhere.

When one realizes the complexities of the process just discussed, it is obvious why the search for a bone induction principle has been unrewarding so far. As mentioned in the discussion of the problem of accelerating or measuring changes in the blood supply of a "delayed" skin flap, it is not likely that a specific accelerator of such processes will be developed until basic processes have been elucidated. In the meantime, accurate reduction, stabilization, protection of blood supply (particularly in the endosteum of long bones), and the use of isogenic cancellous bone grafts to provide a stable lattice work and possibly produce bone induction are the clinical adjuvants which appear to be most soundly based on present biological knowledge.

Joints

Fundamental biological processes involved in the development of stiff joints appear to be found almost entirely within the collagen-ground substance system. The joint capsule and collateral ligaments are the structures primarily involved, and the basic process appears to be remodeling so that previously redundant tissues become shorter and do not permit movement of the articular surfaces of long bones. Recent studies suggest that changes in the elasticity of joint structures are not involved and that decrease in the length of structures is the fundamental process leading to joint immobility (Peacock, 1966). Why inactivity should increase collagenolytic activity and result in some collagen synthesis and deposition in strategic areas so that a shortened configuration is maintained has not been elucidated. The fundamental processes of increased collagen synthesis and deposition and accelerated collagenolytic activity in the joint capsule and collateral ligaments strongly suggest, however, that remodeling of the joint capsule and collateral ligaments, while they are in shortened positions, is the fundamental process leading to development of a stiff joint.

The studies described above suggest that methods of controlling intermediary collagen metabolism may be the most likely adjuvants for developing clinical control of joint stiffness. It has been shown in rats and dogs that control of the formation of inter- and intramolecular cross links by inducing controlled lathyrism can prevent development of joint stiffness following immobilization and can shorten the time required to mobilize a joint with a flexion contracture (Furlow and Peacock, 1967). It should be emphasized, however, that the time required for animals to recover from a stiff joint is so short that the results of experiments showing a mathematically significant decrease in the time required to mobilize a joint may not necessarily be transferable to human beings. The concept that intermediate collagen metabolism is involved in the development of stiff joints does suggest several methods by which joint stiffness could be controlled. However, the only experiments based on these data—induction of lathyrism—strongly suggest that a significant effect in human beings can be obtained.

Clinical transplantation of joints—particularly non–weight-bearing joints—has a sound biological basis. Actually, the initial work in this area was done 50 years ago and strongly suggests that both allografts and isografts of joints are biologically sound in human beings (Lexer, 1925). In the author's opinion, there is a sound biological basis for proceeding with more clinical experiments in human beings, but, for some reason, the development of artificial joints has preoccupied surgeons working in this area.

Again, however, the most promising biological reasoning is that the best joint substitute will not be an artificial joint as such but a spacer which induces a specific mesenchymal tissue reaction, producing a product not unlike a joint capsule. Reference, of course, is made to the recent use of Silastic implants, which are being modified at present to produce an adequate spacer between two bones and to take advantage of the rather remarkable organization of the loose and dense connective tissue induced by Silastic material. The implants do not mechanically mimic a normal joint. In effect, a reasonably stable pseudoarthrosis or nonunion is the objective of such experiments. The biological basis for producing controlled pseudoarthrosis appears sound, and the reaction which Silastic produces is consonant with the objective of producing a controlled fibrous tissue connection between two bone ends.

REFERENCES

Bullough, W. S., and Lawrence, E. B.: The control of epidermal mitotic activity in the mouse. Proc. R. Soc. Lond., *B151*:517, 1970.

Dunphy, J. E., and Udupa, K. N.: Chemical and histochemical sequences in the normal healing of wounds. New Engl. J. Med., *253*:847, 1955.

Fujimoto, D., and Tamiya, N.: Incorporation of ^{18}O from air into hydroxyproline by chick embryo. Biochem. J., *84*:333, 1962.

Furlow, L. T., Jr., and Peacock, E. E., Jr.: The effect of beta-aminopropionitrile on joint stiffness in rats. Ann. Surg., *165*:442, 1967.

Gabbiani, G., Ryan, G. B., and Majno, G.: Presence of modified fibroblasts in granulation tissue and their possible role in wound contraction. Experimentia, *27*:549, 1971.

Gillman, T., and Penn, J.: Studies on the repair of cutaneous wounds. Med. Proc., *2*(Suppl. 3):121, 1956.

Glimcher, M., François, C., and Krane, S. M.: *In* Jackson, S. F., et al. (Eds.): Studies on the Mechanism of Calcification in Structure and Function of Connective and Skeletal Tissues. London, Butterworth & Co., 1965, p. 344.

Grillo, H. C.: Origin of fibroblasts in wound healing. An autoradiographic study of inhibition of cellular proliferation by local X-irradiation. Ann. Surg., *157*:453, 1963.

Grillo, H. C., and Gross, J.: Studies in wound healing. III. Contraction in vitamin C deficiency. Proc. Soc. Exp. Biol. Med., *101*:268, 1959.

Grillo, H. C., and Gross, J.: Collagenolytic activity and epithelial-mesenchymal interaction in healing mammalian wounds. J. Cell Biol., *23*:39A, 1964.

Grillo, H. C., and Gross, J.: Collagenolytic activity during mammalian wound repair. Dev. Biol., *15*:300, 1967.

Hutton, J. J., Tappel, A. L., and Udenfriend, S.: Cofactor and substrate requirements of collagen proline hydroxylase. Arch. Biochem. Biophys., *118*:231, 1967.

Levene, C. L.: Structural requirements for lathyrogenic agents. J. Exp. Med., *114*:295, 1961.

Levene, C. L., and Gross, J.: Alterations in state of molecular aggregation of collagen induced in chick embryos by aminopropionitrile (lathyrus factor). J. Exp. Med., *110*:771, 1959.

Lexer, E.: Substitution of whole or half joints from freshly amputated extremities by free plastic operation. Surg. Gynecol. Obstet., *40*:782, 1925.

Madden, J. W., Davis, W. M., Butler, C., and Peacock, E. E., Jr.: Experimental esophageal lye burns. II. Correcting established strictures with beta-aminopropionitrile and bougienage. Ann. Surg., *178*:297, 1973.

Madden, J. W., Morton, D., and Peacock, E. E., Jr.: Contraction of experimental wounds. I. Inhibiting wound contraction by using a topical smooth muscle antagonist. Surgery, *76*:8, 1974.

Millesi, H., Meissl, G., and Berger, A.: The interfascicular nerve grafting of the median and ulnar nerves. J. Bone Joint Surg., *54*:727, 1972.

Nimni, M. E., Deshmukh, K., and Gerth, N.: Changes in collagen metabolism associated with the administration of penicillamine and various amino and thiol compounds. Biochem. Pharmacol., *18*:707, 1969.

Peacock, E. E., Jr.: Some biochemical and biophysical aspects of joint stiffness: Role of collagen synthesis as opposed to altered molecular bonding. Ann. Surg., *164*:1, 1966.

Peacock, E. E., Jr.: Dynamic aspects of collagen biology. Part I. Synthesis and assembly. J. Surg. Res., *7*:433, 1967a.

Peacock, E. E., Jr.: Dynamic aspects of collagen biology. Part II. Degradation and metabolism. J. Surg. Res., *7*:481, 1967b.

Peacock, E. E., Jr.: Thomas Orr Memorial Lecture: Biologic frontiers in the control of healing. Am. J. Surg., *126*:708, 1973.

Peacock, E. E., Jr., and Madden, J. W.: Some studies on the effects of beta-aminopropionitrile in patients with injured flexor tendons. Surgery, *66*:215, 1969.

Peacock, E. E., Jr., and Van Winkle, W.: Surgery and Biology of Repair. Philadelphia, W. B. Saunders Company, 1970.

Phillips, J. L., and Peacock, E. E., Jr.: Importance of horizontal plane cell mass integrity in wound contraction. Proc. Soc. Exp. Biol. Med., *117*:534, 1964.

Pinkus, H.: Examination of the epidermis by the strip method of removing horny layers. J. Invest. Dermatol., *16*:383, 1951.

Riley, W. B., and Peacock, E. E., Jr.: The identification, distribution, and significance of a collagenolytic enzyme in human tissues. Proc. Soc. Exp. Biol. Med., *124*:207, 1967.

Schofield, J. D., and Prockop, D. J.: Formation of interchain disulfide bonds and helical structure during biosynthesis of procollagen by embryonic tendon cells. Biochemistry, *13*:1801, 1974.

Skinner, N. S., and Costen, J. C.: Tissue metabolites and regulation of blood flow. Fed. Proc., *27*:1426, 1968.

Sullivan, G. J., and Epstein, W. S.: Mitotic activity of wounded human epidermis. J. Invest. Dermatol., *41*:39, 1963.

Uitto, J., and Prockop, D. J.: Hydroxylation of peptide-bound proline and lysine before and after chain completion of the polypeptide chains of procollagen. Arch. Biochem., *164*:210, 1974.

Urist, M. R., Dowell, T. A., Hay, P. H., and Strates, B. S.: Inductive substrates for bone formation. Clin. Orthoped., *59*:59, 1968.

Watts, G. T., Grillo, H. C., and Gross, J.: Studies in wound healing. Part II. The role of granulation tissue in contraction. Ann. Surg., *148*:153, 1958.

White, B. N., Shetlar, M. R., and Schilling, J. A.: The glycoproteins and their relationship to the healing of wounds. Ann. N. Y. Acad. Sci., *94*:297, 1961.

CHAPTER 4

CONGENITAL MALFORMATIONS: GENERAL CONSIDERATIONS

CHESTER A. SWINYARD, M.D., PH.D.

In the first edition of this book, the emphasis of this chapter was on the historical and conceptual aspects of malformations with a brief review of genetic principles and their utilization in genetic counseling.

The contributors to these volumes have discussed genetic considerations pertinent to specific subjects being considered. The objective of this chapter is to present some basic concepts concerning developmental defects, to provide a brief introduction to some genetic mechanisms, to discuss the principles of genetic counseling, and to mention some contemporary problems which concern reconstructive plastic surgeons working with severely disabled children.

Discussions of a large variety of congenital malformations of interest to the reconstructive plastic surgeon are provided in many sections of these volumes. It is neither possible nor desirable to include in this chapter extensive descriptions of the history, etiology, incidence, diagnosis, and management of all the anomalies that have special significance to the plastic surgeon.

In this review of basic concepts of congenital malformations and pertinent genetic considerations, an effort has been made to select from the literature examples that illustrate certain points of interest. The breadth of the considerations that must at least be acknowledged makes it necessary, in some instances, to limit the consideration to nothing more than a tabulation with reference to a source for further reading. It is hoped that the references will provide those interested with greater detail.

HISTORICAL CONSIDERATIONS

Congenital malformations (or congenital anomalies) are structural defects apparent at birth. These malformations have probably occurred since the dawn of human history. The antiquity of the problem is indicated by the Egyptian paintings that depict achondroplasia, prehistoric Peruvian pottery ornamented with pictures of congenital malformations of limbs, and the finding of Egyptian mummies with cleft lip. Man's interest in congenital defects has changed through the ages and may arbitrarily be divided into several overlapping periods of time:

The Period of Curiosity. This period extended from man's first awareness of these phenomena through at least the sixteenth century. This period was characterized by curiosity and speculation regarding the etiology of the defect. The curiosity and speculation usually took the form of attributing the condition to an act of theistic beings who created the defect in retribution for parental transgressions, or else these anomalies were considered to be related to meteorologic phenomena or maternal impressions. The interpretation of the anomalies varied with the cultural background of the population concerned.

The Period of Compilation and Description. During this time, biologists were concerned with morphologic description of the many varieties of anomalies and, in the latter part of the period, with compiling statistics on the frequency of malformations. This period culminated with the comprehensive eight volume work in descriptive teratology by Taruffi (1881–1895), the large monograph of Gould and Pyle (1898), and the classic work of Schwalbe in 1906.

The Period of Descriptive Morphologic Embryology. During this time, German investigators began the embryologic study of congenital malformations. Among the outstanding investigators of this period were Wilhelm His and his student, Franklin P. Mall. Mall's work resulted in his magnificent monograph (1908), in which he described the pathologic findings in 163 of the 434 human embryos in his collection. Mall described embryos with spina bifida, anencephaly, limb deformity, and cleft lip.

The Period of Experimental Embryology. Although Mall made important suggestions that reflected his interest in experimental embryology, this type of study of congenital anomalies should, perhaps, be attributed to Geoffroy Saint-Hilaire (1822), who produced spina bifida and anencephaly in chick embryos by needling the shell or varnishing the shell to cut off the oxygen supply to the developing embryo. In this area, the early, significant contributions of Thomas Hunt Morgan (1893), Jacques Loeb (1907), Charles R. Stockard (1921), and E. B. Wilson (1925) provided the background for this imaginative and fruitful type of investigation of congenital anomalies. As an outgrowth of this approach, the awareness that one could produce congenital malformations by deficiencies or excesses of vitamins, hormones, and many chemicals has resulted in numerous publications on what

might be called experimental teratogenesis. Comprehensive reviews of this subject are provided by J. G. Wilson (1959) and Warkany (1947, 1961, 1971).

In 1960, investigators interested in congenital malformation formed The Teratology Society, which holds annual meetings.

The Genetic Period. During the last half century, developments in human genetics have provided the teratologists with new tools and techniques of investigation. This period may be considered to begin with the demonstration by Muller (1927) that ionizing radiation would induce mutations in the fruit fly, Drosophila. This observation led to the use of ionizing radiation in the production of mutations and congenital anomalies in vertebrates. Impetus to the additional study of the genetic aspect of teratology was provided by Barr and Bertram, in 1949, when they demonstrated that somatic cells of the male and female could be distinguished by the presence or absence of a small tag of chromatin found in the female autosomal cell, and by the accurate counting of chromosomes by Tjio and Levan (1956). Other landmarks of this period are the transmissibility of the hereditary material (deoxyribonucleic acid) by Lederberg (1959); the definition of its biochemistry by Ochoa and his coworkers (Grunberg-Manago, Ortiz, and Ochoa, 1955, 1956); the contribution of Watson and Crick (1953), who determined the molecular configuration of deoxyribonucleic acid; and Wilkins' (1956) demonstration of its structure by x-ray diffraction studies. The tremendous impact of the contributions of these five investigators upon the entire biological world was appropriately recognized by making them Nobel laureates.

The descriptive embryologists accurately described the invaginations, evaginations, foldings, and fusion of tissues in the complex morphologic changes that are associated with development. There was, initially, a natural reaction to describe an embryologic anomaly in terms of failure of closure or a failure of fusion. However, recent advances in genetics indicate that these failures of fusion may have their basic deficit in the genetic material (deoxyribonucleic acid) and that the failure of fusion may be an expression of a single or polygenic defect coupled with environmental influences. It is thus impossible to give any general consideration to congenital malformations without, at the same time, acknowledging the recent advances in genetics.

INCIDENCE OF CONGENITAL ANOMALIES

One of the difficulties in arriving at true incidence figures for the entire gamut of congenital anomalies is related to the decision as to what comprises a congenital malformation. Spina bifida manifesta with myelomeningocele is a serious, easily visible malformation; on the other hand, a pilonidal cyst, an undescended testis, or an enlarged internal inguinal ring, which later results in an indirect hernia, may be overlooked. The small junctional nevus is a malformation that may become life-threatening years later. Internally, the duodenal stricture or the tracheoesophageal fistula may become apparent early in the neonatal period. On the contrary, a biliary tree anomaly, a ureteral duplication, a circle of Willis aneurysm, or a bicornuate uterus may not be of significance until certain physiologic or pathophysiologic events occur.

When one considers both the externally visible malformations and the internal ones, it is quite possible that every individual is born with one or more congenital malformations. It is fortunate that only a relatively small percentage are or become of clinical significance.

Consideration of the full range of malformations is important. Some writers have considered only what they term major malformations, while others have included lesser anomalies. For example, Malpas (1937) included minor auricular malformations in his study. Stevenson, Worcester, and Rice (1950) included pilonidal cyst and supernumerary nipples. Shapiro, Eddy, Fitzgibbon, and O'Brien (1958) included polydactyly in their study and noted that the incidence of this anomaly is greater in Negro than in Caucasian babies. Warkany (1971) has pointed out that 53 per cent of Shapiro's study population were Negro, and only 0.06 per cent of Stevenson's study were Negro. Thus there are racial differences in the incidence of congenital anomalies, and a predominance of a given race in an incidence study results in biased conclusions. There are also geographic differences in incidence. Coffey and Jessop (1955) recorded an incidence of 1:196 births for anencephaly in the Irish population, which is several times higher than other incidence figures (Malpas, 1937). Searle (1959) reported the incidence of anencephaly to be nine times higher among the Sikhs of Singapore than among other Indians; however, this has not been verified.

The influence of inclusion of minor anomalies in such studies is demonstrated by the data of McIntosh and coworkers (1954), who computed an incidence of 7.54 per cent but whose data included many minor malformations. Warkany (1971) estimated that 21 per cent of the malformations included in the above study were of minor clinical importance.

The incidence figures derived from birth registration records result in figures close to 1.0 per cent (Deporte and Parkhurst, 1945, 1.16%; Wallace, Baumgartner, and Rich, 1953, 0.92%). Similar studies in England resulted in higher incidence figures (McKeown and Record, 1960, 1.73%). Warkany (1971) suggested that 2 to 3 per cent of all live-born infants show one or more significant congenital anomalies (those generally requiring attention shortly after birth) and that the incidence rises to 4 to 6 per cent at the end of the first year by the discovery of malformations not noted at birth.

A concept of the magnitude of the birth defect problem can be obtained by referring to the following monumental volumes: Warkany (1971) or Bergsma (1973), a compendium which provides 641 photographs, 904 summaries of specific defects, and more than 2000 references to the pertinent literature.

There has been speculation that the incidence of congenital anomalies has been rising in recent years. Comparison of old (Malpas, 1937) with new statistics indicates this may be so. Fogh-Andersen (1942) found a slightly increasing frequency of cleft lip in Denmark during the past twenty years (see Chapter 38). A factor that may contribute to an increasing frequency is the improved surgical repair of the cleft with virtually normal chance that affected individuals may marry and, for the same reason, chances are increased that two affected individuals may marry. However, the increase may be more apparent than real because in earlier years many anomalies were not recognized or given clinical diagnoses. On the other hand, there is some evidence that natural radiation may vary significantly in certain geographic areas, and some feel that fall-out from nuclear explosions will soon be a factor (Stevenson, 1961; UN Committee report, 1958; Penrose, 1957). Certainly, the iatrogenic, thalidomide-related deformities of the limbs (Lenz and Knapp, 1962a, b) have caused physicians everywhere to take a new and careful look at the possible teratogenic effect of many drugs now in common usage.

ETIOLOGY OF CONGENITAL ANOMALIES

It has been previously emphasized that most congenital anomalies represent the interaction product of genetic constitution (nature) with environment (nurture). There are a few anomalies, such as those resulting from maternal rubella, from toxoplasmosis, and from thalidomide ingestion in the first trimester, that appear to be primarily environmental. At the other extreme, there are a few malformations, such as syndactyly, recessive-type epidermolysis bullosa, and Marfan's syndrome, that appear to be largely genetic and result from a single or polygenic mutation. These mutations may be transmitted in classic mendelian ratios as autosomal-dominant or recessive traits, or as sex-linked traits. On the other hand, the vast majorities of anomalies are seen as sporadic cases in which there is no simple mendelian pattern of inheritance. This latter group, which is by far the largest, may be due to predisposing genes which make the embryonic or fetal developing patterns unstable so that minor environmental disturbances produce developmental anomalies (Fraser, 1961).

It is important to realize that, in many conditions considered in these volumes, the problem arises as a product of genetic and environmental influences. Patients are prone to conceive of the hereditary influence in an all or none sense. It is more appropriate, however, to think of a continuum of hereditary influence ranging from conditions which are almost wholly genetically determined (progressive muscular dystrophy) to damage resulting from ionizing radiation, which is largely environmental in its origin (Fig. 4–1). This concept helps patients realize that many defects not inherited in mendelian ratio may still have a strong genetic influence.

In an effort to sort out the genetic and environmental contributions to a given congenital anomaly, the geneticist makes use of the four following methods:

1. The contingency method. Propositi (affected individuals) with the abnormality are identified without reference to affected relatives; then the frequency of the malformation is measured in various groups of relatives.

RELATIONSHIP OF ENVIRONMENT AND HEREDITY TO HUMAN DISEASE

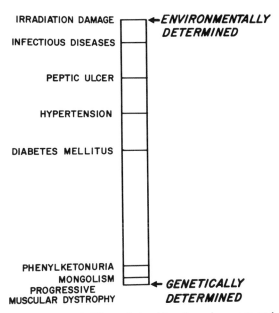

FIGURE 4–1. The relationship of environment and heredity to human disease.

Fraser (1961) has pointed out that this method is not usually successful but may result in data useful for genetic counseling.

2. The twin method. Twin pairs in which one member of the pair has the anomaly are studied without reference to whether the co-twin is affected, and concordance rates are measured. A higher concordance rate in monozygotic than in dizygotic pairs reflects the genetic factor. Most malformations show a higher concordance in monozygotic twins, but it is virtually always less than 100 per cent, which indicates nongenetic influences. For example, Metrakas, Metrakas, and Baxter (1958) found concordance of monozygotic pairs with cleft lip (with or without cleft palate) to be 40 per cent as compared with 5 per cent in dizygotic pairs.

3. The consanguinity method. The rate of blood relationship in parents of children with a given congenital anomaly has been studied. Fogh-Andersen (1942) found no increase of parental consanguinity in children with cleft lip.

4. Racial comparisons. Comparison of frequencies of given malformations in different races has been made. A significant difference would suggest a genetic factor but does not eliminate an environmental influence. Neel (1958) has made a comprehensive study of Japanese children and compared the incidence of malformation with that in Caucasian children.

There are major problems with, and deficiencies in, each of the above methods. These pitfalls have been discussed by Roberts (1959) and Fraser (1961). The techniques of determining the strength of genetic influence in the production of malformations are mentioned only to emphasize that mere observation of the occurrence of the same anomaly in two or more members of the same family does not necessarily indicate genetic transmission. The possibility of the same detrimental environmental abnormality being continuously present must be considered. Penrose (1957), for example, has observed significant geographic variation in the frequency of anencephaly. Several writers (Holmes, 1956; Stevenson, Dudgeon, and McClure, 1959; Wilson and Harris, 1961) have called attention to the high frequency of congenital malformations produced by mothers who have a malformation of the uterus. Another, little understood, environmental factor concerns fetal inanition. The presence of adequate amounts and types of protein, carbohydrate, fat, minerals, and vitamins in the mother's diet does not necessarily guarantee that these substances are digested, absorbed, and transported to the fetus in adequate amounts. Several writers (Stevenson, 1960, 1961; Edwards and associates, 1960) have pointed out that a significant percentage of the pregnancies resulting in malformed children are accompanied by hydramnios. Hydramnios also occurs in association with mongolism but appears not to be associated with anomalies attributable to a single gene (Edwards and associates, 1960).

It appears that there are few clear-cut data on the genetic mechanism involved in the large number of congenital malformations that are due neither to single gene defects nor to aberration in chromosomal number or morphology. It is also in this large group of gross malformations that the interaction of genetic and environmental contributions to the defect is most difficult to assess.

Chromosomal Abnormalities and Congenital Malformations. Although for years plant and invertebrate cytogeneticists had been studying chromosome number and morphology in relationship to the traits that they transmit, comparatively little attention was paid to human chromosomes. In 1949, Barr and Bertram, by a chance observation, made the significant discovery that female somatic cells of the cat could be distinguished from male cells by the presence of a small chromatin mass just under the nuclear membrane of the cell. This observation initiated an avalanche of human chromosomal studies (Fig. 4–2).

Barr and his colleagues soon extended this observation to man, and it is known that 30 to 60 per cent of the nuclei of female cells contain the sex chromatin (chromatin-positive). It was soon discovered (Grumbach and Barr, 1958) that two-thirds of the true hermaphrodites were chromatin-positive; that male pseudohermaphrodites were chromatin-negative; and female pseudohermaphrodites were chromatin-positive. In 1954, Polani, Hunter, and Lennox found female patients with gonadal aplasia (Turner's syndrome) to be chromatin-negative. In 1956, Plunkett and Barr reported that male patients with testicular aplasia (Klinefelter's syndrome) are chromatin-positive. The sex chromatin body is largely DNA and is thought to be a heteropyknotic portion of one of the female X chromosomes. Thus, the important

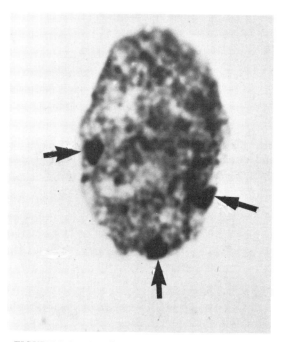

FIGURE 4–2. A cell with three Barr bodies, taken from a male patient with four X chromosomes and one Y chromosome. (From Guide to Human Chromosome Defects. Birth Defects—Original Article Ser., Vol. IV, No. 4, 1968, p. 5. Courtesy of The National Foundation and Drs. A. Redding and K. Hirschhorn.)

observation of Barr and Bertram led directly to evidence that congenital anomalies of the reproductive system of man could be related to a morphologic abnormality of chromatin material. The syndromes are discussed in detail in Chapter 100.

In 1962, Lyon hypothesized that the Barr bodies represent a condensed, randomly inactivated X chromosome. There has been extensive discussion of the hypothesis, but the available evidence supports this concept. There is a definitive relationship between the number of X chromosomes and the number of Barr bodies (sex chromatin) in a given cell. Since all X chromosomes beyond one are partially deactivated and, in stained preparations, appear as dark masses under the nuclear membrane, the number of Barr bodies in a given cell is one less than the number of X chromosomes in that cell (see Fig. 4–2). The following data will clarify this relationship:

SEX CHROMOSOMAL CONSTITUTION	NUMBER OF BARR BODIES (SEX CHROMATINS)
XY, XY	0
XX, XXY, XXYY	1
XXX, XXXY, XXXYY	2
XXXX, XXXXY	3
XXXXX	4

Thus, in a patient with ambivalent genitalia, abnormal sexual development, infertility, mental retardation, hypogonadism, and so forth, a buccal cell study of the Barr bodies (sex chromatins) is a quick and inexpensive method of detecting abnormality in the number of X chromosomes.

A second landmark in the understanding of the relationship between human cytogenetics and congenital malformation had its origin in the accidental discovery that the use of hypotonic solutions would separate the chromosomes for more accurate counting and morphologic study (Makino and Nishimura, 1952). This technique enabled Tjio and Levan (1956) to count human chromosomes correctly and establish the human karyotype of 46 chromosomes.

In 1959, Lejeune, Gautier, and Turpin described an extra autosome in patients with mongolism (47 chromosomes). Very shortly after this, it was established that congenital malformations of the male reproductive system (Klinefelter's syndrome) (Jacobs and Strong, 1959; Bergman and others, 1960) and the female reproductive system (Turner's syndrome) (Fraccaro, Kaijser, and Linsten, 1959; Ford and others, 1959) were characterized by chromosomal abnormalities. Because these two conditions present reconstructive problems of interest to the plastic surgeon, the principal clinical features and chromosomal abnormalities are summarized at the bottom of the page. Patients in either category may consult the reconstructive surgeon with reference to problems of the secondary sexual characteristics or other associated features.

There is much more to the story of congenital malformation of the reproductive system and chromosomal abnormalities. Comprehensive reviews are provided by Hirschhorn and Cooper (1961) and Harnden and Jacobs (1961).

It has been 27 years since the description of sexual dimorphism in interphase nuclei (Barr and Bertram, 1949), 20 years since the first karyotype display was made (Tjio and Levan, 1956), and 17 years since Lejeune, Gautier, and Turpin (1959) described a chromosomal anomaly in a patient with Down's syndrome. During this period thousands of manuscripts have described hundreds of varieties of chromosomal defects. There is now general agreement that about 1 per cent of all newborns have gross chromosomal defects, of which 75 per cent involve the autosomes and 25 per cent are in the sex chromosomes. There is also evidence that the incidence of chromosomal abnormality is many times higher in a population of spontaneous abortuses (Carr, 1967).

Two Significant Chromosomal Abnormalities

SYNDROME	CLINICAL FEATURES	NUCLEAR SEX	NO. AND CHROMOSONAL CONSTITUTION
Klinefelter's syndrome	Look and behave like males; gynecomastia; high voice; small prostate and testes without spermatozoa.	Chromatin-positive	$44 + XXY = 47$
Turner's syndrome	Stunted, infantilistic girls; lack secondary sex characteristics; primary amenorrhea; webbing of the neck.	$^4/_5$ Chromatin-negative; $^1/_5$ Chromatin-positive	$44 + X = 45$

110 General Principles

A large number of the chromosomal abnormalities result in physical disproportions or malformations which are of special concern to the reconstructive plastic surgeon. Specifics of a number of chromosomal abnormalities will be mentioned in those chapters detailing particular malformations. The objectives of this chapter would not be served by detailing any group of malformations related to a chromosomal defect; however, a brief review of recent techniques and concepts which have advanced knowledge in this field will be provided.

The remarkable advances which have been achieved in chromosomal analysis in recent years are due largely to two factors: first, organization of periodic conferences attended by leading international experts in chromosomal morphology for review and updating of chromosomal nomenclature. Four major conferences have been held (Denver, Puck, 1960; London, Penrose, 1963; Chicago, Bergsma, 1966; Paris, Hamerton Jacobs and Klinger, 1971). The conferences plus interpersonal

communication between experts have avoided what could have resulted in nomenclature chaos which would have retarded progress in the field. Nevertheless, a formidable new genetic language has developed, and two dictionaries of genetics have appeared (Reiger, Michaelis, and Green, 1968; King, 1972). The former dictionary is the first English edition of *Genetisches und Cytogenetisches Worterbuch,* initially printed in Germany (1954 and 1958), and in 461 pages it contains 2500 entries.

The second area of progress has resulted from the development of new techniques for studying chromosomal morphology. Techniques which enable one to be more certain about the identification of specific chromosome pairs are proliferating rapidly (Pardue and Gall, 1970; Caspersson and coworkers, 1971; Chen and Ruddle, 1971; Drets and Shaw, 1971; Dutrillaux and Lejeune, 1971). The approaches to this problem may be listed categorically as follows:

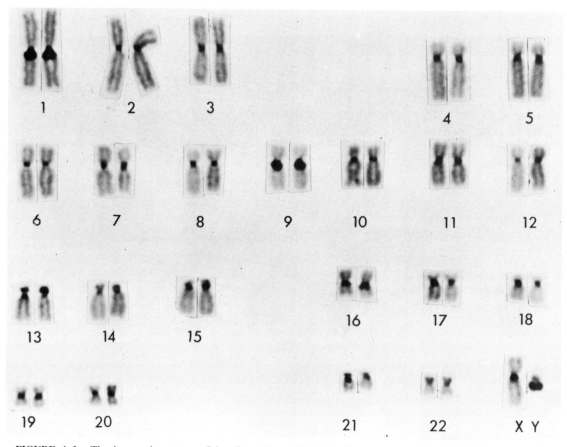

FIGURE 4–3. The human karyotype: C-banding. (From Paris Conference: Standardization in Human Genetics. Birth Defects—Original Article Ser., Vol. VIII, No. 7, 1972, pg. 5. Courtesy of The National Foundation and Dr. F. Ruddle.)

1. Conventional staining technique in which all chromosomes are quite uniformly dark.

2. Autoradiographic procedures in which tritiated thymidine is incorporated by the DNA. The beta emissions from the isotope produce a photographic record.

3. Banding techniques: with these procedures part of a chromosome is clearly identifiable from an adjacent segment by its lighter or darker color. There are a number of different banding techniques.

   (a) Staining of the C-band (constitutive heterochromatin) (Chen and Ruddle, 1971) (Fig. 4–3).

   (b) G-band obtained by use of the Giemsa stain (Drets and Shaw, 1971) (Fig. 4–4).

   (c) Q-band obtained by application of quinacrine mustard and studying the preparation with fluorescence microscopy (Caspersson and coworkers, 1971) (Fig. 4–5).

   (d) R-band: a modification of the Giemsa technique which gives the reverse picture of the G-band (reverse-staining Giemsa method) (Dutrillaux and Lejeune, 1971) (Fig. 4–6).

In addition to the above procedures, several alkali heating techniques give results similar to the quinacrine fluorochrome patterns (Sumner and coworkers, 1971). The use of proteolytic enzymes gives the chromosomes a different appearance (Finaz and de Grouchy, 1971), and finally a group of protein denaturing substances has recently been used (Lee and coworkers, 1973).

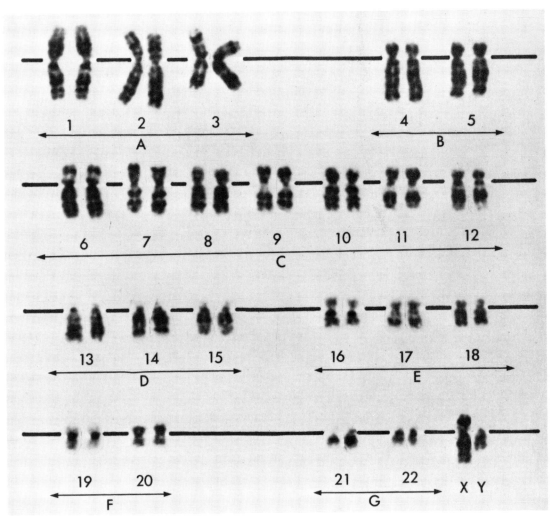

FIGURE 4–4. The human karyotype: G-banding. (From Paris Conference: Standardization in Human Genetics. Birth Defects—Original Article Ser. Vol. VIII, No. 7, 1972, p. 14. Courtesy of The National Foundation and Dr. H. J. Evans.)

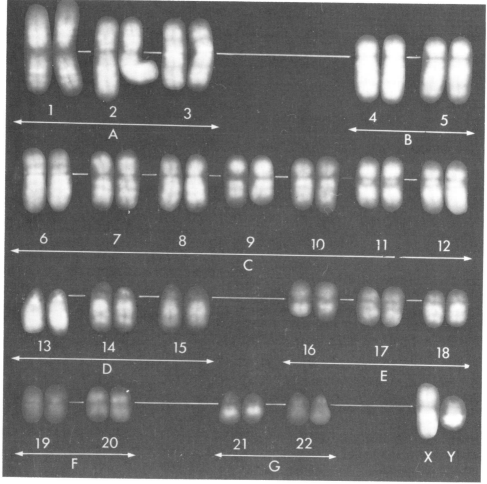

FIGURE 4–5. The human karyotype: Q-banding showing type "A" features. (From Paris Conference: Standardization in Human Genetics. Birth Defects — Original Article Ser., Vol. VIII, No. 7, 1972, pg. 6. Courtesy of The National Foundation and Dr. K. Patau.)

A diagrammatic representation of some of the banding techniques is shown in Figure 4–7. Collectively, the foregoing techniques now enable the geneticist unequivocally to identify each of the 23 pairs of human chromosomes.

An excellent guide, useful to those beginning a study of human chromosomal defects, has been prepared by Redding and Hirschhorn (1968).

Hundreds of publications have displayed, in a uniform format, both normal and numerous varieties of abnormal sets of chromosomes (karyotypes). The abnormal karyotypes show variation in either the number or morphology of one or more chromosomes. The general references provided should enable the reader to find the details concerning syndromes of par-

ticular interest; however, the following concepts, briefly presented, may be helpful.

Abnormality of either chromosome number or morphology generally occurs during the process of gametogenesis, and the end result is the production of mature sex cells with aberration in chromosome number or morphology. Errors in the process of cell division may also occur during the segmentation process as the blastula is making its three-inch, seven-day journey from the middle one-third of the uterine tube to the intrauterine implantation site. There is evidence (Hertig and coworkers, 1954) that approximately 50 per cent of the preimplantation human embryos (blastulae) are abnormal and that 32 per cent of the postimplantation embryos recovered prior to the 17th

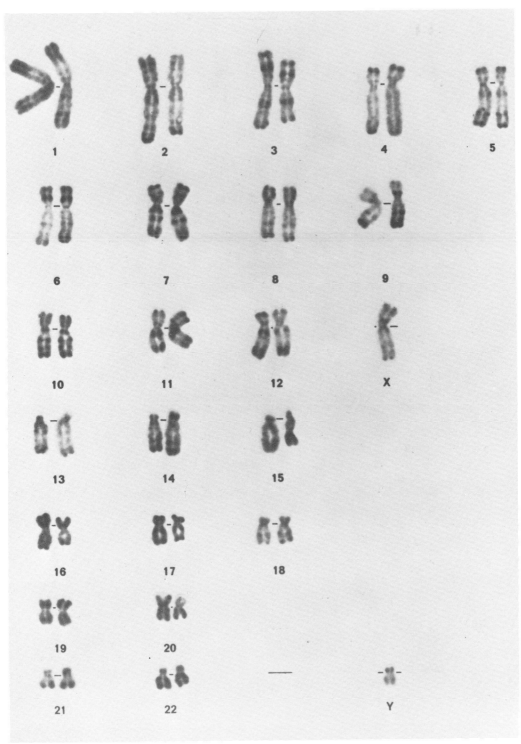

FIGURE 4–6. The human karyotype: R-banding. (From Paris Conference: Standardization in Human Genetics. Birth Defects—Original Article Ser., Vol. VIII, No. 7, 1972, p. 15. Courtesy of The National Foundation and Dr. B. Dutrillaux.)

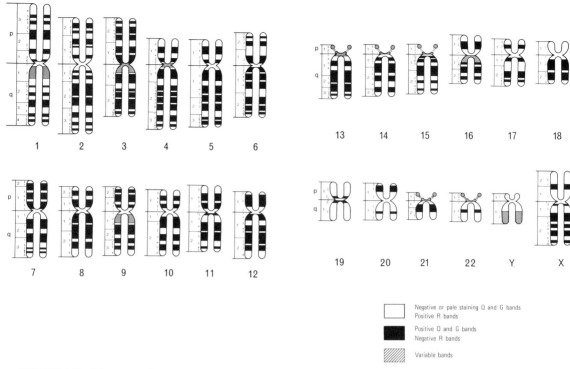

FIGURE 4–7. Diagrammatic representation of chromosome bands as observed with the Q-, G-, and R-staining methods; the centromere is representative of Q-staining method only. (From Paris Conference: Standardization in Human Genetics. Birth Defects—Original Article Ser., Vol. VIII, No. 7, 1972, pp. 18–19. Courtesy of The National Foundation.)

day of gestation are abnormal. It is not known what fraction of these large losses is related to chromosomal defects; however, Hertig and associates observed that the commonest abnormality was multinucleated blastomeres.

The fundamental objective of gametogenesis is a reduction of the quantity of hereditary material by one-half (reduction of chromosome number from 46 to 23). Since fertilization restores the chromosome number to 46, the quantity of the hereditary material in terms of normal chromosome number remains constant.

Geneticists refer to this process as reducing the diploid number of chromosomes to the haploid number (found only in the mature normal ovum and spermatozoon), and fertilization converts the haploid to the diploid chromosome number. The suffix "ploidy" is used extensively to indicate differences in the numbers of chromosomes. The term "eploidy" is used to designate the condition in which chromosome number is either the haploid number (n) or an exact multiple of the haploid number. Thus diploidy is 2n and polyploidy may be 3n or 4n, etc. Aneuploidy is characterized by somatic nuclei that do not contain an exact multiple of the haploid number of chromosomes. A tri-

somy karyotype would therefore be designated as 2n+1 and monosomy as 2n−1. These aneuploidies are sometimes referred to as hyperploidy and hypoploidy, respectively.

The foregoing errors in transfer of genetic material to daughter cells during the process of gametogenesis or early embryonic segmentation may be categorized as follows:

Chromosome deletions:	Loss of part of a chromosome.
Duplications:	An extra piece of chromosome usually resulting from an unequal crossing over during the meiotic division of gametogenesis (more common and less harmful than deletions).
Inversions:	Two breaks in a chromosome in which the free segment inverts (ABCDEFG becomes ABCFEDG). These do not generally result in phenotypic change.

Nondysjunction: Failure of two chromosomes to separate during meiosis.

Translocation: A fragment of a chromosome becomes attached to the broken end of another nonhomologous chromosome (reciprocal: two heterologous chromosomes exchange fragments).

The etiology of the above aberrations in number and/or morphology of the chromosomes is by no means completely understood; however, the following factors have been implicated in causation: late maternal age, autoimmune disease (high thyroid autoantibodies and chromosomal abnormalities), radiation, and virus infection. Chromosomal abnormalities themselves lead to abnormal segregation (transmission of translocation).

The late maternal age factor is presumed to be related to the following differences between gametogenesis in the two sexes. In the male the spermatogonia remain in their primary state throughout fetal life and until puberty. At puberty the maturation process begins (spermatogenesis) and continues throughout the male reproductive period. Primary spermatocytes are formed and proceed with reduction, division, and subsequent stages of spermatogenesis in a continuous cycle of 70 to 80 days. On the other hand, in the female, the primary oocytes are formed in the female fetus at about 60 days of gestation. These cells go into the prophase of the meiotic division and remain in this state until puberty; then one meiotic division is completed each month throughout the reproductive cycle. The second meiotic division occurs when the ovum is penetrated by the spermatozoon. Although this aging factor has been implicated in nondysjunction, there may be hormonal and other factors related to this problem.

Interest in chromosome morphology has stimulated many to expect chromosomal abnormalities in many malformations; however, Harnden (1961) prepared a table of 33 congenital abnormalities which showed normal chromosomal number and morphology. Such results do not mean there are not genetic aspects to many of these abnormalities. It may mean that the abnormalities are too small to be recognized with available cytologic techniques or that the abnormalities are at a molecular level (genic) far below the current range of the light or electron microscope.

Nature of the Hereditary Material. During the 70 odd years since Mendel's work was rediscovered, thousands of experiments with plants and animals have proved beyond doubt that the basic organic units controlling heredity are located in the chromosomes. These units are known as genes, and there are thousands of them arranged in linear fashion in a given chromosome. The location of a gene in the chromosome is known as the locus.

The brilliant work of Kornberg (1950) and Lederberg (1951, 1959) advanced the understanding of the biochemical nature of deoxyribonucleic acid, and Grunberg-Manago, Ortiz, and Ochoa (1955) were the first to synthesize RNA from precursor molecules. In 1953, Watson and Crick, aided by the x-ray diffraction studies of Wilkins (1956), proposed the double helix configuration for DNA.

The DNA molecule is 30,000 angstrom units long and only 20 angstrom units wide (1500 times as long as wide) with a molecular weight of approximately 6,000,000. This large, complex molecule may be described as a polymer, which is a giant molecule whose size is produced by linking many small units together. In this case, the units are nucleotides. There are thousands of nucleotides in the DNA molecule, and each one consists of a nitrogenous base (a purine—adenine or guanine; or a pyrimidine—cystosine or thymine), a sugar (deoxyribose), and phosphate. The nucleotides are aranged in a double strand and are tied to their neighbors by ester linkages and paired to each other by hydrogen bonds (Fig. 4–8). The two strands of the double helix separate at the point of the weak hydrogen bond. During cell division, the DNA molecule figuratively unzips itself along the series of weak hydrogen bonds, and the single chains then attract complementary bases that are circulating freely in the nucleus. It has been suggested that mutations may occur by the escape of a hydrogen atom from the parent base and the resultant joining of noncomplementary bases.

DNA appears to provide the universal coding mechanism that synthesizes amino acids in a specific arrangement to form a particular protein. The arrangement must be a coding mechanism, because the four nucleotides of the DNA molecule must identify more than 20 amino acids. It probably does this in the same way that 26 letters of the English alphabet can form thousands of combinations, each of which indicates a word. Thus, a certain group of nucleotides encodes a particular amino acid. The plan of amino acid arrangement that must be followed to synthesize a given protein is

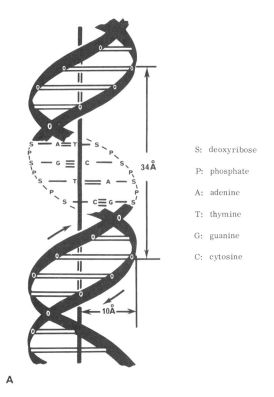

S: deoxyribose

P: phosphate

A: adenine

T: thymine

G: guanine

C: cytosine

A

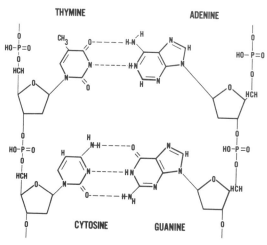

B

FIGURE 4–8. *A*, Diagrammatic representation of the Crick-Watson spiral helix model of the DNA molecule. *B*, Structural formula of the base pairing in DNA molecules. Splitting of the molecule occurs at the point of the hydrogen bonds. (From Calvert, A. F.: Chemical basis of inheritance. *In* Bartalos, M. (Ed.): Genetics in Medical Practice. Philadelphia, J. B. Lippincott, 1968, pp. 30–31.)

cies but also regulates the synthesis of the enzymes that function at the cellular level. In other words, DNA not only carries the code information for its own protein assembly line but also makes it available to the cell's offspring by replicating itself. The replication of the DNA molecule occurs during the metabolic interphase in those cells that later divide, and the DNA is equitably distributed to the daughter cells during metaphase.

DNA is confined to the nucleus, and protein synthesis goes on in cytoplasmic structures. There must, therefore, be a way for the DNA code to be transferred to the cytoplasm. Transfer is accomplished by replication of the DNA code in RNA (ribonucleic acid: same as DNA except the sugar is ribose and uracil replaces thymine). RNA is termed "messenger RNA" because it carries the code from nuclear DNA to the cytoplasmic protein-synthesizing structures (ribosomes). The ribosomes are the machinery that makes protein, but the energy for the synthesis is provided by the oxidative phosphorylation that occurs in the mitochondria of the cytoplasm.

Although the code is brought from the nuclear DNA to the cytoplasmic ribosomes by messenger RNA, there appears to be a smaller molecule of RNA known as "transfer RNA" which reacts with activated amino acids. The transfer RNA probably interprets the code of the messenger RNA. There may be a transfer RNA for each amino acid.

Structure and Function of Chromatin As It Relates to DNA. This is an area of intensive study with remarkable advances derived from sophisticated microchemical and physical-chemical techniques. Although some comment should be made, the objective of this chapter would not be served by even a brief view of this subject. A distinguished investigator in this field (Comings, 1972) has detailed recent advances in this area in 196 pages of text in which he reviewed contributions from 789 publications.

It is apparent that the DNA spiral helix is the principal gene-bearing substance of a chromatin thread; however, the threads are covered with histone and nonhistone protein. For this reason, chromatin in metaphase chromosomes contains 13 to 17 per cent DNA, 8 to 15 per cent RNA, and 68 to 79 per cent protein. Since most chromatin fibers are about 250 Å in diameter and the threads in chromosome 13 are over 30,000 μ in length, it is obvious that a number of foldings of the fiber are

recorded in DNA code. DNA, therefore, governs both enzymatic and nonenzymatic protein formation. Since almost all cellular reactions are enzymatic, DNA not only provides the code for the proteins characteristic of the spe-

required to pack it into a chromosome of given size. The number of foldings required (pack ratio) is related to the thickness of the fiber and the pitch of the coils; hence, packing ratios appear to vary considerably. Evidence strongly suggests that a single strand of chromatin fiber, surrounded by histone and nonhistone proteins, is coiled to form the width of a chromatid.

Apparently, the histone and nonhistone protein coatings of DNA in the chromatin threads are synthesized by multiple gene action, and the proteins seem to have the ability to suppress or activate some gene action. There is evidence that DNA is quite heterogeneous, and in the genome there is a surplus of DNA which appears to be genetically inactive. Although the term "junk DNA" has been applied to the surplus DNA, one must consider the possibility that, under certain circumstances, it may become genetically active and very likely has other presently unknown functions. A number of animal species appear to have a much higher haploid genome content of DNA than that which has been found in man. It has been suggested that the mutational load would be too great if all of the DNA were composed of essential genes.

Although single genes of lower forms have been seen and photographed under the electron microscope, human gene dimensions have not yet been accurately quantitated. Comings (1972) considered the amount of DNA in the haploid genome in man as 3.0 picograms and suggested that a haploid cell could contain 3 million genes, each 1000 base pairs long; however, he estimated that 200,000 genes are adequate to make and sustain one human being.

This elementary discussion of highly complex biochemical reactions and morphologic relationships indicates that much progress has been made during the last 20 years in understanding hereditary mechanisms. There is little doubt that, when further progress is made in our understanding of congenital malformations, it will be learned that in many instances the template from which enzymatic proteins are made is defective. The nature of the defective template, the way it is handed to the gametes and the gametic recombination will determine the genetic aspect of the expression of the malformation.

Essential Factors in Mendelian Ratios. Space limitations do not permit any discussion of the types of mendelian inheritance; however, these ratios are discussed in all textbooks of genetics. This subject is especially well presented for the unsophisticated by Bartalos

(1968), Emery (1968), Roberts (1973), and Thompson (1973). Advanced students should consult Harris and Hirschhorn (1974), McKusick (1971), Stern (1973), and Steinberg and Bearn (1974). The following criteria for recognizing several types of mendelian inheritance are summarized from Roberts. References must be consulted to understand the factual bases of these criteria.

CRITERIA FOR RECOGNIZING SEVERAL TYPES OF MENDELIAN RATIOS

A. Simple dominant inheritance.

1. Every affected person has an affected parent, unless dominance is incomplete or it is a mutation.
2. Affected persons married to normal persons have affected and normal offspring in equal proportions.
3. Normal children of affected parents, when married to normals, have only normal children.
4. An affected parent is assumed to be heterozygous, and inheritance from one parent only is assumed.
5. Whenever the defective gene is present, its effect is produced.
6. When two affected persons marry, the ratio of affected to normal children is 3:1.

B. Recessive inheritance.

1. The trait appears only if the individual received the defective gene from both parents (i.e., is homozygous).
2. If the trait is at all rare, the great majority of affected persons have normal parents.
3. The affected person must have received the defective gene from both parents.
4. Mating of heterozygous parents produces a ratio of three normal (one without the defective gene and two heterozygous for the defective gene) and one affected individual (homozygous for the defective gene).
5. Affected individuals who marry affected individuals have only affected children—provided the abnormality is due to the same gene defect.
6. Generally speaking, the average defects due to recessive genes are more serious than those of dominant gene defects.

C. Sex-linked inheritance.

1. There are many ordinary genes in the X chromosomes affecting many structures and functions not related to sex.
2. For practical purposes, sex-linked transmission is related to X chromosome. Evidence for Y gene inheritance is poor.
3. Since the male has only one X chromosome, the defective gene is unpaired and no question of homozygous or heterozygous state exists.
4. If the male carries the defective gene on the X chromosome, he is abnormal.
5. The female has two X chromosomes; therefore the sex-linked trait may express itself in either the single dose (heterozygous) or double dose (homozygous) situation, depending on its degree of dominance.
6. Most of the human sex-linked genes are recessive.

7. Marriage of a heterozygous female (normal) to a normal male produces: all normal females, 50 per cent of whom are heterozygous; normal males and affected males in equal proportions.
8. Marriage of an affected male to a normal female results in all normal children, but the females are heterozygous carriers. An affected male cannot transmit to a son, nor to a subsequent generation through the son, but only through the unaffected daughter.
9. Marriage of affected men and heterozygous (carrier) women produces the following ratio: 25% affected males, 25% affected females, 25% normal males, 25% unaffected females (heterozygous carriers).
10. Marriage of an affected female and a normal male results in normal females, but all are heterozygous carriers. Males are all affected.
11. Marriage of affected men and affected women produces all children affected.

The previously summarized criteria of three types of mendelian inheritance are not meaningful without an understanding of gametic formation, gene frequency in the population, mutation rates, and problems of dominant and intermediate X-borne genes.

It is essential to go beyond familiarity with transmission ratios in the several types of mendelian inheritance. The genes code specific enzymes which are essential for developing certain amino acid sequences necessary for a particular protein. If a gene base pair substitution occurs, this leads to an amino acid substitution in the gene-determined protein. If the altered protein results in a pathophysiologic effect, then the responsible gene may be detected as mutant.

In McKusick's catalogue (1975) of mendelian inheritance in man, a total of 2336 different conditions are listed, among which 1218 are transmitted as autosomal dominant traits, 947 are autosomal recessive traits, and 171 are sex-linked traits.

Very few of the congenital anomalies with which the reconstructive plastic surgeon is concerned represent clear-cut examples of simple mendelian inheritance. The complexities of the genetic modifying factors cannot be discussed here; however, several of the environmental factors that influence genetic expression have been mentioned.

PRINCIPLES OF GENETIC COUNSELING

Genetic counseling is a form of therapy for those with hereditary disease and should be an integral part of comprehensive medical care. There are three fundamental prerequisites for effective genetic counseling: an accurate diagnosis, a comprehensive family history, and an awareness of the basic principles and recent advances in genetics. The need for an accurate detailed diagnosis can be illustrated by reference to a diagnosis such as "progressive muscular dystrophy." Such a diagnosis may be inherently accurate but is inadequate for genetic counseling because there are no less than five clinical types of progressive muscular dystrophy transmitted by at least three different genetic mechanisms, with great variation in prognosis (Swinyard, 1968).

Even greater variability is found with reference to a diagnosis of hereditary deafness. Nance, Sweeney, and McLeod (1970) have made comprehensive studies of hereditary deafness and have pointed out that there are nearly 40 varieties. Alexander Graham Bell first pointed out that deaf couples may have children with normal hearing. There is a high degree of assortative mating among deaf mutes, and normal children from such parents may result when the parents are homozygous for two different mutant genes for deafness. Thus, when one counsels deaf couples, it becomes important to know specifically what type of hereditary deafness each member of a couple has (Konigsmark, 1969; Nance and coworkers, 1970).

Children born with many types of disfiguring and disabling congenital anomalies are referred to the plastic surgeon shortly after birth. The prolonged contact the surgeon has with these children and their parents elicits a firm, confidential relationship in which the parents explore with the surgeon the reasons for occurrence of the anomaly, the chances of recurrence in future children, and the possibility of the child's transmitting the defect to his own children. It is hoped that the brief and elementary discussion of genetics previously presented will indicate some of the difficulties involved in answering such questions and counseling the parents. Details of genetic counseling are readily available (Lynch and coworkers, 1970; Stevenson and Davidson, 1970; Gordon, 1971; Swinyard, 1971).

The multiple facets of disability presented by many of the congenital anomalies have, perforce, brought together trained personnel who work as a group to evaluate, plan, and provide medical treatment, and to assist the patient and his family in accepting the residual disability and in making an optimal psychologic adjustment to the circumstances. The necessity for such group effort is epitomized by the diverse personnel now considered essential to an effective cleft palate clinic or craniofacial anomaly center. The questions that parents ask are inextricably bound to the anxieties and psychologic problems, and these comprise an important aspect of the overall rehabilitation problem. For these reasons, such clinics should also include a consulting geneticist, who should counsel the parents about genetic problems and who should be available for consultation with other staff members, particularly the social service staff and the psychologists.

One of the first questions asked by parents of a child born with a congenital anomaly is, "What are the chances of having another child like this one?"; or "Would you advise us to have more children?" There is a distressing tendency for some physicians, who lack understanding or appreciation of the genetics of the problem, to take a chance with the parent with a quick response such as "not a chance in a million," or "lightning never strikes the same place twice." It is a sober fact that parents who have had one child with a congenital anomaly may be much more likely to produce a second, similarly involved child than parents who have not produced such a child. For example, unaffected parents in the general population have approximately a 0.10 to 0.15 per cent chance of having a child with a cleft lip. If unaffected parents have a child with a cleft lip, there is a 5.0 per cent chance of each subsequent child being affected. If a second child is born with cleft lip, the chances of a subsequent child being so affected rise to about 10 per cent (Fraser, 1958, 1961). Such figures imply a considerable risk and are actually socalled risk figures which are empirically determined average figures. Carefully computed risk figures have clinical usefulness, but there are many pitfalls to be avoided in their use.

Empiric Risks and Their Use. Herndon (1962) defines empiric risk as the probability of occurrence of a specified event based on prior experience and observation, rather than upon theoretical prediction. Such figures are useful in genetic research and in hereditary counseling.

Risk figures are essential in an analysis of the method of genetic transmission. The proportion of affected and nonaffected individuals in many family units is observed and tested for appropriateness to a genetic hypothesis. If the data fit, then it is possible to apply the risk figures to populations. If the risk figures fail to fit the genetic hypothesis, then one's attention should be drawn to modifying environmental factors, unknown mechanisms, or defects in sampling techniques. Risk figures are also useful in studying a disease in which the genetic mechanism of transmission is known but the observed number of affected individuals is consistently different from the expected number of affected individuals. This variation is expressed in terms of *penetrance* (the frequency with which the characteristic expression of a gene is manifest among those who possess it).

As mentioned in the discussion of the etiology and frequency of congenital malformations, data from Stevenson (1961) have shown that the largest group of malformations were those of a complex genetic and environmental etiology. It is in this group, where environmental influences may modify the genetic expression, that risk figures must be used cautiously. For example, galactosemic children lack or have an alteration in the enzyme (galactose 1-phosphate uridyl transferase) that is essential for galactose metabolism. Absence of the enzyme leads to accumulation of glucose 1-phosphate in the cells, with resultant lesions in the liver, kidney, lens, and brain. Clinical signs and symptoms are malnutrition, liver enlargement, jaundice, and mental retardation. This condition is transmitted as a single, autosomal recessive trait (Stevenson, 1961). The clinical manifestations appear at the end of the first week of life after milk feeding occurs. Elimination of milk sugar from the diet prevents the expression of the gene defect.

Another single or compound gene (three closely linked loci) in which environmental factors must, apparently, be present in order for the genetically determined factor to receive clinical expression is the Rh factor. First, the mother must be Rh-negative and the father Rh-positive. Second, a transplacental hemorrhage, large enough to cause a significant antigenic response, must occur (Clarke, 1962). Finn and coworkers (1961) have shown that a minority of pregnant women experience what might be called large (over 10 ml) transplacental fetal hemorrhages; hence, not all of the women with the appropriate genetic circumstances produce erythroblastotic infants.

The total genetic environment may also modify the expression of certain genetic and environmental influences. For example, the blood group ABO incompatibility of the Rh-negative mother and the Rh-positive fetus has a protective effect with reference to Rh interaction. Immunization to Rh usually occurs only in pregnancies in which the ABO blood group of the fetus is compatible with that of the mother. The mother is sensitized to Rh by fetal erythrocytes that leak through gaps in the placental villi. It has been suggested that ABO incompatible red cells do not survive long enough in the maternal circulation to allow maternal sensitization. Therefore, immunization to Rh factor occurs only when the fetus is ABO compatible with the mother.

This discovery that hemolytic disease of the newborn is caused by maternal isoimmunization which results from special mother-fetus combinations of inherited traits is also a good example of immunogenetics, which has very special importance to the surgeon. Immunogenetics is the basic foundation for allograft rejection and autograft acceptance. The successful transplantation of kidneys between monozygotic twins and rejection of these transplants between dizygotic twins indicates that the present practical limitations to allografting are immunogenetic rather than surgical (see Chapter 5).

Another example of the interaction of genetic and environmental factors is that of the sex-linked hereditary deficiency of glucose-6-phosphate dehydrogenase. The lack of this enzyme causes no clinical signs or symptoms unless the individual consumes fava beans or takes primaquine or sulfonamide drugs; then a dangerous, acute hemolytic anemia develops. The enzyme deficiency rests on a clear-cut genetic basis, but the disease appears only when such individuals are exposed to a special environment (fava beans or certain drugs).

These examples of the interaction of hereditary traits with environmental factors, which give clinical expression to the defect, stimulate one to speculate how many other diseases there may be that are single gene mutations but do not have a mendelian pattern of expression because the metabolic defects become clinical problems only under specific environmental circumstances. It is quite likely that many of the malformations mentioned in these volumes will ultimately be found to be the product of an interaction of environmental and genetic factors. It is the diverse environmental influences that bring uncertainty into the use of empiric risk figures.

No specific answer can or should be given to the question, "What are the chances of my having another child like this one?" If empiric risk figures are available, they should be given only as a guide. Frequently, such figures are reassuring to parents because they have in mind higher risks.

Another essential aspect of counseling is an explantation of the chance of occurrence of the genetic trait and the factors that relate to mutant production. If parents have an elementary understanding of these factors, the problems of guilt and self-incrimination will be more easily managed by the clinical psychologist.

The physician or geneticist should never attempt to tell the family what an acceptable risk for the family should be. Nor should he tell an individual to marry or not to marry, or advise prospective parents of normal intelligence, carrying a known defective gene, how to regulate their progeny. Such decisions are influenced by religious, psychologic, moral, and personal reasons. The probabilities should be presented, and the decision for marriage and/or progeny should be left to the individual.

Positive and Negative Accents in Genetic Counseling

When one discusses with parents risk figures for recurrence of a given condition or the percentage of expected affected children transmitted in mendelian ratios, one can give the advice in either a positive or negative fashion. Perhaps the simple anecdote about the optimist who states, "My glass is half full," or the pessimist who observes, "My glass is half empty," is pertinent. There are meaningful differences to parents when these two approaches are made in genetic counseling. For example, with an autosomal recessive trait when one would expect 25 per cent of the offspring to be affected, the positive approach would indicate the chance that 75 per cent of the offspring would be normal. One can turn to simple examples to emphasize the risks involved. For example, a baseball batter who is batting .250 comes to bat with a 25 per cent chance of hitting safely and a 75 per cent chance of striking out. There are many such examples which help parents achieve the concept of the problem. In general, it is our opinion that parents with sufficient intelligence to seek genetic counseling are also able to understand the information that is presented.

One might ask what evidence is available to suggest that parents act on the advice given. There are several avenues of evidence which suggest that they do: first, the large percentage of at-risk patents who have requested amniocentesis when the problem is fully explained to them; and second, the percentage who request a therapeutic abortion when prenatal diagnostic techniques indicate the mother is carrying a defective child. A second line of evidence can be derived from analysis of the behavior of parents who have received genetic counseling.

In a follow-up of 455 couples who received counseling at the Hospital for Sick Children (London) it was found (Carter and coworkers, 1971) that the parents understood the information provided and made responsible decisions based on the counseling. The risk figures given were also found to be accurate.

Amniocentesis and Genetic Counseling

It has been nearly 40 years since amniocentesis was developed as a clinical technique (in an effort to evalute prenatally the Rh syndrome). Since then increasing interest has been shown in the study and culture of the cells in amniotic fluid and quantitation of enzymes and chemical compounds in the fluid to detect genetic disorders prenatally (Lieberman, 1971; Motulsky and coworkers, 1971; Nadler and Gerbie, 1971; Nadler, 1972). Nearly 30 different enzymes have been detected in either uncultured or cultured amniotic fluid cells. At the present time, it is possible by light and electron microscopic study of uncultured and cultured cells to determine sex and more than 20 genetically transmitted metabolic disorders.

In the early investigations of this technique, it was feared that there might be an unacceptably high frequency of pregnancy complications in terms of abortion, fetal morbidity, or mortality. However, analysis of over 20,000 amniocenteses performed at 20 weeks or over indicates that the pregnancy complications occur in less than 1 per cent of the cases.

Amniocentesis has added a new dimension to genetic counseling. Obviously, prenatal genetic diagnosis will comprise a medical advance only if therapy can be provided once a diagnosis has been made. Therapy at the present time is limited to termination of the pregnancy to spare the family from the birth of a child with a serious developmental disorder. However, there have been recent attempts to treat some disorders by an injection of hormones into the intrauterine fetus. The outlook for the future use of amniocentesis is promising Many additional potentially fruitful approaches are possible which will undoubtedly increase the number of disorders which may be detected prenatally. The future holds the possi-

bility for prenatal treatment of genetic disease detected in utero.

The remarkable advances in genetics which have been briefly outlined in this chapter have created much greater public and medical profession awareness and interest in the genetic aspects of human disease. The result is a great increase in the need for genetic counselors.

The American Society of Human Genetics has recently considered the urgent need for more genetic counselors and has also discussed the training required for this specialty (Fraser, 1974). One point of discussion was related to the advantages of a counselor having an M.D. degree versus a Ph.D. degree in human genetics. Regardless of the path taken for qualification, accurate counseling is dependent upon an accurate diagnosis, a complete family history, and familiarity with the basic principles of human inheritance. Since genetic counseling usually requires repetitive sessions, which frequently reach into areas of clinical problems related to the syndrome, counseling needs in this area now unmet could be managed if reconstructive plastic surgeons prepare themselves to counsel patients and families about syndromes with which they are frequently concerned.

No one can be expected to be familiar with all of the 2336 catalogued conditions transmitted by mendelian ratios (McKusick, 1975), the many varieties of chromosomal defects, and the hundreds of recognizable malformation syndromes. However, available monographs and catalogues enable one to learn and to add to one's reservoir of knowledge. It is important that all physicians doing counseling learn the fundamentals of human genetics, recognize their limitations, and seek advice from professional geneticists and/or refer patients with complex genetic problems to those qualified to provide expert advice.

Medical Ethics, Law, and Genetic Counseling

During the last several years, there have been increasing public awareness of the universality of genetic disease and increasing requests for counseling. This intensified interest has been fostered largely by advances in genetic knowledge and refinements in the techniques of amniocentesis. These advances coupled with social changes have led to the desire, in a large segment of the public, to sponsor liberalization of abortion laws to enable mothers carrying genetically defective fetuses to obtain therapeutic abortions within the law and under ideal medical circumstances (Peter, 1971). These vital and contemporary considerations were reviewed in a conference sponsored jointly by the Institute of Society, Ethics and the Life Sciences and the John H. Fogarty International Center of the National Institutes of Health (Bergsma, 1972; Callahan, 1972) and have recently been reviewed by Hilton, Callahan, Harris, Condliffe, and Burkley (1973).

There are over 60 genetically determined conditions which can now be detected prenatally, and additions to the list are made almost monthly. This means increasing public pressure for the right to obtain therapy and increasing responsibilities for the physician and/or genetic counselor in handling the information acquired. For example, the law does not require a counselor to make known the fact that a disease is genetic in origin, nor does it require the physician to make this known to other members of the family. On the other hand, good medical practice does require that the physician give complete medical information to the patient to enable him or her to understand the rationale of available or recommended therapeutic procedures.

The debate surrounding these highly charged emotional, social, and legal issues has recently been aggravated by discussions in the medical literature (Lorber, 1971; Cook, 1972; J. M. Freeman, 1972) and lay press (Freeman, 1972) concerning the quality of life which is in store for severely defective children, such as those with Down's syndrome, myelomeningocele, and other disorders which are described in these volumes. In these discussions, the view is taken that some infants with severe developmental defects should be deprived of medical care with the thought that they would soon die. It has been suggested that patients selected for passive euthanasia should be chosen by a group composed of a pediatrician, surgeon, clergyman, and lawyer.

The author believes this philosophy is based on two important misconceptions. First, the fallacy that one can predict the time when an infant might die under a passive euthanasia program based on deprivation of medical care. We have seen many such children in institutions living almost a vegetative existence for many years after a decision was made to withhold a cerebrospinal fluid shunting procedure for congenital hydrocephalus.

The second fallacy of such a program is the assumption that a professional committee can determine for a given set of parents what an acceptable quality of life would be for them.

It is the author's personal opinion that a parent should be given the risk figures for recurrence of the condition and, if it can be detected prenatally, the mother should be informed about amniocentesis and provided the procedure if it is requested. In the event the fetus is defective, the parent should have the right to obtain legal therapeutic abortion performed under ideal medical circumstances. If, on the other hand, a defective child is born, the parent expects and should receive the best medical care available for both acute and chronic problems.

The objectives of comprehensive multidisciplinary programs, which are essential to a large proportion of the conditions discussed in these volumes, are to capitalize on the child's assets and minimize his disabilities, to enable the patient to achieve maximal independence, and to provide the required personalized educational and vocational program that would enable the patient to contribute to society and enjoy the highest quality of life possible.

Progress in the medical aspects of human welfare is not made by turning one's back on the difficult problems but rather by encouraging clinical research devoted to improved methods of caring for the patient. This approach should be coupled with basic research which will lead to detection of the etiology and ultimately to prevention of the problem.

The social, ethical, and medical concerns which confront those doing genetic counseling in these times of rapid social change and genetic advances are not wholly unique to our times. Perhaps the response given more than 70 years ago to these same problems by the distinguished Scottish obstetrician John William Ballantyne (1902) is pertinent today:

> The goal of the medical man's ambition, and the limits of his usefulness to his patient, are not reached when the diagnosis of the malady from which the latter is suffering has been made.
>
> The most exact diagnosis is unsatisfactory if unaccompanied by effective treatment.
>
> The end and aim of all medical practice is prevention; and, failing that, cure; and, failing that, amelioration.

REFERENCES

Ballantyne, J. W.: Manual of Antenatal Pathology and Hygiene. Ch. XXVI, The Fetus. Edinburgh, William Green and Sons, 1902.

Barr, M. L., and Bertram, E. G.: A morphological distinction between neurones of the male and female; the behavior of the nucleolar satellites during accelerated nucleoprotein synthesis. Nature, *163*:676, 1949.

Bergman, S., Reitalu, J., Nowakowski, H., and Lenz, W.: Chromosomes in two patients with Klinefelter's syndrome. Ann. Hum. Genet., *24*:81, 1960.

Bergsma, D. (Ed.): Chicago Conference: Standardization in Human Cytogenetics. (National Foundation – Birth Defects–Original Article Ser.) Vol. II, No. 2, 1966.

Bergsma, D. (Ed.): Advances in human genetics and their impact on society. Proc. Symposium Assoc. Advanc. Sci. (National Foundation–Birth Defects–Original Article Ser.) Vol. VIII, No. 4, 1972.

Bergsma, D. (Ed.): Birth Defects Atlas and Compendium. (National Foundation–Birth Defects–Original Article Ser.) Baltimore, Williams and Wilkins Company, 1973.

Callahan, D.: Ethics, law and genetic counseling. Science, *176*:197, 1972.

Carr, D. H.: Chromosome anomalies as a cause of spontaneous abortion. Am. J. Obstet. Gynecol., *97*:283, 1967.

Carter, C. O., Roberts, J. A. Fraser, Evans, K. A., and Buck, A. R.: Genetic clinic: A follow-up. Lancet, *1*:281, 1971.

Caspersson, T., Lomakka, G., and Zech, L.: The 24 fluorescence patterns of human metaphase chromosomes–distinguishing characters and variability. Hereditas (Lund), *67*:89, 1971.

Chen, T. R., and Ruddle, F. H.: Karyotype analysis utilizing differentially stained constitutive heterochromatin of human and murine chromosomes. Chromosoma, *34*:51, 1971.

Clarke, C. A.: Genetics for the Clinician. Springfield, Ill., Charles C Thomas, Publisher, 1962.

Coffey, V. P., and Jessop, W. J. E.: Congenital abnormalities. Irish J. Med. Sci., p. 30, 1955.

Comings, D. E.: The structure and function of chromatin. *In* Harris, H., and Hirschhorn, K. (Eds.): Advances in Human Genetics. New York, Plenum Press, 1972.

Cook, R. E.: Whose suffering? J. Pediatr., *80*:906, 1972.

Deporte, J. V., and Parkhurst, E.: Congenital malformations and birth injuries among children born in New York State, outside New York City, in 1940–1942. N. Y. State J. Med., *45*:1097, 1945.

Drets, M. E., and Shaw, M. W.: Specific banding patterns of human chromosomes. Proc. Natl. Acad. Sci. U.S.A., *68*:2073, 1971.

Dutrillaux, B., and Lejeune, J.: Sur une nouvelle technique d'analyse du caryotype humain. C. R. Acad. Sci., *272*:2638, 1971.

Edwards, J. H., Harnden, D. G., Cameron, A. H., Crosse, V. M., and Wolff, O. H.: A new trisomic syndrome. Lancet, *1*:787, 1960.

Finaz, C., and de Grouchy, J. de: Le caryotype humain après traitement par l'α-chymotrypsine. Ann. Genet. (Paris), *14*:309, 1971.

Finn, R., Clarke, C. A., Donohue, W. T. A., McConnell, R. B., Sheppard, P. M., Lehane, D., and Kulke, W.: Experimental studies on the prevention of Rh hemolytic disease. Br. Med. J., *1*:1486, 1961.

Fogh-Andersen, P.: Inheritance of Harelip and Cleft Palate. Copenhagen, Arnold Busck, 1942.

Ford, C. E., Jones, K. W., Polani, P. E., DeAlmeida, J. C., and Briggs, J. H.: A sex-chromosome anomaly in a case of gonadal dysgenesis (Turner's syndrome). Lancet, *1*:711, 1959.

Fraccaro, M., Kaijser, K., and Linsten, J.: Chromosome complement in gonadal dysgenesis (Turner's syndrome). Lancet, *1*:886, 1959.

Fraser, F. C.: Genetic counseling in some common paediatric diseases. Pediatr. Clin. North Am., *5*:475, 1958.

Fraser, F. C.: Congenital malformations. *In* Steinberg, A. G. (Ed.): Progress in Medical Genetics. Vol. 1. New York, Grune and Stratton, 1961.

Fraser, F. C.: Genetic counseling. Am. J. Hum. Genet., *26*:636, 1974.

Freeman, E.: The "God Committee." The New York Times Magazine, May 21. New York, The New York Times Company, 1972.

Freeman, J. M.: Is there a right to die – quickly? J. Pediatr., *80*:904, 1972.

Geoffroy Saint-Hilaire, E.: Philosophie Anatomique. Des monstruosités humaines. Vol. 3, Paris, 1822.

Gordon, H.: Genetic counseling: Considerations for talking to parents and prospective parents. J.A.M.A., *217*:1215, 1971.

Gould, G. M., and Pyle, W. L.: Anomalies and Curiosities of Medicine. Philadelphia, W. B. Saunders Company, 1898, p. 968.

Grumbach, M. M., and Barr, M. L.: Cytologic tests of chromosomal sex in relation to sex anomalies in man. Recent Progr. Horm. Res., *14*:255, 1958.

Grunberg-Manago, M., Ortiz, P. J., and Ochoa, S.: Enzymatic synthesis of nucleic acid-like polynucleotides. Science, *122*:907,1955.

Grunberg-Manago, M., Ortiz, P. J., and Ochoa, S.: Enzymic synthesis of polynucleotides. Biochim. Biophys. Acta, *20*:269, 1956.

Hamerton, J. L., Jacobs, P. A., and Klinger, H. P. (Eds.): Paris Conference: Standardization in Human Genetics. (National Foundation – Birth Defects – Original Article Ser.) Vol. III, No. 7, 1971.

Harnden, D. G.: Congenital abnormalities with an apparently normal chromosome complement. *In* Davidson, W. M., and Robertson Smith, D. (Eds.): Human Chromosomal Abnormalities. Springfield, Ill., Charles C Thomas, Publisher, 1961.

Harnden, D. G., and Jacobs, P. A.: Cytogenetics of abnormal sexual development in man. Br. Med. Bull., *17*:206, 1961.

Herndon, C. N.: Methodology in human genetics. *In* Burdette, W. J. (Ed.): Empiric Risks, 1962, pp. 144–155.

Hertig, A. T., Rock, J., Adams, E. C., and Mulligan, W. J.: On the preimplantation stages of 4 normal and 4 abnormal specimens ranging from the second to the fifth day of development. Contrib. Embryol. Carneg. Inst., *35*:199, 1954.

Hirschhorn, K., and Cooper, H. L.: Chromosomal aberrations in human disease. A review of the status of cytogenetics in medicine. Am. J. Med., *31*:442, 1961.

Holmes, J. A.: Congenital abnormalities of the uterus and pregnancy. Br. Med. J., *1*:1144, 1956.

Jacobs, P. A., and Strong, J. A.: A case of human intersexuality having a possible XXY sex-determining mechanism. Nature, *183*:302, 1959.

King, R. C.: A Dictionary of Genetics. 2nd Ed. New York, Oxford University Press, 1972.

Konigsmark, B. W.: Hereditary deafness in man. New Engl. J. Med., *281*:713, 774, 827, 1969.

Kornberg, A.: Reversible enzymatic synthesis of diphospyridine nucleotide and inorganic pyrophosphate. J. Biol. Chem., *182*:779, 1950.

Lederberg, J.: Genes and antibodies. Science, *129*:1649, 1959.

Lederberg, J., Lederberg, E. M., Zinder, N. D., and Lively, E. R.: Recombination analysis of bacterial heredity. Cold Spring Harbor Symposium Quant. Biol., *16*:413, 1951.

Lee, C. L. Y., Welch, J. P., and Lee, S. H. S.: Banding of human chromosomes by protein denaturation. Nature [New Biol.], *241*:142, 1973.

Lejeune, J., Gautier, M., and Turpin, R.: Etude des chromosomes somatiques de neuf enfants mongoliens. C. R. Acad. Sci., *248*:1721, 1959.

Lenz, W., and Knapp, K.: Thalidomide embryopathy. Arch. Environ. Health, *5*:100, 1962a.

Lenz, W., and Knapp, K.: Die Thalidomid-Embryopathie. Dtsch. Med. Wochenschr., *87*:1232, 1962b.

Lieberman, E. J.: Psychosocial aspects of selective abortion. *In* Bergsma, D. (Ed.): Intrauterine Diagnosis. (National Foundation–Birth Defects–Original Article Ser.) Vol. VII, No. 5, 1971.

Loeb, J.: The chemical character of the process of fertilization and its bearing upon the theory of life phenomena. Univ. Calif. Pub. Physiol. (Berkeley), *3*:61, 1907.

Lorber, J.: Results of treatment of myelomeningocele. Dev. Med. Child Neurol., *13*:279, 1971.

Lynch, H. T., Mulcahy, J. M., and Krush, A. J.: Genetic counseling and the physician. J.A.M.A., *211*:647, 1970.

Lyon, M.: Sex chromatin and gene action in the mammalian X chromosome. Am. J. Hum. Gent., *14*:135, 1962.

Makino, S., and Nishimura, I.: Water pre-treatment squash technique. Stain Technol., *27*:1, 1952.

Mall, F. P.: A study of the causes underlying the origin of human monsters. J. Morphol., *19*:1, 1908.

Malpas, P.: Incidence of human malformations and significance of changes in maternal environment in their causation. J. Obstet. Gynaecol. Br. Emp., *44*:434, 1937.

McIntosh, R., Merritt, K. K., Richards, M. R., Samuels, M. H., and Bellows, M. T.: Incidence of congenital malformations. Study of 5,964 pregnancies. Pediatrics, *14*:505, 1954.

McKeown, T., and Record, R. G.: Malformations in population observed for five years after birth. *In* Wolstenholme, G. E. W., and O'Connor, C. M. (Eds.): Ciba Foundation Symposium on Congenital Malformations. Boston, Little, Brown and Company, 1960, pp. 2–16.

Metrakas, J. D., Metrakas, K., and Baxter, H.: Clefts of the lip and palate in twins. Including a discordant pair whose monozygosity was confirmed by skin transplants. Plast. Reconstr. Surg., *22*:109, 1958.

Morgan, T. H.: Experimental studies on teleost eggs. Anat. Anz., *8*:803, 1893.

Motulsky, A. G., Frazer, G. R., and Felsenstein, J.: Public health and long term genetic implications of intrauterine diagnosis and selective abortion. *In* Bergsma, D. (Ed.): Intrauterine Diagnosis. (National Foundation — Birth Defects — Original Article Ser.) Vol. VII, No. 5, 1971.

Muller, H. J.: Artificial transmutation of the gene. Science, *66*:84, 1927.

Nadler, H. L.: Prenatal detection of genetic disorders. *In* Harris, H., and Hirschhorn, K. (Eds.): Advances in Human Genetics. New York, Plenum Press, 1972.

Nadler, H. L., and Gerbie, A.: Present status of amniocentesis in intrauterine diagnosis of genetic defects. Obstet. Gynecol., *38*:789, 1971.

Nance, W. E., Sweeney, A., and McLeod, A.: Hereditary deafness: A presentation of some recognized types. Modes of inheritance. Technic and aids in counseling. South. Med. Bull., *58*:41, 1970.

Neel, V.: A study of major congenital defects in Japanese infants. J. Hum. Genet., *10*:398, 1958.

Pardue, M. L., and Gall, J. G.: Chromosomal localization of mouse satellite DNA. Science, *168*:1356, 1970.

Penrose, L. S.: *In* World Health Organization: The effect of radiation on human heredity. WHO, Geneva, 1957a, p. 101.

Penrose, L. S.: Genetics in anencephaly. J. Ment. Def. Res., *1*:4, 1957b.

Penrose, L. S.: The London Conference on the Normal Human Karyotype (ABA Foundation Guest Symposium sponsored by the Association for the Aid of Crippled Children). Cytogenetics, *2*:264, 1963.

Peter, W. G., III: Ethical perspectives in the use of genetic knowledge. Bioscience, *21*:1133, 1971.

Plunkett, E. R., and Barr, M. L.: Testicular dysgenesis. Lancet, *2*:853, 1956.

Polani, P. E., Hunter, W. F., and Lennox, B.: Chromosomal sex in Turner's syndrome with coarctation of the aorta. Lancet, *2*:120, 1954.

Puck, T. T.: Report of the Denver Conference on Chromosomal Nomenclature. Am. J. Hum. Genet., *24*:319, 1960.

Redding, A., and Hirschhorn, K.: Guide to human chromosome defects. (National Foundation–Birth Defects–Original Article Ser.) Vol. IV, No. 4, 1968.

Reiger, R., Michaelis, A., and Green, M. M.: A glossary of Genetics and Cytogenetics. 3rd Ed. New York, Springer-Verlag, 1968.

Roberts, J. A. Fraser: An Introduction to Medical Genetics. 2nd Ed. London, Oxford University Press, 1959.

Schwalbe, E.: Die Morphologie d. Missbildungen des Menschen und der Thiere. Jena, Pt. 1, 1906; Pt. II, 1907.

Searle, A. G.: The incidence of anencephaly in a polytypic population. Ann. Hum. Genet., *23*:279, 1959.

Shapiro, R. N., Eddy, W., Fitzgibbon, J., and O'Brien, G.: Incidence of congenital anomalies discovered in the neonatal period. Am. J. Surg., *96*:396, 1958.

Stern, C.: Principles of Human Genetics. 2nd Ed. San Francisco, W. H. Freeman and Company, 1960.

Stevenson, A. C.: *In* Wolstenholme, G. E. W., and O'Connor, C. M. (Eds.): Ciba Foundation Symposium on Congenital Malformations. Boston, Little, Brown and Company, 1960.

Stevenson, A. C.: Frequency of congenital and hereditary disease. Br. Med. Bull., *17*:254, 1961.

Stevenson, A. C., Dudgeon, M. Y., and McClure, H. I.: Observations on the results of pregnancies in women resident in Belfast. Ann. Hum. Genet., *23*:395, 1959.

Stevenson, S. S., Worcester, J., and Rice, R. G.: Six hundred seventy-seven malformed infants and associated gestational characteristics. I. General considerations. Pediatrics, *6*:37, 1950.

Stockard, C. R.: Developmental rate and structural expression: Experimental study of twins, "double monsters" and single deformities, and interaction among embryonic organs during their origin and development. Am. J. Anat., *28*:115, 1921.

Sumner, A. T., Evans, H. J., and Buckland, R. A.: A new technique for distinguishing between human chromosomes. Nature [New Biol.], *232*:31, 1971.

Swinyard, C. A.: Muscular dystrophies. Hospital Med., September, 1968, pp. 57–67.

Swinyard, C. A.: Genetic counseling in rehabilitation medicine. Int. Rehab. Review, *23*:3, 1971.

Taruffi, C.: Storia della teratologia. Eight volumes. Bologna, 1881–1895.

Tjio, J. H., and Levan, A.: The chromosome number of man. Hereditas (Lund), *42*:1, 1956.

United Nations Scientific Committee Report on the Effects of Atomic Radiation. General Assembly Official Records: Thirteenth Session, Suppl. 17 (A/3838), 1958.

Wallace, H. M., Baumgartner, L., and Rich, H.: Congenital malformations and birth injuries in New York. Pediatrics, *12*:525, 1953.

Warkany, J.: Etiology of congenital malformations. Advances Pediatr., *2*:1, 1947.

Warkany, J.: Congenital malformations. New Engl. J. Med., *265*:993, 1046, 1961.

Warkany, J.: Congenital Malformations. Notes and Comments. Chicago, Year Book Medical Publishers, 1971.

Watson, J. D., and Crick, F. H. C.: The structure of DNA. Cold Springs Harbor Symposium Quant. Biol., *18*:123, 1953.

Wilkins, M. H. F.: Physical studies of the molecular structure of deoxyribose nucleic acid and nucleoprotein. Cold Spring Harbor Symposium Quant. Biol., *21*:75, 1956.

Wilson, D., and Harris, G. H.: Congenital abnormalities of the uterus and associated malformations. J. Obstet. Gynaceol. Br. Emp., *68*:844, 1961.

Wilson, E. B.: The Cell Development and Heredity. New York, Macmillan, 1925.

Wilson, J. G.: Experimental studies on congenital malformations. J. Chronic Dis., *10*:111, 1959.

SELECTED GENERAL INTEREST READING LIST

Birth Defects, Principles and Technics of Teratology, Syndrome Identification, Drugs and Malformation, Principles of Genetics and Genetic Counseling, Cytogenetics, Antenatal Diagnoses, and Ethical Issues in Genetics. The volumes listed range considerably in their detail and comprehensiveness.

Bartalos, M. (Ed.): Genetics in Medical Practice. Philadelphia, J. B. Lippincott Company, 1968, 244 pages.

Bergsma, D. (Ed.): The Third Conference on the Clinical Delineation of Birth Defects. Part 11. Orofacial Structures. 322 pages. Part 12. Skin, Hair, Nails. 357 pages. (National Foundation–Birth Defects–Original Article Ser.) Vol. 7. Baltimore, Williams and Wilkins Company, 1971.

Bergsma, D. (Ed.): Birth Defects—Atlas and Compendium. (National Foundation–Birth Defects–Original Article Ser.) Baltimore, Williams and Wilkins Company, 1973. 1006 pages.

Buckston, K. E., and Evans, H. J. (Eds.): Methods for the Analysis of Human Chromosome Aberrations. World Health Organization, 1973. 66 pages.

Carter, C. O., and Fairbank, T. J.: Genetic Disorders of the Locomotor System. New York, Oxford University Press, 1974. 230 pages.

Cavalli-Sforza, L. L., and Bodmer, W. F.: The Genetics of Human Populations. San Francisco, W. H. Freeman Company, 1971. 965 pages.

de Grouchy, J., Ebling, F. J., and Henderson, I. W. (Eds.): Human Genetics. Proceedings of the 4th International Congress of Human Genetics, Paris, 1971. Amsterdam, Excerpta Medica, 1972. 500 pages.

Emery, A. E. H.: Heredity, Disease and Man: Genetics in Medicine. Berkeley, University of California Press, 1968. 247 pages.

Emery, A. E. H. (Ed.): Antenatal Diagnosis of Genetic Disease. Baltimore, Williams and Wilkins Company, 1973. 169 pages.

Ford, E. H. R.: Human Chromosomes. New York, Academic Press, 1973. 381 pages.

Harris, H., and Hirschhorn, K.: Advances in Human Genetics. Vol. 4. New York, Plenum Publishing Corporation, 1974. 388 pages.

Hilton, B., Callahan, D., Harris, M., Condliffe, P., and Burkley, B (Eds.): Ethical Issues in Human Genetics. New York, Plenum Publishing Corporation, 1973. 445 pages.

McKusick, V. A.: Mendelian Inheritance in Man. 4th Ed. Baltimore, The Johns Hopkins University Press, 1975. 837 pages.

McKusick, V. A., and Claiborne, R. (Eds.): Medical Genetics. New York, H. P. Publishing Company, Inc., 1974. 318 pages.

Michison, J. M.: The Biology of the Cell Cycle. Cambridge, Cambridge University Press, 1971. 313 pages.

Milunsky, A.: The Prenatal Diagnosis of Hereditary Disorders. Springfield, Ill., Charles C Thomas, Publisher, 1973. 253 pages.

Motulsky, A. J., and Lenz, W. (Eds.): Birth Defects. Proceedings of the 4th International Conference, Vienna, Sept., 1973. Amsterdam, Excerpta Medica, 1974.

Nishimura, H., and Miller, J. R. (Eds.): Methods for Teratological Studies in Experimental Animals and Man. Tokyo, Igaku Shoin, Ltd., 1969. 316 pages.

Pratt, R. T. C.: The Genetics of Neurological Disorders. New York, Oxford University Press, 1967. 310 pages, 2814 references.

Roberts, J. A. Fraser: An Introduction to Medical Genetics. 6th Ed. New York, Oxford University Press, 1973. 320 pages.

Sharma, A. K., and Sharma, A.: Chromosome Technics: Theory and Practice. 2nd Ed. Baltimore, University Park Press, 1972. 575 pages.

Shepard, T. H.: Catalogue of Teratogenic Agents. Baltimore, The Johns Hopkins University Press, 1973. 211 pages.

Slater, E., and Cowie, V.: The Genetics of Mental Disorders. New York, Oxford University Press, 1971. 413 pages.

Smith, D. W.: Recognizable Patterns of Human Malformation. Philadelphia, W. B. Saunders Company, 1970. 368 pages.

Steinberg, A. G., and Bearn, A. (Eds.): Progress in Medical Genetics. Vol. X. New York, Grune and Stratton, 1974. 288 pages.

Stern, C.: Principles of Human Genetics. 3rd Ed. San Francisco, W. H. Freeman Company, 1973. 891 pages.

Stevenson, A. C., and Davidson, B. C. C.: Genetic Counseling. Philadelphia, J. B. Lippincott Company, 1970. 355 pages.

Swinyard, C. A. (Ed.): Limb Development and Deformity: Problems of Evaluation and Rehabilitation. Springfield, Ill., Charles C Thomas, Publisher, 1969. 672 pages.

Sybenga, J.: General Cytogenetics. New York, American Elsevier Publishing Company, 1972. 359 pages.

Thompson, G. S., and Thompson, M. W.: Genetics in Medicine. 2nd Ed. Philadelphia, W. B. Saunders Company, 1973. 400 pages.

Warkany, J.: Congenital Malformations: Notes and Comments. Chicago, Year Book Medical Publishers, 1971. 1309 pages.

Wilson, J. G.: Environment and Birth Defects. New York, Academic Press, 1973. 305 pages.

Wilson, J. G., and Warkany, J. (Eds.): Teratology Principles and Techniques. Chicago, The University of Chicago Press, 1965. 279 pages.

Zbinden, J.: Progress in Toxicology. Vol. I. Special Topics. New York, Springer-Verlag, 1973. 88 pages, 844 references.

CHAPTER 5

TRANSPLANTATION BIOLOGY

ALAN R. SHONS, M.D., PH.D.,
JOHN MARQUIS CONVERSE, M.D.,
AND FELIX T. RAPAPORT, M.D.

Genetics of Transplantation
Fritz H. Bach, M.D.

The replacement of diseased, injured, or worn-out parts has been a dream of man for centuries. In Greek mythology, there are accounts of transplants from animals to man. Folk tales of the Middle Ages recount the transplantation of limbs between different persons. Many of the early legends and much of the original scientific investigation in transplantation are relevant to the work of contemporary plastic surgeons.

Bert, in a thesis in 1863, recognized differing success rates in skin grafts within the same animal (autografts), between animals of the same species (allografts), and between animals of different species (xenografts). Medawar (1958), in a description of tumor experiments in mice, attributed to Jensen (1903) the concept that the allograft rejection is mediated by active immune response. Lexer (1911) reported that skin allografts were rejected in man. This observation provided the first affirmation that skin allografts differed from autografts in man.

Schöne (1912) also suggested that allografting was unsuccessful owing to a phenomenon termed "Transplantationsimmunität," i.e., transplantation immunity. Shawan (1919) described a series of skin graft experiments in man and suggested that erythrocyte blood groups were important in transplantation, since grafts between individuals of the same blood groups were accepted, whereas grafts between individuals with different blood groups were rejected. His conclusion that blood groups are important was correct; unfortunately, his period of follow-up was too short, and he failed to realize that the problem of histocompatibility testing is more complex than simple matching of red blood cell groups. Holman (1924) made several observations whose significance was largely unappreciated at the time. He recognized that the first set skin grafts between human beings sensitized the recipient and that second set grafts from the same donor precipitated a more extreme and rapid form of rejection. He also observed the specificity of sensi-

126

tization produced by grafts from a single donor.

Paralleling the observations in skin graft experiments during the early period were the studies of workers in the field of tumor research. There were two postulates to explain the failure of a tumor to grow following transplantation into another animal. Ehrlich (1906) believed that each animal provided vital substances necessary for the growth of its tissues. The tissues, when transplanted, survived only a few days owing to exhaustion of the special nutrient. An alternative theory of immunity was proposed by Bashford, Murray, and Haaland (1908) and by Russell (1912). They observed a shortened survival of second set tumor transplants and believed that an active immunity had developed as a result of the first transplant. Murphy (1914) advanced the immunity theory by identification of the small lymphoid cell as the primary cellular element involved in tumor rejection reactions in mice.

Though many of the significant observations and conclusions regarding the immunologic basis of transplantation rejection were made in the first half of the twentieth century, many doubts persisted as to the true nature of the process. Loeb, as late as 1945, stressed that individuality differentials between the donor and recipient, and *not* an immune process, were responsible for transplant rejection.

It is no accident that plastic surgeons played a definitive role in the elucidation of allograft rejection, and among them should be listed Brown, Converse, Conway, Edgerton, Gibson, McDowell, Murray, Padgett, Peer, Rogers and Stark (Murray, 1971).

The conclusions of Loeb concerning "individuality differentials" appeared to be confirmed by the demonstrations of Padgett (1932), Brown (1937), and Converse and Duchet (1947) that skin grafts transplanted between monozygotic twins survived permanently. Brown and McDowell (1942) described the clinical application of life-saving large skin allografts in massive burns and had published (1943) biopsy studies of rejecting allografts. They also suggested that the dissolution of the grafts was an "allergic reaction" or an "immune response."

During the early part of World War II one of the authors (J.M.C.) was serving in the Plastic Surgery Center directed by Sir Harold Gillies in England. One day Sir Harold came into the operating room with a tall, thin, masked gentleman, who was introduced as a zoologist from Oxford interested in the "homograft problem."

The operative procedure was explained, and the fate of skin allografts was described. This was a first meeting with Peter Medawar, who returned to Oxford with a piece of the patient's skin and separated the epidermis from the dermis with trypsin in the hope that the absence of blood vessels in the epidermis might prevent its rejection when grafted. However, when transplanted to a granulating area on another patient, the epidermis gradually melted away. This was probably Sir Peter Medawar's first clinical experiment in transplantation and may well have sparked his lifelong interest in transplantation which led to the classic studies for which he was later awarded the Nobel Prize for Medicine in 1956. In his own words: "... but for some of us, the impulsion behind our research had always been the determination that one day the transplantation of tissues and organs should become an ordinary clinical procedure."

Searching for an opportunity to study the behavior of skin allografts in man, Medawar went to Glasgow, where many burn victims from sea warfare were being treated by Gibson. Gibson and Medawar (1943) described the events which led to the rejection of allografts and the more rapid rejection of second set allografts in man. These experiments were the beginning of Medawar's subsequent experimental work (1946, 1948) which marked the beginning of the modern era of transplantation. Among the major conclusions of these studies were the following: (a) resistance to skin allografts is not innate; first set allografts have a brief latent period of acceptance; (b) allograft sensitivity, once developed, is systemic; (c) second set allografts are rejected in an accelerated fashion; and (d) allograft rejection is donor-specific.

A number of other developments quickly followed. By this time, Jerome Webster had become interested in the subject of allotransplantation and suggested to Rogers that he collect the first comprehensive bibliography on the subject, which was published in 1951. Rogers, working with Converse, also grafted skin allografts on volunteers at New York University Medical Center where Taylor and Lehrfeld (1953) began experiments on laboratory animals, leading to the first method of detection of allograft rejection by stereomicroscopic observation.

Prior to the first International Conference at the New York Academy of Sciences in 1954, with Converse and Rogers serving as co-chairmen, the pleadings with immunologists to participate were generally unsuccessful. Paradoxically, subsequent rapid progress in transplantation research triggered a renaissance in orthodox immunology, and the successive biennial conferences held between 1954 and 1966 and the monographs which were published and the papers read at the conferences attracted increasing numbers of immunologists and scientists from other disciplines. The multidisciplinary nature of the conferences was at the origin of the Transplantation Society in 1966, a unique interdisciplinary society which proved a common forum for many divergent interests.

In 1955 Murray, Merrill and Harrison performed the first successful renal allotransplantation in identical (monozygotic) twins. Peer's *Transplantation of Tissues* (1959) was the first book reviewing the rapidly growing field of transplantation.

In 1956 Converse and Rapaport defined allograft survival in man, and the transfer of transplantation hypersensitivity done in collaboration with Lawrence was a direct result of the efforts of the new team (Lawrence, Rapaport, Converse and Tillett, 1960). This work led to the definitive demonstration of allograft rejection in man by the transfer of extracts of leukocytes obtained from specifically sensitized donors; it also provided a concordance between the events of allograft rejection and other cellular hypersensitivity responses mediated by transfer factor (Lawrence, 1974). During this period the team's continued studies of skin allograft rejection also provided the first evidence of the sharing of transplantation antigens by unrelated human subjects.

The discovery of the first tissue type, MAC, by Dausset in 1958 added a new dimension to human transplantation. Classical genetic methods of analysis, already employed in histocompatibility studies in the mouse by the earlier pioneering studies of Gorer (1937), Snell and coworkers (1955), and Amos, Gorer, and Mikulska (1955), were applied to studies of tissue types in man, particularly by van Rood and his associates (1972).

Clinical application of HLA typing has produced significant improvements in the results of kidney transplantation in living-related donor situations, particularly in HLA identical siblings. However, the results with cadaver organs have not been as successful, and the worldwide surgical consensus is that HLA serology may not be as useful in cadaver transplantation as it is in living-related donor transplants.

The "Gold Rush era" of HLA serology underwent a healthy, albeit abrupt and agonizing, reappraisal at the 1970 Hague Congress of the Transplantation Society. Largely through the efforts of Terasaki (1968), it was noted that, even under immunosuppression, HLA serology was not the final answer in clinical organ transplantation. That this should indeed be so was not surprising to those familiar with the earlier studies of Billingham, Brent, Medawar, and Sparrow (1954), Snell and coworkers (1955), and many others who had provided concrete evidence that, once the *major* histocompatibility barriers between donor and recipient were removed, the cumulative effects of minor and possibly as yet undetected histoincompatibilities could have just as harmful an influence upon allograft survival as a major incompatibility.

At first glance one might wonder whether each of the countless genetic differences between two individuals has a part to play in the systemic rejection of all grafts from one person to another, a phenomenon which occurs in all instances except in monozygotic twins. Although many differences do intervene, they appear to be limited in scope. The vast majority of these differences appear to be neutral or to have barely perceptible effects. Some differences, however, which may be governed by a limited number of genetic loci, have a very important role. They are components of the so-called histocompatibility systems.

It is generally agreed that the long-term success of human allotransplantation will depend upon providing each potential recipient with a preselected, optimally histocompatible donor. For this reason it has become essential to acquire additional knowledge of the antigens composing the various systems capable of influencing the fate of human allografts. Likewise, methods must be developed to assess the relative strengths of the different antigens in order to establish a priority system for the selection of the most compatible donor. This facet of the field of transplantation will be discussed in a subsequent section on transplantation genetics.

SKIN ALLOGRAFT REJECTION REACTIONS

Autografts survive indefinitely; allograft survival is inversely proportional to the genetic disparity between the donor and the recipient; the most rapid rejection is accorded to xenografts. Because much of the immunologic and genetic knowledge of transplantation has been derived from skin graft experiments, the skin allograft reaction in man will be described.

Full thickness skin grafts (11 mm in diameter) are used in a standardized transplant technique (Converse and Rapaport, 1956). In the first two days after grafting, skin allografts and autografts appear similar. There are multiple dilated capillaries on the graft surface without evidence of blood flow. By the third or fourth day, the dilated capillaries are replaced by small-caliber vessels with rapid blood flow. These vessels persist and mature in the autografts. In the allografts, blood flow ceases on the eighth or ninth day. Dilated vessels, thrombi, and punctate hemorrhages develop over the next two days. There is an infiltration by leukocytes of the perivascular spaces beginning at two to five days. Escharification and slough of the graft follows.

Second grafts from the same donor are rejected in accelerated fashion. If the second set grafts are applied within one week of first set rejection, a "white graft reaction" develops, in which revascularization of the graft fails to occur. A second set graft applied between 8 and 80 days after the first set rejection results in a compressed first set type of rejection taking only four or five days. Late application of second set grafts, three months or more after first set rejection, results in rejection similar to that of a first set graft (Rapaport and Converse, 1957, 1958).

TRANSPLANTATION ANTIGENS

Tissue rejection is based upon the recipient's ability to recognize the transplanted tissue as foreign. Foreignness implies the existence in the graft of antigens that are not present in the recipient. Antigens which can stimulate graft rejection are called histocompatibility antigens, and these range from very weak (e.g., between closely related members of the same species) to very strong (as between members of different species).

Serologic studies have indicated the existence of a cross reactivity or similarity between histocompatibility antigens on the endothelium of the glomerular basement membrane and the arteries. There is a similar sharing of antigens by man and bacterial membranes (Rapaport and associates, 1971). These studies indicate that histocompatibility antigens are composed of a wide range of determinants, which may be individually specific or ubiquitous throughout nature.

Histocompatibility antigens are present in all tissues, but the relative amounts vary between tissues. They are present in high concentration in spleen, liver, and lymphoid tissues and in small concentration in brain and muscle. Within the tissue of a vascularized organ, the distribution of histocompatibility antigens varies a great deal. Immunofluorescence studies of human kidneys have shown a localization of histocompatibility antigens on the endothelium of the glomerular basement membrane and the arteries. There are smaller amounts of antigens within the interstitial tissue (Sybesma and coworkers, 1974).

Histocompatibility antigens are found primarily on cell surfaces. Möller (1961), using fluorescent antibody techniques, showed a cell membrane localization of mouse alloantigens. Ferritin-labeled antibody in an electron microscopic technique also disclosed cell membrane localization of alloantigens (Davis and Silverman, 1968). In addition, cell fractionation studies have detected alloantigens in microsomal membrane fractions (Dumonde and coworkers, 1963).

The cell membrane is a lipid-protein-glycoprotein-carbohydrate complex arranged in the form of a fluid mosaic (Singer and Nicolson, 1972). Membrane extraction procedures have utilized detergents, sonication, enzymes, and 3-molar KCl. Purification of the extracts have yielded, in the mouse, fragments containing alloantigenic activity of 34,000 and 55,000 molecular weight; the fragments are composed of 70 to 90 per cent protein and 4 to 7 per cent carbohydrate (Shimada and Nathenson, 1969). In man, histocompatibility antigen extraction procedures have yielded an antigen with a sedimentation coefficient S_{20} W of 2.3 and a molecular weight of 31,000 (Reisfeld and coworkers, 1973). Since protein constitutes the largest portion of the antigenically active membrane fragment, it is likely that the antigenic specificity of the fragment lies in the protein structure. Denaturation of protein using heat, phenol, 8-molar urea (Basch and Stetson, 1962), or proteolysis (Kandutsch, 1960) results in a loss of biologic activity.

HISTOCOMPATIBILITY GENETICS

Histocompatibility antigens are the products of a histocompatibility genetic complex. The details of histocompatibility genetics have been thoroughly studied in the mouse, with evidence of great similarity between the major histocompatibility complex (MHC) of the mouse and that of man.

Two methods are currently used to define the MHC phenotype. Serologically defined (SD) antigens present on lymphoid cells may be identified using appropriate antisera in a cytotoxicity assay. Lymphocytes, antisera, and complement are incubated; lymphocytes containing the surface antigen for which the antisera is specific are destroyed.

The mixed leukocyte culture test (MLC), first described by Bach and Hirschorn (1964) and Bain, Vas, and Lowenstein (1964), measures antigenic differences (lymphocyte-defined — LD) between allogeneic or xenogeneic cells (Shons and coworkers, 1973b). In the MLC test (Fig. 5–1), peripheral blood leukocytes from two individuals, A and B, are mixed

in culture. One set of cells (stimulating cells — B) is treated with mitomycin C (Bm) to inhibit DNA synthesis. The other set of cells (responding cells — A) is not treated. In culture (ABm), if B cells are recognized as foreign by A cells, the A cells will enlarge and transform into blast cells. The transformation can be quantitated by measurement of the uptake of radioactive thymidine, which will be no greater than in control isogeneic cultures of A cells stimulated by mitomycin C–treated A cells (AAm) (Shons and coworkers, 1973a).

In the mouse, a genetic region called H-2 is identified as the MHC (Fig. 5–2). At the left and right extremes of H-2 are two polymorphic loci, H-2K and H-2D, alleles of which determine the serum-defined (SD) antigens present on tissues. Between the H-2K and H-2D regions there is an immune response locus, Ir IA–Ir IB, alleles of which control the ability of an animal to respond to a variety of antigens.

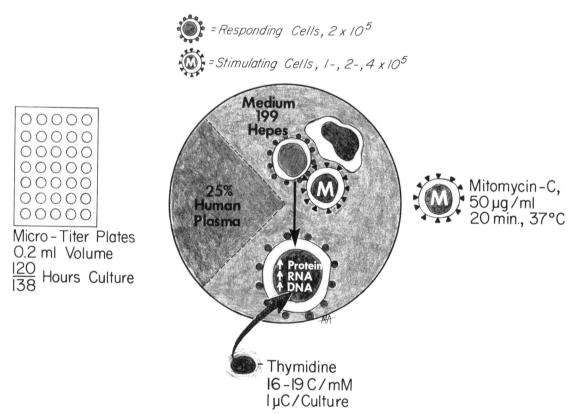

FIGURE 5–1. Schema of a typical MLC test. Leukocytes are obtained from heparinized blood using a ficol-hypaque density gradient sedimentation technique which yields a nearly pure mononuclear cell suspension. Cells are present in culture in microtiter plates at a concentration of 2×10^5 responding cells and 1, 2, or 4×10^5 stimulating cells per 0.2 ml of culture volume. Stimulating cells are inactivated by mitomycin C treatment prior to placement in culture. Cells are cultured in medium 199 buffered with sodium hepes and supplemented with 25% human plasma. Blast transformation of the stimulated leukocytes is quantitated by the addition of radioactive thymidine to the culture at 120 hours of incubation, with harvesting of the cells and radioactivity measurement 18 hours later.

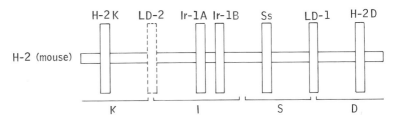

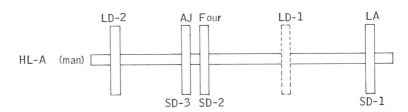

FIGURE 5–2. Diagram of the major histocompatibility complex in man and mouse.

The S region also lies between the H-2K and H-2D regions and controls the level of serum protein.

Until recently the H-2 SD antigens were considered the strong transplantation antigens, recognized as foreign by the host and against which the immune rejection response is aimed. However, there is now evidence that differences only in the I region, and to a lesser extent in the S region, can cause proliferative responses in MLC (Bach and coworkers, 1972). Certain mouse strains which are identical for the SD antigens of H-2K and H-2D, but which differ for H-2 LD factors, can reject skin grafts, presumably due to only H-2 LD differences (Bailey and coworkers, 1971). Klein (1973) has shown that two pairs of mouse strains which are SD-identical can also cause significant graft versus host reactions. This type of evidence suggests that LD differences may be of critical importance in clinical problems of transplantation.

In man, the HLA complex is the MHC. The chromosome complex consists of the SD-1 locus LA at the right and the SD-2 four and SD-3AJ loci left of center. SD-2 and SD-3 have not yet been separated by recombination. In addition, presumably two LD loci exist (see Fig. 5–2).

Amos and Bach (1968) first suggested the possibility that parts of the HLA chromosome, which are genetically separable from the SD loci, may play a role in MLC activation in man. Yunis and Amos (1971) confirmed the existence of HLA LD genes. Although it is difficult to evaluate the role of LD differences in allograft phenomena in man, both SD and LD differences are probably important. Etheredge, Shons, Schmidtke, and Najarian (1974)

have shown a correlation between LD disparity and graft survival in renal transplantation between SD-identical individuals.

Present methods for assaying LD disparity are far more complex and time-consuming than techniques to measure SD differences. LD antigens may eventually be serologically definable or detectable using a battery of standard typing cells. One of the goals in human transplantation is to match donor and recipient as closely as possible. Assay of SD differences measures the number of serologically detectable antigens by which donor and recipient differ, whereas MLC assay of LD differences measures the amount of stimulation between donor and recipient. With improvement of LD typing methods, a more complete definition of the MHC phenotype may be possible.

THE LYMPHOID SYSTEM

A basic hematopoietic stem cell which first arises in the yolk sac eventually differentiates along a number of cell lines to yield all hematopoietic cells. The local microchemical milieu determines the course of differentiation which the cell will take. The multipotential stem cell of the yolk sac differentiates into oligopotential progenitor cells of the myeloid series (eosinophils, neutrophils, basophils), erythroid series (erythrocytes), and lymphoid series. Progenitor cells of the lymphoid series come under the influence of two central lymphoid organs, the thymus and the bursal equivalent tissues. Within the parenchyma of the thymus, lymphoid cells proliferate and differentiate; they then circulate to subserve the functions of cellular immunity (Good and coworkers, 1966). Such immune reactions include allograft rejection, delayed hypersensitivity, graft versus host reactions, destruction of bacterial pyogenic pathogens (Mackaness and Blanden, 1969), and tumor defense (Good and Finstad, 1967). Lymphoid cells which are not influenced by the thymus may differentiate along another pathway controlled by the bursal system. In birds, the bursa of Fabricius is a well-defined anatomical structure (Cooper and coworkers, 1965). Its anatomical location in man has not yet been determined, but it is known to exist, probably along the course of the gastrointestinal tract. Lymphoid cells of the bursa-dependent system produce circulating antibodies.

From the central lymphoid tissue—i.e., thymus and bursal equivalent area—lymphoid cells travel to the peripheral lymphoid tissues, primarily the lymph nodes and the spleen. Within lymph nodes, there is a division into thymus-dependent and thymus-independent morphologic areas. The deep cortical or paracortical areas contain predominantly thymus-dependent populations of lymphoid cells. The far cortical area and medullary cords of the nodes contain the thymus-independent population cells (Parrott and coworkers, 1966) (Fig. 5–3).

MECHANISM OF TRANSPLANT REJECTION

Sensitization and Recognition

The development of immunity and of the rejection process begins by exposure of the host to the histocompatibility antigens of the graft.

The route of administration of the antigen determines the onset and strength of the immunologic response. The intravenous route provokes the earliest but weakest response. Subcutaneous placement produces a stronger immune response, while the intradermal route provides the most pronounced immunity. The strong response produced by intradermal administration is probably the result of prolonged exposure to the antigen in the regional lymph node.

Sensitization to a graft takes place primarily within the peripheral lymphoid tissue of the host. Histocompatibility antigens, being membrane components, are likely shed during membrane maintenance and can be easily separated from the cell surface. Studies have shown antigen release from cells by gentle osmotic shock (Davies, 1966) and from vascularized allografts following transplantation (Najarian and associates, 1966). Antigens reach the lymph nodes by the lymphatics or the bloodstream. It is also probable that sensitization can take place directly by contact of the lymphoid cells of the host with histocompatibility antigens within the graft.

The small lymphocyte is the specific cellular site of immunologic recognition. In their pioneering work, Billingham, Brent, and Medawar (1956) showed that lymph node suspensions from nontolerant animals could produce rejection of long-standing allografts in tolerant animals. The immunologic capability of the lymphoid system was thus demonstrated, but the specific effector cell was not identified. Gowans (1962) showed that a suspension of small lymphocytes of parental strain rats would cause a graft versus host reaction in F_1 (first generation) hybrid animals. Subsequently, Gowans, McGregor, and Cowen (1963) showed that transfused small lymphocytes

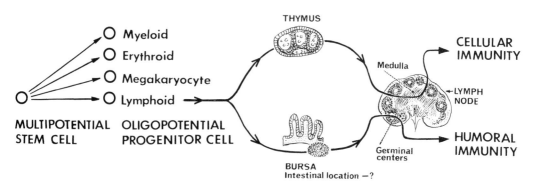

FIGURE 5–3. Lymphoid progenitor cells, which may come under the influence of either thymus or bursal central lymphoid tissue, travel to the peripheral lymphoid tissue to subserve the function of cellular or humoral immunity.

would destroy long-standing skin allografts in rats, thereby implicating the small lymphocyte in the rejection process.

Some type of antigen processing by the macrophage may be necessary prior to lymphocyte recognition. Studies have shown that the macrophage must be present for antibody production in a cell suspension (Feldman and Gallily, 1967; Mishell and Dutton, 1967). The macrophage may simply hold the antigen for recognition by the lymphocyte. It is more probable, however, that there is an actual ingestion of the antigen by the macrophage. Fishman and Adler (1963) demonstrated that an RNA-containing extract of macrophages could stimulate nonsensitized lymphocytes to produce antibodies. Askonsis and Rhodes (1965) showed that the active RNA-containing macrophage extract also contained antigen. Therefore, macrophages may break down antigen to their immunologic essentials and unite them with a cellular RNA that in itself may be preformed and nonspecific.

Recognition by the small lymphocyte begins as a surface phenomenon. There are specific antigen receptor sites on the lymphocyte membrane. On cells of the bursal-dependent system (B cells), the receptor sites are immunoglobulins, as proved by numerous techniques. Pernis, Forni, and Amante (1970) have shown by immunofluorescence studies that there are discrete loci of immunoglobulins on the lymphocyte membrane; antisera to immunoglobulin will stimulate lymphocytes to DNA synthesis and mitosis (Coombs and coworkers, 1969). In addition, as would be expected with an antigen-antibody combination, selective absorption of antigen has been shown on the lymphocyte membrane (Byrt and Ada, 1969). The receptor sites on thymus-dependent cells (T cells) have not been well characterized. These receptor sites may be immunoglobulins or immunoglobulin analogues.

Studies designed to locate antigen receptor sites have been done only on immune cells, which are already programmed for a specific antigen. The mode of development of receptor sites on a truly virgin or noncommitted cell is a matter of speculation. The clonal selection theory (Burnet, 1959) proposes that clones of cells reactive to a specific antigen arise spontaneously prior to antigenic exposure. It is thought that such precommitted cells develop specific surface immunoglobulin as a result of somatic mutation.

The reaction of antigen and specific receptor site will initiate the cellular response necessary for antibody production or cell-mediated immunity. Various cell-cell interactions occur, however, in the development of the complete immune response. The macrophage plays a role in antigen processing. Other studies have demonstrated the requirement for both T (thymus) and B (bursal) cells for some types of antibody response. The T cell may be the initial recognition cell in the response. T cells may also serve a recruitment function for B cells.

The small lymphocyte undergoes numerous morphologic changes in response to an antigenic challenge. Scothorne and McGregor (1955) described the appearance of large RNA-containing lymphoid cells in the lymph nodes draining the site of skin allografts in rabbits. Cell culture techniques have permitted close examination of the structural changes of the stimulated cell. The cells transform from small lymphocytes with dense nuclei and scanty cytoplasm to large cells with open nuclei, prominent nucleoli, and polysome-filled cytoplasm. Radioactive labeling techniques have shown an intracellular increase in DNA production and eventual mitotic division.

The production of immunologically competent T or B cells may be a multistage process. Sercarz and Coons (1962) postulated a three-stage development of immunocompetent cells. The first stage is represented by the responsive but uncommitted "X" cell. Antigen exposure results in the development of the "Y" cell, a memory cell with some immunologic competence. Further antigenic exposure stimulates progression to the "Z" cell, a fully immunocompetent, antibody-producing effector cell.

The end result of antigen-stimulated differentiation of the T cell line is the "killer" lymphocyte, whose functions will be discussed later. The fully differentiated B cell is the plasma cell, which produces antibody. Each plasma cell produces only one specific antibody of one specific immunoglobulin class. In man, five immunoglobulin classes exist: IgG, IgM, IgA, IgD, and IgE. IgG is the most prevalent fraction. Each IgG molecule is composed of four polypeptide chains—two light (MW, 20,000–25,000) chains and two heavy (MW, 50,000) chains linked by disulfide bonds. The complete molecular weight is 145,000. Amino acid analysis reveals that both heavy and light chains have a constant amino acid sequence at the C-terminal end and a variable amino acid sequence at the N-terminal end (Putnam, Titani, Wikler, and Shinoda, 1967; Potter, Appella, and Geisser, 1975). The N-terminal end is the antigen combining site, of which there are two on IgG molecules (Fig. 5–4).

IgM immunoglobulins are larger than IgG molecules (MW, 850,000) and have five antigen combining sites (Franklin and Frangione, 1969). Each of the five subunits of IgM molecules resembles the IgG molecule, possessing two heavy and two light chains. IgG and IgM are the classes of antibodies primarily involved in transplant rejection. The roles of IgA, IgD, and IgE in graft rejection, if any, have not yet been defined.

Mediators of Immunity

Early investigators of skin allograft rejection noted that the cellular infiltrates about the graft were primarily composed of mononuclear cells. It was felt that direct contact with the sensitized cell resulted in destruction of the graft. It is now known that the process is far more complex. The exact roles played by the sensitized T cell and the antibody-producing B cell in graft rejection have yet to be defined. The specifically sensitized T cell can apparently kill by direct cell-to-cell contact. Govaerts (1960) first demonstrated the ability of a sensitized lymphocyte to kill an antigen-bearing target cell in vitro in a medium devoid of antibody. Ginsburg, Ax, and Berke (1969) demonstrated lymphocyte–target cell contact by a projection of the lymphocyte membrane prior to lysis of the target cell. This demonstrated that cell-cell contact was important, but the mechanism of cell lysis is still uncertain. Lymphocytes may kill target cells by the release of a specific lymphotoxin, a substance which destroys target cell membranes (Williams and Granger, 1968).

Sensitized lymphocytes release other factors which initiate nonspecific immune mechanisms. Migration inhibitory factor and chemotactic factor (Bloom, 1969) increase the number of macrophages in the area of the stimulated lymphocyte. A mitogenic factor is produced which will stimulate blast cell transformation in normal lymphocytes. A vascular permeability factor is released to produce the characteristic interstitial edema in the rejecting allograft. Sensitized lymphocytes also release transfer factor—a small non-antigenic molecule of <10,000 molecular weight (MW) which can confer specific sensitivity upon uncommitted lymphocytes (Lawrence, 1969). Transfer factor may serve to increase the number of actively destructive lymphocytes in the area of the allograft.

Antibodies were initially felt to be unimportant in allograft rejection. Mitchison and Dube (1955) showed that specific sensitivity to grafts could be transferred with lymphoid cells but not by high-titered anti-donor serum. Billingham, Silvers, and Wilson (1963) demonstrated that allogeneic cells survived in millipore chambers in hosts sensitized against them. Finally, animals without antibody-producing capability—neonatally bursectomized chickens—can reject allografts (Perey and coworkers, 1967). Later work using more refined techniques, however, has defined a functional participation of antibody in allograft rejection (Cochrum and coworkers, 1969). Immunofluorescence studies have also shown antibody deposits on the endothelium of rejecting allografts (Lindquist and coworkers, 1968).

Antibodies act as the recognition mechanism in their attachment to the allograft. The antigen-antibody complex thus formed activates a number of nonspecific effector and amplification systems. The complement system is one of the effector systems. Complement is a series of circulating protein molecules of nine major subcomponents which react in a sequential fashion. Classic activation of the complement system is triggered by activation of the first component of complement (C1) by the Fc portion of antibody which has combined with the antigen. An alternate activation of complement is possible by the interaction of antigen-antibody complexes and properdin to activate the

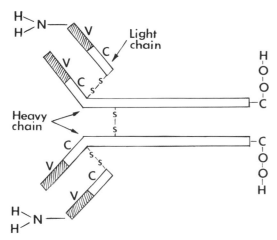

FIGURE 5–4. Schematic diagram of the IgG molecule. The variable and constant regions of the heavy and light chains are shown. The two N-terminal ends are antigen combining sites; the single C-terminal end is the Fc portion which activates complement.

C3 component of the cascade (Ruddy, 1974). Activation of the third component of complement (C3) results in the production of chemotactic factor and anaphylotoxin. Chemotactic factor promotes the movement of polymorphonuclear leukocytes to the graft area. Mobilized neutrophils release acid and alkaline phosphatase, collagenase, and glucuronidase as well as the proteolytic enzymes cathepsins D and E, all of which promote graft destruction. Anaphylatoxin increases capillary permeability and causes smooth muscle contraction and the release of histamine from mast cells. Activation of C5 produces additional chemotactic and anaphylatoxic factors. Further activation through terminal C9 produces an enzymatic system capable of lysing cell membranes and disrupting cells.

Early studies providing morphologic evidence of complement participation in allograft rejection also implicated a second cascade—the clotting system in graft rejection (McKenzie and Whittingham, 1968). The clotting system may be activated by the release of tissue thromboplastin resulting from complement- or lymphocyte-mediated tissue damage. Alternatively, the clotting system may be directly activated by the antigen-antibody complex activation of Hageman factor (Ratnoff, 1969).

A third molecular cascade system which may participate in the rejection process is the kinin system. Activated Hageman factor of the clotting system can activate an enzymatic sequence resulting in the production of kinins with the functional capacity to cause increased vascular permeability and vascular dilatation.

The relative participation of cellular and humoral factors in allograft rejection probably depends largely on the preexisting state of sensitization of the host to antigens present within the graft. The time course and histologic features of first set allograft rejection are consistent with a primary cellular mechanism of rejection. A second set allograft is rejected more quickly, with histologic features such as endothelial disruption and intravascular coagulation indicating a greater participation of complement, clotting, and kinin factors in the rejection. The rejection of grafts between species can be a very rapid process, one which has been shown to be primarily mediated by humoral factors (Shons and coworkers, 1972) (Fig. 5–5).

MODIFICATION OF THE REJECTION PROCESS

The rejection process can be modified by a variety of factors (Fig. 5–6), including immunologically privileged sites, immunologic tolerance, immunologic enhancement, and immunosuppression.

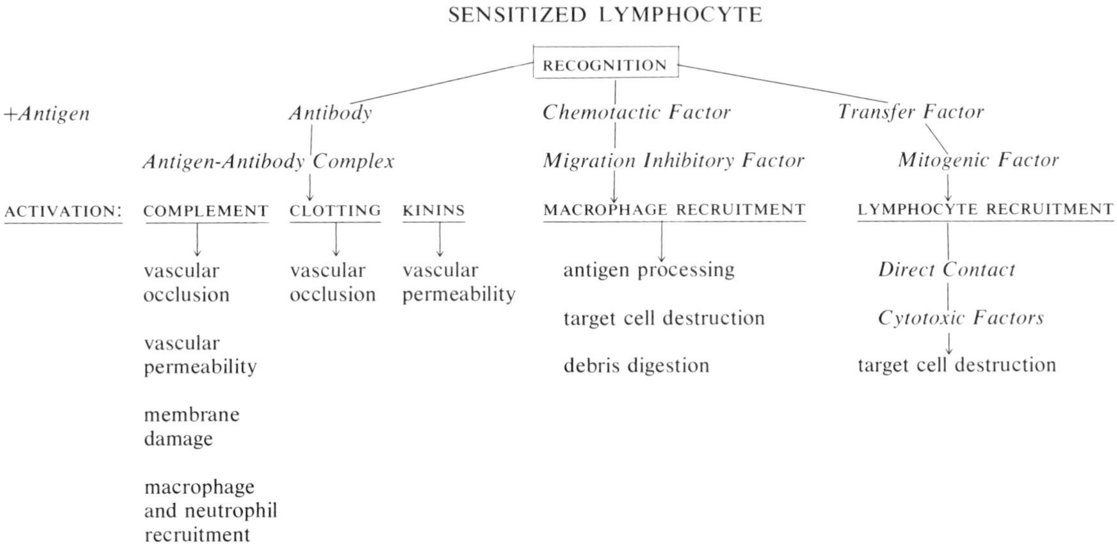

FIGURE 5–5. The sensitized lymphocyte may produce antibody; antigen-antibody complexes may activate the complement, clotting, and kinin cascades through release of chemotactic factors and migration inhibitory factor. The sensitized lymphocyte may recruit macrophages and polymorphonuclear leukocytes which can process antigen, kill target cells, and digest debris. Alternatively, sensitized lymphocytes may release transfer factor and mitogenic factor to recruit additional lymphocytes.

MODIFICATION OF REJECTION

ANTIGEN-SPECIFIC   ANTIGEN-NONSPECIFIC

Privileged Site   Antilymphocyte Serum
  Anatomical area of lesser   *Small lymphocyte destruction*
  immune response
Immunologic Tolerance   Antimetabolite
  Central cellular unresponsiveness   *Enzyme competition*
Immunologic Enhancement   Alkylating Agents
  Antibody-mediated abrogation of rejection   *Intracellular disruption*
                                                             Enzyme
                                                               Amino acid depletion

FIGURE 5-6.   The antigen-specific modifications of rejection are anatomical sites or immunologic phenomena; antigen-nonspecific modifications of rejection are mechanistic phenomena.

Immunologically Privileged Sites. Certain anatomical areas have been defined in which a lesser immunologic response is provoked by foreign tissue. The anterior chamber of the eye was used by Greene (1941, 1943) for extensive xenograft experiments. He found that transplanted mouse tissues grew unrestrained in the anterior chambers of the eyes of rabbits and guinea pigs. The long accepted explanation of the anterior chamber as a privileged site has been that without lymphatic drainage or vascularization both efferent and afferent arms of the immunologic response are blocked. However, experiments by Raju and Grogan (1971) would indicate that anterior chamber allografts may be vascularized and may also lead to a host sensitization. The final explanation of the immunologically incompetent status of the anterior chamber of the eye remains obscure.

The brain lacks lymphatic drainage, an anatomical finding which eliminates a portion of the afferent pathway of the immunologic reflex. Murphy and Sturm (1923) successfully transplanted mouse tumors to the brains of rats, guinea pigs, and pigeons and found that the same tumors were not supported in subcutaneous or intramuscular locations. The grafts had to be placed within the cerebral cortex and could not make contact with the ependymal lining of the ventricle, lest they be rejected.

The cheek pouch of the Syrian hamster is a highly vascular, mucous membrane-lined, backward projection of the cheek cavity. Experiments by Patterson (1968) documented the privileged status of the site. The pouch lacks lymphatic drainage, and egress of antigen from the area is blocked. Furthermore, a barrier of sialomucin partially blocks ingress of immunocompetent cells.

Immunologic Tolerance. The ideal modification of the rejection process would be the in- duction within the host of a specific nonreactivity to the antigen mosaic of the graft. Immunologic tolerance refers to the immunologically unresponsive state produced by controlled exposure to antigen. Owen (1945) showed that, as a result of prenatal exchange of red cell precursors, most twin cattle retain throughout life a mixture of each other's erythrocytes, a condition called chimerism. Subsequently, Billingham, Lampkin, Medawar, and Williams (1952) showed that chimeric cattle would accept skin grafts from each other but not from parents or other siblings. Burnet and Fenner (1948) predicted that specific unresponsiveness could be produced by exposure to the antigen in early life. Billingham, Brent, and Medawar (1956) later demonstrated the induction of immunologic unresponsiveness to histocompatibility antigens in mice by the neonatal injection of allogeneic cells.

Much experimental work has subsequently demonstrated the feasibility of immunologic tolerance in carefully controlled models. The form of the antigen, the dose, and the route of administration are critically important. Immunologic tolerance is most easily induced to substances such as serum proteins, which are small molecules that can be administered intravenously and will equilibrate throughout the body, remaining in circulation for a prolonged time. Particulate antigens such as bacteria cannot be used. Immunologic tolerance is more easily developed in young immunologically incompetent animals. The degree of tolerance induced is inversely proportional to the antigenic disparity of antigen and recipient. Induction of immunologic tolerance to xenogeneic tissue is difficult. Immunologic tolerance to the antigen mosaic of a tissue is accomplished with more difficulty than is tolerance to a single antigenic determinant.

Tolerance to allogeneic tissue grafts can be

produced by the injection of replicating hematopoietic cells into an irradiated host. Prolonged kidney allograft survival has been achieved in selectively bred lines of dogs by initial transplantation of bone marrow, followed by transplantation of a kidney to an irradiated host determined to be identical for the major canine histocompatibility antigens. Hematopoietic chimerism and specific unresponsiveness to the antigen of the donor animal was achieved. The animals remained immunologically competent in that grafts from animals other than the bone marrow donor would be rejected (Rapaport and associates, 1972). Such measures are not yet clinically feasible. Another current line of investigation involves the possible induction of tolerance by the administration of solubilized histocompatibility antigen. Rat kidney allograft survival has been significantly prolonged by the administration to the recipient of papain digest-prepared rat histocompatibility antigen (von Haefen and coworkers, 1973).

Immunologic Enhancement. Immunologic tolerance refers to an antigen-specific absence of immunologic response; immunologic enhancement refers to prolonged graft survival in the presence of demonstrable antigraft antibody within the host. Enhancement may be either active or passive.

Active enhancement follows sensitization of the host with either live or killed tissue of the same histocompatibility antigen configuration as the graft. Accelerated rejection usually follows sensitization. However, under certain carefully controlled conditions, sensitization may be followed by prolonged graft survival, i.e., enhancement. The timing of graft challenge following sensitization is important. Ferrer (1968) obtained enhancement of tumor allografts in mice three weeks following sensitization; allografts placed two or eight weeks following sensitization were rejected in accelerated fashion. The dose of sensitizing antigen is important, large injections being frequently the most effective. The route of administration of the sensitizing antigen is also critical: in mice intraperitoneal injections of spleen cells in Freund's adjuvant prolonged subsequent graft survival, while homografts of spleen cells were less effective (Chutna, 1968).

There has been little correlation between antibody levels as measured by standard techniques (cytotoxicity, leukoagglutination, hemagglutination) and graft survival. It is probable that the enhancement phenomenon is based upon a class of antibodies which may not have the functional capabilities of usual antibodies and which are not measurable by standard techniques.

Passive enhancement may be obtained by transferring immune serum. The enhancing activity lies in the IgG gamma globulin fraction (Irvin and coworkers, 1967). Late hyperimmune sera are the most effective. Prolonged survival of kidney allografts has been produced in certain strains of rats by combined protocols of active sensitization and passively administered antiserum in experiments which indicated that combined therapy was more effective than either active or passive enhancement alone (Stuart and coworkers, 1968).

A possible interrelationship between tolerance and enhancement has been seriously considered since the reports of Hellström and Hellström in 1970. They reported that the cytotoxicity of the lymphocytes of tumor-bearing patients toward their tumor cells could be blocked in vitro by serum factors. The concept arose of a blocking antibody, and the possibility was suggested that tolerance is simply a form of enhancement. It is the opinion of Medawar (1973), however, that the balance of evidence still favors the concept of tolerance as a central state of unresponsiveness, one in which either a specific immune capability or clone of immunologically competent cells becomes depleted or inhibited.

Immunosuppression. In the consideration of privileged sites, immunologic tolerance, and immunologic enhancement, we have dealt with the phenomenon of reduced immunologic response to a specific antigenic stimulus. A variety of techniques are available which will produce a generalized depression of the immune response. Clinical organ transplantation has been made possible by the development of such methods.

ANTILYMPHOCYTE GLOBULIN. Heterologous antilymphocyte serum (ALS) prolongs graft survival by destruction of the small lymphocyte. Metchnikoff (1899) first described the destruction of white cells by such immunologic means. Flexner (1902) reported depletion of lymph nodes in animals treated with rabbit anti–guinea pig serum. Interbitzen (1958) reported the alteration of an immune response (delayed hypersensitivity) by ALS in vivo. Woodruff and Anderson (1963) first reported prolonged skin allograft survival in ALS-treated rats. Monaco, Wood, and Russell

(1967) provided the first demonstration of the immunosuppressive effectiveness of ALS in man.

ALS is produced by the immunization of animals—usually horse, rabbit, or goat—with lymphocytes of the graft host species. The active fraction of the immune sera is the IgG portion, which can be separated to provide antilymphocyte globulin (ALG). ALG probably acts by coating the small lymphocyte with antibody, which leads to destruction of the lymphocyte within the reticuloendothelial system. Evidence supporting the clinical efficacy of ALG in kidney transplantation has been reported (Najarian and Simmons, 1971).

IMMUNOSUPPRESSIVE DRUGS. Many drugs have been found in the laboratory to have immunosuppressive properties. This discussion will be confined to those few which have shown clinical usefulness.

Adrenal Steroids. Corticosteroids are a mainstay in current clinical immunosuppressive regimens; however, little is known of their mechanism of action. They have been shown to have anti-inflammatory effects (Glenn and coworkers, 1963), lympholytic effects (White, 1948), anticomplementing effects (Gewurz and coworkers, 1965), and lysosome-stabilizing effects (Weissmann and Thomas, 1963), and they are capable of producing a fall in serum globulins (Bitler and Rossen, 1973). Early work indicated that steroids could produce prolonged skin graft survival in laboratory animals (Billingham and coworkers, 1951). However, their effects are variable among species, and frequently steroids alone will not prolong graft survival. The effectiveness of steroids as immunosuppressants is based upon a summation of their inhibitory activity on both the acquisition and expression of immunity.

Antimetabolites. The antimetabolites (purine or pyrimidine analogues and folic acid antagonists) act primarily by inhibition of enzyme systems. The most widely used immunosuppressant, azathioprine, is a purine analogue. Azathioprine is a derivative of 6-mercaptopurine (6–MP). Schwartz, Stack, and Dameshek (1958) first noted the immunosuppressive properties of 6–MP. Numerous subsequent studies have confirmed its ability to prolong graft survival in varied species. Azathioprine is converted in the liver to 6–MP, which resembles inosine monophosphate. Thus, 6–MP competes with inosine in the synthetic pathway of RNA and DNA. Azathioprine is most effective against rapidly proliferating cells, such as lymphocytes responding to an antigenic stimulus. The drug has bone marrow and liver toxicity.

Alkylating agents. The alkylating agents combine with cellular components, frequently DNA, to interfere with cellular function. Cyclophosphamide is an example of this class of drug. Stender, Ringlieb, Strauch, and Winter (1959) first reported inhibition of the immune response by cyclophosphamide. Cyclophosphamide binds to the guanine molecule in DNA, an action which may result in mispairing, ring cleavage, depurination, and DNA chain breakage or cross linking. Cyclophosphamide has recently been used in place of azathioprine in selected renal transplant patients in whom the hepatotoxic effect of azathioprine is a problem (Starzl and associates, 1973).

Enzymes. L-Asparaginase is an example of a new class of immunosuppressive drugs (Hersh, 1971). L-Asparaginase depletes the nonessential amino acid L-asparagine in the milieu outside the cell. It has inhibitory effects on the rapidly proliferating lymphocyte. L-Asparaginase has been shown to have immunosuppressive properties in vitro (Shons and coworkers, 1971), and it can prolong skin allograft survival (Shons and coworkers, 1970). It has inhibitory properties against both cellular and humoral immunity. The effects of the enzyme appear to be short-lived, probably due to the induction of asparagine synthetase in lymphoid tissue. While its clinical efficacy in graft prolongation has yet to be shown, the concept of amino acid depletion in the armamentarium of immunosuppression is intriguing. The drug has found wide clinical usefulness in the treatment of childhood leukemias.

Genetics of Transplantation

FRITZ H. BACH, M.D.

Tissue transplanted from one individual to another will be rejected if the new host recognizes that tissue as foreign. Foreignness is equated with the presence on the transplanted cells of antigens which the new host does not possess and recognizes as nonself. Graft rejection is associated with a cellular immunologic reaction which involves lymphocytes and perhaps other cells. While relatively little is understood about the nature and specificity of recognition by the lymphocyte of foreign antigens in the allograft response, and while at present the actual mechanism of graft rejection remains largely obscure, the ability of the host to differentiate self from nonself antigens must be considered the basic tenet of immunologic reactions.

Antigens are considered histocompatibility antigens if they can be related to graft rejection. It is presumed that, in the absence of treatment protocols designed to delay or prevent graft rejection, any histocompatibility antigen will lead to graft rejection if it is present on donor tissue and absent from the host. In fact, some histocompatibility differences are probably present in all donor-recipient combinations, with the exception of identical twins in man and inbred strains in other animal species. However, the "strength" of different antigenic incompatibilities can vary widely in that some can lead to graft rejection in eight days, and others permit graft survival of well over a hundred days.

This section is concerned with the basic principles underlying the genetic control of transplantation antigens and with the biological situation as we presently understand it. For more detailed information, the reader is referred to a review by Bach and van Rood (1976).

BASIC GENETICS

There are 46 chromosomes made up of 23 pairs in man; 22 pairs are *autosomes* and one pair consists of the *sex chromosomes* (see Chapter 4). In the male an X chromosome is inherited from the mother (included in the C group of chromosomes) and a Y chromosome is inherited from the father. If we consider any one pair of chromosomes, one member of that pair will have been inherited from the father and one member from the mother. Two such chromosomes are called *homologous chromosomes*.

Chromosomes are homologous, i.e., fit into a pair, because the genetic information on one concerns itself with the same phenotypic traits as the genetic information on the other (see Chapter 4). For instance, one pair of homologous chromosomes contains the genetic information (*genes*) which determines eye color. On one member of that pair a person can inherit the gene for blue eyes, perhaps from the father, and on the homologous chromosome the gene for brown eyes, from the mother. The region on the chromosome (which is small compared to the entire length of the chromosome) associated with that given trait is called a *locus* or location on the chromosome. The genetic material at that locus is referred to as a gene or allele. The latter term, allele, is used to refer to the alternate forms of the gene which can exist at a locus. Thus in our example, the individual in question has a "blue" allele and a "brown" allele.

While one individual can have only two alleles at a given genetic locus, more than two alleles can exist in the population. An example of this is the ABO genetic system, in which one individual can have, for example, the A allele from one parent and the B allele from the other parent. Such an individual would be blood type AB. On the other hand, another individual can have the O allele on both of his homologous chromosomes and thus be blood type O. These are three different alleles of the ABO locus. An individual who has the same gene at a given locus on the homologous chromosomes is said to be *homozygous* at that locus; if there are different alleles on the homologous chromosomes, the individual is *heterozygous*. *Polymorphism* refers to the existence in the population of more than one allele at a given locus.

Let us consider first a single genetic locus in a mating in which the father and mother are both heterozygous for different alleles. The possible offspring of such a mating are given in Table 5–1. If we call the two alleles of the father a and b, and those of the mother c and d, then the four possible offspring are as follows: If a child inherits the $\underline{a}$ allele of the father, he can inherit either the $\underline{c}$ or the $\underline{d}$ allele of the mother, giving rise to the allelic combinations $\underline{ac}$ or $\underline{ad}$. Similarly, the alleles $\underline{b}$ and $\underline{c}$ or $\underline{b}$ and $\underline{d}$ can be inherited. The inheritance of these alleles is random; thus, the four genotypes in the children should be present in equal numbers. It should be noted that no matter how many alleles there are in the population at this one locus, there can be only four alleles in the two parents; and thus, barring genetic recombination (discussed below), only four genotypes are possible for the children. Even with an infinite number of alleles in the population, a minimum of 25 per cent of siblings will still be identical at that locus. The probability that both parents will be heterozygous for different alleles depends on the gene frequencies in the population. As the frequency for each allele increases, the probability increases that at least one parent will be homozygous or that they will share one allele. In these two latter cases, there will be only two and three possible sibling groups, respectively. The inheritance of alleles as discussed above is referred to as *segregation*.

If we consider two separate loci, A and B, on different chromosomes, and again designate the parents as heterozygous for different alleles at each locus, another genetic principle can be demonstrated. Let us call the alleles of the father at the A locus $\underline{a}$ and $\underline{b}$, and his alleles at the B locus $\underline{w}$ and $\underline{x}$. The corresponding alleles of the mother can be designated $\underline{c}$ and $\underline{d}$ and $\underline{y}$ and $\underline{z}$. Since we have already discussed segregation of alleles at one locus, let us consider only siblings who inherit alleles $\underline{a}$ and $\underline{c}$ at locus A. Inheritance of alleles of locus B is independent of inheritance of locus A (*independent* assortment). Siblings with alleles $\underline{ac}$ can thus inherit alleles $\underline{wy}$, $\underline{wz}$, $\underline{xy}$, or $\underline{xz}$. The possible combinations for segregation and independent assortment of the alleles at these two

loci is shown in Table 5–2. With two independently segregating loci, a minimum of 1 in 16 sibling pairs is identical for both loci.

So far only loci on different chromosomes which segregate independently of one another have been considered. If two loci are very close together on a chromosome, they will usually segregate as a unit. Two such loci are considered *linked*.

During meiosis, homologous chromosomes pair prior to reduction of the number of chromosomes from 46 (the *diploid* number) to 23 (the *haploid* number). During this time it is possible for *recombination* to occur, in which homologous regions of the paired chromosomes exchange parts. After the crossover, the haploid set of chromosomes will include a chromosome of which part was inherited from the father and part from the mother. The frequency of recombination is proportional to the distance separating the loci. Two very closely linked loci are thus usually inherited as a unit; two loci relatively far apart on the chromosome may show essentially independent assortment, with a recombination frequency of 50 per cent.

In the unrelated population, alleles of two linked loci will, with time, come to "equilibrium." That is, a given allele of locus A will be found on the same chromosome with a given allele at locus B, with a frequency not significantly different from the product of the two gene frequencies. If the two genes in question are found together more frequently, they are said to be in *linkage disequilibrium*.

GENES AND ANTIGENS

When dealing with antigens, one tends to equate an "allele" with an "antigen." Howev-

TABLE 5–2. *Segregation of Parental Alleles at Two Independently Segregating Loci*

		Father (ab;wx)			
		aw	ax	bw	bx
Mother (cd;yz)	cy	ac;wy	ac;xy	bc;wy	bc;xy
	cz	ac;wz	ac;xz	bc;wz	bc;xz
	dy	ad;wy	ad;wy	bd;wy	bd;xy
	dz	ad;wz	ad;xz	bd;wz	bd;xz

TABLE 5–1. *Segregation of Parental Alleles at a Simple Genetic Locus*

Father ab	×	Mother cd
ac	ad bc	bd
	Siblings	

er, if the allele determines a polypeptide chain, and it is the polypeptide chain itself, in its tertiary configuration, which is the "antigen," then complexity arises. An antigen, i.e., the moiety recognized by an antibody combining site, is a relatively small site on a molecule so that even a relatively small polypeptide chain, when folded, could have many different antigenic sites. Thus the several antigens associated with any given genetic region may be parts of one or more distinct molecules. In addition, it should be mentionted that alleles are codominant (i.e., they are both phenotypically expressed).

Our present understanding of the role of transplantation antigens is based mainly on work in inbred animal species, such as the mouse. It appears that the genetic control of histocompatibility antigens in the mouse and in man is quite similar, and as such a discussion of the genetics of histocompatibility in the mouse is of value.

Inbreeding, the mating of two individuals who are more closely related than two individuals chosen at random from the population, leads to a decrease in genetic heterogeneity. Thus, brother-sister mating and repeated mating of their offspring would eventually result in a strain of animals each member of which would be genetically identical except for the sex chromosomes. Such a strain of animals is called an *inbred strain*. Two animals of the same sex from such an inbred strain will accept skin grafts from one another.

A refinement of this procedure is to obtain two strains of animals that are identical to each other except for the alleles at a single genetic locus. If this locus is a histocompatibility locus, then animals of the two strains will reject skin grafts from each other because of the incompatibility for antigens determined by the alleles at that locus. Two such strains are called coisogenic. *Syngeneic* refers to two members of the same inbred strain, *allogeneic* to members of two different strains—genetically different animals.

Let us consider two inbred strains, animals of the first being homozygous for allele A at a histocompatibility locus, and animals of the second being homozygous for allele B at the same locus. We are interested in having mice that are genetically identical to the first strain, except that they should have allele B at the locus in question. Progeny of a mating of mice of the two strains will be heterozygous AB at the locus in question. A mating of such heterozygotes with parental mice is called a *backcross*. Fifty per cent of the progeny of the backcross mating to the first parental strain will be AB and 50 per cent AA. The heterozygous progeny can be identified, since they will accept skin from the B parent, whereas the homozygous AA mice will not. In addition to being AB, the progeny of the backcross will, by random segregation of the parental chromosomes, have additional chromosomes of the genotype of the first parent. Repeated backcrosses of the AB progeny to animals of strain one will eventually result in AB progeny in which all the chromosomes are those of the first strain, except that chromosome on which the B allele is retained. Those portions of the chromosome carrying the B allele which are not involved in the determination of the B allele antigen(s) are eventually also eliminated by recombination—being replaced by genes of the homologous chromosome carried by the first strain. The eventual new coisogenic strain will thus be genetically identical to the first strain except for the allele which has been intentionally retained in all of the matings. Depending on the degree to which one wants to eliminate the genetic material adjacent to the allele in question, one can obtain the homozygous coisogenic strain carrying the B allele by matings between the AB backcross offspring, in each mating choosing the B homozygous progeny.

The concept that a tissue is rejected because that tissue carries antigens which are foreign to the recipient, i.e., not possessed by the recipient, can be illustrated by grafting experiments between two inbred parental strains and their F_1 hybrid offspring. In such a situation, the F_1 animal carries antigens which are foreign to either parent—given that the two inbred parents differ in their histocompatibility genotypes. Thus, either parent will reject a graft from the F_1 animal, but the F_1 offspring will not reject grafts from either parental strain because there will be no antigens foreign to the F_1 on the graft.

Many histocompatibility systems have been discovered in the mouse (named H-1 through H-13, H-Y, and H-X); incompatibility at any one of these will lead to graft rejection. One of these, the H-2 system, seems to be of greater importance than any of the other systems and has been termed the "major" histocompatibility system in the mouse. Similarly, in the rat and chicken a single major histocompatibility system has been identified. A detailed description of the phenotypic expression of the H-2 system and its genetic control is given below.

In the mouse, a genetic region called H-2 (see Fig. 5-2) is identified as the major histocompatibility complex (MHC). At the presently known left and right "extremes" of H-2 are two highly polymorphic loci, H-2K and H-2D, respectively, alleles of which determine serologically defined (SD) antigens present on essentially all tissues. H-2K and H-2D are separated by a recombination frequency of about 0.5 per cent and serve as "markers" for the K and D regions of H-2. Between K and D are the I region, marked by the immune response locus Ir-1A (its alleles control the ability of an animal to respond to a variety of antigens), and the S region, marked the S_s locus (its alleles control the quantitative levels of a serum protein).

There are essentially two methods used to define the MHC phenotype of a mouse or an individual as it relates to histocompatibility antigens: first, definition with antisera of antigens present on essentially all lymphoid cells and most other tissues or serologically defined (SD) antigenic differences; second, measurement of "antigenic" differences between cells in the mixed leukocyte culture (MLC) test, which are known as lymphocyte-defined (LD) differences.

In the mixed leukocyte culture (MLC) test, blood leukocytes from two allogeneic individuals, A and B, are mixed in culture (see Fig. 5-1). One set of cells (stimulating cells) is treated with mitomycin C, designated by the subscript "m" (e.g., B_m), so that the cells cannot synthesize DNA. The other set of cells, A (responding cells), is not treated, and in mixed culture (AB_m), it responds to the presence of foreign H-2 antigens (or HLA antigens in man) on the stimulating cells by enlargement and division as indicated by the incorporation of tritiated thymidine into DNA. If the stimulating cell presents no foreign antigens to the responding cell, the rate of incorporation of tritiated thymidine by A cells will not exceed that obtained in a culture of A cells mixed with its own mitomycin C–treated cells, AA_m—the isogeneic control culture.

The H-2 serologically defined antigens have for years been considered the strong transplantation antigens recognized as foreign by the host, against which the immune rejection response is aimed. Recently, evidence has been obtained that the proliferative response in MLC when H-2 differences are recognized is not due to H-2 SD differences, but rather to differences in the I region which stimulate

strong MLC activation; or differences in the region between Ss and D are weaker with respect to MLC activation. These differences are termed LD differences, and the loci in the mouse are called Hld, as indicated in Figure 5-2. There are thus the H-2 SD and H-2 LD systems. The situation in man is analogous. There are three SD loci and presumably two LD loci (one strong and one weak locus). One major reason for presenting the situation in the mouse before considering that in man is that in the mouse in vivo experiments can be done to test the relative roles of LD and SD in allograft phenomena.

The HLA Serologically Defined (SD) System. HLA-A and HLA-B are highly polymorphic loci, while HLA-C has been defined more recently, and fewer antigens are known. Table 5-3 lists the antigens of these loci. Numbers such as 1, 2, and 3 refer to the HLA antigens which have been officially accepted by the World Health Organization Committee on HLA nomenclature; W numbers refer to antigens designated at International Histocompatibility Workshops.

The serologic definition of "single" antigens is exceedingly difficult; some of the "official" HLA "SD antigens" designated only two years ago have now been "split" with the development of new antisera.

The HLA Lymphocyte-Defined (LD) Systems. Except for the presumed existence of the HLA-LD loci and the knowledge that these loci must be relatively polymorphic, little information has yet been gained regarding the different alleles of the two loci. Since LD-2 (the LD locus occurring in close proximity to HLA-B) is relatively stronger than LD-1, most attention has been focused on it. New methods are

TABLE 5-3. *Antigens of the HLA SD Loci*

LA (1ST) LOCUS	FOUR (2ND) LOCUS	AJ (3RD) LOCUS
HL-A1	HL-A5	W20 (SA-AJ) (T1)
HL-A2	HL-A13	FJH (170) (T2)
HL-A3	W17	UPS (T3)
HL-A9	W27	TW (T5)
HL-A10	HL-A12	P1.16 (T6)
HL-A11	W5	
W19	W15	
W28	W16	
	W21	
	HL-A7	
	HL-A8	
	W10	
	W14	
	W18	
	W22	

now being developed to define the HLA-D alleles. The best assay is still the MLC test; it must be remembered, however, that quantitative MLC results, while providing a measure of the amount of LD disparity (which may well be the practical answer desired), do not indicate which LD alleles are involved.

Definition of MHC–LD Alleles—LD Typing Cells. An approach that has recently evolved for the identification of LD alleles is based on the following scheme. If cells are obtained from individuals who are homozygous for at least the D locus, and these cells, to be called "typing cells," are used as stimulating cells in the MLC test, responding cells which share either in homozygous or heterozygous form the LD allele in question will not respond to the homozygous stimulating cell. This approach was first described by Bradley and associates (1972) and was further developed in several laboratories (Mempel and associates, 1973; van den Tweel and associates, 1973; Jørgensen, Lamm and Kissmeyer-Nielsen, 1973; Keuning and associates, 1975) (Table 5–4).

Mempel and associates (1973) used typing cells that were phenotypically homozygous for the SD loci; such cells might also be homo-zygous for the strong LD alleles secondary to linkage disequilibrium. Keuning and co-workers (1975) have worked with genotypically homozygous typing cells obtained from offspring of first cousin marriages (which essentially assures LD and SD identity). In considering the use of homozygous typing cells for matching individuals, one cannot necessarily equate the identical response of cells of two individuals to the typing cells with MLC identity; the regular MLC test serves here as a "cross-matching" procedure for all MHC LD differences. Also, in considering a "low" response in MLC it should be realized that such a response can result from at least two mechanisms: first, sharing of LD antigens, and second, an intrinsic incapacity on the part of the responder to react vigorously to MHC LD differences present on the stimulating cells.

Homozygous typing cells were used as part of the 1975 Histocompatibility Workshop. The results showed that six different LD clusters (HLA–DW1 through HLA–DW6) could be identified by homozygous typing cells; at least two different typing cells identified each LD cluster. The six clusters are listed in Table 5–5 together with the gene frequencies for the clusters (Thorsby and Piazza, 1975). Two other potential clusters (LD 107 and LD 108) were less clearly identifiable.

The conclusion that a responding cell carries a given LD cluster is based on the low or zero response of that cell to the appropriate homozygous typing cell (see Table 5–4). In any given LD cluster, some typing cells give near identical results, while others show only a pattern of partial identity. These differences may be due to technical problems or to the influence on MLC stimulation of determinants coded for by loci other than HLA-D. Alternatively, a single haplotype may code for more than one LD determinant, and an LD cluster defined by a homozygous typing cell may thus include several LD determinants (Bach and coworkers, 1975; Dupont and coworkers, 1975).

A more recently described method for detecting the LD antigen that has been informative in this regard is the primed LD typing (PLT) test. The test is based on the finding in mouse (Häyry, Andersson and Nordling, 1973) that lymphocytes, stimulated in an MLC and left for 9 to 14 days (beyond their peak proliferative activity), give a rapid and strong (secondary type) proliferative response if restimulated with the cells of the original stimulating cell donor. Sheehy and associates

TABLE 5–4. *Typing for LD Typing Cells Homozygous for the HLA System Including LD and SD Components**

PATTERN NUMBER	RESPONDER	STIMULATOR	MLC REACTION	LD TYPE OF X†
1	X	a/a$_m$‡	Negative	a/a a/b or a/c etc.
2	X	a/a$_m$	Positive	b/c etc.
3	a/a	X$_m$	Negative	a/a
4	a/a	X$_m$	Positive	a/b or a/c or b/c etc.
Result	1 + 3	X = a/a		
	2 + 3	should not occur		
	1 + 4	X = a/b or a/c etc.		
	2 + 4	X = b/c, d/e etc.		

*Lymphocytes obtained from cousin marriage offspring, homozygous for HLA-A, HLA-B and LD loci, can be used to type for the LD determinants on the assumption that a negative MLC test implies that stimulator and responder have (at least) one LD determinant in common. In general, cells to be typed are used first as responder cells against selected typing cells homozygous for the LD determinants. If a negative reaction is found, the procedure is reversed (pattern number 3 and 4). When the cell to be typed is identical with the typing cell, if it is negative only as responder, it implies that it has one LD determinant in common with the typing cell. (Reproduced with permission of authors and publisher from van den Tweel and associates, Transplant. Proc., 5:1535, 1973.)

†X = cell to be typed for the LD determinants.

‡a/a = homozygous typing cell; m = mitomycin-C treated.

TABLE 5–5. *Frequency of HLA–D Specificities as Defined by The Sixth International Histocompatibility Workshop**

HLA–D SPECIFICITY GROUP	ANTIGEN FREQUENCY (%)	GENE FREQUENCY† (p)	MOST SIGNIFICANT HLA–B ASSOCIATION	DELTA VALUE‡
DW 1	19.3	0.102	BW35 (W5)	0.021
DW 2	15.2	0.078	B7	0.031
DW 3	16.4	0.085	B8	0.044
DW 4	15.6	0.082	BW15	0.017
DW 5	14.6	0.075	BW16	0.013
DW 6	10.5	0.054	——	——
"Blank"	——	0.524	——	——

*Frequencies for the six provisional HLA–D "clusters" calculated from the pooled data of the Sixth International Histocompatibility Workshop. The responses of 171 random Caucasian donors were available for analysis. A specificity was assigned to a responder if at least 50 per cent of the typing cells belonging to a specific DW-group elicited typing responses from the responder. DW1–DW6: Provisional HLA–D specificities ("clusters"). "Blank": Haplotypes that were not assigned a DW number. (We thank A. Piazza and E. Thorsby for permission to publish these data from the Joint Report. *In* Kissmeyer-Nielsen (Ed.): Histocompatibility Testing 1975. Munksgaard, Copenhagen, 1975, pp. 414–458.)

†Gene Frequency (p) calculated using the method of maximum likelihood.

‡Delta value, the coefficient of linkage disequilibrium, was calculated using the formula of Mattiuz and associates (1970).

(1975a) have used this priming of lymphocytes and restimulation to study the genetic control of the restimulating antigens in man. The findings indicate that the HLA LD antigens are primarily responsible for restimulation; the SD antigens appear to be neither essential for, nor capable of causing a secondary type proliferative response. The secondary response can be assayed with radioactive thymidine within 24 hours and at an even earlier time with radioactive uridine (Sheehy and associates, 1975b). These, findings have been further extended (Bach and associates, 1975; Bradley and co-workers, 1976).

The PLT test appears to measure the same factors that are measured by the homozygous typing cells in that PLT cells sensitized to a given LD cluster in a primary MLC are restimulated strongly by those cells carrying that cluster (Hirschberg, Kaakinen and Thorsby, 1976; Bach and coworkers, 1976) (Table 5–6). The PLT test may, however, have certain advantages in that PLT cells can be generated against any LD haplotype, whereas homozygous typing cells may be difficult to find for the rare LD cluster. Furthermore, results of PLT tests are available within a few hours.

Other H Loci and Practical Considerations. Aside from HLA in man, compatibility for the ABO blood group system is of great importance to transplantation. In addition there are many H loci in man (as there are in the mouse) which may be minor H loci as compared with HLA, the major system. One practical

consideration must be noted in this regard: it is of the utmost importance to do a "cross-match" before transplantation, in an attempt to ensure that the recipient does not have any antibodies against donor tissue, especially the HLA SD antigens.

The eventual goal is to reduce any incompatibilities. By SD typing and matching one seeks to minimize the number of antigens by which the donor and recipient differ, while by MLC testing and matching one seeks to minimize the amount of stimulation between donor and recipient.

The Relative Importance of the Major Histocompatibility Complex LD and SD components. In the mouse there are congenic strains which, because of their breeding history, are presumed to be genetically identical except for the H-2 complex, or even, in some cases, for only certain regions of the H-2 complex. Any genetic difference between such congenic strains can thus, with high probability, be ascribed to their H-2 disparity. By testing the appropriate strain combinations, one can make a rather direct evaluation of the role of H-2 LD and SD factors in allograft phenomena. In studies of the graft versus host (GvH) reaction in mice using both the Simonsen splenomegaly assay (Livnat and coworkers, 1973) and the donor cell proliferation assay of Elkins and coworkers, 1973, it has been established that GvH reactions correlate with LD disparity (MLC activation) to a much greater extent than with SD disparity. Rodey, Bortin, Bach,

TABLE 5–6. *Primary MLC with Homozygous Cells**

	STIMULATING CELLS	
RESPONDING CELLS	HB (DW2/DW2)	RR (DW2/DW2)
NK (DW2 neg.)	42,030	21,057
BB (DW2 neg.)	79,713	41,223
BKJ (DW2 hetero.)	11,185	6,202
MT (DW2 hetero.)	4,863	3,251
RR (DW2 homo.)	1,073	364
HB (DW2 homo.)	667	447

PLT–Homozygous Typing Cell Correlation

	RESPONDING PLT
RESTIMULATING CELLS	Primary MLC A (RR)$_m$ (DW2 neg.) (DW2 homo.)$_m$
A (DW2 neg.)	588
BB (DW2 neg.)	3,097
BKJ (DW2 hetero.)	13,059
MT (DW2 hetero.)	12,997
RR (DW2 homo.)	20,778
KJ (DW2 homo.)	21,110

*In the top part of the table, six responding cells are tested for their response to two homozygous typing cells defining the DW2 cluster. The first two cells (based on analysis as per Table 5–3) are DW2 negative; the others are DW2 heterozygous and DW2 homozygous, respectively. In the second half of the table, a PLT cell was prepared in which the cells of an individual negative for DW2 were used as the responding cells, and the homozygous typing cell (RR) was used as a sensitizing cell. The restimulating cells are as indicated in the table. In addition to differentiating between individuals who carry the DW2 cluster and those who do not, a gene dosage effect appears to be detected in the PLT test, in that DW2 heterozygous cells stimulate less than DW2 homozygous cells. (We thank Dr. Arne Svejgaard of Copenhagen, Denmark, for permission to publish these results of a collaborative study.)

and Rimm (1972) have demonstrated that, in H-2 SD-identical mouse strains, there is an excellent correlation between the degree of MLC activation (LD disparity) and the percentile mortality from secondary (runt) disease. In addition, congenic mouse strains identical for the SD antigens of H-2K and H-2D but differing for H-2 LD factors *can* reject skin grafts, presumably due to H-2 LD differences, although this is not true in every H-2 SD-identical, LD-different combination (Livnat and coworkers, 1973). One must thus conclude that MHC LD differences, despite H-2 SD identity, can stimulate GvH reactions, including fatal secondary disease, and skin graft rejection.

It is more difficult to evaluate the role of SD antigenic disparity in GvH and skin graft rejection. This is because we have not completely identified the LD loci and therefore cannot be sure that the MLC reactivity seen between SD-different individuals is not due to a simultaneous LD difference for which we cannot type rather than to the SD differences which we know to be present. As more sensitive MLC assays have been developed, it has been found that all SD-different mouse strain combinations can, under some conditions, lead to MLC activation. The concept of two strains (or two individuals) differing for an *SD region* (where one cannot rule out possible accompanying LD differences) must be differentiated from two strains differing for the *SD locus* as demonstrated by their having SD antigens, where one cannot rule out accompanying LD differences. From studies to date, it would appear that SD region disparity plays a relatively minor role in MLC and GvH reactions; skin grafts are rejected with only SD region disparity, although relatively slowly.

With this background in the mouse, let us turn our attention to man. The evidence that the HLA chromosomal region is the major histocompatibility complex (MHC) in man is based on the striking similarity in the genetic organization of the MHC in mouse and man, and on the demonstration that the various LD and SD loci appear to subserve the same biological functions, at least in vitro.

The overriding importance of HLA compatibility is demonstrated in siblings who have inherited the same HLA haplotypes from their parents. Between such individuals, there is markedly prolonged skin graft survival, essentially 100 per cent long-term renal graft survival under immunosuppression, and the possibility of establishing chimerism following bone marrow transplantation without fatal GvH (graft versus host) disease. The reason why pairing for the HLA SD antigens in unrelated combinations does not have the same salutary effect can be discussed by considering our knowledge regarding the importance of LD factors.

The possibility that parts of the HLA chromosome (now called LD) genetically separable from the SD loci may play a role in MLC activation was first suggested in studies in man by Amos and Bach (1968) and Bach and colleagues (1969). It remained for Yunis and Amos (1971) and Eijsvoogel and collaborators (1972) to provide the convincing evidence for the existence of such HLA LD genes. It is much more difficult to evaluate the influence of MHC LD differences upon allograft phenomena in man. Sibling transplants are not useful because, in the vast majority of cases, identity for either SD (assayed serologically) or LD (assayed by MLC) will guarantee *both* SD and LD identity, since the HLA haplotype is inherited as a unit. This is not so in the case of unrelated individuals, because the same LD and SD antigens are not necessarily linked in the general population. Thus two unrelated subjects may inherit chromosomes which differ for LD, even though they determine the same SD antigens.

If we examine the data in unrelated pairs and limit ourselves to nonimmunized recipients, there is disagreement as to whether typing for the SD antigens significantly improves graft survival (Dausset and associates, 1974; Belzer and associates, 1974). Disparity for LD has only recently been evaluated in large series, although Hamburger and his colleagues (1971) have for some years pointed out an association between low MLC stimulation and improved kidney graft survival. Cochrum and associates (1973) found that low MLC stimulation (a stimulation index less than 8) was correlated with improved graft survival. These authors have extended their series, and most important, for reasons discussed below, their correlation·between LD disparity (MLC stimulation) and graft survival still obtains when they compare donor-recipient pairs in the two groups (those with "low" MLC stimulation indices and those with "higher" ones) who differ by the same number of SD antigens. Segall and coworkers (1975) have obtained similar preliminary data. Koch and coworkers (1972) have done skin grafts between unrelated individuals who are HLA SD-identical and have found a significant correlation between low or zero MLC activation and prolonged graft survival.

Could one critically make the argument, given the present data, that the importance of MHC disparity in graft survival in nonimmunized recipients may be solely due to LD differences? While we do not favor this conclusion in its entirety, it does offer a provocative argument for further studies. It has been demonstrated in man that there is linkage disequilibrium between the two SD loci and between the SD and LD loci A and B (Bach and van Rood, 1976). In the presence of linkage disequilibrium, an allele at one locus, say B, will be present on the same haplotype (chromosome) with a given allele of another locus, say LD-2, more frequently than predicted by chance alone, given the gene frequencies. To state this in another way, assuring donor-recipient HLA–B locus identity by SD typing will to a significant degree reduce LD-2 disparity by increasing the probability that donor and recipient share one or both LD-2 locus alleles. One could thus explain any beneficial effect of SD pairing for graft survival, if such does exist in unrelated pairs, by the argument that the SD identity per se is not important, but that pairing for SD actually reduces LD disparity secondary to linkage disequilibrium. The opposite argument, i.e., that any effect of LD matching is due to concomitant reduction in SD disparity, could also be made, except for two findings. First, there is the evidence that LD differences, with SD identity, can lead to allograft phenomena in mice, as noted earlier. Second, Cochrum's and van Rood's preliminary findings of correlations between LD disparity and graft survival are valid, even where there are equal numbers of SD differences in the LD-"mismatched" and LD-"matched" groups.

There is little question that the SD antigens are histocompatibility antigens. Their role, however, may be more or less important, depending on the transplant in question and the state of immunization of the recipient, as stressed by Bach and van Rood (1976). The successful bone marrow transplant in Copenhagen (Dupont and associates, 1973), in which donor and recipient showed HLA LD identity but extensive SD disparity, argues powerfully that, for some forms of transplantation, SD may be relatively unimportant.

Recent in vitro studies using MLC reactions to generate cytotoxic lymphocytes (Schendel and Bach, 1974) may provide some clues for understanding at least one role of the SD antigens and interplay between LD and SD. Effector cells generated in the MLC test are specifically cytotoxic to target cells obtained from the donor of the stimulating cells (Miggiano and associates, 1972). It appears from studies in man (Eijsvoogel and associates, 1972) and mouse (Schendel and Bach, 1974) that, whereas it is the LD differences which stimulate lymphocytes in MLC, these LD differences do not serve as a target for the cytotoxic lymphocytes. Rather, the SD antigens, or presumed cell surface products determined by genes very closely linked to those which determine the SD antigens (i.e., genes in the SD region), serve as a target. Further, the cytotoxic reaction against SD is significantly enhanced by the concomitant presence of an LD difference. At the present time, we do not understand what in vivo role there is for this "cytotoxic reaction aimed at SD components" and must remember that SD disparity is not essential for graft rejection.

What of the practicalities of assaying LD disparity? For kidney transplantation, the length of time required for the MLC assay is still too long for preoperative application, except in the case of living donors. However, an assay which takes only a few hours may be possible in the future. A better definition of the HLA–D genetic system may come from the attempts by several laboratories to use homozygous "typing cells" or the PLT test to define the LD alleles (Bach and van Rood, 1976). This might allow "LD matching" without actual mixing of the cells of donor and recipient, since the LD types of both subjects could then be determined. The most hopeful note comes from the preliminary findings of van Leeuwen, Schuit, and van Rood (1973), who suggest that the LD antigens may be serologically definable.

The evidence that the HLA system is the major histocompatibility complex in man, i.e., that it has an enormous import on graft survival, is commanding. Two components of HLA have been defined, LD and SD. The LD factors, since they are defined by allograft phenomena, are certainly of importance; it would seem most probable that the SD factors play a role in the rejection process, over and above their very likely importance in hyperacute rejection.

REFERENCES

Amos, D. B., and Bach, F. H.: Phenotypic expressions of the major histocompatibility locus in man (HL-A): Leukocyte antigens and mixed leukocyte culture reactivity. J. Exp. Med., *128*:623, 1968.

Amos, D. B., Gorer, P. A., and Mikulska, Z. B.: An analysis of an antigenic system in the mouse (the H-2 system). Proc. Roy. Soc. [B], *144*:369, 1955.

Askonsis, B. A., and Rhodes, J. M.: Immunogenicity of antigen-containing ribonucleic acid preparations from macrophages. Nature (Lond.), *205*:470, 1965.

Bach, F. H., and Hirschorn, K.: Lymphocyte interaction: A potential histocompatibility test in vitro. Science, *143*:813, 1964.

Bach, F. H., and van Rood, J. J.: The major histocompatibility complex—Its genetics and biology. New Engl. J. Med., *295*:806; 872; 927, 1976.

Bach, F. H., Albertini, R. H., Amos, D. B., Ceppellini, R., Mattiuz, P. L., and Miggiano, V. C.: Mixed leukocyte culture studies in families with known HL-A genotypes. Transplant Proc., *1*:339, 1969.

Bach, F. H., Widmer, M. B., Bach, M. L., and Klein, J.: Serologically defined and lymphocyte defined compo-

nents of the major histocompatibility complex in the mouse. J. Exp. Med., *136*:1430, 1972.

Bach, F. H., Sondel, P. M., Sheehy, M. J., Wank, R., Alter, B. J., and Bach, M. L.: The complexity of the HL-A system: A PLT analysis. *In* Kissmeyer-Nielson, F. (Ed.): Histocompatibility Testing 1975. Munksgaard, Copenhagen, 1975, p. 576.

Bach, F. H., Valentine, E. A., Alter, B. J., Svejgaard, A., and Thomsen, M.: Typing for HLA-D: Primed LD typing and homozygous typing cells. Tissue Antigens, *8*:151, 1976.

Bailey, D. W., Snell, G. D., and Cherry, M.: Complementation and serological analysis of a H-2 mutant. *In* Lengerova, A., and Vojtiskova, M. (Eds.): Proceedings of the Symposium on Immunogenetics of the H-2 System. Basel, S. Karger, 1971, p. 155.

Bain, B., Vas, M. R., and Lowenstein, L.: The mixed leukocyte reactions. Science, *145*:1315, 1964.

Baronio, G.: Degli Innesti Animati, Milan, 1804.

Basch, R. S., and Stetson, C. A., Jr.,: The relationship between hemagglutinogens and histocompatibility antigen in the mouse. Ann. N. Y. Acad. Sci., 97:83, 1962.

Bashford, E. F., Murray, J. A., and Haaland, M.: Resistance and susceptibility to inoculated cancer. Third Sci. Rep. Cancer Res. Fund, 1908, p. 359.

Belzer, F. O., Perkins, H. A., Fortmann, J. L., et al.: Is HL-A typing of clinical significance in cadaver renal transplantation? Lancet, *1*:774, 1974.

Bert, P.: Thèse pour le doctorat en médecine de la greffe animale. Paris, E. Martinet, 1863.

Billingham, R. E., Krohn, P. L., and Medawar, P. B.: Effect of cortisone on survival of skin homografts in rabbits. Br. Med. J., *1*:1157, 1951.

Billingham, R. E., Lampkin, G. H., Medawar, P. B., and Williams, H. L.: Tolerance to homografts, twin diagnosis, and the freemartin condition in cattle. Heredity, 6:201, 1952.

Billingham, R. E., Brent, L., Medawar, P. B., and Sparrow, E. M.: Quantitative studies in tissue transplantation immunity. I. The survival times of skin homografts exchanged between members of different inbred strains of mice. Proc. Roy. Soc. [B], *143*:43, 1954.

Billingham, R. E., Brent, L., and Medawar, P. B.: Quantitative studies on tissue transplantation immunity. III. Actively acquired tolerance. Philos. Trans. R. Soc. Lond. [Biol. Sci.], *239*:375, 1956.

Billingham, R. E., Silvers, W. K., and Wilson, D. B.: Further studies on adoptive transfer of sensitivity to skin homografts. J. Exp. Med., *118*:397, 1963.

Bitler, W. T., and Rossen, R. D.: Effects of corticosteroids on immunity in man. II. Alterations in serum protein components after methylprednisolone. Transplant. Proc., 5:1215, 1973.

Bloom, B. R.: Biological activities of lymphocyte products. *In* Lawrence, H. S., and Landy, M. (Eds.): Mediators of Cellular Immunity. New York, Academic Press, 1969, p. 253.

Bradley, B. A., Edwards, J. M., Dunn, D. C., and Calne, R. Y.: Quantitation of mixed lymphocyte reaction by gene dosage phenomenon. Nature New Biol., *240*:54, 1972.

Bradley, B. A., Sheehy, M. J., Keuning, J. J., Termijtelen, A., Franks, D., and van Rood, J. J.: The phenotyping of HLA–D region products by negative and positive mixed lymphocyte reactions. Immunogenetics, *3*:573, 1976.

Brown, J. B.: Homografting of skin. Report of success in identical twins. Surgery, *1*:559, 1937.

Brown, J. B., and McDowell, F.: Epithelial healing and

transplantation of skin. Ann. Surg., *115*:1166; 1177, 1942.

Brown, J. B., and McDowell, F.: Massive repairs of burns with thick split-skin grafts; emergency "dressings" with homografts. Ann. Surg., *115*:658, 1942.

Burnet, F. M.: The Clonal Selection Theory of Acquired Immunity. Nashville, Vanderbilt University Press, 1959.

Burnet, F. M., and Fenner, T.: Genetics and immunology. Heredity, *2*:289, 1948.

Byrt, P., and Ada, G. L.: An in vitro reaction between labelled flagellin or hemocyanin and lymphocyte-like cells from normal animals. Immunology, *17*:503, 1969.

Chutna, J.: Enhancement of skin homografts and dissociation of immune response in mice immunized with lyophelized tissues in Freund adjuvant. Nature (Lond.), *217*:175, 1968.

Cochrum, K. C., Davis, W. C., Kountz, S. L., and Fudenberg, H. H.: Renal rejection initiated by passive transfer of immune plasma. Transplant Proc., *1*:301, 1969.

Cochrum, K. C., Perkins, H., Payne, R., Kountz, S. L., and Belzer, F. O.: The correlation of MLC with graft survival. Transplant Proc.,5:391, 1973.

Converse, J. M., and Duchet, G.: Successful homologous skin grafting in a war burn using an identical twin as donor. Plast. Reconstr. Surg., *2*:342, 1947.

Converse, J. M., and Rapaport, F. T.: The vascularization of skin autografts and homografts. An experimental study in man. Ann. Surg., *143*:306, 1956.

Coombs, R. R. A., Feinstein, A., and Wilson, A. B.: Immunoglobulin determinants on the surface of human lymphocytes. Lancet, *2*:1157, 1969.

Cooper, M. D., Peterson, R. D. A., and Good, R. A.: Delineation of the thymic and bursal lymphoid system in the chicken. Nature (Lond.), *205*:143, 1965.

Dausset, J.: Iso leuco anticorps. Acta Haematol. (Basel), *20*:156, 1958.

Dausset, J., Hors, J., Festenstein H., et al.: Serologically defined HL-A antigens and longterm survival of cadaver kidney transplants. New Engl. J. Med., *290*:979, 1974.

Davies, D. A. L.: Mouse histocompatibility isoantigens derived from normal and from tumor cells. Immunology, *11*:115, 1966.

Davis, W. C., and Silverman, L.: Localization of mouse H-2 histocompatibility antigen with ferritin-labelled antibody. Transplantation, *6*:535, 1968.

Dumonde, D. C., Al-Askari, S., Lawrence, H. S., and Thomas, L.: Microsomal factors as transplantation antigens. Nature (Lond.), *198*:598, 1963.

Dupont, B., Andersen, V., Ernst, P., et al.: Immunologic reconstitution in severe combined immunodeficiency with HL-A incompatible bone marrow graft: Donor selection by mixed lymphocyte culture. Transplant Proc., *5*:905, 1973.

Dupont, B., Yunis, E. J., Hansen, J. A., Reinsmoen, N., Suciu–Foca, N., Michelson, E., and Amos, D. B.: Evidence for three genes involved in the expression of the mixed lymphocyte culture reaction. *In* Kissmeyer-Nielsen, F. (Ed.): Histocompatibility Testing 1975. Munksgaard, Copenhagen, 1975, p. 547.

Ehrlich, P.: Experimentelle Karzinomstudien an Mausen. Arb. Inst. Exp. Ther. Frankfurt, *1*:77, 1906.

Eijsvoogel, V. P., van Rood, J. J., du Toit, E. D., and Schellekens, P. T. A.: Position of a locus determining mixed lymphocyte reaction distinct from the known HL-A loci. Eur. J. Immunol., *2*:413, 1972.

Elkins, W., Kavathas, P., and Bach, F. H.: Activation of T cells by H-2 factors in the graft versus host reactions. Transplant Proc., *5*:1759, 1973.

Etheredge, E. D., Shons, A. R., Schmidtke, J. R., and

Najarian, J. S.: Mixed leukocyte culture reactivity and rejection in renal transplantation in HL-A identical siblings. Transplantation, *17*:537, 1974.

Feldman, M., and Gallily, R.: Cell interactions in the induction of antibody formation. *In* Frisch, L. (Ed.): Cold Spring Harbor Symposia on Quantitative Biology (Vol. XXXII, Antibodies). Cold Spring Harbor, Cold Spring Harbor Laboratory of Quantitative Biology, 1967, p. 415.

Ferrer, J. F.: Enhancement of the growth of sarcoma 180 in splenectomized and sham-operated AKR mice. Transplantation, 6:160, 1968.

Fishman, M., and Adler, F. L.: Antibody formation initiated in vitro. II. Antibody synthesis in x-irradiated recipients of diffusion chambers containing nucleic acid derived from macrophages incubated with antigen. J. Exp. Med., *117*:595, 1963.

Flexner, S.: The pathology of lymphotoxic and myelotoxic intoxication. Univ. Penn. Med. Bull., *15*:287, 1902.

Franklin, E. C., and Frangione, B.: Immunoglobulins. Ann. Rev. Med., *20*:155, 1969.

Gewurz, H., Wernick, P. R., Quie, P. G., and Good, R. A.: Effects of hydrocortisone succinate on the complement system. Nature (Lond.), *208*:755, 1965.

Gibson, T., and Medawar, P. B.: The fate of skin homografts in man. J. Anat., *77*:299, 1943.

Ginsburg, H., Ax, W., and Burke, G.: Graft reaction in tissue culture by normal rat lymphocytes. Transplant. Proc., *1*:551, 1969.

Glenn, E. M., Miller, W. L., and Schlagel, C. A.: Metabolic effects of adrenocortical steroids in vivo and in vitro: Relationship to anti-inflammatory effects. Recent Progr. Hormone Res., *19*:107, 1963.

Good, R. A., and Finstad, J.: The Gordon Wilson Lecture: The development and involution of the lymphoid system and immunologic capacity. Trans. Am. Clin. Climatol. Assoc., *79*:69, 1967.

Good, R. A., Gabrielson, A. E., Peterson, R. D. A., Finstad, J., and Cooper, M. D.: The development of the central and peripheral lymphoid tissues — Autogenetic and phylogenetic consideration. *In* Wolstenholme, G. E., and Porter, R. (Eds.): CIBA Foundation Symposium on Thymus and Autoimmune Disease. London, Churchill, 1966, p. 81.

Gorer, P. A.: Genetic and antigenic basis of tumor transplantation. J. Pathol. Bacteriol., *44*:691, 1937.

Govaerts, A.: Cellular antibodies in kidney homotransplantation. J. Immunol., *85*:516, 1960.

Gowans, J. L.: The fate of parental strain small lymphocytes in F1 hybrid rats. Ann. N. Y. Acad. Sci., *99*:432, 1962.

Gowans, J. L., McGregor, D. D., and Cowen, D. M.: The role of small lymphocytes in the rejection of homograft skin. *In* Wolstenholme, G. E., and Knoght, J. (Eds.): The Immunologically Competent Cell. Ciba Foundation Study Group No. 16, London. Boston, Little, Brown and Company, 1963, p. 20.

Greene, H. S. N.: Heterologous transplantation of mammalian tumors. I. The transfer of rabbit tumors to alien species. J. Exp. Med., *73*:461, 1941.

Greene, H. S. N.: The heterologous transplantation of mammalian tissues. Cancer Res., *3*:809, 1943.

Haefen, U. von, Shaipanich, T., Wren, S., Busch, G., Kim, J. P., and Wilson, R. E.: Immune responsiveness and active enhancement of rat renal allografts with soluble specific antigen. Transplant Proc., *5*:573, 1973.

Hamburger, J., Crosnier, J., Decamps, B., and Rowinska, D.: The value of present methodology used for selection of organ donors. Transplant Proc., *3*:260, 1971.

Häyry, P., Andersson, L. C., and Nordling, S.: Electrophoretic fractionation of mouse T and B lymphocytes. Efficiency of the method and purity of separated cells. Transplant. Proc., 5:87, 1973.

Hellström, K. E., and Hellström, I.: Immunological enhancement as studied by cell culture techniques. Annu. Rev. Microbiol., 24:373, 1970.

Hersh, E. M.: Immunosuppression by L-asparaginase and related enzymes. A review. Transplantation, 12:368, 1971.

Hirschberg, H., Kaakinen, A., and Thorsby, E.: Typing for HLA–D determinants. Comparison of typing results using homozygous stimulating cells and primed lymphocyte typing PLT. Tissue Antigens, 1976 (in press).

Holman, E.: Protein sensitization in iso skin grafting. Is the latter of practical value? Surg. Gynecol. Obstet., 38:100, 1924.

Interbitzen, T.: Histamine in allergic responses of the skin. *In* Shaffer, J. H., LoGrippe, G. A., and Chase, M. W. (Eds.): Mechanisms of Hypersensitivity. Boston, Little, Brown and Company, 1958, p. 493.

Irvin, G. L., Eustace, J. C., and Faber, J. L.: Enhancement activity of mouse immunoglobulin classes. J. Immunol., 99:1085, 1967.

Jensen, C. O.: Transplantation of mammary gland carcinoma in mice. Zentralbl. Bakteriol., 34:28, 1903.

Jørgensen, F., Lamm, L. U., and Kissmeyer–Nielsen, F.: Mixed lymphocyte cultures with inbred individuals: an approach to MLC typing. Tissue Antigens, 3:323, 1973.

Kandutsch, A. A.: Intracellular distribution and extraction of tumor homograft enhancing antigens. Cancer Res., 20:264, 1960.

Keuning, J. J., Termijtelen, A., Blussé van Oud Alblas, A., Gabb, B. W., D'Amaro, J., and van Rood, J. J.: LD (MLC) population and family studies in a Dutch population. *In* Kissmeyer–Nielsen, F. (Ed.): Histocompatibility Testing 1975. Munksgaard, Copenhagen, 1975, p. 533.

Klein, J.: The H-2 system: Past and present. Transplant. Proc., 5:11, 1973.

Koch, C. T., van den Tweel, J. G., van Rood, J. J., van Hooff, J. P., van Leeuwen, A., Frederiks, E., van der Steen, G., and Schippers, H. M. A.: The relative importance of matching for the MLC versus the HL-A loci in organ transplantation. *In* Dausset, J., and Colombani, J. (Eds.): Histocompatibility Testing. Copenhagen, Munksgaard, 1972, pp. 521–524.

Lawrence, H. S.: Transfer factor. *In* Lawrence, H. S., and Landy, M. (Eds.): Mediators of Cellular Immunity. New York, Academic Press, 1969, p. 145.

Lawrence, H. S.: Transfer factor in cellular immunity. Harvey Lectures Series 68. New York, Academic Press, 1974.

Lawrence, H. S., Rapaport, F. T., Converse, J. M., and Tillett, W. S.: Transfer of delayed hypersensitivity to skin homografts with leukocyte extracts in man. J. Clin. Invest., 39:185, 1960.

Lexer, E.: Ueber freie Transplantation. Arch. Klin. Chir., 95:827, 1911.

Lindquist, R. R., Guttmann, R. D., and Merrill, J. P.: Renal transplantation in the inbred rat. II. An immuno-histochemical study of acute allograft rejection. Am. J. Pathol., 52:531, 1968.

Livnat, S., Klein, J., and Bach, F. H.: Graft versus host reactions of strains of mice identical for H-2K and H-2D antigens. Nature [New Biol.], 243:42, 1973.

Loeb, L.: The Biological Basis of Individuality. Springfield, Charles C Thomas, Publisher, 1945.

Mackaness, G. B., and Blanden, R. V.: Cellular immunity. *In* Mudd, S. (Ed.): Infection, Agents and Host Reactions. Philadelphia, W. B. Saunders Company, 1969, p. 22.

Mattiuz, P., Ihde, D., Piazza, A., Ceppellini, R., and Bodmer, W. F.: New approaches to the population. Genetic and segregation analysis of the HLA System. *In* Terasaki, P. I. (Ed.): Histocompatibility Testing 1970. Monksgaard, Copenhagen, 1970, pp. 193–205.

McKenzie, I. F. C., and Whittingham, S.: Deposits of immunoglobulin and fibrin in human allografted kidneys. Lancet, 2:1313, 1968.

Medawar, P. B.: The behavior and fate of skin autografts and skin homografts in rabbits. J. Anat., 78:176, 1944.

Medawar, P. B.: Second study of behaviour and fate of skin homografts in rabbits. J. Anat., 79:157, 1945.

Medawar, P. B.: Immunity to homologous grafted skin. I. The suppression of cell division in grafts transplanted to immunized animals. Br. J. Exp. Pathol., 27:9, 1946a.

Medawar, P. B.: Immunity to homologous grafted skin. II. The relationship between the antigens of blood and skin. Br. J. Exp. Pathol., 27:15, 1946b.

Medawar, P. B.: Immunity to homologous grafted skin. III. The fate of skin homografts transplanted to the brain, to subcutaneous tissue, and to the anterior chamber of the eye. Brit. J. Exp. Pathol., 29:58, 1948.

Medawar, P. B.: Immunology of transplantation. Harvey Lect., 52:144, 1958.

Medawar, P. B.: Tolerance reconsidered—A critical survey. Transplant. Proc., 5:7, 1973.

Mempel, W., Grosse-Wilde, H., Baumann, P., Netzel, B., Steinhauer–Rosenthal, I., Scholz, S., Bertrams, J., and Albert, E. D.: Population genetics of the MLC response: typing for MLC determinants using homozygous and heterozygous reference cells. Transplant. Proc., 5:1529, 1973.

Metchnikoff, E.: Recherches sur l'influence de l'organisme sur les toxines. Ann. Inst. Pasteur, 13:737, 1899.

Miggiano, V. C., Bernoco, D., Lightbody, J. J., Trinchieri, G., and Ceppellini, R.: Cell-mediated lympholysis in vitro with normal lymphocytes as target, specificity and cross-reactivity of the test. Transplant. Proc., 4:231, 1972.

Mishell, R. I., and Dutton, R. W.: Immunization of dissociated spleen cell cultures from normal mice. J. Exp. Med., 125:423, 1967.

Mitchison, N. A., and Dube, O. L.: Studies on the immunological response to foreign tumor transplants in the mouse. II. The relation between hemagglutinating antibody and graft resistance in the normal mouse and mice pretreated with tissue preparations. J. Exp. Med., 102:179, 1955.

Möller, G.: Demonstration of mouse isoantigens at the cellular level by the fluorescent antibody technique. J. Exp. Med., 114:415, 1961.

Monaco, A. P., Wood, M. L., and Russell, P. S.: Some effects of purified heterologous anti-human lymphocyte serum in man. Transplantation, 5:1106, 1967.

Murphy, J. B.: Factors of resistance to heteroplastic tissue graftings. Studies in tissue specificity III. J. Exp. Med., 19:513, 1914.

Murphy, J. B., and Sturm, E.: Conditions determining the transplantability of tissue in the brain. J. Exp. Med., 38:183, 1923.

Murray, J. E.: Organ transplantation (skin, kidney, heart) and the plastic surgeon. Plast. Reconstr. Surg., 47:425, 1971.

Murray, J. E., Merrill, J. P., and Harrison, J. H.: Renal homotransplantation in identical twins. Surg. Forum, 6:432, 1955.

Najarian, J. S., and Simmon, R. L.: The clinical use of

antilymphocyte globulin. New Engl. J. Med., *285*:158, 1971.

Najarian, J. S., May, J., Cochrum, K. C., Baronberg, N., and Way, L. W.: Mechanism of antigen release from canine kidney homotransplants. N.Y. Acad. Sci., *129*:76, 1966.

Owen, R. D.: Immunogenetic consequences of vascular anastomoses between bovine twins. Science, *102*:400, 1945.

Padgett, E. C.: Is iso-skin grafting practicable? South. Med. J., *25*:895, 1932.

Parrot, D. M. V., deSoussa, M. A. B., and East, J.: Thymus dependent areas in the lymphoid organs of neonatally thymectomized mice. J. Exp. Med., *123*:191, 1966.

Patterson, W. B.: Transplantation of human cancers to hamster cheek pouches. Cancer Res., *28*:1637, 1968.

Peer, L. A., Transplantation of tissues. Cartilage, Bone, Fascia, Tendon and Muscles. Vols. I & II. Baltimore, The Williams & Wilkins Co., 1955, 1959.

Perey, D. Y., Cooper, M. D., and Good, R. A.: Normal second set wattle homograft rejection in agammaglobulinemic chickens. Transplantation, *5*:615, 1967.

Pernis, B., Forni, L., and Amante, L.: Immunoglobulin spots on the surface of rabbit lymphocytes. J. Exp. Med., *132*:1001, 1970.

Potter, M., Appella, E., and Geisser, S.: Variations in the heavy polypeptide chain structure of gamma myeloma immunoglobulins from an inbred strain of mice and a hypothesis as to their origin. J. Mol. Biol., *14*:561, 1975.

Putnam, F. W., Shinoda, T., Titani, K., and Wikler, M.: Immunoglobulin structure: variations in amino acid sequence and length of human lambda light chains. Science, *157*:1050, 1967.

Raju, S., and Grogan, J. B.: Immunology of the anterior chamber of the eye. Transplant. Proc., *3*:605, 1971.

Rapaport, F. T., and Converse, J. M.: Observations on immunological manifestations of the homograft rejection phenomenon in man: The recall flare. Ann. N. Y. Acad. Sci., *64*:836, 1957.

Rapaport, F. T., and Converse, J. M.: The immune response to multiple-set skin homografts. An experimental study in man. Ann. Surg., *147*:273, 1958.

Rapaport, F. T., Chase, R. M., Markowitz, A. S., McCluskey, R. T., Shimada, T., and Watanabe, K.: Cross-reactions in mammalian transplantation—with particular reference to streptococcal antigens and antibodies. Transplant. Proc., *3*:89, 1971.

Rapaport, F. T., Watanabe, K., Matsuyama, M., Cannon, F. D., Mollen, N., Blumenstock, D. A., and Ferrebee, J. W.: Induction of immunological tolerance to allogeneic tissues in the canine species. Ann. Surg., *176*:329, 1972.

Ratnoff, O. D.: Some relationships among hemostasis, fibrinolytic phenomena, immunity and the inflammatory response. Adv. Immunol., *10*:145, 1969.

Reisfeld, R. A., Pellegrino, M. A., Ferrone, S., and Kahan, B. D.: Chemical and molecular nature of HL-A antigens. Transplant Proc., *5*:447, 1973.

Rodey, G., Bortin, M. M., Bach, F. H., and Rimm, A. A.: Mixed leukocyte culture reactivity and chronic graft versus host reactions (secondary disease) between allogeneic H-2^k mouse strains. Transplantation, *17*:84, 1972.

Rogers, B. O.: Guide and bibliography for research into skin homograft problem. Plast. Reconstr. Surg., *7*:169, 1951.

Ruddy, S.: Chemistry and biologic activity of the complement system. Transplant Proc., *6*:1, 1974.

Russell, B. R. G.: The manifestation of active resistance to the growth of implanted cancer. Fifth Sci. Rep. Cancer Res. Fund, 1912, p. 1.

Schendel, D. J., and Bach, F. H.: Genetic control of cell-mediated lympholysis in mouse. J. Exp. Med., *140*:1534, 1974.

Schöne, G.: Ueber Transplantationsimmunität. Munch. Med. Wochenschr., *59*:457, 1912.

Schwartz, R. S., Stack, J., and Dameshek, W.: Effect of 6-MP on antibody production. Proc. Soc. Exp. Biol. Med., *99*:164, 1958.

Scothorne, R. J., and McGregor, I. A.: Cellular changes in lymph nodes and spleen following skin homografting in the rabbit. J. Anat., *89*:283, 1955.

Segall, M., Bach, F. H., Bach, M. L., Hussey, J. L., and Uehling, D.: Correlation of MLC stimulation and clinical course in kidney transplants. Transplant. Proc., *7*:41, 1975.

Sercarz, E., and Coons, A. H.: *In* Hasek, M., Lingeiova, A., and Vojtiskova, M. (Eds.): Mechanisms of Immunological Tolerance. New York, Academic Press, 1962, p. 73.

Shawan, H. K.: The principle of blood grouping applied to skin grafting. Am. J. Med. Sci., *157*:503, 1919.

Sheehy, M. J., Sondel, P. M., Bach, M. L., Wank, R., and Bach, F. H.: HL-A LD (lymphocyte defined) typing: A rapid assay with primed lymphocytes. Science, *188*:1308, 1975a.

Sheehy, M. J., Sondel, P. M., Bach, F. H., Sopori, M. L., and Bach, M. L.: Rapid detection of LD determinants: The PLT assay. *In* Kissmeyer–Nielsen, F. (Ed.): Histocompatibility Testing 1975. Munksgaard, Copenhagen, 1975b, p. 569.

Shimada, A., and Nathenson, S. G.: Murine histocompatibility-2 (H-2) alloantigens. Purification and some chemical properties of soluble products from H-2 genotypes released by papain digestion of membrane fractions. Biochemistry, *8*:4048, 1969.

Shons, A. R., Jetzer, T., and Najarian, J. S.: Prolongation of skin homograft survival by L-asparaginase. Transplantation, *10*:280, 1970.

Shons, A. R., Etheredge, E. E., and Najarian, J. S.: The effect of L-asparaginase in mixed leukocyte culture. Transplantation, *12*:85, 1971.

Shons, A. R., Moberg, A. W., and Najarian, J. S.: Xenotransplantation. *In* Najarian, J. S., and Simmons, R. L. (Eds.): Transplantation. Philadelphia, Lea and Febiger, 1972, p. 729.

Shons, A. R., Etheredge, E. E., and Najarian, J. S.: Mixed leukocyte response in human renal transplantation. Transplant Proc., *5*:330, 1973a.

Shons, A. R., Kromrey, C., and Najarian, J. S.: Xenogeneic mixed leukocyte response. Cell. Immunol., *6*:420, 1973b.

Singer, S. J., and Nicolson, G. L.: The fluid mosaic model of the structure of cell membranes. Science, *175*:720, 1972.

Snell, G. D., Counce, S., Smith, P., Dube, LeR., and Kelton, D.: A 5th chromosome histocompatibility locus identified in the mouse by tumor transplantation. Proc. Am. Assoc. Cancer Res., *2*:46, 1955.

Starzl, T. E., Groth, C. G., Putnam, C. W., Corman, J., Halgremson, C. G., Penn, I., Husberg, B., Gustafsson, A., Cascardo, W., Geis, P., and Iwatsuki, S.: Cyclophosphamide for clinical renal hepatic transplantation. Transplant. Proc., *5*:511, 1973.

Stender, H. S., Ringlieb, D., Strauch, D., and Winter, H.: Die Beeinflussung der Antikorperbildung durch Zytostatika und Röntgenbestrählung. Strahlentherapie, *43*:392, 1959.

Stuart, F. P., Saitoh, T., Fitch, F. W., and Spargo, B. H.: Immunological enhancement of renal allografts in the rat. Surgery, *64*:17, 1968.

Sybesma, J. P., Kater, L., Borst-Eilers, E., de Planque, B.

A., Van Soelen, T., and Tuit, G.: HL-A antigen in kidney tissue. Transplantation, *17*:576, 1974.

Taylor, A. C., and Lehrfeld, J. W.: Determination of survival time of skin homografts in rat by observation of vascular changes in graft. Plast. Reconstr. Surg., *12*:423, 1953.

Terasaki, P. I., Thrasher, D. L., and Hauber, T. H.: Stereotyping for homotransplantation. XIII. Immediate kidney transplant rejection and associated preformed antibodies. First International Congress on Transplantation Society, Paris, 27–30 June, 1967. J. Dausset (Ed.). Copenhagen, Munksgaard, 1968, pp. 225–229.

Thorsby, E., and Piazza, A.: Joint report from the Sixth International Histocompatibility Workshop Conference. II. Typing for HLA–D (LD-1 or MLC) determinants. *In* Kissmeyer–Nielsen, F. (Ed.): Histocompatibility Testing 1975. Munksgaard, Copenhagen, 1975, p. 414.

Van den Tweel, J. G., Blussé an Oud Alblas, A., Keuning, J. J., Goulmy, E., Termijtelen, A., Bach, M. L., and van Rood, J. J.,: Typing for MLC (LD). I. Lymphocytes from cousin marriages offspring as typing cells. Transplant. Proc., *5*:1535, 1973.

Van Leeuwen, A., Schuit, J. J., and van Rood, J. J.: Typing for MLC (LD). II. The selection of non-stimulator cells by MLC inhibition tests using SD identical stimulator cells (MISIS) and fluorescent antibody studies. Transplant. Proc., *5*:1539, 1973.

Van Rood, J. J., van Leeuwen, A., and Balner, H.: HL-A and CHL-A: Similarities and differences. Transplant. Proc., *4*:55, 1972.

Weissmann, G., and Thomas, L.: Studies on lysosomes. II. The effect of cortisone on the release of acid hydrolases from a large granule fraction of rabbit liver induced by an excess of vitamin A. J. Clin. Invest., *42*:661, 1963.

White A.: Influence of endocrine secretions on the structure and function of lymphoid tissue. Harvey Lect., *43*:43, 1948.

Williams, T. W., and Granger, G. A.: Lymphocyte in vitro cytotoxicity: Lymphotoxins of several mammalian species. Nature (Lond.), *219*:1076, 1968.

Woodruff, M. F. A., and Anderson, N.: Effect of lymphocyte depletion by thoracic duct fistula and administration of antilymphocyte serum on the survival of skin homograft in rats. Nature (Lond.), *200*:702, 1963.

Yunis, E. J., and Amos, D. B.: Three closely linked genetic systems relevant to transplantation. Proc. Natl. Acad. Sci. U. S. A., *68*:3031, 1971.

CHAPTER 6

TRANSPLANTATION OF SKIN: GRAFTS AND FLAPS

JOHN MARQUIS CONVERSE, M.D.,
JOSEPH G. MCCARTHY, M.D.,
RAYMOND O. BRAUER, M.D.,
AND DONALD L. BALLANTYNE, JR., PH.D.

Dermal Overgrafting
  Noel Thompson, F.R.C.S.
Reinnervation of Skin Transplants
  Joan M. Platt, M.D.

Transplantation of Hair-Bearing Scalp
  Jerome E. Adamson, M.D.

SKIN ANATOMY

Skin, or integument, envelops the entire surface of the body, and its epithelium is continuous with that of the digestive, respiratory, and urogenital systems. It is an indispensable organ inasmuch as its destruction is incompatible with survival. Skin serves as a barrier against the environment and is also the principal site of communication with the environment.

Skin plays an important role in regulating body temperature. Vasoconstriction of the skin capillaries reduces heat loss; vasodilation facilitates it. In addition, facultative heat loss occurs by evaporation of sweat. The entire cutaneous system can be considered a large glandular system (Montagna, 1962) because of the presence of holocrine (sebaceous) glands. Cells die as the epidermis is replaced, and keratin and sebum represent accumulations of these dead cells. The skin also contains many sensory nerve endings.

Skin is a compound organ. The two layers of the skin are derived from different embryonic layers and differ in character (Fig. 6–1). The outermost thinner layer is the epidermis; the innermost thicker layer is the dermis, which consists of connective tissue. The two layers are intimately connected by means of fine protoplasmic processes and elastic fibers which can be dissolved by a trypsin preparation (Medawar, 1941). The epidermis contains no blood vessels; the dermis, acting as the nutrient membrane of the epidermis, is thus indispensable. This relationship is well demonstrated by the fact that epithelial cells grown in sheets on tissue culture rarely survive permanently when transplanted back to the original donor.

152

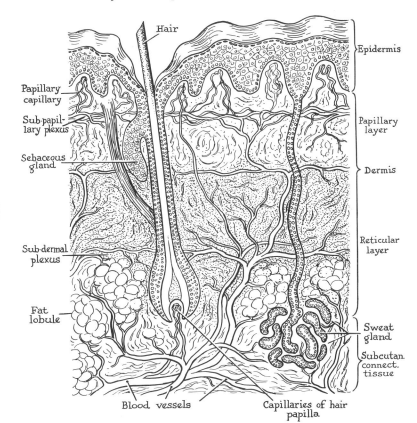

FIGURE 6–1. Section of human skin. (From Kazanjian and Converse.)

Epidermis

The epidermis is a stratified squamous epithelium that covers the entire surface of the body. It differentiates early, having been recognized by Medawar (1953) in a 12 week old human embryo. The epidermis is composed of living malpighian stratum which rests upon the dermis and a desquamating dead superficial layer known as the stratum corneum. The cells of the malpighian stratum are arranged in layers which are not clearly defined and which can probably be considered as separate steps in a continuous evolution from the basal to the outer cornified squamous layer. The basal layer, also called the stratum germinativum, is located adjacent to the dermis and its blood supply. In the stratum spinosum or prickle cell layer, which is superficial to the basal layer, the cells are larger and are joined by tiny fibrils known as tonofibrils. More superficially, the cytoplasm of the cells contains granules; the area is known as the stratum granulosum. The stratum lucidum, a clear band, separates this layer from the outer layer of the epidermis,

which is the cornified stratum corneum. All these layers can be demonstrated in the thick skin of the palms and soles; the epidermis is considerably thinner elsewhere. The stratum corneum and stratum germinativum are the only layers consistently present in all parts of the body.

Epidermis undergoes growth and replacement throughout life (Storey and Leblond, 1951). New cells produced by mitosis in the basal layer exert a pressure which results in movement of the cells to the surface (Flemming, 1884); extruded cells are transformed into a horny material which forms the keratinized layers. The keratinization may be soft, as in the skin, or hard, as in the nails or hair cortex. It has been calculated that the renewal time of the malpighian layer is about 19 days. Thus, each epidermal cell spends an average of 19 days in its migration to the surface. The epidermis shows topographic differences which are remarkably persistent after transplantation. In the experimental animal, when the epithelium of the foot pads is transplanted to regions where it is not subject to stress, it retains its characteristic features. The transparency of the epithelium of the cornea is not lost after transplantation to the chest wall in the guinea pig. As the characteristics of transplanted skin do not change, the matching of skin from other areas of the body with the skin of the face is always difficult.

Epidermal tissue is subjected to trauma more often than other tissues of the body. The epidermis usually withstands environmental trauma, such as periodic exposure to solar radiation, wide variations in temperature, cuts, scratches, burns, bacteria, and viruses. The insoluble and tough keratinized superficial layers of the epidermis protect the body from the environment. Keratin does not cover the soft, stratified squamous epithelium of the oral and nasal cavities.

Dermis

The dermis consists of two layers, a superficial or papillary layer and a deep or reticular layer.

The papillary layer, characteristic of man and less distinct in many mammals, contains widely separated, delicate, collagenous elastic and reticular fibers, enmeshed with capillaries and surrounded by ground substance.

The reticular layer is formed by dense, coarse, branching, collagenous fibers arranged in layers mostly parallel to the surface. Many fine furrows form a close network on the surface of facial skin. The small rhomboid ridges in which the orifices of the sweat glands are grouped, separated by fine grooves, depend on the arrangement of the dermal papillae in the dermis (Unna, 1883). The surface elevations are associated with the higher papillae and the furrows with the lower papillae.

Elastic tissue is distributed throughout the dermis and is closely interlaced in the reticular layer. The ground substance and interstitial fluid consist of extracellular fluid, derived largely from the blood plasma, and mucopolysaccharides, chiefly hyaluronic acid, chondroitin sulfates, and glycoproteins, in a varying degree of polymerization. The ground substance ordinarily has a gel-like consistency; the proportion of ground substance decreases with age, being replaced by fibrous intercellular tissue.

Connective tissue cells are sparsely distributed among the fibers. Fibroblasts are usually associated with mast cells. Pigment-bearing cells, melanocytes, are sparingly distributed in the dermis of normal skin.

Dermoepidermal Junction

The dermoepidermal junction of human skin appears as an irregularly wavy line; the ridges or rete pegs project into the dermis, enclosing between them the vascularized dermal papillae, as mentioned earlier in the chapter. The keratinocytes, keratin-producing cells of the epidermis, which comprise the majority of the epidermal cells, are attached to each other by desmosomes. Desmosomes are plaquettes of thickened cell membrane, each joined to the plaquette on the neighboring cell by three intermediary plaquettes seen by electronmicroscopy (Eriksson, 1972). The cells of the basal layer of the epidermis are attached to the basement membrane, a connective tissue layer, by half-desmosomes, so called because they have half the number of plaquettes. The basement membrane, on its dermal side, leads into a disorganized arrangement of "anchoring" fibrils (Braun-Falco, 1969).

Hair Follicles

Cells of the developing epidermis invade the dermis during embryonic development to form intradermal epithelial structures: the hair follicles, sebaceous glands, and sweat glands. These structures, principally the omnipresent sebaceous glands, are the source of an additional epidermal layer when the covering epidermis has been removed or destroyed, as in burns, abrasions, and donor areas of split-thickness skin grafts.

The downgrowth of epidermis into the underlying dermis begins early in the third month of fetal life. The fetus at about the sixth month has become covered with delicate hair (lanugo). This hair is shed before birth except in the eyebrows, eyelashes, and scalp, where it persists and becomes somewhat stronger. These hairs are replaced by coarser ones a few months after birth. A new hairy growth occurs over the rest of the body, covering it with a downy coat, the vellus. Coarse hair develops at puberty in the axilla, in the pubic region, and on the face in males and to a lesser extent on other parts of the body. A small bundle of smooth muscle fibers, the arrector pili, is attached to the connective tissue sheath of the hair follicle and extends upward to reach the papillary layer of the dermis near the mouth of the hair follicle. Muscle contraction pulls upon the hair follicle and acts upon the sebaceous glands, expressing an oily secretion (Hamilton, 1951).

In transplanted skin the growth of hair in an area which should be hairless creates problems. Hair grows according to hair growth characteristics in the donor site and is also known to grow in skin grafts transplanted from a hairless donor site.

The skin of the eyelids contains no hair follicles. Hairs do not grow vertically from the skin but assume a slanting direction. This fact merits consideration when hair is being transplanted for the reconstruction of an eyebrow; the incisions should be oblique in order to parallel the direction of the hair follicles.

Sebaceous Holocrine Glands

Most sebaceous glands are appendages of hair follicles and open inside the pilosebaceous canal (see Fig. 6–1). These racemose or saccular glands are generally found on the underside of the hair follicles, but away from the hairs on the lips, buccal mucosa, and lacrimal caruncles. Sebaceous glands are at their largest size and greatest density in the skin of the forehead, nose, and cheeks, where their density attains 400 to 900 per sq cm of skin surface; in other areas of the body there may be fewer than 100 per sq cm. The lobules of sebaceous glands are solid masses of cells which gradually become filled with fat granules and finally disintegrate, giving forth an oily secretion known as sebum, which provides a lubricant for the hair and keeps the skin supple, protects it against friction, and makes it more impervious to moisture.

Doupe and Sharp (1943) have shown that the secretion of the sebaceous glands is the end product of cellular disruption and, in contradistinction to the secretion of sweat glands, is not under control of the nervous system.

Sweat (Eccrine and Apocrine) Glands

Eccrine sweat glands are found over the general body surface of man except in the lips and some parts of the external genitalia; apocrine sweat glands tend to be concentrated in a number of areas, including the eyelids and axillae.

These are simple, tubular glands, usually coiled at the base of the dermis (see Fig. 6–1). The ducts of the sweat glands pass through the epidermis and open either at the sweat pores on the skin surface or above the opening of the sebaceous glands in the walls of the hair follicles.

The density and distribution of sweat glands vary in different parts of the body. There are two distinct types of eccrine glands: those located in the palms of the hands and soles of the feet, and those of the whole body surface. The former are phylogenetically older and respond to emotional and mental stress, while the latter, which are found in significant numbers only in man and higher primates, are concerned with temperature regulation. The apocrine glands which become active at puberty secrete continuously. This activity is varied by emotion and hormonal changes (menstruation, pregnancy). The secretions of eccrine glands are odorless, whereas those of the apocrine glands undergo bacterial decomposition and produce a characteristic odor.

Transplanted skin, temporarily severed from the nerve connections, lacks the lubrication normally supplied by the eccrine and apocrine glands and is therefore dry and more susceptible to injury. Bland creams, such as lanolin or coconut ointment, should be applied to grafted skin until reinnervation and function of the secreting glands are restored.

Hypodermis

Beneath the dermis is a fatty layer or panniculus adiposus. Deep to the fatty layer is a discontinuous flat sheet of muscle, the panniculus carnosus, the main vestigium of which in man is represented by the platysma of the cervical region. The area of junction of dermis and subcutaneous adipose tissue is irregular. Domes of fat, the columnae adiposae, project between the retinacula cutis into the lower layers of the dermis. Collagenous fiber bundles extend perpendicularly into the hypodermis and branch loosely to form the retinaculum cutis, which separates the lobules of fat. When sections of skin are cut in a plane parallel to the surface of the skin at the level of the junction between dermis and fat, the pattern is that of a collagen network, the fat protruding through the interspaces.

Many hair follicles, with their arrector pili muscles, are implanted into the summits of the fat domes, two or three to each dome. Most of the sweat glands are situated between the fat domes and the collagen bundles. They are usually placed at a deeper level than the hair follicles; in the bearded area of the male face, however, hair follicles are implanted into the subcutaneous fat below the level of junction with the dermis. The irregular line of junction between dermis and fat and the presence of deeply situated epidermal structures account for the epithelization which follows burns of the face in which the cutaneous layer is apparently destroyed.

The blood supply of the skin is discussed later in the chapter under Skin Flaps.

Skin Grafts

Skin is transplanted by completely detaching a portion of integument from its donor site and transferring it to a host bed, where it acquires a new blood supply to ensure the viability of the transplanted cells. Such a method of transplantation is known as *skin grafting*. Another method of transplanting skin is by the skin flap. A *flap* consists of a portion of skin and subcutaneous tissue which is raised from the donor site; the flap is left attached to the surrounding skin by a vascular pedicle. The vascular supply maintained through the pedicle en-

sures the viability of the flap until it acquires a new blood supply from the host bed.

A skin graft consists of epidermis and dermis, the dermal component comprising either the entire thickness or only a portion of the dermis (Fig. 6–2); thus skin grafts can be either full-thickness or split-thickness. A skin autograft (autogenous graft) is a graft transferred from a donor to a recipient site in the same animal; an allograft (homograft) is a transplant between genetically disparate individuals of the same species; a xenograft (heterograft) is a graft transplanted between individuals of different species. The term "isograft" is a term employed in experimental transplantation to designate an allograft between highly inbred (genetically pure) strains of animals.

Although Bünger in 1823 had applied a skin graft from the thigh to the nose and Baronio (1804) had previously performed experimental skin grafts in sheep, the clinical importance of skin grafting was not appreciated until the latter part of the 19th century (see Chapter 1, p. 9).

The first split-thickness grafts used clinically were of the thin split-thickness type. Ollier

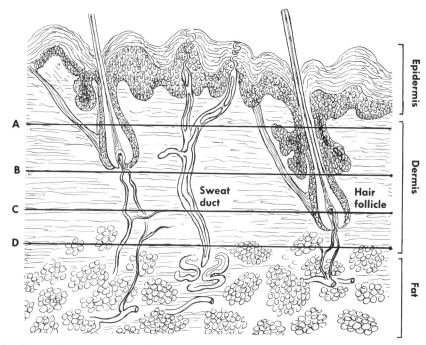

FIGURE 6–2. Schematic representation of a section of the skin to illustrate the comparative thickness of skin grafts. *A*, Line of section of the thin split-thickness (Thiersch) graft. *B*, Line of section of the split-thickness graft. *C*, Line of section of the thick split-thickness or three-quarter thickness graft. *D*, Line of section of the full-thickness graft. Note that the junction between the dermis and the subcutaneous tissue is irregular. The protrusions of the subcutaneous fat into the dermis are known as the columnae adiposae.

(1872) appears to have been one of the first surgeons who appreciated the importance of the dermal component of the graft, as he opposed the term *epidermic* graft employed by Reverdin and suggested the term *dermoepidermic* graft; Thiersch (1874) extended the size of the dermoepidermic graft, using large sheets of thin split-thickness grafts to cover wounds. The clinical importance of the thicker split-thickness graft was first emphasized over 50 years later by Blair and Brown (1929), who described the removal of thicker (intermediate) split-thickness skin grafts. The introduction by Padgett (1939) of the dermatome, a mechanical means of removing calibrated skin grafts, and the subsequent development of other mechanical devices have facilitated the removal of skin grafts of varying thickness.

The full-thickness graft, comprising the entire thickness of the dermis as well as the epidermis, was employed by Lawson (1870), Le Fort (1872) and Wolfe (1875) for the correction of eyelid ectropion; Krause in 1893 reported in detail his technique for full-thickness skin grafting. The full-thickness graft is often designated as a Wolfe graft in the English-speaking world.

Prior to describing the technique of removal of skin grafts and their clinical applications, the revascularization and mode of survival (or "take," a common clinical term), which are permanent in autografting and temporary in allografting, will be reviewed. The fate of xenografts will also be considered separately.

Vascularization of Skin Grafts, Autografts, and Allografts

The biologic fate of skin grafts has intrigued clinicians and researchers since the technique was first employed.

Transplantation of living tissues involves the surgical removal of viable cells from a donor area and subsequent transfer to a recipient site. Whether or not the transplanted cells survive and propagate a lineage of living cells in the recipient site depends on the following factors: (1) the accessibility of nutritive materials; (2) the resources for disposing of metabolic waste products; (3) the anatomic distinction between the tissue of the donor and recipient; and (4) the taxonomic and immunogenetic relationships between the donor and recipient.

Because of its accessibility, skin has enjoyed considerable study as a transplantation model. The mode of vascularization and subsequent vascular changes during the life span of grafted tissue have been extensively investigated. Much of the basic understanding of the biological laws of tissue transplantation has been derived primarily from the study of skin grafts.

At the time of surgical excision from its donor area, a graft of skin is completely severed from the surrounding skin and subjacent connective tissue layer; the circulation, lymphatic drainage, and nerve continuity are abruptly terminated.

It is recognized that the survival of a skin graft is dependent on rapidly acquiring a blood supply adequate for nutrition and for the disposal of metabolic waste products. In the time interval between transplantation and the process of revascularization, survival of the anoxic graft cells appears to be ensured by the absorption of fluids from the host (Converse and co-workers, 1957, 1969). The process of imbibition of exudate from the host bed, first noted by Hübscher in 1888 and Goldmann in 1890 and termed by them "Die Plasmatische Zirkulation" (plasmatic circulation), appears to play an important role in assuring an interim period of nourishment before the establishment of a definitive vasculature; it is not capable, however, of indefinitely maintaining the survival of a skin graft which fails to become successfully vascularized.

The mode of vascularization of skin grafts is still a subject of legitimate debate. Revascularization of skin grafts has been attributed to one or a combination of three processes: (1) direct connection of the graft and host vessels, referred to as "inosculation"; (2) ingrowth of host vessels into the endothelial channels of the graft; and (3) penetration of the host vessels into the graft dermis, creating new endothelial channels. The available data supporting the roles of the three processes in the revascularization of various types of skin transplants will be reviewed.

From a technical standpoint, the conditions necessary for the success of a skin graft are (1) a favorable and well-vascularized host bed; (2) rapid serum imbibition occurring soon after grafting; (3) adequate immobilization of the skin graft on the host site to assure the exchange of nutrient fluids and to reduce to a minimum any tendency to disrupt newly formed, delicate, vascular communications between the donor and host; and (4) rapid vascularization from the recipient site.

The Phases of Skin Graft Survival

The Phase of Serum Imbibition. Hübscher (1888) and Goldmann (1890) suggested that Thiersch grafts in human patients were nourished by fluid from the host prior to the establishment of new vascular and lymphatic channels in the graft. They termed this early process of fluid nourishment the "plasmatic circulation" of a graft.

Using a modification of the Algire tissue chamber technique for evaluating skin grafts in mice, Conway, Stark, and Joslin (1951) observed profuse flow of extracellular fluids from the surrounding area of the host into the transparent chamber during the first 24 hours. They stressed the importance of early plasmatic circulation, by which the grafts were able to be sustained during the first postoperative week.

Observations by Converse, Ballantyne, Rogers, and Raisbeck (1957) on a series of skin xenografts removed from the rabbit and placed upon the chorioallantois of the chick embryo indicated a rapid fluid uptake in the graft. The rabbit skin grafts were removed from the surface of the chorioallantoic membrane at time intervals varying from one to 20 postoperative hours. These grafts were weighed prior to transplantation and again after their removal by traction from the membrane. A progressive weight increase with ensuing time was observed in 165 grafts; the average increase in graft weight, which was 10 per cent after one hour, progressed steadily to 38.2 per cent after 10 hours and to 52 per cent after 20 hours. It has been suggested that skin grafts are capable of absorbing fluid from the host bed because of the spongelike structure of their dermis, which is canalized by innumerable endothelial spaces in addition to the self-contained lumina of blood vessels and lymphatics.

Most investigators have generally accepted Hübscher's original concept of the plasmatic circulation as an important factor in the early nourishment of skin grafts before the restoration of an adequate blood supply. However, Clemmesen (1962) believed that the main role of the plasmatic circulation is not nutritional. He felt it serves to prevent desiccation of the graft and to keep the graft vessels patent. Henry, Marshall, Friedman, Dammin, and Merrill (1962), working with human skin grafts, reported that the donor skin derives its nutrition and oxygenation from the process of plasmatic circulation for the first two postoperative days. Thereafter, this type of nourishment is inadequate for maintaining the viability of full-thickness grafts unless it is supplemented by an adequate vascular supply.

BIOCHEMICAL STUDIES. In several series of experimental studies involving biochemical determinations of skin autografts in the rat, Marckmann and Zachariae (1964) and Marckmann (1965a,b, 1967) attempted to explain the response of graft dermis to injury from the transplantation procedure. During the first five critical days, the reaction of a graft to surgical trauma is reflected by edema and changes in the metabolic activity of sulfomucopolysaccharides and in the levels of hexosamine, hydroxyproline, uronic acid, and histamine. The authors assumed that the biochemical alterations in the graft are associated in part with the reduced blood supply and accompanying changes in the metabolic equilibrium.

Psillakis and his colleagues (1969), after transplanting auricular skin autografts in rabbits, measured the water and electrolyte composition in the graft during the first five days. The findings indicated a significant increase in water content on the first day, lasting until the fifth day, whereas the sodium concentration, already significantly increased on the first day, showed a subsequent progressive diminution. By contrast, potassium content was significantly reduced during the first two postoperative days but increased considerably over the subsequent three days. The authors attributed the edema in the graft to the changes in the water and electrolyte levels which were reflected by the response of collagen to grafting injury, a finding similar

to that noted in traumatized tissues. As a consequence of injury, the graft dermis is rich in extracellular macromolecules capable of absorbing water and cations from the recipient site without direct vascular continuity with the host blood supply.

STUDIES BY VITAL MICROSCOPY THROUGH A TRANSPARENT CHAMBER AND MICROANGIOGRAPHY. Birch and Brånemark (1969), using full-thickness scrotal skin autografts placed on the perichondrial recipient bed of an auricle in rabbits, which they studied through a transparent ear chamber by vital microscopy, observed graft edema immediately after grafting. The edema attained its maximum on the third postoperative day. The authors attributed the edema to ground substance depolymerization in the graft dermis, to the absorption of tissue fluids into the graft extracellular compartments, and to the increased capillary pressure and the permeability in the inflamed host bed. The gradual subsidence of the graft edema is due to the improved hemodynamics which result from the reestablishment of the blood and lymphatic circulation. In a rabbit study using the same transplantation model as well as microangiography, Birch, Brånemark, and Lundskog (1969a) reached similar conclusions concerning the graft edema.

STUDIES IN EXPERIMENTAL ORTHOTOPIC GRAFTS. A study of plasmatic circulation under experimental conditions more closely approximating the events occurring in orthotopic grafting was undertaken by Converse, Uhlschmid, and Ballantyne (1969) in the rat. They found a 37.34 per cent weight gain in full-thickness autografts at 24 postoperative hours, followed by a drop in the relative weight increase to 25.69 per cent by 48 hours. After this drop, the average weight gain increased gradually to 30.44 per cent by the 96th hour and then steadily returned to its original weight by nine days. The authors suggested that the rise in weight between 48 and 72 hours coincides with the development of a stereomicroscopically visible blood circulation in the grafts. This gain in weight has been attributed to the filling of the graft vascular system and to the inadequate venous and lymphatic drainage, probably the product of engorgement and interstitial edema. With improved venous drainage subsequent to the establishment of an arterial and venous network, the graft attains its original weight by the eighth to ninth day following transplantation. The minus values noticed on the eleventh day may well be attributed to improved venous and lymphatic drainage. The graft is first fixed to the host site by fibrin; thus the fluid penetrating the graft is serum, not plasma. Consequently it was proposed that the term "plasmatic circulation" be replaced by the term "phase of serum imbibition."

STUDIES BY INTRAVENOUS COLLOIDAL CARBON SUSPENSION. Kikuchi and Omori (1970) injected an intravenous colloidal carbon suspension into rabbits at varying time intervals after full-thickness skin autografting. They reported that, during the first two days after grafting, the principal plasma leakage originates from the venules of the graft bed, although capillaries, terminal arterioles, and metarterioles are also leaking. This phenomenon at the graft-host junction has been correlated with the phase of the so-called plasmatic circulation. However, on the third day a different pattern of carbon labeling, being more faint or even absent, appeared and possibly reflected the phase of graft revascularization.

COLOR CHANGES IN THE SKIN GRAFT. The graft when excised from the donor becomes chalk white and blanched. Within a few hours after transplantation it assumes a pinkish hue, which progresses to a bright pink color during the following days. Douglas (1944) noted a faint pink tint in the graft as early as eight hours after grafting. McLaughlin (1954), studying the color changes in a composite graft of cartilage and skin which had been transferred from the ear to reconstruct the border of a nostril, described a change from blanched white to a more harmonious cutaneous coloration within six hours after grafting. Hynes (1954) observed that the blood vessels in a freshly cut human skin graft of a thickness varying from split-thickness to full-thickness are collapsed and empty. The graft vessels, probably as the result of separation from the donor site, undergo spasm and expel most of the formed hemic elements through the severed ends of the vessels on the graft undersurface. Within 24 hours after transplantation, the graft vessels are again dilated, although they contain only a few hemic elements. By 48 hours, the vessels are more distended and contain large numbers of erythrocytes. According to Hynes (1954), the exudate which accumulates at the line of demarcation between the graft and host tissues consists of plasma, erythrocytes, and polymorphonuclear leukocytes. This fluid exudate, after precipitating its fibrinogen in the form of fibrin on the surface of the host site, penetrates the overlying graft vessels as a fibrinogen-free suspension of erythrocytes, thereby nourishing the grafts and explaining the rapid color change which occurs within hours after transplantation.

SUMMARY OF THE PHASE OF SERUM IMBIBITION. The "phase of serum imbibition" may be described, therefore, as a period during which the graft vessels fill with a fibrinogen-free fluid and cells from the host bed. The term "circulation" is actually a misnomer, because the fluid absorbed by the graft from the host bed is passively trapped within the graft. Endothelial ingrowth from the host progresses until a definitive vasculature is established. The stagnant fluid absorbed by the graft during the early phase of serum imbibition is apparently drained off by the newly established blood and lymphatic circulation. Clinically, skin grafts in man usually appear edematous and their surfaces are elevated above the surrounding host skin during the early postoperative period. Within a few days after grafting, however, the graft flattens and edema subsides. This phenomenon reflects the establishment of a plasmatic and hemic flow and the evacuation of the fluid initially trapped in the graft.

The Phase of Graft Revascularization—Autografts and Allografts. Controversy has arisen over the method of graft acceptance and the mode of graft vascularization. Several research techniques have been developed to study the physiology of graft acceptance and vascularization. These have included gross and stereomicroscopic observations of the graft in situ; histologic and histochemical analyses of skin biopsy specimens; in vivo transparent chambers and microangiography; and the injection of dyes or radioactive isotopes into the vascular system of the recipient animals. However, an ideal in vivo method of studying these processes still does not exist; this fact partially explains the persistent controversies surrounding the exact mode of revascularization.

Bert in 1865 first noted an early connection between the blood vessels of the graft and host and employed the term "abouchement" to illustrate the mouth-to-mouth apposition of the vessels. In 1874 Thiersch, studying the histologic sections of experimental full-thickness skin grafts in man, used the term "inosculation" to signify the direct connection between the graft and host vessels.

Garré (1889), studying human skin grafts, reported evidence of endothelial mitosis in the host bed 5½ hours after grafting, inflammatory cells in the grafts by nine hours, and active invasion of wandering white cells into the donor vessels at 11 hours. He discounted the importance of the inosculatory process and described actual invasion of the graft by host capillary buds, which commenced on the third or fourth day, after most of the original graft vessels had become obliterated. Garré's conclusions coincided with those of Hübscher (1888), and a similar opinion was expressed by Goldmann (1890). Jungengel (1891) and Enderlen (1897) maintained that most of the preexisting graft vessels degenerated, but that some of the endothelial cells were able to survive and form new vessels which eventually connected with the ingrowing host vessels.

Braun (1899) assumed that graft revascularization was achieved by a dual process of ingrowth of host vessels and anastomoses between the host and original graft vasculature. Henle (1899), after injecting various dyes into rabbit recipients of full-thickness grafts, arrived at conclusions similar to those expressed by Garré (1889), i.e., early evidence of endothelial mitosis followed by rapid capillary ingrowth from the recipient site. An extensive vascular network in the donor skin was reconstituted without the cooperation of the original graft vessels, which rapidly underwent degenerative changes. Henle (1899) felt that in time some of the invading host capillaries may penetrate and grow along the channels formed by the necrosed original graft vessels.

Most of the pioneer studies on the origin and development of the blood supply in skin grafts have been derived from experiments on split-thickness grafts during the years 1888 to 1897 (Enderlen, 1897; Garré, 1889; Goldmann, 1890; Hübscher, 1888; Jungengel, 1891). Subsequently there have been many reports concerning the process of vascularization in transplanted skin, but *no serious efforts* were made to study the nature of vascularization in skin of varying thicknesses.

In 1925 Davis and Traut, using intracardiac injections of China ink in dogs, described the anastomosis of graft and host vessels, which began as early as 22 hours and persisted up to 72 hours after application of the graft. They also stressed subsequent host capillary growth, occurring by the fourth day, and concluded it was the decisive factor involved in establishing the definitive vascular system of the graft. Mir y Mir (1951), experimenting with postmortem dye injection into the aorta, considered the thickness of skin grafts in dogs an important factor controlling the mode of vascularization; according to Mir y Mir the restoration of blood supply in the thin split-thickness grafts is achieved mainly by the establishment of direct vascular continuity between the respective vessels of the graft and host. The sequence of vascular changes in full-thickness skin grafts, as reported by Mir y Mir (1951), parallel those of Davis and Traut (1925), in which the vitality of such grafts is initially assured by the direct vascular connections between the two tissues, followed, in turn, by extensive host vascular ingrowth. From his classic study, Medawar (1944) observed that the revascularization of skin grafts in the rabbit was achieved four days after grafting by the ingrowth of capillaries from the host bed; the original graft vessels, which he designated as "wound vessels," disappeared between the fourth and eighth postoperative days.

Peer and Walker (1951) believed that the restoration of the circulation in skin grafts is achieved mainly by direct connection between the severed ends of the blood vessels in the graft and host tissues and stressed the importance of the early processes of vascular anastomosis for survival of the centrally located cells in the grafted tissue.

Conway, Stark, and Joslin (1951), using a transparent tissue chamber, found that the vascularization of skin *autografts* in the mouse was achieved by capillary budding in the host site and by subsequent vascular ingrowth of capillary sprouts into the grafts. In 1952 Conway, Joslin, Rees, and Stark, using a similar mouse chamber technique, and

Ham (1952), who injected pigs with India ink suspensions, stated that skin *allografts* did not become vascularized, offering this finding as an explanation of allograft rejection. However, Taylor and Lehrfeld (1953), by means of the direct skin stereomicroscopic method, found that allografts in rats were successfully vascularized prior to the rejection reaction; their findings that autografts and allografts were both vascularized have been confirmed in man by Converse and Rapaport (1956). These findings are consistent with the histologic evidence of the vascularization of skin allografts in man, as reported by Gibson and Medawar (1942) and McGregor (1955a,b). After injecting India ink or bromophenol blue into the circulatory system of rabbits, Scothorne and McGregor (1953) cited evidence of vascularization in allografts, but did not specify the actual mode. Following the criticism of Scothorne and McGregor (1953) and of Taylor and Lehrfeld (1953), Conway, Griffith, Shannon, and Findley (1957) and Conway, Sedar, and Shannon (1957) modified their transparent apparatus technique and described evidence of active blood circulation in murine skin allografts.

THE REVASCULARIZATION OF SKIN GRAFTS IN MAN. The technique for observing cutaneous blood vessels in vivo was described by Lombard in 1911 and developed by Lewis in 1927.

The stereomicroscopic technique for the direct observation of the vascularization of grafts was modified for experimental studies in man by Converse and Rapaport (1956). The stereomicroscopic appearance of autografts and allografts has been fully described, with particular attention to vascular changes, by Taylor and Lehrfeld (1955) in the rat and by Converse and Rapaport (1956) in man. These changes may be summarized as follows: immediately after application to the recipient bed and during the subsequent 24 hours, the blood vessels of the grafts appear less filled with blood and are not readily detected when compared with those in the neighboring recipient areas. On the day after grafting, many vessels in the donor tissue show early evidence of distention and rapid filling with static blood. On the second day vessel distention continues, but blood circulation has not commenced. A sluggish flow of blood occurs in the graft vasculature on the third or fourth day and continues to improve until the fifth or sixth day. During the subsequent days, a return of all blood vessels to normal caliber and circulation occurs in all *autografts*.

In *allografts*, the similarity persists only until the onset of the allograft rejection. This is heralded by increased distention in the vascular system, followed by sluggish circulation with clumped elements. Complete cessation of blood flow and vascular disruption in most skin allografts usually occur between seven to ten postoperative days. The direct observation of the vessels in skin transplants by means of a dissecting microscope, as practiced by Converse and Rapaport (1956), has also been used by Ceppellini and associates (1966) for assessing vascularization and survival end-points of human skin grafts. While the use of skin stereomicroscopy is a useful tool for determining changes in the appearance and state of blood circulation in the grafted tissue from the time of transplantation to the rejection reaction, the direct method is not adequate for defining the actual source of vascular supply and the mode of vascularization in various types of skin grafts.

HISTOLOGIC STUDIES. Henry and coworkers (1961, 1962), following their histologic studies in humans, attributed the vascularization of auto- and allografts of skin to the "inosculation" of the patent original capillaries in the deeper layers of the graft dermis with the capillary loops from the host bed. As a consequence of even a few initial vascular connections, the superficial graft capillaries, whose endothelial linings have degenerated during the first few postoperative days, are supplied with blood and become dilated. The authors infer that this feature persists until the superficial channels are reconstituted by endothelial cells growing along the existing vessels. Their histologic study showed no vascular connections between the donor and host skin for two days following transplantation; during this time, the superficial capillaries in the graft collapse and the endothelial cells degenerate, leaving the basement membrane intact. While the graft vascular system appears dilated and engorged with static blood by the second or third postoperative day, the superficial vessels continue to demonstrate an intact basement membrane, with the endothelial nuclei either pyknotic or entirely absent; in the meantime the original vessels located in the deep dermal layers of the graft seem histologically patent. The process of graft vascularization is completed on the sixth or seventh day.

FURTHER EXPERIMENTAL STUDIES. A modification of the Algire transparent chamber was developed by Edgerton and Edgerton (1955) to evaluate the vascular activity of mouse skin grafts. Their findings are somewhat similar to those recorded by Taylor and Lehrfeld (1953) and Converse and Rapaport (1956). In the chamber, Edgerton and Edgerton (1955) noted vigorous vascular ingrowth from the host to the graft as early as the second or third day, filling the original graft vascular system with static blood. During the ensuing time, flow velocity, which is sluggish soon after the establishment of some vascular connections between the host and graft, progressively increases to a normal rate after the third or fourth postoperative day. They concluded that the vascular continuity between the original graft vessels and host vessels plays an important role in the establishment of a definitive vasculature with active circulation in the graft. A similar opinion was expressed by Kamrin (1960, 1961), who held that, in rat auto- and allografts, the ingrowth of capillary buds from the recipient site achieves contact with the original graft vessels by the end of the fourth day or the beginning of the next day, as evidenced by the histologic appearance of sudden emptying of the crenated (deformed) erythrocytes from the clotted graft vascular system and their subsequent replacement by normal host cellular blood elements.

In a previous study by Egdahl, Good, and Varco (1957), attention was called to the disappearance of intradermally injected fluorescein during the early stages of vascularization in 50 free full-thickness rat allografts. These workers found the disappearance of intradermal fluorescein as early as 12 hours prior to the onset of blood circulation, as shown by the direct skin stereomicroscopic method of Taylor and Lehrfeld (1953). "The removal of fluorescein test" and the capacity to develop localized Shwartzman reactions in first set allografts are considered as strong evidence of successful vascularization via direct connections between the vessels of the graft and those of the recipient. Castermans (1957), who applied vital microscopic methods to skin autografts and allografts in mice, obtained results somewhat similar to those previously reported. As seen by Castermans (1957), the graft capillaries commence to fill with formed hemic elements and dilate as early as 24 hours after grafting, followed by initial blood flow at 48 hours; at six or seven postoperative days the capillary network is well developed and functional, although still distended.

In an attempt to evaluate the source of blood supply in the autologous and allogeneic transplants of mouse and rat skin, Rolle, Taylor, and Charipper (1959) utilized a combination of four criteria: direct skin microscopy, routine histologic methods, cardiac injections of India ink suspensions into the vascular system, and intravenous injections of a diffusible dye, bromophenol blue. In all grafts studied many of the graft vessels, empty at the time of removal from the donor, begin to acquire stagnant blood and appear distended by the end of 24 hours after surgery. At three days, the blood circulation within the graft vasculature is restored and resumes the normal velocity of blood flow the following day; there is no histologic evidence of degenerative changes in the original graft vessels. Rolle and her coworkers (1959), as well as Hildeman and Haas (1960), concluded that the definitive vasculature in the graft capable of supporting an active circulation appears to depend on the establishment of direct vascular continuity between the host and graft, not on the ingrowth of newly formed vessels from the host.

A combined stereomicroangiographic and histologic method used at varying time intervals after transplantation was undertaken by Ljungqvist and Almgård (1966) to determine the vascular changes in skin auto- and allografts placed on the auricles of rabbits. The results indicated that the ingrowth of precapillary and capillary vessels from the underlying host bed, first noted at two postoperative days, invades the graft and extends in a perpendicular and spiral fashion toward the dermoepidermal surface, replacing the degenerated graft vessels. Such ingrowing vessels form the definitive vasculature of the graft. While there is some evidence of direct connection between the graft and host blood systems, the degenerative changes with thrombosis in the preexisting graft vessels suggest the *minor* and *temporary* role of these vascular connections.

HISTOCHEMICAL STUDIES. Until 1961, relatively few histochemical methods (Scothorne and Tough, 1952; Scothorne and Scothorne, 1953; Thompson, 1962; Russell and Monaco, 1965) had been employed to evaluate the metabolic changes occurring in skin transplants, and no efforts were expended to define the vascular pattern of grafts. In order to study the problem under experimental conditions that more closely approximated the events occurring in orthotopic grafting, skin autografts and allografts placed on mammalian recipients were studied by Converse and Ballantyne (1962), using an enzyme-histochemical method.

The reagents employed, neotetrazolium chloride (NT) and reduced diphosphopyridine nucleotide (DPNH), indicate the presence of DPNH dehydrogenase (diaphorase) in fresh frozen sections (Antopol and coworkers, 1950). Histochemical sections of full-thickness skin autografts and allografts in rats have shown that the ingrowth of host capillaries into a skin transplant is essential for the establishment of the definitive vasculature of the graft. The structural differences between the preexisting graft and new host blood vessels permit identification of the two types of vasculature. The process of graft revascularization by the host is very rapid; the host capillaries have penetrated through the demarcation line into the graft dermis by 12 hours and reach the dermoepidermal junction by 48 hours. The data in this study also indicate a progressive decline of enzymatic activity, accompanied by degenerative changes, in the original graft vasculature during the first four days after grafting. In contrast to the vasculature of the surrounding host tissue, the vascular pattern in the graft has changed. The vessels are numerous, exhibit greater ramification and distention, and show a purposeful and parallel ingrowth in a perpendicular direction from the recipient bed to the dermoepidermal junction of the graft. The new vasculature progressively resumes a finer pattern during the following days. These findings appear to corroborate the stereomicroscopic observations of a progressive distention of the vessels and an increase in their number during the first few postoperative days (Taylor and Lehrfeld, 1953; Converse and Rapaport,

1956; Ballantyne and Converse, 1957). The dilated vessels resume a fine caliber and become less numerous during the ensuing days. For the first six postoperative days, the vascular changes associated with revascularization by the host in both the full-thickness skin autografts and allografts are similar. However, during the following days the extent of the vascular pattern in allografts depends largely upon the time of the changes associated with the rejection reaction of skin.

The histochemical studies of Converse and Ballantyne (1962), showing the rapid vascular ingrowth from the host into the graft, strongly suggest that the new vessels are capable of establishing an adequate blood circulation in the graft within a short time. Although their findings confirmed that an ingrowth of new vessels from the host occurs, it was not inferred that inosculation does not take place.

In subsequent histochemical studies using various hydrolytic and oxidative enzymes in porcine split-thickness skin grafts, Wolff and Schellander (1965, 1966) confirmed the enzymatic findings of Converse and Ballantyne (1962) and the original thesis of Garré (1889) that the definitive skin graft vasculature is derived from the ingrowth of host capillaries.

EARLY FILLING OF THE VESSELS. Haller and Billingham (1967) studied the origin of the vasculature in skin grafts using the cheek pouch of Syrian hamsters. Being devoid of pigmentation and appendages, the skinlike tissue constituting the highly vascular cheek pouch is almost transparent. When transplanted to genetically compatible hosts, it offers a window through which serial observation on the developing circulation can be studied. The authors reported that the blood vessels of the graft filled immediately following transplantation, but no flow was noted before the fourth or the fifth day; the blood vessel patterns in the healed isografts were identical to the original graft vessels. They noted that, when these vessels were blocked by previous injections of silicone rubber, the grafts became necrotic, strongly suggesting that the intrinsic vessels of the graft are reutilized for its survival.

REVASCULARIZATION FROM THE HOST BED MARGINS. Rees, Ballantyne, Hawthorne, and Nathan (1968) inserted silicone rubber sheeting between a suprapannicular skin autograft and the host bed in rats. The insertion of the silicone rubber sheets failed to prevent the development of blood supply in these small skin grafts. This finding supports the concept that, while vessels in the host bed may well be the main source of graft revascularization, the ingrowth of new vessels from the host bed margins can also play an important role in the vascularization of skin transplants.

STUDIES IN MICROCIRCULATION. A modification of the mouse skin transparent chamber of Merwin and Algire (1956) was used by Zarem, Zweifach, and McGehee (1967) to evaluate the development of the microcirculation in full-thickness skin autografts in mice. Their microscopic findings indicated that endothelial budding arises from the small arteries and veins in the host bed rather than from the capillaries or arterioles and venules. The endothelial buds then progress along the original graft vessels, which serve as nonviable conduits, and develop into an immature plexus of thin-walled, irregular channels with an oscillatory or slow unidirectional flow. By the eighth postoperative day the immature plexus differentiates into arterioles, capillaries, and venules. On the basis of their observations, the authors believed that the reestablishment of the graft vasculature occurs primarily as a vascular ingrowth from the host.

More recently, O'Donoghue and Zarem (1971), using the same chamber technique in mice, evaluated the differences in the angiogenic properties of fresh skin autografts, fresh skin allografts, lyophilized autografts, and freeze-thawed autografts. It was reported that, despite a consistent difference in the *angiogenic properties* of various types of grafts, all grafts are capable of inducing hyperemia in the host beds and neovascularization, consisting of the formation of host vascular buds and the development of sausage-shaped vessels extending toward the graft. In both fresh auto- and allografts, hyperemia is apparent on the third or fourth day after transplantation, neovascularization by the sixth day, and complete graft revascularization by the eighth day. The authors concluded that the presence of grafted tissue plays an important role in stimulating host vascular budding, either to anastomose with the original graft vessels or to penetrate the entire graft tissue.

Birch and Brånemark (1969) placed a full-thickness scrotal skin autograft over a thin vascular bed of outer auricular perichondrium and used the modified ear chamber of Brånemark and Lindström (1963) for vital microscopic evaluation. Immediately after surgery, the authors observed a shunting to-and-fro movement of blood within the preexisting graft vessels. Between 24 and 28 hours postoperatively, slow, irregular blood circulation appeared in the original graft vessels. During the subsequent 24 hours most of the grafts had resumed nearly normal circulation. Vascular proliferation was observed to commence soon after the development of circulation and to originate from the preexisting graft vessels, reaching a peak six to ten days after grafting. The investigators concluded that the blood flow noted in the graft depends on the vascular connection between the graft and recipient bed and on the host circulation.

In a subsequent study Birch, Brånemark, and Lundskog (1969) repeated the procedure of transplanting rabbit scrotal skin autografts to the auricular host bed for microangiographic study and reached similar conclusions. Microangiograms showed that the initial graft circulation appears to result from connections between vessels in the recipient bed and large dilated graft vessels. Between 48 and 72 hours following transplantation, capillaries in the host bed penetrate the lower layers of the graft; at the graft periphery, capillary invasion is even more pronounced. However, the authors stated that the host invasion does not explain the increased number of small blood vessels noted in the superficial layers of the graft. Instead, the new vessels in these layers originate from the original graft vessels.

Infrared thermography supplemented by macrophotography has been used by Birch, Brånemark, and Nilsson (1969) to study the heat emission patterns by vessels of the scrotal skin autograft and its auricular recipient bed. The findings indicate normal heat emission from the host bed vessels under the graft immediately after transplantation. According to the authors the dilated proliferating vessels in the recipient site slightly increase the temperature of the graft area within the first few days after surgery, provided that the heat emission is not masked by the graft edema.

Another method for assessing the vascular condition and circulation in skin grafts was devised by Marckmann (1966). With a live rat positioned under a microscope and with a television screen amplifier for projection onto a monitor, it is possible to visualize the status of blood circulation in skin autografts and to obtain cinematographic and photographic records. Slow flow could be seen in some areas of the graft at two postoperative days, becoming normal in flow velocity by the seventh postoperative day. The authors concluded that the restoration of the microcirculation is attained by connections of the graft blood vessels with those in the recipient bed.

SOURCE OF BLOOD SUPPLY. Many investigative attempts have been made to define the actual source of new blood supply in orthotopic skin grafts by the administration of various dyes, colloidal suspensions, or radioactive substances into the animal vascular system. The conclusions of some authors, including Jungengel (1891), Enderlen (1897), Henle (1899), Davis and Traut (1925), Mir y Mir (1951), and Ham (1952), have already been described.

After intravenous injections of ^{32}P into rabbits, Ohmori and Kurata (1960) noted the onset of blood circulation in full-thickness skin autografts and allografts on the fourth day after grafting. The velocity of the hemic flow is normal in autografts by the twentieth day, whereas in allografts the flow diminishes by the sixth day and ceases on the ninth day. Later, Pihl and Weiber (1963) measured the impulse frequencies over the skin and full-thickness grafts in rabbits after the intravenous administration of radioactive ^{32}P, partly in the form of a crystalloid and partly in the form of radiolabeled red corpuscles. The data indicate a progressive increase in the vascularity of auto- and allografts until the maximal activity is attained by the fifth day. During the ensuing time the activity gradually subsides in the autografts, persisting above the normal level noted in normal skin at 11 days, whereas in the allografts the values diminish with degeneration and the rejection reaction. Ohmori and Kurata (1960) and Pihl and Weiber (1963) did not describe the actual mode of vascularization.

In vivo microangiographic techniques were employed by Bellman and Velander (1957) and Bellman, Velander, Frank, and Lambert (1964) to define the vascular events in the full-thickness skin graft removed from the auricle of the rabbit and then replaced on its bed. In one experiment (1957) all grafts were rotated 90° before being replaced, and in another experiment (1964) the grafts were not rotated but replaced with exact adaptation. After analyzing the results obtained from both experiments, the authors were unable to state definitely whether the original blood vessels of the transplanted skin participated in the establishment of the definitive vasculature of the graft; however, they wrote that "incorporation of graft vessels into the ambient vessel network is a function of the local hemodynamic status."

Šmahel (1962, 1967) used intracardiac injections of a mixture of gelatin and India ink in an attempt to determine the exact mode of vascularization of skin grafts in rats. He reported that, during the first two postoperative days, the host capillaries formed a rich arcade-like network in the host bed. On the following day endothelial sprouts originated from this dense network and invaded the graft through the union line; during the subsequent days the host vessels linked with the original vascular system of the graft. It has been implied by Šmahel (1962) that, if the sprouting of the arcade-like network in the host bed does not develop, the definitive vasculature of the graft will not develop. According to Šmahel and Ganzoni (1970), the revascularization of the skin graft is largely dependent upon the original graft vasculature. However, they were also convinced that under certain conditions the host vessels furnished the major definitive vasculature of the graft. More recently, Šmahel and Clodius (1971) have stated that the degree of vascularization of the human skin graft is primarily dependent upon the vascularity of the donor site and secondly upon the thickness of the graft.

Smith, Ringland, and Wilson (1964) injected siliconed rubber at a high pressure into the vascular system of the rabbit hosts of auricular skin grafts between one and 30 postoperative days; their histologic sections indicated, as did those of Converse and Ballantyne (1962), an early and profound sprouting of capillaries in the host bed underlying the graft, numerous capillary sprouts growing in a parallel direction into the graft undersurface at about 48 hours, and rapid revascularization of the transplant between 48 hours and eight days.

INOSCULATION: A FORTUITOUS ENCOUNTER? A study by Converse. Šmahel, Ballantyne, and Harper (1975) suggested that inosculation between vessels of the host and graft is spotty and fortuitous. Full-thickness suprapannicular grafts in rats were removed at hourly intervals after grafting. The host bed showed bleeding points after 24 hours, and these were situated in varying areas of the host bed. This observation suggests that inosculation occurs in a spotty fashion. The data suggest that the revascularization of skin grafts is an orderly sequence of events, which include: active invasion of the graft dermis by the ingrowing host capillary sprouts; development of anastomoses between the graft and host vasculature; entry of blood into the graft through the vascular anastomoses by 48 hours after transplantation.

SPLIT-THICKNESS GRAFTS. It has been generally assumed that thin grafts of skin are revascularized more rapidly than thicker grafts. The histologic appearance of thin and thick grafts shows that degenerative changes in the transplant depend on the rate of vascularization; the degenerative changes in the transplant appear to be inversely proportional to the rapidity of vascularization. The changes are less apparent in split-thickness grafts, because the invading blood vessels have a shorter distance to traverse through the entire thickness of donor dermis.

A study employing combined methods of vital skin microscopy and enzyme histochemistry with neotetrazolium chloride and reduced diphosphopyridine nucleotide as reagents was conducted by Converse, Filler, and Ballantyne (1965) in rats. They attempted to define the actual source and development of the blood supply in split-thickness skin grafts which were removed, rotated 180°, and immediately replaced on the dermal bed. Before commencing the experiment, the authors had presumed that the revascularization of a split-thickness skin graft transplanted to a suprapannicular bed would be more rapid than that of a full-thickness graft for two reasons: (1) the split-thickness graft is thinner, and the invading vessels from the host have a shorter distance to travel; and (2) the suprapannicular host site contains a rich supply of vessels. Their histochemical data, however, indicated that the new host capillaries originate as endothelial buds from deep-lying distended blood vessels in the upper epimysium of the panniculus carnosus rather than from the host vessels in close proximity to the graft undersurface. The vascular pattern in the host bed has changed; in contrast to the vasculature noted in the surrounding host tissue, the vessels are more numerous and show greater ramification and dilatation. The new vessels exhibit parallel ingrowth from the upper epimysium overlying the pannicular layer to the host-graft junction. The complete revascularization with active circulation of the split-thickness graft occurs at the same rate as in the full-thickness graft on a suprapannicular bed. In contrast to an early rapid decrease of enzymatic activity in the vessels of full-thickness grafts placed on a suprapannicular bed (Converse, Filler, and Ballantyne, 1965), the delayed and slower loss of activity in such vessels of split-thickness grafts implies that the onset and rate of degenerative changes in the graft vessels vary with the thickness of the graft dermis. In thin grafts, nutrient fluids have a shorter distance to diffuse, and the thinner graft has fewer cellular elements requiring nourishment. As emphasized by Mir y Mir (1951), the rapidity of vascularization and the state of nutrition of the skin graft are controlled by the dermal thickness of the graft and the state of the host site. Woodruff (1960) supported the hypothesis of Mir y Mir (1951) that, in thin grafts, serum

imbibition is adequate to maintain the viability of the grafted tissue for several days, and early vascularization is not essential; in thicker grafts, however, early or rapid vascularization is essential for survival.

As mentioned in a previous section Wolff and Schellander (1965, 1966), in somewhat similar enzyme histochemical studies, noted that the definitive vasculature of split-thickness skin grafts in pigs is formed entirely by the ingrowing capillaries from the host, and the original vessels degenerate. These investigators confirmed the histochemical studies of Converse and Ballantyne (1962) employing full-thickness suprapannicular skin grafts in rats. Their findings also coincided with those of Converse, Filler, and Ballantyne (1965) on split-thickness grafts in rats.

In 1964 Clemmesen, after introducing India ink suspension into the vascular system of pigs under forced intracardiac pressure, deduced from his histologic examination that the revascularization of thin split-thickness skin autografts depends largely on the sinus like channels between the vessels of the underlying host tissue and the graft vessels. He concluded that, during the ensuing time, the sinuslike communications formed by the interstice in the fibrin network at the host-graft junction are transformed into thin-walled vessels, permitting the reestablishment of active hemal flow in the original graft vasculature. Various studies (stereomicroscopy, histology, or histochemistry) of the behavior and fate of skin transplants in animals, chick embryos, and man failed to confirm Clemmesen's findings of sinuslike channels at the host-graft junction. Presumably, excessive intracardiac pressure of the India ink injectant ruptures the newly formed blood vessels at the surface of the recipient areas or at the junction line between the two tissues, thus liberating the solution to form the ink-filled areas.

SUMMARY OF PHASE OF GRAFT VASCULARIZATION. The present interpretation is that the early filling of the graft's endothelial spaces with serumlike fluid (previously thought to be plasmalike fluid) is accompanied by the infiltration of erythrocytes, as a result of the anastomosis of graft vessels with host vessels, coupled with the early ingrowth of host endothelium. These events may account for the pinkish tint which appears in human skin within the first 12 hours after transplantation. The color changes progress to a cherry-red hue in vascularized grafts with well-established blood circulation. The cyanotic color of more slowly revascularized grafts, which reflects poorly oxygenized hemoglobin, may be due to incomplete or inadequate hemic flow caused by an embarrassed venous return or drainage from the graft. With ensuing time and the development of an improved circulation, the color progresses to a cherry-red hue.

Types of Skin Grafts

THE FULL-THICKNESS SKIN GRAFT

The full-thickness skin graft comprises the entire thickness of the skin (see Fig. 6–2). The fat must be trimmed from the undersurface of the dermis in order to facilitate vascularization of the graft. Because of its thickness, the full-thickness graft is more slowly revascularized than the split-thickness graft and requires optimal conditions, such as an adequate blood supply and complete immobilization, in order to survive.

Because the full-thickness graft contains the

entire dermal layer, its characteristics approximate more closely those of normal skin than does a split-thickness graft. The full-thickness graft has the following advantages over the split-thickness graft: (1) there is less tendency to contract, particularly when it is transplanted to an area consisting of loose soft tissue, such as the face, neck, and axilla; (2) there is less tendency to pigment postoperatively; (3) the cover is functionally superior; and (4) there is less tendency to develop a smooth sheen, a characteristic which resists the use of cosmetics.

Use of the Full-Thickness Graft. The full-thickness graft is generally employed for the definitive repair of a defect on the face when it is estimated that a better appearance can be obtained by this method than by means of a local flap, or when a local flap is not available or easily obtainable. Grafts taken from areas of the head and neck give a good color match in the repair of facial defects. The full-thickness graft is ideal for the replacement of the lower eyelid skin, for example, where the color and texture match renders it practically indistinguishable from normal eyelid skin. It can also be used as an interim cover following the excision of basal cell carcinoma of the face, where the use of a flap would mask a recurrence. In many patients the grafts will blend so well after a year that later flap coverage is not required. Full-thickness skin grafts are also indicated in resurfacing defects on the volar aspect of the hand and fingers.

Donor Sites for Full-Thickness Skin Grafts

RETROAURICULAR AREA. Large sections of full-thickness skin can be removed from the posterior aspect of the helix and mastoid area (Fig. 6–3). The wound can usually be closed primarily and, when the donor defect exceeds 3 cm, the retroauricular sulcus may be obliterated with primary closure. The sulcus can be reconstructed with a split-thickness skin graft, especially if the entire retroauricular area from helical rim to hairline has served as a donor site. Retroauricular skin, after an initial period of increased vascularity, is thin and provides a suitable match in resurfacing a facial defect.

SUPRACLAVICULAR AREA. When larger full-thickness skin grafts are required, such as for a large forehead defect or the upper lip esthetic unit, the supraclavicular area is preferred. Color and texture are nearly as acceptable as in the retroauricular graft. The supraclavicular area is

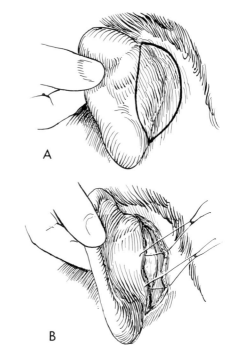

FIGURE 6–3. Retroauricular area as a donor site for a full-thickness skin graft. *A*, Proposed graft, including portion of retroauricular sulcus. *B*, The defect can usually be closed primarily.

contraindicated if a neck dissection or cervical flap is planned in the future. The supraclavicular donor site is cosmetically less desirable in the female.

UPPER EYELIDS. This area provides ellipses of full-thickness skin and is the donor site of choice in the reconstruction of small eyelid defects.

ABDOMEN AND THIGH. Full-thickness grafts may also be removed from the abdomen or thigh, but the color-texture match is poor when this type of skin is grafted to the face. Because the skin is so thick, the abdomen or thigh is preferred as a donor site for split-thickness skin grafts. Full-thickness grafts from the abdomen have been employed in grafting areas predisposed to contracture, such as the cervical and axillary areas. The presence of the entire thickness of the dermis in full-thickness grafts counteracts the tendency to contraction following the release of a contracture in these areas. The full-thickness graft has been largely replaced for this purpose by the thick split-thickness graft (called the three-quarter thickness graft by Padgett); the thick split-thickness graft has advantages similar to those of the full-thickness graft and is easier to remove. Cronin (see Chapter 34) has demonstrated that prolonged immobilization is effective in preventing long-term graft contracture. When a thick split-thickness graft is required—in grafting a defect in the axilla, for example—the donor area of the split-thickness graft should be grafted with a thin split-thickness graft to avoid delayed healing and hypertrophic scarring.

OTHER SITES. The antecubital flexor crease, volar wrist crease, and inguinal crease provide alternative donor sites. The former is particularly suited for the resurfacing of finger or hand defects, since it obviates the need for a second operative field.

Preputial skin in the male and labia majora skin in the female are occasionally used as full-thickness grafts. The former is used for the reconstruction of the urethra in hypospadias reconstructive surgery (see Chapter 95). Labial skin, because of its color and pigmentation, has been used in nipple-areolar reconstruction. Wexler and Oneal (1973) hemisected and removed half of a nipple and areola; both semi-areolas are approximated to form two smaller nipple-areolar complexes.

Removal of the Full-Thickness Graft. The full-thickness graft is generally cut according to a pattern of the defect to be grafted (Fig. 6–4). A cloth flannel pattern or transparent pliable plastic material can be employed, the outline

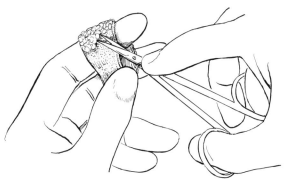

FIGURE 6–5. Defatting the undersurface of a full-thickness skin graft with a pair of scissors.

being designed either before or after excision of the lesion or scar. It is preferable to make the pattern after the excision, as the final defect is often larger than the pre-excision defect. Following excision, the edges of the wound retract, thus enlarging the size of the defect. Following excision and hemostasis, the defect is outlined by means of a blood imprint on moistened cotton cloth.

The pattern of the graft should be oriented by means of an ink mark or small cut made with scissors. The pattern is then applied to a donor site and an outline made around the pattern with ink. It is usually useful to inject a solution of procaine and epinephrine immediately beneath the dermal layer of the donor site and balloon the whole area with the anesthetic fluid. This assists in the separation of the dermal layer from the underlying fat and facilitates the surgical removal of the graft. Excision of the full-thickness graft without the inclusion of the fat is a tedious procedure. It is preferable to excise the graft rapidly along a plane situated immediately below the junction of the dermis and the fat and trim the fat from the graft after the removal of the graft. The removal of the fat from the graft must be accomplished with a pair of sharp-cutting scissors in order to avoid injury to the base of the dermis with the crushing action of dull-cutting scissors (Fig. 6–5).

The donor site is closed by undermining the skin edges and closing the wound primarily. For larger defects a rotation flap or a split-thickness skin graft may be required.

The Pressure Dressings. The full-thickness skin graft is sutured into the recipient site after meticulous hemostasis with electrocoagulation. Certain sutures are left long to be used to tie over a bolster of gauze, cotton, or lamb's wool for immobilization (Fig. 6–6). These bolsters

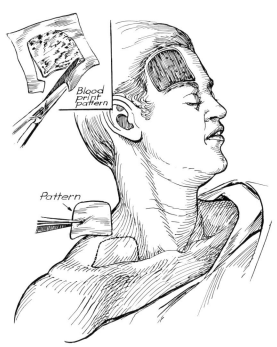

FIGURE 6–4. Removal of a full-thickness skin graft from the supraclavicular area. Graft was cut according to a pattern of the forehead defect.

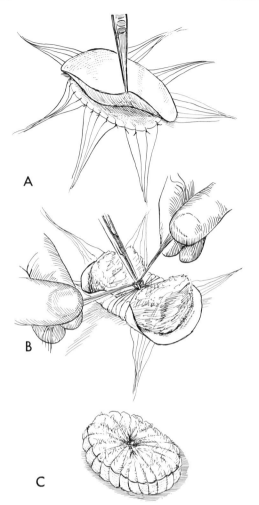

A

B

C

FIGURE 6–6. Bolus dressing used to immobilize a full-thickness skin graft. *A,* Inner layer of petrolatum gauze applied. Sutures are kept long. *B,* Layer of fluffed gauze is applied and the sutures are tied. Assistant holds first loop of the tie to prevent slippage. *C,* Final appearance. (From Chase, R. A.: Atlas of Hand Surgery. Philadelphia, W. B. Saunders Company, 1973.)

THE SPLIT-THICKNESS SKIN GRAFT

The split-thickness graft is the most widely used method of skin grafting for covering raw areas resulting from trauma and burns and for the immediate replacement of a cutaneous defect following excision for malignancy. Split-thickness grafts may be employed either as definitive treatment or as temporary skin graft dressings to be replaced at a later date by a more definitive type of graft or a flap.

Split-thickness skin grafts are cut at various thicknesses (see Fig. 6–2). The thin type of split-thickness grafts are often referred to as Thiersch grafts. They extend through the skin at a level immediately below the epidermis and comprise only a thin layer of dermis. Most split-thickness grafts extend through the dermis at a level about halfway through the dermis, and thick split-thickness or three-quarter thickness grafts are removed at a level that extends across the deeper layers of the dermis.

Removal of the Split-Thickness Skin Grafts. Plastic surgeons prior to World War II had become experienced at removing skin grafts freehand and at controlling the skin depth by varying the angle of the knife in relation to the skin. Large grafts representing a major portion of the inner aspect of the thigh were removed freehand with great skill by these experts. Consequently, the removal of skin grafts was restricted to a few surgeons.

One of the first attempts at developing an instrument that would permit more precise control of the thickness of the graft was that of Finochietto (1920). The first widely used in-

should be kept low and are left in place for five to ten days, though the graft can be inspected after four to six days by cutting a few of the ties.

It should be emphasized that circumferential scarring will occur in every area in which a graft is placed. If the graft is too long and improperly defatted or if the recipient area is too shallow, the graft may persist as a raised knob, giving a cobblestone-like effect. Arteriovenous fistulas, neuromas, and scarring are complications which have been observed in the donor site. Similarly, arteriovenous fistulas, the cobblestone effect, and lack of hair growth in the transferred graft have been complications noted in recipient areas.

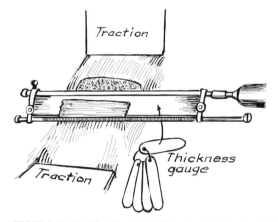

FIGURE 6–7. The Humby knife. A roller is attached to the knife. The distance between the roller and the blade of the knife can be varied by means of a calibration device to permit the cutting of skin grafts of varying thicknesses.

strument permitting depth control was that developed by Humby, who was working at the Hospital for Sick Children, Great Ormond Street, London, prior to World War II. Humby added a roller to the Blair knife. The distance between the roller and the blade of the knife could be varied by means of a calibration device. The Humby knife, with various modifications by Bodenham, Braithwaite, and Marcks, is a popular instrument, often preferred to the dermatome (Fig. 6–7).

The development by Padgett and Hood (1939) of a superior instrument, the dermatome (Fig. 6–8), permitting the removal of split-thickness grafts with increased precision and with minimal risk of failure, was a major contribution to surgery. This instrument became available immediately before World War II and rendered great service to the war wounded, since it made possible the cutting of skin grafts not only by the expert plastic surgeon but also by any well trained surgeon. During World War II, Reese (1946) of Philadelphia designed a more refined instrument that permitted greater accuracy and control of the thickness of the graft. The technical details of the Reese dermatome (see Fig. 6–11) are discussed later in the chapter.

Also during World War II, a young American surgeon, Harry M. Brown, conceived the idea of a new instrument, the electric dermatome (Fig. 6–9). Brown was taken prisoner of war during the Bataan campaign in the Philippines and conceived the idea of the new instrument while a prisoner. After the war he was able to develop the instrument but, unfortunately, did not live to witness the magnitude

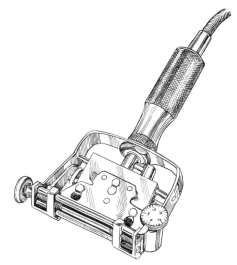

FIGURE 6–9. The Brown electric dermatome. (Drawing courtesy of Dr. D. Wood-Smith.)

of his clinical contribution, as he died in a tragic accident shortly after completing his surgical residency. The original Brown electric dermatome and various modifications of the instrument developed in the United States, England, and France permit the rapid removal of long strips of split-thickness skin, a distinct advantage in the grafting of the burned patient. The use of the Padgett or Reese dermatome, which requires painting the surface of the skin with cement prior to the removal of the graft, is more time consuming when a large amount of skin is needed to cover a large defect, as is often the case in the burned patient. The rapid removal of skin grafts made possible by the electric dermatome has been responsible for the routine use of this instrument in the removal of split-thickness skin grafts in burn patients.

A more recent development (Fig. 6–10) in the evolution of dermatomes has been the introduction of the air-driven (liquid nitrogen) dermatomes.* They are easily managed and are capable of removing long strips of skin with a precision approaching that of the Padgett and Reese dermatomes.

DRUM DERMATOMES. Since World War II the drum dermatomes have enjoyed wide popularity and have been employed when a precisely cut split-thickness graft is desired.

Reese Dermatome. The Reese dermatome† (Fig. 6–11), a carefully machined instrument, is a modification of the Padgett-

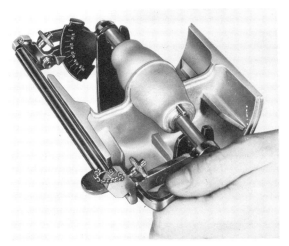

FIGURE 6–8. The Padgett-Hood dermatome. (Courtesy of Padgett Dermatome, Kansas City Assemblage Company, Kansas City, Mo. 64111)

---

*Stryker Corporation, Kalamazoo, Michigan 49001, and Hall Instrument, Inc., Santa Barbara, California 93103.
†Bard Parker Company, Danbury, Connecticut.

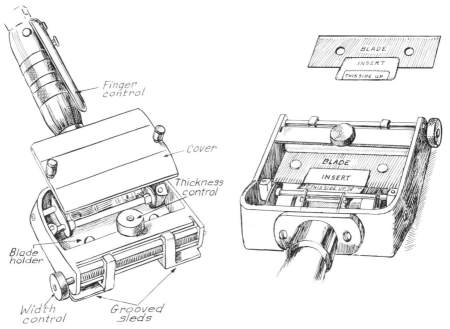

FIGURE 6–10. Air-driven dermatome. There are separate knobs to control the width and depth of the skin graft. A disposable blade is also provided.

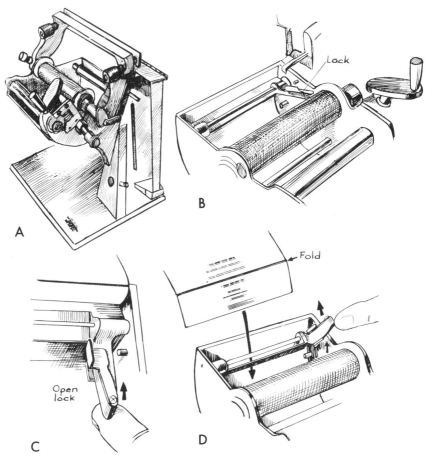

FIGURE 6–11. The Reese dermatome. *A*, Dermatome on stand. *B*, Handle of dermatome and lock of clamp bar. *C*, Opening the lock. *D*, The folded end of the dermatape is inserted under the clamp bar.

Illustration continued on opposite page.

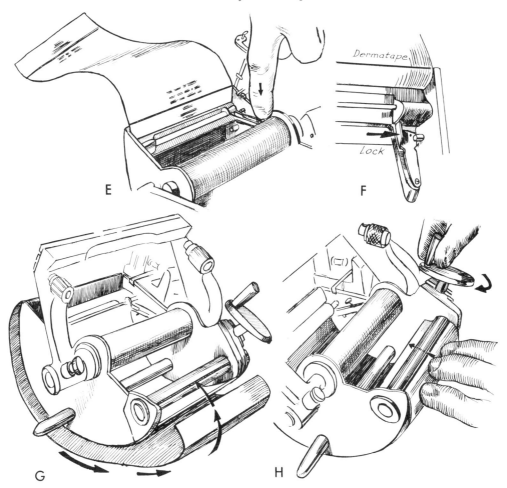

FIGURE 6–11 *Continued.* *E, F*, Locking the clamp bar to secure one end of the dermatape. *G*, The opposite folded end is inserted into a slot of the tightening spool. *H*, Tightening the spool with a key.

Illustration continued on following page.

Hood dermatome. An accompanying set of shims permits careful calibration of the thickness of the graft. There is a disadvantage in that, if the graft is too thick or thin, it is difficult to change the calibration in the middle of a skin graft removal.

The skin is prepared by applying a topical antiseptic to the donor site, followed by a defatting agent, such as ether. The donor site is painted with the dermatome cement, care being exercised that the glue on the brush is not allowed to dry so there is no lumping of the prepared surface. If less than a full drum or a pattern graft is required, the desired shape can be outlined with ink and the pattern painted with dermatome glue. Vaseline ointment can be applied around the pattern to avoid cutting into the surrounding tissue with the dermatome.

While the prepared donor site is drying (three minutes should elapse), the dermatome can be assembled. The dermatome sits in a stand which holds the full set of shims (Fig. 6–11, *A*). The clamp bar which secures the laminated dermatape is opened. The dermatape is carefully folded at both ends along the black lines (Fig. 6–11, *B, C*). One end of the dermatape is inserted beneath the clamp bar (Fig. 6–11, *D*) so that the folded edge fits over the face margin of the drum. The clamp bar is returned to secure the dermatape and is locked in position (Fig. 6–11, *E, F*). The opposite end of the dermatape is inserted into a slot in the tightening spool (Fig. 6–11, *G*). The crank is then rotated to turn the spool and tighten the dermatape against the drum surface (Fig. 6–11, *H*). The tape is incised along both free surfaces of the drum, and the outer cover is peeled back to expose the adhesive surface of the dermatape (Fig. 6–11, *I*). A disposable blade and a shim of desired thickness are inserted into the blade clamp. Round nuts are tightened at either end

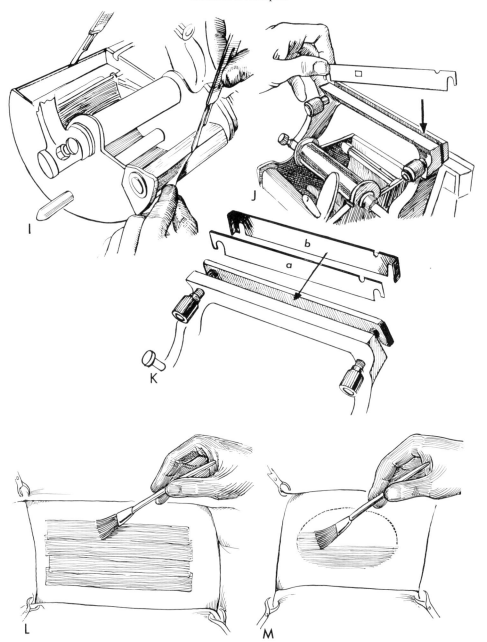

FIGURE 6–11 *Continued.* *I*, The tape is incised on both edges prior to removal of the outer layer to expose the adhesive surface. *J*, *K*, Insertion of disposable blade (a) and shim (b). *L*, *M*, Painting of skin surface with glue in single strokes.

Illustration continued on opposite page.

to secure the blade clamp (Fig. 6–11, *J*, *K*). While the instrument is being assembled, the skin is painted with glue in single strokes. Three minutes should elapse for drying of the adhesive (Fig. 6–11, *L*, *M*).

To remove the skin, the instrument is first pressed against the donor site along its free edge (Fig. 6–11, *N*) and then rotated slowly until the skin begins to fall away at the margins of the drum but still does not become detached (Fig. 6–11, *O*, *P*). The cutting is started with almost no more forward force than is present in the weight of the blade assembly. The blade is moved from side to side while the drum is rotated slowly (dorsiflexion of the wrist) but held steady; at no time is the blade forced forward (Fig. 6–11, *Q*). If there is any tendency for the skin to pull away at the margins, the drum is

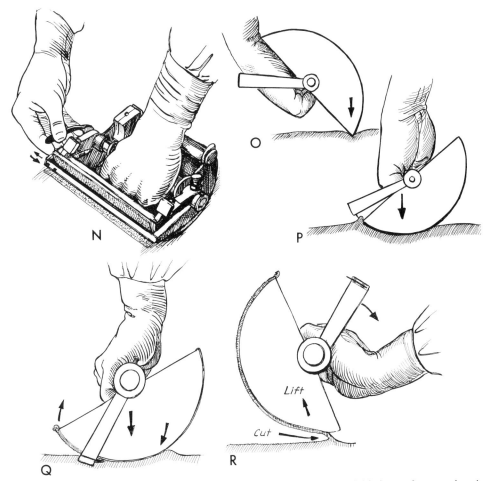

FIGURE 6–11 *Continued.* *N*, Removal of the graft. *O*, Cross-sectional view of initiating graft removal at the edge of the drum. *P*, Incorrect way of starting graft removal. *Q*, Proper way of advancing drum. Note direction of forces (arrows). *R*, The drum is lifted prior to cutting the graft through. (From Chase, R. A.: Atlas of Hand Surgery. Philadelphia, W. B. Saunders Company, 1973.)

pressed more firmly against the skin and, in addition, is rotated slightly toward the cutting blade to roll the skin up in front of the cutting edge. If the blade tends to cut beyond the width of the drum, this is remedied by vertically lifting the drum away from the skin and/or having the assistant hold the skin away from the drum at each margin with a pair of hemostats. This complication can also be avoided by spreading some paraffin ointment or mineral oil over the edges of the drum. The completion of the cutting can be effected by lifting the drum and graft away from the donor site and, with a few deft strokes of the blade, cutting the graft through (Fig. 6–11, *R*); alternatively, the dermatome may be turned back and the graft severed from the bed with a knife.

The instrument is returned to the rack and the blade turned back to the protected posi-

tion. The disposable blade should be removed to avoid injury to any member of the operating personnel. The dermatape is removed and covered with a sponge gauze soaked in normal saline solution.

When it becomes necessary to use the neck, chest, flank, or other area of the body where there may be a depression or bony prominence, it is helpful to fill out such a depression or pad the prominence by injecting normal saline with the Pitkin automatic refilling syringe until it becomes level with the surrounding area. This technique will permit the removal of grafts from any part of the body.

Padgett Dermatome. The Padgett dermatome,* although lacking the precision of the

---

* Kansas City Assemblage Company, 3953 Broadway, Kansas City, Missouri 64111.

Reese dermatome, is lighter and can be used more rapidly (see Fig. 6–8). It is built on the drum principle but lacks any shims. The distance between the blade and drum is calibrated in thousandths of an inch and is adjusted by turning a ratchet on one side of the blade arm. There is now available for the Padgett dermatome a plastic tape with glue on both surfaces. The outer protective cover is removed from the tape, and the latter is applied to the drum of the dermatome. The thickness of the cut must be increased approximately 0.004 inch to compensate for the thickness of the tape. The graft can be removed as outlined above for the Reese dermatome, and the skin graft can be easily pulled from the tape.

In cutting grafts with the Reese or Padgett dermatome, it is important to cut transversely to the part rather than parallel to a convex surface, that is, transversely across the thigh, abdomen, or trunk. There will be less tendency for the skin to pull away at the sides of the instrument, and a greater amount of skin can be removed in this manner.

ELECTRIC DERMATOME. The Brown dermatome* (see Fig. 6–9) was the first of the electric dermatomes to be developed and is especially valuable because a large amount of skin can be rapidly cut. The electric dermatome has largely replaced the Vacutome, developed by Barker (1948), another instrument that permits rapid removal of skin grafts. These instruments do not require the use of cement. The blades are sterilized by soaking in Zephiran or other suitable sterilizing solution, while the cutting head and rubber-covered cable are autoclaved. Individually wrapped, sterile blades are also available.

The blade is inserted with the blade adjustment set screws opened. The blade is carefully slid into place and dropped over the three rivets before the three anchoring screws are tightened. Both adjustable set screws are then turned down as far as they will go toward zero. They are opened simultaneously to the desired thickness of the graft calibrated in thousandths of an inch.

There is now available an air-driven modification of the Brown dermatome, which eliminates any hazards inherent in an electrically operated instrument.

After the instrument has been adjusted to the desired setting, sterile mineral oil is applied to the donor site. With the assistant holding the extremity, the surgeon applies counterpressure with his left hand while pushing the instrument forward with the right. As the dermatome moves away and out of the range of the counterpressure, the instrument is stopped to allow the left hand to move forward to reapply counterpressure. If the graft appears to be too thick, the calibration is reset without removing the instrument from the donor site.

When multiple grafts are removed, they are stretched out, raw (dermal) surface up, on sterile cellophane or gauze strips covered with a thin layer of petrolatum. Each new graft is taken as close to the previous donor site as possible in order to utilize all the available donor skin. The grafts are covered with a moist sponge until they are ready to be applied.

It is important to become acquainted with the cutting characteristics of the instrument, which vary from instrument to instrument by 0.002 to 0.005 inch in depth of skin penetration. The thickness of the graft is also influenced by the degree of pressure applied by the operator. When cutting over an area with underlying bone, such as the anterior aspect of the thigh or leg, only slight pressure is required or the graft will be too thick. Ordinarily, with the setting at 0.0018 inch, one will obtain a graft of about 0.0016 inch, which is considered a medium-thick split-thickness skin graft. A nick or irregularity in the blade will produce a longitudinal split in the graft; the blade should be inspected before it is inserted and the setting viewed to be sure the cut will be even and correct.

A good rule is to limit the use of this instrument to the extremities, except in an obese individual. Care should be taken when cutting on the inside of a baby's thigh, as there is a tendency for the instrument to skip and jump over the irregular fat bulges. Indiscriminate and improper use of the Brown dermatome may render the trunk useless as a donor site for subsequent skin graft removal.

Electric dermatome in shaving of scars. The electric dermatome can also be used for removal of flat scar plaques when there is no contracture. By setting the instrument at about 0.0025 inch to 0.0030 inch, the scar can be shaved off gradually by repeated strokes with the instrument until all that remains is a thin layer of scar overlying the fat; the resulting bed provides a smooth base on which to apply a graft. The graft can be applied at the time of the scar excision if adequate hemostasis is obtained, or it can be applied as a delayed procedure.

*Zimmer, Warsaw, Indiana 46580.

Electric dermatome in removal of burn eschar. Another use of the electric dermatome is for debridement in a third degree (full-thickness) burn. If there is some question as to the thickness of the eschar, the dermatome is set for about 0.0020 inch, and the outer layers of the eschar are excised. If there is no question as to the depth of the burn, the instrument can be opened to 0.0030 inch and the full thickness of the eschar excised down to normal fat. This should be done with a pneumatic tourniquet or a sterile Esmarch bandage in place to decrease blood loss. Its use for this purpose should be limited to smaller burns because of the danger of producing a significant hypovolemia secondary to blood loss. Blood replacement is an almost inevitable consequence. Newer methods such as tangential excision are associated with less blood loss.

The electric dermatome can also be used for removal of tattoos, but, where the margins are irregular, it may be easier to use the Padgett dermatome.

HALL AND STRYKER ROLLO TURBINE DERMATOMES. The Hall* and Stryker† turbine dermatomes are similar to the electric model except that they are driven by liquid nitrogen. They are extremely smooth and produce an even graft with thickness control approaching that of the Reese drum dermatome. A technique similar to that described for the Brown electric dermatome is employed in taking the graft.

CASTROVIEJO DERMATOME. This instrument is useful for cutting mucous membrane grafts for the treatment of eyelid and socket deformities (Fig. 6–12). The instrument is powered by a Norelco shaving motor and has a tiny cutting head with special blades and shims to control the thickness of the cut. The instrument has also been useful as an adjunct in the removal of tattoos after the initial excision has been accomplished by either the Brown or the Padgett dermatome. If small areas of tattoo remain, the Castroviejo dermatome can be used to shave off the residual areas.

DISPOSABLE DERMATOMES. Davol* has marketed a disposable dermatome (Fig. 6–13) that will cut a graft that is almost 0.15 inch thick and 1½ inches wide. The cutting head is dispensed in a sterile plastic bag. The motor is an Oral B rechargeable toothbrush motor, which can be inserted in a plastic bag and sealed. The sterile cutting head is pushed through the bag into the motor to ensure a sterile unit.

BLAIR AND HUMBY KNIVES. Before the electric Padgett and Reese dermatomes were developed and became popular, all grafts were cut freehand with a sharp knife. Knives

---

*Hall Instrument, Inc., Santa Barbara, California 93103.
†Stryker Corporation, Kalamazoo, Michigan 49001.

*Davol, Inc., Providence, Rhode Island 02901.

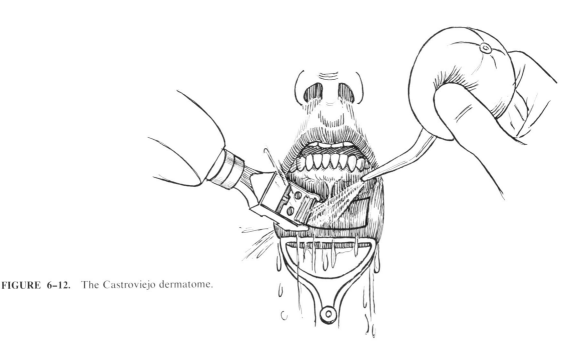

FIGURE 6–12. The Castroviejo dermatome.

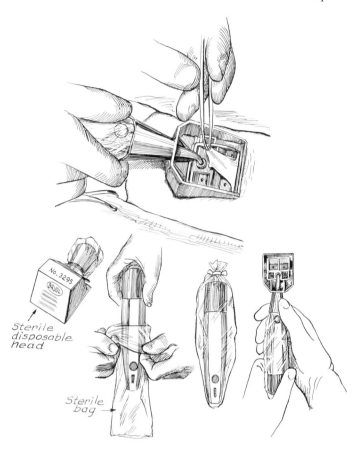

Sterile
disposable
head

Sterile
bag

FIGURE 6-13. Disposable head derma-tome (Davol). The instrument is powered by a rechargeable toothbrush motor, which can be stored in a sterile bag.

used for this purpose have long, sharp blades, usually with an adapter over the blade to facili-tate the cutting of the graft and to control the thickness of the graft. Large pieces of skin may be cut from a thigh or even from the trunk after one becomes adept with their use. They may be used with suction boxes which are designed to keep the skin taut during the cut-ting of the graft, or with a flat board or tongue blade to hold the skin taut while counterpres-sure is maintained by the assistant. Sterile petrolatum or mineral oil is applied to the donor site to facilitate the forward progression of the blade.

A very sharp blade is requisite; it is held flat against the skin and is moved back and forth with short strokes and very little forward pres-sure. If one attempts to press forward too rap-idly, the blade will cut through the skin and the continuity of the graft will be broken. All students or residents in plastic surgery should familiarize themselves with the cutting of a freehand graft, since there are many occasions when small or moderate-sized grafts must be cut in the office, outpatient clinic, or even at the bedside.

Mesh Grafts. Mesh grafts are thin split-thickness skin grafts in which multiple tiny slits have been made to allow the graft to be stretched or expanded in two directions to many times its original size (Tanner and co-workers, 1964). These grafts, held in place by sutures, sterile tape, or suitable dressings, are indicated as a cover in extensive burns and fol-lowing extensive traumatic defects (Fig. 6–14).

Mesh grafts can also be used in wounds of trauma for temporary early coverage, often before all the slough has cleared. The slits fa-cilitate drainage and should be used when hemostasis in the recipient bed is not com-plete.

There are two devices available to produce these grafts. One is made by Zimmer; the grafts are run through the instrument and a series of blades on a rotary shaft cuts the slits (Fig. 6–15). The other is made by Padgett (Fig. 6–16); the grafts are placed over the exposed blades and a roller presses the skin against the blades.

The Zimmer instrument will provide a long, narrow (8 inches × 2⅞ inches) strip of skin. The grafts must also be kept thin (0.012 to

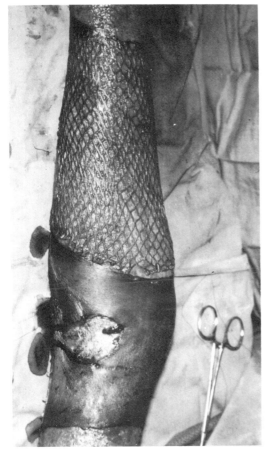

FIGURE 6–14. Mesh graft used to cover an extensive defect of the lower extremity.

0.015 inch) or they tend to jam in the rotor. The Padgett instrument will easily handle a wide or thick graft, but the grafts must be lifted

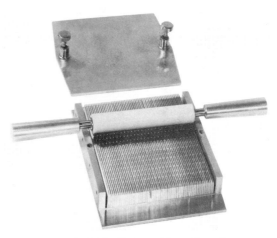

FIGURE 6–16. Padgett skin graft mesher.

from the blades and repositioned after each cutting.

The Zimmer instrument has four variations, and the expansion ratio ranges from $1\frac{1}{2}$ to 1 to 9 to 1.

SPLIT-THICKNESS SKIN GRAFTING

When a defect of the skin, whether produced by trauma, by a burn, or by a surgical excision, covers a surface that is too wide for the use of a full-thickness graft, the split-thickness graft is indicated, as it does not leave in its wake a full-thickness defect and the donor area is capable of resurfacing itself by secondary epithelization.

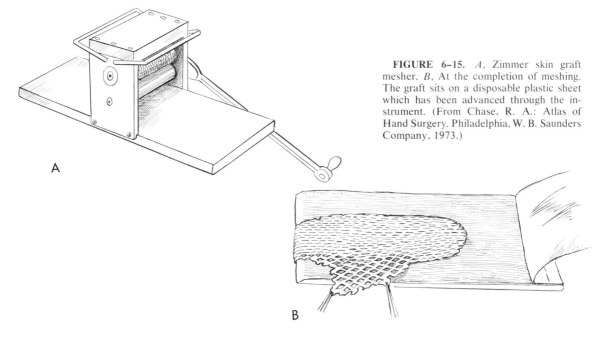

FIGURE 6–15. *A*, Zimmer skin graft mesher. *B*, At the completion of meshing. The graft sits on a disposable plastic sheet which has been advanced through the instrument. (From Chase, R. A.: Atlas of Hand Surgery. Philadelphia, W. B. Saunders Company, 1973.)

A

B

The excision of large pigmented nevi or burn scars or the release of burn scar contractures, as well as certain other surgical excisions, may result in a defect that cannot be closed primarily and must be covered with a skin graft. When the defect is small and located on the face or upper neck, a full-thickness graft is indicated. In some instances the area of primary excision is covered by a transposition flap and the secondary defect is covered by a split-thickness skin graft. Once the decision has been made to apply a split-thickness graft, the surgeon must decide on the donor site, the cutting instrument, and the method of dressing.

Choice of the Donor Site. For the average graft, the abdomen provides the best donor site unless it is riddled with striae (Fig. 6–17). This area is superior to the thigh or buttock for several reasons. It is covered by most bathing suits or other clothing, and its use allows the patient to be ambulatory with a minimum of pain. When the graft is placed in the facial or cervical area, the chest or upper back is superior as a donor site in terms of color match.

When grafting large surface defects resulting from skin loss, such as in thermal burns, the surgeon must consider multiple donor sites. The unburned areas on the leg can be used for cutting thin grafts with the electric and turbine dermatomes. However, for covering the flexion areas, such as the cervical, knee, ankle, axillary, or inguinal regions, the abdomen, back, or buttocks should be used as donor sites and a thick split-thickness graft taken. These thicker grafts containing a relatively larger amount of dermis will give a superior functional result with less contracture (see Chapter 34). The donor site of the thick graft can, in turn, be covered with a thin split-thickness (0.008 inch) graft.

Mucosal Grafts. Mucosal grafts are required to replace the lining of the conjunctival sac and nasal cavity. They are also used in eye socket reconstruction.

Calibrated split-thickness mucosa can be ob-

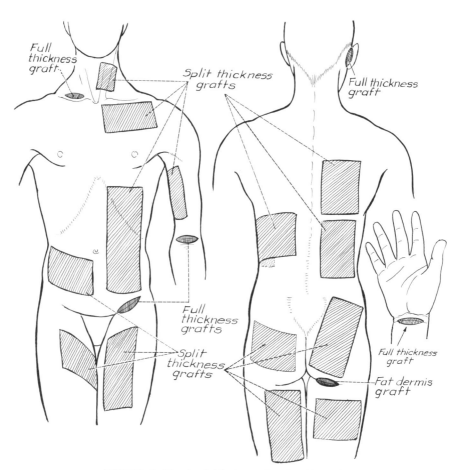

FIGURE 6–17. Available donor sites for skin grafts.

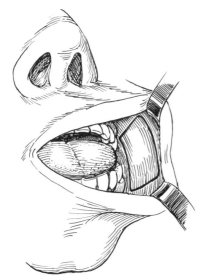

FIGURE 6–18. Full-thickness mucosal grafts can be procured from the inner aspect of the cheek.

tained from the inner aspect of the lower lip with a small electrical or air-driven dermatome (see Fig. 6–12) (Castroviejo, 1959).

Full-thickness mucosal grafts can be removed from the inner aspect of the cheek (Fig. 6–18). An incision is made above the buccal groove, and a piece of full-thickness mucosa measuring 2.5 by 5.0 cm can be procured with preservation of the opening of Stensen's duct. The graft is defatted in a manner similar to that used in full-thickness skin grafts.

Application of the Skin Graft. The usual split-thickness skin graft which is applied to a surgically clean wound is stretched out over the bed and sutured with 4–0 or 5–0 silk or nylon. In most instances the best fixation is provided by a tie-over bolus dressing. The sutures are placed about 1.5 to 2.5 cm apart and are left long in order to facilitate tie-over suturing over the dressing (see Fig. 6–6). The graft is cut flush with the skin edge with no overlap; the skin edges may overlap when esthetic considerations are not primary. Puncture holes in the graft are avoided, and it is not necessary to quilt or suture the graft in the bed. A few interrupted sutures sufficient to prevent the skin from retracting at the margins are placed between the long tie-over sutures.

An ideal material to be used as the tie-over dressing is fluffed gauze. Fluffed cotton, Acrilan, wool, or mechanic's waste are also satisfactory materials. The selected material is worked back and forth over the graft to hold it evenly in the bed, and the sutures are tied in place. It is advisable to keep the tie-over dressing from rocking and disturbing the graft. This dressing can then in turn be covered with Elastoplast or an Ace bandage.

The Pressure Dressing. A great deal of importance was formerly attributed to the pressure dressing in the success of a skin grafting procedure. It is realized today that the main object of the pressure dressing is to maintain contact between the graft and the host bed.

After the graft has been fixed in position, care should be taken to express any collection of blood or serum which may have become interposed between the graft and the bed. It is obvious that the thinner the fibrin layer between the graft and the host bed, the quicker the host vessels can penetrate the graft. The pressure dressing, however, does not necessarily hasten the fibrin fixation of the graft. Furthermore, Polk (1966) showed that the rate of graft adherence was greatest in the first eight hours and continued at a slower rate through the fourth day. After 24 hours only the most careless dressing change results in any significant displacement of the graft.

The pressure dressing has considerable value in skin grafting of the extremities by assuring a uniform pressure over the entire grafted area and the portion of the extremity distal to the grafted area. Venous congestion and edema are prevented, and the circulation in the grafted area is improved. The extremity should always be elevated as an added precaution to enhance circulation in the limb. Adequate immobilization of the grafted region should be assured, and the grafted extremity should always be provided with a plaster splint to prevent joint motion in the grafted area. Movements of flexion and extension would result in displacement of the graft from the host bed and tearing of the ingrowing capillaries, with subsequent hemorrhage and hematoma formation under the graft.

Before the compression dressing is applied, verification that there are no blood clots under the graft should be made. It is useful to leave one area of the junction of the graft to the wound edge unsutured in order to permit removal of any blood clots by means of cotton tip applicators or irrigation with a rubber bulb syringe. Patient hand compression over the graft until adhesion of the graft has taken place, prior to the completion of the suturing and the application of the pressure dressing, prevents the recurrence of blood clots beneath the graft.

Skin Graft Inlay (Stent). In resurfacing defects in the oral, nasal, or orbital cavities, the mucosal or skin graft can be secured and immobilized by a mold of dental compound. The latter was discovered by Stent, an English dentist, and the term "Stent" has come to mean a splint. This technique was called the "epidermic inlay" by Esser (1917) and was used in reconstructing an obliterated oral vestibular sulcus through a cutaneous incision.

Waldron, working with Gillies at Sidcup, developed the technique of introducing the skin graft–covered stent through the mouth. The scarred tissue in the obliterated sulcus is incised, and a defect, greater in size than a normal sulcus, is created (Fig. 6–19). An impression is taken of the resulting cavity with softened dental compound. The latter is allowed to harden and is covered with the skin graft (dermal surface exposed). With the aid of a prosthodontist, the dental compound mold can be secured to a metal plate fitted to a dental cap splint. As there is a tendency toward contraction, splinting must be maintained for six months.

Skin Graft Outlay. The skin graft inlay technique was modified by Gillies for securing a skin graft following correction of burn ectropion of the eyelid. The edges of the defect are undermined and the softened dental compound

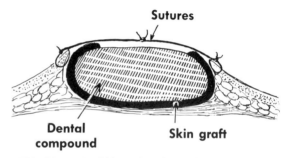

FIGURE 6–20. Skin graft outlay technique (cross section).

is spread under the undermined edges of the defect (Fig. 6–20). After the mold hardens, the skin graft is applied. The technique provides an excess of skin to accommodate late wound contraction.

Postoperative Care of a Skin Graft. The postoperative care is as important as the technique of application of the graft for the successful vascularization of the graft. Within 48 hours, and preferably after 24 hours, the graft is inspected in its entirety. The sutures are cut over the center of the dressing and the tie-over dressing gently teased from the bed. To prevent the graft from being torn off the host bed, one of the sutures is grasped near the knot and held firmly while the dressing is lifted away from the graft in this area. This maneuver is repeated along the margin of the graft until the tie-over dressing can be turned back like a page of a book. Often a "peek" can be obtained by cutting sutures only along one edge. It is not necessary to remove the dressing completely from the bed unless something must be done to the graft.

Seromas, hematomas, or clots under the graft should be immediately evacuated. This can be done in the patient's room. A stab incision is made in the graft overlying the hematoma, clot, or seroma. A sterile eyedropper is attached to the nasal suction machine, and the margin of the graft is lifted at the stab wound; the sterile eyedropper is inserted under the graft, and the collection is evacuated. If this is done within the first 24 hours, the graft can be salvaged and a 100 per cent take of the graft is assured. The dressing is carefully folded back over the graft and dressed with a wrap-around bandage. It may be advisable to inspect the graft the following day or within two days, depending on the condition of the graft at the initial dressing.

Skin Grafting by the Open Method: Grafts Without Dressings. Split-thickness grafts, when applied to an extremity or to other parts

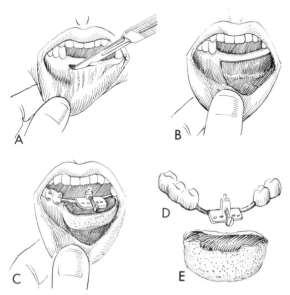

FIGURE 6–19. Skin graft inlay technique. *A*, The obliterated sulcus is incised. *B*, Resulting defect. *C*, Dental compound impression of defect is covered with the skin graft and secured to a metal plate fitted to a dental splint. *D*, Metal plate attached to dental splint. *E*, Dental compound covered with skin graft (dermal side exposed).

of the body, are usually covered with a pressure dressing, which is considered an important and necessary part of the procedure. The primary purpose of a dressing is to protect and hold the graft so that it will not be disturbed during the first days while the graft develops its blood supply and becomes adherent. It should be kept in mind that the pressure dressing is not essential for a split-thickness graft to "take," become vascularized and incorporated into the recipient by the establishment of vascular continuity between the graft and host.

In certain areas of the body a dressing is contraindicated; these areas are the chest, abdomen, shoulder, back, and neck (see Chapter 34). These anatomical areas are in constant motion from breathing, turning, and other movements of the body, and it is practically impossible to apply a satisfactory dressing that will not cause friction and movement at the graft-host interface. Constant movement of the graft produces seromas, hematomas, or a loss of contact between graft and host. All these factors impair the vascularization of the skin graft.

In preparation of the recipient bed after the surgical excision in the above areas, the bed is inspected for oozing or bleeding points. These are controlled by a combination of warm saline compresses, 5–0 catgut ties, and needle tip electrocoagulation.

After the grafts have been excised, the undersurface of the graft and the bed are gently dried with a cotton sponge. Care is taken not to rub the recipient area, as this will produce additional bleeding. As the graft is applied, it becomes adherent to the bed, and this will prevent further bleeding.

When grafts are applied by this technique, few if any sutures are required. The graft should not be shifted, pulled, or otherwise moved in the bed to avoid disrupting the early fixation of the graft to the bed. It is most important that the host bed be dry, and irrigations under the graft cannot be permitted or the graft will be washed off. For best results the grafts should be cut thin (0.10 to 0.15 inch), or they will curl at the margins and pull away from the bed. Breathing and limited movement by the patient do not result in slipping or shifting of the graft, as occurs under a dressing.

If the skin is to be applied under maximum tension, it must be sutured at the margins in order to prevent it from pulling away from the bed. However, regardless of the method of application and fixation of the graft, no dressing is used in these critical areas.

The donor site is dressed in the desired manner, and the patient is sent to the recovery room with no dressing over the grafted area. A large cradle or a fenestrated paper container taped to the area is used to keep the bed clothes from touching the graft; the patient is restrained until he is awake and cooperative. The patient is advised to limit his movement in the bed for one to two days until the graft becomes adherent. The graft is open to inspection, and its progress is easily followed. As seromas and hematomas appear, a stab incision is made over these sites and their contents drained or removed by "rolling" with a cotton-tipped applicator.

The skin graft will usually be pink, adherent, and viable in 48 hours. Crusts appearing around the margins are removed with forceps, keeping the margins clean. In grafting by the open method, the postoperative care is relatively simple, as there are no dressings to change. When the grafts have become adherent, a dressing may be applied if marginal infection and drainage are problems.

The mesh graft is less amenable to the open method of treatment, as it tends to become desiccated; the closed method is therefore preferable. Mesh grafts are vascularized in a manner similar to other types of autografts. Epithelization spreads from the edges of the graft, and epithelization of the nongrafted interstices is completed by the eighth postoperative day (Šmahel and Ganzoni, 1972).

Delayed Skin Grafting. The term "delayed skin grafting" refers to the application of a skin graft over a wound as a delayed procedure after allowing time for an improvement in the recipient bed. The delay permits more successful grafting. The technique is particularly indicated following the excision of burn scars or the excision of any lesion where hemostasis is not complete. It should also be considered for an avascular recipient bed.

One obvious disadvantage of the technique is that the patient is subjected to an additional anesthesia. This can be obviated by using any of the methods discussed under the section Storage of Skin Grafts.

After a delay of at least 48 hours there should be no active bleeding in the recipient site. An early, smooth, granulating bed provides more favorable conditions for successful grafting. Furthermore, Šmahel (1969) has observed that skin graft vascularization is more rapid when the delayed technique is employed.

Causes of Failure of "Take" of a Skin Graft. The one most important cause of failure of a take of any graft is *bleeding and hematoma* beneath the graft. A skin graft survives by the rapid ingrowth of host vessels, and the interposition of blood clots or serum will prevent this ingrowth. Consequently, hemostasis must be complete before application of the graft. Any clots or seromas that accumulate must be evacuated before there is permanent loss of the graft. If adequate hemostasis cannot be obtained, the skin graft should be applied as a delayed procedure.

The second most important cause of graft failure is *external mechanical factors*. These include an improperly applied dressing, failure to apply a plaster splint where immobilization of the extremity is necessary, and the use of a dressing when complete immobilization cannot be assured, as on the trunk and shoulders.

The third cause of loss is *necrosis* in the bed. This is particularly true when the bed is composed primarily of fat or when there has been a crush-avulsion type of injury. Exposed bone, tendon, and nerves without their associated periosteum, paratenon, or epineurium provide an unsuitable bed for successful grafting.

When the graft is to be applied over fat, except possibly on the face, one can anticipate bleeding under the graft together with the presence of avascular areas where the large fat lobules undergo necrosis from lack of blood supply. If a graft is to be applied at the time of the excision, one takes a calculated risk in losing certain areas of the graft. Delayed grafting is preferred in this situation.

When adequate hemostasis has been obtained, an excellent take of the graft can be anticipated with a graft placed on deep fascia, muscle, the deep layers of the dermis, or even over a layer of de-epithelized scar tissue.

The fourth and the least common cause of graft failure is *infection*. All too often in the past, the surgeon has blamed the failure of the graft on infection. It is true that, in certain instances, partial or even complete loss of a graft has resulted from a particularly severe infection. Group A beta-hemolytic streptococcal infections have resulted in rapid and complete loss of a skin graft. In most instances the wound is sterile within 18 to 24 hours after the application of the graft. In addition, one does not expect an infection in a clean, surgically excised wound.

Postoperative Care of the Donor Area.   Care of the donor site varies from surgeon to surgeon, but the aim is to stop drainage and to secure a dry wound as soon as possible. This is particularly important in regions where the humidity is high.

One routine that has proved satisfactory begins immediately after the cutting of the graft. The donor site is covered with moist sponges, which are either turned over or replaced until most, if not all, of the oozing has stopped. It is then covered with a layer of nonadherent gauze, such as xeroform gauze. The latter is covered with Kerlix or gauze compresses without cotton. Cotton, which obstructs drainage and dries on the outside, gives the impression that the whole dressing is dry, while beneath the cotton there may be drainage that is trapped. This can lead to delayed healing or even infection of the donor site.

On the first postoperative day, the dressing is removed down to the first layer (xeroform gauze). A hair dryer is employed on the exposed area until a dry coagulum is formed. The gauze is not disturbed and is allowed to separate spontaneously, an event which usually occurs in seven to ten days. If this has not occurred in ten to 12 days, one may anticipate delayed healing and some residual scarring in the donor area.

Careful attention to the donor site is important to prevent scar hypertrophy occurring where the graft was either deliberately or inadvertently cut rather thick, leaving a residual thin dermal bed. Should the graft have been cut too thick, it is best to take a thin split-thickness graft and cover the donor site immediately.

If a Pseudomonas overgrowth of the donor area occurs, it is best managed with the frequent changing of gauze dressings soaked in either 0.5 per cent silver nitrate solution or 0.25 per cent acetic acid. A split-thickness donor site can be converted to a full-thickness defect following a Pseudomonas infection.

The initial enthusiasm for porcine xenograft dressings of donor sites has waned with reports of increased inflammation, delay of healing, and incorporation of the porcine xenogenic collagen in the subepithelial layer of the donor site (Salisbury and coworkers, 1973).

Healing of Donor Sites.   In 1944 Converse and Robb-Smith, after an investigation of the healing of split-thickness graft donor sites, concluded that the thinner the graft, the more rapid the healing of the donor site; the quality of the repair was proportional to the rapidity of healing. Thin (Thiersch) graft donor sites healed within ten days and left merely a faintly visible scar with a soft pliable base. However, thick split-thickness donor sites, which included 70 to 90 per cent of the dermis, required three to eight weeks to heal and often left permanent disfigurement in the form of retracted hypertrophic scars. The healed donor site, following the removal of such thick split-thickness grafts, was found on histologic examination to be covered by thin atrophic epithelium incapable of providing adequate surface protection. Under the atrophic epithelium was a thick layer of dense scar tissue almost five times the thickness of normal dermis and completely deficient in elastic tissue.

A study of the healing of split-thickness donor sites by Sawhney, Subbaraju, and Chakravarti (1969) showed that the regenerated epidermis is fully differentiated and normal looking in 21 to 30 days. The dermis shows little evidence of regeneration, and the portion of the dermis removed with the graft represents a net loss of dermis to the skin.

By comparing ungrafted split-thickness graft donor sites with grafted donor sites, Thompson (1960) noted that prolonged periods were required for complete healing of ungrafted sites and that there was an associated high incidence of hypertrophic scarring. In contrast to the flat epidermis with a greatly increased depth of dense subepidermal scar tissue, which even after 20 months was devoid of elastic tissue, the grafted donor site after a similar period presented an epidermis showing normal surface corrugations and rete peg formation. Beneath the epithelium there was delicate dermal tissue with normal elastic tissue content. There was also evidence of advanced regeneration of elastic tissue in the organized layers intermediate between the graft and host tissue. Tests done by the technique described by Guttman (1947), using quinizarin powder, showed that in the grafted donor site sweating was demonstrated as early as ten weeks after grafting, though the active sweat pore population never approached the density found in ungrafted donor sites (except at the site of hypertrophic scarring where sweating was virtually absent). Histologic examination of grafted donor sites, however, showed an apparently normal distribution of secretory coils in and beneath the deep dermis of the host. Thompson (1960), by histochemical investigation, demonstrated unimpaired intracellular enzyme activity of the sweat glands and concluded that they continue to survive and function. Sweat gland secretion is probably resorbed internally into the local circulation.

Repeated Removal of Skin Grafts from the Same Donor Site. A second crop of split-thickness skin may be removed from the same donor site two or three weeks after the first crop, and a third crop may be removed at a later date. Gillman, Penn, Bronks, and Roux (1955) pointed out that the regenerating epithelium covering a split-thickness graft donor site attains its maximum thickness in 14 to 16 days after the operation.

STORAGE OF SKIN GRAFTS

The simplest method of storing split-thickness skin grafts is by suturing the grafts to the donor site. Shepard (1972) has shown that skin grafts can be stored without complications on their donor sites and transferred at the bedside without the need for an anesthetic for up to ten days. The technique lends itself to delayed grafting whenever hemostasis is incomplete or there is an avascular recipient bed.

Perry (1966) has reviewed the different cryobiologic methods of skin preservation.

Skin Storage Above 0° C in Saline or Serum. Marrangoni (1950) recommended storage of skin autografts in 10 per cent serum in a standard refrigerator. Skin grafts can be wrapped in a saline-soaked sponge and stored in a sterile Petri dish. Actual immersion in saline or Ringer's solution tends to macerate the graft. Feller and DeWeese (1958) felt that skin stored in a refrigerator (4° C) remained viable for up to 23 days. After 14 days of storage in saline, skin graft respiratory activity is halved (Lawrence, 1972). After 20 days skin cellular respiration had ceased, and this corresponds with a progressive decrease in clinical viability of skin stored in a refrigerator at 3° C over a three-week period (Georgiade and co-workers, 1956).

Preservation of Skin in the Frozen State (Below 0° C). Frozen skin must be pretreated with a protective agent, slowly frozen, and rapidly thawed. Lawrence (1972) reported that glycerol was preferable to dimethyl sulfoxide (DMSO) as a cryoprotective agent. The successful take of deep-frozen skin autografts was 40 per cent (Santoni-Rugiu, 1962). The metabolic activity of skin stored in liquid nitrogen was 60 to 70 per cent of the prestorage rate and did not vary for periods of 1 to 28 days (Lawrence, 1972). Bondoc and Burke (1971) showed that skin grafts could be stored in liquid nitrogen for up to six months.

Preservation of Freeze-Dried Skin at Room Temperature. The vascularization of freeze-dried skin is insignificant and of poor quality (Santoni-Rugiu, 1962). Being nonviable, freeze-dried skin serves only as a biologic dressing.

Stereomicroscopic observations were made by Taylor, Gerstner, and Converse (1956) to follow the course of vascular changes in mammalian transplants preserved at temperatures below freezing. Ingrowth of vessels was always delayed and incomplete, occurring as late as five to seven days after grafting. In contrast, revascularization occurred within three days in untreated skin grafts.

Nonviable, freeze-dried skin grafts removed from bovine embryo and placed on the chorioallantois of the chick embryo are readily penetrated by the membranal blood vessels, but at a reduced rate when compared to that seen in viable and untreated skin xenografts (Converse and coworkers, 1958). Rogers and Converse (1958) observed in histologic sections of fresh and freeze-dried embryonic bovine skin applied to experimental defects in man that endothelial buds from the host bed had grown into the graft; they disintegrated within ten days.

Using gross and stereomicroscopic methods, Berggren and Lehr (1965) reported that some split-thickness autografts and allografts, after treatment with 10 per cent dimethyl sulfoxide solution and storage in the frozen state, became effectively vascularized. On the other hand, if the grafts were not viable, they exhibited no evidence of vascularization and as a consequence became soft, white, and nonadherent.

According to O'Donoghue and Zarem (1971) from the direct examination of blood vessels within the mouse transparent chamber, the preserved isografts are capable of inducing hyperemia and neovascularization in the recipient bed and of becoming vascularized. Hyperemia appears in the host beds of the lyophilized grafts and the freeze-thawed grafts by the fifth day after transplantation, but neovascularization occurs on the seventh and eighth days in the respective host beds; the vascularization of the grafts is completely achieved by the tenth and eleventh days, respectively. It should be noted that lyophilized grafts seem to be more effective in inducing the host vascular budding and to be vascularized, when compared with that of freeze-thawed grafts. With the same mouse chamber technique, Pandya and Zarem

in 1974 were not able to demonstrate vascularization in either the vacuum-dried or frozen xenografts of porcine split-thickness skin on mice.

In summary, the findings appear to support the concept that the revascularization of frozen or freeze-dried skin grafts applied to man or animals is not entirely dependent upon the viability of the original graft vasculature. As demonstrated by the study of Ballantyne, Hawthorne, Rees, and Seidman (1971), vascular ingrowth from the host site can occur readily, provided that the vascular pattern of tissue grafts after preservation at low temperature is not unduly disorganized. However, Bromberg, Song, and Mohn (1965), working with freeze-dried split-thickness pig skin xenografts transplanted to mice, found no evidence of revascularization.

BEHAVIOR OF THE SPLIT-THICKNESS SKIN GRAFT

Growth and Contraction. Although surgically created defects in growing minipigs resurfaced with either a full-thickness skin graft or skin flap grew at approximately the same rate as normal uninjured skin, similar defects covered with split-thickness skin grafts showed considerable contraction (Baran and Horton, 1972). Ragnell (1952) demonstrated in rabbits that contraction of full-thickness skin grafts reached a maximum at one month and had subsided after two months. The full-thickness grafts then expanded to their original size and kept pace with the animal's subsequent growth.

Contraction of grafted skin has been a source of disappointment for plastic surgeons, particularly if there is resultant wrinkling or corrugation of the graft in an exposed facial or neck wound.

Primary Contraction. Skin grafts possess an inherent tendency toward contraction because of the contained elastic fibers. The only variable in skin grafts of different thickness is the amount of dermis and its contained elastic tissue. Consequently, primary contraction or shrinkage of skin grafts prior to application to the recipient bed ranges from 41 per cent of body surface area (full-thickness) to 9 per cent for thin split-thickness grafts of the Ollier-Thiersch variety (Davis and Kitlowski, 1931).

Secondary Contraction. Secondary contraction defines the shrinkage of a skin graft after it has been revascularized. While it is true that the thicker a skin graft, the less tendency toward shrinkage, secondary contraction follows biological changes in the host bed and *not* in the transplanted skin. For example, a skin graft transplanted to a relatively fixed site, such as the pericranium, will show less contraction than a skin graft on a mobile site, such as an eyelid. The work of Majno and associates (1971) identifying the presence of the myofibroblast (see Chapter 3) explains that the transplanted skin is a passive victim of a contracting recipient bed.

Some measures can be taken to decrease the contraction phenomenon following skin grafting. Full-thickness or thick split-thickness grafts resist contraction better than thin grafts. Splinting of a relatively mobile recipient bed (e.g., the neck) is helpful. Darts extended out into the surrounding tissue also serve to splint the grafted area and decrease the degree of contraction.

Color Changes. Obtaining a satisfactory color match between the grafted skin and the surrounding cutaneous surface can be a difficult problem. As mentioned earlier in the chapter, donor sites below the neck should be avoided in skin grafting defects of the facial region. Superior results are obtained with local (e.g., retroauricular, supraclavicular, or upper eyelid) full-thickness grafts; color differences are minimal. If split-thickness skin must be used, the neck is the preferred donor site. Split-thickness skin, especially the thin Ollier-Thiersch type, tends to develop pigmentation changes with time. Dark-skinned individuals are also more prone to pigmentation problems.

Mir y Mir (1961) has recommended serial dermabrasions to correct hyperpigmentation of a skin graft. It has also been noted that skin removed from a previously used donor site is less likely to show undesirable pigmentation changes (Lopez-Mas and associates, 1972). In the absence of an old donor site, a thin graft can be removed before a second "crop" is cut at a later date to resurface a critical area such as on the face. Hyperpigmentation can also be avoided by applying commercially available sun screen ointments to block the ultraviolet rays which, along with hormones, are the exogenous factors in melanogenesis.

Sweat gland and sebaceous gland function in transplanted skin is discussed later in the chapter under Reinnervation of Skin Grafts and Flaps.

SKIN GRAFTING ON A DERMAL BED: DERMAL OVERGRAFTING*

The application of split-thickness skin grafts to a host bed of dermis or scar tissue following preliminary removal of the surface epithelium was first described by Webster in 1954 and published by Webster, Peterson, and Stein in 1958. The method was applied solely to the treatment of unstable scars of the lower limb, dermal overgrafting being regarded as a simple and rapid substitute for repair by skin flaps. In one patient as many as three separate grafts were serially applied at three separate operations, each graft surviving on the bleeding, abraded surface of the graft or scar beneath it.

Hynes (1956, 1957, 1959) independently investigated the technique and developed the full spectrum of the applications under the title of "shaving and skin grafting." Dermal overgrafting constitutes one of the most valuable contributions to plastic surgery made during the past two decades and is the treatment of choice in the operative management of chronic radiodermatitis, certain extensive unstable scars, giant nevi, and many lower limb injuries formerly treated by staged skin flaps.

Principle of the Method. As described earlier in the chapter, the split-thickness skin graft becomes vascularized within 48 to 72 hours after transfer. Hynes (1957) has shown that mature scars possess a much freer capillary circulation, which is capable of vascularizing skin grafts with more certainty than subcutaneous fat or fascia. If the epidermal covering of a scar is removed, despite the relatively impaired vascularity, there remains a multitude of minute but freely bleeding capillary points visible to the naked eye; these facilitate vascular anastomoses between the graft and host to such a degree that active blood flow to the entire dermal capillary plexus of the graft is restored. This is visible clinically and histologically, but it is more precisely demonstrable by recording the clearance rate of sterile technetium-99m as pertechnetate ion, used as a measure of local blood flow following its injection into a scar preoperatively and at intervals after dermal overlay grafting. Thus, the scar shown in Figure 6–21, *A* showed circulatory clearance rates of injected radioactive isotope reduced to one-fifth of the rate in the contralat-

*Contributed by Noel Thompson, F.R.C.S.

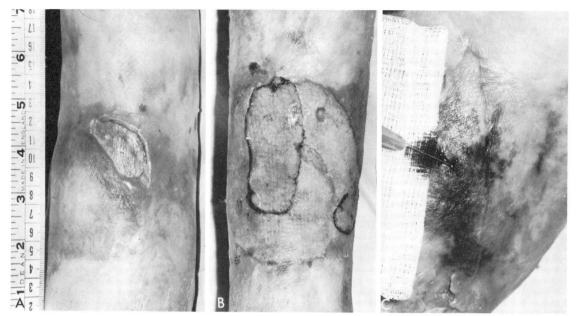

FIGURE 6–21. Dermal overgrafting technique. *A*, Unstable scar of the lower extremity. *B*, Following application of two layers of dermal onlay. *C*, Demonstration of dermal lymphatic plexus in the graft by patent blue violet dye. Note that the lymphatics are continuous with the surrounding tissue.

eral normal limb preoperatively. However, blood flow increased to almost double the normal value three months after the serial application of two layers of dermal overgrafts (Fig. 6–21, *B*). Over the succeeding months there was a progressive reduction to normal levels (Thompson, 1970; Thompson and Ell, 1974).

The formation of lymphatic connections between the graft and the surrounding host tissues is of almost equal importance in obtaining a stable repair by skin grafting. By injecting a suitable dye into the dermis of split-thickness skin grafts, Butcher and Hoover (1955) were able to demonstrate lymphatic connections between the dermal plexus of the graft and host tissue at two to four months after skin grafting. After they injected patent blue violet dye in 10 per cent isotonic solution into the subepithelial scar tissue, no lymphatic plexus could be demonstrated. However, after resurfacing the scar with dermal overlay grafts, a dermal lymphatic plexus was present in the grafted tissue, and this was also continuous with the dermal lymphatic plexus of the surrounding host tissues (Fig. 6–21, *C*) (Thompson, 1970; Thompson and Ell, 1974).

In scars, the dermal pad, which is the most important element in giving weight-bearing protection, does not regenerate, and the surface epithelium, which is thin and devoid of papillae, can be readily stripped from the underlying fibrous tissue (Brown and McDowell,

1958). The application of thick split-thickness skin grafts restores the dermal pad with its content of collagen and numerous interlacing elastic fibers, components essential to providing adequate tissue resilience to withstand surface trauma, together with a normally papillated and firmly adherent epidermis. By repeated dermal overlay grafting, the dermal pad can be built up to almost any required thickness.

Histologic Studies of Dermal Overgrafting. The technique of overgrafting involves the burying of epidermal appendages — hair follicles and sebaceous and sweat glands. The theoretical possibility of widespread and recurrent complications from epidermoid cyst formation has been considered a contraindication to such a procedure. The burying of epithelial elements is routinely followed by the formation of microscopic epidermoid cysts, which undergo spontaneous dissolution within a year in the vast majority of cases (Thompson, 1960). Scattered cysts of pinhead size may appear following grafting and disappear spontaneously within three to six months. Simple incisions without anesthesia evacuate these collections of sebaceous material. The prompt evacuation of the sebaceous collection is necessary to prevent large collections which may undermine the grafted skin.

Thompson (1960) has made a histologic

study of grafted donor sites and has reported the following findings:

1. Elastic tissue is present in the dermis of the graft and host in the biopsies studied. In the intermediate layers between the graft and host bed, elastic tissue appears late, being absent at three months but plentiful at 20 months.

2. Hair follicles for the most part undergo epidermoid cyst formation and subsequent disintegration, whether situated in the graft or the host dermis.

3. Sebaceous gland cells are found in relation to epidermoid cysts formed from pilosebaceous units as late as six weeks after grafting. None persists after this time.

4. Sweat gland elements persist as functioning units only if continuity is reestablished between the superficial and deep sweat gland structures. The remainder of the epithelial elements buried under the split-thickness graft form microscopic epidermoid cysts, which undergo spontaneous dissolution within a year in the majority of cases.

It is a chief function of squamous epithelium to produce keratin (Montagna, 1956). Such keratinized epithelial debris thrown off by the squamous epithelial wall into the lumen of the cyst increases tension inside the cyst cavity, causing necrosis of the epithelial wall and allowing direct contact with the dermis. As first indicated by Stewart (1912) and later by Peer and Paddock (1937), direct contact of this debris with the surrounding dermal tissue results in the replacement of the cyst by granulation tissue and foreign body giant cells. When phagocytosis of the epithelial products is complete, microscopic cysts are replaced by fibrous tissue, and the foreign body giant cell and round cell infiltration disappears.

Technique. The surface epidermis can be removed by sandpapering (Webster and co-workers, 1958), dermabrasion (Serafini, 1962), dermatome (Rees and Casson, 1966), or free-hand graft knife or scalpel blade (Hynes, 1956). It is essential that the removal of epidermis be meticulous and complete. A light circumferential incision is made to demarcate clearly the area to be shaved of epidermis. The free capillary host bleeding that results is readily controlled by pressure with a gauze swab moistened with warm saline or topical adrenalin solution (1:100,000). Persistent bleeding points can be controlled by fine electrocoagulation, for hemostasis must be absolute before the surface graft is applied.

The split-thickness skin graft is cut thickly where surface protection on a weight-bearing surface is required, the thickness of the dermal element being increased by applying the graft without tension in a state of maximum relaxation; this does not adversely affect graft "take" and appreciably increases the bulk of transplanted tissue. Where cosmetic values only are to be considered, as in extensive facial scars, the graft is cut thinly. Some correction of depressed scars can be effected by marking out the size and shape of the graft required at the donor site. The donor site pattern is manipulated by an assistant in order to alter the convexity of the surface, so that on cutting the graft the body of the graft will be thick, whereas its margins remain thin.

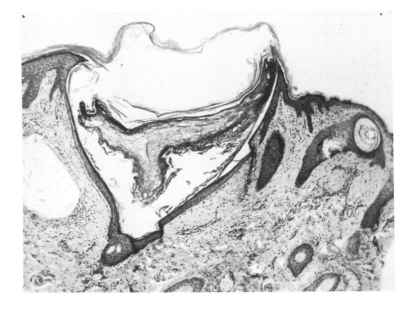

FIGURE 6–22. Microscopic section of epidermoid cyst at the graft surface following dermal overgrafting.

The margins of the graft are accurately coapted to the skin edges at the margins of the recipient site, sutured in situ, and a suitable pressure dressing applied; the "take" of the grafts is so certain that elaborate immobilization is unnecessary.

When laminated dermal overgrafts are used to build up a thick, protective dermal pad, an interval of at least one month is allowed to elapse between stages of overgrafting.

Complications. Failure of survival of the grafts is almost unknown in the absence of hematoma formation or infection.

It is not rare, in early weeks, for minute miliary cysts to appear at the graft surface. These are invariably epidermoid cysts (Fig. 6–22) arising from epidermal appendages (usually hair follicles) in the graft or in the underlying host dermis (Thompson, 1960). They respond to simple unroofing of the cysts and show no tendency to recur after a few months. In scars and radiodermatitis, the absence of epithelial elements in the host bed at the recipient site greatly reduces the incidence of cyst formation.

Indications for Dermal Overgrafting. (1) *Extensive pigmented moles,* if planed off along the deepest layers of the dermis, lose most of their pigmented cells, while a healthy capillary bed remains in the residual host dermis sufficient to nourish the dermal overlay graft (Hynes, 1956). The latter is cut thickly so that any remaining islands of pigment are usually successfully camouflaged. If small pigmented outcrops become visible later, limited local excisions may be used to produce further improvement. Since the dermoepidermal junctional area is entirely removed, the possibility of late malignant change in surviving cells must be slight.

(2) *Extensive scars* which are unstable, contracted, depressed, pigmented, or hypertrophied can be treated with a speed and simplicity unequalled by skin flap replacement. There is also a certainty of graft take unapproached by skin grafting following full-thickness scar excision (Hynes, 1957). Its use should be limited to mature scars, since active or florid scars, although accepting the graft with certainty, tend to become thickened and raised again. Mature hypertrophic scars, with irregularly corrugated or hyperpigmented surface, can be greatly improved in appearance by shaving them flat and applying a thin sheet of split-thickness skin graft. Satisfactory cosmetic results are obtained in extensive facial burns by extending the circumference of the treated area widely to the hairline, jawline, nasolabial groove, and eyebrows (Serafini, 1962).

The blood supply in these regions of reduced vascularity is restored to normal levels. Even if the volume of protective tissue reconstituted on exposed parts is less than in skin flap reconstruction, the surface is almost routinely adequate to sustain normal levels of activity. When used as laminated layers of dermal overgrafts successively applied in the manner advocated by Webster, Peterson, and Stein (1958), especially on weight-bearing areas of the foot, the dermal onlay stands up to use better than a skin flap and lacks the unstable mobility of the latter. In addition, dermal overgrafting offers a simple and effective alternative to the cross-leg flap (see Chapter 86) in traumatic and ulcerative lesions of the lower limb, including those cases in which granulation tissue has formed over exposed tibial bone and bare, stripped tendons after repeated thin shaving-down of the exposed surface.

Chronic venous stasis ulcers respond better

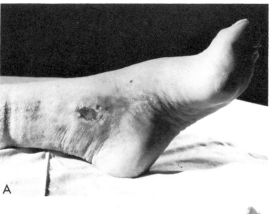

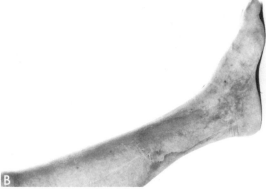

FIGURE 6–23. Dermal overgrafting for venous ulcers. *A,* Appearance of chronic venous ulcer of the medial malleolar area. *B,* Following serial application of dermal overgrafts. The perforating veins were also ligated.

to management if the initial skin graft is followed by wide dermal overlay grafting of the entire medial malleolar region following appropriate vein ligation (Fig. 6–23).

Thin adherent scars can be denuded of epidermis without exposure of the underlying bone or other deep tissue, and following maturation the dermal onlays develop a considerable amount of resilience and mobility. The method has particular applicability in the treatment of scars contiguous with important structures (exposed meninges, major vessels of the neck or extremities, exposed pleura, and so forth).

(3) *Chronic radiodermatitis* is associated with discomfort and local irritation accompanied by scaling and cracking of unstable surface epithelium; in the later stages there can be malignant epithelial changes (see Chapter 20). As with scars, removal of the surface epidermis reveals a freely bleeding capillary bed which effectively nourishes any applied skin graft. This affords immediate relief of all symptoms, and, since the entire surface epithelium is inevitably completely removed, the possibility of late malignant change is eliminated (Hynes, 1959). It is of interest that, with improved vascularization and restoration of normal tissue at the surface, the histologic appearances of the deeper tissue beneath the graft revert towards normal (Fig. 6–24).

(4) There are a number of *miscellaneous uses* of dermal overgrafting. The superficial removal of epidermis can be used at the site of insetting of a migrated tube flap and at the site of application of composite auricular grafts by applying a generous flange of graft skin at the periphery of the composite graft to a corresponding shaved rim of skin at the recipient site. This will increase the surface area through which vascularization of the graft can occur (Hynes, 1959). Dermal overgrafting has also been employed to resurface the skin of xeroderma pigmentosum (Converse, 1964).

(5) *Tattoos* can be treated successfully by removing a thick split-thickness skin graft from the site of the tattoo and applying a thick dermal overgraft to the defect (Rees and Casson, 1966). It is often possible to excise any small

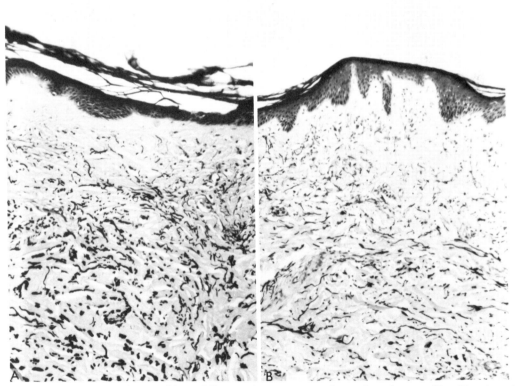

FIGURE 6–24. Chronic radiodermatitis. *A*, Microscopic appearance prior to dermal overgrafting. Note hyperkeratinization, atrophy of epidermis, and absence of epidermal appendages. Dermal collagen is replaced by coarse hyaline fibrous tissue with hypertrophic elastic tissue. Elastic stain. × 100. *B*, Two years after dermal overgrafting. Note epidermis with normal papillae and papillary dermis. There is improved vascularization and normal distribution of the elastic fibers of the underlying host bed. Elastic stain. × 100.

surviving islands of pigmentation in the host bed (Bailey, 1967) before applying the dermal overgraft, with a resulting improvement in the final appearance.

SKIN ALLOGRAFTS

Réverdin recommended the use of skin allografts in 1872, and Brown and associates (1953) advocated their use as biological dressings for extensive burn wounds and denuded areas.

The initial vascularization of skin allografts and the ultimate immunologic rejection have already been discussed. In order to avoid a rejection response, skin allografts, if used as biological dressings, should be changed every two to three days.

The chief handicap in the use of skin allografts is availability. They can be obtained fresh, usually from relatives, and either used immediately or stored after rapid freezing, as discussed above. Large crops of allograft skin can also be obtained from disease-free cadavers.

When used as biological dressings, skin allografts, as noted by Artz, Rittenbury, and Yarbrough (1972), can serve several functions:

1. Clean up granulating areas prior to autografting.
2. Protect open wounds from water and protein loss until autografts are available.
3. Decrease pain at the site of an open wound.
4. Facilitate early motion of the affected part.
5. Decrease surface bacterial counts.
6. Cover exposed vital structures.
7. Enhance the growth of any underlying epithelium (questionable).

Skin allografts are used chiefly as temporary coverage in patients who have sustained massive, full-thickness burns. Until permanent coverage can be obtained by autografting, skin allografts will serve to decrease the water and protein loss from the open wound, increase the patient's comfort, and decrease surface bacterial counts.

In burn patients the survival of skin allografts is fortunately prolonged (Rapaport and associates, 1964). Allergic responses of the delayed hypersensitivity type are also depressed by thermal injury (Casson and associates, 1966). Immunologic paralysis, antigen competition, and the chance sharing of histocompatibility antigens by randomly selected unrelated individuals are probably factors accounting for these phenomena following thermal injury.

Batchelor and Hackett (1970) showed that if the HL-A antigen incompatibility of the allograft donor is limited to one or less, allograft survival of two months or more can be expected in patients with third-degree burns involving more than 40 per cent of the body surface area.

The technique of alternating skin auto- and allografts for obtaining skin coverage for areas of extensive skin loss, such as occur in deep burns, was proposed by Mowlem and described by Jackson (1954). The technique has been largely replaced by the application of skin allografts under which "seeds" of autografts are placed. The technique of alternating autografts and allografts has been described by Colson and associates (1959), who have also studied the histology of the progressive replacement of the allografts by the autograft.

The Chinese (Burns Unit, 1973) reported remarkable improvement in survival rates following massive burns involving more than 70 per cent of the body surface area (third-degree burn exceeding 50 per cent BSA). After early debridement of the eschars, minute-sized skin autografts were introduced through button holes in large sheets of skin allografts which covered the burn wounds. The allografts provided favorable wound conditions for the spread and growth of the islands of skin autografts.

Skin allografts have also been recommended for coverage of second-degree burns (Miller and associates, 1967; Miller and White, 1972). In addition to providing relief of pain and inhibition of evaporative and exudative water loss, skin allografts promote healing with an improved cosmetic result.

Miller (1974) has cautioned against coverage of split-thickness skin donor sites with a viable skin allograft, as rejection of the latter results in conversion of the donor site from a partial thickness to a full-thickness defect.

SKIN XENOGRAFTS

Biological Behavior. The mode of vascularization and the changes of vascular pattern following the application of skin xenograft have not been extensively investigated. It has been generally held that the survival time of xenografts is too restricted to permit a successful reestablishment of blood circulation. According to Ribbert (1905), who transplanted skin from humans and guinea pigs on the subcutaneous tissue of rabbits, the xenografts were rejected within three days after transplantation. Loeb and Addison (1909, 1911) reported that skin xenografts interchanged between various animals inclusive of rats, mice, guinea pigs, rabbits, dogs, cats, and even pigeons eventually became necrotic between six and 11 postoperative days and occasionally even more rapidly. They did not provide information regarding either the vascularization or the vascular pattern of the xenografts.

In 1917 Kiyono and Sueyasu were apparently the first to report the transplantation of tissue, including skin, on the chorioallantoic membrane of the chick embryo and described absorption of nutrient fluids by the graft from the embryonic tissue and the actual entry of avian blood vessels into the grafts. Goodpasture, Douglas, and Anderson (1938) reported the revascularization and growth of split-thickness human skin grafts transplanted to the chorioallantois of the chick embryo; the presence of nucleated chick red blood cells in the graft was considered presumptive evidence of vascular ingrowth, an observation originally described by Murphy (1912). The chorionic capillaries penetrated the undersurface of the human skin dermis within 48 hours after grafting, and by three or four days the network of endothelial channels in the graft contained avian nucleated erythrocytes. Goodpasture, Douglas, and Anderson (1938) accepted the concept of the direct connection of host and graft vessels, because their histologic sections demonstrated a mixture of human and chick red blood cells, suggesting such a connection. However, they implied that, while there is ample evidence favoring anastomoses between the vasculatures of the human skin transplant and avian membrane as well as capillary ingrowth from the host into the undersurface of the graft, it does not permit active blood flow in the graft. The nourishment of the graft is therefore primarily derived from the "plasmatic circulation" through the temporary vascular communication between the two vascular systems.

Further attempts to define the mode of vascularization of skin xenografts from man and various animal species transplanted to the surface of the chorioallantoic membrane were undertaken by Converse, Ballantyne, Rogers, and Raisbeck (1958), who adopted the modified chick chorioallantois method of Goodpasture, Douglas, and Anderson (1938). Differences in structure between the mammalian erythrocytes and the nucleated avain erythrocytes made it possible to suggest that the definitive vasculature of the full-thickness skin xenografts of rabbit, rat, and bovine embryo was provided mainly by the host vascular ingrowth into the graft, while the original vessels of the grafts degenerated. When human skin of varying thickness was applied to the chorioallantois of the chick, the major definitive vasculature capable of supporting an active circulatory function between graft and host was similarly derived from the progressive ingrowth of avian endothelial cells into the graft. There was also rapid deterioration of most of the original graft vessels. In addition, histologic studies by Ballantyne and Converse (1958) of composite grafts taken from the auricles of rabbits and transferred to the chorionic membrane of chick embryos showed that the embryonal blood vessels made a tortuous course around the cartilage barrier and eventually penetrated into the dermis above the cartilage. Meanwhile, most of the preexisting vessels in the auricular grafts degenerated.

Blood flow was observed in the vasculature of skin xenografts removed from the rabbit or mouse and transferred to a recipient rat (Egdahl and associates, 1957, 1958), whereas transplants from rat, mouse, or guinea pig to rabbit never became effectively vascularized. According to the authors, who used the in vivo stereomicroscopic method of Taylor and Lehrfeld (1953) and an intradermal fluorescein test as their criteria for hemic circulation, the donor skin of mouse or rabbit placed on rat recipients was vascularized slower and had a shorter period of circulatory function when compared to that normally seen in skin allografts. Blood flow in the xenografts is usually initiated on the fourth or fifth day after grafting, attains the maximal rate of circulation soon thereafter, continues at this velocity for only a few hours, and suddenly ceases on or around the sixth day. It has been suggested that the vasculature of the xenografts capable of bearing blood flow was not newly formed but represented the original graft vascular system which had established direct connection with that of the host.

Rolle, Taylor, and Charipper (1959) exchanged skin grafts between mice and rats and found that the early sequence of vascular events occurring in the xenografts is similar to that in autografts and allografts. As shown by stereomicroscopy, histology, and the injection of dyes, the onset and restoration of circulation as well as other vascular changes prior to the rejection reaction are identical to those seen in allografts of mice or rats. The authors concluded that the blood supply in xenografts is restored by the establishment of continuity between the host and graft vessels.

Woodruff (1960) maintained that xenografts show little or no evidence of vascularization and that ischemia rather than rejection is responsible for the lack of success of the xenografts. Despite adherence to the wound and minimal inflammatory cell infiltration into the lower dermal collagen fibril networks of the graft, neither fresh porcine nor human skin xenografts showed evidence of vascularization by the India ink injection technique (Silverstein and associates, 1971).

Bromberg, Song, and Mohn (1965) injected Evans blue dye into the femoral veins of recipient mice after porcine split-thickness skin grafts had been applied on defects of the lower extremity. Following sacrifice of the animals, histologic study failed to show any evidence of revascularization of the xenografts. In contrast, murine skin autografts and allografts demonstrated functional revascularization by the third day.

With microangiographic techniques, Toranto, Salyer, and Myers (1974) demonstrated vascularization and viability of porcine skin xenografts on both rat and rabbit recipient sites by the fourth day. However, in the human host they were unable to distinguish between xenograft vascularization and invasion of the graft-host interface by granulation tissue. At 14 days there was no evidence of vascularization or viability of any xenografts, a finding consistent with rejection. Consequently, when porcine skin is used as a biological dressing, the authors recommended removing the xenograft to minimize the risk of host sensitization.

According to Ben-Hur, Solowey, and Rapaport (1969a), the response of mice to rat skin xenografts was characterized by early cellular infiltration of the xenografts, varying degrees of vascularization and blood circulation, and rapid epidermal destruction. Such grafts, which had become successfully vascularized by the third day following transplantation, showed abrupt cessation of blood flow, thrombosis, and hemorrhage on the third and fourth days; the other grafts, which failed to be vascularized, underwent the typical features of avascular white graft reaction with rapid progression into tan-colored eschars. In contrast to the rat xenografts, most of the guinea pig grafts applied to mouse recipients were characterized by absence of vascularization; in a few grafts the vessels and blood flow were stereomicroscopically evident on the third or fourth day. Although rabbit xenografts on mice exhibited an active process of vascularization, there was no stereomicroscopic evidence of active blood flow within the graft vasculature by the fourth postoperative day. However, the authors did not explain the mode of graft revascularization.

The nature of the vascular response was converted to that of guinea pig hosts to skin xenografts taken from mouse, rat, and rabbit by Ben-Hur, Solowey, and Rapaport (1969b) in a subsequent work. They found that xenograft reactivity in all three species studied was bascially a white graft (avascular) type of rejection.

The skin window technique was employed in human burn recipients who had received successive applications of porcine skin xenografts (McCabe and associates, 1973). An initial nonimmune, inflammatory cellular response during the first week following grafting was followed by an increasingly immunocompetent cellular reaction that peaked at 30 days. Anti-pigskin humoral factors could not be detected. While there was no clinical manifestation of any host sensitization, such symptoms could have been masked by the usual stormy clinical course of severely burned patients.

Clinical Use of Skin Xenografts. Rogers and Converse (1958) initially used experimental fetal calf skin xenografts as biological dressings in humans and observed a surprising lack of host reaction to the xenografts even after 12 to 17 days of graft retention. Bromberg and associates (1965) popularized the use of porcine xenografts as temporary biological dressings. The properties of skin xenografts as biological dressings are similar to those outlined in the section on Skin Allografts.

Burleson and Eiseman (1973) felt that the efficacy of biological dressings could be attributed to their ability to adhere to tissue, and the adherence was due to a fibrin-elastin biological bonding system. The same authors (1972) demonstrated that the unique adherent qualities of porcine skin were responsible for its antibacterial effect. They also questioned the role of neomycin and Betadine, used in the commercial preparation of porcine xenografts, and felt these agents might be responsible for reducing surface bacterial counts.

While xenografts have been most extensively used in covering large burn wounds prior to autografting, the use of xenografts has also been extended to the temporary coverage of exposed vessels, tendons, leg ulcers, flap donor sites, and skin graft donor sites (Elliott and Hoehn, 1973).

Salisbury and associates (1973) have cautioned against the use of porcine skin as temporary biological dressings of skin graft donor sites because of incorporation of porcine collagen in the subepithelial area of the donor site. In the authors' series there was a significant incidence of donor site inflammation and delayed repair following the application of porcine xenografts.

Two cases of neomycin-induced nephrotoxicity and ototoxicity following the application of commercially prepared porcine skin xenografts have been reported. High neomycin blood levels had been documented in both patients (Sugarbaker, Sabath and Morgan, 1974).

Porcine skin* is currently available in several forms: (1) fresh porcine skin can be used for up to 14 days after harvesting if stored in a refrigerator (4° C); (2) lyophilized (dried) porcine skin has an 18-month shelf-life, requires no refrigeration, and can be reconstituted with a sterile saline solution; (3) fresh frozen porcine skin can be stored three months at or below common freezer temperature (−18°C) and, once thawed, can be stored in a refrigerator for up to seven days; (4) frozen irradiated porcine skin can be stored indefinitely at −78° C or for six months at freezer temperature (−18° C).

COMPOSITE GRAFTS

Composite grafts of skin and cartilage from the auricle, of mucosa and cartilage from the septum, and of skin and fat from the ear lobe, and full-thickness nasal alar tissue are employed in the reconstructive surgery of the nose and auricle. Sweeney (1973) claimed remarkable success in transplanting composite grafts of skin and fat which had been pretreated with beating until ecchymosis and erythema had resulted. Composite grafts are discussed in Chapters 29 and 35.

Skin Flaps

In clinical practice some surface defects are not amenable to skin graft coverage; in such situations skin flaps are preferred. The relative

indications for the use of skin grafts and flaps are discussed later in the chapter.

Skin flaps are a composite of skin and subcutaneous tissue transferred from a donor to a recipient site. Survival is ensured by a vascular pedicle. The flap can have a random vasculature pattern or a specific arteriovenous sytem (axial pattern). The pedicle may remain attached during the transfer, or microsurgical anastomosis of the pedicle vessels of an axial pattern flap may be required (free flap). The flap may be transferred to an adjacent defect (local flap) or to a distant site (distant flap). The term "pedicle flap" is redundant, as a flap of skin must have a base or pedicle. "Skin flap" is the preferred term and will be used exclusively in the text. Delay of a flap is an expression designating a means of augmenting the surviving length of a flap by sympathetic denervation.

Vascular Anatomy

The blood supply of a flap must be carefully considered in planning a flap, and it is the critical factor in the survival of the flap. Knowledge of the blood supply not only avoids disastrous results but also permits resurfacing of defects with larger flaps and fewer staged surgical procedures. The vascular supply of the skin has three components: (1) segmental or major vessels arising from the aorta, (2) perforators, and (3) cutaneous vessels (Daniel and Williams, 1973).

Segmental Vasculature. The segmental vessels are large vessels arising from the aorta and

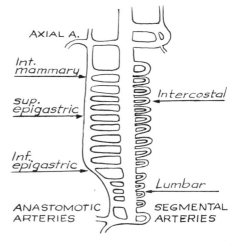

FIGURE 6–25. Vascular anatomy of a 5-mm human embryo. (From Daniel, R. K., and Williams, H. B.: The free transfer of skin flaps by microvascular anastomosis. An experimental study and a reappraisal. Plast. Reconstr. Surg., *52*:16. Copyright 1973, The Williams & Wilkins Company, Baltimore.)

---

*Burn Treatment Skin Bank, Inc., Phoenix, Arizona 85034.

lying deep to the muscle mass. The segmental pattern is determined in the developing embryo along the course of the underlying peripheral nerves (Fig. 6–25). In the 5-mm embryo there are 30 rows of dorsal segmental branches of the aorta, and their ventral rami become the intercostal lumbar arteries (Daniel and Williams, 1973). Intercommunications between the ventral segmental branches develop into the internal mammary and epigastric arteries. In the ex-

tremities the vascular pattern (e.g., lying along the limb axis) reflects the unsegmented mesodermal development of the extremity. Axial vessels, such as the femoral or branchial arteries, lie in close approximation to the major nerves in a location both deep and superficial to the musculature.

Perforators. The perforators are vessels connecting the segmental and cutaneous vas-

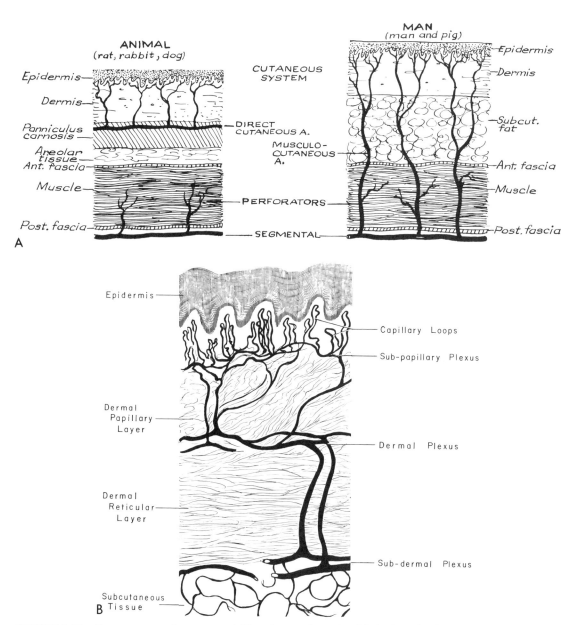

FIGURE 6–26. Cutaneous vascular system. *A,* Vascular supply to the skin in the animal and man (and pig). (From Daniel, R. K., and Williams, H. B.: The free transfer of skin flaps by microvascular anastomosis. An experimental study and a reappraisal. Plast. Reconstr. Surg., *52:*16. Copyright 1973, The Williams & Wilkins Company, Baltimore.) *B,* Vascular supply to the skin superficial to the subdermal plexus.

cular systems. They also supply the muscles through which they pass.

Cutaneous Vasculature. The cutaneous blood supply is considered the vasculature superficial to the deep fascia (Fig. 6–26). After penetrating the deep fascia, the arteries run for varying distances within the deep layer of the superficial fascia. Branches arise from these vessels to penetrate the superficial layer of the fascia and to join the subdermal arterial plexus. The latter consititues the major conduit of the arterial supply to the skin and is a characteristic of the "skin bleeders" encountered during a surgical procedure (Fujino, 1967). Branches pass from the subdermal plexus to supply the skin appendages and end in a plexus located in the superficial layer of the papillary layer of the dermis. From the latter plexus capillary loops pass to lie within the dermal papillae. Because of the interlacing network any area of skin is not solely dependent on the proximal ascending artery.

Venous drainage of the skin commences at the efferent portion of the capillary loops. The latter connect with narrow endothelium-lined spaces in the superficial layer of the papillary layer of the dermis. Venous drainage occurs through the entire thickness of the dermis and finally empties into the subdermal venous plexus. The latter is drained by the segmental veins.

The cutaneous circulation is supplied by two types of arteries—the musculocutaneous and the direct cutaneous systems (Daniel and Williams, 1973).

The musculocutaneous arteries (Fig. 6–27) receive their blood supply from segmental ves-

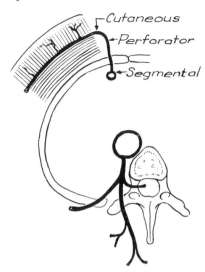

FIGURE 6–28. Diagram of the direct cutaneous system. (Modified from Daniel, R. K., and Williams, H. B.: The free transfer of skin flaps by microvascular anastomosis. An experimental study and a reappraisal. Plast. Reconstr. Surg., *52*:16. Copyright 1973, The Williams & Wilkins Company, Baltimore.)

sels lying deep to the underlying muscle, with a perforator vessel serving as a link between the two. The musculocutaneous artery lying in the subcutaneous fat terminates in the subdermal plexus and supplies a relatively small surface area.

The direct cutaneous arteries (Fig. 6–28) course parallel rather than perpendicular to the surface of the skin and lie superficial to the underlying muscle fascia. They receive their blood supply from the segmental vessels via perforators which penetrate the muscle. The direct cutaneous arteries terminate in the dermal-subdermal plexuses.

Direct cutaneous arteries supply greater areas of the skin surface. Direct cutaneous arteries are accompanied by paired venae comitantes, as the direct cutaneous veins lie in a subdermal position.

Corso (1961) demonstrated progressive arteriosclerotic changes in these vessels with increasing age of the patient and cautioned against the use of long flaps beyond the seventh decade. The importance of including the above vessels when designing the pedicle or base of the flap had been previously emphasized (Corso, 1961; Fujino, 1967; Patterson, 1968).

Classification of Skin Flaps

As in most attempts at categorization, there is no simple and all-encompassing system which is suitable for classifying skin flaps. It is now generally agreed that the anatomical vascular basis of the flap provides the most accurate approach for classification.

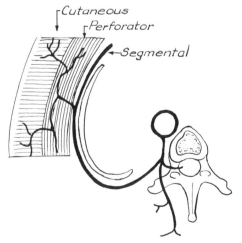

FIGURE 6–27. Diagram of the musculocutaneous system. (Modified from Daniel, R. K., and Williams, H. B.: The free transfer of skin flaps by microvascular anastomosis. An experimental study and a reappraisal. Plast. Reconstr. Surg., *52*:16. Copyright 1973, The Williams & Wilkins Company, Baltimore.)

Random and Axial Pattern Flaps. McGregor and Morgan (1973) divided skin flaps into two general types—the random pattern flap and the axial pattern flap.

The random pattern flap lacks an anatomically recognized arteriovenous system. Such a flap is subject to the classic restrictions, such as length-width ratio, delays, and the age of the patient.

Axial pattern flaps contain at least one axial arteriovenous system, e.g., deltopectoral or groin flap. Studies in pigs (Milton, 1970) have shown the fallacy of the traditional concept of length-width ratios in flap planning. It is the contained vasculature and not the width or bulk of the pedicle that is critical and determines the surviving length of the flap. The only effect of decreasing the width is to reduce the chance of the pedicle containing a large vessel. Experimental studies of porcine island flaps based solely on the segmental vessels (after division of the skin, fat, and panniculus carnosus of the pedicle) showed that such flaps survive to at least the same length as a flap with a cutaneous pedicle containing segmental vessels (Milton, 1971). They survive to a 50 per cent greater length than cutaneous flaps of the random pattern type.

After injecting fluorescein intra-arterially, McGregor and Morgan (1973) studied the surface territories subserved by specific axial pattern vascular systems. They demonstrated that the clinically safe length of the deltopectoral, groin, hypogastric, and temporal flaps exceeded the territory of their axial system. It was postulated that the distal portions of such flaps represented a random pattern flap (distal) attached to a more proximal axial pattern flap. Any boundaries which may exist between adjacent vascular areas result from a dynamic pressure equilibrium existing in the blood vessels of each vascular area. Consequently, if a deltopectoral flap is extended around the shoulder or a groin flap around the flank, delays are indicated to ensure the viability of the distally attached random pattern segment of the flap.

Cutaneous, Arterial, and Island Flaps. An alternative classification of skin flaps based on vascular supply was proposed by Daniel and Williams (1973). The three main types were (1) cutaneous, (2) arterial, and (3) island flaps.

The vast majority of *cutaneous flaps*, especially local flaps, lack a specific vascular supply (random pattern flap of McGregor). Such flaps (Fig. 6–29) are perfused by musculocutaneous arteries (see Fig. 6–27) located in the pedicle of the flap and connected to the

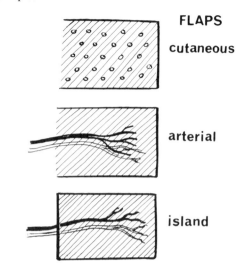

FIGURE 6–29. Classification of skin flaps on the basis of their vascular supply. (Modified from Daniel, R. K., and Williams, H. B.: The free transfer of skin flaps by microvascular anastomosis. An experimental study and a reappraisal. Plast. Reconstr. Surg., *52*:16. Copyright 1973. The Williams & Wilkins Company, Baltimore.)

dermal-subdermal plexuses. Such flaps are subject to restrictions in length design, and delays are often indicated. Care must be exercised in raising such flaps to avoid damage to the all-important subdermal plexus.

Arterial flaps contain at least one specific direct cutaneous artery within their longitudinal axis (see Fig. 6–28). As the latter lies in the subcutaneous layer just superficial to the muscular fascia (see Fig. 6–28), the flap thickness should include the subcutaneous fat and deep fascia (i.e., pectoralis fascia in the deltopectoral flap). Arterial flaps are lengthened at the distal end by an attached random pattern flap, as previously mentioned (McGregor and Morgan, 1973).

Examples of arterial flaps are the forehead (superficial temporal artery) flap (McGregor, 1963); median forehead (supraorbital and supratrochlear arteries) flap (Kazanjian, 1946; Converse and Wood-Smith, 1963); deltopectoral (internal mammary arteries) flap (Bakamjian, 1965); hypogastric (superficial epigastric artery) flap (Shaw and Payne, 1946); thoracoepigastric (long thoracic artery and superficial inferior epigastric artery) flap (Webster, 1937); groin (superficial circumflex iliac artery) flap (McGregor and Jackson, 1972); dorsum of the foot (dorsalis pedis artery) flap (McCraw and Furlow, 1975).

Island flaps have a pedicle devoid of skin and consisting only of the nutrient artery and vein. Island flaps survive to at least the same length as flaps with a cutaneous pedicle containing segmental vessels (Milton, 1971).

Dunham (1893) replaced a cheek defect with a flap based on the anterior temporal vessels and is credited with being the first surgeon to describe a vascularized island flap with identifiable blood vessels. Monks (1898) restored an eyelid with a flap of skin and scalp supplied by the anterior branch of the temporal artery advanced through a subcutaneous tunnel. Esser (1917) advocated the transfer of an island of skin detached except for the vascular pedicle; he called this type of flap the "biologic flap."

Clinical examples of the island flap technique are those based on the digital artery (Littler, 1960) for finger reconstruction and the superficial temporal artery for eyebrow reconstruction (Esser, 1917).

Microvascular Free Flap. A recent variation of the island flap has been the development of microsurgical techniques (see Chapter 14) and the transfer of island flaps between distant sites. This type of island flap is called the microvascular free flap. Reestablishment of the vascular supply is achieved by microvascular anastomosis and was first accomplished by Harii and his associates (1974). Daniel and Taylor (1973) and O'Brien and coworkers (1973) also reported similar results. This new technique should reduce multistaged surgical procedures to a single operation. The donor island flaps are removed from cutaneous territories with a well-defined axial pattern vasculature, e.g., superficial circumflex iliac artery. The techniques are discussed in Chapter 14.

Tests of Flap Circulation

Various tests have been devised to assess the viability of flaps which have been elevated. They have also been employed to study the circulation in flaps and the optimum time to transfer a flap following a delay procedure.

Originally popularized by Gillies, the simplest method of evaluating the circulation of a flap is by blanching the distal end of a flap by finger pressure and noting the rate of capillary filling or disappearance of the "comet streak." Color should return to a blanched area within four seconds and any delay is indicative of vascular insufficiency. Observing the rate of dermal bleeding at the distal end of a flap, which has been elevated, is another commonly employed technique but is not totally reliable. Although both methods are simple, they lack precision and fail to give any information on the venous circuit. Consequently, several tests have been

designed and have been used experimentally and clinically in the evaluation of skin flap viability.

1. Fluorescein dye tests. Fluorescein absorbs light in the ultraviolet range and emits light in the visible range with a yellow hue. The dye is injected intravenously, and the subserved vasculature is outlined by a fluorescence if an ultraviolet light is used in a darkened room. The test was first described by Lange and Boyd in 1942 and is simple and reliable (Myers, 1962; Goode and Linehan, 1970). One case of nonfatal anaphylactoid reaction to the dye has been reported (Thorvaldsson and Grabb, 1974).The test is easily performed and represents a simple and accurate method of evaluating skin flap circulation.

2. Saline wheal test. A small amount of 0.85 per cent saline solution is injected intracutaneously (Stern and Cohen, 1926). Normal disappearance time exceeds 60 minutes but can be as low as five minutes with arterial circulatory embarrassment.

3. Disulphine blue dye. This dye has been used to evaluate flap circulation. The flap will be quickly and intensely colored in the presence of brisk flap hemodynamics. A delay in the disappearance of the dye indicates insufficient venous return (Patterson, 1968; Teich-Alasia, 1971).

4. Atropine absorption test. Atropine injected into the flap is used as an indicator of venous return in the flap by recording the time of onset of symptoms attributable to the presence of atropine in the systemic circulation (dryness of the mouth, tachycardia, and reading problems). The test was described by Hynes in 1948.

5. Histamine scratch test. The distal surface of the flap is scratched and several drops of the phosphate salt of histamine (1:1000) are applied. Conway, Stark, and Joslin (1951) recommended transferring the flap if a wheal formed within eight minutes.

6. Liquid crystallometry. Liquid crystals change color in a 3 to 5°C scale. Consequently, during the performance of the test the flap must be shielded from the core temperature. The changes in color are helpful in evaluating flap viability (Freshwater and Krizek, 1970; Hoehn and Binkert, 1970).

7. Photoplethysmograph. The photoelectric principle is used to evaluate flap pulsatile blood flow by recording the changes in the amount of light reflected by the tissues (Hayes and associates, 1967; Thorne and associates, 1969b). The recording equipment, however, is expensive and cumbersome, and motion and extraneous light are a source of artifacts of measurement.

8. *Infrared thermography.* Infrared scanning is reliable in monitoring and prognosticating the viability of skin flaps (Bloomenstein, 1968, 1973). If the proximal pedicle of a tube flap is clamped, the technique can be used to determine if the opposite pedicle is adequate to maintain the viability of the flap during transfer. With the thermography technique, temperature changes on the surface of the tube flap can be recorded (Thorne and coworkers, 1969a).

9. *Mass spectrometer.* Flap tissue gas tensions have been recorded by a mass spectrometer to predict the extent of flap viability (Guthrie and coworkers, 1972). No part of the flap survived if the oxygen tension was less than 50 mm Hg or the carbon dioxide tension exceeded 80 mm Hg. No part became necrotic if the oxygen tension was greater than 83 mm Hg or the carbon dioxide tension was less than 64 mm Hg. Because of anaerobic metabolism and the accumulation of lactate ion in inadequately perfused tissue, Glinz and Clodius (1972) measured flap tissue pH as an indicator of viability following elevation of a flap. Adjacent subcutaneous tissue was used as a control.

10. *Radioactive isotope clearance studies.* Various radioactive isotopes, including sodium (Barron and coworkers, 1952; Hauser and associates, 1961; Fujino, 1967) and pertechnetate (Tauxe and associates, 1970), have been used to evaluate the functional vascular supply of a skin flap. The rate of disappearance or clearance of the isotope from the flap is recorded as an index of the flap circulation. If the donor end of a tube flap is clamped, the optimum and earliest time for flap division can be determined.

The Delay of Flaps

The blood supply of a flap may be enhanced by a preliminary procedure consisting of partially dividing the blood supply to the flap before its transplantation. If a flap is raised in two or more stages, it has been noted that a greater length will survive than if the flap is raised and transferred at the same procedure. The purpose of the delay is to condition a flap to be able to survive in a state of relative hypoxia after it is raised and transferred.

Mechanism of Delay. Although practiced by Tagliacozzi, Blair (1912) appears to have been

the first surgeon to employ the term "delayed flap," and the term has come into common usage in the English-speaking world. After a flap has been outlined by incisions and raised, the vessels in the flap increase in size and in number and become reoriented in the direction of the long axis of the flap. German, Finesilver, and Davis (1933) showed that these changes in the vessels of the flap occur within seven days. Braithwaite (1950) used microradiography after the injection of pyelosil or 20 per cent colloidal silver iodide to study the vascular channels in human skin. He demonstrated that the dermal and subdermal vascular plexuses play a dominant role in maintaining the circulation of a skin flap. Peskova (1955) in a histologic study showed that, four to five weeks after transfer of a tube flap, the number of blood vessels increases in the flaps that have been repeatedly transferred, as compared with the number and caliber of blood vessels in a flap that has been tubed for the first time. Bardach and Kurnatowski (1961) noted that the main role of the blood supply of the flap is played by the vessels in the dermis and those situated in the subdermal layer at the junction between the skin and the subcutaneous fat. The blood supply of the skin was evaluated by counting the number of blood vessels in three fields of each slide at the same magnification and measuring the diameter of the vessels with a special eyepiece fitted with a measuring scale. Histologic examination of excised tissue from two skin flaps in man showed that the blood supply of the skin of a tube flap is superior to that of the abdominal skin at the site in which the flap was formed. These authors also confirmed the findings of Peskova that the number of vessels in a skin flap increases after each transfer or delay procedure.

McFarlane and associates (1965), using methylmethacrylate casts of the flap vasculature, demonstrated that, after a delay, longitudinal anastomoses were added to the basic transverse disposition of the flap vessels. In addition, the number of vessels at each end of the flap increased. By the twelfth day after delay, the arterial pattern had returned to the normal or predelay state. Consequently, the change in the arterial pattern from a transverse to a longitudinal direction was temporary. They were unable to demonstrate any significant increase in the size or number of vessels on histologic examination following delay.

Myers, Cherry, and Milton (1972) implanted Silastic tubing in skin flaps and recorded tissue gas tensions as an index of the adequacy of the flap circulation. A flap with a higher P_{CO_2} level (reflecting higher ischemia) after a delay procedure showed a greater area of survival. The conclusions of the study were that ischemia is the stimulus of the delay phenomenon and that only a relatively short period of ischemia (as measured by elevated Pco_2 levels) is required to stimulate the development of collateral circulation. Estimates of the increase in the area of flap survival over the expected survival length in experimental animals ranged from 60 per cent (Milton, 1969b) to 100 per cent (Myers and Cherry, 1971).

In a study of the delay phenomenon, Reinisch (1974) noted that necrosis of the distal end of the flap may not be the result of ischemia in the usual sense but may represent a microcirculatory alteration in which necrosis results despite the presence of blood flow in the ischemic portion of the flap. In a study of flaps elevated on pigs, Reinisch demonstrated that circulation persisted in the ischemic portion of the flap (as determined by the presence of radioactively tagged red blood cells). However, radioactively tagged microspheres were used to determine the presence of patent arteriovenous anastomoses, and these could not be demonstrated in the ischemic portion of the flap. These data support the concept that the sympathetic denervation caused by raising a flap (Hynes, 1950) opens the sympathetically innervated, normally present arteriovenous channels. Consequently, blood flow in the raised flap is directed through these vessels, which are thick-walled and nonnutritive. This finding explains the apparently avascular nature of the distal end of the flap.

Following delay, however, there was a higher degree of microsphere trapping, and fewer microspheres were able to escape the capillary bed. As the arteriovenous connections are closed over a period of 10 to 14 days following delay, there is a greater percentage of flap blood flow through the nutritive capillary bed.

Optimum Time for Transfer after Delay. The optimum time for transfer of a flap following a delay procedure has been the subject of much controversy. Gillies and Millard (1957) estimated that most flaps could be safely transferred ten days after the delay procedure. In the laboratory the problem has been extensively studied. Hoffmeister (1957) studied the rates of clearance of radioactive sodium (^{22}Na) in canine flaps. In the immediate period following delay, there was an initial decrease in circulatory efficiency. However, the initial decrease was followed by an increase in circulatory efficiency, ranging from a 98 per cent to a 150 per cent increase over the controls. The interval between the delay and the circulatory peak ranged from 10 to 21 days. The circulatory peak was followed by a rapid decline to normal predelay values over a three-day period. Consequently, the authors concluded that raising a flap during the first week after the delay procedure is hazardous and is best performed about two to four weeks after the delay.

Studies designed to measure the cutaneous pulsatile blood flow in skin flaps with photoelectric pulse pickup (PEPP) have shown that blood flow increases rapidly during the first week after delay with little change thereafter (Hayes and associates, 1967). The maximum blood flow in canine bipedicle tube flaps, as recorded by thermocouples, was at four to nine days after surgery, after the edema had subsided. While the beneficial effects of delay were apparent in all animals by four days, the time interval required between delay and transfer for maximum survival was seven days in the rabbit and pig but 42 days in the rat (Myers and Cherry, 1971). Milton (1969b) showed that delay of porcine skin flaps by undermining and constructing bipedicled flaps is maximal at about two weeks.

The decision to delay a flap depends upon the area from which the flap is removed and upon the age of the patient. In flaps of the lower extremity, delay procedures are more frequently required than in the region of the head and neck. Delays are also less frequently indicated for axial pattern flaps. In the older patient, a delay procedure is nearly always a necessity, especially for a cross-leg flap; in the young, healthy adult, in contrast, such a flap, if it is of adequate proportions, may be transferred without a preliminary delay.

Types of Delay. The type of delay varies according to the area in which the flap is being prepared and also the position of the flap during the transfer. A simple outline delay (Fig. 6–30), making incisions around the flap without raising the flap, is adequate in the forehead and the scalp region, where none of the vessels are of the perforating type but instead originate from the periphery of the flap. In the abdominal wall, where perforating vessels are numerous, such a delay would not be satisfactory, and the preliminary raising of the flap is necessary. Silastic sheets can be inserted beneath a flap at the time of delay to prevent the growth of capillaries across the delayed surface. In addition to maintaining the

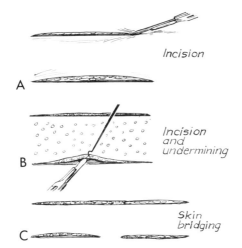

Incision

A

*Incision
and
undermining*

B

*Skin
bridging*

C

FIGURE 6–30. Type of delay. *A,* Simple outline or incision delay. *B,* Combination of outline and undermining. *C,* A skin bridge can decrease the anoxic stimulus in a particularly long flap.

anoxic stimulus to the flap, it is reported that such a maneuver also reduces the incidence of bleeding or hematoma formation when the flap is finally transferred (Williams, 1973).

In the delay of random pattern or cutaneous flaps (see Classification of Skin Flaps), the flap should be undermined in a plane that leaves sufficient subcutaneous fat on the flap to protect the subdermal plexus. Axial pattern or arterial flaps (e.g., deltopectoral flap) should be elevated deep to the muscular fascia to avoid injury to the direct cutaneous artery.

Delaying a flap is no substitute for adequate design and proportions of the flap. In the lower extremity, most cross-leg flaps should have a square shape; such a broad pedicle not only serves to assure adequate blood supply but also provides a flap of sufficient dimension to overlap the defective area in every direction. The cross-leg flap becomes rapidly revascularized from the adequately vascularized area on each side above and below the exposed bone.

Flap delay has certain inconveniences. For example, if a forehead flap is raised and reapplied to its bed prior to its transfer, it will be found that the flap has stiffened considerably as a result of fibrosis during the period of healing. Such changes make molding of the flap to construct a columella or alar rim, as required in nasal reconstruction, extremely difficult. Since there are no perforating vessels in the forehead, this problem can be obviated by simply performing an outline delay.

The most obvious inconvenience of a delay procedure is the added hospitalization. Often, however, stages of the delay can be performed on an outpatient basis. With the development of microsurgical free flap techniques, many reconstructions previously requiring multiple stages may be reduced to a single procedure.

Vascular Augmentation or Enhancement of Survival of Skin Flaps

There has been a search for a substance or technique which, if used at the time of flap reconstruction, would augment the vascular supply of the flap and enhance the ultimate survival of the flap.

DeHaan and Stark (1961) reported that histamine iontophoresis, while augmenting the afferent circulation, did not improve the efferent circulation of the flap. Histamine iontophoresis did not increase the survival of flaps with a longer and narrower pedicle. In a study by Milton and Corbett (1969), histamine iontophoresis failed to increase the survival of experimental flaps in rabbits. Ketchum and associates (1967) reported that, while pretreatment of the pedicle tissue with histamine iontophoresis increased flap survival, the effect was not predictable.

Systemic hypertension, i.e., hypertensive perfusion, resulted in a larger portion of the flap surviving (Ketchum and associates, 1967), but the finding could not be duplicated in another study (Milton and Corbett, 1969).

Dimethyl sulfoxide (DMSO) was reported as being effective in enhancing flap survival (Adamson and associates, 1966). However, other studies reported only a marginal positive effect (Arturson and Khanna, 1970) or more extensive sloughing following treatment with DMSO (Myers and Cherry, 1968; Koehnlein and Lemperle, 1970).

An adrenergic blocking agent, phenoxybenzamine, is effective, when injected subcutaneously into the flap (Myers and Cherry, 1968), in augmenting the length of flap survival. It has been postulated that the agent causes the opening of collateral vessels, with improvement in the perfusion of the distal portion of the flap.

Recently Reinisch (1974) augmented the surviving length of flaps by chemical treatment (6-hydroxydopamine and dilute epinephrine) and electrical manipulation prior to elevating the flaps. It was speculated that both types of pretreatment closed the sympathetically innervated arteriovenous channels of the flap which shunt blood from the nutritive vessels in the distal end of the flap and are responsible for distal flap necrosis.

Principles of Flap Surgery

Design of the Flap. After the extent of the true defect has been determined and the flap to be utilized has been planned, an accurate design of the future flap may be obtained by the method described by Gillies (1932). The recipient and donor areas are brought into the positions they will assume during the transfer of the flap (Fig. 6–31, *A, B*). A pattern is cut to shape and fitted as though the operation of flap transfer had been finished (Fig. 6–31, *B, C*). It is important that a larger pattern is used than is finally required for covering the defect. The pattern is held to the donor area while the recipient limb is displaced, and it is then spread over the donor area (Fig. 6–31, *C*).

Location of the Flap. Local flaps are preferred, as reconstruction can be restricted to one procedure, transfers are not required, and adjacent tissue provides better texture and color match. Axial pattern flaps, based on a specific arteriovenous system, are superior to random pattern or cutaneous flaps, as discussed earlier in the chapter. The Doppler flowmeter can be used to determine the direction of the contained axial vasculature. Old traumatic or surgical scars, which could interfere with the blood supply of the flap, must also be considered in flap planning. In general, any flap should be free of cutaneous scars. Because of a difference in blood supply, flaps in the head and neck region can be designed with a relatively narrower pedicle and can be transferred with less consideration for a delay procedure. Theoretically, flaps should not be designed so that the midline of the torso is transgressed,

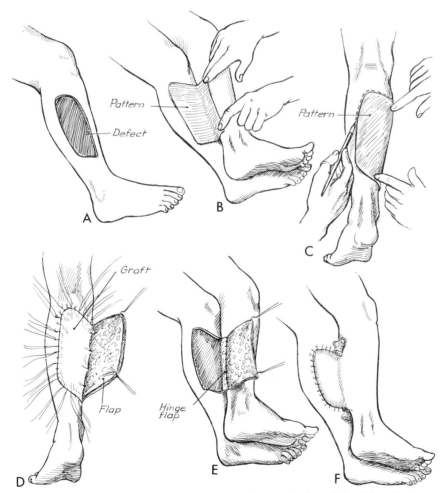

FIGURE 6–31. Flap design. The technique of the cross-leg flap. *A*, Outline of the defect. *B*, A pattern is placed, simulating the flap transfer procedure in the cross-leg position. *C*, The legs are separated and the pattern outline made on the donor leg. *D*, A split-thickness skin graft is applied to the defect on the donor leg. Donor site ready to receive a tie-over pressure dressing. *E*, The cross-leg flap is raised, and the hinge flap is sutured to the base of the pedicle of the cross-leg flap. *F*, Cross-leg flap operation completed.

because of the segmental arrangement of the vasculature.

Age of the Patient. Elderly patients are poor risks in terms of large flaps because of arteriosclerotic changes in the flap vasculature (Conway, 1960; Corso, 1961).

Mechanical Factors. Suturing the flap under excessive *tension* is a major factor in flap necrosis. If a flap is sutured in the recipient bed under tension, a white, avascular line can be seen from the flap pivot point to the most distal portion of the flap (i.e., the line of greatest tension) (Fig. 6–32). However, a study of flaps closed under tension showed that skin sloughs are primarily due to devascularization of the flap. Flaps with an adequate blood supply can be inserted under tension without fear of necrosis (Myers and coworkers, 1965).

The effect of *gravity* is usually seen in a large tube flap, a portion of which will be in a relatively dependent position. The latter has been held responsible for an impairment of venous return within the flap and the development of engorgement and flap necrosis. An experimental study in rabbits and pigs (Myers and coworkers, 1973) failed to show any effect of gravity on either the blood supply or the survival of tube flaps.

Kinking or unusual angulation of the flap is seen more often in long tube flaps and can be responsible for compromise of the blood supply. Such problems can be obviated by proper design of the flap or positioning of the patient. This is one area in which the nursing staff should be alert.

Pressure on the flap should be avoided. Dressings over the flap are not necessary, and the open method allows continuous observa-

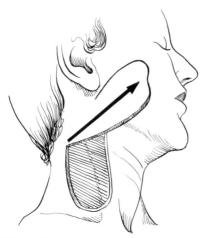

FIGURE 6–32. Line of greatest tension extends from the pivot point to the most distal portion of the flap.

tion of the color of the flap and prevents unnoticed pressure. Care should also be taken in securing a tracheostomy with an umbilical tape, as the latter can occlude the pedicle of a deltopectoral flap which has been transferred to the neck region.

Hematoma formation can be the "bête noire" of flap reconstruction. A large underlying hematoma can distend a flap sufficiently to interrupt the vascular supply and interfere with vascularization of the flap. It is a common cause of morbidity associated with flap reconstruction. Complete hemostasis, the use of suction drainage, and delay of flap transfer when hemostasis is a problem in the recipient bed are measures which can reduce the incidence of hematoma formation. If a hematoma forms, the patient should be immediately returned to the operating room for evacuation of the hematoma.

Delay Procedure. The mechanism and role of the delay procedure were discussed earlier in the chapter.

Transfer of Flaps from a Distance. Certain points of technique are common to all flap transfers; others are specific to certain particular flaps.

With all flaps, one should endeavor to make direct flap transfer a closed operation by eliminating the raw areas produced by the raising of the flap. This can be done in the following manner:

1. By bringing the recipient area as close as possible to the donor area along the line of attachment to the flap.

2. By skin grafting immediately or closing by direct approximation the raw area produced by the raising of the flap. A split-thickness skin graft, held to the edges of the defect by a continuous running lock stitch and maintained by a pressure tie-over dressing over the defect, gives a satisfactory repair (Fig. 6–33). When moderate-sized flaps from the abdomen are employed, one can close the defect by carefully suturing the wound after undermining the edges. It is preferable, however, to skin graft the donor defect rather than to attempt to close it with undue tension.

3. By employing the hinge flap. As stated previously, the portion of the flap situated between the recipient area and the attachment of the flap should be as short as possible. However, in order to eliminate completely the raw area under the flap, it is advantageous to make an additional flap with normal skin on the side of the defect opposite the attachment of the

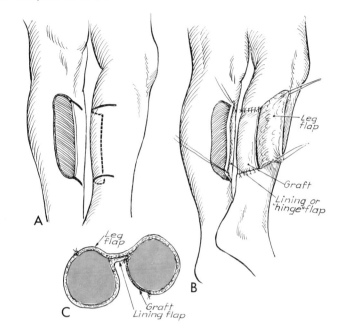

FIGURE 6-33. Use of a skin graft and hinge flap to cover all surface defects in the transfer of a cross-leg flap.

flap as shown in Figure 6-33. The hinge flap is sutured to the undersurface of the main flap, thus completely closing the intervening open area. The hinge flap has been shown to present the following four advantages:

a. The avoidance of infection and suppuration on the undersurface of the flap, particularly when the defect contains exposed tendons, which are especially vulnerable to infection.

b. The avoidance of inflammatory reaction after section of the pedicle and insetting of the distal portion of the flap into the defect, because of the absence of raw area under the pedicle of the flap.

c. The elimination of tension, and thus of inflammation and of delayed healing, along the line of suture of the sectioned pedicle. It has been repeatedly noted that, when there is an excess of healthy tissue, such as is provided by the hinge flap, healing occurs satisfactorily. Delayed healing due to tension along the line of section of the pedicle is seen particularly in flap repairs of the foot. The adoption of the hinge flap greatly accelerates the healing time of such wounds.

d. The hinge flap, made with healthy tissue, provides the main flap with additional vascular connections, particularly when the latter is applied to a poorly vascularized area.

Division and Insetting of the Flap. The optimum time of division of a flap was discussed under The Delay of Flaps. Under ordinary circumstances, flaps may be separated after the fourteenth day. When conditions are unfavorable for the revascularization of the flap, as when the flap is placed over denuded bone at an irradiated area, approximately 21 days should elapse before the separation of the flap. When the entire defect cannot be covered in one stage, the portion of the flap applied in the first stage must serve as the base for the vascular supply of the entire flap in the second stage. It is prudent to postpone the sectioning of the flap more than 21 days, in order to permit the newly transplanted flap to acquire an adequate vascularization.

While in clinical practice it has become traditional to divide a flap after two or three weeks, there are exceptions based on regional anatomical differences. The head and neck area has a rich vascular supply, and a local flap can be divided at ten days. Similarly, local finger flaps can be divided at two weeks. At the other end of the spectrum, a cross-leg flap should not be divided before three weeks after the preliminary procedure, and serial division may be indicated. However, Klingenström and Nylén (1966) showed that flaps can be divided earlier than generally believed. They successfully divided four tube flaps, five cross-leg flaps, and two cross-finger flaps at an interval of 7 to 14 days.

Velander (1964), using microangiographic techniques, noted the first anatomical signs of vascular contact between the recipient bed and the transferred flap about four to five days after transposition. Initially veins of small caliber were noted; arteries did not become apparent until one week after transfer and then increased rapidly in capacity. Vascular connections were noted at an earlier stage (two to three days) if there had been a delay procedure. At seven days circulatory function between a flap and the recipient bed is well established, although there is some depression with recovery at 21 days after flap transposition (Hugo, 1972).

There can also be a "delayed" or serial division of the flap, a technique in which the pedicle is only partially severed initially. Several days later the division can be completed. This is often practiced in the division of cross-leg flaps.

The work of Segarra and Bennett (1972) has shown that a delay of several days between division and inset of the flap pedicle may be indicated to decrease distal necrosis of flaps with marginal circulation.

Salvaging the Flap of Marginal Viability. The flap with inadequate vascularization inevitably reflects poor planning; mechanical problems play only a secondary role.

Last-ditch efforts include releasing the sutures to relieve any tension which may be compromising the circulation. Venous congestion can be relieved by elevating the flap or changing it from a dependent position. Hynes (1951) designed a mechanical intermittent venous occluder device, which could be applied to the distal end of the flap. The use of leeches for the treatment of venous congestion in a flap is practiced in Europe (Derganc and Zdravic, 1960).

Cooling is commonly employed for the treatment of a flap of doubtful viability in an attempt to decrease its metabolic requirements. Cooling of flaps so that the surface temperature of the pedicle was maintained at 20° C did not prevent necrosis; rather, it postponed the onset of necrosis and made it less severe (Kiehn and Desprez, 1960).

Hyperbaric oxygen has been successfully employed in increasing the survival of experimental flaps (Champion, McSherry and Goulian, 1967). Another study on porcine flaps failed to show any significant beneficial effect of hyperbaric oxygen on experimental (porcine) flaps (Kernahan, Zingg and Kay, 1965).

Low molecular weight dextran has been reported to decrease blood viscosity, diminish red cell sludging, and increase capillary flow.

However, a study by Myers and Cherry (1967) showed that treatment with low molecular weight dextran did not increase the vascularity or survival of experimental skin flaps.

Types of Flaps

In the discussion of flaps that follows, the classification of McGregor and Morgan (1973) will be used as follows:

Random Pattern Flaps

Advancement flaps
Transposition flaps
Rotation flaps
Tube flaps
Flaps from a distance

Axial Pattern Flaps

Island flaps, myocutaneous, and microvascular free flaps are variations, which will also be discussed.

RANDOM PATTERN FLAPS

Advancement Flaps. Advancement flaps were first employed by Celsus in ancient Rome but

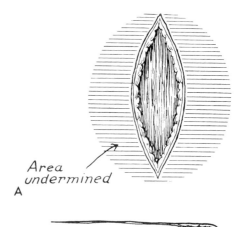

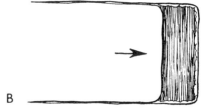

FIGURE 6–34. Advancement flap. *A,* The simplest advancement flap is that produced by the closure of a defect following undermining of the skin, facilitating linear closure of the defect. *B,* Example of a straight advancement flap. (From Kazanjian and Converse.)

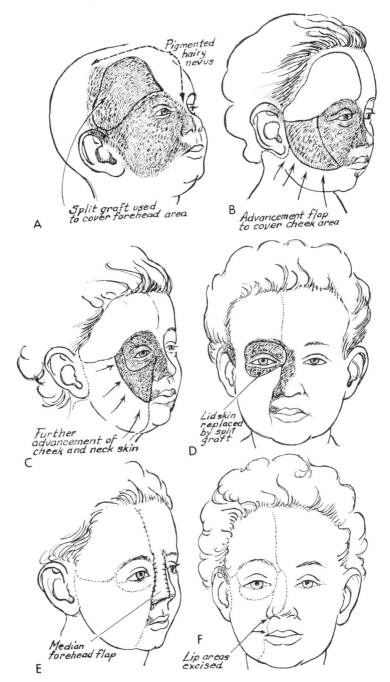

FIGURE 6–35. Excision and coverage of a facial hairy nevus. *A*, Preoperative appearance. Forehead defect to be covered with split-thickness skin graft. *B*, Cheek defect resurfaced by advancement flap from cheek and neck. *C*, Further advancement of cheek and neck skin. *D*, Resurfacing of eyelid skin with skin grafts. *E*, Median forehead flap used to resurface nasal defect. *F*, Residual nevus of upper lip excised and defect closed by approximation.

were popularized by the French surgeons during the first half of the nineteenth century; they were called sliding flaps (lambeaux par glissement) (Fig. 6–34).

A simple advancement flap is possible in areas of the body where there is an excess of skin. It is also more feasible in the very young and the aged. In infants, the highly elastic skin may be stretched. In the patient shown in Figures 6–35 and 6–36, a hairy nevus covered nearly half of the face and scalp. Progressive advancement and rotation of the skin of the neck onto the cheek was achieved in stages. After each stage, the stretched skin appeared to progressively lose its tenseness. In the aged, because of the loss of elasticity and the progressive relaxation of the skin, considerable excess is present in the adjacent area and may be utilized to cover the defect.

Another application of the advancement flap

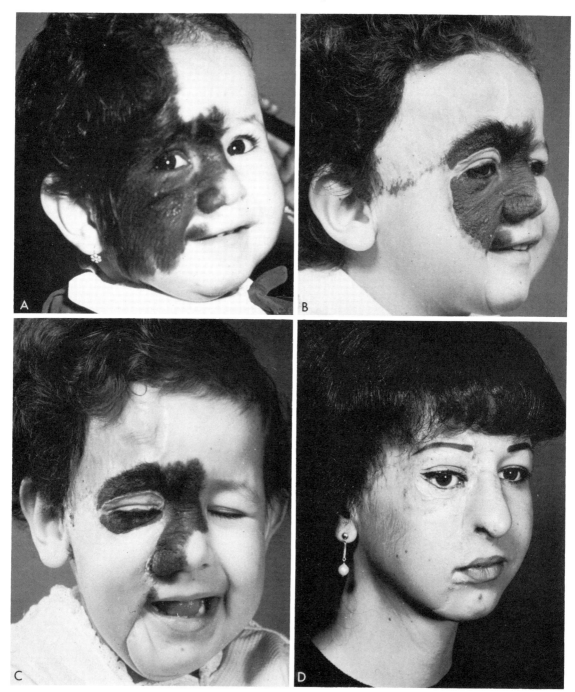

FIGURE 6–36. Same patient as in Figure 6–35. *A*, Hairy nevus of face in an 8 month old child. *B*, Following excision and skin grafting of forehead and upper eyelid and advancement flap of cheek and neck. *C*, After additional advancement of cheek and neck flap. *D*, Nevus has been completely excised. Eyebrow defect closed by primary closure. Skin graft was applied to the lower eyelid, and the nose was resurfaced with a median forehead flap. (From Converse, J. M., Guy, C. L., and Molenaar, A.: The treatment of giant pigmented naevi of the face. Br. J. Plast. Surg., *22*:302, 1969.)

is the deliberate placing of the flap under tension, releasing it in a second stage after vascularization of the flap from the host bed has taken place (Fig. 6–37). Converse (1967) has utilized this procedure and refers to it as the "1–2" flap. Figure 6–38 is a drawing of a patient with a burn ectropion of the lower lip. The scarred tissue is excised, and the cervical skin is widely undermined and advanced to cover the defect. The patient is maintained

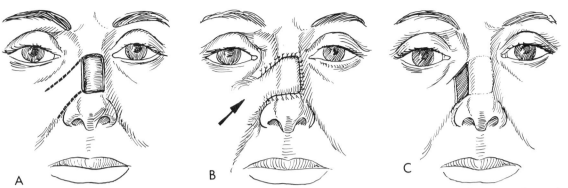

FIGURE 6-37. The 1–2 advancement flap. *A*, Advancement flap prepared. *B*, The advancement flap covers the nasal defect. *C*, In a second stage after healing of the flap, the pedicle is severed and the resultant defect is covered by a full-thickness retroauricular graft.

with his neck in a position of flexion, and, for this reason, the technique is indicated only in younger patients without degenerative changes of the cervical spine. As a second-stage procedure, two to three weeks later, the portion of the advancement flap that is to remain on the lower lip is detached from the adjacent cervical skin, and the cervical skin is allowed to retract into the position it previously occupied. A split-thickness skin graft is placed over the secondary defect in the suprahyoid area.

Most advancement flaps are made by outlining three sides of the flap by incisions, leaving a pedicle on one side to preserve the blood supply. The inherent elasticity of the skin permits a certain amount of advancement, particularly if the flap is taken from an area where the skin is loose. Various procedures have been devised to facilitate the advancement of the flap. When a flap is stretched, it will be noted that two folds of skin form on each side of the base of the pedicle. Burow (1838) devised the method of excising triangles of skin from this area, thus further facilitating advancement (Fig. 6–39, *A*). Advancement is also facilitated by incisions cut transversely into the flap, a dangerous method unless the flap has an excellent blood supply (Fig. 6–39, *B*). Elongation of the flap is obtained by lateral incisions outlining the flap cut in an angular fashion (Fig. 6–39, *C*) or along a curved line (Fig. 6–39, *D*). An additional method is to elongate the flap by the Z-plasty technique (Fig. 6–39, *E*).

Other types of advancement flaps are the V-Y advancement closure (Fig. 6–40) and bipedicle advancement flaps (Fig. 6–41). The latter have only limited clinical application because they lack significant mobility.

Transposition Flaps. The tissues in the area adjacent to the defect may be loose in a plane different from that in which the defect is situat-

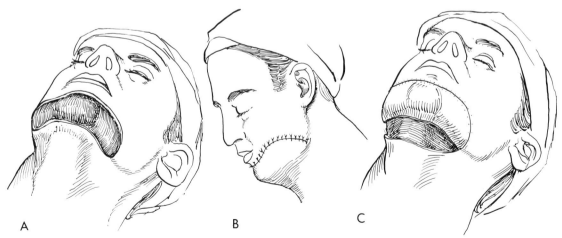

FIGURE 6-38. Another example of the 1–2 advancement flap. *A, B,* Straight advancement flap of the cervical skin to cover a defect of the lower portion of the face. *C,* In a second stage, a submandibular incision severs the pedicle of the flap. The resultant raw area is covered with a thick split-thickness skin graft. This technique covers the chin with hair-bearing skin.

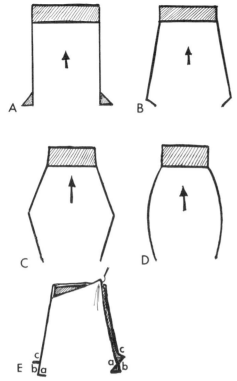

FIGURE 6–39. Various methods of facilitating the advancement of a flap. *A*, Excision of Burow's triangle. *B*, Counterincision made in the base of a flap. *C*, Triangular design of the flap. *D*, Curvilinear design of the flap. *E*, Elongation by Z-plasty technique at the base of the flap.

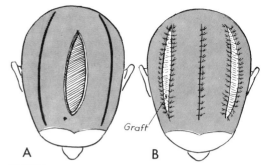

FIGURE 6–41. Example of bipedicle advancement flaps. *A*, Midline scalp defect. *B*, Both bipedicle flaps are advanced to the midline and the resulting defects covered with split-thickness skin grafts.

ed. A flap may be raised from this area and submitted to a transposition through an angle to the defect (Fig. 6–42). In this manner the flap is removed and transposed to an area where tissue is deficient. If adequately designed, the flap fits into the defect without tension (Fig. 6–42).

Various types of transposition flaps have been designed, some taken from the area immediately adjacent to the defect, others being transposed over an area of intact skin, such as advocated by Limberg (1946) (Fig. 6–43). The special design of the transposition flap shown in Figure 6–44 permits closure of the second-

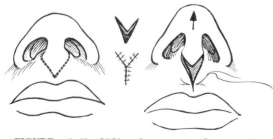

FIGURE 6–40. V-Y advancement flap used to elongate the columella.

ary defect in a different plane from that of the primary defect by the V-Y method. Transposition flaps can also be employed in conjunction with skin grafts which cover the secondary defect. In designing such flaps, it is well to remember that the maximum tension on the flap is on the edge of the flap distal to the defect (see Fig. 6–42, *A*).

It is often possible after transferring a flap to close the secondary defect by an additional neighboring flap. This is made possible by the fact that considerable laxity may be present in the tissues at a right angle to the defect. The bi-lobed flap of Zimany (1953) consists of a large lobe (Fig. 6–45), which is transposed into the primary defect, and a smaller second lobe, which is transposed to fill the secondary defect produced by the mobilization of the larger component.

Rotation Flaps. The rotation flap, usually semicircular in shape, is designed adjacent to the defect and is rotated about a fixed pivot point to resurface the defect (Fig. 6–46). The donor site can be closed by primary approximation, by removal of a triangle of tissue, or by a split-thickness skin graft. In order to facilitate the transposition of a flap, it is tempting to make an incision extending part of the way through the base of the pedicle on the edge which is distal to the defect. The incision increases the mobility of the flap but diminishes the width of the pedicle and endangers the blood supply (Fig. 6–46, *A*). In a rotation flap, the width of the flap is increased by transforming the edge of the flap distal to the defect into a curved line. The flap is submitted to a movement of rotation, and a counterincision at the base of the curved incision increases the mobility of the flap. Esser (1917) popularized this type of rotation flap. Imre (1928) designed a rotation flap

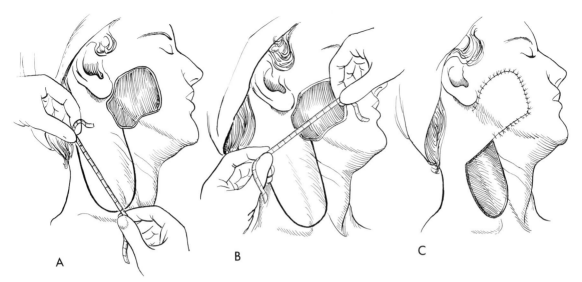

FIGURE 6–42. Example of transposition flap. *A*, *B*, Defect of the cheek area. Flap designed in the cervical region. Measure denotes line of greatest tension and assures adequate flap length. *C*, Flap has been transposed.

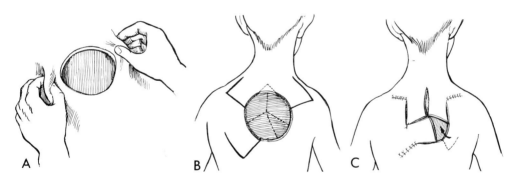

FIGURE 6–43. Limberg (1946) technique of multiple transposition flaps for closure of a circular defect. *A*, The amount and position of loose tissue around the defect are evaluated by pinching the skin. *B*, Design of transposition flaps. Limberg technique requires conversion of the circular to a 60° rhomboid defect with all sides equal and 60° angles at the end of the long axis of the defect. The far angle of the flap is also 60°. *C*, Closure of defect. (From Kazanjian and Converse.)

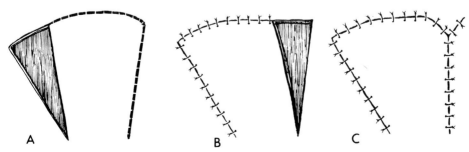

FIGURE 6–44. Example of a transposition flap. *A*, Design of transposition flap. *B*, Transposition of flap and resulting donor defect. *C*, Closure of the secondary defect by the V-Y advancement method.

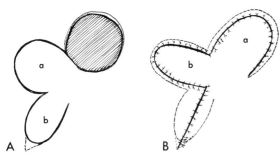

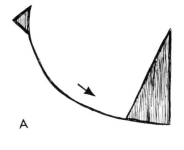

FIGURE 6–45. The bilobed flap (Zimany). *A*, Flap a is outlined in preparation for transfer to the defect. Flap b is outlined and transferred to cover the secondary defect. *B*, Position of the flap after the transfer of the bilobed flap. The donor area of flap b is closed by direct approximation.

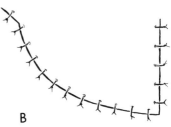

in which additional advancement was obtained by excision of a Bürow triangle from the lateral aspect of the base of the pedicle (Fig. 6–47).

Tube Flaps. For purposes of discussion, the tube flap is classified under random pattern flaps. However, certain tube flaps are true axial pattern flaps, as they are based on a specific arteriovenous axis, e.g., the thoracoepigastric flap of Webster (1937), which is based on the superior thoracic and superficial inferior epigastric arteries. The tube flap is a bipedicle flap, the edges of which are rolled under to form a tube. The tube flap was described almost concomitantly by Filatov (1917), Ganzer (1917), Gillies (1920), and Aymard (1917). In describing the history of the development of the tube flap, Milton (1969a) noted that Dieffenbach (1845–1848) used tube flaps from the arm to reconstruct noses. Gillies popularized the method and described its various applications. His description of the technique of the tube flap (Gillies

FIGURE 6–47. Example of a rotation flap. *A*, Burow's triangle excised from the base of the flap to facilitate rotation. *B*, Following rotation.

and Millard, 1957) is both instructive and entertaining reading.

The tube flap (Fig. 6–48) is prepared by making two parallel incisions through the skin and subcutaneous tissue to the deep fascia. A ratio of $2\frac{1}{2}$ to 1 between length and breadth of the tube is generally considered to be a safe ratio. In children, the length of the tube may be increased; in obese adults, prudence should be exerted, as the tissues are less well vascularized. The adipose layer is then separated from the deep fascia by sharp dissection, and tubing of the skin is accomplished. In thin individuals, the tubing generally is done without difficulty. If a considerable layer of adipose tissue is present, closure is impossible or can be done only by compressing the fat. Fat should be trimmed from the undersurface of the flap until the tube can be closed without tension. However, defatting, if excessively performed, will cause injury to the vital vasculature of the flap. After careful hemostasis the tube is closed, first by an interrupted suture placed at each extremity of the tube. The remainder of the tube can then be closed by a continuous running suture.

Closure of the donor site is accomplished by direct approximation whenever possible; an advancement flap facilitates closure of the donor site. When closure by direct approximation is not possible because of the size of the tube, the wound edges are advanced and sutured to the deep fascia. The remainder of

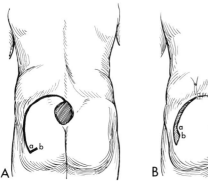

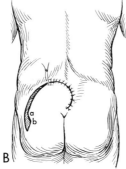

FIGURE 6–46. Example of a rotation flap. *A*, Rotation flap to cover a sacral defect. Line a-b increases the mobility of the flap but jeopardizes the safety of the flap by decreasing the pedicle. *B*, Flap after rotation.

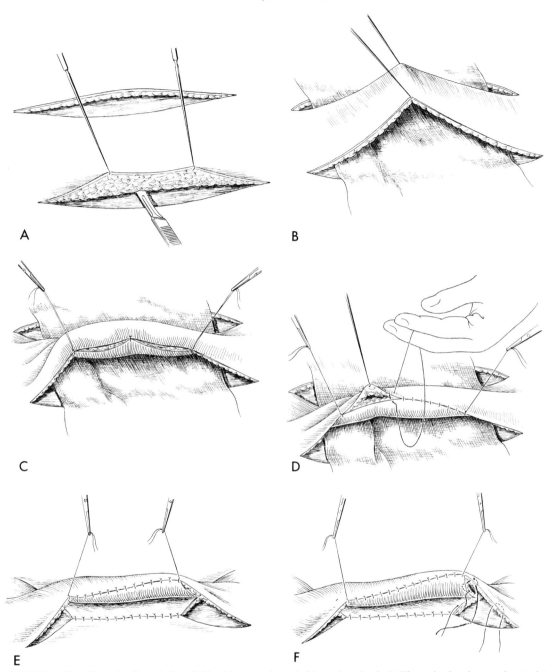

FIGURE 6–48. The tube flap. *A*, Parallel incisions made and skin undermined. *B*, Flap raised and gauze inserted to cover raw area. *C*, The tubing is started by placing sutures at each end of the flap. *D*, Tube closed with a continuous suture. *E*, The tubed portion of the flap is raised with traction sutures, exposing the triangular defect remaining at each end after approximation of the edges of the donor area. *F*, Method of closure of the triangular defect at the end of the flap. (From Kazanjian and Converse.)

the donor defect is covered by a split-thickness skin graft.

When the wound edges are closed by direct approximation, a triangular suture, recommended by Gillies (see Fig. 6–48, *F*), is employed to close the open triangle. When a skin graft covers the raw surface, the open triangle at the extremity of the tube is sutured to the raw surface prior to the application of the skin graft. Alternatively, the graft can be applied to this triangular raw area on the underside of the pedicle flap. This will add to the mobility of the flap and prevent the revascularization of this part of the flap from the donor side. The skin graft should be held by a bolster to ensure adequate healing.

The tube flap is best used when the patient and the surgeon are not in a hurry. Tube flaps cannot be rushed, and complete healing and softening of the flap tissue are essential prior to transfer. If a tube flap shows signs of inadequate circulation, there is always the danger that progressive necrosis will develop. The tube should be opened and the flap reinserted into its donor bed. Each stage requires many weeks of waiting before the next stage can be undertaken. The adage of Gillies—"Never do today what you can possibly do tomorrow"—finds its best application in the surgery of tube flaps. In recent years the development of axial pattern flaps and microvascular free flaps has reduced the use of tube flaps, because of the possibility of immediate transfer of the former.

VARIETIES OF TUBE FLAPS. Tube flaps may be constructed in any area of the body, but it is obvious that their chance of survival is greater if the long axis of the tube is parallel to the direction of the direct cutaneous vasculature. Gillies stated that a tube flap placed in series with recognized vascular and lymphatic channels can be as long as 18 cm if it is at least 5 cm in width. The largest tube flaps have been constructed by the thoracoepigastric technique of Webster (1937). This tube, extending from

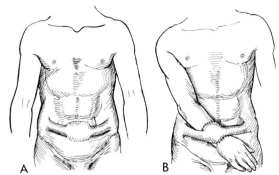

FIGURE 6–50. After construction of two oblique abdominal tube flaps *(A)*, the intermediary portion is delayed, then attached to the wrist *(B)* for later migration to the recipient site.

the inner wall of the axilla and curving down around the abdomen to the pubic region, is situated in an area where the skin is generally abundant and nonhairy; there is an excellent venous and lymphatic system draining into the axilla and the groin.

The most commonly employed tubes (Fig. 6–49) are the oblique abdominal, the transverse cervical, the acromiopectoral and the dorsal tubes, and, particularly in male patients, the arm and thigh tube flaps.

ELONGATION OF THE TUBE. Elongation of the tube flap can be achieved by various methods. The simplest is to construct a tube, then elongate it by a second tube made in continuity with the first. Another method is to construct two tubes, leaving an intermediary untubed portion of skin. When crossing the midline, extra precautions should be taken, and tubing of the intermediary skin should be delayed. A useful method is to attach the intermediary portion, after delay, to a carrier such as the wrist (Fig. 6–50).

TRANSFER OF TUBE FLAPS. The transfer of skin tubes may be either *direct,* such as in the detachment of the sternal end of the acromiopectoral flap and its insertion into a facial defect, or *indirect,* when, for example, a dorsal pedicle is moved by detaching its lower end and attaching it to the shoulder (Fig. 6–51). In a later stage the tube may be transferred to the neck. This procedure of detaching one extremity of the tube and attaching it to an area nearer the defect is often referred to as "waltzing."

Another type of indirect transfer is one that requires a "carrier," usually the upper extremity. In transferring an abdominal tube flap to the face, the favorite method of transfer in the United States and in Great Britain has been the detachment of the lower extremity of the

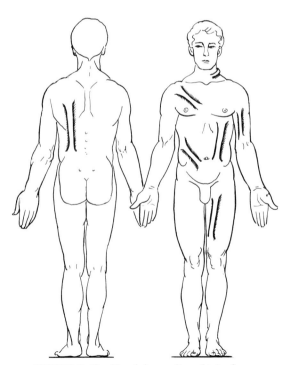

FIGURE 6–49. Usual donor sites of tube flaps.

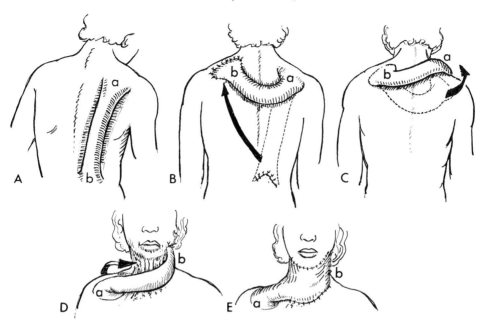

FIGURE 6–51.   Transfer of a scapular tube flap to the neck. *A*, Large scapular tube flap. *B*, The lower end (b) of the flap is transferred to the upper portion of the left scapular area. *C*, The upper end (a) of the tube flap is transferred to the right supraclavicular area. *D*, The extremity (b) of the tube flap is transferred over the right shoulder to the anterior aspect of the neck, being implanted into the left side of the neck. *E*, The flap is opened and is spread over the neck.

abdominal flap, its attachment to the radial aspect of the wrist (Fig. 6–52, *A*), and its transfer to the face after detachment of the remaining abdominal attachment, the hand resting on the patient's shoulder (Fig. 6–52, *B*).

The "salute" position of Kilner (Fig. 6–52, *C*, *D*) is another position of transfer which utilizes the radial aspect of the wrist as the carrier. Schuchardt (1944) preferred to attach the upper extremity of an oblique abdominal flap to the

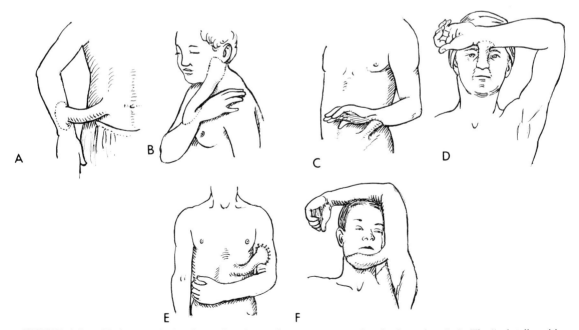

FIGURE 6–52.   Various methods of transfer of tube flaps. *A, B*, Transfer via the wrist. *C, D*, The "salute" position of Kilner, *E, F*, Transfer via the arm (Schuchardt).

arm. The position of transfer to the face is then obtained by placing the forearm over the patient's head (Fig. 6–52, *E, F*). For transfers to the lower extremity (for example, coverage of a cutaneous defect of the knee), one end of an abdominal tube flap is detached and carried on the wrist to the defect (Fig. 6–53).

When effecting the transfer of one end of a tube flap it is important to avoid detaching the tube beyond a line represented by X-Y in Figure 6–54, for fear of exceeding the limits of the vascular supply. An extension of the tube (a larger "paddle") should be delayed by raising the flap in a preliminary stage. Insertion of the end of a tube flap into a new site in the course of the transfer from one area of the body to another is usually accomplished by a trap door flap (Fig. 6–55).

It has been traditional to wait approximately three weeks before transferring a tube flap, and the efficacy of this time interval has been experimentally confirmed (Winster, Manalo and Barsky, 1961). However, studies by Tauxe and associates (1970) indicate that a possible severance time as short as ten days is safe.

Regardless of the method of attachment, the inset should represent between ¼ and ⅓ of the total length of the flap in order to prepare for a safe and early detachment of the other end, especially when more than the tubed portion of the pedicle is to be transferred. In certain instances, this will mean opening a part of the tubed portion of the pedicle, as in Fig. 6–56.

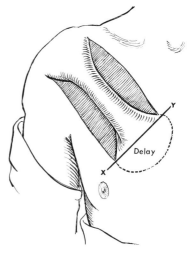

FIGURE 6–54. The safety line X-Y in detaching one end of a tube flap. Beyond this line the flap is not delayed. (From Kazanjian and Converse.)

Direct Flaps from a Distance. Flaps can be constructed in one area and transferred directly to another region of the body. The flaps are usually open, and an extremity, because of the mobility it affords, is usually involved, either as the donor or as recipient site.

TRUNK. The trunk can be used as a donor site in resurfacing defects in the upper extremity, particularly in the elbow area (Fig. 6–57). Abdominal flaps have also been used for repair of defects of the dorsum of the hand and forearm. The flap can usually be transferred directly and the abdominal donor site closed primarily after the wound margins are undermined.

Theoretically, a flap taken from the upper part of the abdomen should have its pedicle based above, so as to receive the blood supply from the branches of the internal mammary artery; a flap taken from the lower part of the abdomen should have its pedicle based inferiorly, so as to receive the branches of the superficial epigastric artery (Fig. 6–58). Practically speaking, the position of the base is determined by the site to be repaired. In defects of the dorsum of the hand and of the dorsal aspect and radial border of the forearm, an abdominal flap based above is used. In repairs of the volar aspect of the forearm and its ulnar border, a flap based inferiorly is applied. Flaps which are inferiorly based tend to be less edematous in the postoperative period because of a more favorable position for venous drainage.

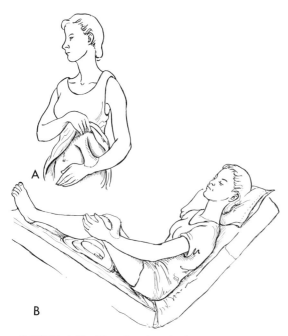

FIGURE 6–53. Transfer of a tube flap to the lower extremity. *A,* Inferior end of an oblique abdominal tube flap is attached to a wrist carrier. *B,* Transfer of flap via the wrist to a defect of the knee region.

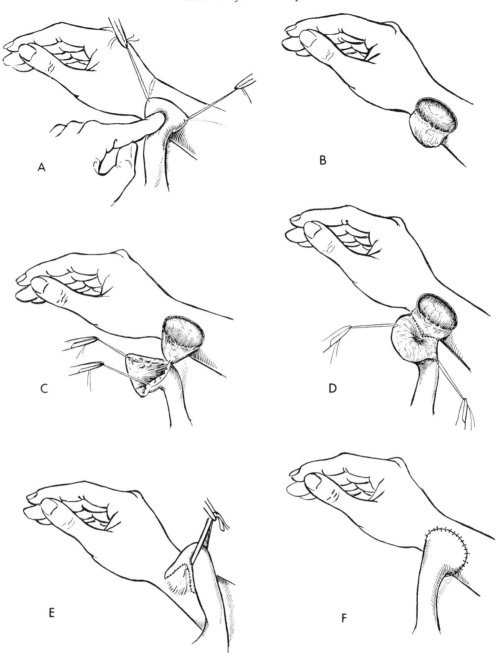

FIGURE 6–55. Technique of implantation of the end of a tube flap into the wrist. *A*, The raw area at the end of the flap is pressed against the wrist, thus making a blood stain. *B*, Trap door flap raised. *C*, The end of the trap door flap is sutured to the edge of the raw area at the end of the tube flap. *D*, Suture of the trap door flap to the tube flap is completed. *E*, Junction of the trap door flap with the tube flap. *F*, Illustrates suture of the end of the tube flap into the defect of the wrist. (From Kazanjian and Converse.)

Abdominal flaps to the hand and forearm are often thick and usually require subsequent thinning. Many weeks after the flap has healed, one-half of the flap is raised, and a layer of fat is excised. The other half of the flap is left attached, so as to ensure the vascularization of

the flap. A few weeks later, the same procedure is done in the latter half.

For defects of the elbow region, a flap raised just above the iliac crest can be employed (see Fig. 6–57). In the lower abdomen, the superficial fascia contains elastic tissue in sufficient

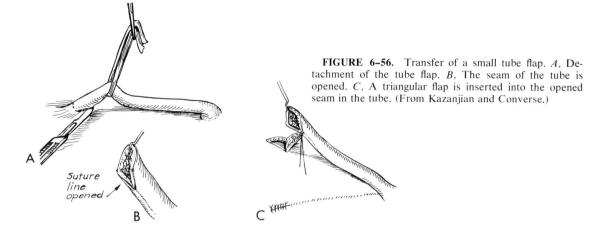

FIGURE 6–56. Transfer of a small tube flap. *A*, Detachment of the tube flap. *B*, The seam of the tube is opened. *C*, A triangular flap is inserted into the opened seam in the tube. (From Kazanjian and Converse.)

abundance to comprise a separate stratum, the fascia of Scarpa. Flaps taken from this region have a natural elasticity and are particularly suitable as a covering for a mobile region, such as the elbow. In repairing the medial surface of the elbow, a flap with a superiorly based pedicle is used. When the lateral surface requires a flap repair, the base of the flap is placed in-

feriorly. When flap repair is needed on both the lateral and medial aspects of the elbow, a flap based inferiorly is used to cover the lateral surface, and the olecranon is buried in a pocket produced by undermining the base of the flap (Fig. 6–59). The upper edge of the abdominal skin defect is sutured to the edge of the defect on the medial aspect of the elbow. In a second-

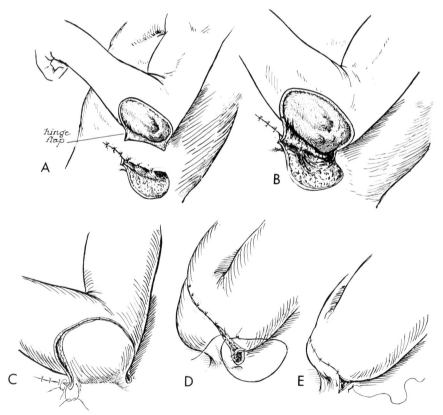

FIGURE 6–57. Direct abdominal flap repair of the elbow. *A*, The abdominal flap has been raised, and the abdominal defect has been closed. The flap is ready to be applied to the elbow defect. *B*, Suture of the hinge flap, *C*, *D*, *E*, Suture of the flap to the defect.

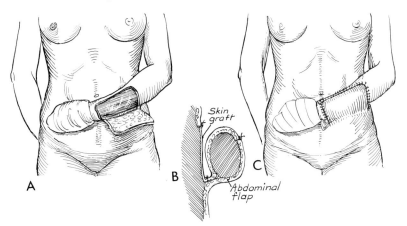

FIGURE 6-58. Example of direct abdominal flap from a distance to cover a defect of the extensor surface of the forearm. *A,* Forearm defect. Abdominal flap has been raised. *B,* The donor defect can be covered with a split-thickness skin graft but usually can be primarily closed after undermining of the wound margins. *C,* Flap sutured into the defect. The upper extremity is held in a comfortable position.

stage operation two or three weeks later, another flap, based upon the portion already inserted upon the lateral aspect of the elbow, covers the medial aspect.

Thoracobrachial flaps present relatively little discomfort during transfer. These flaps are based posteriorly for the repair of the posterior aspect of the arm (Fig. 6–60) and anteriorly for the anterior aspect of the arm.

The infraclavicular area has also been used in resurfacing defects of the thumb, fingers, and dorsum of the hand. While the skin is thinner than in the abdominal wall and the contralateral infraclavicular area is a comfortable position during immobilization of the upper extremity, the donor site offers a distinct cosmetic disadvantage, particularly in the female patient.

During the period of immobilization prior to division of the flap, it is sufficient to use only 6-inch Ace bandages wrapped around the arm and trunk. Plaster dressings are unnecessary.

The deltopectoral, groin (superficial circum-

flex iliac artery), and hypogastric (superficial inferior epigastric artery) flaps are discussed in the section on Axial Pattern Flaps.

UPPER EXTREMITY. Flaps of the upper extremity are often used to cover defects of the contralateral hand. The cross-arm flap is particularly suited for providing coverage on the contralateral hand and fingers. The donor skin is relatively devoid of subcutaneous tissue and

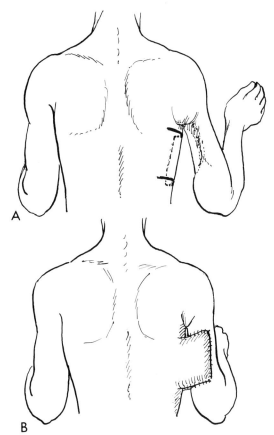

FIGURE 6-60. Example of trunk flap to resurface a defect of the upper arm. *A,* Outline of flap. *B,* Insertion of flap into the defect.

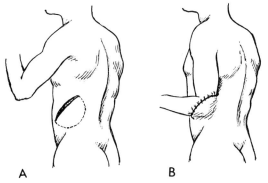

FIGURE 6-59. Abdominal flap repair of the elbow. *A,* Incisions used to delimit the flap destined to cover the elbow region when the joint is ankylosed in a 90° position. *B,* The elbow is placed in a pocket established by undermining the abdominal skin.

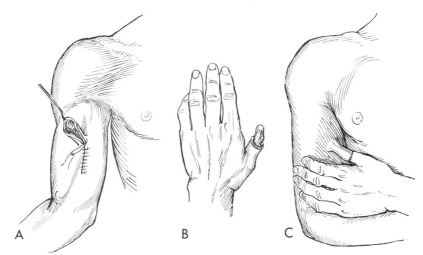

FIGURE 6–61. Cross-arm flap. *A*, Flap has been raised and the donor defect primarily closed. *B*, Avulsion injury of thumb. *B*, Thumb resurfaced by cross-arm flap.

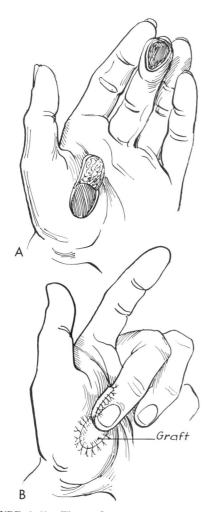

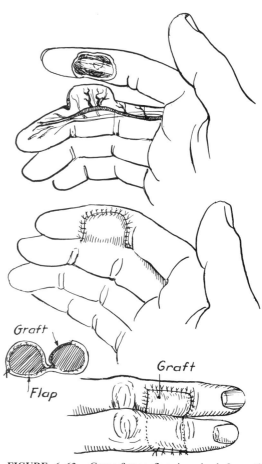

FIGURE 6–62. Thenar flap. *A*, Tip defect of middle finger. Thenar flap has been raised. *B*, Flap sutured to the finger. Donor defect covered with full-thickness skin graft (removed from volar wrist crease).

FIGURE 6–63. Cross-finger flap is raised from the dorsum of an adjoining finger without injury to the neuro-vascular bundle. The donor site is covered with a skin graft.

is an ideal match of the skin of the thumb and fingers. A flap (either a single or double pedicle) can be raised from the relatively hairless area of the biceps region (Fig. 6–61). The pedicle can be safely divided at 2½ to 3 weeks.

The upper arm was also used to reconstruct the nose in the classic method of Tagliacozzi (see Chapter 29). The flap is based proximally and can be elevated and transferred at the same time.

Defects of the fingers and thumbs are best covered with the thenar or cross-finger flaps. The thenar flap (Fig. 6–62) provides tissue coverage which is a near match of that of the fingers and thumb. Its one disadvantage is that immobilization of the PIP joint of the recipient finger in acute flexion for two to three weeks can result in disabling joint problems, especially in the older patient.

The cross-finger flap is particularly suited for covering defects of the volar aspect of the fingers (Fig. 6–63).

The donor sites can be covered with full-thickness skin grafts, which can be removed from the area of the volar wrist crease. The latter defect can be primarily closed with the wrist in a flexed position.

LOWER EXTREMITY. Cross-leg flaps are usually performed to procure stable skin coverage of the bones and exposed tendons of the contralateral lower extremity.

The calf is the usual donor site, but the thigh can also be used. It should be noted that, in young children, flexibility of the limb is such that a foot defect can be resurfaced from the upper thigh or buttock.

The usual flap is based along the medial aspect of the tibia (see Fig. 6–31). As the base of the flap is proportionately broad, a delay procedure, especially in the younger patient, is not necessary. The donor site is covered with a split-thickness skin graft.

Immobilization, so essential to prevent kinking and to ensure the vascularity of the flap, presents a problem in the patient with a cross-leg flap. Interconnected plaster of Paris casts of both legs, connected to an overhead balanced suspension system, have been traditionally used. In recent years the trend has been away from this technique to one of threaded Steinman pin fixation (Adams and coworkers, 1969).

The details of the cross-leg flap and other methods of resurfacing lower extremity defects are discussed in Chapter 86.

AXIAL PATTERN FLAPS

Axial pattern flaps, as noted earlier, are supplied by a direct cutaneous artery. The safe

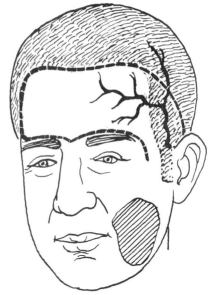

FIGURE 6–64. Forehead flap based on the superficial temporal artery can be used to cover a buccal defect (McGregor, 1963).

length of the flap is related to the length of the direct cutaneous vessel plus an attached random pattern segment supplied by the dermal-subdermal plexuses (McGregor and Morgan, 1973). Traditional length-width ratios play no role in the planning of arterial flaps (Smith, 1973).

Arterial flaps are distinguished from island flaps in that the pedicle consists of skin, subcutaneous tissue, and the direct cutaneous artery and vein. The pedicle of an island flap consists solely of the artery and vein (see Fig. 6–29).

The superficial temporal artery forms the vascular basis of the forehead flap (McGregor, 1963). The flap is outlined along the hair line and eyebrows (Fig. 6–64) and is tunneled into an intraoral location to resurface buccal, pharyngeal, and floor of the mouth defects (see Chapter 62). The same axial vascular system forms the basis of other forehead and scalping flaps (Converse, 1942).

Median forehead flaps (Kazanjian, 1946); a variation is the "island flap" with a subcutaneous pedicle (Converse and Wood-Smith, 1963). Both flaps can be employed for nasal and medial canthal defects. See Chapter 29 for further details.

The deltopectoral flap, described by Bakamjian (1965), is based on the second, third, and fourth anterior perforating branches of the internal mammary arteries (Fig. 6–65). The flap can be lengthened by random-pattern "paddle" extensions over the deltoid area. It has found

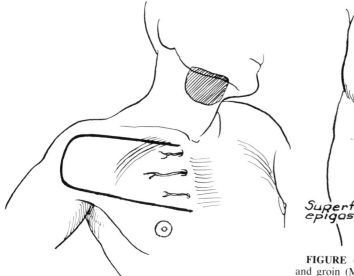

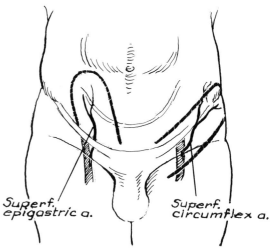

FIGURE 6–67. Hypogastric (Shaw and Payne, 1946) and groin (McGregor and Jackson, 1972) flaps as examples of axial pattern or arterial flaps.

FIGURE 6–65. Deltopectoral flap (Bakamjian, 1965) is an arterial or axial pattern flap utilized to reconstruct oral defects.

wide application in reconstruction of the pharyngoesophageal area, cheeks, and neck. The flap is discussed in detail in Chapter 63. The forehead and deltopectoral flaps, used together, can provide two-layer closure of a cheek defect (Fig. 6–66).

The superficial inferior epigastric artery provides the vascular axis of the hypogastric or lower abdominal flap (Shaw and Payne, 1946).

The flap has been used in resurfacing defects of the contralateral hand, such as thumb web space contracture (Fig. 6–67).

The groin flap (Fig. 6–68) (superficial circumflex iliac arteriovenous system) was recently described by McGregor and Jackson (1972). Its unusually long design permits resurfacing of defects of the hand and forearm, pubic and perineal area, or head and neck area via a hand carrier. The anatomical vascular basis of the flap is discussed by Smith

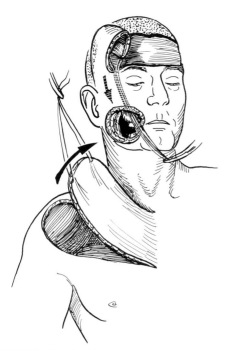

FIGURE 6–66. Combination of forehead and deltopectoral flaps to reconstruct a full-thickness cheek defect.

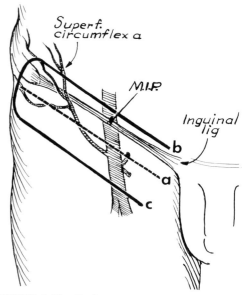

FIGURE 6–68. Design of the groin flap. Central axis (a) of the flap lies on a line 2.5 cm below the anterior superior iliac spine and the midinguinal point (M.I.P.). (Adapted from Smith, P. J., Foley, B., McGregor, I. A., and Jackson, I. T.: The anatomical basis of the groin flap. Plast. Reconstr. Surg., *49*:41, 1972.)

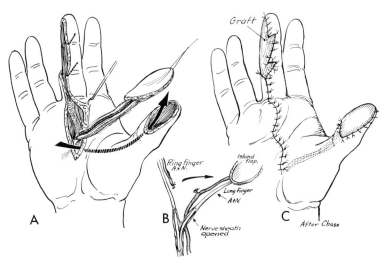

FIGURE 6-69. Neurovascular island flap (after Littler, 1960). *A,* Island of skin has been raised on its neurovascular pedicle. *B,* Details of the pedicle. *C,* Flap sutured into thumb defect. Donor site covered with a skin graft. (From Chase, R. A.: Atlas of Hand Surgery. Philadelphia, W. B. Saunders Company, 1973.)

and associates (1972). The flap is based medially, and the central axis of the flap lies on a line lying 2.5 cm below the mid-inguinal point (half-way between the pubic tubercle and the anterior superior iliac spine) and a point 2.5 cm below the anterior superior iliac spine (Fig. 6–68).

Taylor and Daniel (1975) have described the vascular anatomy of the iliofemoral region.

A flap designed and raised on the dorsum of the foot (dorsalis pedis artery and vein) is useful in resurfacing ankle and foot defects (McCraw and Furlow, 1975) (see Chapter 86).

Island Flaps. Similar to axial pattern flaps in design and location, island flaps represent a variation in that they have pedicles containing only the direct cutaneous artery and vein. Conversion of an arterial flap to an island flap does not reduce the surviving length of the flap (Daniel and Williams, 1973).

An example of an island flap is the neurovascular island flap (Littler, 1960). An island of skin can be removed from the ulnar aspect of the ring finger and transferred on its neurovascular pedicle (Fig. 6–69) for coverage on the thumb or index finger.

Eyebrow reconstruction can be accomplished by an island of hair-bearing scalp supported by a superficial temporal arterial pedicle and transferred to the supraorbital area (Fig. 6–70).

Myocutaneous Flaps. There are few known independent cutaneous vascular territories, a fact which limits the clinical application of axial pattern flaps. Previously it was suggested by Manchot (1889) that all of the skin was sup-

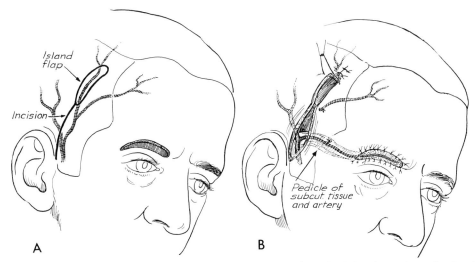

FIGURE 6-70. Island flap reconstruction of the eyebrow. *A,* Island flap of hair-bearing scalp outlined on branch of the superficial temporal artery. *B,* Flap transferred to right supraorbital area. The donor defect can be directly approximated.

SECONDARY MYOCUTANEOUS AND CUTANEOUS AREAS

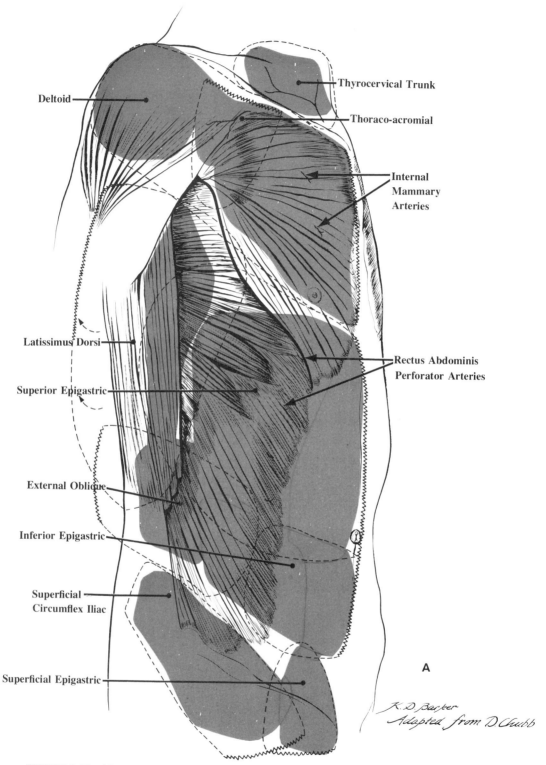

FIGURE 6–71. Myocutaneous vascular territories. *A*, Anterior trunk. (Courtesy of Dr. John McCraw.)

Illustration continued on opposite page.

SECONDARY MYOCUTANEOUS AND CUTANEOUS AREAS

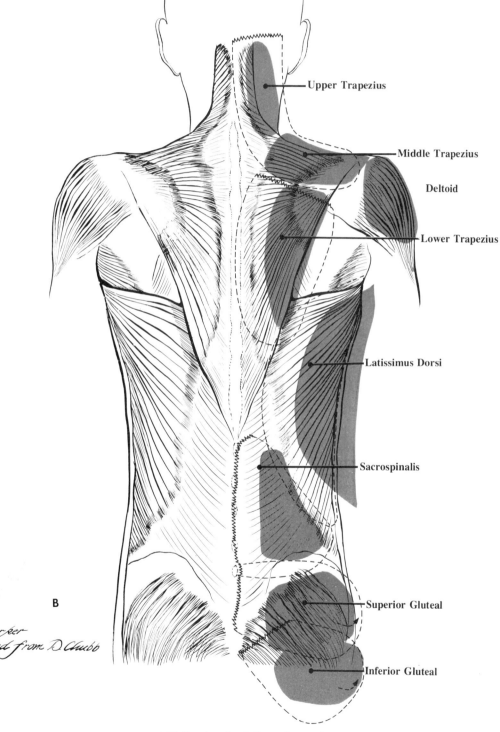

Upper Trapezius

Middle Trapezius

Deltoid

Lower Trapezius

Latissimus Dorsi

Sacrospinalis

Superior Gluteal

Inferior Gluteal

B

K. D. Barper
Adapted from D. Chubb

Figure 6–71 *Continued. B*, Posterior trunk.

plied by specific arterialized cutaneous vascular territories. Manchot's anatomical study described existing cutaneous vascular areas in a remarkably accurate fashion, but it has since been found that few of these are supplied by existing longitudinal cutaneous vessels which act as "independent cutaneous vascular territories." As there are few independent cutaneous vascular territories, one must ask, "What is the blood supply to the remaining skin?" By deduction, this must be the perforating muscular vessels (see Fig. 6–27).

Since axial pattern flaps are scarce, and since muscular perforators supply the remaining skin, the random pattern flap must be considered a "dissociated" myocutaneous flap, because the random flap receives essentially all of its blood supply from the underlying muscle. The definition of independent myocutaneous vascular territories has thus become pertinent.

The concept that skin is sustained, primarily, by its underlying muscle has not been clinically exploited. Owens (1955) and later Bakamjian (1963) pioneered the application of compound myocutaneous flaps. Supraclavicular skin was carried by the sternocleidomastoid muscle and used to repair defects of the cheek and palate, respectively. Later, Orticochea (1972) introduced the gracilis compound skin-muscle flap. Initially, the flap was raised in several stages to reconstruct the penis; subsequently, the flap was elevated and immediately inset as a cross-leg flap. In both instances the muscle was used to augment the blood supply of a cutaneous thigh flap, but this did demonstrate that muscle is capable of supporting a certain portion of its overlying skin without any cutaneous "delay" or staged reduction of existing blood supply.

All of the authors recognized the principle of a certain cutaneous dependence upon the underlying muscle. None recognized the "primary" island myocutaneous flap as an integral skin-muscle unit which is supported by a single muscle neurovascular pedicle. When elevated as a compound flap, this discrete and definable area of skin and muscle will survive completely because its blood supply is essentially unchanged.

McCraw and associates (1976), following experimental work in dogs, have defined multiple myocutaneous vascular territories (Fig. 6–71). These myocutaneous territories, surrounding the territories of the known arterialized flaps, expand the sources of arterialized flaps available to the plastic surgeon.

Each of the myocutaneous vascular territories is discrete and definable and is affected by each adjacent myocutaneous vascular territory. In the anterior trunk, the largest territory is that of the upper rectus abdominis, which extends to the anterior axillary line from the midline; superiorly it impinges on the pectoralis major territory, and inferiorly it impinges on the external oblique and the lower rectus abdominis territories. The perforators of this territory allow one to elevate a transverse flap that is axial to the anterior axillary line and random to the posterior axillary line. Remarkably, it is also possible to raise the entire shaded area of the upper rectus abdominis area depicted in Figure 6–71 on the superior epigastric vessels as an island flap. As one moves caudally, the external oblique territory becomes dominant and such a transverse flap is not possible. Because of the importance of the external oblique area, it is preferable to base flaps posteriorly in the lower abdomen rather than anteriorly. Similarly in the latissimus dorsi area, it is more important to base flaps superiorly rather than inferiorly in the axillary line.

On the back, the sacrospinalis flap is a viable myocutaneous area, but it is less dominant than the external oblique myocutaneous area when the posterior axillary line is encountered. Superiorly, the latissimus dorsi area is the most prominent area of the back and provides the largest available myocutaneous flap of the trunk. Above this, the only available myocutaneous flap is the upper trapezius myocutaneous flap, based on the trapezius muscle in the neck. This is the only usable trapezius myocutaneous flap because of its mobility (the middle and lower trapezius musculature also supply well arterialized flaps, but neither one is movable). Finally, in the lower back the superior and inferior gluteal vessels supply myocutaneous flaps which have limited application because of their rotational deficits.

Additional applications of myocutaneous flaps are discussed in Chapters 86 and 99.

Microvascular Free Flaps. A variation of the island flap has been the development of the microvascular free flap technique, in which composites of tissue based on a specific arteriovenous system are detached and transferred to another anatomical area. The arteriovenous vessels of the flap are then anastomosed to the recipient vessels by microvascular techniques (see Chapter 14).

Experimental studies in animals proved the feasibility of transplanting composite blocks of tissue by microvascular anastomoses (Goldwyn, Lamb and White, 1963; Krizek and associates, 1965; Strauch and Murray, 1967).

Harii, Ohmori, and Ohmori (1974), Daniel and Taylor (1973), and O'Brien and associates (1973) reported the first successful human transfer of an island flap by microvascular anastomosis (microvascular free flap). Free scalp transplants were anastomosed to the superficial temporal system, and other types of free flaps were first accomplished in 1973 (Harii and coworkers, 1974). In the case reported by Daniel and Taylor (1973), the vessels of an iliofemoral island flap were sutured to the posterior tibial artery, a single vena comitans of the posterior tibial artery, and the saphenous vein in the region of a medial malleolar defect of the ankle. Subsequent arteriograms confirmed the success of the microsurgical anastomosis.

O'Brien and coworkers (1973) transferred a large island flap from the groin to the foot. A preoperative arteriogram established the presence of adequate vasculature in the proposed flaps. O'Brien and coworkers (1974) have subsequently extended the technique to achieve coverage in various anatomical areas.

COMPOSITE FLAPS

Composite flaps can be defined as skin flaps which also carry adjacent muscle, bone, or cartilage. The best known example is the Stein-Abbé lip flap, containing skin, subcutaneous tissue, and orbicularis muscle. O'Brien (1970) used a neck flap of skin and sternocleidomastoid muscle to reconstruct a defect of the lower lip. Snyder and associates (1970) popularized reconstruction of mandibulofacial defects with "osteocutaneous" flaps. Conley (1972) reported a variety of composite flaps in various combinations (sternocleidomastoid muscle and attached clavicle; trapezius and scapula, and so forth). Long-term evaluation of the transplanted bone by microscopic analysis and radioactive bone scans showed a wide spectrum of changes dependent on the vascular supply of the bone (Conley and coworkers, 1973). Ketchum, Masters, and Robinson (1974) reconstructed a mandibular defect with a composite island rib flap based on the intercostal vessels. With refinements in microsurgical techniques, free musculocutaneous compound flaps, including the gracilis muscle, have been transferred in one stage (Harii, Ohmori and Sekiguchi, 1976).

OVERFLAPPING

The term "overflapping" may be used to designate the placing of one flap over another. This procedure may be required to build up the thickness of the cutaneous layer in a depressed area or to compensate for the deficiency in bulk of a previously applied flap. Overflapping may be done by means of an advancement flap placed over an adjacent area of skin which has been deprived of its surface epithelium by shaving or by dermabrasion. Prior to the removal of the epithelium, an incision is made through the skin outlining the area that is to receive the covering flap.

Overflapping may also be practiced to cover a previously transplanted flap that has shrunk in dimension and is not adequate to achieve a satisfactory reconstruction. An example of such a case is that of a patient who underwent a forehead flap for reconstruction of the upper half of the nose. The flap was of inadequate dimension, and further shrinking reduced it to an even smaller size. The epithelium was removed by dermabrasion, and a second forehead flap was applied over the first, achieving a satisfactory result.

OVERGRAFTING A FLAP

Such a procedure may be required for a flap from a distance placed in the facial area which has undergone color changes, rendering the flap unsightly. The surface epithelium is removed, and the abraded dermis of the flap is covered with a split-thickness skin graft taken from the cervical area; should the flap be of insufficient size, a full-thickness graft from the retroauricular or supraclavicular area may be employed.

The crane principle is a term (Millard, 1969) describing a technique of transporting subcutaneous tissue to cover exposed bone, nerve, blood vessels, and tendon. Initially the area is covered with a flap. After seven days the flap is shaved off, leaving a 7-mm margin of subcutaneous tissue over the original defect. The skin and a small amount of fat from the flap are returned to the original donor site. The transported subcutaneous tissue should be sufficiently vascularized by the twelfth day to receive a split-thickness skin graft.

THE SUITABILITY OF SKIN GRAFTS AND FLAPS

Skin grafts are unsuitable in five clinical situations:

1. For covering densely scarred areas. Permanent repair by a skin graft cannot be assured when it is applied over a poorly vascularized surface containing scar tissue which has not been entirely resected, either because the scar merges onto a joint capsule or bare bone or because it incorporates large vessels or nerves. In such cases, even after an immediate "take," the skin graft may secondarily break down. This complication is seen particularly when the skin graft covers an area of functional stress, such as the weight-bearing area of the foot.

2. For covering bone. Skin grafts survive when transplanted over healthy periosteum and will resist ordinary trauma, if they are not placed in positions of functional stress. A skin graft, however, does not provide a covering that will permit a secondary operation, such as bone grafting or arthroplasty. A skin graft receives little blood supply from the surrounding tissue, so that it cannot be raised from its bed without danger of necrosis. Bone denuded of periosteum, if it is to survive, must be covered by well vascularized integument. It should be covered at the earliest moment by a skin flap to prevent ischemic necrosis, elimination of bone, osteitis, and sequestration. Dermal overgrafting, as discussed earlier, is an alternative technique in such a situation.

3. For covering tendons. Tendons must be placed among tissues which permit gliding—tendon sheath, paratenon, loose areolar tissue, or fat. In repairing tendons or freeing tendons that are bound in an overlying cutaneous scar, the importance of removing all the surrounding scar tissue and of covering the tendons with the adipose tissue of a flap cannot be overstressed. Tendons, even when they have been carved out of a solid block of scar tissue, may glide if they are surrounded by fat or loose areolar tissue.

4. In peripheral nerve surgery. Penetrating injuries affect not only bone, tendons, muscles, skin, and subcutaneous tissue but also adjacent peripheral nerves. It has become increasingly apparent that the covering of the nerve by normal, well vascularized skin and subcutaneous tissue is an essential part of peripheral nerve repair for the following reasons:

    a. A nerve constricted by scar tissue loses its conductivity. If the nerve is anatomically intact, freeing it from the constricting extrinsic scar usually hastens its recovery and will seldom retard it. If the severed nerve must be sutured, it is essential that the return of conductivity be unhampered by adjacent scar (see Chapter 76).

    b. The covering scar tissue may provide inadequate protection to the nerve, when it is superficial. The injured nerve may become superficial in position as a result of the destruction of overlying muscles. In healed wounds of the posteromedial aspect of the elbow, the ulnar nerve may lie immediately beneath the scar tissue or may even be incorporated in the scar itself.

    c. Pain may be caused by the presence of scar tissue around a nerve. Sensory fibers from the nerve may become incorporated in the overlying scar, and a painful scar results. Such intracutaneous neuromas can be cured only by total excision of the scar containing the constricted sensory nerve endings. A flexor tendon may become adherent to the median curve, causing pain by pulling on the nerve in the course of its excursion, until the nerve is freed from the binding scar. Many nerve injuries are associated with causalgia-like pain, which may be relieved by the dissection of the extrinsic scar and placement of the nerve in a new bed, where it is surrounded by nonscarred tissues. Skin flaps, transplanted over the nerve, give the latter a well-vascularized protective covering, a property which skin grafts fail to provide.

5. When secondary operations are necessary in the repaired area. An area in which an operation upon bone, tendons, ligaments, or joints is to be performed or through which a peripheral nerve is to be explored must be covered by a skin flap, which alone will be sufficiently resistant to withstand the incisions, undermining, and unavoidable manipulations associated with the operation. The use of a skin flap also permits combined simultaneous operative procedures on tendons or nerves, the overlying skin defect being immediately covered by a flap.

TIMING OF SKIN REPLACEMENT

So much emphasis has rightly been placed on early skin replacement that often it is not appreciated that the optimum time for repair may not be immediately after injury. The timing of operation for skin closure or skin replacement in acute wounds merits careful consideration, and the method of skin replacement and its integration with early and late treatment of injury to bones, tendons, or nerves are of the greatest importance.

In avlusion injuries with extensive skin loss, careful examination of the base of the wound will show that conditions are far from ideal for the immediate reception of skin grafts. Edema is often present, a hematoma may fill the subcutaneous area, and poorly vascularized tissues such as tendon or bone may be exposed. It may be preferable in a wound of this sort to delay the definitive operation after a primary operation for the careful assessment of the state of the wound, debridement, and application of a pressure dressing, with immobilization and elevation of the injured extremity. In the interval, the open wound can be covered with commercially available porcine skin. After a short time edema will subside, and the wound will fill with granulation tissue; skin grafting at this stage with a split-thickness graft results in complete and immediate healing, with an eventual stable graft.

Compound fractures of the limbs offer difficult problems in skin closure. At the primary operation for assessment of the injury, debridement, and immobilization of the fracture, there is often considerable edema of the skin and soft tissues. Closure of wounds of this sort by suturing, or of wounds with skin loss and exposure of bone by a transposition or rotation flap, may lead to breakdown or sloughing of the skin because of increased postoperative edema and a progressive increase in flap tension. In such cases, the closure of the wound by skin grafts or flaps is best delayed until edema has subsided. These considerations are important because skin replacement is an essential part of the treatment of compound fractures of the leg (see Chapter 86). The healing of a fracture cannot take place unless the consolidating fracture area is covered by well vascularized soft tissue.

Closure of a wound by a flap should not be done when the wound is discharging pus, as this usually indicates the presence of infected and necrotic tissue in the depth of the wound. Such a wound can be closed by a flap only after complete excision of all devitalized tissue. In compound fractures of the leg, one should be particularly careful to obtain control of the suppuration before covering the wound with a flap, as there is no adequate posterior drainage route for the shaft of the tibia. Before plaster is applied, all necrotic tissue and loose bone fragments should be removed, recesses in the wound should be opened, and the wound should be packed open with gauze. When bone is devitalized through exposure, it should be surgically removed before the remaining bone is covered by a flap; necrotic bone should not be left buried under the flap.

As discussed in the section on delayed skin grafting, there is also merit in delaying the transfer of a flap for several days after excision of a lesion when hemostasis is not complete.

FAILURES IN FLAP TRANSFER

The failures that follow the transfer of skin flaps may be due to necrosis, to infection of the flap, or to improper postoperative care.

Failure Due to Necrosis. Necrosis of the whole flap or of a portion of the flap, generally the distal end, because of a deficiency in the blood supply is caused by various planning and technical errors. It is usually caused by improper planning and failure to incorporate an adequate vascular supply in the flap. Survival of flap length is not related to the width of the pedicle (Milton, 1970). A flap with sharp angles survives with difficulty. The flap may also be designed too small.

The flap must not be sutured into position under tension in an effort to provide a covering for the defect. Twisting, kinking of the flap, or placing the flap under tension may result from poor designing and planning of the flap or from the position of transfer, which is inadvertently changed when the immobilization of the donor limb is secured. This is a frequent complication during the application of a plaster cast for the immobilization of a cross-leg flap. To obviate this danger, the two limbs should be firmly immobilized on an orthopedic table before the plaster is applied, or Steinman pin fixation should be employed.

Not more than moderate pressure should be applied over a flap, lest the venous return is obstructed, and superficial necrosis, blistering, epidermal desquamation, or even a loss of a portion of the dermis results.

A frequent mistake in the covering of poorly vascularized areas is the employment of a flap that is too small. It is essential that the scar tissue of such areas be widely excised; moreover, a flap that is to cover an area devoid of a normal blood supply should extend widely into the normal tissue around the defect. In this manner, the flap will derive a sufficient blood supply from the surrounding well-vascularized tissue. Failure to provide a wide area of insertion of the flap may result in necrosis of a portion of the flap when the pedicle is sectioned. Prior to designing a flap, the recipient lesion or defect should be excised. Often the true defect is larger than the apparent defect, and a larger flap will be required.

Separation and gaping over the secondary suture line after the section of the pedicle of the flap are frequent complications when the design of the flap was too small. The hinge flap procedure assists in obtaining a vascularized base of insertion.

Failure Due to Infection. Skin flaps show resistance to infection, even when applied over a septic area. However, the covering of a grossly suppurating wound by a skin flap is a mistake. The flap tends to convert an open wound into a closed one and impede drainage. Flaps are rarely lost because of infection.

Failure Due to Improper Postoperative Care. After a successful flap transfer, complications may occur because of the imprudent treatment of the freshly transplanted tissue. This tissue has been severed from its nerve connections and is insensitive; in addition, the inactive sebaceous and sweat glands fail to provide the skin with its normal lubrication. The patient may unduly traumatize the transplanted skin by exposing it to heat and burning. The burn sustained by laying the foot, newly covered by a flap, over a hot radiator is a typical complication. Even prolonged exposure to the ultraviolet rays of the sun may cause further desquamation of the already dry and scaly skin.

The vascular connections are delicate for weeks after transplantation; slight trauma may cause ecchymosis, hematoma, blistering, and ulceration of the flap.

Because of the peripheral barrier of scar tissue, the venous drainage is sluggish, and the lymphatic circulation is only gradually reestablished. The venous return from the flap is improved by wearing a pressure bandage over the flap for months after the flap transfer. Physiotherapy will improve the circulation and hasten the softening of the peripheral scar.

After the transfer of a flap to a weight-bearing area, the patient should avoid full weight-bearing for several months, until the peripheral scar has softened and normal circulation has been reestablished within the flap.

Care should be exercised in placing secondary incision lines and in undermining flaps at the time of a subsequent operative procedure, such as bone grafting. Necrosis of the flap may occur if an incision is placed in the center of the flap and if the latter is undermined laterally. The flap is then left hinged upon lines of scar tissue, and the blood supply is inadequate. Furthermore, even if healing takes place without incident, the presence of three scar lines instead of two interferes with the circulation of the flap. It is essential that the secondary incisions be placed in former suture lines and that not more than one half of the flap is raised at one time, the other half being left attached to maintain an adequate blood supply.

REINNERVATION OF SKIN TRANS-PLANTS*

The reinnervation of skin grafts and flaps has been extensively studied by both clinical observation and experimental design. For a review of the early literature, the reader is referred to an article by Pontén (1960).

Neurohistologic Basis of Cutaneous Sensation

The exact neurohistologic basis of sensation and the pathways taken by new nerve axons in the reestablishment of innervation are still not entirely clear. The theory of von Frey (1895), which held that each of the four sensory modalities had a corresponding end organ (pain: free nerve endings; touch: networks around hair follicles and Meissner's corpuscles; warmth: Ruffini endings; cold: Krause's end bulbs), was refuted by Sinclair, Weddell and Zander (1952). These investigators found that all modalities are equally represented in the fingertip and the skin of the ear. The fingertip contains organized nerve endings of the Meissner, Krause, and Ruffini types, as well as the nerve plexus, while the skin of the ear contains only free nerve endings and nerve nets surrounding individual hair follicles. It was demonstrated that the nerve fiber enters the skin from below, dividing repeatedly and forming branches which spread to form a nerve plexus supplying an approximately circular area. The fibers end as fine filaments, both freely in the dermis and epidermis and in association with skin appendages, such as the vessels, sweat glands, and hair follicles. Such nerve plexuses are found throughout the skin in varying densities, and the free nerve endings are considered the receptors for all stimuli, with the possible exception of touch, the receptor for which is believed to be the basketlike nerve net surrounding the hair follicles. Weddell, Palmer, and Pallie (1955) believed that these nerve nets are formed from several different fibers which intermingle without contact and end as free axoplasmic filaments.

Reinnervation of Skin Grafts and Flaps

In a histologic study of the reinnervation of skin grafts and flaps, Santoni-Rugiu (1966)

---

*Contributed by Joan M. Platt, M.D.

described the sequence of events which occurs following skin transplants in rabbits. Histologic sections of full-thickness grafts taken ten days after grafting showed evidence of damage in the fibrils of Langerhans and the free nerve endings, although the larger nerve structures of the deeper layers appeared relatively normal. Later, degeneration occurred in these structures; 30 days after grafting, no nerve structures could be identified, with the exception of what appeared to be empty Schwann tubes, occasionally containing fragmented, pale fibers. Forty days after grafting, delicate new fibrils were found, particularly in the deep layers of the graft. Such fibrils were seen more frequently at 50 or 60 days, and by three months, the number of fibrils had increased and nerve fibers could be seen in the deep layers of the graft.

Degenerative changes in the nerves in skin flaps occurred earlier but were less complete than in free grafts. Regeneration appeared to occur earlier and more closely resembled the nerve structure of normal skin.

Controversy still exists concerning the pathways taken by new nerve axons innervating skin transplants. Davis and Kitlowski (1934) and Napier (1952) believed that reinnervation takes place by contact between the ingrowing axons and the nerve plexus of the graft, the empty Schwann tubes and the associated nerve endings connected with them becoming reinnervated.

Kredel and Evans (1933), Davis (1934), Hutchison, Tough, and Wyburn (1949), and Folkerts, Sneep, and Meijling (1959) were of the contrary opinion, i.e., that the new axons grow into the graft independently of preexisting Schwann sheaths.

Adeymo and Wyburn (1957), studying grafts in rabbits, described two types of nerve penetration of the grafts: marginal invasion, in which regenerating axons enter the periphery of the graft, and subdermal invasion, in which the divided ends of nerve trunks in the graft bed enter the deep surface of the graft. In the former, the regenerating axons must penetrate scar tissue, and many fail to do so; of those that succeed, a majority have no cellular sheath and terminate as free nerve endings. A minority appear to enter preexisting Schwann tubes. In subdermal invasion, it was found that new axons were distributed at random, some finding their way into existing Schwann tubes, others ending as independent filaments before reaching the superficial layers of the graft. The authors concluded that "the final result is, in terms of crude structure, a reformation of the

cutaneous nerve plexuses and endings characteristic of the grafted skin, particularly so in the central regions of the graft . . ., supplemented by a marginal fringe of 'abnormal' nerve fibers for the most part made up of 'independent' axons invading from the side and from below."

Fitzgerald, Martin, and Paletta (1967), using the pig as an experimental animal, transferred nasal skin grafts to the dorsum of the animal. They also replaced dorsal skin grafts, with and without rotation, and transferred dorsal skin grafts to the opposite side of the body. Since the nerve structure of the dorsal skin of the pig differs in several respects from that of nasal skin, the patterns of reinnervation of transplanted skin from these areas could be objectively compared. It was found in this study that, in the dorsal skin grafts, nerves enter the graft through the sides and base by following the course of blood vessels or collagen bundles. Once within the graft, 90 per cent appear to enter vacant neurilemmal sheaths; the remainder apparently follow the new blood vessels, their axis cylinders appearing to be naked.

In the nasal skin grafts, the method of nerve invasion is apparently the same as is seen in dorsal skin grafts. The majority enter neurilemmal sheaths, by which they are conducted to blood vessels, vibrissae, and epidermis. The size and disposition of nerve fibers were found to be typical of nasal innervation. The authors concluded that the pattern of innervation of the *donor* skin is reproduced and is determined primarily by the disposition of the neurilemmal cell pathways within the graft and their accessibility to the ingrowing nerve fibers, being most accessible in flaps and least accessible in split-thickness skin grafts. In the latter, the ingrowing fibers must first cross a thick scar.

Grafts of all types are devoid of sensation immediately after transplantation, but recovery of sensation begins as early as one to two months after surgery. Sensation during the first year or two may be abnormal. Pain is frequently more intense than in the surrounding skin (Davis, 1934; Guttman, 1938; Pontén, 1960), and the stimuli of touch, heat, and cold may be experienced as painful (Guttman, 1938). The phenomenon of hypersensitivity may be explained, as suggested by Santoni-Rugiu (1966), by the higher than normal number of nerve fibers and fibrils present in grafts during the process of reinnervation.

Although skin transplants rarely attain the high sensory quality of normal skin, the ability to appreciate pain, touch, warmth, and cold returns to some extent in both free grafts and flaps. The degree, quality, and time of sensory return depend on a number of factors. In general, sensation returns earliest and most completely in skin flaps. Full-thickness skin grafts usually acquire more adequate innervation than split-thickness grafts. Several explanations have been given for this fact: (1) the denser fibrosis developing between thin grafts and their recipient beds (Kredel and Evans, 1933; Davis and Kitlowski, 1934; Kernwein, 1948; Fitzgerald, Martin and Paletta, 1967); (2) the smaller number of nerve endings in split-thickness skin grafts (Davis and Kitlowski, 1934); (3) the fact that split-thickness grafts are often used in circumstances in which the recipient bed is of poor quality, as in deep thermal burns and crushing injuries (Pontén, 1960).

The recipient site is of considerable importance in the ultimate quality of sensation in transplants. Free grafts placed directly on periosteum or muscle usually do not acquire good sensation. Deep cutaneous injury, nerve damage in the surrounding skin, infection, or hematoma may seriously impair the speed and quality of reinnervation.

Of the sensory modalities, pain develops most rapidly, with the ability to appreciate touch, heat, and cold returning later. While reinnervation is still incomplete, there may also be a spatial dissociation in which pain is appreciated over a greater area than touch. Tactile discrimination and touch were found by Pontén (1960) to be the most reliable indices for evaluating return of sensory function, since grafts were frequently found to be hypersensitive to both pain and cold and testing for the sensation of warmth was so variable as to be inconclusive. Hutchison, Tough, and Wyburn (1949), Folkerts, Sneep, and Meijling (1959), and Pontén (1960) all found that tactile discrimination in the graft approached that of the recipient site. Pontén (1960) further noted that, in contrast to the other sensory modalities, there was no difference among the various types of grafts and that none of the factors determining the degree of return of other sensory modalities seemed to affect the final result of tactile discrimination.

In a study of 16 patients one to ten years following neurovascular island flap reconstruction of finger defects, it was found that sensation was reduced in those flaps carried on only one neurovascular pedicle (Murray, Ord, and Gavelin, 1967). Two-point discrimination was absent in the flaps of 12 patients; seven patients complained of hyperesthesia symptoms in the area of the flap.

Maquieira (1974) dissected full-thickness skin units and their corresponding sensory nerve for a variable distance. The donor nerve was then sutured to a sensory nerve in the recipient area. Innervated skin grafts may be particularly indicated in resurfacing the heel and fingertip.

In a critical evaluation of sensory and functional return in a series of fingertip avulsion injuries, Sturman and Duran (1963) reported that the group of patients resurfaced with cross-finger flaps had less subjective complaints and better objective testing than patients covered with split-thickness or full-thickness skin grafts and palmar flaps.

Sweat Gland Function

Since split-thickness skin grafts rarely contain functioning sweat glands, such grafts almost never acquire the ability to sweat. Full-thickness grafts usually contain a variable number of glands, and skin flaps contain all the sweat glands originally present in the donor site. McGregor (1950) found that 70 to 80 per cent of the original glands in the ten flaps he studied became reinnervated and functional. Some degree of reinnervation is necessary for sweat glands to become active (Kredel and Phemister, 1939; Löfgren, 1952; Moberg, 1958; Pontén, 1960), and there is apparently a close relationship between the return of sensory innervation and the secretion of sweat.

McGregor (1950) established that skin grafts assumed the characteristic pattern of sweating of the recipient site; skin transferred from the abdomen, for example, where sweat glands respond primarily to thermogenic stimuli, when transferred to an area of primarily neurogenic sweating (e.g., palm of the hand), assumes the latter pattern. This finding was confirmed by Pontén (1960).

Pilomotor and Vasomotor Function

Kredel and Phemister (1939) and Löfgren (1952) demonstrated that pilomotor function can return in skin flaps. Kredel and Phemister (1939) also showed that vasomotor function returned in flaps, although it was abnormal; there was prolonged redness when the graft was exposed to warmth and prolonged contracture when exposed to cold. This finding was confirmed by Löfgren (1952).

Sebaceous Gland Function

Sebaceous gland function was studied by Pontén (1960), who found that all skin grafts, including split-thickness grafts, contained functioning sebaceous glands and that their ability to secrete and express sebum was independent of sensory innervation or pilomotor function.

HAIR TRANSPLANTATION FOR CORRECTION OF BALDNESS*

Since Orentreich (1959) described a technique for treating baldness with small full-thickness scalp autografts, the effectiveness of correction of male pattern baldness and baldness related to trauma has been accepted as a standard form of treatment.

It is estimated that a sex-linked dominant gene is responsible for varying degrees of baldness in over 80 per cent of American males. Many accept this fact gracefully, while increasing numbers desire treatment for the psychosocial or simple cosmetic problems associated with baldness.

With any individual who seeks assistance, great care must be taken to determine his psychologic motivation. As in any type of corrective surgery, if the motivations are not sound and personality instability is evident, the result will not be satisfactory to the patient, regardless of the surgeon's own evaluation of his work.

It is important to determine the pattern of the patient's forebears' baldness so that a suitable donor site, usually from the occipital or parietal regions, can be chosen. If the patient's father had extensive baldness with only a rim

of hair in these regions, one must realize that grafts taken from a donor site which will eventually become bald will also become bald. It has been the clinical experience of those utilizing the punch graft technique that the full-thickness graft carries the genetic capability to produce hair associated with the area from which it is obtained. The graft is not affected by the area in which it is placed. If, ten years after a graft has been taken from the occipital area, this region becomes bald, it can be anticipated that the graft will lose its hair in the same time interval.

The Punch Graft Technique

A hairline which is acceptable and reasonable is carefully discussed with the patient with the aid of mirrors before any operative procedure is performed. This usually turns out to be a compromise between the bald patient's hairline and his previous hairline with a full growth of hair. In most instances it is not practical to try to reestablish the former hairline which the individual had in his early twenties. With the aid of a marking pencil, a satisfactory curved hairline, which is acceptable to the patient and surgeon, is outlined on the scalp.

The technique is a simple one and is best performed by utilizing one of the 4-mm Orentreich punches on a slowly revolving handpiece (Fig. 6–72).* This punch, which was originally used as a hand instrument, is very effective, but the hand technique is quite laborious to both patient and surgeon. By using the slowly revolving handpiece run by an electric motor, the time of the procedure is greatly shortened, with

---

*Contributed by Jerome E. Adamson, M.D.

*Punch and handpiece are manufactured by the Robbins Instruments Inc., Chatham, New Jersey 07928.

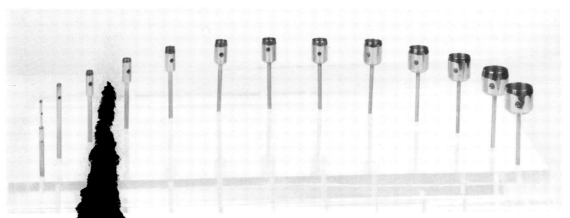

FIGURE 6–72. [P]unch biopsies of increasing caliber. (Courtesy of Robbins Instruments Inc., Chatham, N.J.)

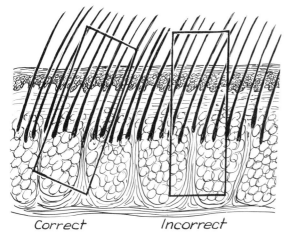

FIGURE 6-73. Correct and incorrect angles for removing donor scalp plugs. The punch must be introduced in a direction parallel to the hair follicles. (From Rees, T. D., and Wood-Smith, D.: Cosmetic Facial Surgery. Philadelphia, W. B. Saunders Company, 1973.)

an average of 45 minutes necessary to transfer approximately 50 plugs.

Under local anesthesia and sterile technique, full-thickness grafts are obtained, using the rotating punch, from the occipital or parietal donor areas. It is important to run the punch slowly to prevent "coneing" of the graft from the too-rapid action of the revolving punch. It is also important to angle the approach of the punch to parallel that of the shafts of the hair follicles (Fig. 6-73). This prevents obliquely cutting off the hair shafts in the midportion of the graft. It is conceivable that, if the angle of the cutting instrument is not appropriately placed, the graft would have no growth of hair, since all of the transferred follicles would be damaged. Approximately 10 to 15 hairs are present in each graft.

One usually obtains 40 to 50 plugs in two rows across the occipital scalp region. The depth of the plugs is slightly greater than the length of the hair follicle and varies from 4½ to 7 mm in length. The grafts are carefully defatted to the base of the follicle and are placed in a beaker upon a saline-soaked gauze. In most of our patients the donor sites are sutured with a running 3-0 black silk suture, which controls any postoperative bleeding.

The forehead and anterior scalp regions are prepared in the usual manner, and local anesthesia by means of local infiltration for hemostasis and a field block is performed. Recipient plugs of non-hair bearing scalp are removed along the preplanned forehead hairline, with care being taken to space the defects approximately 4 to 5 mm apart. This provides equal-sized intervals between the grafts, so at a sec-

ond stage other 4-mm plugs can be placed between the grafts transferred initially. This technique will establish a satisfactory hairline. At the first sitting at least two or more rows of grafts are transferred. Bleeding is controlled by digital pressure. Rarely will it be necessary to use a through and through suture to control bleeding in the recipient area.

A Telfa pad with a circumferential helmet type of head dressing is left in place for 48 hours. The grafts are then exposed and daily gentle showering begun. Mild analgesics are rarely employed postoperatively. Vigorous showering and normal activity are recommended by 2½ to 3 weeks after grafting.

The usual plug will contain approximately 10 to 15 hairs, depending upon the density of hair growth in the individual. Approximately 95 per cent of the hairs should be expected to survive. After transfer of the graft, the hair follicles immediately go into a resting (telogen) state for approximately 2½ to 3 months. After this period hair growth occurs at the same rate as that seen in the donor site (Fig. 6-74).

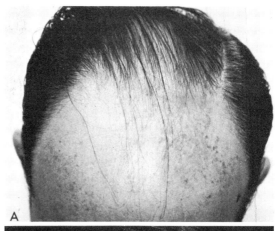

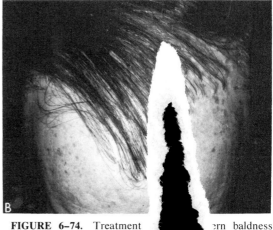

FIGURE 6-74. Treatment ⟨...⟩ ern baldness with full-thickness scalp autog⟨...⟩ reatment. *B,* Following treatment.

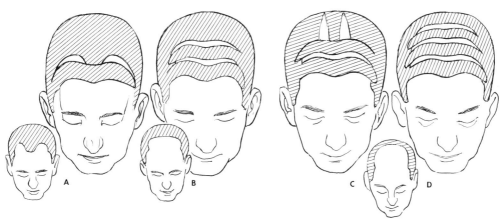

FIGURE 6–75. Types of male pattern baldness treated by scalp flaps. *A*, Type I: a single parieto-occipital flap has been transposed. *B*, Type II: bilateral parieto-occipital flaps have been transposed. *C*, Type III: correction by bilateral parieto-occipital flaps and a third flap from the occipito-parietal region. *D*, Type III: correction by two parieto-occipital flaps on one side and a third from the contralateral side. (Figs. 6–75 and 6–76 after Juri, J.: Use of parieto-occipital flaps in the surgical treatment of baldness. Plast. Reconstr. Surg., 55:456. Copyright 1975, The Williams and Wilkins Company, Baltimore.)

Further stages of grafting are deferred until growth is demonstrated in the previous grafts. Eade (1969) has reported doing massive grafting, with over 100 grafts transferred at one time, under general anesthesia.

Other Techniques

Vallis (1967) has obtained successful results by transferring a long strip of full-thickness hair-bearing scalp to establish a forehead hairline.

This strip, which measures approximately $\frac{1}{8}$ to $\frac{3}{16}$ of an inch in width, is then supplemented by punch grafts placed behind it to fill out the remaining balding areas.

Glanz (1968) has reported using blocks of full-thickness grafts obtained in a similar fashion from occipital donor areas. These blocks, which measure approximately 0.6 cm in width by 1.25 cm or larger in length, are placed in a bricklike fashion in stages over the scalp to provide hair coverage.

With strip grafts or block grafts, the possibil-

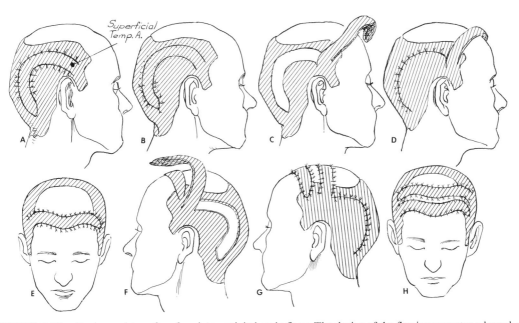

FIGURE 6–76. Design and transfer of parieto-occipital scalp flaps. The design of the flap incorporates a branch of the superficial temporal artery which serves as the central axis; the flap is approximately 4 cm wide. The distal portion is often delayed. The donor area can be closed by direct approximation.

ity of hematoma formation beneath the graft preventing growth of hair from inadequate circulation is a real one. These techniques are reserved for use by surgeons who are especially skilled in the fine points of full-thickness skin grafting and are well aware of the loss of hair growth which may occur from an underlying hematoma. The technique is also used in eyebrow reconstruction following thermal burns.

The patient must be informed of the probable final appearance of the punch graft in the initial interview. It must be emphasized that hair growth will not be absolutely normal because of the difficulty in obtaining as dense a growth of hair as normal by the punch graft technique. Small irregular areas between the grafts will remain bald unless a smaller 2-mm size punch is used to obtain grafts containing three or four hair follicles to fill in the regions. Even with this meticulous technique, the density of the hair will never be normal.

Parieto-occipital scalp flaps have been used for the correction of baldness. Juri (1975) has described a variety of flaps usually encompassing the superficial temporal artery (Figs. 6–75 and 6–76); delay procedures were often employed. After a lapse of 30 days, the contralateral flap is elevated and transposed.

REFERENCES

Adams, W. M., Wisner, H. K., Larson, D. L., Lynch, J. B., and Lewis, S. R.: Steinman pin fixation of extremities for cross-leg flaps. Plast. Reconstr. Surg., 44:364, 1969.

Adamson, J. E., Horton, C. E., Crawford, H. H., and Ayers, W. T.: The effects of dimethyl sulfoxide on the experimental pedicle flaps: A preliminary report. Plast. Reconstr. Surg., 37:105, 1966.

Adeymo, C., and Wyburn, G. M.: Innervation of skin grafts. Transplant. Bull., 4:152, 1957.

Antopol, W., Glaubach, S., and Goldman, L.: The use of neotetrazolium as a tool in the study of active cell processes. Trans. N.Y. Acad. Sci., 12:156, 1950.

Arturson, G., and Khanna, N. N.: The effects of hyperbaric oxygen, dimethyl sulfoxide and complamin on the survival of experimental skin flaps. Scand. J. Plast. Reconstr. Surg., 4:8, 1970.

Artz, C. P., Rittenbury, M. S., and Yarbrough, D. R.: An appraisal of allografts and xenografts as biologic dressings for wounds and burns. Ann. Surg., 175:934, 1972.

Aymard, J. L.: Nasal reconstruction, with a note on nature's plastic surgery. Lancet, 2:888, 1917.

Bailey, B. N.: Treatment of tattoos. Plast. Reconstr. Surg., 40:361, 1967.

Bakamjian, V. Y.: A technique for primary reconstruction of the palate after radical maxillectomy for cancer. Plast. Reconstr. Surg., 31:103, 1963.

Bakamjian, V. Y.: A two-stage method for pharyngoesophageal reconstruction with a primary pectoral skin flap. Plast. Reconstr. Surg., 36:173, 1965.

Ballantyne, D. L., Jr., and Converse, J. M.: The relation of hair cycles to the survival time of suprapannicular and subpannicular skin homografts in rats. Ann. N.Y. Acad. Sci., 64:958, 1957.

Ballantyne, D. L., Jr., and Converse, J. M.: Vascularization of composite auricular grafts transplanted to the chorio-allantois of the chick embryo. Transplant. Bull., 5:373, 1958.

Ballantyne, D. L., Jr., Hawthorne, G. A., Rees, T. D., and Seidman, I.: An experimental evaluation of skin graft preservation with silicone fluid. Cryobiology, 8:211, 1971.

Baran, N. K., and Horton, C. E.: Growth of skin grafts, flaps and scars in young minipigs. Plast. Reconstr. Surg., 50:487, 1972.

Bardach, J., and Kurnatowski, A.: Blood supply of a Filatov's skin flap. Acta Chir. Plast. (Praha), 3:290, 1961.

Barker, D.: Vacutome, a new machine for obtaining split-thickness skin grafts. Plast. Reconstr. Surg., 4:492, 1948.

Baronio, G.: Degli Innesti Animali. Stamperia e Fonderia del Genio, Milan, 1804.

Barron, J. N., and Emmett, A. J. J.: Subcutaneous pedicle flaps. Br. J. Plast. Surg., 18:51, 1965.

Barron, J. N., Veall, N., and Arnott, D. G.: The measurement of the local clearance of radioactive sodium in tubed skin pedicles. Br. J. Plast. Surg., 4:16, 1952.

Batchelor, J. R., and Hackett, M.: HL-A matching in treatment of burned patients with skin allografts. Lancet, 2:581, 1970.

Bellman, S., and Velander, E.: Vascular reaction following experimental transplantation of free full thickness skin grafts. Trans. Internatl. Soc. Plast. Surg., First Congress. Stockholm and Upsala, 1955. Baltimore, The Williams & Wilkins Company, 1957, p. 493.

Bellman, S., Velander, E., Frank, H. A., and Lambert, P. B.: Survival of arteries in experimental full thickness skin autografts. Transplantation, 2:167, 1964.

Ben-Hur, N., Solowey, A. C., and Rapaport, F. T.: The xenograft rejection phenomenon. I. Response of the mouse to rabbit, guinea pig and rat skin xenografts. Israel J. Med. Sci., 5:1, 1969a.

Ben-Hur, N., Solowey, A. C., and Rapaport, F. T.: The xenograft rejection phenomenon. II. Response of the guinea pig to mouse, rat and rabbit xenografts. Israel J. Med. Sci., 5:322, 1969b.

Berggren, R. B., and Lehr, H. B.: Clinical use of viable frozen human skin. J.A.M.A., 194:129, 1965.

Bert, B.: Expériences de greffe animale. C. R. Soc. Biol., 1:172, 1865.

Birch, J., and Brånemark, P.-I.: The vascularization of a free full thickness skin graft. I. A vital microscopic study. Scand. J. Plast. Reconstr. Surg., 3:1, 1969.

Birch, J., Brånemark, P.-I., and Lundskog, J.: The vascularization of a free full thickness skin graft. II. A microangiographic study. Scand. J. Plast. Reconstr. Surg., 3:11, 1969.

Birch, J., Brånemark, P.-I., and Nilsson, K.: The vascularization of a free full thickness skin graft. III. An infrared thermographic study. Scand. J. Plast. Reconstr. Surg., 3:1969.

Blair, V. P.: Surgery and Diseases of the Mouth and Jaws. St. Louis, Mo., C. V. Mosby Company, 1912.

Blair, V. P., and Brown, J. B.: Use and uses of large split skin grafts of intermediate thickness. Surg. Gynecol. Obstet., 49:82, 1929.

Bloomenstein, R. B.: Viability prediction in pedicle flaps by infrared thermometry. Plast. Reconstr. Surg., 42:252, 1968.

Bloomenstein, R. B.: Follow-up clinic. Plast. Reconstr. Surg., 52:185, 1973.

Bondoc, C. C., and Burke, J. F.: Clinical experience with viable frozen human skin and a frozen skin bank. Ann. Surg., *174*:371, 1971.

Braithwaite, F.: Preliminary observations on the vascular channels in tube pedicles. Br. J. Plast. Surg., *3*:40, 1950.

Brånemark, P.-I., and Lindström, J.: A modified rabbit's ear chamber, high power, high-resolution studies in regenerating and preformed tissues. Anat. Rec., *145*:533, 1963.

Braun, W.: Klinisch-histologische Untersuchungen über die Anheilung ungestielter Hautlappen. Beitr. Klin. Chir., *25*:238, 1899.

Braun-Falco, O.: The Pathology of Blister Formation (1969 Year Book of Dermatology). Kopf, A. W., and Andrade, R. (Eds.), Chicago, Year Book Medical Publishers, 1969.

Bromberg, B. E., Song, I. C., and Mohn, M. P.: The use of pig skin as a temporary biological dressing. Plast. Reconstr. Surg., *36*:80, 1965.

Brown, J. B., and McDowell, F.: Skin Grafting. 3rd Ed. Philadelphia, J. B. Lippincott Company, 1958.

Brown, J. B., Fryer, M. P., Randall, P., and Lu, M.: Post-mortem homografts as "biological dressings" for extensive burns and denuded areas. Immediate and preserved homografts as life-saving procedures. Ann. Surg., *138*:618, 1953.

Bünger, C.: Gelungener Versuch einer Nasenbildung aus einem vollig getrennten Hsutstuck aus dem Beine. J. Chir. Augenh., *4*:569, 1823.

Burleson, R., and Eiseman, B.: Nature of the bond between partial-thickness skin and wound granulations. Surgery, *72*:315, 1972.

Burleson, R., and Eiseman, B.: Mechanisms of antibacterial effect of biologic dressings. Ann. Surg., *177*:181, 1973.

Burns Unit, First Affiliated Hospital of Number 245 Unit, Chinese PLA: A review of the management of extensive third degree burns in 14 successive years. Chinese Med. J., *11*:148, 1973.

Bürow, A.: Zur Blepharoplastik. Monatsschr. Med. Augenh. Chir., *1*:57, 1838.

Butcher, H. R., and Hoover, A. L.: Abnormalities of human superficial cutaneous lymphatics associated with stasis ulcers, lympho-edema, scars and cutaneous autografts. Ann. Surg., *142*:633, 1955.

Casson, P. R., Solowey, A. C., Converse, J. M., and Rappaport, F. T.: Delayed hypersensitivity status of burned patients. Surg. Forum, *17*:268, 1966.

Castermans, A.: Vascularization of skin grafts. Transplant. Bull., *4*:154, 1957.

Castroviejo, R.: Plastic and reconstructive surgery of the conjunctiva. Plast. Reconstr. Surg., *24*:1, 1959.

Ceppellini, R., Curtoni, E. S., Mattiuz, P. L., Leigheb, G., Visetti, M., and Colombi, A.: Survival of test skin grafts in man: Effect of genetic relationship and of blood groups incompatibility. Ann. N.Y. Acad. Sci., *129*:421, 1966.

Champion, W. M., McSherry, C. K., and Goulian, D.: Effect of hyperbaric oxygen on the survival of pedicle skin flaps. J. Surg. Res., *7*:583, 1967.

Clemmesen, T.: The early circulation in split skin grafts. Acta Chir. Scand., *124*:11, 1962.

Clemmesen, T.: The early circulation in split skin grafts. Restoration of blood supply to split skin autografts. Acta Chir. Scand., *127*:1, 1964.

Colson, P., Leclercq, P., Gangolphe, M., Houot, R., Janvier, H., and Prunieras, M.: Utilisation des homogreffes alternées avec des autogreffes dans le traitement des grands brulés. II. Étude histo-biologique. Ann. Chir. Plast., *4*:177, 1959.

Conley, J.: Use of composite flaps containing bone for major repairs in the head and neck. Plast. Reconstr. Surg., *49*:522, 1972.

Conley, J., Cinelli, P. B., Johnson, P. M., and Koss, M.: Investigation of bone changes in composite flaps after transfer to the head and neck region. Plast. Reconstr. Surg., *51*:658, 1973.

Converse, J. M.: New forehead flap for nasal reconstruction. Proc. R. Soc. Med., *35*:811, 1942.

Converse, J. M.: Transplantation of skin—overgrafting. *In* Reconstructive Plastic Surgery. Philadelphia, W. B. Saunders Company, 1964, p. 39.

Converse, J. M.: Burn deformities of the face and neck. The 1–2 advancement flap. Surg. Clin. North Am., *47*:345, 1967.

Converse, J. M., and Ballantyne, D. L., Jr.: Distribution of diphosphopyridine nucleotide diaphorase in rat skin autografts and homografts. Plast. Reconstr. Surg., *30*:415, 1962.

Converse, J. M., and Rapaport, F. T.: The vascularization of skin autografts and homografts; an experimental study in man. Ann. Surg., *143*:306, 1956.

Converse, J. M., and Robb-Smith, A. H. T.: The healing of surface cutaneous wounds; its analogy with the healing of superficial burns. Ann. Surg., *120*:873, 1944.

Converse, J. M., and Wood-Smith, D.: Experiences with the forehead island flap with a subcutaneous pedicle. Plast. Reconstr. Surg., *31*:521, 1963.

Converse, J. M., Ballantyne, D. L., Rogers, B. O., and Raisbeck, A. P.: Plasmatic circulation of skin grafts. Transplant. Bull., *4*:154, 1957.

Converse, J. M., Ballantyne, D. L., Jr., Rogers, B. O., and Raisbeck, A. P.: A study of viable and non-viable skin grafts transplanted to the chorio-allantoic membrane of the chick embryo. Transplant. Bull., *5*:108, 1958.

Converse, J. M., Filler, M., and Ballantyne, D. L., Jr.: Vascularization of split-thickness skin autografts in the rat. Transplantation, *3*:22, 1965.

Converse, J. M., Šmahel, J., Ballantyne, D. L., Jr., and Harper, A. D.: Inosculation of vessels of skin graft and host bed: A fortuitous encounter. Br. J. Plast. Surg., *28*:282, 1975.

Converse, J. M., Uhlschmid, G. K., and Ballantyne, D. L., Jr.: "Plasmatic circulation" in skin grafts. The phase of serum imbibition. Plast. Reconstr. Surg., *43*:495, 1969.

Conway, H.: Arteriosclerosis, age and the transplantation of tissue. Plast. Reconstr. Surg., *26*:558, 1960.

Conway, H., Stark, R. B., and Joslin, D.: Cutaneous histamine reaction as a test of circulatory efficiency of tubed pedicles and flaps. Surg. Gynecol. Obstet., *93*:185, 1951.

Conway, H., Joslin, D., Rees, T. D., and Stark, R. B.: III. Morphologic changes observed in homologous skin grafts. Plast. Reconstr. Surg., *9*:557, 1952.

Conway, H., Sedar, J. D., and Shannon, J. E.: Re-evaluation of the transplant chamber techniques in the study of the circulation in autografts and homografts of skin. Transplant. Bull., *4*:62, 1957.

Conway, H., Griffith, H., Shannon, J. E., Jr., and Findley, A.: Re-examination of the transparent chamber technique as applied to the study of circulation in autografts and homografts of the skin. Plast. Reconstr. Surg., *20*:103, 1957.

Corso, P. F.: Variations of the arterial, venous and capillary circulation of the soft tissue of the head by decades as demonstrated by the methyl methacrylate injection technique, and their application to the construction of flaps and pedicles. Plast. Reconstr. Surg., *27*:160, 1961.

Daniel, R. K., and Taylor, G. I.: Distant transfer of an island flap by microvascular anastomosis. A clinical technique. Plast. Reconstr. Surg., 52:111, 1973.

Daniel, R. K., and Williams, H. B.: The free transfer of skin flaps by microvascular anastomosis. An experimental study and a reappraisal. Plast. Reconstr. Surg., 52:16, 1973.

Davis, J. S., and Kitlowski, E. A.: The immediate contraction of cutaneous grafts and its course. Arch. Surg., 23:954, 1931.

Davis, J. S., and Kitlowski, E. A.: Regeneration of nerves in skin grafts and skin flaps. Am. J. Surg., 24:501, 1934.

Davis, J. S., and Traut, H. F.: Origin and development of the blood supply of whole-thickness skin grafts. Ann. Surg., 82:871, 1925.

Davis, L.: The return of sensation to transplanted skin. Surg. Gynecol. Obstet., 59:533, 1934.

DeHaan, C. R., and Stark, R. B.: Changes in efferent circulation of tubed pedicles and in the transplantability of large composite grafts produced by histamine iontophoresis. Plast. Reconstr. Surg., 28:577, 1961.

Derganc, M., and Zdravic, F.: Venous congestion of flaps treated by application of leeches. Br. J. Plast. Surg., 13:187, 1960.

Dieffenbach, J. F.: Die operative Chirurgie. Leipzig, F. A. Brockhaus, 1845–1848.

Douglas, B.: The treatment of burns and other extensive wounds with special emphasis on the transplanted jacket system. Surgery, 15:96, 1944.

Doupe, J., and Sharp, M. E.: Studies in denervation: sebaceous secretion. J. Neurol. Psychiatr., 6:133, 1943.

Dunham, T.: A method for obtaining a skin flap from the scalp and a permanent buried vascular pedicle for covering defects of the face. Ann. Surg., 17:677, 1893.

Eade, G.: Personal communication, 1969.

Edgerton, M. T., and Edgerton, P. J.: Vascularization of homografts. Transplant. Bull., 2:98, 1955.

Egdahl, R. H., Good, R. A., and Varco, R. L.: Studies in homograft and heterograft survival. Surgery, 42:228, 1957.

Egdahl, R. H., Varco, R. L., and Good, R. A.: Local reactions and lymph node response to skin heterografts between rabbits and rats. Int. Arch. Allergy Appl. Immunol., 13:129, 1958.

Elliott, R. A., and Hoehn, J. G.: Use of commercial porcine skin for wound dressings. Plast. Reconstr. Surg., 52:401, 1973.

Enderlen: Histologische Untersuchungen über die Einheilung von Pfroplungen nach Thiersch und Drause. Dtsch. Z. Chir., 14:453, 1897.

Eriksson, G.: Studies in Regeneration and Autotransplantation of Epidermis in Man. Uppsala, Almqvist and Wiksell, 1972.

Esser, J. F. S.: Studies in plastic surgery of the face. Ann. Surg., 65:297, 1917.

Feller, I., and DeWeese, M. S.: The use of stored cutaneous autografts in wound treatment. Surgery, 44:540, 1958.

Filatov, V. P.: Plastic procedure using a round pedicle (in Russian). Vestn. Oftal., 34:149, 1917.

Finochietto, E.: Presentacion de instrumentos. Prensa Méd. argent., 6:256, 1920.

Fitzgerald, M. S. T., Martin, F., and Paletta, F. X.: Innervation of skin grafts. Surg. Gynecol. Obstet., 124:808, 1967.

Flemming, W.: Zur Kenntniss der Regeneration der Epidermis bein Säugethier. Arch. Mikr. Anat., 23:148, 1884.

Folkerts, J. F., Sneep, A. J., and Meijling, H. A.: A comparative investigation on the return of sensations to skin

grafts. In Biemond, A. (Ed.): Recent Neurological Research. Amsterdam, Elsevier Publishing Company, 1959.

Freshwater, M. F., and Krizek, T. S.: Liquid crystallometry: A new technique for predicting the viability of pedicle flaps. Surg. Forum, 21:497, 1970.

Frey, M., von: Beiträge zur Sinnesphysiologie der Haut. Ber. d. Verhand. d. k. Sachs. Gesellsch d. Wissensch., 47:166, 1895.

Fujino, T.: Contribution of the axial and peforator vasculature to circulation in flaps. Plast. Reconstr. Surg., 39:125, 1967.

Ganzer, H.: Weichteilplastik des Gesichts bei Kieferschusverletzungen. Dtsch. Monatsschr. Zahnheilkd., 35:348, 1917.

Garré, C.: Über die histologischen Vorgänge bei der Auheilung der Thiersch'schen Granulationen. Beitr. Klin. Chir., 4:625, 1889.

Georgiade, N., Peschel, E., Georgiade, R., and Brown, I.: A clinical and experimental investigation of the preservation of skin. Plast. Reconstr. Surg., 17:267, 1956.

German, W., Finesilver, E. M., and Davis, J. S.: Establishment of circulation in tubed skin flaps. Arch. Surg., 26:27, 1933.

Gersuny, R.: Kleinere mittheilung. Plastischer Ersatz der Wangen-Schleimhaut. Zentralbl. Chir., 14:706, 1887.

Gibson, T., and Medawar, P. B.: The fate of skin homografts in man. J. Anat., 77:299, 1942.

Gillies, H. D.: The tubed pedicle in plastic surgery. N.Y. Med. J., 111:1, 1920.

Gillies, H. D.: Design of direct pedicle flaps. Br. Med. J., 2:1008, 1932.

Gillies, H. D., and Millard, D. R., Jr.: Principles and Arts of Plastic Surgery. Boston, Little, Brown & Co., 1957.

Gillman, T., Penn, J., Bronks, D., and Roux, M.: A reexamination of certain aspects of the histogenesis of the healing of cutaneous wounds: A preliminary report. Br. J. Surg., 43:141, 1955.

Glanz, S.: "Brick Laying" Technique in Hair Strip Transplantation for Baldness, A New Method. Presented at the American Society of Plastic and Reconstructive Surgeons, October 2, 1968, New Orleans, Louisiana.

Glinz, W., and Clodius, L.: Measurement of tissue pH for predicting viability in pedicle flaps: Experimental studies in pigs. Br. J. Plast. Surg., 25:111, 1972.

Goldmann, E. E.: Die künstliche Überhautung offener Krebse durch Haut-transplantationen nach Thiersch. Zentralbl. Allg. Pathol., 1:505, 1890.

Goldwyn, R. M., Lamb, D. L., and White, W. L.: An experimental study of large island flaps in dogs. Plast. Reconstr. Surg., 31:528, 1963.

Goode, R. L., and Linehan, J. W.: The fluorescein test in post irradiation surgery. A preliminary report. Arch. Otolaryng., 91:526, 1970.

Goodpasture, E. W., Douglas, B., and Anderson, K.: A study of human skin grafted upon the chorio-allantois of chick embryos. J. Exp. Med., 68:891, 1938.

Guthrie, R. H., Goulian, D., and Cucin, R. L.: Predicting the extent of viability in flaps by measurement of gas tensions, using a mass spectrometer. Plast. Reconstr. Surg., 50:385, 1972.

Guttmann, L.: Zur Frage der Widerherstellung der Schweissdrusen function in Hauttransplantaten. Dermatol. Z., 77:73, 1938.

Guttmann, L.: Management of quinizarin sweat test. Postgrad. Med. J., 23:353, 1947.

Haller, J. A., and Billingham, R. E.: Studies of the origin of the vasculature in free skin grafts. Ann. Surg., 166:896, 1967.

Ham, A. W.: Some histophysiological problems peculiar to calcified tissues. J. Bone Joint Surg., *34A*:701, 1952.

Hamilton, J. B.: Patterned loss of hair in man; types and incidence. Ann. N.Y. Acad. Sci., *53*:708, 1951.

Harii, K., Ohmori, K., and Ohmori, S.: Successful clinical transfer of ten free flaps by microvascular anastomoses. Plast. Reconstr. Surg., *53*:259, 1974.

Harii, K., Ohmori, K., and Sekiguchi, J.: The free musculo-cutaneous flap. Plast. Reconstr. Surg., *57*:294, 1976.

Hauser, W. H., Tauxe, W. N., Owen, C. A., and Lipscomb, P. R.: Determination of the vascular status of pedicle skin grafts by radioactive tracer studies. Surg. Gynecol. Obstet., *112*:625, 1961.

Hayes, J. E., Robinson, D. W., Schloerb, P. R., and Masters, F. W.: A simple method of testing the circulation of pedicle flaps. Surg. Forum, *18*:516, 1967.

Henle, A.: Klinische und experimentelle Beiträge zur Lehre von der transplantation ungestielter Hautlappen. II. Experomenteller Teil. Beitr. Klin. Chir., *24*:615, 1899.

Henry, L., Marshall, D. C., Friedman, E. A., Goldstein, D. P., and Dammin, G. J.: A histologic study of the human skin autograft. Am. J. Pathol., *39*:317, 1961.

Henry, L., Marshall, D. C., Friedman, E. A., Dammin, G. J., and Merrill, J. P.: The rejection of skin homografts in the normal human subject. Part II. Histological findings. J. Clin. Invest., *41*:420, 1962.

Hildemann, W. H., and Haas, R.: Comparative studies of homotransplantation in fishes. J. Cell. Comp. Physiol., *55*:227, 1960.

Hoehn, F., and Binkert, B.: Cholesterol liquid crystals: A new visual aid to study flap circulation. Surg. Forum, *21*:499, 1970.

Hoffmeister, F. S.: Studies on timing of tissue transfer in reconstructive surgery. Plast. Reconstr. Surg., *19*:283, 1957.

Hübscher, C.: Beitrage zur Hautverpflanzung nach Thiersch. Beitr. Klin. Chir., *4*:395, 1888.

Hugo, N. E.: Vascular anastomoses vs. circulation across the junction, after transfer of a pedicle. Plast. Reconstr. Surg., *50*:216, 1972.

Hutchison, J., Tough, J. S., and Wyburn, G. M.: Regeneration of sensation in grafted skin. Br. J. Plast. Surg., *2*:82, 1949.

Hynes, W.: A simple method of estimating blood flow with special references to the circulation in pedicled skin flaps and tubes. Br. J. Plast. Surg., *1*:159, 1948.

Hynes, W.: The blood vessels in skin tubes and flaps. Br. J. Plast. Surg., *3*:165, 1950.

Hynes, W.: The "blue flap": A method of treatment. Br. J. Plast. Surg., *4*:166, 1951.

Hynes, W.: The early circulation in skin grafts with a consideration of methods to encourage their survival. Br. J. Plast. Surg., *6*:257, 1954.

Hynes, W.: The treatment of pigmented moles by shaving and skin graft. Br. J. Plast. Surg., *9*:47, 1956.

Hynes, W.: The treatment of scars by shaving and skin graft. Br. J. Plast. Surg., *10*:1, 1957.

Hynes, W.: "Shaving" in plastic surgery with special reference to the treatment of chronic radiodermatitis. Br. J. Plast. Surg., *12*:43, 1959.

Imre, J.: Lidplastik, und Plastische Operationen und anderer Weichteile des Gesichts. Budapest, Stadium Verlag, 1928.

Jackson, D.: A clinical study of the use of skin homografts for burns. Br. J. Plast. Surg., *7*:26, 1954.

Jungengel, M.: Die Hauttransplantation nach Thiersch. Verhandlungen der physikalischer medicinischen. Gesellschaft zu Wurzburg, *25*:87, 1891.

Juri, J.: Use of parieto-occipital flaps in the surgical treatment of baldness. Plast. Reconstr. Surg., *55*:456, 1975.

Kamrin, B. B.: Studies on the healing of successful skin homografts in albino rats. Ann. N.Y. Acad. Sci., *87*:323, 1960.

Kamrin, B. B.: Analysis of the union between host and graft in the albino rat. Plast. Reconstr. Surg., *28*:221, 1961.

Kazanjian, V. H.: The repair of nasal defects with the median forehead flap: Primary closure of the forehead wound. Surg. Gynecol. Obstet., *83*:37, 1946.

Kernahan, D. A., Zingg, W., and Kay, C. W.: The effect of hyperbaric oxygen on the survival of the experimental skin flaps. Plast. Reconstr. Surg., *36*:19, 1965.

Kernwein, G. A.: Recovery of sensation in split-thickness skin grafts. Arch. Surg., *56*:459, 1948.

Ketchum, L. D., Ellis, S. S., Robinson, D. W., and Masters, F. W.: Vascular augmentation of pedicled tissue by combined histamine iontophoresis and hypertensive perfusion. Plast. Reconstr. Surg., *39*:138, 1967.

Ketchum, L. D., Masters, F. W., and Robinson, D. W.: Mandibular reconstruction using a composite island rib flap. Plast. Reconstr. Surg., *53*:471, 1974.

Kiehn, C. L., and Desprez, J. D.: Effects of local hypothermia on pedicle flap tissue. I. Enhancement of survival of experimental pedicles. Plast. Reconstr. Surg., *25*:349, 1960.

Kekuchi, I., and Omori, M.: Demonstration of leaking vessels under skin grafts. Plast. Reconstr. Surg., *45*:66, 1970.

Kiyono, K., and Sueyasu, Y.: The experimental study in avian embryo after inoculation of tissues from various animals. I. Further classification of species for inoculation. Kyoto Igakkai Zasshi, *14*:68, 1917.

Klingenström, P., and Nylén, B.: Timing of transfer of tubed pedicles and cross-flaps. Plast. Reconstr. Surg., *37*:1, 1966.

Koehnlein, H. E., and Lemperle, G.: Experimental studies on the effect of dimethyl sulfoxide on pedicle flaps. Surgery, *67*:672, 1970.

Krause, F.: Über die transplantation grosser, ungestielter Hautlappen. Verh. Dtsch. Ges. Chir., *26*:46, 1893.

Kredel, F. E., and Evans, J. P.: Recovery of sensation in denervated pedicle and free skin grafts. Arch. Neurol. Psychiatr., *29*:1203, 1933.

Kredel, F. E., and Phemister, D. B.: Recovery of sympathetic nerve function in transplants. Arch. Neurol. Psychiatr., *42*:403, 1939.

Krizek, T. J., Tasaburo, T., Desprez, J. D., and Kiehn, C.: Experimental transplantation of composite grafts by microsurgical vascular anastomoses. Plast. Reconstr. Surg., *36*:538, 1965.

Lange, K., and Boyd, L. J.: Use of fluorescein to determine adequacy of circulation. Med. Clin. North Am., *26*:943, 1942.

Lawrence, J. C.: Storage and skin metabolism. Br. J. Plast. Surg., *25*:440, 1972.

Lawson, G.: On the successful transplantation of portions of skin for the closure of large granulating surfaces. Lancet, *2*:708, 1870.

Le Fort, L.: Blépharoplastie par un lambeau complètement détaché du bras et reporté à la face. Insuccès. Bull. Soc. Chir. Paris, *1*:39, 1872.

Lewis, T.: The Blood Vessels of the Human Skin and Their Responses. London, Shaw & Sons, Ltd., 1927.

Limberg, A. A.: Matematicheskie Osnovuy Mestnoy Plastiki Na Poverchnosti Chelovecheskogo Tela. Medgiz, 1946.

Littler, J. W.: Neurovascular skin island transfer in reconstructive hand surgery. Trans. Internatl. Soc. Plast. Surg., 2:175, 1960.

Ljungqvist, A., and Almgård, L. E.: The vascular reaction in the free skin allo- and autografts. A stereomicroangiographic and histological study in the rabbit. Acta Pathol. Microbiol. Scand., 68:553, 1966.

Loeb, L., and Addison, W. H. F.: Beitrage zur Analyse des Gewbewachstums. II. Transplantation zur Haut des Meerschweinschens in Tiere verschiedener Species. Arch. Entwickl.-Mech. Org., 27:73, 1909.

Loeb, L., and Addison, W. H. F.: Beitrage zur Analyse des Gewebewachstums. V. Über die Transplantation der Tauberhaut in die Taube und in andere Tierarten. Arch. Entwickl.-Mech. Org., 32:44, 1911.

Löfgren, L.: Recovery of nervous function in skin transplants with special reference to the sympathetic functions. Acta Chir. Scand., 102:229, 1952.

Lombard, W. P.: The blood pressure in the arterioles and small veins of the human skin. Am. J. Physiol., 29:335, 1911–1912.

Lopez-Mas, J., Ortiz-Monasterio, F., Viale de Gonzalez, M., and Olmedo, A.: Skin graft pigmentation. A new approach to prevention. Plast. Reconstr. Surg., 49:18, 1972.

Majno, G., Gabbiani, G., Hirschel, B. J., Ryan, G. B., and Stratkov, P. R.: Contraction of granulation tissue in vitro: Similarity to smooth muscle. Science, 173:548, 1971.

Manchot, C.: Die Hautarterien des menschlichen Corters. Leipzig, 1889.

Maquieira, N. O.: An innervated full-thickness skin graft to restore sensibility to fingertips and heels. Plast. Reconstr. Surg., 53:568, 1974.

Marckmann, A.: Autologous skin grafts in the rat. Uptake of ³⁵S-sulfate. Proc. Exp. Biol. Med., 119:557, 1965a.

Marckmann, A.: Autologous skin grafts in the rat. Biochemical analysis of mucopolysaccharides and hydroxyproline. Proc. Soc. Exp. Biol. Med., 119:794, 1965b.

Marckmann, A.: Autologous skin grafts in the rat: Vital microscopic studies of the microcirculation. Angiology, 17:475, 1966.

Marckmann, A.: Biology of skin autografts. Dan. Med. Bull., 14:135, 1967.

Marckmann, A., and Zachariae, H.: Histamine in full-thickness skin autografts of rat. Proc. Soc. Exp. Biol. Med., 117:705, 1964.

Marrangoni, A. G.: An experimental study in refrigerated skin grafts stored in 10 per cent homologous serum. Plast. Reconstr. Surg., 6:425, 1950.

McCabe, W. P., Rebuck, J. W., Kelly, A. P., Jr., and Ditmars, S. M., Jr.: Cellular immune response of humans to pigskin. Plast. Reconstr. Surg., 51:181, 1973.

McCraw, J. B., and Furlow, L. T.: The dorsalis pedis arterialized flap. Plast. Reconstr. Surg., 55:177, 1975.

McCraw, J. B., Dibbell, D. G., Horton, C. E., Adamson, J. E., and Carraway, J. H.: Definition of new arterialized myocutaneous vascular territories. Submitted for publication, Plast. Reconstr. Surg. Presented before American Association of Plastic Surgeons, May, 1976.

McFarlane, R. M., Heagy, F. C., Rodin, S., Aust, J. C., and Wermuth, R. G.: A study of the delay phenomenon in experimental pedicle flaps. Plast. Reconstr. Surg., 35:245, 1965.

McGregor, I. A.: The regeneration of sympathetic activity in grafted skin as evidenced by sweating. Br. J. Plast. Surg., 3:12, 1950.

McGregor, I. A.: The vascularization of human skin. Br. J. Plast. Surg., 7:331, 1955a.

McGregor, I. A.: Vascularization of homografts of human skin. Transplant. Bull., 2:11, 1955b.

McGregor, I.A.: The temporal flap in intraoral cancer; its use in repairing the post-excisional defect. Br. J. Plast. Surg., 16:318, 1963.

McGregor, I. A., and Jackson, I. T.: The groin flap. Br. J. Plast. Surg., 25:3, 1972.

McGregor, I. A., and Morgan, G.: Axial and random pattern flaps. Br. J. Plast. Surg., 26:202, 1973.

McLaughlin, C. R.: Composite ear grafts and their blood supply. Br. J. Plast. Surg., 7:274, 1954.

Medawar, P. B.: Sheets of pure epidermal epithelium from human skin. Nature, 148:783, 1941.

Medawar, P. B.: Behavior and fate of skin autografts and skin homografts in rabbits. J. Anat., 78:176, 1944.

Medawar, P. B.: The micro-anatomy of mammalian skin. Quart. J. Microscop. Sci., 94:481, 1953.

Merwin, R. M., and Algire, G. H.: The role of graft and host vessels in the vascularization of normal and neoplastic tissue. J. Natl. Cancer Inst., 17:23, 1956.

Millard, D. R.: The crane principle for the transport of subcutaneous tissue. Plast. Reconstr. Surg., 43:451, 1969.

Miller, T. A.: The deleterious effect of split-skin homograft coverage on split-skin donor sites. Plast. Reconstr. Surg., 53:316, 1974.

Miller, T. A., and White, W. L.: Healing of second degree burns. Comparison of effects of early application of homografts and coverage with tape. Plast. Reconstr. Surg., 49:552, 1972.

Miller, T. A., Switzer, W. E., Foley, F. D., and Moncrief, J. A.: Early homografting of second degree burns. Plast. Reconstr. Surg., 40:117, 1967.

Milton, S. H.: The tubed pedicle flap. Br. J. Plast. Surg., 22:53, 1969a.

Milton, S. H.: The effects of "delay" on the survival of experimental pedicled skin flaps. Br. J. Plast. Surg., 22:244, 1969b.

Milton, S. H.: Pedicled skin flaps: The fallacy of the length-width ratio. Br. J. Surg., 57:502, 1970.

Milton, S. H.: Experimental studies on island flaps. 1. The surviving length. Plast. Reconstr. Surg., 48:574, 1971.

Milton, S. H., and Corbett, J. L.: Failure to increase the survival of experimental flaps by histamine and hypertension. Plast. Reconstr. Surg., 43:235, 1969.

Mir y Mir, L.: Biology of the skin graft. New aspects to consider in its revascularization. Plast. Reconstr. Surg., 8:378, 1951.

Mir y Mir, L.: The problem of pigmentation in the cutaneous graft. Br. J. Plast. Surg., 14:303, 1961.

Moberg, E.: Objective methods for determining the functional value of sensibility in the hand. J. Bone Joint Surg., 40A:454, 1958.

Monks, G. H.: The restoration of a lower eyelid by a new method. Boston Med. Surg. J., 139:385, 1898.

Montagna, W.: Histology and cytochemistry of human skin. X-irradiation of the scalp. Am. J. Anat., 99:415, 1956.

Montagna, W.: The structure and function of skin. 2nd Ed. New York, Academic Press, 1962.

Murphy, J. B.: Transplantability of malignant tumors to the embryos of a foreign species. J.A.M.A., 59:874, 1912.

Murray, J. F., Ord, J. V. R., and Gavelin, G. E.: The neurovascular island pedicle flap. An assessment of late results in 16 cases. J. Bone Joint Surg., 49A:1285, 1967.

Myers, M. B.: Prediction of skin sloughs at the time of operation with the use of fluorescein dye. Surgery, 51:158, 1962.

Myers, M. B., and Cherry, G.: Design of skin flaps to study vascular insufficiency. Failure of dextran 40 to improve tissue survival in devascularized skin. J. Surg. Res., *7*:399, 1967.

Myers, M. B., and Cherry, G.: Enhancement of survival in devascularized pedicles by the use of phenoxybenzamine. Plast. Reconstr. Surg., *41*:254, 1968.

Myers, M. B., and Cherry, G.: Mechanism of the delay phenomenon. Plast. Reconstr. Surg., *44*:52, 1969.

Myers, M. B., and Cherry, G.: Differences in the delay phenomenon in the rabbit, rat and pig. Plast. Reconstr. Surg., *47*:73, 1971.

Myers, M. B., Combs, B., and Cohen, G.: Wound tension and wound sloughs: A negative correlation. Am. J. Surg., *100*:711, 1965.

Myers, M. B., Cherry, G., and Milton, S.: Tissue gas levels as an index of the adequacy of circulation: The relation between ischemia and the development of collateral circulation (delay phenomenon). Surgery, *71*:15, 1972.

Myers, M. B., Cherry, G., and Bombet, R.: On the lack of any effect of gravity on the survival of tubed flaps. An experimental study in rabbits and pigs. Plast. Reconstr. Surg., *51*:428, 1973.

Napier, J. R.: The return of pain sensibility in full thickness skin grafts. Brain, *75*:147, 1952.

O'Brien, B.: A muscle-skin pedicle for total reconstruction of the lower lip. Plast. Reconstr. Surg., *45*:395, 1970.

O'Brien, B., MacLeod, A. M., Hayhurst, J. W., and Morrison, W. A.: Successful transfer of a large island flap from the groin to the foot by microvascular anastomoses. Plast. Reconstr. Surg., *52*:271, 1973.

O'Brien, B., Morrison, W. A., Ishida, H., MacLeod, A. M., and Gilbert, A.: Free flap transfers with microvascular anastomoses. Br. J. Plast. Surg., *27*:220, 1974.

O'Donoghue, M. N., and Zarem, H. A.: Stimulation of neovascularization—Comparative efficacy of fresh and preserved skin grafts. Plast. Reconstr. Surg., *48*:474, 1971.

Ohmori, S., and Kurata, K.: Experimental studies on the blood supply to various types of skin grafts in rabbits using isotope P³². Plast. Reconstr. Surg., *25*:547, 1960.

Ollier, L.: Greffes cutanées ou autoplastiques. Bull. Acad. Med., *1*:243, 1872.

Orentreich, N.: Autografts in alopecias and other selected dermatological conditions. Ann. N.Y. Acad. Sci., *83*:463, 1959.

Orticochea, M.: The musculo-cutaneous flap method. Br. J. Plast. Surg., *25*:106, 1972.

Owens, N.: A compound neck pedicle designed for the repair of massive facial defects. Plast. Reconstr. Surg., *15*:369, 1955.

Padgett, E. C.: Calibrated intermediate skin grafts. Surg. Gynecol. Obstet., *69*:799, 1939.

Pandya, N. J., and Zarem, H. A.: The absence of vascularization in porcine skin grafts on mice. Plast. Reconstr. Surg., *53*:211, 1974.

Patterson, T. J. S.: The survival of skin flaps in the pig. Br. J. Plast. Surg., *21*:113, 1968.

Peer, L. A., and Paddock, R.: Histologic studies on fate of deeply implanted dermal grafts. Arch. Surg., *34*:268, 1937.

Peer, L. A., and Walker, J. C.: The behavior of autogenous human tissue grafts; comparative study. Plast. Reconstr. Surg., *7*:73, 1951.

Penn, J.: Zigzag modification of tubed-pedicle flap. Br. J. Plast. Surg., *1*:110, 1948.

Perry, V. P.: A review of skin preservation. Cryobiology, *3*:109, 1966.

Peskova, H.: Tubed flap according to Filatov (title translated from the Czech.). Prague, 1955.

Pihl, B., and Weiber, A.: Studies of the vascularization of free full-thickness skin grafts with radio-isotope technique. Acta Chir. Scand., *125*:19, 1963.

Polk, H. C.: Adherence of thin skin grafts. Surg. Forum, *17*:487, 1966.

Pontén, B.: Grafted skin: Observations on innervation and other qualities. Acta Chir. Scand., Suppl. 257, 1960.

Psillakis, J. M., deJorge, F. B., Villardo, R., Albano, A. M., Martins, M., and Spina, V.: Water and electrolyte changes in autogenous skin grafts. Discussion of the so-called "plasmatic circulation." Plast. Reconstr. Surg., *43*:500, 1969.

Ragnell, A.: The secondary contracting tendency of free skin grafts. An experimental investigation on animals. Br. J. Plast. Surg., *5*:6, 1952.

Rapaport, F. T., Converse, J. M., Horn, L., Ballantyne, D. L., and Mulholland, J. H.: Altered reactivity to skin homografts in severe thermal injury. Ann. Surg., *159*:390, 1964.

Rees, T. D., and Casson, P. R.: The indications for cutaneous dermal overgrafting. Plast. Reconstr. Surg., *38*:522, 1966.

Rees, T. D., Ballantyne, D. L., Jr., Hawthorne, G. A., and Nathan, A.: Effects of Silastic sheet implants under simultaneous skin autografts in rats. Plast. Reconstr. Surg., *42*:339, 1968.

Reese, J. D.: Dermatape: a new method for management of split skin grafts. Plast. Reconstr. Surg., *1*:98, 1946.

Reinisch, J. F.: The pathophysiology of skin flap circulation. The delay phenomenon. Plast. Reconstr. Surg., *54*:585, 1974.

Réverdin, J. L.: De la Greffe épidermique. Arch. Gén. Méd., *19*:276, 555, 703, 1872.

Ribbert, H.: Über Transplantation auf Individuen anderer Gattung. Verh. Dtsch. Ges. Pathol., *8*:104, 1905.

Rogers, B. O., and Converse, J. M.: Bovine embryo skin zoografts as temporary biologic dressings for burns and other skin defects. Plast. Reconstr. Surg., *22*:471, 1958.

Rolle, G. K., Taylor, A. C., and Charipper, H. A.: A study of vascular changes in skin grafts in mice and their relationship to homograft breakdown. J. Cell Comp. Physiol., *53*:215, 1959.

Russell, P. S., and Monaco, A. P.: The biology of tissue transplantation. Boston, Little, Brown and Company, 1965.

Salisbury, R. E., Wilmore, D. W., Silverstein, P., and Pruitt, B. A.: Biologic dressings for skin graft donor sites. Arch. Surg., *106*:705, 1973.

Santoni-Rugiu, P.: Compared studies in the viability of skin stored by different methods. Plast. Reconstr. Surg., *30*:586, 1962.

Santoni-Rugiu, P.: An experimental study on the reinnervation of free skin grafts and pedicle flaps. Plast. Reconstr. Surg., *38*:98, 1966.

Sawhney, C. P., Subbaraju, G. V., and Chakravarti, R. N.: Healing of donor sites of split skin graft. Br. J. Plast. Surg., *22*:359, 1969.

Schuchardt, K.: Der Rundstiellappen in der Wiederherstellungs-chirurgie des Gesichtskieferbereiches, Leipzig, Georg Thieme Verlag, 1944.

Scothorne, R. J., and McGregor, I. A.: The vascularization of autografts and homografts of rabbit skin. J. Anat., *87*:379, 1953.

Scothorne, R. J., and Scothorne, A. W.: Histochemical studies on human skin autografts. J. Anat., *87*:22, 1953.

Scothorne, R. J., and Tough, J. S.: Histochemical studies of human skin autografts and homografts. Br. J. Plast. Surg., *5*:161, 1952.

Segarra, J. A., and Bennett, J. E.: Distal necrosis of dorsal pedicle flaps in the rat: Immediate versus delayed terminal inset. Surg. Forum, *23*:520, 1972.

Serafini, G.: Treatment of burn scars of the face by dermabrasion and skin grafts. Br. J. Plast. Surg., *15*:308, 1962.

Shaw, D. T., and Payne, R. L.: One stage tubed abdominal flaps. Surg. Gynecol. Obstet., *83*:205, 1946.

Shepard, G. H.: The storage of split-skin grafts on their donor sites. Clinical and experimental study. Plast. Reconstr. Surg., *49*:115, 1972.

Silverstein, P.: American Burn Association Conference. San Antonio, Texas, 1971.

Silverstein, P., Raulston, G. L., Walker, H., Foley, F. D., and Pruitt, B. A.: Evaluation of formalin-fixed skin as a temporary dressing for granulating wounds. Surg. Forum, *22*:60, 1971.

Sinclair, D. C., Weddell, G., and Zander, E.: The relationship of cutaneous sensibility to neurohistology in the human pinna. J. Anat., *86*:402, 1952.

Šmahel, J.: Revascularization of a free skin autograft. Acta Chir. Plast., *4*:102, 1962.

Šmahel, J.: The revascularization of a free skin autograft. Acta Chir. Plast., *9*:76, 1967.

Šmahel, J.: Paper read at the European Congress of Plastic and Reconstructive Surgery. Bristol, England, 1969.

Šmahel, J., and Clodius, L.: The blood vessel system of free human skin grafts. Plast. Reconstr. Surg., *47*:61, 1971.

Šmahel, J., and Ganzoni, N.: Contribution to the origin of the vasculature in free skin autografts. Br. J. Plast. Surg., *23*:322, 1970.

Šmahel, J., and Ganzoni, N.: Experiments with mesh grafts. Acta Chir. Plast., *14*:90, 1972.

Smith, J. W., Ringland, J., and Wilson, R.: Vascularization of skin grafts. Surg. Forum, *15*:473, 1964.

Smith, P. J.: The vascular basis of axial pattern flaps. Br. J. Plast. Surg., *26*:150, 1973.

Smith, P. J., Foley, B., McGregor, I. A., and Jackson, L. A.: The anatomical basis of the groin flap. Plast. Reconstr. Surg., *49*:41, 1972.

Snyder, C. C., Bateman, J. M., Davis, C. W., and Warren, G. D.: Mandibulofacial restoration with live osteocutaneous flaps. Plast. Reconstr. Surg., *45*:14, 1970.

Stern, W. G., and Cohen, M. B.: The intracutaneous salt solution wheal test. J.A.M.A., *87*:1355, 1926.

Stewart, M. J.: On the occurrence of irritation giant cells in dermoid and epidermoid cysts. J. Pathol. Bacteriol., *17*:502, 1912.

Storey, W. F., and LeBlond, C. P.: Measurement of rate of proliferation of epidermis and associated structures. Ann. N.Y. Acad. Sci., *53*:537, 1951.

Strauch, B., and Murray, D. E.: Transfer of composite graft with immediate suture. Anastomosis of its vascular pedicle measuring less than 1 mm. in external diameter using microsurgical technique. Plast. Reconstr. Surg., *40*:325, 1967.

Sturman, M. J., and Duran, R. J.: Late results in finger-tip injuries. J. Bone Joint Surg., *45A*:289, 1963.

Sugarbaker, P. H., Sabath, L. D., and Morgan, A. P.: Neomycin toxicity from porcine skin xenografts. Ann. Surg., *179*:183, 1974.

Sweeney, N. V.: Composite grafts of skin and fat. Br. J. Plast. Surg., *26*:72, 1973.

Tanner, J. C., Vandeput, J., and Olley, J. F.: The mesh skin graft. Plast. Reconstr. Surg., *34*:287, 1964.

Tauxe, W. M., Simons, J. N., Lipscomb, P. R., and Hamamoto, K.: Determination of vascular status of pedicle skin flaps by use of radioactive pertechnetate (^{99m}Tc). Surg. Gynecol. Obstet., *130*:87, 1970.

Taylor, A. C., and Lehrfeld, J. W.: Determination of survival time of skin homografts in rats by observation of vascular changes in grafts. Plast. Reconstr. Surg., *12*:423, 1953.

Taylor, A. C., and Lehrfeld, J. W.: Definition of survival time of homografts. Ann. N.Y. Acad. Sci., *59*:351, 1955.

Taylor, A. C., Gerstner, R., and Converse, J. M.: Preservation of skin grafts by refrigeration for reconstructive surgery. Plast. Reconstr. Surg., *18*:275, 1956.

Taylor, G. I., and Daniel, R. K.: The anatomy of several free flap donor sites. Plast. Reconstr. Surg., *56*:243, 1975.

Teich-Alasia, S.: Vascularization of pedicle flaps using disulphine blue. Br. J. Plast. Surg., *24*:282, 1971.

Thiersch, C.: Ueber die feineren anatomischen Veränderungen bei Aufheilung von Haut auf Granulationen. Arch. Klin. Chir., *17*:318, 1874.

Thiersch, C.: Ueber Hautverpflanzung. Verh. Dtsch. Ges. Chir., *15*:17, 1886.

Thompson, N.: A clinical and histological investigation into the fate of epithelial elements buried following the grafting of "shaved" skin surfaces. Br. J. Plast. Surg., *13*:219, 1960.

Thompson, N.: The role of succinic dehydrogenase and sulfhydryl groups during epidermal rejection in skin homografts. A preliminary histochemical study in rats. Transplant. Bull., *30*:113, 1962.

Thompson, N.: Unpublished work, 1970.

Thompson, N., and Ell, P. J.: Dermal overgrafting in the treatment of venous stasis ulcers. Plast. Reconstr. Surg., *54*:290, 1974.

Thorne, F. L., Georgiade, N. G., and Mladick, R.: The use of thermography in determining viability of pedicle flaps. Arch. Surg., *99*:97, 1969.

Thorne, F. L., Georgiade, N. G., Wheeler, W. F., and Mladick, R. A.: Photoplethysmography as an aid in determining the viability of pedicle flaps. Plast. Reconstr. Surg., *44*:279, 1969.

Thorvaldsson, S. E., and Grabb, W. C.: The intravenous fluorescein test as a measure of skin viability. Plast. Reconstr. Surg., *53*:576, 1974.

Toranto, I. R., Salyer, K. E., and Myers, M. B.: Vascularization of porcine skin heterografts. Plast. Reconstr. Surg., *54*:195, 1974.

Trevaskis, A. E., Rempel, J., Okunski, W., and Rea, M.: Sliding subcutaneous pedicle flaps to close a circular defect. Plast. Reconstr. Surg., *46*:155, 1970.

Unna, P. G.: Handbuch der Hautkrankheiten. Leipzig, F. C. W. Vogel, 1883.

Vallis, C.: Surgical treatment of the receding hairline. Plast. Reconstr. Surg., *40*:138, 1967.

Velander, E.: Vascular changes in tubed pedicles: An experimental study. Acta Chir. Scand., Suppl. 322, 1964.

Webster, G. V., Peterson, R. A., and Stein, H. L.: Dermal overgrafting of the leg. J. Bone Joint Surg., *40A*:4, 796, 1958.

Webster, J. P.: Thoraco-epigastric tubed pedicles. Surg. Clin. North Am., *17*:145, 1937.

Weddell, G., Palmer, E., and Pallie, W.: Nerve endings in mammalian skin. Biol. Rev., *30*:159, 1955.

Wexler, M. R., and Oneal, R. M.: Areolar sharing to reconstruct the absent nipple. Plast. Reconstr. Surg., *51*:176, 1973.

Williams, C.: Delaying of flaps. A useful adjunct. Br. J. Plast. Surg., *26*:61, 1973.

Winster, J., Manalo, P. D., and Barsky, A. J.: Studies on the circulation of tubed flaps. Plast. Reconstr. Surg., *28*:619, 1961.

Wolfe, J. R.: A new method for performing plastic operations. Br. Med. J., *2*:360, 1875.

Wolff, K., and Schellander, F. G.: Enzyme-histochemical studies on the healing process of split skin grafts. I.

Aminopeptidase, diphosphopyridine nucleotidediaphorase and succinic dehydrogenase in autografts. J. Invest. Dermatol., *45*:38, 1965.

Wolff, K., and Schellander, F. G.: Enzyme-histochemical studies on the healing process of split skin grafts. II. 5-Nucleotidase, adenosinetriphosphatase, acid and alkaline phosphatase in autografts. J. Invest. Dermatol., *46*:205, 1966.

Woodruff, M. F. A.: The Transplantation of Tissues and Organs. Springfield, Ill., Charles C Thomas, Publisher, 1960.

Woodruff, M. F. A., and Simpson, L. Q.: Experimental skin grafting in rats with special references to split skin grafts. Plast. Reconstr. Surg., *15*:451, 1955.

Zarem, H. A., Zweifach, B. W., and McGehee, J. M.: Development of microcirculation in full thickness autogenous skin grafts in mice. Am. J. Physiol., *212*:1081, 1967.

Zimany, A.: The bi-lobed flap. Plast. Reconstr. Surg., *11*:423, 1953.

CHAPTER 7

TRANSPLANTATION OF DERMIS

NOEL THOMPSON, F.R.C.S.

The dermis graft is a free graft containing all layers of the skin remaining after removal of the epidermis as a thin split-thickness (or Thiersch) graft. It therefore contains the deeper layers of the papillary, and all the reticular layer of the dermis, together with a minimal amount of adherent subcutaneous fat. It includes within it as its only epithelial constituents the epidermal appendages: hair follicles, sebaceous glands, and sweat glands, in their subepidermal extensions.

The advantages of autogenous dermis as a graft are its ready availability, its ease of manipulation, its limited postoperative absorption which does not usually exceed 20 per cent of the bulk of the graft (Fig. 7–1), and its strength, stability, and capacity to survive adverse conditions and heal rapidly. Inserted subcutaneously as a buried graft to correct defective surface contours, it has been described as "the most useful transplant for the correction of nonrigid regions—nose, eyelids, face, lips, and supraorbital region" (Smith, 1950), and "the only tissue with a real clinical merit" in elevating small depressed scars (Padgett and Stephenson, 1948) (Fig. 7–2). The bulk of the graft and the area of dermal contact with host tissues can be doubled by the expedient of folding the graft upon itself. The simplicity of the procedure lends itself to repetition as often as necessary at intervals of six months—by which period almost all absorption that is going to occur has taken place—or even

less, until adequate restoration of contour is obtained. In addition, the future use of other graft material at the same site is not prejudiced inasmuch as the blood supply of the dermal graft is so satisfactory.

Its usefulness in the correction of saddle nose deformities may be considered to illustrate the graft's special virtues. It constitutes a simple method of correcting the minimal deformity when the use of autogenous bone or cartilage may not seem justified (Fig. 7–3). It can safely be used when extensive scarring from chronic infection (see Fig. 7–2) or severe trauma (Fig. 7–4) might jeopardize the survival of skeletal or synthetic implants. In children it offers a simple means of early correction which can be repeated as often as necessary with the patient's growth, until a final permanent graft of bone or cartilage can be inserted at the time of completion of nasal development.

Finally, brief mention may be made of its use together with attached subcutaneous fat as a composite dermal-fat graft in the correction of larger concavities. By acting as a vasoinductive agent for the rapid vascularization of the adipose element in the graft, especially when the surface area of the dermis is large in relation to the thickness of the attached fat (Watson, 1959), the late absorption of fat cells is so greatly limited that accurate permanent correction of the deformity can be readily obtained by only slight overcorrection at the time of operation (Fig. 7–5). In a review of 23 major

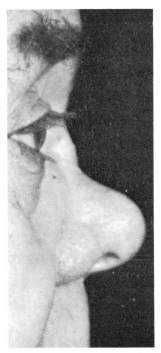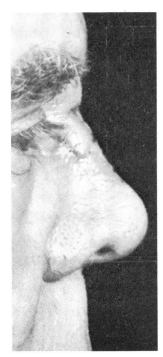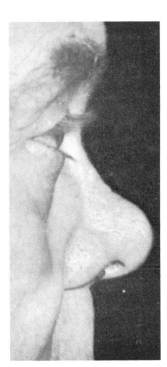

FIGURE 7–1. Male, aged 62 years, with syphilitic saddle nose. *Left,* Preoperative nasal profile. *Center,* Early postoperative profile, 16 days after the insertion of a doubled dermis graft. *Right,* Late postoperative profile 3½ years after the operation, illustrating the relatively slight degree of absorption (about 20 per cent) occurring with consolidation of the graft.

dermal-fat grafts applied to extensive facial defects (17 grafts) and the hypoplastic breast (six grafts) and observed for periods of one to five years, it was found that 21 grafts (91.3 per cent) survived to produce successful correction (Thompson, 1968). Although experimental work in the pig showed absorption of one-third of the volume of the graft following complete

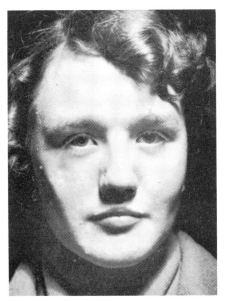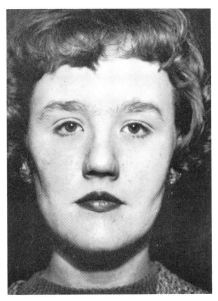

FIGURE 7–2. Female, aged 18 years, with depressed scars of the right malar region following prolonged suppuration from a retained foreign body (wood splinter) in childhood. *Left,* Preoperative appearance. *Right,* Postoperative appearance 1½ years after the insertion of a doubled dermis graft into the right cheek.

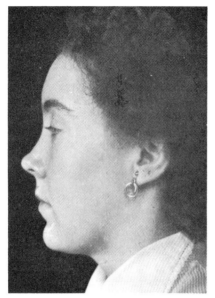 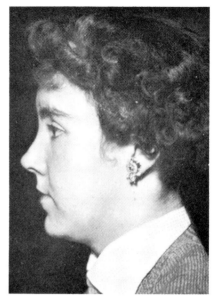

FIGURE 7–3. Female, aged 18 years, with a minor saddle nose deformity resulting from a comminuted nasal fracture two years previously. *Left,* Preoperative profile. *Right,* Postoperative profile two years after the insertion of a dermis graft into the nose.

replacement of the fat cells by fibrous tissue (Sawhney and coworkers, 1969), this is not in accordance with human tissue findings, and the buried dermal-fat graft continues to preserve its place in the treatment of facial asymmetry (Boering and Huffstadt, 1967; Thompson, 1968).

HISTORY

Autogenous dermal grafts were first introduced as a substitute for transplants of fascia or tendon in the repair of hernias and severed hand tendons and in reconstructive operations where

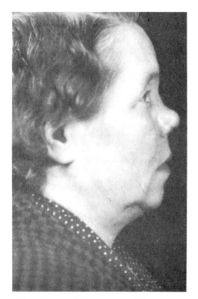 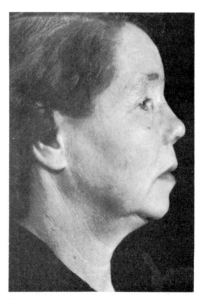

FIGURE 7–4. Female, aged 50 years, with a traumatic saddle nose following extensive injuries to the middle third of the face, including severe comminution of the nasal bones with overlying skin lacerations. *Left,* Preoperative appearance six months after injury. *Right,* Postoperative appearance one year after the insertion of a doubled dermis graft into the nose.

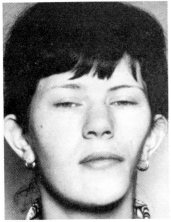 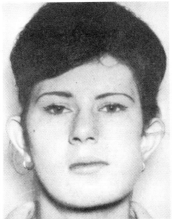 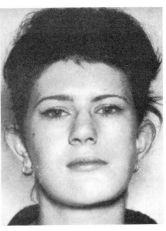

FIGURE 7–5. Female, aged 21 years, with congenital facial asymmetry. *Left,* Preoperative appearance. *Center,* Early postoperative appearance 17 days after the insertion of a dermal-fat graft, taken from the lower abdomen, into the left cheek through a preauricular incision, with limited overcorrection of the defect. *Right,* The appearance six months after transplantation.

appreciable tensile strength was required in the grafted tissue. Their successful clinical use for this purpose was first reported in 1913 by Loewe from Frankfurt-on-Main, who abraded the epidermis from grafts of full-thickness skin by scraping their surface with a knife. Independently, Rehn (1914) in Jena utilized dermis for the same purposes but improved the technique of removing the surface epidermis by shaving it off as a thin Thiersch graft with the aid of a suitable razor or graft knife.

The use of buried dermis grafts to fill out depressions in the correction of facial contour was first reported by Lexer (1914), who used them on the nasal tip and alae as well as the helix "to build up an entire auricle, constructing a solid elastic plate." Subsequently Eitner (1920) reported his use of the method to correct two cases of sunken cheeks and found the results more permanent than those obtained using fat or fascia.

In 1929, Loewe reported the clinical use of dermis grafts in more than a hundred cases, including all those in which fascia had hitherto been used: the repair of hernias and dura mater, internal fixation of fractures of long bones, arthroplasties of the knee, hip, and elbow, and recurrent dislocation of the shoulder.,

Having seen the use of buried dermis grafts during a visit to the clinic of Blair in 1932, Straatsma first reported the use of the method in the successful correction of three cases of minor saddle nose deformity.

Widespread interest outside Germany in the use of dermis grafts followed the review by Uihlein (1939) of 104 cases completed in Rehn's clinic during the previous ten years. These were chiefly concerned with the repair of hernias (80 cases) but the report included examples of reinforcement of extra-articular ligaments in the unstable knee joint and in recurrent dislocations of the patella, temporomandibular joint, and fingers, as well as in elbow arthroplasty and the repair of ruptured and lacerated tendons. In the United States the method was thereafter adopted by Cannaday (1942, 1943) for the repair of hernias and later extended (Cannaday, 1945) to the treatment of ankylosis of the mandible by inserting a dermis graft into the line of a high osteotomy—a method revived by Georgiade, Altany, and Pickrell (1957). Other applications included the staged ligation of the common carotid artery and repair of herniation of the buccinator muscle. In later years many surgeons reported favorably on the use of dermis grafts in hernia repair (Harkins, 1945; Swanker, 1948; May and Spann, 1948; Swenson, 1950), and the grafts were also extended to the repair of stenosed bronchi (Gebauer, 1950) and major diaphragmatic defects (Metheny, Lundmark and Morcom, 1952).

An ingenious variation on the use of dermis has been designed by Hynes (1954), who, by using it as a surface graft, avoided the use of distant skin flaps in the repair of adherent and unstable scars of the limbs. The lesion was excised down to vascular tissue, allowed to granulate, and a dermis graft then applied to the defect in a reversed position, i.e., "upside down," with the normally superficial surface of the dermis (papillary layer) in contact with the wound. Vascularization of the graft became much more certain than in conventional full-thickness skin grafts used under similar conditions, because of the elimination of all adherent subcutaneous fat between host and graft. Experimental work has confirmed this observation, for when full-thickness, split-thickness, and reversed dermis skin grafts were applied to the bare skull bones of the cat, the reversed dermis graft survived to double the extent of the survival of the other types of skin graft (Stallings and coworkers, 1969). Indeed, the blood supply to the reversed dermis graft on occasion became so rapidly established that the thin split-thickness skin graft applied to it as a biological surface dressing at the time of operation not infrequently also healed successfully; more usually, however, a final thick split-thickness skin graft had to be applied to the surface of the fully "taken" reversed dermis graft at a subsequent operation. Although representing an advance in the grafting of persistently ulcerating adherent scars, the method is now superseded in all but the most avascular lesions by the technique of shaving and skin grafting (Hynes, 1957), whereby successive layers of thick split-thickness skin grafts may be applied at intervals to build up as thick a protective dermal pad as may be required, with remarkable certainty (see section on dermal overgrafting in Chapter 6). The reversed dermis graft has, however, continued to find a useful place in the treatment of decubitus ulcers (Wesser and Kahn, 1967).

In recent years dermis grafts have been used to relieve the stigmata of leprosy in the hand by augmenting the wasted thenar muscles (Johnson, 1961) and to replace the articular disc following meniscectomy of the temporomandibular joint for intractable pain (Georgiade, 1962). Dermis has also been found to be suitable material for sealing defects in the dura mater (Guiot and coworkers, 1967).

OPERATIVE PROCEDURE

The basic principles have been clearly defined by Ferris Smith (1950). As an example of their specific application, the modification devised by Hynes (1962) for the correction of saddle deformities of the nose is illustrated (Fig. 7–6).

A suitable subcutaneous bed for the graft is prepared over the nasal bridge, using blunt scissors dissection through a midcolumellar incision, throughout the full extent of the saddle deformity. The graft is planned to occupy fully the undermined area in order to exclude the possibility of dead space and to provide a double layer of dermis graft over the area of maximum concavity with only a single layer elsewhere. A small pack of ribbon gauze soaked in dilute epinephrine solution may be left in the subcutaneous pocket prepared as a recipient site, while the graft is being procured, to assist hemostasis.

A donor site for the dermis graft is selected where the skin is thick but relatively free from hair. In the female the submammary skin fold, the lateral buttock, and the lower abdomen constitute such sites; in the male, where visible scars may cause less concern, the lateral thigh and deltoid region of the arm offer convenient alternatives. The graft is outlined and tattooed at intervals along its periphery, a surface area excess of about 25 per cent being planned to allow for the linear contraction which follows excision. No attempt is made to preserve normal tissue tension in the completed graft, which, being inserted in its contracted state, results in the implantation of an increased quantity of dermis. The overlying epidermis is shaved off as a thin split-thickness skin graft by means of a freehand graft knife or dermatome, and the underlying dermis (as outlined by the persisting tattoo marks) is excised as a free graft, with as little adherent subcutaneous fat as possible. The donor site is closed by direct suture.

The dermis graft is inserted into the prepared subcutaneous bed in the nose, being guided into position by sutures passed through each extremity of the graft and threaded into long straight needles. Each needle is introduced beneath the undermined skin—a maneuver facilitated by the use of specially constructed split metal tubes, readily prepared in the dental laboratory—and brought out through the skin of the nasal bridge at appropriate points. Gentle traction on the guide sutures draws the graft into precise position, with its shaved subepithelial surface in contact with the host tissues. After excision of any redundant graft material left protruding from the columellar incision, the guide sutures are tied over small bolsters of petrolatum gauze and the incison closed without drainage. A firm dressing is applied for five days to assist preliminary vascularization of the graft.

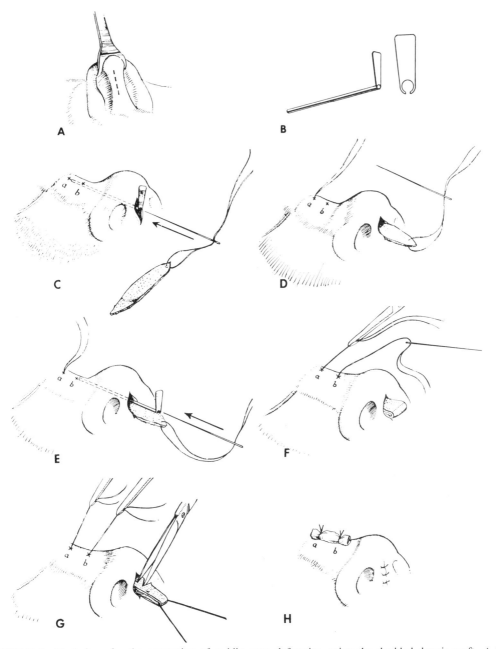

FIGURE 7–6. Technique for the correction of saddle nose deformity, using the doubled dermis graft. *A*, Site of midcolumellar incision. *B*, Split metal tubes for the introduction of the guide sutures. *C*, Introduction of the first guide suture. The point a represents the highest point of the saddle, and b the upper limit of the region of maximum concavity in the deformity. *D*, Traction on the first guide suture has drawn the upper end of the graft into the recipient bed. *E*, Introduction of the second guide suture. *F*, Traction on the second guide suture draws the lower end of the graft into the prepared bed, with doubling of the graft upon itself. *G*, Traction on the graft from below is exerted before excision of the redundant dermis, to allow spontaneous retraction of the implanted graft into its bed. *H*, Guide sutures tied over a small petrolatum gauze bolster. Columellar incision sutured.

Postoperative Complications. These have become increasingly rare since the introduction of antibiotics. Hematoma and wound infection were reported as occurring in 5 per cent and 14 per cent, respectively, in 1939 (Uihlein), in 3.5 per cent and 5.4 per cent in

1945 (Cannaday), and in 1.25 per cent each in 1949 (Schuessler and Steffanoff).

In 80 cases of dermal implants to the face, clinical cyst formation or necrosis was reported as occurring in only 2.5 per cent (Schuessler and Steffanoff, 1949).

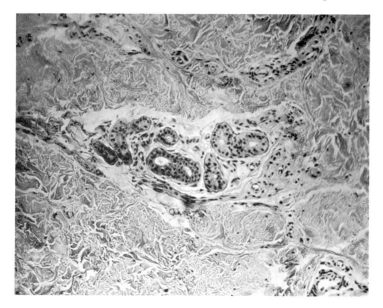

FIGURE 7–7. Human autogenous dermis graft, buried subcutaneously for four years. The essentially normal secretory coil of a sweat gland is shown. Hematoxylin-eosin, × 120.

In a series of 43 subcutaneous dermis grafts (Thompson, 1960a), it was found that about 90 per cent of grafts survived satisfactorily without any complication; no evidence of clinical epidermoid cyst formation occurred, the usual cause of failure being necrosis followed by complete absorption of the graft—presumably the result of failure of the dermis implant to "take" as a free graft.

HISTOLOGIC CHANGES IN DERMIS GRAFTS

Animal Experiments. Rehn (1914) described the successful experimental use in dogs of plaited strips of dermis to replace the Achilles tendon. It was claimed that under the influence of tension the epithelial elements disappeared and the dermis became replaced by connective tissue microscopically indistinguishable from tendon in about 10 weeks; this was confirmed by Schwartz (1922). Similarly reasonable claims for mesodermal metaplasia in response to functional stimulus—this time, of pressure—have been made by Georgiade (1962), who found that dermis implanted in the mandibular joint of monkeys developed the histologic appearances of an articular disc within six months.

The fate of the epithelial elements in dermal implants in animals has limited significance in the context of human grafts, in view of the relatively hairless condition of man and the absence of eccrine sweat glands in all

mammals used. In the dog, dermal grafts showed no surviving epithelial cells after 15 weeks in a subcutaneous site (Swenson, 1950) and only slightly longer survival at intraperi-

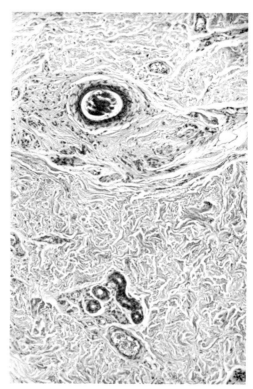

FIGURE 7–8. From the same section as Figure 7–7. The greatly dilated excretory duct containing a secretion cast in its lumen (above) is shown with its associated sweat gland (below). Hematoxylin-eosin, × 75.

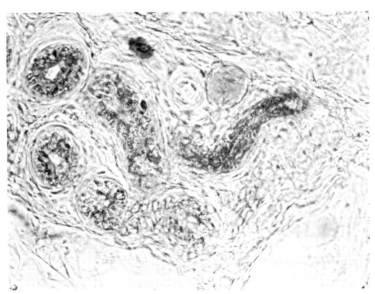

FIGURE 7–9. Human autogenous dermis graft, buried subcutaneously for four years. The dark granules represent sites of succinic dehydrogenase activity inside the cells of a surviving sweat gland. Succinic dehydrogenase, an enzyme in the Krebs citric acid cycle, is essential for the vital processes of mammalian cells. Neo-tetrazolium method, × 300.

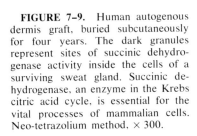

toneal (Horton and coworkers, 1953; Armistead, 1956), intrathoracic (Horton and coworkers, 1955), and intracranial (Crawford, 1957) sites.

In pigs, sebaceous glands disappeared in two weeks and hair follicles in eight weeks, but sweat glands survived throughout the observation period of eight weeks; dermal collagen and elastic tissue showed no abnormality (Sawhney and coworkers, 1969).

Human Material. In 1937 Peer and Paddock, finding that the buried dermis graft "has achieved little popularity because of the theoretical possibility of the formation of cysts from sweat glands, hair follicles and sebaceous glands in the dermis, or from remnants of epidermis incompletely removed from the surface of the dermis," completed the first thorough investigation of the histologic changes following the burying of autogenous dermis grafts for periods up to one year in human subjects. They found that usually remnants of the epidermis had survived on the graft surface, and epidermoid cysts rapidly formed at these points. Such cysts were, however, of microscopic proportions and appeared to have lost all epithelial lining in the later sections. Sebaceous glands were absent after two weeks, and hair follicles after two months; sweat glands were still present after one year but showed marked degenerative changes and appeared to be "undergoing slow but continuous replacement by fibrous tissue." Uihlein (1939) biopsied two dermis grafts buried for four years and failed to demonstrate cysts or

surviving epidermal elements, but found occasional "large cells with rather large nuclei, deep staining and lying in rows or in rings," whose significance was unknown.

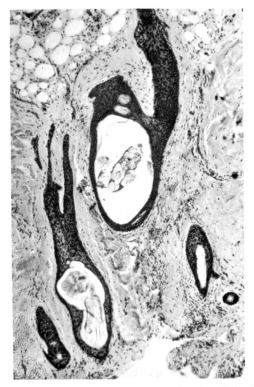

FIGURE 7–10. Human autogenous dermis graft, buried subcutaneously for two weeks. An early stage in the formation of epidermoid cysts from degenerating hair follicles. Hematoxylin-eosin, × 60.

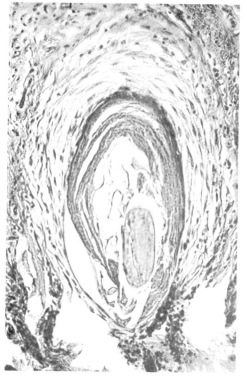

FIGURE 7–11. Human autogenous dermis graft, buried subcutaneously for five months. An epidermoid cyst derived from a hair follicle is shown at an intermediate stage of disintegration. The epithelial lining is becoming thinned following the accumulation of keratohyaline debris inside the cyst. There is considerable surrounding reactive fibrosis. Hematoxylin-eosin, × 210.

In a detailed study of autogenous human dermis grafts implanted subcutaneously for periods of from one week to five years,

Thompson (1960a) confirmed the early disappearance of sebaceous glands (usually within two weeks) and hair follicles (within two months), but established that most of the sweat glands survive seemingly permanently and continue to function (Figs. 7–7, 7–8 and 7–9). The excretory sweat duct ends blindly at the surface of the graft, the sweat gland secretion being internally resorbed into adjacent capillaries; preservation of function is clearly demonstrable by histochemical means, for not only do the graft sweat glands contain succinic dehydrogenase and other enzymes in considerable amounts, but also glycogen depletion follows upon secretory stimulation as in normal glands (Thompson, 1960b). There is no evidence to suggest that the surviving sweat glands are liable to malignant, or other deleterious, change. The formation of microscopic epidermoid cysts is common after the second week, deriving occasionally from sebaceous glands but much more commonly from hair follicles (Fig. 7–10). The natural history of such cysts is to end in spontaneous dissolution in the overwhelming majority of cases. Keratinized epithelial debris thrown off by the squamous epithelial lining into the lumen of the cyst so increases internal tension that the epithelial wall becomes thinned (Fig. 7–11), undergoes necrosis, and allows direct contact of the retained epithelial products with the surrounding mesodermal stroma, thereby eliciting (Stewart, 1912) an intense foreign body giant cell and granulomatous reaction (Fig. 7–12). The end result is complete replacement fibrosis at that site.

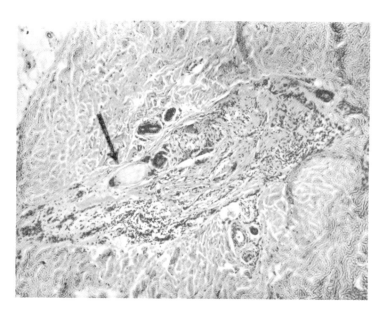

FIGURE 7–12. Human autogenous dermis graft, buried subcutaneously for 15 months. An epidermoid cyst originating from a hair follicle is shown at a late stage of disintegration. All epithelial elements have disappeared, but a hair shaft fragment (arrow) persists. The cyst has become replaced by organizing granulation tissue with many foreign body giant cells and appreciable lymphocytic infiltration. Hematoxylin-eosin, × 60.

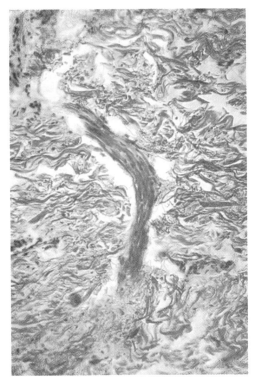

FIGURE 7-13. Human autogenous dermis graft, buried subcutaneously for five years. Surviving arrector pili muscle in the graft dermis. Hematoxylin-eosin, × 120.

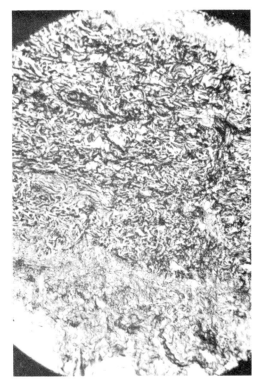

FIGURE 7-14. Human autogenous dermis graft, buried subcutaneously for five years. Elastic tissue showing a pattern of distribution resembling that found in normal skin. Orcein, × 50.

It seems certain that the dermis graft survives as a true tissue transplant, as suggested by Peer (1955), without being subjected to creeping fibrous replacement by host cells. Not only sweat glands but also the pilomotor muscles (Fig. 7-13) survive, while the elastic tissue fibers are preserved in a distribution and quantity comparable to those found in normal skin (Fig. 7-14).

Removal of the surface epidermis ensures early vascularization of the graft on all its aspects, anastomosis of host and graft vessels, and/or ingrowth of host vessels occurring by the fourth day (Peer, 1959). The revascularization, upon which survival of the graft depends, is evidently facilitated by placing the rich subpapillary plexus exposed on the superficial surface of the dermis graft, in direct contact with the most vascular tissue available, i.e. in a subcutaneous recipient site, with the subcutaneous vascular plexus of the host skin. When the dermis is buried with attached subcutaneous fat as a composite dermal-fat graft, the immediately subcutaneous position of the dermal element of the graft is preserved, since the dermis serves its chief function in establishing an early blood supply to both elements of the graft, with consequent increased survival of the adipose cells.

REFERENCES

Armistead, W. W.: The experimental use of skin autografts intraperitoneally. Plast. Reconstr. Surg., *18*:9, 1956.

Boering, G., and Huffstadt, A. J. C.: The use of dermal fat grafts in the face. Br. J. Plast. Surg., *20*:172, 1967.

Cannaday, J. E.: The use of the cutis graft in the repair of certain types of incisional herniae and other conditions. Ann Surg., *115*:775, 1942.

Cannaday, J. E.: Some of the uses of the cutis graft in surgery. Am. J. Surg., *59*:409, 1943.

Cannaday, J. E.: An additional report on some of the uses of cutis graft material in reparative surgery. Am. J. Surg., *67*:238, 1945.

Crawford, H.: Dura replacement. An experimental study of derma autografts and preserved dura homografts. Plast. Reconstr. Surg., *19*:299, 1957.

Eitner, E.: Über Unterpolsterung der Gesichtshaut. Med. Klin., *16*:93, 1920.

Gebauer, P. W.: Plastic reconstruction of tuberculous bronchostenosis with dermal grafts. J. Thoracic Surg., *19*:604, 1950.

Georgiade, N. G.: The surgical correction of temporomandibular joint dysfunction by means of autogenous dermal grafts. Plast Reconstr. Surg., *30*:68, 1962.

Georgiade, N. G., Altany, F., and Pickrell, K.: An experimental and clinical evaluation of autogenous dermal grafts used in the treatment of temporomandibular joint ankylosis. Plast. Reconstr. Surg., *19*:321, 1957.

Guiot, G., Rougerie, J., and Tessier, P.: La greffe dermique. Procédé de protection cérébro-méningée et de blindage duremerien. Ann. Chir. Plast., *12*:93, 1967.

Harkins, H. N.: Cutis grafts: clinical and experimental studies on their use as reinforcing patch in repair of large ventral and incisional herniae. Ann. Surg., *122*:996, 1945.

Horton, C., Georgiade, N., Campbell, F., Masters, F., and Pickrell, K.: The behaviour of split thickness and dermal skin grafts in the peritoneal cavity. An experimental study. Plast. Reconstr. Surg., *12*:269, 1953.

Horton, C., Campbell, F., Connar, R., McWhirt, J., and Pickrell, K.: Behavior of split-thickness, dermal, and full-thickness skin grafts in the thoracic cavity; experimental study. A.M.A. Arch. Surg., *70*:221, 1955.

Hynes, W.: The skin-dermis graft as an alternative to the direct or tubed flap. Br. J. Plast. Surg., *7*:97, 1954.

Hynes, W.: The treatment of scars by shaving and skin graft. Br. J. Plast. Surg., *10*:1, 1957.

Hynes, W.: Personal communication, 1962.

Johnson, H. A.: Dermis graft for post-leprosy muscular wasting in the hand. Plast. Reconstr. Surg., *27*:624, 1961.

Lexer, E.: Free transplantation. Ann. Surg., *60*:166, 1914.

Loewe, O.: Ueber Haut Implantation on Stelle der freien faszien plastik. München. Med. Wochenschr. *60*:1320, 1913.

Loewe, O.: München. Med. Wochenschr., *76*:2125, 1929. Cited by Cannaday (1942).

May, H., and Spann, R. G.: Cutis grafts for repair of incisional and recurrent hernias. Surg. Clin. North Am., *28*:517, 1948.

Metheny, D., Lundmark, V. O., and Morcom, T.: Use of dermal graft to supply defect in the diaphragm. West. J. Surg., *60*:156, 1952.

Padgett, E. C., and Stephenson, K. L.: Plastic and Reconstructive Surgery. Springfield, Ill., Charles C Thomas, Publisher, 1948.

Peer, L. A.: Cell survival theory versus replacement theory. Plast. Reconstr. Surg., *16*:161, 1955.

Peer, L. A.: Transplantation of Tissues. Vol. 2. Baltimore, Williams & Wilkins Company, 1959.

Peer, L. A., and Paddock, R.: Histologic studies on the fate of deeply implanted dermal grafts; observations on sections of implants buried from one week to one year. Arch. Surg., *34*:268, 1937.

Rehn, E.: Das kutane und subkutane Bindegewebe als plasticsches Material. München. Med. Wochenschr., *61*:118, 1914.

Sawhney, C. P., Banerjee, T. N., and Chakravarti, R. N.: Behaviour of dermal fat transplants. Br. J. Plast. Surg., *22*:169, 1969.

Schuessler, W. W., and Steffanoff, D. N.: Dermal grafts for correction of facial defects (series of 80 cases). Plast. Reconstr. Surg., *4*:341, 1949.

Schwartz, E.: Ueber die anatomischen Vorgange bei der Sehnenregeneration und dem plastischen Ersatz von Sehnendefekten durch Sehne, Fascie und Bindegewebe; eine experimentelle Studie. Dtsch. Ztschr. Chir., *173*:301, 1922.

Smith, F.: Plastic and Reconstructive Surgery. Philadelphia, W. B. Saunders Company, 1950.

Stallings, J. O., Huffman, W. C., and Bernstein, L.: Skin grafts on bare bone. Plast. Reconstr. Surg., *43*:152, 1969.

Stewart, M. J.: On the occurrence of irritation giant cells in dermoid and epidermoid cysts. J. Pathol. Bacteriol., *17*:502, 1912.

Straatsma, C. R.: Use of the dermal graft in the repair of small saddle defects of the nose. Arch. Otolaryngol, *16*:506, 1932.

Swanker, W. A.: Repair of fascial defects with whole skin grafts. Am. J. Surg., *75*:677, 1948.

Swenson, S. A., Jr.: Cutis grafts; clinical and experimental observations. Arch. Surg., *61*:881, 1950.

Thompson, N.: The subcutaneous dermis graft. Plast. Reconstr. Surg., *26*:1, 1960a.

Thompson, N.: Tubular resorption of secretion in human eccrine sweat glands. Based on a histochemical study of buried autogenous dermis grafts in man. Clin. Sci., *19*:95, 1960b.

Thompson, N.: The surgical camouflage of facial deformities by subcutaneous autogenous tissue transplants. *In* Longacre, J. E. (Ed.): Craniofacial Anomalies: Pathogenesis and Repair. Philadelphia, J. B. Lippincott Company, 1968.

Uihlein, A., Jr.: Use of the cutis graft in plastic operations. Arch Surg., *38*:118, 1939.

Watson, J.: Some observations on free fat grafts: with special reference to their use in mammaplasty. Br. J. Plast. Surg., *12*:263, 1959.

Wesser, D. R., and Kahn, S.: The reversed graft in the repair of decubitus ulcers. Plast. Reconstr. Surg., *40*:252, 1967.

CHAPTER 8

TRANSPLANTATION
OF FAT

LYNDON A. PEER, M.D.

In perusing the controversial literature concerning the transplantation of fat or adipose tissue, investigators find that this subject has been relatively neglected.

The pioneer in the field of fat transplantation was Neuber, who made the first attempt in humans in 1893. Lexer (1910, 1919, 1925) employed grafts of adipose tissue extensively and reported successful results in transplanting fat to establish normal contour in hemifacial atrophy, in small breasts, and in other deficiencies. Many contemporary plastic surgeons, however, prefer silicone, cartilage, bone, or dermal grafts to fat grafts because they believe that fat grafts either become infected and fail to survive or, if successful, undergo a large amount of absorption, rendering their clinical value negligible.

CELL BEHAVIOR IN FAT GRAFTS

The behavior of fat cells after transplantation in man remains a controversial subject. Some investigators believe that none of the fat in free fat grafts survive and that host histiocytes take on the lipid released from the broken

down fat cells and become the new adipose cells (host cell replacement theory). Others maintain that some adipose cells survive as living entities and that these cells collectively represent the fatty tissue ultimately remaining in the transplant (cell survival theory) (Peer, 1955, 1959).

The behavior of fat grafts after transplantation is complex; a complicated chain of events is observed in sections of human autogenous fat grafts stained and examined histologically from a few days to a year after transplantation (Figs. 8–1 to 8–9). The evidence in the author's series of 60 experimental free human autogenous fat grafts and fat-dermis transplants favors the theory of fat cell survival. Circulation is established in the grafts about four days after transplantation in the same manner as observed in surface skin grafts and other vascular transplants. The host histiocytes, which invade all fat grafts, appear to serve only as scavengers in removing fat from broken down fat cells. In support of the cell survival theory is the fact that traumatized fat grafts lose much more weight and volume than gently handled transplants; thus factors favoring cell survival are associated with the presence of a larger fat cell population in the area of transplantation.

In dermis-fat grafts the hairs and glands tend to degenerate and disppear, so that epidermal cyst formation rarely occurs (Peer and Paddock, 1937; Peer, 1950, 1959).

Drawings throughout this chapter are from Peer, L. A.: Transplantation of Tissues. Vol. II. Copyright © 1959, The Williams & Wilkins Company, Baltimore.

EXPERIMENTAL DERMIS-FAT GRAFTS

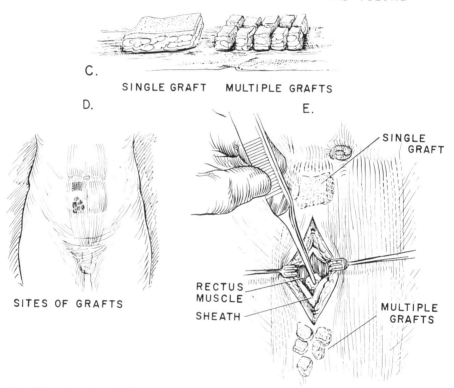

FIGURE 8–1. Transplantation within the rectus sheath. *A*, Dermis-fat grafts are weighed on a sterile scale tray. *B*, Bulk of grafts is determined by immersing them in normal saline solution and recording level of fluid displacement. *C*, One of the equal sized grafts is cut into multiple small segments. *D*, The single graft and the multiple grafts are transplanted within the rectus sheath where fat is not usually present. *E*, At selected intervals the grafts are removed, reexamined for weight and volume, and examined histologically. The removals were accomplished during secondary operations with the full consent of the patients.

The fat grafts in the author's series lost approximately 50 per cent of their weight and volume one year or more following transplantation. Normal appearing adipose cells were present in all the transplants. Eight months after transplantation the grafts appear like normal adipose tissue with normal connective tissue stroma, except for the presence of occasional walled-off cystic cavities containing free lipid from fat cells that had failed to survive transplantation.

AUTOGRAFTS

Autografts of fat with the overlying dermis provide the best available grafting material to substitute for soft tissue deficiencies in the

EXPERIMENTAL DERMIS-FAT GRAFTS

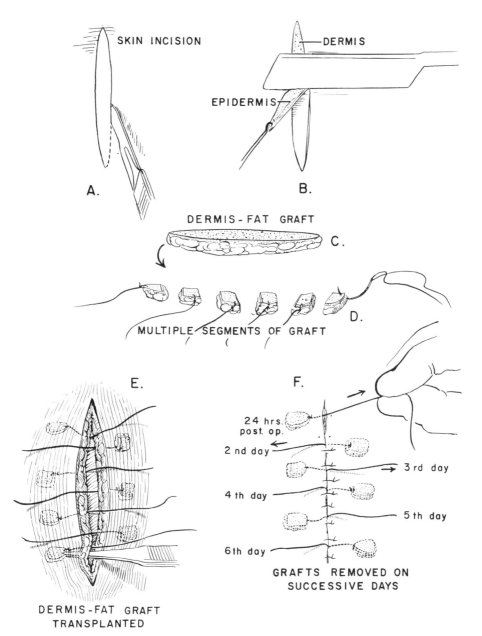

FIGURE 8–2. Subcutaneous transplantation with attached sutures. *A*, Skin incision in abdominal region. *B*, The epidermis with a thin layer of dermis is removed with a razor or knife. *C*, The ellipse of fat and dermis is removed by sharp dissection. *D*, Fat and dermis are cut into multiple segments, and a silk suture is attached to the dermal layer of each segment. *E*, Dermis-fat segments are reintroduced in the donor site with long suture ends extending out through the wound to the skin surface. *F*, On successive days a suture holding the wound edges together is removed and a dermis-fat graft is withdrawn by pulling on the attached silk. This method was suggested by Dr. Alvin Mancuse-Ungaro.

cheeks, arms, and legs. In these locations dermal grafts alone do not have sufficient bulk and must be used in a number of successive operations; bone and cartilage are unsuitable beneath the skin, where a soft consistency is more desirable, and foreign implants often become marblelike in consistency if they are not extruded.

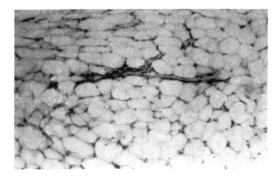

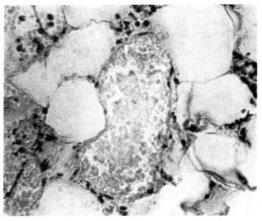

FIGURE 8–3. *Above,* Autogenous human dermis-fat graft buried four days on pull-out sutures. Note the absence of cell infiltration, unruptured fat cells, and empty graft blood vessel. × 100. *Below,* The same graft showing an area with two blood vessels engorged with red blood cells and the adjacent adipose cells. × 400.

ALLOGRAFTS

The grafting of fatty tissue from one patient to another is a useless procedure. In fresh allografts, the fat cells, the fibroblasts in the stroma, the endothelial cells in the blood vessels, and all other living elements fail to survive, and the transplant is replaced by host fibrous tissue (Peer, 1950, 1956). Host tissue cells do not appear to take on fat and portions of the foreign fat graft are replaced, as stated in Neuhof's book (1923). The host connective tissue that replaces the fat allograft is small in bulk and does not serve as a satisfactory substitute for the transplanted fat. Thus a clinical consideration of free fat grafts is concerned with only one type of transplant, the autograft.

INDICATIONS FOR ADIPOSE TISSUE GRAFTS

Transplants of adipose tissue have been employed to establish normal contour in

hemifacial atrophy (Fig. 8–10) (Stevenson, 1949), in underdevelopment of the soft tissues of the face associated with microtia, and in lipodystrophy. Superior results have been obtained in hemifacial atrophy (Romberg's disease) by the technique of the buried de-epithelized flap (see Chapter 53) and by serial subcutaneous injections of medical-grade silicone fluid (see Chapters 15 and 53).

Dermis-fat grafts have been employed instead of foreign implants for establishing normal contour in moderately small breasts and in retracted areola (Fig. 8–11). Bames (1953) and Watson (1959) reported a series of cases in which dermis-fat transplants taken from the buttocks were utilized to establish contour in deficient breasts with good success. The success of dermis-fat grafts is explained by the revascularization of the fat through the dermal vessels, thus explaining the lesser amount of absorption than in fat grafts without dermis attached. Inorganic breast implants have largely replaced dermis-fat grafts for breast augmentation (see Chapter 89).

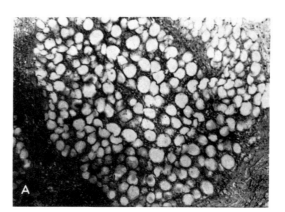

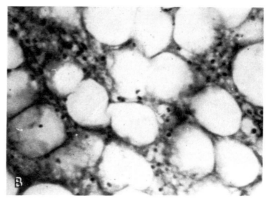

FIGURE 8–4. *A,* Autogenous human fascia-fat graft buried within the rectus sheath 12 days. A rather dense cellular infiltration has appeared with numerous host histiocytes. × 80. *B,* Higher magnification showing fat cells and host histiocytes. × 320.

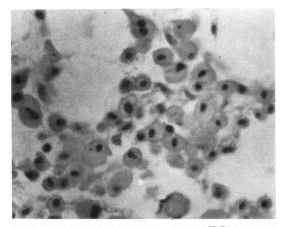

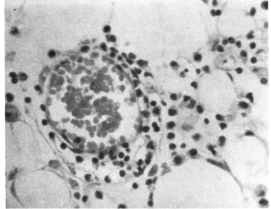

FIGURE 8–5. *Above,* Autogenous human fascia-fat graft buried within rectus sheath 38 days. Note characteristic host histiocytes and adipose cells. × 400. *Below,* Another area of the same graft showing a large blood vessel containing red and white blood cells. The white blood cells can be seen in the process of passing through the blood vessel wall. × 400.

Dermis-fat transplants are especially indicated to fill defects caused by the removal of benign tumors or cysts; *they should not be used after radical mastectomy for cancer.* The preferred techniques for reconstructing the breast after radical mastectomy are discussed in Chapter 89.

CONTRAINDICATIONS TO THE USE OF ADIPOSE TISSUE GRAFTS

An absolute contraindication to fat transplantation is *infection.* When dermis-fat transplants become infected the fat becomes liquefied, and the more resistant dermal portion of the transplant will usually be extruded as a necrotic

mass with some attached fat; fortunately the wound heals, and another dermis-fat transplant can be subsequently introduced. Fat grafts are therefore no longer used in infected bone cavities or draining pulmonary sinus tracts.

Fat grafts are not as satisfactory for the repair of dural defects as are fascial or dermal transplants. Fat grafts were formerly employed to prevent the recurrence of adhesions between the brain and meninges in patients with traumatic epilepsy. A critical analysis of the reported results indicates failure to relieve the epileptic seizures. In some patients the seizures became more severe, and the fat grafts were removed with subsequent improvement in the epilepsy. It is probable that the postoperative swelling in and about fat grafts and the later partial breakdown and prolonged host-cell reaction increase pressure, causing injury to delicate brain cells.

Fat transplants have been used extensively to obviate the formation of adhesions around sutured nerves and sutured tendons. The fat,

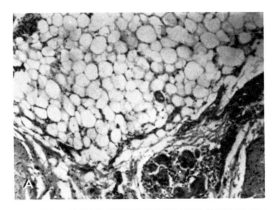

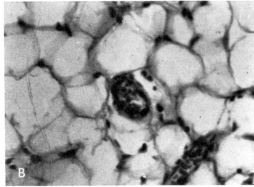

FIGURE 8–6. *A,* Autogenous human fat graft buried within the rectus sheath 60 days. Note the unruptured fat cells. × 80. *B,* Higher magnification of same transplant showing blood vessels containing blood cells and unruptured adipose cells.

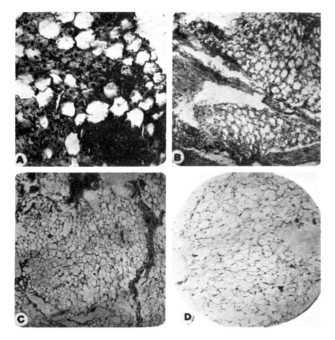

FIGURE 8–7. *A*, Autogenous human fat graft buried in muscle for 21 days. Note the surviving fat cells and large histiocytes. The histiocytes are absorbing fat cells that have failed to survive. *B*, Autogenous human fat graft buried in muscle for 40 days. Note surviving fat cells and large histiocytes are removing broken down fat. *C*, Autogenous human fat graft buried in muscle for 14 months. Note normal appearing fatty tissue. Graft loss was about 50 per cent of its volume. *D*, Autogenous human fat graft buried in muscle for 13 years. Its appearance is that of normal fatty tissue. Graft loss was about 50 per cent of its volume.

however, serves as a barrier to revascularization of the nerves and tendons, and the procedure is no longer employed. If adhesions do occur, fat on a pedicle shifted at a later operation is preferable to a free fat graft to provide a gliding channel for the tendons.

In the field of intra-abdominal surgery, free grafts or flaps of omentum are preferable to fat transplants. The omentum contains some fat, but the surface is covered by flat mesothelial pavement cells, which are physiologically constituted to cover the intestines and other intra-abdominal organs.

Fat, like cartilage, bone, and tendons, lives buried within other body tissues. It does not survive when transplanted on a free surface.

MANAGEMENT OF FAT AUTOGRAFTS

Technique

The successful management of fat autografts, whether for clinical use or experimental transplantation, is similar. The host site should be well vascularized, but all bleeding and even moderate oozing of blood must be controlled. This can best be accomplished by hemostasis obtained by clamping of bleeding vessels and

the application of epinephrine followed by thrombin. Ligatures of silk, catgut, and other foreign materials are to be avoided except when large blood vessels are involved, and the ligature should include only the end of the vessel to avoid necrosis of host tissue. The dissection is made with sharp instruments and, if possible, follows natural lines of cleavage to prevent injury and subsequent breakdown of tissue in the host bed.

The graft is removed with a layer of dermis, and the latter is exposed by removing a thin split-thickness skin graft with the dermatome and later the split-thickness graft is used as a covering for the defect (Fig. 8–12). Whenever surgically feasible it is preferable to discard the skin graft and close the defect by direct approximation. The exposed dermis and the required amount of underlying fat are removed by sharp scalpel dissection, and the graft is immediately transplanted into its bed.

When using dermis with a thin layer of fat, or no fat at all, for small depressions, the graft should be cut about one-third larger in surface area than the surface area of the depression. Contraction of the dermis after removal from the donor site will increase the thickness of the dermis and thus provide a larger transplant to fill out the depression. Mattress sutures holding the graft in place should not stretch it out to its original surface

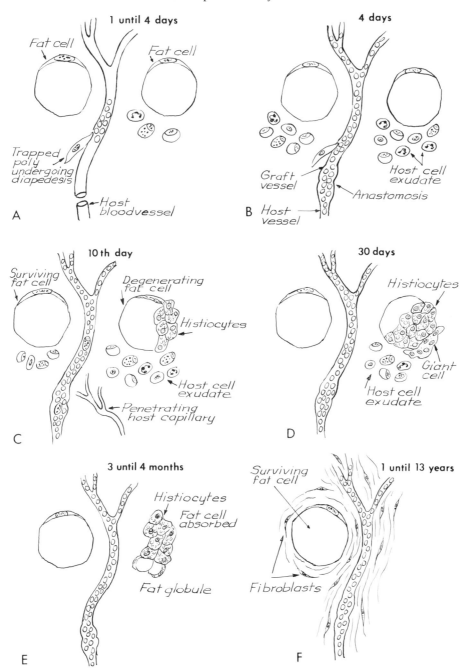

FIGURE 8–8. The contrasting fate of two adipose cells in an autogenous human fat transplant. The fat cell on the right fails to survive transplantation, and its fatty content is removed by host histiocytes and other host cells. The fat cell on the left survives transplantation and constitutes one of the apparently normal adipose cells seen in the grafted area one year or more following transplantation. Drawings are based on a series of 60 autogenous human fat grafts removed and examined histologically.

area, since this would reduce the thickness of the dermis.

Dermis-fat grafts should always overcorrect the depression, because reduction in the bulk of the transplant will occur some months after operation.

Postoperative Care and Complications

After suture of the incision, a firm but not tight supporting dressing is applied over the graft; this is left in place for one week and then reapplied for another week.

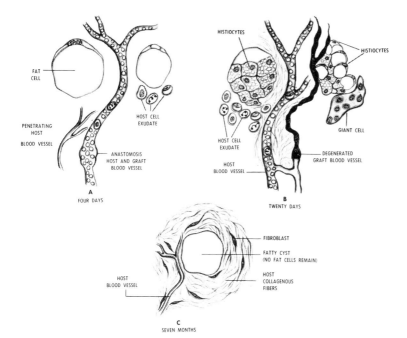

FIGURE 8–9. The fate of adipose cells in human fat allotransplants. The two fat cells in the drawing indicate the behavior of all adipose cells in fat allotransplants. Circulation is established in the graft blood vessels at about four days, as in autografts. By seven to eight days, however, the circulation in the graft vessels stagnates and a new circulation is established through ingrowing host capillaries, which supply the infiltrating host fibroblasts and host exudate cells. The endothelial cells in the graft blood vessels, the fibroblasts in the stroma, and all other cellular components in allotransplants are destroyed, and the graft is replaced by host fibrous tissue. Drawings are based on a series of six allohuman fat grafts which were removed and examined histologically.

Survival of the fat cells in autografts depends on early revascularization, which has been observed the fourth day after transplantation.

Preoperative and postoperative antibiotic therapy is indicated to reduce the possibility of infection. If infection occurs, all or almost all of the graft will probably be lost. With good management, however, this should not often happen, and in locations where a soft filling substance is required, one must accept this calculated risk. If the graft does become infected, it should be removed. Another graft can be introduced after the area has healed. About 80 per cent of our fat grafts have been successful in regard to absence of drainage and later infection requiring removal of the transplant.

About 20 per cent of the tolerated fat grafts have become reduced in size to such an extent

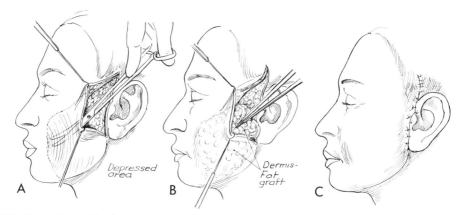

FIGURE 8–10. *A*, An incision is made and a pocket formed in the depressed area. This may extend over the body of the mandible and down into the cervical region. In some cases it may extend around the angle of the mouth and over to the midline of the chin. *B*, Insertion of large dermis-fat graft which should be sufficient in size to overcorrect the depression. *C*, Wound sutured.

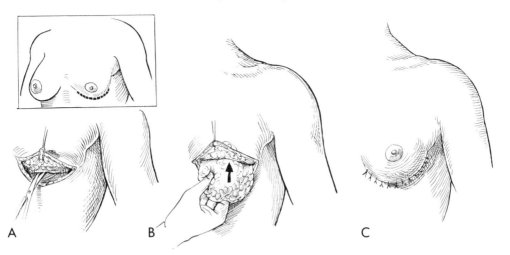

FIGURE 8–11. *A,* An incision has been made down to the deep fascia or, in congenital absence of the pectoralis muscles, down to the chest cage. A pocket is formed to receive the dermis-fat graft. *B,* Insertion of dermis-fat graft. *C,* Incision sutured.

that a second operation was required to transplant another dermis-fat graft or a dermal graft without fat to fill the remaining depression.

Size of Grafts

Moderately large fat grafts appear to lose less bulk after transplantation than smaller multiple grafts (Peer, 1950, 1956). If the procedure is properly managed, massive abdominal or gluteal fat grafts with attached dermis may "take" almost as well as moderately small adipose grafts. There is a breakdown of some fat cells, however, in all adipose grafts, and in large transplants there will be more free lipid material than in small grafts. This free fat in combination with other materials may become encapsulated if the host cells are unable to remove it. Cystic inclusions in large fat grafts have been noted for as long as ten months after transplantation. In one patient in whom a second operation was performed to remove what was thought to be excess fat, a rather large amount of encapsulated fluid material was evacuated, and normal contour was established without actually removing any fatty tissue.

Two-Stage Procedure

The author has also used two-stage transfers of fat grafts. In a first stage the transplant is raised as a flap and replaced in situ at the donor site for one to two months. In a second stage this "conditioned" adipose tissue is transplanted as a graft to the recipient area. Observations are not sufficient at this time to determine the clinical value of the two-stage procedure. Thus far none of the delayed (or "conditioned") dermis-fat transplants have been lost.

Diet as a Factor in Fat Grafting

It may be advantageous to put patients on a fat-free reducing diet before operation. This ensures that the patient's specific fat synthesized from carbohydrates and proteins will be present in the fat cell unmodified by dietary fat. Some fat cells in all fat grafts will break down and release their lipid content, and the individual's own specific fat may be less of an irritant for host tissues than modified food fat.

A reducing diet also serves to diminish the fat content in fat cells, perhaps enabling the cells to withstand better the manipulation and surgical trauma that are unavoidable during the transplantation procedure. When normal diet is resumed postoperatively, both the patient's abdominal fat cells and the surviving cells in the abdominal fat transplants may gain in lipid content, so that the bulk of the graft is increased. Probably about one-half of the fat cells in the grafts fail to survive, but the viable

DERMIS-FAT GRAFTS

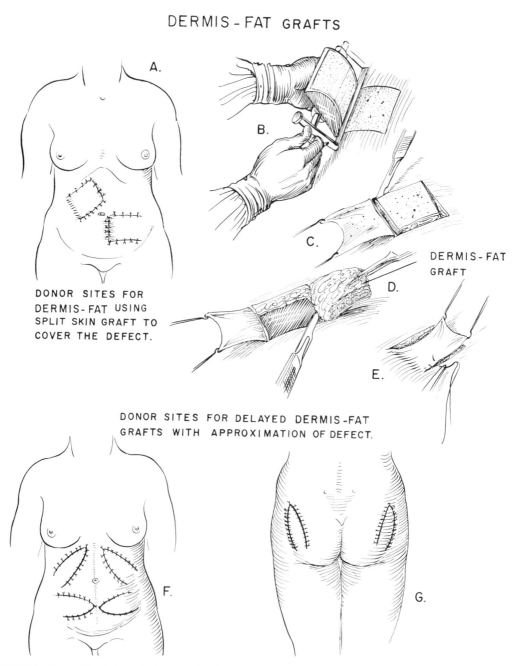

DONOR SITES FOR
DERMIS-FAT USING
SPLIT SKIN GRAFT TO
COVER THE DEFECT.

DERMIS-FAT
GRAFT

DONOR SITES FOR DELAYED DERMIS-FAT
GRAFTS WITH APPROXIMATION OF DEFECT.

FIGURE 8–12. *A,* Usual abdominal donor sites for dermis-fat grafts showing split-thickness skin grafts sutured back to cover the defect. *B,* Removing the thin split-thickness graft with the dermatome. *C* and *D,* Excising the segment of dermis and fat. *E,* Suturing the split-thickness graft to recover the depressed donor site. *F* and *G,* Donor sites for delayed dermis-fat grafts, allowing two months or longer between delay and transfer. Two half sections of the transplant are removed to permit undermining and direct approximation of the wound margins. The two sections may be sutured together to form a single large transplant.

cells in some patients may partly compensate for this loss by increased fat storage.

It is our clinical experience that abdominal fat grafts in lean individuals retain more of their original bulk than transplants in the obese if the former take on an increase in abdominal fat following operation.* Indeed, some of our large transplants to the cheek region in lean patients who gained weight after operation lost so little bulk that secondary operations were necessary to remove excess adipose tissue in the grafts.

In effect, a viable transplanted abdominal fat cell grafted to the cheek will still follow its tribal custom and behave like an abdominal fat cell in the abdominal wall; if increased lipid is taken on by one, it will also be taken on by the other. This observation favors "the cell survival theory" in regard to the fate of fat cells in human adipose grafts. If all of the abdominal fat cells in the graft die and are replaced by host cells which take on lipid and become the new fat cells in the transplantation site, why should they behave like abdominal fat cells?

FLAPS OF DERMIS AND FAT

In selected cases it may be expedient to use fat, or fat and dermis, as a flap that carries its own blood supply, instead of a dermis-fat graft (Neumann, 1953; Longacre, 1953; Maliniac, 1953). Flaps of fatty tissue tend to retain their original bulk after the pedicle is severed, provided adequate circulation has been established from the host tissues at the recipient site. Fat may also be undermined and shifted with a permanent pedicle from adjacent fatty areas to fill small depressions, such as depressed scars; the marginal skin and subcutaneous fat are then undermined and sutured over the transplanted flap to provide an even contour. Shallow depressions may be obliterated by shaving off the thin epidermis over the scar

and covering it by direct approximation of the undermined marginal subcutaneous fat.*

In general the indications for undermining and shifting the fat locally or transplanting dermis fat on a temporary or permanent pedicle are similar to those that govern the shifting of local or distant skin flaps to cover defects. The simplest method is always the best method, and fat grafts, like skin grafts, should be used largely as a procedure of necessity rather than one of choice.

---

*This is a very old but useful procedure, described by Celsus and by Galen during the first century A.D. Galen was the foremost surgeon of his day and the first experimental physiologist. Celsus was not a physician, but he wrote extensively on medical subjects and in *De Re Medicina* gives a full account of skin and fat rotations, which have been discovered as original observations many times by later surgeons.

REFERENCES

Bames, H. O.: Augmentation mammoplasty by lipo-transplant. Plast. Reconstr. Surg., *11*:404, 1953.

Lexer, E.: Freie Fettgewebstransplantation. Dtsch. Med. Wochenschr., *36*:640, 1910.

Lexer, E.: Fettgewebstransplantation, in Die Freien Transplantationen. Part I. Neue Deutsche Chir., *25*: 272, 1919.

Lexer, E.: Zwanzig Jahre Transplantationsforschung in der Chirurgie. Arch. Klin. Chir., *138*:294, 1925.

Longacre, J. J.: Use of local pedicle flaps for reconstruction of breast after subtotal or total extirpation of mammary gland and for correction of distortion and atrophy of breast due to excessive scar. Plast. Reconstr. Surg., *11*:380, 1953.

Maliniac, J. W.: Use of pedicle dermo-fat flap in mammoplasty. Plast. Reconstr. Surg., *12*:110, 1953.

Neuber, G. A.: Fetttransplantation. Verh. Dtsch. Ges. Chir., 1893. Kong. Verh., *22*:66, 1893.

Neuhof, H.: The Transplantation of Tissues. New York, D. Appleton & Company, 1923.

Neumann, C. G.: The use of large buried pedicled flaps of dermis and fat; clinical and pathological evaluation in treatment of progressive hemiatrophy. Plast. Reconstr. Surg., *11*:315, 1953.

Peer, L. A.: Fate of buried skin grafts in man. Arch. Surg., *39*:131, 1939.

Peer, L. A.: Loss of weight and volume in human fat grafts. Plast. Reconstr. Surg., *5*:217, 1950.

Peer, L. A.: The neglected "free fat graft." Its behavior and clinical use. Am. J. Surg., *92*:40, 1956.

Peer, L. A.: Transplantation of Tissues. Baltimore, Williams & Wilkins Company. Vol. I, pp. 396, 397, 404, 406, 1955. Vol. II, pp. 25, 26, 229, 230, 1959.

Peer, L. A., and Paddock, R.: Histologic studies on the fate of deeply implanted dermal grafts. Arch. Surg., *34*:268, 1937.

Stevenson, T. W.: Free fat grafts to the face. Plast. Reconstr. Surg., *4*:458, 1949.

Watson, J.: Some observations on free fat grafts with reference to their use in mammaplasty. Br. J. Plast. Surg., *12*:263, 1959.

---

*This may be explained by the fact that fat in a lean individual contains a greater density of vessels than the fat of the obese; in the latter the vessels are more widely distributed. Thus the revascularization of the lean fat is more rapid than in the obese fat, which explains the lesser degree of absorption in the lean individual (JMC).

CHAPTER 9

TRANSPLANTATION OF FASCIA

REUVEN K. SNYDERMAN, M.D.

During the past 75 years fascia has been used in various surgical procedures. Its popularity has waxed and waned, and it has been regularly rediscovered.

McArthur (1901, 1904) first used strips of the aponeurosis of the external oblique muscles as biologic sutures to repair inguinal hernias. Murphy (1904), using a flap of fascia, performed arthroplasties in the knee and other joints. Other investigators subsequently used transplants of fascia for repairing severed ligaments, tendons, and hernias, as well as pleural, dural, chest wall, tracheal, and esophageal defects, and for strengthening the walls of aneurysms.

Lexer in 1914 claimed that allotransplants of fascia functioned like autotransplants.

Kirschner (1909, 1913), Busch (1913), and Stein (1913) used slings of autogenous fascia lata to correct facial paralysis, a technique that was improved by Blair (1926).

Beginning about 1921, many surgeons in the United States and Canada employed fascia lata in the form of sutures and also as sheets to repair hernias. Gallie and LeMesurier (1924) reported a large series of hernias repaired with fascia lata. Fascial sutures were also employed in the treatment of dislocation of joints, and Lowman in 1932 used fascial slings to compensate for the paralysis of abdominal muscles following poliomyelitis.

Various authors have described the use of fascia for correction of bladder and anal incontinence.

Edwards (1969) and Ionescu and Ross (1969) employed fascia for aortic valve replacement. They believed that autogenous living fascia maintained its structure unchanged after transplantation. The fascia matrix is formed by living fibroblasts, and since it is under continuous mechanical stimulation, its functional property is maintained. Rambo, Newcombe and Gryska (1969) tried autogenous fascia as an arterial graft but found that it was subject to aneurysmal dilatation. Crawford (1968) and others have made use of fascia lata in a number of ophthalmic surgical procedures.

While the general surgeon has employed fascia for various procedures during the past 60 years, the plastic surgeon has utilized fascia mainly in operations for the repair of facial paralysis. These operations are described in Chapter 36 and consist of providing a static support by inserting slings of fascia, or attempting to hook strips of fascia to active muscles, in the hope that some movement of the face can be attained. Fascia lata is also a useful tissue to transplant as interposition material between bony edges, such as after the resection of bone for temporomandibular ankylosis. The fascia prevents the postoperative reunion of the resected bone edges (see Chapter 31).

Lewis, Lynch and Blocker (1968) and others have described a technique of looping a strip of fascia lata for stabilization of the tongue in the treatment of the Pierre Robin anomalad.

Fascia lata is also an excellent contour-restoring tissue for small soft tissue depressions, particularly when the depressed area is caused by scar tissue joining the soft tissue to the underlying bone.

Fascia for these procedures has been removed mainly from the fascia lata of the thigh by means of fascial strippers. Direct dissection of the fascia lata in the thigh has also been practical.

Occasional mention of the use of animal fascia can be found in the literature, and it has undoubtedly been used many times without documentation.

It is the general opinion today that autogenous fascial grafts remain viable after transfer. Fresh fascial allograft cells may also survive. However, the cells of preserved freeze-dried fascia grafts are dead at the time of transfer and are replaced by infiltrating host fibroblasts. Fascial xenografts give rise to a greater cellular reaction, and it is believed that the foreign graft is replaced by host tissue, probably scar tissue, which lacks the tensile strength of true fascia.

From a clinical standpoint freeze-dried allografts or xenografts are of dubious value when used as supporting strips in patients with facial paralysis.

TENSILE STRENGTH OF FASCIA LATA

Crawford (1968, 1969) discussed earlier reports on the physical properties of fascia which showed the specific gravity of fascia lata to be about 1.31 and its average tensile strength approximately 7000 lb per square inch. One can compare this with soft steel, which has a specific gravity of 7.83 and a tensile strength of 45,000 lb per square inch. Thus, in a weight for weight comparison, fascia lata is nearly as strong as soft steel. However, the stress on fascia must be placed longitudinally—that is, in the direction of the fibers—for it has very little strength in a transverse direction. Fresh fascia lata was found to have an average strength of 10.73 lb when measured in quater-inch strips, compared with 10.33 lb for frozen fascia and 10.70 lb for freeze-dried fascia. The mean strength of male fascia was 12.02 lb and that of female fascia 6.92 lb, but in the reported series the mean age of the females was much greater than that of the males. The tensile strength of fascia was also found to decrease with advancing age.

PRESERVED FASCIA

Fascia has been preserved by many methods, including irradiation, heat treatment, and freeze-drying. In the 1950's, a tissue bank was established at the National Naval Medical Center in Bethesda. This bank processes bone, skin, cartilage, dura, fascia, and blood vessels; the tissues are freeze-dried and vacuum-packed. In Czechoslovakia a tissue bank has been in operation for approximately 20 years, and one has been functioning in Poland for over ten years.

In 1954 a tissue bank was established at the Memorial Sloan-Kettering Cancer Center in New York. Since that time approximately 200 freeze-dried fascia lata grafts have been used, mainly to repair chest wall and abdominal wall defects and hernias. Some were also used to repair facial paralysis.

In Czechoslovakia and Poland a large number of patients have been treated with freeze-dried fascia lata. In the author's experience freeze-dried fascia has proved to be as satisfactory as autogenous fascia in supporting the face.* There appears to be no additional amount of stretching, and there has been no increase in the infection rate.

Because of the difficulty in obtaining a sufficient quantity of human freeze-dried fascia, freeze-dried calf fascia has been transplanted in chest wall defects. Koszarouski and coworkers (1969), working in Poland, have reported covering chest wall defects after radical mastectomies with bovine fascia sterilized with gamma rays. A two-year period of observation showed that the xenografts functioned with a complication rate comparable to that of autogenous fascia, and hospitalization was not prolonged.

TECHNIQUE OF REMOVAL OF FASCIA LATA

When a small piece of fascia lata is needed, a short incision over the lateral aspect of the thigh will expose the fascia for removal. When a wide sheet of fascia is required, it is removed through two horizontal incisions suitably placed on the lateral aspect of the thigh.

Fascial strips are obtained by means of a fascial stripper, which obviates the need for a long incision along the lateral aspect of the thigh. The fascial stripper was popularized by Gallie, whose version did not have a guillotine attachment. An additional incision was required to section the upper portion of the fascia. Later fascial strippers, such as those of Wilson and Castroviejo (Fig. 9–1, *A*) have a

---

*This has not been the experience of many surgeons, who prefer autogenous fascia (JMC).

guillotine which permits removal of the fascia through a short incision over the iliotibial band above the knee joint (Fig. 9–1, *B*).

The incision exposes the fascia, which is incised transversely (Fig. 9–1 *C*). Two short incisions made parallel to the fibers of the fascia lata and joining at right angles with the transverse incision permit raising the fascia as a small flap (Fig. 9–1, *C*). The fascial flap is then passed through the distal end of the stripper and is seized by a heavy clamp (Fig. 9–1, *D*). Gallie had designed a square clamp which furnished a strong area of purchase on the fascia lata. Maintaining downward traction upon the fascia with the clamp, the fascia lata is stripped by an upward movement of the stripper, tension being constantly maintained downward upon the fascia in order that the stripper severs the fascia as it moves upward, parallel to the fibers (Fig. 9–1, *E*). The fascial stripper is pushed by a steady upward movement (downward tension still being maintained on the fascia by the clamp) until it reaches the belly of the tensor of the fascia lata. The guillotine mechanism is then used to sever the upper end of the fascia, and the fascia is withdrawn.

The removal of a strip 10 to 15 mm wide does not result in herniation of the muscles of the thigh through the fascia lata, but this complication may occur when wider strips of fascia are removed.

The cutaneous wound is sutured and a pressure dressing and circular bandage are applied in order to avoid hematoma. Edema is prevented by applying a circular bandage from the toes to the upper thigh.

In order to separate narrower strips from the removed fascial strip, the fascia is carefully examined in order to identify the direction of

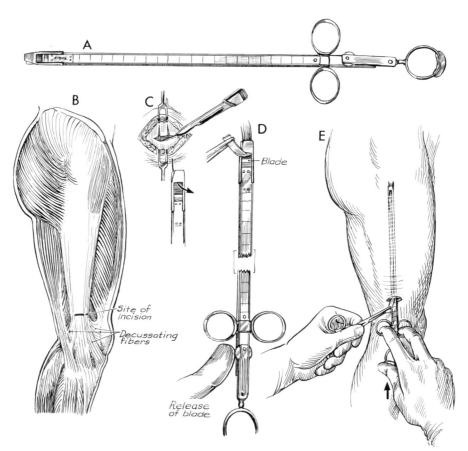

FIGURE 9–1. Method of obtaining a strip of fascia lata. *A*, Fascia stripper. *B*, Anatomy of the fascia lata and the incision site. Note decussation of fascial fibers. *C*, A flap of fascia is raised parallel to the direction of the fibers. *D*, The flap of fascia is introduced into the stripper and held by a heavy clamp. *E*, The stripper is advanced while downward traction is maintained on the clamp. The knee should be flexed, thus maintaining the fascia lata under tension. When a fascial strip of sufficient length is obtained, the upper end of the strip is severed by means of the guillotine.

its fibers. A cut is then made with scissors parallel to the fibers at one end of the strip. With the aid of two pieces of wet gauze, a narrow strip of fascia is stripped off the main graft. Depending on the width of the removed fascial strip, three to five narrow strips can be obtained by this maneuver; the strips can then be used for suspension of the paralyzed face, as described in Chapter 36.

REFERENCES

Blair, V. P.: Notes on the operative corrections of facial palsy. South. Med. J., *19*:116, 1926.

Busch, H., von: Kosmetische Besserung der durch Fazialis-lähmung bedingten Enstellung. Z. Ohrenheilkd., *68*: 175, 1913.

Crawford, J. S.: Fascia lata: Its nature and fate after implantation and its use in ophthalmic surgery. Trans. Am. Ophthalmol. Soc., *66*:673, 1968.

Crawford, J. S.: Nature of fascia lata and its fate after implantation. Am. J. Ophthalmol., *67*:900, 1969.

Edwards, W. S.: Aortic valve replacement with autogenous tissue. Ann. Thorac. Surg., *8*:126, 1969.

Gallie, W. E., and LeMesurier, A. B.: The transplantation of the fibrous tissues in the repair of anatomical defects. Br. J. Surg., *12*:289, 1924.

Ionescu, M. I., and Ross, D. N.: Heart-valve replacement with autologous fascia lata. Lancet, *2*:335, 1969.

Kirschner, M.: Ueber freie Shenen-und Faszientransplantation. Bietr. Klin. Chir., *65*:472, 1909.

Kirschner, M.: Der gegenwartige Stand und die nachsten Aussichten der autoplastischen freien Fascien—Uebertragung. Beitr. Klin. Chir., *86*:5, 1913.

Koszarouski, T., Lewinski, T., Zurakowski, W., and Klein, A.: Application of bovine fascia and aponeurosis in plastic repair of the chest wall after radical mastectomy. Bull. Pol. Med. Sci. Hist., *12*:114, 1969.

Lewis, S. T., Lynch, J. B., and Blocker, T. G.: Fascial slings for tongue stabilization in the Pierre Robin syndrome. Plast. Reconstr. Surg., *42*:237, 1968.

Lowman, C. L.: The relation of the abdominal muscles to paralytic scoliosis. J. Bone Joint Surg., *14*:763, 1932.

Lexer, E.: Free transplantation. Ann. Surg., *60*:166, 1914.

McArthur, L. L.: Autoplastic sutures in hernia and other diseases. Preliminary report. J.A.M.A., *37*:1162, 1901.

McArthur, L. L.: Autoplastic sutures in hernia and other diseases. J.A.M.A., *43*:1039, 1904.

Murphy, J. B.: Ankylosis, arthroplasty, clinical and experimental. Trans. Am. Surg. Assoc., *22*:315, 1904.

Rambo, W. M., Newcombe, J. F., and Gryska, P. F.: Autologous fascia lata femori. Arch. Surg., *98*:760, 1969.

Snyderman, R. K.: Clinical use of tissue bank material. Plast. Reconstr. Surg., *19*:40, 1957.

Stein, A. E.: Die kosmetische Korrektur der Fazialislähmung dur freie Faszienplastik. Munch. Med. Wochenschr., *60*:1370, 1913.

CHAPTER 10

TRANSPLANTATION OF TENDON

D. A. CROCKFORD, F.R.C.S.

A tendon is a collagenous cord forming the dynamic link between muscles and their insertion into bone or other structures. It is a specialized structure with specific physiologic and biomechanical properties which serve to translate bodily energy into effective action.

If a tendon is divided and the free end which remains attached to the muscle is attached to a different bone or other structure, a *tendon transfer* has been effected. However, if the "donor" tendon is entirely separated from all its original attachments before removal to its "recipient" site, then a *tendon transplantation or graft* has been performed. Significant variation in the behavior of a tendon transfer vis-à-vis a tendon transplant will be noted later in the text.

Tendon transplants are used in a number of reconstructive situations. When they are used to restore movements, for example, as a flexor digitorum profundus replacement graft, they are called *dynamic* transplants. The opposite, a *static* type of transplant, may be employed to reconstruct a destroyed tendon sling of the digital theca or to support the angle of the mouth in facial paralysis.

MORPHOLOGY, HISTOLOGY, AND ULTRASTRUCTURE OF TENDON

A tendon is a glistening whitish strip or ribbon of mesodermal tissue joining a muscle to its insertion, usually a bone. It may lie in loose areolar tissue called a paratenon (Mayer, 1916), or pass through a sheath of condensed fibrous tissue, where it is invaginated into a bursa or synovial sheath (see the Gliding Mechanism of Tendon, p. 271). The surface of a tendon shows the longitudinal striations of its component fasciculi, and, when it is not under tension, a regular pattern of oblique intersecting lines can be seen which have been likened to watered silk (Schäfer, 1912). Tendon is composed principally of collagen, together with various intercellular substances and cellular elements in the forms of intrinsic fibrocytes (or tenocytes), blood vessels, lymphatics, and nerves.

Extracellular Components

Collagen. Collagen is a complex protein with properties which make it the ideal major component of tendon—flexibility, great tensile strength, and relative inextensibility (Elliott, 1965). Tendon has a higher content of collagen than any other tissue, approximately 30 per cent on a wet weight basis, and 70 per cent on a dry weight basis (Harkness, 1968).

There is no uniform method to describe tendon, but the following one presented by Elliott (1965) is reasonably comprehensive. All collagenous tissue is composed of fibrils (see also p. 269. The Biochemistry and Physiology of Tendon), which in adult tendon have a width of about 500 to 5000 Å and a considerable but unknown length. The collections of fibrils lying together between rows of tenocytes and encircled by their anastomosing processes are called tendon fibers or primary tendon bundles. These are approximately 300 μ in diameter. The exact pattern of arrangement of these primary tendon bundles is still debated; it is probable that they are arranged parallel to the long axis of the tendon as waves of planar shape (Diamant and coworkers, 1972). The primary tendon bundles are themselves grouped into secondary bundles, the "fasciculi," which have a diameter of about 600 μ and a cross-sectional area of about 0.125 to 0.375 mm² (Edwards, 1946). The aggregation of fasciculi into larger (tertiary) bundles is variable, as there is considerable cross-branching, but a basic helical arrangement with interweaving is fairly constant.

Elliott (1965) has also summarized current understanding of the transfer of tension from myofibril to tendon fibril through an interposition of condensed sarcolemma, the tendon fibril being invaginated into the myofibril, thereby gaining a greater area of attachment. At the osteotendinous junction, the primary tendon bundles gain attachment to bone through four characteristic zones—tendon, fibrocartilage, mineralized fibrocartilage, and the bone itself (Cooper and Misol, 1970).

In tendons which have a straight course, the collagen bundles run longitudinally. However, when abrupt changes of direction occur, spiraling of the bundles around each other prevents deformation and ensures equal distribution of tension to the whole area of insertion (Mollier, 1937; Field, 1971). Various complexities of weave occur in special situations. For example, the decussation of the flexor digitorum superficialis tendon proximal to its insertion allows continued mobility of the flexor digitorum profundus tendon passing through it, while both tendons are under tension. The superficial "pressure"-bearing surfaces of tendons show closely packed bundles (Potenza, 1962a; Sick, 1970) and the absence of a capillary network, in contradistinction to the deeper "traction" bundles (Sick, 1970).

Ground Substance. In addition to collagen, tendon contains other extracellular components. Probably the most important of these is the ground substance. It is likely that it has both mechanical and biological functions (see The Biochemistry and Physiology of Tendon).

Elastin Fibers. These occur in the endo-

tenon in man, lying between the various tendon bundles. Their numbers decrease after birth (Nageotte, 1936). They form about 0.8 per cent of the wet and 2 per cent of the dry weight of the tendo calcaneus in man (Lowry, Gilligan and Katezsky, 1941).

Cellular Components

Tenocytes. Besides the cells of the supportive structures, tendon contains only tenocytes. These are the intrinsic cells of tendon and are mature fibroblasts (see also p. 270). Ranvier (1889) described their processes, which insinuate themselves between what are now called primary tendon bundles. Under the optical microscope they are seen as rows of cells lying between these bundles.

The tendon fasciculus, or secondary tendon bundle, is the smallest structural unit with its own blood supply and lymphatic drainage. The surface of a tendon is covered by a fine condensation of connective tissue called the epitenon (see p. 271). The Gliding Mechanism of Tendon), which is continuous on its "deep" surface with the endotenon, which separates the fasciculi and through which the blood and lymphatic vessels run. At the musculotendinous junction, the endotenon is continuous with the perimysium covering the muscle fibers connected to the collagen fibers of a fasciculus, while at the osteotendinous junction the endotenon is continuous with the periosteum (Mayer, 1916; Edwards, 1946).

Supportive Structures

Blood Supply. The cross-sectional area of a fasciculus is probably determined by the metabolic requirements of its components and the diffusion gradients between the interfascicular vascular bundles. The interfascicular bundles, which usually consist of an arteriole and one or two accompanying venules, communicate with each other and hence with the vessels of the mesotenon by transverse running vessels of similar caliber (Mayer, 1916; Edwards, 1946; Brockis, 1953; Smith, 1965) (Fig. 10–1). The capillary loops from these vessels do not penetrate into the fasciculi. Some of the complexities of this basic pattern have been demonstrated by Schatzker and Brånemark (1969), who used injection studies and vital microangiographic techniques, but the latter allowed visual access to only the

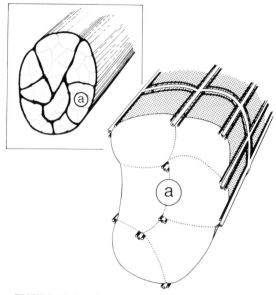

FIGURE 10-1. Cross section of a tendon showing the arrangement of the fasciculi and vascular bundles. (Modified from Braithwaite, F., and Brockis, J. G.: The vascularization of a tendon graft. Br. J. Plast. Surg., 4:130, 1951. Reproduced by permission of E & S Livingstone.)

superficial vessels. They showed that, except in the parts of a tendon subjected to pressure in a sheath, there was a rich capillary plexus just deep to the epitenon, and this plexus communicated with the mesotenon and the interfascicular vessels of the endotenon. They further showed that the capillary loops appeared to be of three different lengths, for reasons unknown.

Sick (1970) found complex, transverse running arteriolar-capillary-venular complexes passing into the deep aspect of the "pressure" layer of a tendon surface from the longitudinal vascular bundles in the core of "traction" fibers. He also noted that the pressure surface itself is devoid of blood vessels and that the clusters of two or four capillaries run parallel to the gliding surface before draining into venules which are variously dilated, so that some appear to be vascular reservoirs. These are similar to those described in the menisci of the knee joint.

Longitudinal tension will eventually cause cessation of superficial blood flow (Schatzker and Brånemark, 1969), though whether this tension was in the physiologic range was not recorded. These vascular specializations may have evolved in order to compensate for changes of tension. They may also be concerned with the production of synovial fluid. Whether they are distributed in paratenon-

covered tendons is not known (see also p. 271, Synovial Sheath).

The blood supply of a tendon is essentially segmental (Smith, 1965; Schatzker and Brånemark, 1969), passing through the mesotenon—a structure analogous to the mesentery of the bowel (Mayer, 1916) (Fig. 10-2). Connections with the periosteal and epimysial vessels at each end of the tendon serve only local needs (Peacock, 1959c); a tendon isolated from either end and other attachments apart from the mesotenon will survive (Peacock, 1957, 1959c; Colville, Callison and White, 1969; Schatzker and Brånemark, 1969). In the mesotenon the vessels are arranged in arcades (Smith, 1965) and individually run in curves or spirals to accommodate the longitudinal excursion of the tendon (Brockis, 1953; Schatzker and Brånemark, 1969). The mesotenon is always attached to the tendon on the surface which is not subjected to pressure (Mayer, 1916).

Most investigators have found no evidence of communication between paratendinous and epitendinous vessels in areas where the tendon is not surrounded by a sheath (Edwards, 1946; Nisbet, 1960; Smith, 1965; Colville, Callison and White, 1969; Schatzker and Brånemark, 1969). However, in the tendo calcaneus of the rabbit (Bergljung, 1968) and in other tendons of the same animal (Chaplin, 1973), such communications have been seen. In the specialized area of a tendon sheath, such as in the digital theca or that surrounding the flexor hallucis longus, the mesotenon is condensed into narrow bands of tissue called vincula, the vessels of which communicate with relatively large channels running longitudinally in the hilus of the tendon (Mayer, 1916; Brockis, 1953). The vincular network of vessels furnishes the sole blood supply in such areas. Obstruction of these vessels by extrinsic pressure as the tendon is angulated across a joint or over a tendon sling is prevented partly by the position of the vessel on the tendon surface opposite to the site of pressure, and partly by the weave of the collagen fasciculi in these regions, preventing deformation of the tendon (Brockis, 1953; Field, 1971). Chaplin (1973), in a microradioangiographic study of the tendons in the hind legs of rabbits, found that, in comparison to the tendons covered with paratenon, those within sheaths were relatively avascular. The vincular arteries arise from transversely running vessels, which leave each digital artery at the level of the neck of the proximal phalanx and pass medially deep to the lateral arcuate

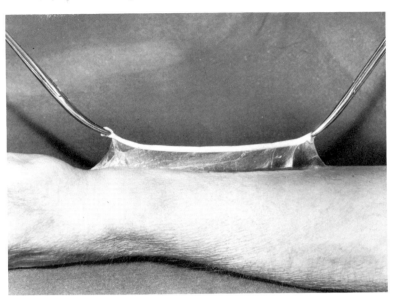

FIGURE 10–2. A segment of palmaris longus raised from its bed with its mesotenon attached.

attachment of the volar plate (Rank, Wakefield and Hueston, 1968; Field, 1971, Lefferty, Weiss and Athanasoulis, 1974). The plicae, or preputial folds, at the ends of a synovial sheath where the parietal layer is reflected onto the tendon as the visceral layer or epitenon are also richly vascular (Verdan, 1972). There is yet a third variation in the blood supply of a tendon which lies somewhat between these two. In this variation the synovial bursa is not so specialized, the visceral layer being less closely applied to the tendon, and the mesotenon is not condensed into vincula. Such an arrangement is found in the palmar bursa.

In tendon transfer surgery, the collateral circulation through the ordinary mesotenon is not sufficient to sustain more than 1 to 2 cm of tendon nearest to the musculocutaneous junction, the remainder surviving as a graft (Smith, 1965; Schatzker and Brånemark, 1969). Even if the transfer is of a tendon from a sheath, the longitudinal vessels are not sufficient to sustain the tendon (Potenza, 1963).

Lymph Drainage. Edwards (1946) found that four lymph channels, with frequent interconnections, accompanied the interfascicular vascular bundles and passed out into the mesotenon. He was unable to establish the connections of this system in the musculocutaneous and osteotendinous areas. The efferent lymph channels drain into the regional lymph nodes (Ssawwin, 1935). After repeated attempts, Schatzker and Brånemark (1969) were unable to demonstrate any lymphatics using vital microangiography.

Nerve Supply. Tendons are innervated both by nerves from the attached muscles and by neighboring cutaneous or deeper nerves, which form a plexus about the tendon and its investing tissues (Stillwell, 1957). Several types of nerve endings within the tendon have been demonstrated. Neurotendinous endings of Golgi are principally found near the musculotendinous junctions and are concerned with the myotactic reflex (Gray, 1973). Free endings are found everywhere but particularly in the proximal third of the tendon (Stillwell, 1957). They have also been found to be concentrated about the vincula of the digital flexor tendons and the extensor hood over the joints (Becton Winkelmann and Lipscomb, 1966). Besides proprioception, these nerves are concerned with exteroception (Stillwell, 1957) and possibly with vasomotor activity, as some endings are intimately associated with blood vessels (Becton and coworkers, 1966).

THE BIOCHEMISTRY AND PHYSIOLOGY OF TENDON

Extracellular Components

Collagen. Collagen may be regarded as the principal structural material of vertebrates, its primary function being mechanical (Cooper and Russell, 1969). It is generally agreed that collagen fibrils are composed of basic tropocollagen macromolecules, each of which consists of three dissimilar polypeptide chains containing about 1000 amino acid residues. In tendon, these are combined in a triple helix about 3000 Å long and 15 Å in diameter. These fibrils have prominent cross striations with a periodicity of 680 Å (Grant and Prockop, 1972). About one-third of these amino acid residues are lysine, and another third are hydroxyproline (14 per cent of total) and proline.

The protean manifestations of collagen throughout the body could suggest that its basic composition is as variable. In fact, its constituent amino acid chains vary little from species to species; rather it is in their morphogenesis that the differences lie (Jackson, 1968). Polypeptide chains are assembled on ribosomes from free amino acids which, by the addition of more amino acids, become the triple helical structure, procollagen, which is extruded from the cell. In the extracellular environment, the procollagen in turn becomes tropocollagen (Bellamy and Bornstein, 1971; Grant and Prockop, 1972).

The molecules form fibrils by the interaction of adjacent side groups. Maturation to full tensile strength comes with cross linking, the intercellular microenvironment composed of the ubiquitous ground substance principally causing this aggregation. The concept of induction, that of "like breeding like," and the variation of collagen structure by changes in ground substance have obvious importance in tendon healing (see below).

The maturation of collagen has the effect of decreasing the stimulus for the synthesis of collagen, so that in mature tendon synthesis may almost stop unless injury or disease supervenes. Thus mature collagen is subjected to incubation at 38° C for the life of the individual, but this exceeds the half-life of most native collagens under these conditions (Sinex, 1968). Furthermore, collagen in vivo is subjected to stress. That tendon collagen is in a state of dynamic equilibrium has been shown using different amino acids labeled with radioisotopes (Neuberger and Slack, 1953; Birdsell, Tustanoff and Lindsay, 1966).

Ground Substance. This has been defined as "a hydrophilic colloid having a continuous nonaqueous component held together by linkages which are disintegrated by trypsin. It therefore belongs to the category of organized proteins" (Day, 1949). In tendon, it is characterized essentially by the presence of glycosaminoglycans (or acid mucopolysaccharides), glycoproteins, and noncollagenous protein (Jackson and Bentley, 1968). It is probably synthesized principally by fibroblasts (Gray, 1973). It is more active, metabolically, than collagen, some of its components (in animal skin) having a half-life of a few days (Schiller and coworkers, 1956).

Glycosaminoglycans form the main component of the ground substance. They are large molecular-weight carbohydrates composed of amino sugars and uronic acids (Jackson and Bentley, 1968). They may, in tendon, be considered to have both biological and mechanical functions which overlap. They have been shown to be connected with the maturation of collagen in the avian embryo (Jackson, 1956), the aggregation of tropocollagen molecules (Wood and Keech, 1960), and the cementing together of collagen fibrils and fibers (Jackson, 1953; Edwards and Dunphy, 1958). Other work has shown that during tendon regeneration, and therefore presumably in tendon healing, the proportions of glycosaminoglycans present vary with the stage of healing (Dorner, 1968). Mechanically, they lubricate the movements of fibrils and fibers, one upon the other, during deformation. They are also thought to produce a "sheath" effect during repeated angulation, thus distributing compression stress away from the area of deformation along the lengths of the fibrils and fibers (Harkness, 1968).

Cellular Components

Tenocytes. This name has been given to the fibrocytes of mature tendon to indicate their role of maintenance in a way analogous to chondrocytes and osteocytes. They are relatively inactive cells with minimal if any capacity for division or protein synthesis (Weiner and Peacock, 1971). Yet slight activity does exist, since Lindsay and Birch (1964) found evidence of occasional mitoses in presumptive tenocytes in the flexor tendons within the digital sheath of the rat foot. This observation, together with the slow turnover of collagen (see above), would appear to fit in with the low range of metabolic activity suggested by a blood flow of about 0.10 ml per g per minute and an oxygen uptake of 0.1 μl per mg of dry weight per hour, reported by White, Ter-Pogossian and Stein (1964) and Peacock (1957, 1959c). Immobility decreases metabolic activity, as suggested by the associated reduction in the capillary bed of tendon (Rothman and Slogoff, 1967) and glycosaminoglycan content (Akeson, 1964; Munro, Lindsay and Jackson, 1970).

Fibroblasts, in one life cycle, can change from making hyaluronic acid to the production of collagen and chondroitin sulfate before eventually ceasing synthetic activity and dying (Sinex, 1968). The exact controlling factors that initiate and modify this pattern are not fully understood, but it seems certain that the microenvironment of the cell is important. During the development of tendon, the fibroblasts are initially close together. As their products, collagen and elastin, accumulate in the intercellular spaces, the cell bodies become separated, yet maintain contact by their processes lying between the primary bundles (Greenlee and Ross, 1967). The final orderly arrangement of cells and collagen varies from tendon to tendon; there may also be differences between areas of the same tendon. The factors controlling this variation in organization are not understood.

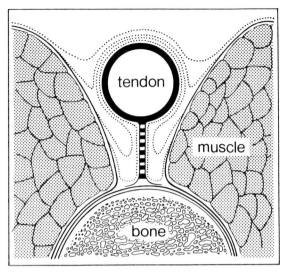

■□■□ Mesotenon

·········· Paratenon

FIGURE 10–3. Schematic diagram of a nonsheath tendon in cross section to show the multilayered nature of paratenon. (Modified from Colville, J., Callison, J. R., and White, W. L.: Role of mesotenon in tendon blood supply. Plast. Reconstr. Surg., *43*:53. Copyright 1969. The Williams & Wilkins Company, Baltimore.)

THE GLIDING MECHANISM OF TENDON

During its course, a tendon may lie entirely in loose areolar tissue called paratenon, or partly in paratenon and partly in a synovial sheath or bursa. The latter specialized tissues have evolved so that, under load, tendon excursions of 4 to 5 cm may occur across a summation of joint angles of more than 200°. Straight excursions of up to 7 cm occur in the forearm (Bunnell, 1970).

Paratenon. This word was suggested by Mayer (1916) in place of the more cumbersome "peritoneum externum," to distinguish it from the connective tissue covering a tendon within a synovial sheath, for which he proposed the word epitenon (see below). Paratenon is the connective tissue that surrounds a tendon which is traversing a straight course and which is not subject to pressure. It has been briefly described by many observers as loose, elastic, areolar, fatty tissue forming the mobile elastic medium joining the surrounding tissues to the epitenon. However, it appears that paratenon is not a single but a multilayered structure (Nisbet, 1960; Colville and coworkers, 1969; Winkler 1970) (Fig. 10–3).

Deep to these layers, occupying the space between the paratenon and epitneon, is a semifluid substance retained in a filmy homogenous material (Nisbet, 1960). It is not difficult to imagine how movement of a tendon is permitted by the sliding of these loosely adherent layers upon each other, particularly as they have a mucopolysaccharide component which favors motion (Peacock, 1971). Paratenon contains fine collagen fibers, which are loosely arranged parallel to the surface of the tendon, in marked contrast to the collagen of tendon (Potenza, 1964a).

Synovial Sheath. When a tendon is required to change direction, it does so by being confined in a condensation of fibrous tissue which is usually attached to bone. This osseofascial canal is designed to bear the resultant pressure and prevent "bowstringing" of the tendon away from the bone, which would decrease its effective excursion. In order for friction and wear on the tendon to be reduced to a minimum in the region of angulation, there is a synovial sheath or bursa. Between the fully developed sheath, such as is found in the digital theca of the hand and the paratenon previously described, there is the arrangement found in the palmar bursa lying deep to the flexor retinaculum. In this area the mesotenon is not condensed into vincula; yet the tendons are fully invaginated into a bursa, the proximal and distal limits of which are reflected onto the tendon. In this way the bursa is closed.

Where the demands of angulation are greater, the synovial sheath becomes more specialized, as around the flexor tendons of the fingers. The parietal layer is closely applied to the walls of this osseofascial tunnel, being reflected onto the vincula and so to the hilus of the tendon. In this area the visceral layer or epitenon is loosely applied (Brockis, 1953), but beyond the confines of the hilus its structure varies. In "nonsheath" tendon, covered with paratenon, the epitenon is an adherent but distinct layer in man (Nisbet, 1960). In the sheath area, however, its characteristics vary from species to species. In chickens, the epitenon is one or two cell layers thick (Lindsay and Mc-Dougall, 1961); in dogs no distinct layer is visible (Potenza, 1962a); in man the epitenon is closely applied (Brockis, 1953).

The synovial sheath is closed at each end by richly vascular folds of synovial membrane (Mayer, 1916), from which project villi or synovial fringes analogous to those seen in synovial joints (Winkler, 1970). The lining of the sheath, the parietal layer, is microscopically similar to the synovial lining of a joint. Consequently, it is likely that the traces of fluid found in these sheaths are also similar to, if not the same as, the synovial fluid of a joint. Such fluid is clear and yellow and it contains only a few cells. Its viscous, elastic, and thixotropic (plastic) qualities depend upon its content (0.02 to 0.5 per cent) of hyaluronate. Synovial fluid varies in composition from joint to joint and species to species, but its characteristics are consistent with the view that it is a dialysate of blood plasma, the mucinous component probably being secreted by the synovial cells (Ghadially and Roy, 1969; Gray, 1973).

Winkler (1970) has described complex arteriolar-capillary-venular structures which he found in the paratenon, synovial fringes, and visceral synovial layers about the flexor tendons of the human hand. Some of these had a distinctly glomerular appearance. It seems probable, therefore, that these structures are concerned with the production of synovial fluid (see also Blood Supply, p. 267).

THE DONOR TENDON

The Ideal Tendon

The ideal donor tendon has the following characteristics: (1) it is always present; (2) it is consistent in all its dimensions; (3) it is of sufficient length to bridge completely the defect at the recipient site; (4) it is superficially located

for ease of access; (5) its loss does not affect the function of the donor area; and (6) it is thin enough for adequate revascularization, yet sufficiently strong for its new task.

Available Donor Tendons

The following tendons are commonly used as grafts: the palmaris longus tendon; the plantaris tendon; the extensor digitorum longus tendons to the second, third, and fourth toes; and any undamaged tendon of an otherwise irreparable part or extremity.

Other structures are less commonly used: the extensor indicis tendon; the ulnar half of the extensor digiti minimi; a flexor digitorum superficialis tendon; parts of the fascia lata, tendo calcaneus, and triceps tendon; and the brachioradialis tendon, particularly if a four-tailed graft is needed (Bunnell, 1970).

None of these possesses all the ideal attributes of the perfect donor tendon, but each has some of them, and these are considered later in the text.

Almost any tendon of either the upper or lower extremity may be divided, and the resultant tendon-muscle motor unit may be used as a tendon transfer to restore active movement across a mobile joint or joints.

Description of the Commonly Used Donor Tendons

PALMARIS LONGUS TENDON

Anatomy.   Showing the features of phylogenetic degeneration, this vestigial muscle (Last, 1966), like the plantaris, has a long tendon and short muscle belly. It lies immediately deep to the deep fascia of the forearm between the flexor carpi radialis and flexor carpi ulnaris and is one of the superficial flexor group of forearm muscles; its nerve supply is from the median nerve (C6, C7) (Gray, 1973). The tendon, usually 10 to 12 cm long, 3 to 5 mm wide, and 1 or 2 mm thick, emerges from the muscle belly at the mid-forearm level and passes distally to be inserted partly into the volar aspect of the flexor retinaculum and partly into the central part of the palmar aponeurosis (Fig. 10–4). In the distal forearm the tendon is enclosed in a duplicature of the deep fascia (Quain, 1923). In addition to these commonly described attachments, slender fibers may diverge from the distal part of the tendon to

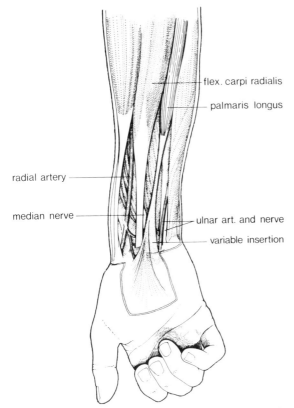

FIGURE 10-4. The principal relations of the palmaris longus tendon and its insertion into the palmar fascia and flexor retinaculum.

nance. Either general or regional (brachial block) anesthesia may be used.

THE OPEN APPROACH. An incision is marked out over the probable course of the tendon. A linear incision may be used, but the so called "lazy S" incision leaves a slightly less conspicuous but still obvious scar. Following exsanguination and the application of a tourniquet, the incision is started at the wrist crease and extended for 2 to 3 cm in a proximal direction. Blunt dissection through the subcutaneous fat will reveal the tendon lying immediately deep to the deep fascia. The fascia is gently incised, avoiding any damage to the underlying tendon. The tendon may be differentiated from the more deeply lying median nerve by its glossy, more slender appearance and by its lack of an accompanying median

gain attachment to the deep fascia of the forearm (Fig. 10-5).

Just proximal to the wrist the palmaris longus tendon lies superficial to the median nerve, covering its medial side. The tendon of the flexor carpi radialis, a thicker structure, lies on the radial side of the tendon. Both these structures have been mistaken for the palmaris longus tendon.

The palmaris longus tendon may be demonstrated by forcible opposition of the tips of the thumb and little finger, with the wrist in slight flexion. If present in a slim wrist, the tendon will project clear of the deeper structures, raising a ridge on the overlying skin in the median line of the wrist region; if the arm is fat, the presence of the tendon may be confirmed by palpation.

Techniques of Removal. The choice of limb will depend on the preoperative demonstration of the presence of the tendon, any associated surgery to the same extremity, and hand domi-

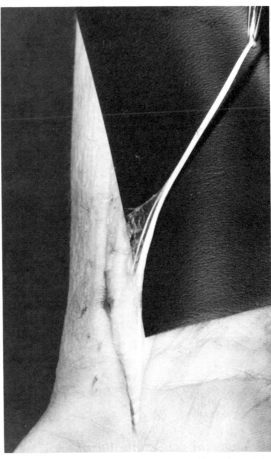

FIGURE 10-5. A common variation of insertion of the palmaris longus. The tendon has been lifted from its bed and laid across contrasting material to show a tendinous slip passing radially to be attached to the deep fascia.

volar blood vessel, which is an almost constant characteristic of the median nerve.

When positively identified, the tendon is traced proximally and displayed, the incision being extended as required until a suitable length of tendon is available. One end is then divided, the securing hemostat being used to raise the tendon from its bed as it is freed by sharp dissection. Paratenon is removed with it if required, and the blood vessels in the mesotenon—which may have some importance in relation to revascularization—are divided (see The Fate of Autograft Tendon, p. 278). Following hemostasis after release of the tourniquet, the wound is closed in two layers.

THE CLOSED APPROACH. After exsanguination and application of a tourniquet, a transverse incision 1 to 2 cm long in or just proximal to the wrist crease is made in the median line of the limb. After the skin is incised, a combination of blunt and sharp dissection will soon reveal the tendon lying just deep to the deep fascia. Dissection is extended distally to deliver all available tendon in that direction. If necessary, and when positive identification of the tendon is assured, it is divided just distal to a hemostat. Traction on this instrument will then allow palpation of the course of the tendon.

A transverse incision 1 to 2 cm long is made over the tendon at about the mid-forearm level and is deepened down to the deep fascia by blunt dissection, avoiding damage to the subcutaneous veins. The tendon will be seen moving just deep to the deep fascial envelope; the latter is incised. If the paratenon is not required, and avulsion of the mesotenon is not considered disadvantageous, the proximal end of the tendon is divided and the tendon is withdrawn through the distal incision. The tendon is transferred to the recipient site immediately, thus preventing damage to its surface from desiccation or manipulation.

However, if transfer of paratenon or sharp division of the mesotenon is desired, an intermediate transverse incision will be required. Each incision must be a little longer to allow full visual access to the tendon by elevation of the skin with a suitable retractor. Thus the tendon may be dissected free with the aid of a long, slender pair of scissors without risk of damage. When it lies free, the proximal end is divided, and the graft is ready for transplantation to the recipient site. Another method of removal is by the use of a stripper, in a way analogous to the procurement of the plantaris tendon (White, 1960a).

Possible Anomalies. The palmaris longus is one of the most variable muscles in the human body. The considerable literature on this subject prior to 1897 was summarized by Le Double (1897). Since then a number of further surveys have been done, the results of which vary, slightly higher percentages of agenesis being recorded by clinical (Rank, Wakefield and Hueston, 1968) than by anatomical (Reimann and coworkers, 1944) observation. Bilateral agenesis is recorded in about 15 per cent, while unilateral absence varies from about 4 to 8 per cent, with an agreed preponderance of left over right. Variations due to sex are less consistent.

It is probable that some of these variations are due to racial differences. Machado and DiDio (1967), in an exhaustive analysis of many surveys, have shown that in Caucasians the incidence of bilateral or unilateral agenesis averages 23.3 per cent, whereas in Negroes it is 6.5 per cent, in Asiatics 4.0 per cent, and in Amerinds 6.6 per cent. No association between absence of the palmaris longus and plantaris tendons has been established (Alexandre, 1970).

The incidence of an anomaly other than agenesis is about 9 per cent (Reimann and coworkers, 1944). The muscle belly may stretch from origin to insertion or be present only in the central or distal parts of its course. It may be digastric or bifid. There are other rarer anomalies (Quain, 1923; Reimann and coworkers, 1944).

Advantages. Its presence may be confirmed by observation and palpation. It is often considered the ideal donor for replacement of the long flexors of the fingers by the "short graft" method (in which the proximal anastomosis is performed in the palm), and for replacement of the flexor pollicis longus tendon. It is also ideal for use as a simple static support in the treatment of facial paralysis, one end being split to enclose the affected half of the mouth.

Access is excellent, and its removal causes no permanent functional sequelae. Indeed, if the recipient site is the same hand or forearm as the donor forearm, all immediate postoperative symptomatology is localized to the same area of the body. It is not too thick to prevent adequate revascularization; yet it is rarely too thin and weak to act as a flexor tendon replacement graft.

Disadvantages. Absence can be detected

preoperatively, but any anomalous malformation rendering the tendon unsuitable as a graft is usually discovered only at operation. It is too short for use as a "long" (digit to wrist) flexor tendon replacement graft, except for the little finger and for the thumb.

PLANTARIS TENDON

Anatomy. The plantaris is also a vestigial muscle showing the characteristics of phylogenetic degeneration—a short muscle belly and a long tendon (Last, 1966). It forms, with the gastrocnemius and soleus, the superficial group of the posterior crural muscles. The small fusiform muscle belly of the plantaris, usually 7 to 10 cm long (Gray, 1973), arises from the lower part of the lateral supracondylar line and the oblique popliteal ligament. The long, slender tendon passes distally between the gastrocnemius and soleus to lie on the medial side of the tendo calcaneus, gaining insertion with it into the calcaneum (Fig. 10–6). It is innervated by the tibial nerve (S1, S2)

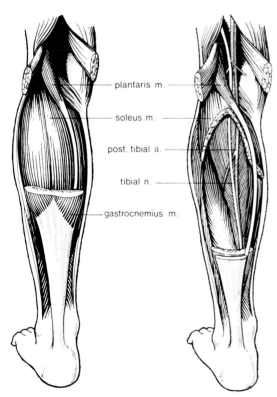

plantaris m.

soleus m.

post. tibial a.

tibial n.

gastrocnemius m.

FIGURE 10–6. The anatomical relationships of the plantaris tendon. (Modified from White, W. L.: Tendon grafts: A consideration of their source, procurement and suitability. Surg. Clin. North Am., *40*:403, 1960.)

(Gray, 1973). Owing to the arrangement of its collagenous fasciculi, this tendon has the unusual property of being able to be expanded into a wide ribbon.

Techniques of Removal. Although preoperative determination of the presence of the tendon is sometimes possible (Pilcher, 1939), choice of the limb will usually depend upon such factors as coincidental lower limb disability and ease of access in conjunction with the main part of the operation. The operation is performed under general anesthesia preferably following exsanguination of the limb. The transverse or curved longitudinal incision of about 2 to 3 cm in length is made just anterior to the tendo calcaneus on the medial aspect of the ankle region, about 1 or 2 fingerbreadths proximal to the most proximal palpable part of the calcaneus.

Deep to the skin, blunt dissection will easily penetrate the loosely knit subcutaneous fat to reveal the tendo calcaneus, with the plantaris tendon usually lying closely applied to its medial aspect. This should be differentiated from an accessory slip of the tendo calcaneus, which will show tendon fibers devoid of paratenon on dissection, and movement of the tendo calcaneus with traction (White, 1960b). Following isolation by blunt dissection, a hemostat is applied close to its insertion, and the tendon is divided.

Using the hemostat as a retractor, the tendon is gently isolated from the surrounding tissue until, proximally, an "edge" of the deep fascia is reached. A Brand tendon stripper designed for this purpose (Brand, 1961), is then slipped over the free end of the tendon, which is again gripped by a hemostat. In order to ensure security of this grip, the tendon should be wound around the end of the hemostat and gripped again by another hemostat (Fig. 10–7).

As tension is maintained on the tendon by traction on the hemostats, the stripper is advanced, gently at first, until it has passed deep to the inferior "edge" of the superior extensor retinaculum. With the knee in extension, the stripper is advanced further along the tendon until resistance is felt at about 20 to 25 cm; this resistance indicates impaction of the cutting edge into the muscle belly. This impaction, with the maintenance of full knee extension, will prevent damage to deep structures (Fig. 10–8).

Firmer movement of the stripper will cut through the muscle and allow the tendon to be

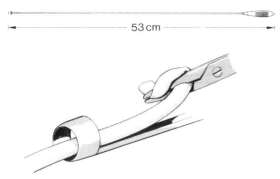

FIGURE 10-7. The Brand plantaris tendon stripper. Inset shows a method of winding the tendon end securely around a hemostat prior to advancement of the stripper. The second hemostat suggested in the text is omitted for clarity. (Modified from White, W. L.: Tendon grafts: A consideration of their source, procurement and suitability. Surg. Clin. North Am., *40*:403, 1960.)

withdrawn through the ankle incision; it is then placed in gauze soaked with saline solution to await trimming. The skin wound is closed, a dressing is applied, and the leg, from popliteal fossa to toes, is firmly bandaged with a pressure dressing and an elastic bandage prior to release of the tourniquet. To decrease the chance of thromboembolism, ambulation is encouraged on the first or second postoperative day.

If a Brand stripper is not available or if it is feared that the stripper may damage the tendon, then it may be freed proximally by division through the musculotendinous region via a direct approach. A longitudinal incision is made just posterior to the subcutaneous border

of the tibia at about the junction of the superior and middle thirds. Damage to the long saphenous vein and nerve is avoided, and the deep fascia is reached by blunt dissection. It is incised in the region where the gastrocnemius overlaps the soleus. Further dissection in the plane between these muscles will reveal the plantaris tendon (Glissan, 1932).

Damage to the tendon is very rare if the stripper is used correctly. A firm tension must be maintained on the tendon during the entire period that the stripper is being advanced. Indeed, it is usual to remove a considerable amount of paratenon in addition to part of the muscle belly. Before transplantation the tendon is stretched horizontally between two hemostats so that surplus paratenon may be trimmed off, extreme care being taken to preserve the surface of the tendon intact from damage and desiccation.

Possible Anomalies. The tendon is absent in about 7 per cent of extremities. It is bilaterally absent in about 2 per cent of the population. When present, 60 per cent of the tendons are inserted with the tendo calcaneus, while about 30 per cent gain their insertion directly to the calcaneus, 0.5 to 2.5 cm anterior to the tendo calcaneus. Of the remaining anomalous insertions, the least uncommon is that into the distal end of the tendo calcaneus itself (Daseler and Anson, 1943). It is possible to palpate the tendon only if its course is separate from that of the tendo calcaneus (Pilcher, 1939).

Advantages. It is nearly always present. It is long enough for use as a "long" flexor tendon replacement graft (wrist to digit) or as two

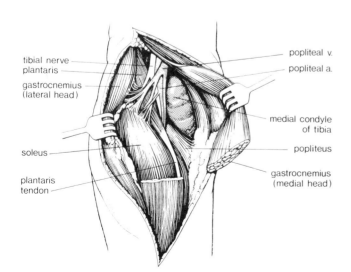

FIGURE 10-8. The anatomical relationships of the plantaris muscle and tendon in the popliteal fossa illustrated to emphasize the importance of ensuring impaction of the stripper into the plantaris muscle belly to avoid injury to the adjacent vessels and nerves. (Modified from White, W. L.: Tendon grafts: A consideration of their source, procurement and suitability. Surg. Clin. North Am., *40*:403, 1960.)

"short" grafts. Its loss does not affect function of the limb. Its strength is usually adequate for flexor tendon replacement grafting, and it is not too thick for adequate revascularization. The tendon can be stretched laterally. Owing to the parallel arrangement of the fibers, the tendon may be split into two or more slips or tails if necessary. Splitting or lateral stretching will interfere with the integrity of the intact tendon surface, thus encouraging collagenous adhesions. The latter will be a factor only if the graft is used in a dynamic situation requiring a long excursion.

Disadvantages. It is not always possible to determine its presence prior to operation. It is uncommon for the prospective recipient site to be on the same extremity; thus there are two operative sites. It may be anomalous.

EXTENSOR DIGITORUM LONGUS TENDONS TO THE SECOND, THIRD, AND FOURTH TOES

Anatomy. The extensor digitorum longus arises in the proximal part of the anterior compartment of the leg, where it is innervated by the deep peroneal (anterior tibial) nerve (L5, S1) (Gray, 1973). The tendon forms over the lower part of the tibia deep to the superior extensor retinaculum. The tendon divides into four slips which pass distally in a compartment of the inferior extensor retinaculum, emerging to spread out over the dorsum of the foot, immediately deep to the deep fascia. As they reach the dorsal aspects of the metatarsophalangeal joints, the tendons to the second, third, and fourth toes are joined on their lateral sides by the tendons of the extensor digitorum brevis before passing distally to their insertions.

As both of these muscles are extensors of the toes, loss of the extensor digitorum longus to the second, third, and fourth toes produces no disability. If the long extensor tendon to the fifth toe is required, then its distal stump should be anastomosed to the tendon of the extensor digitorum brevis supplying the fourth toe.

Technique of Removal. General anesthesia and tourniquet control are employed. Serial transverse incisions are made over the course of the tendon, but if more than one is required, a curved oblique incision is preferred. Care should be taken to avoid damage to the branches of the superficial peroneal (musculocutaneous) nerve lying in the subcutaneous fat, the dorsal veins of the foot being ligated. The deep peroneal nerve and anterior vascular bundle lie on a plane slightly deep to the tendons in the ankle region, and on the dorsum of the foot the tendons diverge laterally (Fig. 10–9).

The prospective tendon graft is removed in a manner similar to that for the palmaris longus tendon (closed method), any accessory slips being divided with care. The skin is closed in one layer; a pressure and elastic bandage is applied prior to release of the tournical.

Possible Anomalies. The arrangement of the tendons on the dorsum of the foot varies in that they may be duplicated, or extra slips may pass to the corresponding metatarsal bones (Quain, 1923).

Advantages. The extensor digitorum longus is always present and easily demonstrable preoperatively. A graft containing up to three tendon slips arising from a common tendon can be provided. The average length of the graft is 12 to 15 cm. Access is excellent. The slips are slender enough for full revascularization, and yet are sufficiently strong for all purposes.

Disadvantages. The division of the frequently present accessory slips leaves the tendon surface devoid of epitenon, thus encouraging adhesions (see The Fate of Autograft Tendon, p. 278). Although the demands of reconstruction may require that this risk be taken, the common tendon stump, if two or

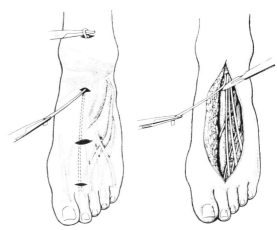

FIGURE 10–9. The anatomical relationship between the long and short toe extensors, and the "closed" and "open" methods of tendon removal. (Modified from White, W. L.: Tendon grafts: A consideration of their source, procurement and suitability. Surg. Clin. North Am., *40*:403, 1960.)

three slips are used, may be too thick for satisfactory revascularization. When the foot is used as a donor site, two separate operative fields are necessary. As healing in this region is encouraged by a few days in bed postoperatively, there are slight added risks (e.g., thromboembolism).

EXTENSOR INDICIS TENDON

The extensor indicis is innervated by the posterior interosseous nerve (C7, C8) (Gray, 1973). The tendon, which is approximately 10 to 12.5 cm long, is formed just before the muscle belly reaches the proximal edge of the extensor retinaculum. The tendon passes deep to this structure in the same compartment as the tendons of the extensor digitorum. It is then directed to the dorsum of the metacarpal joint of the index finger, to be joined on its radial side by the appropriate tendon of the extensor digitorum.

Following visualization through an incision over the second metacarpal head, the tendon is divided. Traction applied on it will show its course and indicate where the other incision should be made proximal to the dorsal retinaculum. The tendon is divided at this point and withdrawn.

The tendon is rarely absent. It may occasionally be duplicated, one of the slips sometimes being inserted elsewhere on the dorsum of the hand (Quain, 1923). Its removal will often leave a slight residual extension lag of the index finger, but this deficit is rarely of functional significance.

EXTENSOR DIGITI MINIMI TENDON

The extensor digiti minimi, the other "proprius" tendon, is similar to the extensor indicis. It also emerges from its muscle belly just proximal to the extensor retinaculum, beneath which it passes in its own compartment, lying on the radioulnar joint. It is innervated by the posterior interosseous nerve (C7, C8) (Gray, 1973). As it crosses the dorsum of the hand it divides in two, the radial slip joining with the tendon from the extensor digitorum. They are inserted into the dorsal expansion of the little finger.

Unless this finger is to be amputated, only the ulnar slip should be used; even so, some weakness of extension may result. It is removed in the same manner as the extensor indicis tendon. The tendon is rarely anomalous. However, it may be undivided or may give a slip to the ring finger. The ulnar slip may be inserted into the fifth metacarpal, and even more rarely the muscle may never have differentiated fully from the extensor digitorum (Quain, 1923). Except in the circumstances stated above, it is rarely justifiable to use this tendon for transplantation.

FLEXOR DIGITORUM SUPERFICIALIS TENDON

The flexor digitorum superficialis muscle is one of the two extrinsic flexor muscles of the fingers. Its belly lies in the proximal two-thirds of the forearm superficial to the other extrinsic flexor of the fingers, the flexor digitorum profundus. The median nerve is applied to its deep surface and innervates it (C7, C8) (Gray, 1973). In the distal forearm the muscle belly divides into four slips, which in turn give rise to the four tendons passing beneath the flexor retinaculum to enter the palm, where they spread out toward their respective fingers. In the region of the proximal digital compartment, each tendon decussates around the appropriate tendon of the flexor digitorum profundus to gain insertion by the radial and ulnar slips into the middle phalanx of each finger. They are the primary flexors of the proximal interphalangeal joints. The tendons vary in thickness and, except for the one to the little finger and occasionally that to the index, are, in adults, usually considered too thick for use as a dynamic transplant (see below).

They may be removed via two incisions. The first is placed proximal to the base of the selected digit, and the other is made in the distal forearm, the tendon being withdrawn through either. Interference with the tendon in the finger is more likely to lead to a recurvatum deformity. Its removal from a normal finger may also reduce the efficiency of digital flexion (White, 1960a). The tendons, apart from their variation in size, are rarely anomalous except for occasional tendinous or muscular connections with the flexor digitorum profundus tendons (Quain, 1923). When used as a graft, the thickness of the tendon makes it likely to undergo central avascular necrosis (Bunnell, 1970), thus provoking a severe local inflammatory response.

THE FATE OF AUTOGRAFT TENDON

The fate of transplanted autograft tendon is still debated. In the last 20 years, there has been a great increase in the number of papers on this subject, often with conflicting conclusions. This is not surprising, for there is a plethora of experimental models in different animals and an inevitable paucity of reports on vital human material. Many authors have emphasized that, even if there is no great qualitative difference, there is probably a quantitative difference in the mechanism of healing in different species.

It is proposed to divide this subject into three sections: (1) the revascularization of the autograft; (2) the healing of the tendon ends; and (3) the problem of scar formation and remodeling. Each of these will be considered separately, though it must be understood that they form the parts of a single current of events.

Differences of behavior will be noted between autografts that originate from a synovial sheath—"sheath grafts"—and those that have a paratenon accompanying the graft—"nonsheath grafts." Either of these two groups of donor tendon may be placed orthotopically or heterotopically into a "sheath" or "nonsheath" bed.

For a static graft, the quality of healing is of no great moment, provided functional survival occurs. However, in a dynamic graft where movement is essential, the manner of healing is crucial. This is particularly true in the autografting of tendons in the flexor compartments of the fingers and thumb. Consequently the majority of research has been directed to the understanding of the healing process in this region, in the hope that the notoriously unpredictable results of autografting can be improved.

The Growth of Autogenous Tendon Transplants. Clinical experience indicates that tendons transplanted in children grow at about the same rate as the child, provided that initial healing is uneventful (Hage and Dupuis, 1965; Rank, Wakefield and Hueston, 1968).

The Revascularization of Autograft Tendon

In this section, the changes occurring in the central part of the graft, as distinct from the healing process of the ends, will be considered.

Controversy exists as to whether an autograft survives completely (Mason and Shearon, 1932; Peer, 1955; Lindsay and McDougall, 1961; Cordrey and coworkers, 1963; Potenza, 1964a), or whether the major part becomes reorganized (Mayer, 1916; Skoog and Persson,

1954, Andreef, Dimoff and Metschkarski, 1967; Salamon and coworkers, 1970).

Tendon deprived of its blood supply by an impervious sheath shows evidence of cellular necrosis after nine days (Peacock, 1959c; Potenza, 1963). Even if a millipore sheath is used instead, survival is only extended for a few days (Potenza, 1963). By the second and third weeks, there is a loss of transverse cohesiveness between the collagen bundles (Peacock, 1957). As ground substance has a half-life of only a few days and is produced by fibroblasts (see Ground Substance, p. 267), the physical change is presumably due to failure of the ground substance secondary to tenocyte necrosis. Therefore, in order to survive, the autograft must acquire a new blood supply from the recipient bed. Theoretically, revascularization could occur either by direct anastomosis of the vessels from the bed with those of the graft or by the ingrowth of capillaries with the establishment of a new vascular network. In this description, these different processes will be called "primary revascularization" and "secondary revascularization," respectively. Under differing circumstances, there is evidence that either can occur.

In one of the few reports available on human material, Braithwaite and Brockis (1951) examined a nonsheath to sheath heterotopic autograft. Injection studies showed circumferential revascularization, the pattern within the graft being similar to, but not as profuse as, the normal pattern. Further indirect evidence of primary revascularization was reported by Peacock (1959c), using a radioactive isotope study in the dog. Birdsell, Tustanoff and Lindsay (1966) demonstrated radioisotopic activity in sheathed orthotopic autografts in chickens six days postoperatively.

Direct evidence of primary revascularization was reported by Peer (1955), who noted the appearance of erythrocytes in heterotopically placed nonsheath grafts in man three days after transplantation. Bergljung (1968), in a stereomicroangiographic study of the tendo calcaneus of the rabbit, noticed that this tendon has a circumferential blood supply rather than one localized through a mesotenon. Three days following orthotopic autografting, he saw anastomosis between vessels of the paratenon and the graft, with some filling of an apparently normal vascular network, which became completely normal within three weeks.

Chaplin (1973) found an essentially normal vascular pattern in the nonsheath part of the digital flexor tendons of the rabbit seven days after transplantation into flexor sheaths from which both tendons had been excised. He noted that the adhesions were extensive. Using orthotopic flexor digitorum profundus grafts, he was unable to demonstrate any revascularization of the central parts of the grafts, even after nine weeks, except in three out of 28 rabbits in which vincular reanastomosis had occurred.

With the current interest in the vital and static investigation of the specialized microvascular architecture of tendon (Schatzker and Brånemark, 1969; Winkler, 1970; Sick, 1970) and its possible effects on healing (Winkler, 1970; Verdan, 1972), primary revascularization may be of growing significance, for it is unlikely that such complex structures could be developed from a secondary revascularization in the critical early weeks of tendon graft healing.

It is probable, however, that tendon graft survival usually occurs by secondary revascularization. Lindsey and McDougall (1961), using sutured orthotopic sheath autografts in the chicken, noted some swelling of the collagen fibers and tenoblasts throughout the grafts in the first few weeks. New fibroblasts appeared, followed by capillaries, lysis of old collagen, and production of new collagen by the new fibroblasts at about five weeks. These vascularized areas of repair persisted for at least ten weeks. In the rat, using nonsutured orthotopic sheath autografts, the changes were not so marked (Lindsay and Birch, 1964). In man, swelling of autografts in the second week has also been reported (Bunnell, 1922; Weiner and Peacock, 1971).

In another series of experiments, Salamon and coworkers (1970) examined canine orthotopic nonsheath autografts by both optical and electron microscopy. They found that there was almost complete replacement with new collagen and fibroblasts by eight weeks. However, at three weeks post graft, while the periphery of the central section of the grafts showed fibroblastic activity and new collagen formation, the deeper parts remained virtually unchanged, suggesting that secondary revascularization required several weeks. On electron microscopy, a granular appearance of the ground substance was seen associated with fibroblastic activity. Munro and coworkers (1970), using radioisotopic techniques in sheathed orthotopic chicken autografts, confirmed that the changes in tendon collagen and ground substance during healing are both interrelated and interdependent.

Radioactive labeling of collagen has been used as another method of investigation. Birdsell and coworkers (1966) and Munro and coworkers (1970) showed that some increase in metabolic activity persisted beyond the 84-day postoperative observation period. Using quantitative methods, Klein and Lewis (1972) found that, in fresh rat isografts, there had been a 50 per cent turnover of collagen with a one-to-one replacement by new collagen by the end of the first postoperative month. At three months the loss of original collagen was 64 per cent, with a proportional increase in replacement.

Thus the consensus of recent work indicates that, with exceptions, the middle zone of most autografts becomes revascularized secondarily by the ingrowth of capillaries, and that some replacement of the constituents of the graft takes place, the proportion varying according to circumstances. This replacement exceeds that occurring in the normal state of dynamic equilibrium (Neuberger and Slack, 1953).

The Healing of the Tendon Ends

It is mandatory that a dynamic tendon transplant should be mobile and should be able to withstand longitudinal tension.

Opinion in the past has been divided as to the process of healing between the ends of a tendon graft and its intended attachments, whether these be bone or another tendon. One school has found evidence of active participation by the graft itself (Garlock, 1927; Ashley and coworkers, 1964); another school has felt that the tendon is passive, all the constituents of the healing process arising from the sheath or paratendinous tissues of the recipient bed (Adams, 1860; Skoog and Persson, 1953; Potenza, 1962a, b; Flynn and Graham, 1965; Lindsay and Birch, 1964). A third school considers that both the graft and the recipient bed contribute to healing (Mason and Shearon, 1932; Mason and Allen, 1941; Bunnell, 1955).

Before this matter is discussed further, the reader should be aware that, in addition to the variables already mentioned, two other factors must be considered: the composition of the suture material and the method of suture.

It has been shown that monofilament nylon or wire elicits the least reaction (Lindsay, Thompson and Walker, 1960; Srugi and Adamson, 1972) and that some methods of suturing cause more local pressure effects than others

(Bergljung, 1968). To avoid these further complicating factors, nonsutured grafts have been used when particular aspects of healing have been under investigation (Birch and Lindsay, 1964; Lindsay and Birch, 1964; Birdsell and coworkers, 1966). It is now generally agreed that tendons heal by the migration and ingrowth of surrounding tissues. Because this invasion is associated with the adhesions that prevent subsequent movement of a dynamic graft, much information of the process has come from experimental attempts to prevent such adhesions. Weiner and Peacock (1971) divided the healing process into three phases. The first two, the cellular response to injury and the phase of fibrous protein synthesis, are common to the healing of most wounds, but the third, the phase of secondary remodeling of scar tissue, is peculiarly significant to the ultimate function of a dynamic graft.

The description of tendon healing that follows is based principally on the work of Lindsay, Potenza, Peacock, and their associates.

The Phase of Cellular Reaction to Injury. Following tendon transplantation all connecting parts of the wound, including the space between the tendon ends, are filled with blood clot, which is rapidly invaded by connective tissue elements and capillaries to form typical granulation tissue. The peritendinous tissues—paratenon or sheath—become edematous and hypervascular by the first day, and it is probably from the stem cells around the blood vessels of these tissues that the fibroblasts develop (Edwards and Dunphy, 1958; Ross, Everett and Tyler, 1970). Certainly, new isotope-labeled fibroblasts are visible in these tissues one day after wounding and are beginning to appear between the tendon ends on the third day, their numbers increasing steadily thereafter. A few fibroblasts are seen within the ends of the tendon stumps. Some of the transplanted tenocytes within the loop of a suture may show signs of necrosis.

By the sixth day, the peritendonous tissues within 5 to 10 mm of the wound have lost their histologic identity, as they become merged with the epitenon in a single mass of granulation tissues in which fibroblasts predominate, other cells disappear, and collagen synthesis is isotopically detectable. It is at this period that invasion of the tendon by granulation tissue occurs in sheath tendons wherever the integrity of the epitenon has been disturbed by trauma, such as the passage of a suture. No such exact information is available for nonsheath tendons.

Mason and Allen (1941) confirmed experimentally in tendons the well-known fact that recent trauma adversely affects tissue cohesion, allowing sutures to pull out. They found that this effect was maximal at two days, and that it was five days before the sutured tendon began to acquire strength and 14 days before that strength equaled the strength at operation. Loosening of the texture of the collagen fibers in both the tendon and the graft and a granular appearance of the ground substance were seen histochemically by Salamon and coworkers (1970). It is known that mucopolysaccharide activity achieves its first peak at four to five days and that this is probably associated with the increasing synthesis of collagen. However, the exact relationship between mucopolysaccharide activity and collagen cohesion during tendon suture awaits further elucidation.

The Phase of Fibrous Protein Synthesis. The second phase of tendon healing extends through the second and third week; the limits are not sharply defined. During this phase, the number of fibroblasts reaches a peak at about the thirteenth day, declining thereafter. They synthesize collagen, the young fibrils between the tendon ends being initially oriented at right angles to the long axis of the tendon, thus lying in the same direction as the advancing fibroblasts. However, the collagen formed in relation to the surface of the tendon lies parallel to it. These patterns are visible by about the tenth day, by which time the granulation tissue growing down the suture tracts has reached the cut tendon ends, and there is an increasing vascularity of these ends.

Bergljung (1968), in primarily revascularizing tendon grafts, noted that anastomoses were occurring between the capillaries of the tendon stump and graft end at about 10 to 14 days, provided they were in close apposition. If distraction had occurred, capillary buds could be seen projecting for about 1 mm into the gap adjacent to the tendon stump.

The third week is marked by a steady reduction of the fibroblast count in the wound and a leveling off in the increasing collagen content, after the first peak of activity at 14 days. The continued strengthening of the union (Mason and Allen, 1941) is explained by the changing orientation of the collagen fibers from a transverse to a longitudinal axis, thus bridging the gap between the tendon and graft ends. By the end of this period almost all evidence of the inflammatory reaction has resolved.

It should be noted that, in the parts of the tendon ends enclosed within the sutures, the collagen fibers show evidence of dissolution. It is in these areas where previous tenocyte necrosis may have occurred that new fibroblasts initially congregate and that new collagen is laid down. Although these changes may be due to the pressure of the sutures, they can hardly be called necrosis, as collagen, being extracellular, is not living tissue. It is also possible that the changes visible in the collagen are secondary to changes in the ground substance following local tenocyte necrosis.

The Phase of Secondary Remodeling of Scar Tissue. It is in the third phase that tendon union continues to gain strength and the peritendinous adhesions lose strength. In this way mobility is acquired by the graft. However, as the practicing surgeon knows all too well, clinically significant remodeling of the peritendinous tissues often does not occur, and the dynamic graft becomes, perforce, static.

In the fourth week, the wound continues to mature with a further significant reduction in the vascularity and cellularity of both the intertendinous and peritendinous parts. If primary revascularization has occurred, there will be an increasing number of anastomoses between the ends, so that by the sixth week the arterial systems in the graft and tendon ends are identical (Bergljung, 1968). During the fourth week, the ends are sufficiently firmly bound together to allow guarded movement, the intertendinous collagen fibers continuing to increase in longitudinal orientation with a concomitant decrease in the transverse fibers.

The longitudinal fibers thicken by accretion of further molecules, perhaps accounting for the second peak of collagen activity at 28 days.

At three weeks the second peak in mucopolysaccharide activity occurs, presumably associated with the change in collagen orientation and increase in strength of the union.

The resolution of the peritendinous granulation tissues is marked by the loosening of the physical tethering of the tendon union to its surroundings. The collagen fibers, in contrast to those between the tendon ends, do not aggregate but remain relatively thin, becoming loosely arranged with their long axes parallel to the tendon surfaces, as the peritendinous tissues continue toward their pretraumatized state. By eight weeks, in the most favorable results, the adhesions between the graft and peritendinous tissues are filmy and loose. Yet, it is six to nine months before the intertendinous collagen fibers become arranged into bundles characteristic of normal tendon.

These differing sequences of maturation of collagen fibers appear to fit into current hypotheses of induction. Gillman (1961) has defined *healing* as the reestablishment of tissue continuity. If the end result is complete restoration of the original architecture, *regeneration* is said to have occurred, but if the damaged tissues are replaced by new structures (e.g., scar tissue) with varying degrees of architectural distortion, *repair* has taken place. If the inductive influences are indeed the collagen fibers and ground substance of the injured tissue, then the contrast between the maturation of the longitudinally aligned new collagen fibers joining the tendon ends and the return of the peritendinous tissues to their former loose and filmy state can be more readily understood. Indeed, in the series of orthotopic sheath grafts reported by Potenza (1964a), incised sheath and tendons "regenerate," so that at 160 days there is virtually complete restoration of the synovial layers, only a few filmy adhesions remaining. This experimental model appears to produce the ideal result. However, if a nonsheath graft is used heterotopically in a sheath, then diffuse adhesions persist (Potenza, 1972).

The Problem of Scar Formation and Remodeling

If the healing process is to occur following tendon transplantation, there must be some connection between the tendon and the recipient site to allow development of a blood supply. Most of the factors which determine whether these adhesions will mature by "regeneration" or "repair" are not known. A few are recognized and are discussed below.

One of Bunnell's greatest contributions to the advancement of hand surgery was his emphasis on the importance of reducing tissue damage to a minimum by a respectful gentleness of technique (Bunnell, 1918). "Scar breeds scar" was a favorite aphorism of his (Boyes, 1968), and, as discussed previously, current trends in the understanding of the induction of collagen proliferation serve only to emphasize this. It seems likely that induction toward a regenerative result is capable only of influencing a certain amount of healing reaction; if there is too much stimulus toward healing by repair, regeneration either will not occur or will not be sufficient to ensure a mobile tendon (Weiner and Peacock, 1971).

Certain factors are known to encourage scar production in relation to the tendon and its recipient site:

A hematoma will encourage excessive adhesion formation.

Infection is likely to lead to total loss of the tendon graft.

Some suture materials are more reactive than others (Lindsay and coworkers, 1960; Srugi and Adamson, 1972).

Disturbance of the integrity of a sheath tendon surface, whether by desiccation or mechanical trauma, will result in adhesion formation (Mason and Shearon, 1932; Skoog and Persson, 1954; Lindsay and coworkers, 1960; Potenza, 1962a). This is probably true for nonsheath tendons and chemical trauma as well.

The nature of the interface between the tendon transplant and the recipient site produces varying reactions. An intact sheath-to-sheath tendon interface may not produce any adhesions (Potenza, 1964a). However, if a nonsheath tendon is used in a sheath, some adhesions form in this experimental model (Potenza, 1972).

Because paratenon is the tissue through which a nonsheath tendon glides, it is often recommended that a nonsheath graft be transplanted with a generous covering of it. However, paratenon is richly endowed with fibroblast precursors, the proliferation of which probably outweighs its inductive advantages (Weiner and Peacock, 1971). Scraping off the paratenon leads to increased adhesions (Skoog and Persson, 1954), presumably because this disturbs the integrity of the epitenon. Therefore a compromise, in which as much paratenon as can be is removed without violating the epitenon, appears indicated.

The recipient site should be "soft and succulent" (Bunnell, 1922). Rigid structures, such as damaged volar plate, periosteum, and joint capsule, to which a graft may become adherent and therefore immobilized are better avoided. Such tissues, in addition to often being relatively ischemic, appear to have a strong "malign" inductive influence towards healing by "repair."

Although remodeling can occur without it (Potenza, 1962a), movement is considered to be an important factor in clinical situations. The loose adhesions of a mobile graft that stand in marked contrast to the thick adhesions that restrict motion are due not to elasticity but to the increased length and lack of polarization of the collagen fiber bundles. This lengthening appears to be due in part to some loss of collagen and in part to a longitudinal slipping of various collagen subunits (Peacock, 1962). The relative importance of induction and gentle persistent movements in this process is not known, but it is recognized that forceful passive movement that leads to rupture of adhesions serves only to increase the number of such adhesions.

Dehiscence of a tendon anastomosis, besides reducing the chances of primary revascularization (Bergljung, 1968), increases unfavorable scar formation because the volume of the gap between the tendon ends is increased, encouraging additional scar formation away from the positive inductive influence of the epitenon. Further damage is caused to the tendon if the sutures tear through it (Lindsey and coworkers, 1961; Douglas, Jackson and Lindsay, 1967).

The Contractile Fibroblast. Gabbiani, Ryan and Majno (1971) have reported that in certain circumstances, such as in granulation tissue, a fibroblast may become a "myofibroblast," and develop features typical of a smooth muscle cell. As myofibroblasts contract, collagen may be laid down and may "lock" the contraction. This mechanism may account for scar contraction. The factors that trigger the morphogenesis and the function of these cells are not known, but if they are connected with tendon healing, the microenvironment between the tendon ends appears favorable to them, whereas that on the surface of the epitenon does not.

For the reconstructive surgeon of the future, the control of the fibroblast and its near relatives may be as important as infection control is today (Madden, 1973).

Extrinsic Factors Modifying the Healing Process

Systemic Factors. Tendon transplantation is similar to any other operation in that a systemic disease, such as scurvy, or general debility will adversely affect healing.

Age is another factor that is acknowledged to affect the result of dynamic tendon transplantation. Before the age of 40 the procedure is more consistently satisfactory than it is in older age groups (Thompson, 1967; Boyes and Stark, 1972). The latter authors also rather unexpectedly found that children under 6 had somewhat worse results than the under 40 age group. Whether these results are due primarily to the changes that increasing age bring to tendon is not known.

Attempts to alter restricting adhesions by chemical means may be divided into two groups: nonspecific inhibitors of the inflammatory response, and those agents which have a known inhibitory effect on some stage of collagen production. Steroids fall into the former group, and the reports of their efficacy are conflicting (Wrenn, Goldner and Markee, 1954; Carstam, 1953; Fetrow, 1967; James, 1969; Ketchum, 1971). Other drugs, such as the anabolic steroid norethandrolone and the antihistamine promethazine, are reported to have some beneficial effects (Douglas and coworkers, 1967).

Investigation of the disease osteolathyrism in animals led to the isolation of beta-aminopropionitrile (BAPN), an agent which irreversibly inhibits the cross linking of collagen and prevents the development of mature fibers of normal tensile strength. Although this substance did reduce restricting adhesion formation following tendon transplantation, its side effects have precluded clinical use (Peacock and Madden, 1967; Herzog, Lindsay and McCann, 1970; Bora, Lane and Prockop, 1972). A recent report of other chemicals (D-penicillamine, and α,α'-dipyridyl and cis-hydroxyproline) indicates that the latter, acting as a proline analogue inhibiting intracellular collagen synthesis, was the most promising (Bora and coworkers, 1972). It was as effective in reducing adhesion formation as the others but did not appear to have any harmful side effects.

Local Factors. Numerous attempts at reducing adhesion formation by interposition of biological or physical agents have been reported. Before the importance of adhesion formation in the healing of tendon was accepted, the following were used for interposition by circumferential exclusion: veins (Henz and Mayer, 1914), paratenon and peritendinous fat (Henz and Mayer, 1914; Bunnell, 1918), cartilage, fascia, silver foil (Henz and Mayer, 1914), nylon (Burman, 1944), polyethylene (Gonzalez, 1949; Potenza, 1963), stainless steel (Skoog and Persson, 1954), Teflon (Gonzalez, 1959), millipore (Ashley and coworkers, 1969; Potenza, 1963), and silicone rubber (Ashley and coworkers, 1964). Reis (1969) used silicone rubber sheaths slit longitudinally to allow ingrowth of granulation tissue, which thus formed a mesotenon. In the tendo calcaneus of the rabbit, this technique was reported as encouraging. The use of paratenon

(Bunnell, 1970) and Silastic sheet (Bader and Curtin, 1971) as underlays to separate a tendon transplant from a localized area of unfavorable recipient site is clinically of undoubted benefit. Adamson, Horton and Mladick (1970) reported the use of silicone fluid injected into tendon sheaths in rats following standard trauma to a flexor tendon. Adhesions were reduced, provided the sheaths were repaired and not excised.

Another way of reducing the formation of restricting adhesions in locally unfavorable conditions, which are too extensive to respond to the use of an underlay, is the encouragement of the formation of pseudosheath around an inert rod (Milgram, 1960; Anzel, Lipscomb and Grindlay, 1961; Bassett and Carrol, 1963; Hunter and Salisbury, 1970; Geldmacher, 1971; Farkas and coworkers, 1973). In this technique, following preparation of the recipient site as for a tendon grafting procedure, an inert, flexible, alloplastic rod prosthesis is laid in the bed. After the lapse of some weeks, a pseudosheath will have formed around the prosthesis; because the alloplastic materials used provoke only a very minimal inflammatory reaction, the pseudosheath is thin, highly vascular (Conway and coworkers, 1970), and only loosely attached to the surrounding tissues.

During this period, the previously unfavorable factors have time to improve. The static "former" is then removed, and at the same time the definitive autograft is drawn into place. Following the normal postoperative routine, a result is achieved that is often superior to that expected in an unfavorable case. Revascularization of the tendon graft occurs by both primary and secondary methods through adhesions from the pseudosheath. The adhesions are filmy except at the suture sites, where dense adhesions develop (Conway, Smith and Elliott, 1970). Movement apparently occurs both between the tendon and the pseudosheath and between the pseudosheath and its surroundings. Farkas and coworkers (1973) found that postoperative activity was associated with adhesion reduction and remodeling.

Topical use of various agents has been reported. Cortisone (Carstam, 1953), Gelfoam and Gelfilm (Wrenn and coworkers, 1954), and triamcinolone (Ketchum, 1971) have all given encouraging laboratory results.

THE FATE OF ALLOGRAFT TENDON

The idea of a bank of allogenic tendons ever available for use is attractive. The procurement of autograft tendon nearly always requires an additional operative intervention and even then may not yield adequate or sufficient tendon for a multiple transplant procedure. Considerable effort has been made to elucidate the fate of allografts in the body of the recipient. Attempts have also been made to assess the effects on the allograft tendon of different methods of preservation and any consequent changes of immunologic status that may occur. As is the case with the investigation of autograft tendon behavior, many experimental models have been used, assessment being further complicated by different methods of preservation and the use of xenografts.

Opinion is divided as to the fate of allografts. Some investigators (Peer, 1955; Iselin and Flores, 1963, 1972; Potenza, 1964b; Beringer and Darkshevich, 1969; Seiffert, 1971; Seiffert and Schmit, 1971) consider that, while cellular death occurs, the collagenous structure is little altered. Others have found that there is complete replacement by the host of all, or virtually all, of the graft (Herzog, 1963; Cordrey, McCorkle and Hilton, 1963; Mshvidobadze, 1966; Salamon and coworkers, 1973). Between these two groups, Artomonova (1969) considers that the amount of graft survival is proportional to the degree of histocompatability of donor and host.

The work of Klein and coworkers (1969, 1972), Klein and Lewis (1972), and Tobias and Seiffert (1972) indicates that alloantigenic tendon collagen continues in a state of dynamic equilibrium after transplantation.

Methods of Preservation. These range from various physiologic fluid media to methods that lead to cellular death and denaturation of collagen.

FLUID MEDIA. Storage at $4°C$ in what may be called physiologic solutions, in which varying proportions of protein hydrolysate, glucose, electrolytes, antihistamines, or antibacterial agents are combined, has been advocated by Mshvidobadze (1966), Beringer and Darkshevich (1969), Cameron and his associates (1970), and Andreef and Wladmirov (1972). As allograft cells are antigenic and in one such fluid medium survived for only 18 to 21 days (Demichev, 1969), it is presumably to some of the components of the ground substance that these methods of preservation are directed. However, there seems to have been no laboratory attempt to ascertain what effect these media have on the extracellular tendon components.

The solutions used may be classified accord-ing to the severity of their action upon the tendon constituents. Cialit [2-(ethylmercurimercapto)-benzoxazol-5-carbonic sodium] (Iselin and Flores, 1963, 1972; Herzog, 1963; Seiffert, 1967, 1971) is an organic mercurial compound with strong antibacterial properties. It has the effect of destroying all the cells and the antigenicity of skin, and therefore by analogy of tendon (Seiffert, 1971) (see below). Another mercurial, thiomersal, has not received such a favorable report (Cordrey and coworkers, 1963; Salamon and coworkers, 1973). Cordrey and coworkers (1963) and Peer (1955) also used ethanol, though the former considered its denaturative effect more marked than with thiomersal.

FREEZING. Storage of tendon at various temperatures from -25 to $-183°C$ sometimes in glycerol, or a similar medium, has been reported by Cameron and coworkers (1970), Klein and coworkers (1972), Kovalenko and Demichev (1972), and Salamon and coworkers (1973).

IRRADIATION. Ashley and coworkers (1964) used frozen irradiated tendon grafts in experimental animals, and Salamon and associates (1973) used irradiated (100 R) tendon stored in physiologic saline at $4°C$.

LYOPHILIZATION. This process has been used by Cordrey and coworkers (1963), Potenza (1964b), Flynn and Graham (1965), Cameron and associates (1970), and Kovalenko and Demichev (1972). In their paper of 1969, Kovalenko and Demichev reviewed the Soviet literature on all aspects of tendon allografting with particular reference to lyophilization.

Alloantigenicity of Tendon. Before considering which methods of preservation appear to give the best clinical results, some discussion of the effects of tendon preservation on alloantigenicity is necessary. Although some attempts to demonstrate the antigenicity of whole intact tendon using allografts (Peacock and Petty, 1960; Seiffert, 1967) and xenografts (Peacock and Petty, 1960) were not successful, Flynn and Graham (1965), using lyophilized xenografts, were able to demonstrate circulating antibodies by hemagglutination reactions. However, Crockford, Rapaport, and Converse (1971), using allograft tendon which was homogenized in an attempt to increase the antigenic challenge, were unable to demonstrate unequivocally accelerated second-set rejection times in subsequent skin grafts. Although tendon contains not only tenocytes but also the cells of its mesenchymal supportive structures, it is relatively hypocellular. Since native collagen is species-specific (Adelmann and coworkers, 1968; Michaeli and coworkers, 1970), it is hardly surprising that tendon is antigenically weak.

Nevertheless, there is microangiographic, histologic, and direct immunologic evidence to show that tendon is antigenic. Bergljung (1968), using contrast media injected into calcaneal tendon allografts in the rabbit, reported reestablishment of the circulation in such grafts from the seventh to the fourteenth postoperative days, but in every specimen examined after this period, no circulation was observed until a new vascular network had been established by the recipient. With autografts, primary revascularization (see p. 279) took place from the third day, persisting for at least six months. These results suggest that the normal "first-set" reaction of whole tendon allografts (i.e., 7 to 14 days) may be longer than that of more antigenic tissues, such as skin, in which stereomicroscopy shows thrombosis of vessels by the eighth post-graft day (Taylor and Lehrfeld, 1953).

Histologic observations in support of a local immunologic reaction have been reported by several investigators (Artomonova, 1969; Herzog, 1963; Seiffert, 1971). Seiffert (1971), in particular, has drawn a distinction between the reactions produced by fresh allografts and those produced by preserved allografts. Using skin and the second-set reaction technique, he showed that preservation by deep freezing and lyophilization reduced the antigenicity in increasing degrees. Cialit-stored skin, however, lost all its antigenicity.

As has already been mentioned, native collagen is species-specific (Adelmann, Glynn and Kirrane, 1968; Michaeli, Martin and Benjamini, 1970). However, autoantigenicity in rabbits has been reported following repeated subcutaneous and intramuscular injections of crude saline extracts from homogenized tendon for periods of 12 weeks or more (Heller and Yakulis, 1963). Circulating complement-fixing antitendon extract antibodies were detected, but the relationship of these observations to the effects of the implantation of whole allograft tendons in reconstructive surgery is not clear. Indeed, Peacock (1959a) and Seiffert (1967) have both found that allograft tendon becomes histologically cell-free about three weeks after implantation.

Moreover, there is a surprisingly brisk turnover of transplanted tendon collagen. With radioactive labeling techniques, it has been shown that rat tail tendon and tendo calcaneus grafts used as isografts lost about 65 per cent of their radioactivity six months after implantation. These grafts were stored frozen and were histologically cell-free when transplanted. Allografts showed the same percentage loss (Klein and coworkers, 1969).

In a more recent paper Klein and Lewis (1972) used fresh isografts and allografts. They found that, one month after grafting, there was a relatively greater loss of radioactivity in the isografts than in the allografts, but this difference was less marked at three months. They considered that this greater loss by the isografts was probably due to the continued metabolic activity of the tenocytes, which of course would not occur in the allografts. By radioactive labeling of the host collagen, they were able to show that, while isografts had a 1:1 net change of collagen, the allografts showed a 20 per cent net loss of collagen by three months.

Seiffert (1971), using a different radioactive isotope, found that after six months the grafts, while still recognizable as tendon, had lost almost all their radioactivity. In another investigation using composite flexor tendon allografts which had also been labeled with a radioactive isotope, Tobias and Seiffert (1972) found evidence of radioactivity in the skin and tendons of the recipient animals, suggesting that some, at least, of the labeled metabolites of the grafts are reused by the recipient for collagen synthesis. Presumably the same processes occur when simple tendon allografts are used.

Correlation of Methods of Preservation With the Results of Allograft Transplantation. From a review of the papers on this subject there is a consensus of opinion that, for clinical purposes, the transplantation of fresh allograft tendon produces an unacceptable amount of host reaction and adhesion formation. Different methods of preservation have been reported to have reduced this problem to a reasonable level. However, it must be emphasized that, while an amount of reaction around a transplanted tendon in a nonsheath situation with a short excursional requirement might not interfere with function significantly, the same amount of reaction around a digital flexor tendon replacement graft would be disastrous.

The antigenicity of a tissue lies principally in its cells and, to a lesser extent, in the ground substance. Peacock (1959a) observed that the invasion of fresh xenografts by recipient cells was delayed until virtually all the cells of the graft had ceased to be histologically detectable. Consequently, the period of delay was increased when thicker and older grafts were used but was almost eliminated if the grafts had been previously treated with trypsin to digest cellular elements and ground substance. Herzog (1963) noted that if preserved allografts were stored beyond a critical period (more than 30 days in Cialit solution), loss of histologically detectable allogeneic cell viability was associated with a reduction in the cellular response of the host.

Seiffert (1971) reported that, whereas fresh, deep frozen, or lyophilized skin specimens used as allografts provoked a second-set skin graft rejection time of 5.1, 5.4 and 6.6 days, respectively, skin stored in Cialit solution did not produce accelerated rejection upon subsequent challenge of the host with a skin graft from the same donor. Herzog (1963) and Seiffert (1971) also noted that, after about three weeks, tendon stored in Cialit was histologically cell-free. Three days after subcutaneous implantation of Cialit-preserved allogenic rat tail tendon, Seiffert (1971) was able to detect cells in the grafts which probably originated in the recipient. This time scale correlates with the findings of Peacock (1959). Seiffert (1971) also noted that, in comparison to fresh, deep frozen, or lyophilized tendon allografts, those preserved in Cialit provoked the least recipient reaction (even less than with autografts).

It is well known that increasing storage time for skin, particularly at 4°C and to a lesser extent by freezing, is associated with a loss of cell viability. This has also been demonstrated in tendons (Demichev, 1969). A number of authors have noted that increasing the period of storage by freezing improves clinical results (Kovalenko and Demichev, 1969).

Except for its mention in a report relating to composite grafts (Cameron and his associates 1971) (see below), lyophilization has not been as popular a method of preservation. However, Potenza (1964b), using the dog forefoot, found remarkably little reaction, recellularization apparently occurring by cellular seeding across the synovial space in this model. Following their paper of 1970, Salamon and coworkers (1973) have reported that, by the criteria of light, polarizing, and electron microscopy, tendons stored in physiologic saline at 4°C following irradiation had a healing pattern similar to autografts.

In conclusion, it seems that there is as yet no universally accepted method of preservation of allogeneic tendon. However, certain principles appear to emerge: the process of preservation should reduce or abolish the allograft antigenicity that lies in its cells and ground substance, and should neither affect the physical integrity nor decrease the relative immunologic inertness of the constituent collagen fibrils. It remains to be determined whether the changes in tendon associated with aging affect the latter.

In clinical practice, the method of preservation that has received the most detailed reports is the use of Cialit solution (Herzog, 1963; Iselin and Flores, 1963, 1972; Seiffert, 1967, 1971; Voorhoeve, 1972). It appears to go furthest towards satisfying the above requirements.

Composite Flexor Tendon Allografts. In an attempt at avoiding some of the problems of adhesion formation that complicate flexor tendon replacement grafting in potentially unfavorable cases, Peacock (1959b) investigated the feasibility of transplanting the complete flexor tendon mechanism. Following encouraging animal experimentation, he successfully performed an allograft procedure in man. Subsequent reports of further successful animal and human cases (Peacock and Madden, 1967; Hueston and coworkers, 1967; Furlow, 1969; Cameron and coworkers, 1971) give this procedure a small but definite place in reconstructive surgery of the hand.

In man, the graft consists of both flexor tendons and the digital theca which is removed intact from the donor. To ensure complete integrity of the synovial sheath, the periosteum and the appropriate volar plates are excised with the specimen. In keeping with Peacock's concept, no significant adhesions have been reported to occur within the synovial sheath of the digital theca. The few complete failures have been due to intractable adhesions around the nonsheathed parts of the flexor tendon allografts. It is of interest that in 70 per cent of these grafts (Peacock and Madden, 1967), which were never stored for more than a few days at 4°C, restricting adhesions sufficient to prevent adequate function did not occur.

Revascularization of the nonsheath parts of the composite allograft is by direct invasion of blood vessels, like the secondary revascularization of autograft tendon. The digital theca is also revascularized by the same method, vessels containing cellular elements of blood being visible on the seventh day (Cameron and co-workers, 1971).

The sheathed part of the allograft is revascularized by the ingrowth of capillaries through the vincula. Tobias and Seiffert (1972), using Kiton Fast Green as a vital dye, found green cross banding in one graft at the end of the first week. This may have been an example of primary revascularization as noted by Bergljung (1968). All of the heterotopically placed rat allografts were revascularized by four weeks, whereas Hueston, Hubble and Rigg (1967), using xenografts (man to dog), found that cellular repopulation had only just started by this time, perhaps because of the greater antigenic disparity of their model. Using a radioactive isotope technique to label rat isografts and allografts, Tobias and Seiffert (1972) found that some of the labeled collagen was still present at ten months, residual activity being higher in the allografts. Cameron and associates (1971), using simian allografts, noted that lyophilization did not appear to alter acceptability of the allografts. Hueston and co-workers (1967) failed to note any difference between their fresh xenografts and those that had been stored deep frozen for a few days.

Some of the immunologic implications of the transplantation of tendon allografts have already been discussed. During the use of composite tendon allografts in man, Peacock and Madden (1967) reported that, in two of their first ten cases, enlargement of the epitrochlear nodes was noted two weeks postoperatively. These subsided within ten days. Both they and Cameron and associates (1971) have remarked on the destruction of the tenocytes by the end of the first week. These observations are consistent with an immunologic reaction.

The Delay in Allograft vis-à-vis Autograft Tendon Healing. As has already been noted (see p. 279), the death of tenocytes is associated with loss of transverse cohesiveness due to failure of the ground substance. This occurs in autografts (Peacock, 1957), xenografts (Peacock, 1959a), and allografts (Peacock and Madden, 1967). Recovery of this property, which is critical to the holding power of sutures and is dependent upon the colonization of the allograft by recipient cells, requires a week longer than in an autograft. It is essential to remember this in clinical practice, so that an adequate period of immobilization may be prescribed. Peacock and Madden (1967) have found that 28 days is adequate.

THE FATE OF XENOGRAFT TENDON

Xenograft tendon has been used by a number of investigators, but it has not found favor for clinical use. Allogeneic tendon, once cleared of cells (and ground substance), presents little, if any, antigenic challenge to the host, as collagen is species-specific (Adelmann and co-workers, 1968; Michaeli and coworkers, 1970) (see above). However, this is not so with xenogeneic tendon, which is, therefore, on theoretical grounds, likely to cause greater host reaction. Klein and Lewis (1972) found that radioisotopically labeled xenografts of rat tail tendon, when transplanted into the tendo calcaneus of guinea pigs, not only had lost 88 per cent of their collagen mass at the end of the first month after grafting but also had lost morphologic integrity. These processes were complete by three months and were in marked contrast to the results using allograft rat tail tendon, which remained morphologically intact. Heterotopically placed (subcutaneous) xenografts do not lose this integrity (Peacock, 1959a; Peacock and Petty, 1960; Hueston and coworkers, 1967). The reason for this disparity in results between orthotopically and heterotopically placed tendon remains a matter for speculation.

REFERENCES

Adams, W.: On the Reparative Process in Human Tendons. London, Churchill, 1860.

Adamson, J. E., Horton, C. E., and Mladick, R. A.: Observations on the effect of silicone fluid and flexor tendon healing in the dog. Surg. Forum, *21*:502, 1970.

Adelmann, B. C., Glynn, L. E., and Kirrane, J.: Delayed-type hypersensitivity reactions of native and denatured rat and calf skin-collagen in sensitized guinea pigs. Fed. Proc., *27*:263, 1968.

Akeson, W.: The connective tissue response to immobility. Total mucopolysaccharide changes in dog tendon. J. Surg. Res., *4*:523, 1964.

Alexandre, J. H.: Combined malformations of palmaris longus and plantaris muscles. Ann. Chir. Plast., *15*:233, 1970.

Andreef, I., and Wladimirov, B.: The vascularization of homogenous tendon graft. An experimental study. Acta Orthop. Belg., *38*:312, 1972.

Andreef, I., Dimoff, G., and Metschkarski, S.: A comparative experimental study on transplantation of autogenous and homogenous tendon tissue. Acta Orthop. Scand., *58*:35, 1967.

Anzel, S. H., Lipscomb, P. R., and Grindlay, J. H.: Construction of artificial tendon sheaths in dogs. Am. J. Surg., *101*:355, 1961.

Artomonova, A. I., quoted by Kovalenko and Demichev (1969).

Ashley, F. L., McConnell, D. V., Polak, T., Stone, R. S., and Marmor, L.: An evaluation of the healing process in avian digital flexor tendons and grafts following the application of an artificial tendon sheath. Plast. Reconstr. Surg., *33*:411, 1964.

Ashley, F. L., Stone, R. S., Alonso-Artieda, M., Syverud, J. M., Edwards, J. W., Sloan, R. F., and Mooney, S. A.: Experimental and clinical studies on the application of monomolecular cellulose filter tubes to create artificial tendon sheaths in digits. Plast. Reconstr. Surg., *23*:526, 1959; Follow-up clinic, Plast. Reconstr. Surg., *43*:625, 1969.

Bader, K. F., and Curtin, J. W.: Clinical survey of silicone underlays and pulleys in tendon surgery in hands. Plast. Reconstr. Surg., *47*:576, 1971.

Bassett, C. A. L., and Carrol, R. E.: Formation of tendon sheath by silicone rod implants. J. Bone Joint Surg., *45A*:884, 1963.

Becton, J. L., Winkelmann, R. K., and Lipscomb, P. R.: Innervation of human finger tendons as determined by histochemical techniques. J. Bone Joint Surg. *48A*:1519, 1966.

Bellamy, G., and Bornstein, P.: Evidence for procollagen, a biosynthetic precursor of collagen. Proc. Natl. Acad. Sci., USA, *68*:1138, 1971.

Bergljung, L.: Vascular reactions after tendon suture and tendon transplantation. Scand. J. Plast. Reconstr. Surg., Suppl. 4, 1968.

Beringer, U. V., and Darkshevich, U. N.: Dynamics of morphological changes after homografts of tendons preserved in anticytolytic solutions. Acta Chir. Plast., *11*:187, 1969.

Birch, J. R., and Lindsay, W. K.: Histochemical studies of the fate of autogenous digital flexor tendon grafts in the chicken. Can. J. Surg., *7*:454, 1964.

Birdsell, D. C., Tustanoff, E. R., and Lindsay, W. K.: Collagen production in regenerating tendon. Plast. Reconstr. Surg., *37*:504, 1966.

Bora, F. W., Lane, J. M., and Prockop, D. J.: Inhibitors of collagen biosynthesis as a means of controlling scar formation in tendon injury. J. Bone Joint Surg., *54A*:1501, 1972.

Boyes, J. H.: Personal communication, 1968.

Boyes, J. H., and Stark, H. H.: Flexor-tendon grafts in the fingers and thumb. A study of factors influencing results in 1,000 cases. J. Bone Joint Surg., *53A*:1332, 1972.

Braithwaite, F., and Brockis, J. G.: The vascularization of a tendon graft. Br. J. Plast. Surg., *4*:130, 1951.

Brand, P. W.: Tendon grafting. Illustrated by a new operation for intrinsic paralysis of the fingers. J. Bone Joint Surg., *43B*:444, 1961.

Brockis, J. G.: The blood supply of the flexor and extensor tendons of the fingers in man. J. Bone Jont Surg., *35B*:131, 1953.

Bunnell, S.: Repair of tendons in the fingers and description of two new instruments. Surg. Gynecol. Obstet., *26*:103, 1918.

Bunnell, S.: Repair of tendons in the fingers. Surg. Gynecol. Obstet., *35*:88, 1922.

Bunnell, S., cited by Peer, L. A.: Transplantation of Tissues. Vol. 1. Baltimore, Williams & Wilkins Company, 1955.

Bunnell, S.: *In* Boyes, J. H. (Ed.): Surgery of the Hand. 5th Ed., Philadelphia, J. B. Lippincott Company, 1970.

Burman, M. S.: The use of a nylon sheath in the secondary repair of torn finger flexor tendons. Bull. Hosp. Joint Dis., *5*:122, 1944.

Cameron, R. R., Conrad, R. N., and Latham, W. D.: Preserved composite tendon allografts: A comparative study of changes in length, elasticity and anastomotic and lineal tensile strength. Surg. Forum, *21*:506, 1970.

Cameron, R. R., Conrad, R. N., Sell, K. W., and Latham, W. D.: Freeze-dried composite tendon allografts: An experimental study. Plast. Reconstr. Surg., *47*:39, 1971.

Carstam, N.: The effect of cortisone on the formation of tendon adhesions and on tendon healing. An experimental investigation in the rabbit. Acta Chir. Scand., Suppl. 182, 1953.

Chaplin, D. M.: Vascular anatomy within normal tendons, divided tendons, free tendon grafts and pedicle tendon grafts in rabbits. J. Bone Joint Surg., *55B*:369, 1973.

Colville, J., Callison, J. R., and White, W. L.: Role of mesotenon in tendon blood supply. Plast. Reconstr. Surg., *43*:53, 1969.

Conway, H., Smith, J. W., and Elliott, M. P.: Studies on the revascularization of tendons grafted by the silicone rod technique. Plast. Reconstr. Surg. *46*:582, 1970.

Cooper, D. R., and Russell, A. E.: Intra- and intermolecular cross-links in collagen in tendon, cartilage and bone. Clin. Orthop., *67*:188, 1969.

Cooper, R. R., and Misol, S.: Tendon and ligament insertion. A light and electron microscopic study. J. Bone Joint Surg., *52A*:1, 1970.

Cordrey, L. J., McCorkle, H., and Hilton, E.: A comparative study of fresh autogenous and preserved homogenous tendon grafts in rabbits. J. Bone Joint Surg., *45B*:182, 1963.

Crockford, D. A., Rapaport, F. T., and Converse, J. M.: Unpublished data, 1971.

Daseler, E. H., and Anson, B. J.: The plantaris muscle. An anatomical study of 750 specimens. J. Bone Joint Surg., *25*:822, 1943.

Day, T. D.: The mode of reaction of interstitial connective tissue with water. J. Physiol., *109*:380, 1949.

Demichev, N. P.: Assessing the biological activity of conserved tendon by tissue culture. Acta Chir. Plast., *11*:56, 1969.

Diamant, J., Keller, A., Baer, E., Litt, M., and Arridge, R. G. C.: Collagen; ultrastructure and its relation to mechanical properties as a function of ageing. Proc. R. Soc. Lond. [Biol.], *180*:293, 1972.

Dorner, R. W.: Changes in glycosaminoglycan composition associated with maturation of regenerating rabbit tendon. Arch. Biochem. Biophys., *128*:34, 1968.

Douglas, L. G., Jackson, S. H., and Lindsay, W. K.: The effects of dexamethasone, norethandrolone, promethazine and a tension relieving procedure on collagen synthesis in healing flexor tendons as estimated by tritiated proline up-take studies. Can. J. Surg., *10*:36, 1967.

Edwards, D. A. W.: The blood supply and lymphatic drainage of tendons. J. Anat., *80*:147, 1946.

Edwards, L. C., and Dunphy, J. E.: Wound healing. A. Injury and normal repair. New Engl. J. Med., *259*:224, 1958.

Elliott, D. H.: The structure and function of mammalian tendon. Biol. Rev., *40*:392, 1965.

Farkas, L. G., McCain, W. G., Sweeney, P., Wilson, W. D., Hurst, L. N., and Lindsay, W. K.: An experimental study of the changes following silastic rod preparation of a pseudo tendon sheath and subsequent tendon grafting. J. Bone Joint Surg., *55A*:1149, 1973.

Fetrow, K. O.: Tenolysis in the hand and wrist. A clinical evaluation of two hundred and twenty flexor and extensor tenolyses. J. Bone Joint Surg., *49A*:667, 1967.

Field, P. L.: Tendon fibre arrangement and blood supply. Aust. N.Z. J. Surg., *40*:298, 1971.

Flynn, J. E., and Graham, J. H.: Healing of tendon wounds. Am. J. Surg., *109*:315, 1965.

Furlow, L. T.: Homologous flexor mechanism replacement in four fingers. Plast. Reconstr. Surg., *43*:531, 1969.

Gabbiani, G., Ryan, G. B., and Majno, G.: Presence of modified fibroblasts in granulation tissue and their possible role in wound contraction. Experimentia, *27*:549, 1971.

Garlock, J. H.: The repair process in wounds of tendons, and in tendon grafts. Ann. Surg., *85*:92, 1927.

Geldmacher, J.: Prevention of adhesions in free flexor tendon grafting. Trans. Internatl. Soc. Plast. Surgeons, Fifth Congress, 1971. Australia, Butterworth, 1971.

Ghadially, F. N., and Roy, S.: Ultrastructure of synovial joints in health and disease. London, Butterworth, 1969.

Gillman, T.: Tissue regeneration. *In* Bourne, G. H. (Ed.): Structural Aspects of Ageing. London, Pitman, 1961.

Glissan, D. J.: The use of the plantaris tendon in certain types of plastic surgery. Aust. N.Z. J. Surg., *2*:64, 1932.

Gonzalez, R. I.: Experimental tendon repair within the flexor tunnels. Use of polyethylene tubes for improvement of functional results in the dog. Surgery, *26*:181, 1949.

Gonzalez, R. I.: Experimental use of Teflon in tendon surgery. Plast. Reconstr. Surg., *23*:535, 1959.

Grant, M. E., and Prockop, D. J.: The biosynthesis of collagen. New Engl. J. Med., *286*:194; 242; 291, 1972.

Gray's Anatomy. 35th Ed. Warwick, R., and Williams, P. L. (Eds.): London, Longman, 1973.

Greenlee, T. K., and Ross, R.: The development of the rat flexor digital tendon, a fine structure study. J. Ultrastruct. Res., *18*:354, 1967.

Hage, J., and Dupuis, C. C.: The intriguing fate of tendon grafts in small children's hands and their results. Br. J. Plast. Surg., *18*:341, 1965.

Harkness, R. D.: Mechanical properties of collagenous tissues. *In* Gould, B. S., and Ramchandran, G. S. (Eds.): Treatise on Collagen. Vol. 2A. New York, Academic Press, 1968, p. 254.

Heller, P., and Yakulis, V. J.: Auto-antigenicity of connective tissue extracts. Proc. Soc. Exp. Biol. Med., *112*:1064, 1963.

Henz, C. W., and Mayer, L.: An experimental study of silk-tendon plastics with particular reference to the prevention of post-operative adhesions. Surg. Gynecol. Obstet., *19*:10, 1914.

Herzog, K. H.: Experimentelle Grundlagen der Transplantation von konserviertem Schnengewebe. Langenbecks Arch. Klin. Chir., *303*:313, 1963.

Herzog, M., Lindsay, W. K., and McCann, W. G.: Effect of B-aminopropionitrile on adhesions following digital flexor tendon repair in chickens. Surg. Forum, *21*:509, 1970.

Hueston, J. T., Hubble, B., and Rigg, B. R.: Homografts of the digital flexor tendon system. Aust. N. Z. J. Surg., *36*:269, 1967.

Hunter, J. M., and Salisbury, R. E.: Use of gliding artificial implants to produce tendon sheaths. Techniques and results in children. Plast. Reconstr. Surg., *45*:564, 1970.

Iselin, M., and Flores, A.: Surgical use of homologous tendon grafts preserved in Cialit. Plast. Reconstr. Surg., *32*:401, 1963; Follow-up clinic, *49*:208, 1972.

Jackson, D. S.: Chondroitin sulphuric acid as a factor in the stability of tendon. Biochem. J., *54*:638, 1953.

Jackson, D. S., and Bentley, J. P.: Collagen glycosaminoglycan interactions. *In* Gould, B. S., and Ramchandran, G. S. (Eds.): Treatise on Collagen. Vol. 2A. New York, Academic Press, 1968.

Jackson, S. F.: The morphogenesis of avian tendon. Proc. R. Soc. Lond., Series B, *144*:556, 1956.

Jackson, S. F.: The morphogenesis of collagen. *In* Gould, B. S., and Ramchandran, G. S. (Eds.): Treatise on Collagen. Vol. 2B. New York, Academic Press, 1968.

James, J. I. P.: The value of tenolysis. Hand, *1*:118, 1969.

Ketchum, L. D.: Effects of triamcinolone on tendon healing and function. A laboratory study. Plast. Reconstr. Surg., *47*:471, 1971.

Klein, L., and Lewis, J.: Simultaneous quantification of ³H-collagen loss and ¹H-collagen replacement during healing of rat tendon grafts. J. Bone Joint Surg., *54A*:137, 1972.

Klein, L., Vessely, J. C., and Heiple, K. G.: Quantification of ³H-collagen loss of rat allografted and isografted tendon. J. Bone Joint Surg., *51A*:891, 1969.

Klein, L., Lunseth, P. A., and Aadalen, R. J.: Comparison of functional and nonfunctional tendon grafts. Isotopic measurement of collagen turnover and mass. J. Bone Joint Surg., *54A*:1745, 1972.

Kovalenko, P. P., and Demichev, N. P.: Homoplasty of tendon under experimental and clinical conditions. Ortop. Travmatol. Protez., *7*:75, 1969.

Kovalenko, P. P., and Demichev, N. P.: Homologous tendonplasty of hand and finger tendons. Acta Chir. Plast., *14*:60, 1972.

Last, R. J.: Anatomy, Regional and Applied. 4th Ed. London, J. & A. Churchill, 1966.

Le Double A. F.: Traité des Variations du Système Musculaire de l'Homme. Paris, Schleicher, 1897.

Leffert, R. D., Weiss, M. D., and Athanasoulis, C. A.: The vincula, with particular reference to their vessels and nerves. J. Bone Joint Surg., *56A*:1191, 1974.

Lindsay, W. K., and Birch, J. R.: The fibroblast in flexor tendon healing. Plast. Reconstr. Surg., *34*:223, 1964.

Lindsay, W. K., and McDougall, E. P.: Digital flexor tendons: an experimental study. Part III. The fate of autogenous digital flexor tendon grafts. Br. J. Plast. Surg., *13*:293, 1961.

Lindsay, W. K., Thomson, H. G., and Walker, F. G.: Digital flexor tendons: an experimental study. Part I. The significance of each component of the flexor mechanism in tendon healing. Br. J. Plast. Surg., *12*:289, 1960.

Lindsay, W. K., Thomson, H. G., and Walker, F. G.: Digital flexor tendons: an experimental study. Part II. The significance of a gap occurring at the line of suture. Br. J. Plast. Surg., *13*:1, 1961.

Lowry, O. H., Gilligan, D. R., and Katersky, E. M.: The determination of collagen and elastin in tissues, with results obtained in various normal tissues from different species. J. Biol. Chem., *139*:795, 1941.

Machado, A. B. M., and DiDio, L. J. A.: Frequency of muscularis palmaris longus studied in vivo in some Amazon Indians. Am. J. Physiol. Anthropol., *27*:11, 1967.

Madden, J. W.: On "The contractile fibroblast." Plast. Reconstr. Surg., *52*:291, 1973.

Mason, M. L., and Allen, H. S.: The rate of healing of tendons. An experimental study of tensile strength. Ann. Surg., *113*:424, 1941.

Mason, M. L., and Shearon, C. G.: The process of tendon repair. An experimental study of tendon suture and tendon graft. Arch. Surg., *25*:615, 1932.

Mayer, L.: The physiological method of tendon transplantation. I. Historical; anatomy and physiology of tendons. Surg. Gynecol. Obstet., *22*:182, 1916. II. Operative technique, *22*:298, 1916. III. Experimental and clinical experiences, *22*:472, 1916.

Michaeli, D., Martin, G. R., and Benjamini, E.: Localization of the antigenic determinants of collagen. *In* Balazs, E. A. (Ed.): Chemistry and Molecular Biology of the Intercellular Matrix. Vol. 1. New York, Academic Press, 1970.

Milgram, J. E.: Transplantation of tendons through preformed gliding channels. Bull. Hosp. Joint Dis., *21*:250, 1960.

Mollier, G. (1937), cited by Elliott (1965).

Mshvidobadze, M. V.: Transplantation of homo- and heterogenous tendon stored in meda solution. Acta Chir. Plast. (Praha), *8*:140, 1966.

Munro, I. R., Lindsay, W. K., and Jackson, S. H.: A synchronous study of collagen and mucopolysaccharide in healing of flexor tendons of chickens. Plast. Reconstr. Surg., *45*:493, 1970.

Nageotte, J.: Trame et cellules dans le tendon. Arch. Biol. (Paris), *47*:605, 1936.

Neuberger, A., and Slack, H. G. B.: The metabolism of collagen from liver, bone, skin, and tendon in the normal rat. Biochem. J., *53*:47, 1953.

Nisbet, N. W.: Anatomy of the calcaneal tendon of the rabbit. J. Bone Joint Surg., *42B*:360, 1960.

Peacock, E. E.: Vascular basis of tendon repair. Surg. Forum, *8*:65, 1957.

Peacock, E. E.: Morphology of homologous and heterologous tendon grafts. Surg. Gynecol. Obstet., *109*:735, 1959a.

Peacock, E. E.: Some problems in flexor tendon healing. Surgery, *45*:415, 1959b.

Peacock, E. E.: A study of the circulation in normal tendons and healing grafts. Ann. Surg., *149*:415, 1959c.

Peacock, E. E.: Some aspects of fibrogenesis during healing of primary and secondary wounds. Surg. Gynecol. Obstet., *115*:408, 1962.

Peacock, E. E.: The influence of modern connective tissue biology upon surgery of the hand. *In* Cooper, P., and Nyhus, L. M. (Eds.): Surgery Annual. Vol. 3. London, Butterworth, 1971.

Peacock, E. E., and Madden, J. W.: Human composite flexor tendon allografts. Ann. Surg., *166*:624, 1967.

Peacock, E. E., and Petty, J.: Antigenicity of tendon. Surg. Gynecol. Obstet., *110*:187, 1960.

Peer, L. A.: Transplantation of Tissues. Vol. 1. Cartilage, Bone, Fascia, Tendon and Muscle. Baltimore, Williams & Wilkins Company, 1955.

Pilcher, R.: Repair of hernia with plantaris tendon graft. A.M.A. Arch. Surg., *38*:16, 1939.

Potenza, A. D.: Tendon healing within the flexor digital sheath in the dog. An experimental study. J. Bone Joint Surg., *44A*:49, 1962a.

Potenza, A. D.: Detailed evaluation of healing processes in canine flexor digital tendons. Milit. Med., *127*:34, 1962b.

Potenza, A. D.: Critical evaluation of flexor-tendon healing and adhesion formation within artificial digital sheaths. An experimental study. J. Bone Joint Surg., *45A*:1217, 1963.

Potenza, A. D.: The healing of autogenous tendon grafts within the flexor digital sheath in dogs. J. Bone Joint Surg., *46A*:1462, 1964a.

Potenza, A. D.: Healing and fate of lyophilized homologous flexor tendon grafts within the digital flexor sheath. J. Bone Joint Surg., *46A*:908, 1964b.

Potenza, A. D., cited by Verdan (1972).

Quain's Elements of Anatomy. 11th Ed. Vol. IV. Part II. Myology. Bryce, T. H. (Ed.). New York, Longmans, Green & Company, 1923.

Rank, B. K., Wakefield, A. R., and Hueston, J. T.: Surgery of Repair as Applied to Hand Injuries. 3rd Ed. Edinburgh, Livingstone, 1968, p. 33.

Ranvier, L. (1889), cited by Elliott (1965).

Reimann, A. F., Daseler, E. H., Anson, B. J., and Beaton, L. E.: The palmaris longus muscle and tendon. A study of 1600 extremities. Anat. Rec., *89*:495, 1944.

Reis, N. D.: Experimental tendon repair: Modification of natural healing by silicone rubber sheath. Br. J. Plast. Surg., *22*:134, 1969.

Ross, R., Everett, N. B., and Tyler, R.: Wound healing and collagen formation. VI. The origin of the wound fibroblast studied in parabiosis. J. Cell Biol., *44*:645, 1970.

Rothman, R. H., and Slogoff, S.: The effect of immobilization on the vascular bed of tendon. Surg. Gynecol. Obstet., *124*:1064, 1967.

Salamon, A., Hámori, J., Deák, G., and Mayer, F.: Submicroscopic investigation of autogenous tendon grafts. Acta Morphol. Acad. Sci. Hung., *18*:23, 1970.

Salamon, A., Deák, G., Hámori, J., Mayer, F., and Temes, G.: Submicroscopic investigation of homologous tendon grafts preserved by means of different methods. Acta Morphol. Acad. Sci. Hung., *21*:175, 1973.

Schäfer, E. A. (1912), quoted by Elliott (1965).

Schatzker, J., and Brånemark, P.: Intravital observations on the microvascular anatomy and microcirculation of the tendon. Acta Orthop. Scand., Suppl. 126, 1969.

Schiller, S., Matthews, M. B., Cifonelli, J. A., and Dorfman, A.: The metabolism of mucopolysaccharides in animals. J. Biol. Chem., *218*:139, 1956.

Seiffert, K. E.: Biologische grundlagen der hormologen transplantation konservierter bindegewebe. Hefte Unfallheilk, *93*:1, 1967.

Seiffert, K. E.: Preserved grafts in reconstructive surgery. Trans. Internatl. Soc. Plast. Surgeons, Fifth Congress, 1971. Australia, Butterworth, 1971.

Seiffert, K. E., and Schmit, K. P.: Preserved tendon grafts in hand surgery. Trans. Internatl. Soc. Plast. Surgeons, Fifth Congress, 1971. Australia, Butterworth, 1971.

Sick, H.: Les réservoirs vasculaires au voisinage de la couche de pression des tendons et des ménisques. C.R. Assoc. Anat., *148*:996, 1970.

Sinex, F. M.: The role of collagen in ageing. *In* Gould, B. S., and Ramchandran, G. S. (Eds.): Treatise on Collagen. Vol. 2B. New York, Academic Press, 1968.

Skoog, T., and Persson, B. H.: An experimental study of the early healing of tendons. Plast. Reconstr. Surg., *13*:384, 1954.

Smith, J. W.: The blood supply of tendons. Am. J. Surg., *109*:272, 1965.

Srugi, S., and Adamson, J. E.: Comparative study of tendon suture materials in dogs. Plast. Reconstr. Surg., *50*:31, 1972.

Ssawwin, V. J.: Abführende lymphgefässe der Synovialsehnenscheiden der extremitäten des menschen. Anat. Anz., *80*:119, 1935. Quoted by Jaffe, H. L.: Metabolic, Degenerative, and Inflammatory Diseases of Bones and Joints. Philadelphia, Lea and Febiger, 1972.

Stillwell, D. L.: The innervation of tendons and aponeuroses. Am. J. Anat., *100*:289, 1957.

Taylor, A. C., and Lehrfeld, J. D.: The determination of survival time of skin homografts in the rat by observation of vascular changes in the graft. Plast. Reconstr. Surg., *12*:423, 1953.

Thompson, R. V.: An evaluation of flexor tendon grafting. Br. J. Plast. Surg., *20*:21, 1967.

Tobias, M., and Seiffert, K. E.: Collagen metabolism in iso- and homografts of tendons. Br. J. Plast. Surg., *25*:83, 1972.

Verdan, C. E.: Half a century of flexor-tendon grafting. Current status and changing philosophies. J. Bone Joint Surg., *54A*:472, 1972.

Voorhoeve, A.: The possibility of using homologous preserved tendon material. Chir. Praxis, *16*:1, 1972.

Weiner, L. J., and Peacock, E. E.: Biologic principles affecting repair of flexor tendons. *In* Welch, C. E., and

Handy, J. W. (Eds.): Advances in Surgery. Vol. 5. Chicago, Year Book Medical Publishers Inc., 1971.

White, N. B., Ter-Pogossian, M. M., and Stein, A. H.: A method to determine the rate of blood flow in long bone and selected soft tissues. Surg. Gynecol. Obstet., *119*: 535, 1964.

White, W. L.: Tendon grafts: A consideration of their source, procurement and suitability. Surg. Clin. North Am., *40*:403, 1960a.

White, W. L.: The unique, accessible and useful plantaris tendon. Plast. Reconstr. Surg., *25*:133, 1960b.

Winkler, G.: Caractères des vaisseaux para- et péritendineux des fléchisseurs des doigts. C. R. Assoc. Anat., *148*:581, 1970.

Wood, G. C., and Keech, M. K.: The formation of fibrils from collagen solutions. 1. The effect of experimental conditions: Kinetic and electron microscopic studies. Biochem. J., *75*:588, 1960.

Wrenn, R. N., Goldner, J. L., and Markee, J. L.: An experimental study of the effect of cortisone on the healing process and tensile strength of tendons. J. Bone Joint Surg., *36A*:588, 1954.

CHAPTER 11

TRANSPLANTATION OF SKELETAL MUSCLE

NOEL THOMPSON, F.R.C.S.

In 1874 Zielonko, a Russian pathologist working in Strasbourg, reported the first attempt to transplant free autografts of skeletal muscle in the frog. The thigh muscles were transferred into the lymph sac of the same animal, but rapid necrosis followed without any evidence of regeneration of muscle. Similar failure resulted when Magnus (1890) transplanted segments of quadriceps femoris muscle into a corresponding site in the opposite limb; histologic degeneration and absorption of all grafts occurred over a period of 7 to 60 days.

These results were confirmed by the classic studies of Volkmann (1893). He replaced completely excised pieces of thigh muscle in the same site, or a corresponding site in the opposite limb of both rabbits and dogs. The grafts were later examined microscopically over a period of 3 to 60 days. He concluded that such grafts suffered immediate necrosis with subsequent progressive resorption and fibrous replacement by scar tissue. During subsequent years repeated confirmation of these conclusions has been obtained. Roy (1966), who used free autografts of the dorsal musculature in dogs as transplants into the thigh muscles, found that total replacement of the graft by fibrous tissue occurred within eight weeks. Peer in 1955 stated the position of free autogenous muscle grafts in the field of transplantation: "All such transplants degenerate and lose contractile power almost immediately as a result of loss of blood supply,

but even where vascularity is maintained gradual but progressive atrophy results from loss of motor nerve supply only."

It is, however, well established that by the ingrowth of motor nerve fibers, arising from the original or some other motor nerve cells, a denervated muscle with unimpaired blood supply may have some function restored before complete atrophy occurs. Heineke (1914) first demonstrated that implantation of the central end of an adjacent severed motor nerve into the denervated limb muscles of a rabbit resulted in the restoration of muscular contractions on faradic stimulation of the implanted nerve. Erlacher (1915) obtained successful "muscular neurotization" of a paralyzed muscle in guinea pigs by applying to the muscle a muscle flap carrying normal neurovascular supply. The outgrowing motor axons spread rapidly along the endoneurial tubes of the degenerated nerves. They were also capable of direct spread along the denervated muscle fibers which they then penetrated to form motor end-plates. These findings have been confirmed histologically in dogs (Steindler, 1916) and rabbits (Aitken, 1950). In rats (Hoffman, 1951) direct nerve transplantation into a normal muscle resulted in "hyperneurotization" by the creation of new motor end-plates on already fully innervated muscle fibers. There was even the appearance of a new end-plate zone at the site of implantation of the additional nerve (Gwyn and Aitken, 1964).

RECENT INVESTIGATION OF SKELETAL MUSCLE GRAFTS

The successful transplantation of skeletal muscle as an autogenous graft has resulted from a consideration of two additional factors: retention of full muscle fiber length in the graft, and the effects of preliminary denervation.

Muscle Fiber Length

Peer (1955) suggested that a contributory factor relevant to the lack of success of muscle transplantation might lie in the exceptional length of the myofibrils. The latter can traverse the full length of the muscle belly. Consequently, a graft consisting only of part of a muscle might be expected to fail since it would represent an attempt to transplant segments of cells rather than the complete cell entities. Although the evidence is conflicting, the data certainly suggest the existence of muscle fibers of considerable length. Thus, in the rabbit the gastrocnemius (Huber, 1916) predominantly has fibers extending the full length of the muscle, while the sartorius (Harreveld, 1947) has fibers about one third the length of the muscle. In man, individual fibers traverse the full length of the muscle in the sartorius (Lockhart and Brandt, 1938), as well as the biceps femoris and semimembranosus muscles (Barrett, 1962).

The effect of transplanting the entire muscle as a complete entity in dogs was therefore investigated (Thompson, 1971a) by applying 20 free grafts taken from the foreleg (using the pronator teres muscle in the majority) to the muscles of the face (the masseter and perioral muscles) and the hind leg (the gracilis and sartorius muscles). The grafts were submitted to faradic stimulation and biopsy examination at intervals of up to six months postoperatively. It was found at six months after transplantation that almost routine macroscopic survival of the graft occurred (about 20 per cent of its original volume). However, microscopic examination showed that only $1/4$ to $1/2$ of the surviving graft tissue consisted of recognizable muscle fibers (Fig. 11–1, *A*). Atrophy of muscle fibers was usual, with widespread evidence of de-differentiation of muscle fibers into collagen; nuclei and striations were well preserved and vascularization was good. Axonal reinnervation was demonstrated and motor end-plates were present (Fig. 11–1, *B, C*).

Some of the motor end-plates preserved a functional appearance, though many showed degenerative changes with elongation and diffusion of enzyme outside the subneural apparatus.

It was concluded that the preservation of full fiber length in muscle grafts was of importance in seeking survival of the transplant, and resulted in a 5 to 10 per cent histologic survival of the transplanted muscle tissue. For useful clinical application it was clear that an additional factor assisting graft survival must be sought, and this was found in preliminary denervation of the muscle entity prior to transplantation.

Preliminary Denervation of the Muscle Graft

It is now fully established (Sandow, 1970) that there are two entirely distinct types of skeletal muscle fibers:

1. Type I is rich in myoglobin and in enzymes of lipid and mitochondrial oxidative metabolism, but low in both phosphorylase and myofibrillar ATP-ase; it is the preponderant type of fiber in red, slow muscles, e.g., soleus.
2. Type II ("glycolytic") has the opposite characteristics. It is poor in myoglobin and in lipid and mitochondrial enzymes, but is rich in both phosphorylase and myofibrillar ATP-ase; it is the preponderant type in white, fast muscles, e.g., gastrocnemius.

Recent work on the effects of denervation upon the enzyme constitution of red and white muscle in the rat, using biochemical quantitative estimations (Hogan, Dawson, and Romanul, 1965) and qualitative histochemical staining (Romanul and Hogan, 1965), has demonstrated that in the gastrocnemius muscle there is a progressive loss of glycolytic anaerobic enzymes, while the red fibers of the soleus muscle show a steady decrease of aerobic and lipolytic enzymes. As one would expect, the white fibers of the gastrocnemius muscle become pink in color because of an increase in blood supply and of myoglobin. Using similar histochemical methods, these results on the denervation of white muscle have been confirmed in the rat (Smith, 1965) and the guinea pig (Hogenhuis and Engel, 1965).

Denervation not only produced in white muscle a rapid change in enzyme content which allowed diminished energy requirements to be met by the oxidative metabolism of ketones and fatty acids, but there was also a parallel increase in the density of the capillary

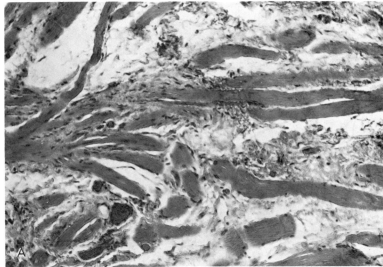

FIGURE 11–1. Dog. Free graft of pronator teres muscle applied to the gracilis and sartorius muscles of the hind leg. *A*, At six months after transfer. There is atrophy and fibrous replacement of the muscle, but many fibers show well-preserved striations and nuclei. Hematoxylin-eosin, × 100. *B*, At six months after grafting. There is terminal arborization of axon over muscle fiber, demonstrating reinnervation. Bodian, × 1000. *C*, At three months after grafting. Cholinesterase staining to show motor end-plates, most of which are degenerative, but a few (*arrows*) show normal contour and peripheral guttering, indicating reinnervation. Koelle, × 100.

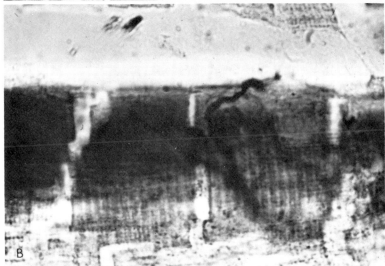

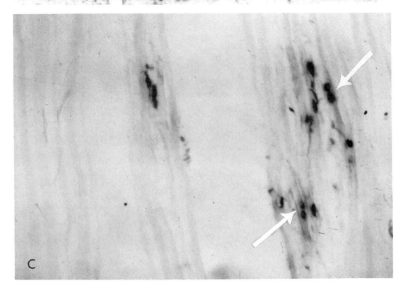

network around each muscle fiber (Romanul and Hogan, 1965). It is clear, therefore, that denervation might constitute a useful preliminary measure in the preconditioning of skeletal muscle for free transplantation. It was assumed that the diminished metabolic requirements might enable graft survival to become possible during the initial period of three or four days of total ischemia which exists before a local blood supply becomes established by the direct anastomosis of graft and host vessels at the graft recipient site (Peer and Walker, 1951). Moreover, revascularization would be accelerated and intensified by the enriched blood vessel content of the graft itself.

It is also known that axonal regeneration is more effective in the presence of preliminary denervation. Gutmann (1942) found that when the rabbit's sciatic nerve was crushed twice at intervals 16 to 42 days apart, axonal regeneration was significantly more rapid than after a single crush. This finding suggested that the improved regeneration might be due to an increase in the number of Schwann cells accessible to the regenerated nerve fibers in the nerve distal to the lesion. Lieberman (1971)

stated that during the first week after nerve injury the protein synthetic machinery of traumatized neurons, as indicated by morphologic and biochemical criteria, is in disarray; over the next week this machinery reorganizes and may hypertrophy to such a degree that the protein content may be doubled. Ducker, Kempe, and Hayes (1969) have suggested that axonal outgrowth would proceed faster after a second nerve lesion than after the first if there were an interval of two to three weeks between the two lesions, a thesis given firm supportive evidence by McQuarrie and Grafstein (1973).

It seems certain that the metabolic processes characteristic of red and white muscle are determined by their nerve supply. In animals the cross-innervation of red and white muscles results in changes whereby red (slow) muscle takes on the characteristics of white (fast) muscle in both its contractile response and its enzyme characteristics; the reverse changes occur in white muscle (Dubowitz, 1967; Prewitt and Salafsky, 1967; Romanul and van der Meulen, 1967; Guth, Watson, and Brown, 1968). It would seem therefore that any free

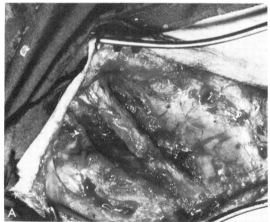

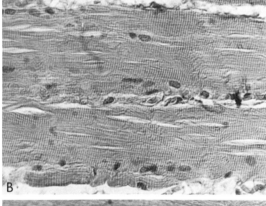

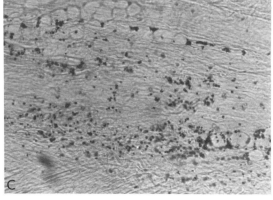

FIGURE 11–2. Dog. Free graft of the complete pronator teres muscle applied 14 days after preliminary denervation to the gracilis and sartorius muscles of the hind leg. *A,* Survival of 70 per cent of the original volume of the graft at six months after transplantation. *B,* Histologically normal muscle at six months after transplantation. Van Gieson, × 450. *C,* Cholinesterase staining showing multiple ectopic motor end-plates of reinnervation six months after transplantation. Koelle, × 200.

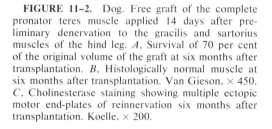

graft of white skeletal muscle, which by virtue of preliminary denervation develops an alien form of metabolism subserving its ultimate survival, will, following its reinnervation by axons from normal muscle in the host recipient site, adopt ultimately the metabolic and physical properties of the recipient site musculature.

In dogs, eight autogenous grafts of the complete pronator teres muscle were transplanted from the foreleg into the hindleg (applied directly to the sartorius and gracilis muscles) 14 to 21 days after preliminary denervation by division of the median nerve (Thompson, 1971b). With preservation of complete muscle fiber length after preliminary denervation, significant survival of the graft was observed in up to 50 to 80 per cent of its original volume after six months (Fig. 11-2, *A*). On microscopic examination the great proportion of surviving graft tissue was normal skeletal muscle, with occasional areas showing evidence of atrophy, fibrosis, and hyaline degeneration (Fig. 11-2, *B*). Silver impregnation staining demonstrated ramifying axons with multiple innervation of muscle fibers, and cholinesterase staining disclosed multiple, spherical, small motor end-plates scattered generally throughout the surviving muscle, suggestive of profuse ectopic and multiple reinnervation of muscle fibers (Fig. 11-2, *C*). Faradic stimulation of the surviving graft produced visible contractions, and stimulation of the adjacent sartorius muscle resulted in the transmission of visible contractions to the contiguous graft tissue. Vascularization of all grafts was in excess of normal.

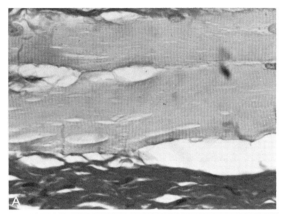
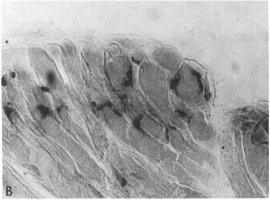

FIGURE 11-3. Man. Muscle graft of extensor digitorum brevis, applied to the temporalis muscle. *A*, At eight months after transplantation. Normal muscle fibers, with fibrous replacement of fibers below. Van Gieson, × 450. *B*, Muscle graft at eight months. Reinnervation of motor end-plates, some showing persisting signs of degeneration. Koelle, × 100.

SKELETAL MUSCLE GRAFTS IN MAN

Skeletal muscle grafts have been used clinically in more than 100 patients, and in four patients there has been opportunity to take biopsy material for histologic examination at intervals of three to nine months after transplantation. All demonstrated survival of myofibrils of normal appearance without nuclear changes or loss of striations (Fig. 11-3, *A*). There were preserved motor end-plates on cholinesterase staining, and silver impregnation stains disclosed exuberant axonal proliferation in the graft (Thompson, 1971b) (Fig. 11-3, *B*).

Clinical Use of Skeletal Muscle Autografts

The volume of muscle capable of successful transplantation is limited by the thickness of muscle tissue capable of surviving the initial period of ischemia before revascularization of the graft becomes established. Peer and Walker (1951) believed that skeletal muscle grafts in man required three to four days to develop an anastomotic blood supply at the recipient site. It seems likely that any myofibrils more than 2 to 3 cm from a source of active circulation at the time of transfer might be expected to undergo fibrous replacement; there is of course no limit to the length of the muscle graft able to be transplanted, provided it is in major contact with normal host muscle at the graft recipient site. This limitation on the volume of muscle capable of successful transplantation to orthotopic sites renders the technique particularly applicable to the reconstruction of small muscles of essential function, e.g., skeletal muscle sphincters whose activity has been impaired by congenital maldevelopment, injury, or disease. Sphincters successfully reconstructed in this way are those of the eyelids and mouth (Thompson, 1971c) in unilateral facial paralysis (see Chapter 36), the palatopharyngeal sphincter (in patients with velopharyngeal incompetence) (see Chapter 52), the external anal sphincter (in cases of anal incontinence), and the bladder neck sphincter (in cases of congenital defects in this region). Movement has been successfully restored to the median element of the upper lip in adult cases of bilateral complete lip clefts primarily repaired in infancy (see Chapters 44 and 47); the movements of opposition and extension have also been restored in the paralyzed thumb.

In almost all cases the muscles used as free grafts have been the extensor digitorum brevis muscles of the foot or the palmaris longus muscle of the forearm; on occasion, the pronator teres muscle of the forearm and the extensor digitorum longus muscles of the leg have served as donor muscles. In all cases the muscles were carefully denervated 14 days before transfer, and at the time of transplantation care was taken to retain the entire length of the constituent graft muscle fibers by removing the complete muscle belly intact. The graft was carefully sutured under normal tension to normal (fully innervated and vascularized) skeletal muscles at the recipient site.

Denervation and Transplantation of Muscle Grafts

Denervation is undertaken 14 days before transplantation. A pneumatic tourniquet is employed to ensure an avascular field for dissection, and an electrical nerve stimulator is used to locate the motor nerve supply which is then excised. It is essential to preserve the vascular supply to the graft.

Extensor Digitorum Brevis Muscles of the Foot. The extensor digitorum brevis muscles of the foot are the grafts of choice in reactivation of paralyzed eyelids, for application as onlay grafts to reinforce the weakened elevators of the angle of the mouth, and for reconstruction of the bilateral cleft lip and palatopharyngeal sphincter. The muscle consists of

four discrete bellies of varied size. As single entities or a combination of two or more selected bellies, a graft unit of appropriate size can be constructed. If the palmaris longus muscles are absent, the short extensors from both feet along with a plantaris (or long toe extensor) tendon, provide sufficient transplant material to treat both eyelids and mouth. The denervation is performed through a 3-cm vertical incision overlying the anterior aspect of the ankle joint at a point midway between the malleoli. The anterior tibial nerve is found on the plane of the bone, after dividing the lower border of the lower extensor retinaculum. The nerve lies just laterally to the extensor hallucis tendon, alongside the dorsalis pedis vessels. If the nerve has divided at this point (a common finding), the lateral branch is divided and a small segment of nerve excised. The medial division should then also be stimulated to ensure that no motor fibers are distributed through it to the short extensor muscles of the toes; if it does react to stimulation, it should also be divided, for motor denervation must be complete. The dorsalis pedis vessels must be carefully protected.

At the time of graft transplantation two weeks later, a pneumatic tourniquet is applied to the thigh. A transverse incision on the dorsum of the foot is made just proximal to the web spaces, and the four tendons of the extensor digitorum brevis muscle are divided at their insertions into the base of the proximal phalanx of the great toe (in the case of the extensor hallucis brevis muscle) and into the lateral aspect of the second, third, and fourth long extensor tendons (in the case of the remaining three muscle bellies). An additional oblique incision extends from the lateral aspect of the dorsum of the foot near the lateral malleolus to within two fingers-breadth of the midpoint of the first incision to expose the muscle bellies of the extensor digitorum brevis. After their associated tendons have been mobilized from beneath the long extensor tendons and brought into the second incision, the muscle bellies are stripped back from their calcaneal insertion using sharp dissection to preserve the entire muscle bellies in continuity with their attached tendons. The muscle graft is then meticulously denuded of all fatty, fascial, or ligamentous tissue. The tourniquet is released, hemostasis obtained, and the wounds sutured with drainage.

Palmaris Longus Muscle. The palmaris longus is the muscle graft of choice in restoring movement to the oral sphincter or the completely paralyzed elevators of the angle of the mouth. It is occasionally absent on one or both sides. In such situations, the extensor hallucis brevis muscle (with or without additional bellies of the extensor digitorum brevis in association), together with a plantaris (or long toe extensor) tendon, may be used as a substitute.

Denervation is completed through a 7-cm incision over the medial aspect of the antecubital fossa of the elbow. The median nerve is exposed and gently dislocated from its bed to demonstrate the medial flowing branches supplying the pronator teres, flexor carpi radialis, and palmaris longus muscles. All of these motor branches are successively stimulated to detect that nerve (or occasionally, nerves) supplying the palmaris longus muscle. Identification is assisted by a small median volar incision in the distal wrist crease, allowing division of the palmaris longus tendon just proximal to its insertion; hemostatic forceps left attached to the proximal tendon after its division will retract into the wrist wound on stimulation of the relevant motor nerve at the elbow. It is essential to divide any nerve whose electrical stimulation causes palmaris longus contraction. Before both wounds are closed, the proximal palmaris longus tendon is transfixed at the level of the wrist by a single buried suture to assist its subsequent identification at the second operation.

Two weeks later, under tourniquet control, the palmaris longus muscle with its associated tendon in continuity is removed after reopening and extending the earlier incisions. A ring tendon stripper inserted through the wrist incision will limit the extension of the antecubital incision required, but it is essential that the palmaris longus muscle belly should be carefully separated by sharp dissection from its origin in order to preserve the entire muscle intact. The muscle graft is carefully cleansed of all adherent fat and fascia, and all wounds closed. Drains are frequently employed.

MUSCLE FLAPS

Muscle can also be transplanted as muscle flaps on a vascular pedicle. The technique has been used in reconstruction for facial palsy (see Chapter 36), coverage of pressure sores (see Chapter 91), and resurfacing defects of the lower extremity (see Chapter 86).

REFERENCES

Aitken, J. T.: Growth of nerve implants in voluntary muscle. J. Anat., *84*:38, 1950.

Barrett, B.: The length and mode of termination of individual muscle fibers in the human sartorius and posterior femoral muscles. Acta Anat., *48*:242, 1962.

Dubowitz, V.: Cross-innervated mammalian skeletal muscle. Histochemical, physiological and biochemical observations. J. Physiol., *193*:481, 1967.

Ducker, T. B., Kempe, L. G., and Hayes, G. J.: The metabolic background for peripheral nerve surgery. J. Neurosurg., *30*:270, 1969.

Erlacher, P.: Direct and muscular neurotization of paralysed muscles. Experimental research. Am. J. Orthop. Surg., *13*:22, 1915.

Guth, L., Watson, P. K., and Brown, W. C.: Effects of cross reinnervation on some chemical properties of red and white muscles of rat and cat. Exp. Neurol., *20*:52, 1968.

Gutmann, E.: Factors affecting recovery of motor function after nerve lesions. J. Neurol. Psychiat., *5*:81, 1942.

Gwyn, D. J., and Aitken, J. T.: New motor end plates and their relationship to muscle fibre injury. Nature, *203*:651, 1964.

Harreveld, A. van: On the force and size of motor units in the rabbit's sartorius muscle. Am. J. Physiol., *151*:96, 1947.

Heineke, H.: Die direkte Einpflanzung des Nerven in den Muskel. Zentralbl. Chir., *41*:465, 1914.

Hoffman, H.: A study of the factors influencing innervation of muscles by implanted nerves. Aust. J. Exp. Biol. Med. Sci., *29*:289, 1951.

Hogan, E. L., Dawson, D. M., and Romanul, F. C. A.: Enzymatic changes in denervated muscle. II. Biochemical studies. Arch. Neurol., *13*:274, 1965.

Hogenhuis, L. A. H., and Engel, W. K.: Histochemistry and cytochemistry of experimentally denervated guinea pig muscle. I. Histochemistry. Acta Anat., *60*:39, 1965.

Huber, G. C.: On the form and arrangement in fasciculi of striated voluntary muscle fibers. Anat. Rec., *11*:149, 1916.

Lieberman, A. R.: The axon reaction. A review of the principal features of perikaryal responses to axon injury. Internatl. Rev. Neurobiol., *49*:124, 1971.

Lockhart, R. D., and Brandt, W.: Length of striated muscle fibers. J. Anat., *72*:470, 1938.

Magnus, R.: Ueber Muskeltransplantation. Munch. Med. Wochenschr., *37*:515, 1890.

McQuarrie, I. G., and Grafstein, B.: Axon outgrowth enhanced by a previous nerve injury. Arch. Neurol., *29*:53, 1973.

Peer, L. A.: Transplantation of Tissues. Vol. 1. Baltimore, Williams & Wilkins Company, 1955.

Peer, L. A., and Walker, J. C.: The behaviour of autogenous human tissue grafts. Part II. Plast. Reconstr. Surg., *7*:73, 1951.

Prewitt, M. A., and Salafsky, B.: Effect of cross-innervation on biochemical characteristics of skeletal muscles. Am. J. Physiol., *213*:295, 1967.

Romanul, F. C. A., and Hogan, E. L.: Enzymatic changes in denervated muscle. I. Histochemical studies. Arch. Neurol., *13*:263, 1965.

Romanul, F. C. A., and Meulen, J. P., van der: Slow and fast muscles after cross-innervation. Enzymatic and physiological changes. Arch. Neurol., *17*:387, 1967.

Roy, P. R.: Behaviour of a free autogenous muscle graft into the skeletal muscles of the dog. J. Exp. Med. Sci., *9*:78, 1966.

Sandow, A.: Skeletal muscle. Ann. Rev. Physiol., *32*: 87, 1970.

Smith, B.: Changes in the enzyme histochemistry of skeletal muscle during experimental denervation and reinnervation. J. Neurol. Neurosurg. Psychiat., *28*: 99, 1965.

Steindler, A.: Direct neurotization of paralysed muscles: Further study of the question of direct nerve implantation. Am. J. Orthop. Surg., *14*:707, 1916.

Thompson, N.: Autogenous free grafts of skeletal muscle. A preliminary experimental and clinical study. Plast. Reconstr. Surg., *48*:11, 1971a.

Thompson, N.: Investigation of autogenous skeletal muscle free grafts in the dog. With a report on a successful free graft of skeletal muscle in man. Transplantation, *12*:353, 1971b.

Thompson, N.: Treatment of facial paralysis by free skeletal muscle grafts. Trans. Fifth Internatl. Congr. Plast. and Reconstr. Surg., Melbourne. Australia. Butterworth & Co., Ltd., 1971c, p. 66.

Volkmann, R.: Über die Regeneration des quergestreiften Muskelgewebes beim Menschen und Sangetier. Ziegler's Beitr. Pathol. Anat., *12*:233, 1893.

Zielonko, J.: Ueber die Entwicklung und Proliferation von Epithelien und Endothelien. Arch. Mikroscop. Anat., *10*:351, 1874.

CHAPTER 12

TRANSPLANTATION OF CARTILAGE

Thomas Gibson, D.Sc., F.R.C.S.

THE POLYMORPHISM OF HUMAN CARTILAGE

In the evolution of animal species, cartilage long preceded bone as a skeletal support and has since acquired many diverse forms and functions. The rib cartilages, for example, are essential for the free but limited range of movement in the thoracic cage and act like torsion bars, returning the bony ribs to a neutral position after inspiration and deep expiration. The intervertebral discs not only act as shock absorbers, preserving the integrity of the brain, but also help to control the range of movements of the spine. Cartilage maintains the prominence of the ears and the nose with just the correct degree of rigidity. The laryngeal cartilages are concerned with the infinite modulation of the voice, while those in the bronchi maintain patency under pressure. In joints, cartilage plays a unique role in allowing friction-free movement.

These "permanent" cartilages have little power of growth or regeneration, yet growth is the prime function of the "temporary" cartilaginous precursors of bone, the most highly and individually specialized of all cartilages. Although their potentials differ widely, they are so precisely ordained that not only do they control exactly the relative length of bones, but growth proceeds symmetrically and synchronously.

These widely different functional adaptations result from variations in the three basic constituents of cartilage: the cells or chondrocytes, the chondromucoprotein ground substance in which they are embedded, and the fibers which interlace the ground substance. The ground substance and fibers constitute the matrix.

The traditional classification of cartilage into hyaline, elastic, and fibrocartilage is based on the kind of fiber present and is valueless for practical purposes. "Hyaline" cartilage, for example, includes the temporary precursors of bone, the articular cartilages, the costal cartilages, the nasal septal and alar cartilages, and those of the trachea and larger bronchi. Each human cartilage should be regarded as a unique structure whose physical and mechanical properties are precisely adapted for a specific function. Nor is there any evidence of metaplasia after transplantation; rib cartilage transplanted to the ear, for example, retains its original character.

Indeed there are good grounds for considering that many individual chondrocytes are uniquely adapted for a task which they alone can perform. The various growth potentials of the chondrocytes in epiphyseal cartilage are one example. Another is the different pressures under which the matrix of rib cartilage is secreted to provide the balanced stress system needed for its function as a torsion spring.

The most fascinating example is the apparent specialization of each chondrocyte in ear cartilage. Papain injected into baby rabbits (Thomas, 1956) causes their ears to collapse and become limp and flabby, an effect due to degradation of the ground substance which becomes soluble and is removed. Within days, however, each chondrocyte will replace in its neighborhood the correct amount of ground substance needed to reproduce exactly the normally convoluted erect ear. This occurs even when various external restraints are applied to distort it into a new shape (De Palma, De Palma and De Forrest, 1964).

The chondrocyte is a very versatile cell. It not only is capable of constructing the complex molecules of chondromucoprotein, collagen, and elastin but also is continually making new matrix around it (Fig. 12–1). The metabolic turnover of the matrix by the chondrocyte can be readily demonstrated by the uptake of ^{35}S, and this is the basis for a useful test of viability (Curran and Gibson, 1956). It is essential, therefore, for the well-being of any cartilage graft that the chondrocytes survive transplantation; otherwise eventual absorption is likely. Fortunately cartilage, whether autograft or allograft, "takes" readily as a free transplant,

provided that the elementary precaution is observed of keeping the graft in contact with the host tissues. A cartilage graft surrounded by blood clot will die, and yet it is surprising how often in clinical practice grafts are inserted loosely into artificially created cavities with no precautions to coapt the graft to its bed. Many apparent discrepancies in the reported behavior of cartilage grafts may be due to this factor; allografts and xenografts are as likely to be dead from nutritional lack as from any immune reaction.

THE DEFORMATION OF CARTILAGE WHEN CUT

Cartilage is a prestressed material; in more precise engineering terms, there exists a system of self-locked stresses which are nicely balanced in intact cartilage but which may be released and cause distortion when cartilage is cut. These inbuilt stresses have been measured accurately in human cartilage (Kenedi, Gibson and Abrahams, 1963; Abrahams and Duggan, 1965). Throughout the thickness of costal cartilage, areas of tension are found to

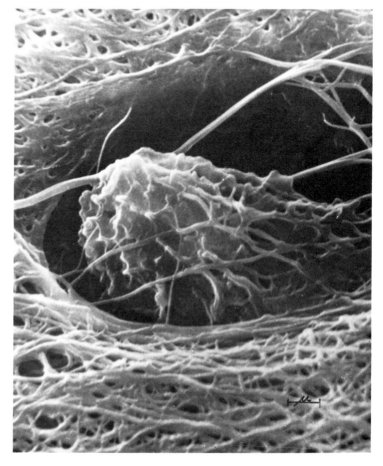

FIGURE 12–1. The chondrocyte is a versatile cell producing all the structures of the cartilage matrix. Through the scanning electron microscope this chondrocyte was observed spinning the fine fibers which are interlaced around it. (Courtesy of Dr. J. G. McCall.)

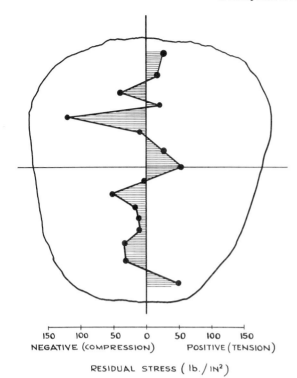

150   100   50   0   50   100   150
NEGATIVE (COMPRESSION)   POSITIVE (TENSION)

RESIDUAL STRESS (lb. / IN²)

FIGURE 12–2. Engineering analysis of the alternating compression and tension stresses in a cartilaginous rib from a 50 year old male, shown graphically and superimposed on the rib's cross-sectional outline. (From Gibson, T.: Cartilage grafts. Br. Med. Bull., *21*:153, 1965.)

alternate with areas of compression (Fig. 12–2). To avoid deformation when carving a cartilage graft, it is obvious that these forces must remain symmetrically balanced. Unfortunately no two cartilaginous ribs have the same distribution or magnitude of forces, and measurement of the individual forces destroys the rib. Absolute precision is therefore impossible.

The "balanced cross sections" (Fig. 12–3) found by trial and error by Gibson and Davis (1958), however, are a useful approximation, although it must be stressed that, even when these principles are strictly adhered to, a small proportion of grafts may still show a tendency to warp, albeit much less so than when the principles are ignored; this is particularly so with tapering sections.

The only absolute way of preventing warping is to carry out no trimming at all. This is rarely feasible, but carving should always be kept to a minimum by selecting for the graft that portion of cartilage which most nearly approaches the size and shape required. For example, in seeking a costal cartilage graft to support the nasal bridge, the lower margin of the rib cage is

explored through a rectus-splitting incision. The free-lying cartilaginous tip of the eighth rib is occasionally so shaped that it may be used intact; more frequently a little trimming is needed (Fig. 12–4). For thicker grafts the lower half of the seventh cartilage usually presents suitably straight segments (Figs. 12–5 and 12–6).

Like most biological tissues, cartilage has visco-elastic properties; in other words, time is required before the maximum deformation occurs. Thus a cartilage graft carved into shape and immediately introduced into a cavity will have warped when the dressings are later removed. In practice the time required for a carved piece of cartilage to reach its maximum deformation is about 30 minutes (Abrahams and Duggan, 1965). It is wise to allow this period to elapse before final insertion. Any warping that has occurred may then be corrected by further trimming or abolished by making small cuts along the curved surfaces. This latter practice, however, weakens the graft.

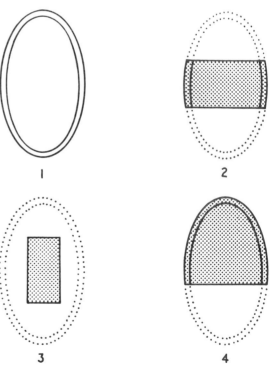

FIGURE 12–3. The four basic balanced cross sections of rib cartilage assuming a symmetrical distribution of stresses. This is not always so, but at the same time adherence to these sections produces nonbending grafts in a high proportion of cases. (From Gibson, T., and Davis, W. B.: The distortion of autogenous grafts: Its cause and prevention. Br. J. Plast. Surg., *10*:257, 1958.)

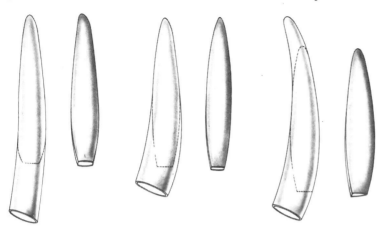

FIGURE 12–4. The tip of the eighth rib is a useful source of cartilage grafts to support the nasal bridge, since very little trimming is usually required. Carving as shown here maintains balanced cross sections. (From Gibson, T., and Davis, W. B.: The distortion of autogenous cartilage grafts: Its cause and prevention. Br. J. Plast. Surg., *10*:257, 1958.)

Of course distortion of cartilage is not always necessarily objectionable. This property may be exploited to obtain a suitable curve in a cartilage graft and also forms the basis of certain techniques for correction of prominent ears (Chongchet, 1963).

The self-locked stress system of cartilage is a vital property which disappears as the chondrocytes die. It is this fact more than any other that has made the use of stored, dead cartilage so attractive to so many plastic surgeons.

THE LIMITED SCOPE OF CARTILAGE AUTOGRAFTS

Because they are so uniquely specialized and so essential to function, few of the human body's cartilages are interchangeable and few are available as autografts. Indeed the only donor sources are the rib cartilages, the nasal septal cartilage, and the ear cartilage.

Rib Cartilage

The cartilages commonly used are the seventh and eighth, the seventh being the longest of all. Occasionally that portion of the sixth adjacent to the seventh near the sternum is excised along with the seventh to give a broader piece of cartilage from which to carve an ear skeleton (see Chapter 35). Older textbooks suggested that the sixth and seventh were fused in this region, but they are in fact discrete, though held together by fibrous tissue. These portions of cartilage lie below the reflection of the pleura, and there is little risk of opening the chest cavity, a hazard with other costal cartilages. They may be exposed through an 8- to 10-cm incision over the lower border of the thoracic cage. The rectus sheath is divided in the line of the incision and the rectus muscle split in the direction of its fibers. Some energetic retraction will disclose the last 6 cm of the eighth and the seventh ribs up to the sternum; the selected portion is then excised and the wound closed in layers.

Such segments of costal cartilage are of convenient size and shape for grafts to the nasal bridge and occasionally to restore other facial contours, particularly in the orbital and zygomatic regions. The skeleton for a missing

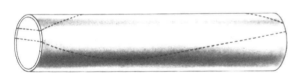

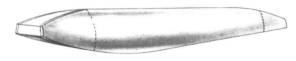

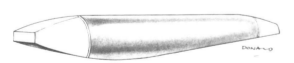

FIGURE 12–5. Thicker nasal bridge supports may be carved as shown from a straight section of the seventh rib, ensuring balanced sections along the length. A complete segment should not be removed, as suggested here. The lower two-thirds is adequate to supply the graft, and the remaining third will maintain the continuity of the rib. (From Gibson, T., and Davis, W. B.: The distortion of autogenous cartilage grafts: Its cause and prevention. Br. J. Plast. Surg., *10*:257, 1958.)

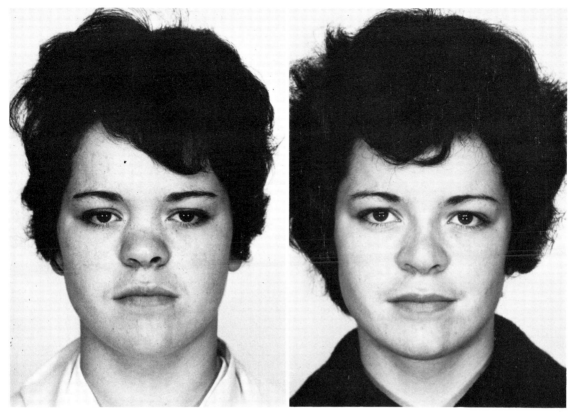

FIGURE 12–6. A graft from the seventh rib shaped as in Figure 12–5 was used to support the nasal bridge in this patient. (From Gibson, T.: Cartilage grafts. Br. Med. Bull., *21*:153, 1965.)

pinna may be carved from one or more pieces, and rods of rib cartilage have been used in the reconstruction of the penis.

Peer in 1943 introduced the technique of dicing rib cartilage — that is, cutting it into small cubes. This effectively overcame both the propensity of cut cartilage to warp and the limitations imposed by the shape and size of the rib. The cartilage cubes could be packed into bony or other defects (Fig. 12–7). Peer's ingenious development of the technique was the introduction of preformed, perforated vitallium, hinged boxes of the exact size and shape of the cartilage graft required; these were filled with diced cartilage and then inserted subcutaneously in the patient. Vascular granulation tissue grew through the perforations until all the cubes were fixed to each other by fibrous tissue and the plastic surgeon had a fibro-cartilaginous graft of the size and shape required, after an interval of five months. Peer (1955) has described molds for ear skeletons and also fibrocartilaginous cover of the femoral head in ankylosis of the hip.

Diced cartilage has two disadvantages. If a large mass is inserted, it is unlikely that a blood supply will reach the central cubes before the chondrocytes are dead, and it can be readily shown that a cartilage graft surrounded by blood clot will also die. Secondly, even if all the cubes survive, some absorption may occur. Davis and Gibson (1956) demonstrated that cartilage grafts invariably showed some degree of erosion and absorption on any cut surface. With larger cubes the process will have little observable effect, but the smaller the segments, the more diminution in bulk would be likely to occur. Chopping the cartilage into pieces small enough to be injected with a syringe and needle, therefore, is unlikely to give a satisfactory reconstruction.

Nasal Septal Cartilage

Peer (1941) showed that autogenous septal cartilage survived as living cartilage. As Millard (1966) pointed out, it is at hand if

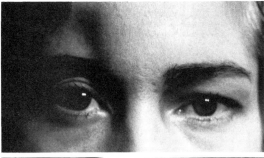

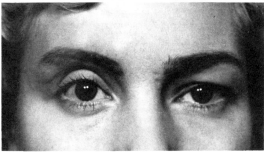

FIGURE 12–7. Bony defect in the supraorbital region reconstructed with diced autogenous cartilage. (From Gibson, T.: Cartilage grafts. *In* Seiffert, K. E., and Geissendorfer, R. (Eds.): Transplantation von Organen und Geweben. Stuttgart, Georg Thieme Verlag, 1967, p. 203.)

required for minor additions to the nasal skeleton during rhinoplasty procedures; he recommended it as a columellar strut support to give definition to the tip. In cases of severe septal deviation, Szabon (1962) recommended the reimplantation of portions of the resected septal cartilage to prevent subsequent collapse of the bridge. Converse (1956) utilized a composite graft of septal cartilage and attached mucoperichondrium as a routine procedure in reconstructing unilateral defects of the nose involving the ala (see Chapter 29). Millard (1962) and Mustardé (1969) also reported the successful use of a composite graft of nasal septal cartilage with mucosa retained on one surface to replace conjunctiva and the tarsal plate in eyelid reconstruction (see Chapter 28).

Ear Cartilage

Small elliptical portions of the patient's own ear may be removed without much deformity and are occasionally valuable in supporting the alae nasi in nasal reconstruction. Barsky and Blinick (1953) inserted strips of ear cartilage, carved into a ring, into the wall of the fallopian tubes to maintain patency. Small pieces are also valuable in middle ear surgery (Duncan,

1962; Brockman, 1965). Composite grafts of ear cartilage sandwiched between two layers of skin are useful in restoring full thickness alar and columellar defects. In order to "take" reliably, composite grafts must be relatively small in size.

THE UNIQUE PRIVILEGE OF CARTILAGE ALLOGRAFTS

Chondrocytes are the only mammalian cells which can be transplanted allogeneically without provoking an immune response. This had been suspected for many years since Leopold in 1881 demonstrated growth in small cartilage allografts in the anterior chamber of rabbits' eyes. The final proof came in 1958 when Gibson, Davis, and Curran made a series of experimental allografts in man and found the chondrocytes actively metabolizing sulfur throughout the two-year period of the observations. Subsequently they had the opportunity of examining portions of two grafts of mothers' ear cartilage transplanted to their children 18 and 23 years previously (Gibson and Davis, 1960). The 18-year specimen was received fresh, and sulfur metabolism was demonstrated in the cells; the 23-year specimen was fixed, but the cells had every appearance of normality. Peer (1958) has also shown by nuclear sexing that these are the original cells; there is no question of allograft rejection of the donor cells and subsequent recolonization by the host.

Two possible factors may be responsible for the immunologic privilege of cartilage: the lack of antigenicity of cells and matrix, or the protective action of the matrix preventing cellular antigens from leaving the cells or cell-bound antibodies from reaching them.

The Lack of Antigenicity of Cartilage

Whole cartilage is only weakly antigenic, if at all. Peacock, Weeks and Petty (1960) were unable to immunize mice with allografts of whole xiphisternum so far as accelerated rejection of subsequent skin grafts was concerned. Craigmyle (1958a, b), however, reported accelerated rejection of skin grafts and enlargement of regional lymph nodes in a few instances when he transplanted finely diced allograft cartilage. The difference in results probably lies in the fact that Craigmyle diced his cartilage and thus not only exposed cells normally enclosed in matrix but also damaged cells with release of antigenic material not usually available.

Chondrocytes per se appear to be nonantigenic. Smith (1965) has been able to separate articular chondrocytes entirely from the matrix, and she found that six weeks after allogeneic transplantation they had arranged themselves in columns and were surrounded by well-stained matrix. It must be assumed, therefore, that either the cells are nonantigenic or they surround themselves so quickly with a mucopolysaccharide barrier that the antigenic stimulus is rendered abortive.

It is not possible to obtain cell-free matrix, but we have made several series of experiments in human volunteers with cartilage implants, the cells of which had been killed by boiling or freezing. The method used was to insert an implant, excise it after two months, insert a second implant at this time, remove it after two months, and so on. Each implant was therefore in the tissues for a standard time, but the total exposure of the tissues to the implanted material increased with each specimen.

Xenografts of ox cartilage showed a progressive reaction with each specimen to such a degree that, after a year's exposure, complete liquefaction of the implant occurred in the two-month period (Gibson and Davis, 1953). On the other hand, allograft cartilage showed no increased reaction, although the experiments were carried on for 18 months (Gibson, 1968). It would seem, therefore, that cartilage matrix may excite an immune response when transplanted xenogeneically but not allogeneically. This finding is in keeping with the work of Loewi and Muir (1965), who have shown that chondromucoprotein extracted from pig cartilage produced specific antibodies when injected in rabbits and guinea pigs; they suggested that chondromucoprotein contains several species-specific proteins as well as a polysaccharide peptide common to several species.

The Protective Matrix

The immunologic protection afforded to the chondrocytes by the intact matrix appears to be very high. Even when the host has been previously immunized with one or more skin grafts, allografts from the same donor are unaffected (Craigmyle, 1960; Peacock, Weeks and Petty 1960). It seems most likely that this is due to the physical barrier which the matrix interposes between the chondrocytes and the cells of the host, a situation analogous to certain experimental conditions, such as allografts floating free in the anterior chamber of the eye (Medawar, 1948) or wrapped in millipore filter paper (Weaver, Algire and Prehn, 1955; Woodruff, 1957), in which prolonged survival occurs. This would seem to fit in with the generally accepted concept that allograft rejection is cell-mediated and does not result from the activity of humoral antibodies.

Even in the case of xenografts, the survival of the chondrocytes may be greatly prolonged; calf xenografts have been found alive two years after transplantation in rabbits (Kluzak, Titibach and Zastava, 1963), and human xenografts 12 months after transplantation in rabbits (Krüger, 1964).

Clinical Scope of Cartilage Allografts

Since allograft cartilage behaves precisely as an autograft, there would seem to be little need for the latter. However, since reliable methods of long-term storage in a viable state have still to be devised, it is often more practical to use the patient's own rib, ear, or nasal septal cartilage as required. In addition to the problem of storage, there are other practical difficulties which limit the use of certain cartilages as allografts. The most important is the intimate association which some have with other tissues which themselves are subject to rejection and without which the cartilage is of little value. The laryngeal and tracheal cartilages would be ideal for reconstruction after excision of the larynx, but the difficulties of recreating the mucous lining, the muscle, and the interconnecting fibrous tissues seem almost insuperable.

Articular cartilage is another case in point. It is too thin and friable to be transplanted alone, but a composite graft of articular cartilage and the underlying bone will survive as long as the bony layer does not exceed 2 or 3 mm in thickness. Cartilage vitality was found to be unimpaired up to six months in such grafts in dogs, and the bone was completely incorporated in the host (Gibson, 1968). The problems of transplanting articular cartilage allografts are now largely those of the techniques of accurate preparation of the thin osseocartilaginous shells and of the bed, so that a near perfect fit is obtained, and also the fixation of the grafts in position without unduly traumatizing them (Gibson, 1967).

Ear Cartilage Allografts. Gillies (1920) introduced the use of mothers' ear cartilage to reconstruct the ear in children with a congenitally absent pinna and in a late survey Gillies and Millard (1957) reported satisfactory results.* On the other hand Greeley (1944) found that such grafts underwent absorption. Bäckdahl, Consiglio and Falconer (1954) reviewed a series of 25 grafts of maternal ear cartilage allografts and noted a complete disappearance of two and partial absorption of seven after an average interval of less than two years.

As noted above Gibson and Davis (1960) demonstrated living chondrocytes in a graft of a mother's ear cartilage transplanted to her child 18 years previously.

The reason for the occasional absorption noted by some workers seems most likely to be patchy take of the graft. Cartilage surrounded by blood clot will die and will be subject to absorption. The introduction of a corrugated mother's ear cartilage into a skin pocket against the smooth surface of the skull creates exactly those conditions in which parts of the graft will live and others die. If a suitable technique could be devised for keeping the whole of the ear cartilage in contact with a vascular bed, the use of living allograft cartilage would be worth reconsidering in ear reconstruction.

STORING CARTILAGE
IN A VIABLE STATE

If the clinical use of cartilage allografts is to be extended, it is preferable that methods of storage can be found to maintain the viability of the cartilage between removal from the donor (usually a cadaver) and its transplantation in the recipient. Cartilage taken from the recently dead is still viable, as demonstrated by the in vitro uptake of ^{35}S, and retains some metabolic activity for at least six weeks when stored at 4° C (Curran and Gibson, 1956). This is not, however, a simple matter of survival for a period and then death. Quantitative studies with ^{35}S or intravital dyes show that

*A review of maternal cartilage allografts for auricular construction in congenital microtia, performed by Gillies in the 1930's, was done in 1941. Only one of these patients showed persistence of the cartilage; in all the other patients the maternal auricular transplant underwent shrinkage and absorption. This was not reported. The editor was present when the follow-up evaluation of 21 patients was done. The survival of one maternal cartilage allograft (and one other observed by Gibson) can be attributed to a close tissue-typing match between mother and child (JMC).

the metabolic activity falls off very rapidly during the first few days of storage and subsequently declines slowly at a much lower level (Hagerty and coworkers, 1960; Gibson, unpublished observations). After transplantation, cartilage which has been stored for more than a few days regains only part of its original metabolic activity. For this reason, the author prefers to use stored cartilage as soon as possible. At the same time, Mikhelson (1962) reported from Moscow the use of cadaver cartilage stored at 3 to 4° C for up to two months; in 1819 cases, he had only three instances of resorption, suggesting that even partial viability may be adequate for survival.

When whole cartilage is cooled below 0° C, the chondrocytes die even when pretreated with glycerol (Curran and Gibson, 1956; Gibson, 1957). Chondrocytes freed from their matrix and protected by dimethyl sulfoxide will survive freezing to −79° C (Smith, 1965) and after transplantation will reconstitute a matrix. It may be that a similar technique will be found for whole cartilage.

THE BEHAVIOR OF DEAD
CARTILAGE IMPLANTS

Throughout the literature of the last three decades there are innumerable references to the clinical use of dead cartilage, killed by prolonged storage in Merthiolate, by boiling, or by formalin fixation, and taken from human cadavers, cattle, pigs, and other mammals. Dead cartilage loses all tendency to warp when cut, it is easily stored in any desired quantity and size, and after implantation it will persist unchanged for sufficient time to give rise to claims of permanent success. It would be tedious and futile to list all the papers written about it; in the great majority there is no adequate follow-up and few real conclusions to be drawn. It is probably highly significant that the flow of papers on preserved cartilage virtually ceased about 1960 at the time when the silicone rubbers were coming into use. Silicone rubber implants have all the advantages of dead cartilage without the disadvantage of a high rate of eventual absorption.

The absorption which overtakes the majority of dead cartilage implants is acknowledged verbally by most of those who have used them but is difficult to document conclusively. There are three reasons for this. First, some so-called "preserved" grafts have undoubtedly been alive when inserted; second, while there are many enthusiastic short-term reports, there are few long-term follow-ups; third, there are at least two biological phenomena which in certain instances will lead to persistence of dead cartilage for many years.

"Preserved" But Living Grafts

Mikhelson, as noted previously, reported only three instances of absorption in 1819 preserved allografts of cadaver cartilage performed in his clinic in Moscow, and he expressed surprise at the high incidence of absorption reported by "foreign authors." His cartilage, however, was stored at 3 to 6° C and never for more than two months. Curran and Gibson (1956) showed that cadaver cartilage stored at this temperature will retain some metabolic activity for at least six weeks, and Mikhelson's implants must be regarded as living homografts.

In the United States most preserved cartilage has been stored in Merthiolate at 3 to 4° C. Hagerty and coworkers (1960) have shown that under these circumstances chondrocytes may survive for a few days. When a fresh batch of such cartilage has been prepared, perhaps for a number of waiting patients, the grafts may again have been used early and have been alive, though if stored for any length of time they would of course be dead.

Long-term Follow-up

The behavior of boiled bovine cartilage is well documented (Gibson and Davis, 1953; North, 1953). With rare exceptions (see below) it undergoes progressive absorption. Furthermore, it is antigenic, and subsequent implants are destroyed more rapidly than the first.

The best followed series of Merthiolate-preserved cartilage grafts was that initiated by Straith and Slaughter (1941), whose results over a five-year period were reviewed by Rasi in 1959. The follow-up was not entirely satisfactory, since of the 353 patients involved, only 49 returned for examination. Fifty-nine implants had been inserted in these 49 patients, and only 19 (32 per cent) showed no loss of bulk. Many were still present in reduced size, and it seems likely that progressive absorption was occurring.

Asked recently to comment on this work, Rasi (1972) wrote, "I have not used preserved human cartilage since 1955. Since that time I have been using Silastic and Ivalon sponge — and occasionally autogenous cartilage and bone."

Prolonged Persistence of Dead Cartilage

Following up cases of bovine cartilage implants, Gibson, Davis and Gillies (1959) found an occasional instance of lack of resorption even after several years. In each case the implant was found lying free in a capsule with a lining resembling an adventitious bursa. The occurrence of such long-term survivals, although unpredictable, undoubtedly encouraged some enthusiasts to persist with use of ox cartilage for longer than it deserved.

A second phenomenon which will lead to persistence of a dead cartilage implant is progressive calcification. Recently Mühlbauer, Schmidt-Tintemann and Glaser (1971) have upset the writer's long-held views that most dead cartilage is absorbed by reporting a follow-up of 40 L-shaped grafts to support the bridges of saddle-shaped noses. The time of follow-up ranged from one to ten years. Thirty had persisted unchanged, eight showed moderate absorption and two, in which the deformity was due to syphilis, almost completely disappeared. The cartilage had been removed from cadavers and stored in 1:5000 Merthiolate at 4° C. In most cases x-ray films showed progressive calcification beginning 1½ to 2 years after insertion (Fig. 12–8), and a biopsy of one implant nine years after insertion showed that this was due to invasion by cancellous bone and not simply to calcium deposition. It is of interest in this connection that Gibson and Davis (1956) reported a case in which an ox cartilage onlay to a mandible was partly replaced by cancellous bone.

REFERENCES

Abrahams, M., and Duggan, T. C.: The mechanical characteristics of costal cartilage. *In* Kenedi, R. M. (Ed.): Biomechanics and Related Bio-engineering Topics. Proceedings of Symposium held in Glasgow. London, Pergamon Press, 1965, p. 285.

Bäckdahl, M., Consiglio, V., and Falconer, B.: Reconstruction of the external ear with the use of maternal cartilage. Br. J. Plast. Surg., 7:263, 1954.

Barsky, A., and Blinick, G.: The use of cartilage grafts to maintain patency of the fallopian tubes. Plast. Reconstr. Surg., 11:87, 1953.

Brockman, S. J.: Cartilage graft tympanoplasty type III. Laryngoscope, 75:1452, 1965.

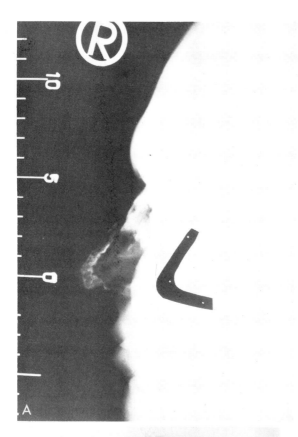

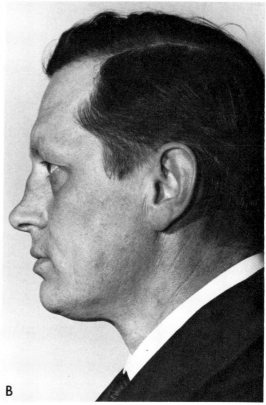

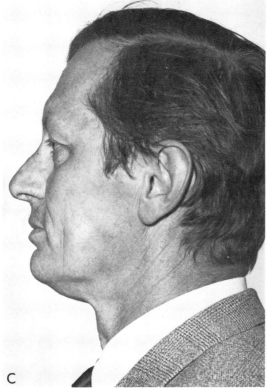

FIGURE 12–8. *A*, Partial calcification in a Merthiolate-preserved allograft 5½ years after insertion. The lead template shows the original size of the transplant. *B*, The patient preoperatively. *C*, The profile has remained unchanged since the operation. (From Mühlbauer, W. D., Schmidt-Tintemann, U., and Glaser, M.: Long-term behaviour of preserved homologous rib cartilage in the correction of saddle nose deformity. Br. J. Plast. Surg., *24*:325, 1971.)

Chongchet, V.: A method of antihelix reconstruction. Br. J. Plast. Surg., *16*:268, 1963.

Converse, J. M.: Composite grafts from the septum in nasal reconstruction. Trans. 8th Latin American Congress of Plast. Surg., *8*:281, 1956.

Craigmyle, M. B. L.: Antigenicity and survival of cartilage homografts. Nature (Lond.), *182*:1248, 1958a.

Craigmyle, M. B. L.: Regional lymph node changes induced by cartilage homo- and heterografts in the rabbit. J. Anat., *92*:467, 1958b.

Craigmyle, M. B. L.: A study of cartilage homografts in rabbits sensitized by a skin homograft from the cartilage donor. Plast. Reconstr. Surg., *26*:150, 1960.

Curran, R. C., and Gibson, T.: The uptake of labelled sulphate by human cartilage cells and its use as a test of viability. Proc. R. Soc. (Biol.), *155*:572, 1956.

Davis, P. K. B., and Jones, S. M.: The complications of Silastic implants. Br. J. Plast. Surg., *24*:405, 1971.

Davis, W. B., and Gibson, T.: Absorption of autogenous cartilage grafts in man. Br. J. Plast. Surg., *9*:177, 1956.

DePalma, R. G., DePalma, M. T., and DeForrest, M.: Experimental alteration of the shape of rabbit ear cartilage. J. Surg. Res., *4*:2, 1964.

Duncan, R. B.: Cartilage grafting in stapes surgery: Report of two cases. N. Z. Med. J., *61*:278, 1962.

Gibson, T.: Viability of cartilage after freezing. Proc. R. Soc. (Biol.), *147*:528, 1957.

Gibson, T.: Cartilage grafts. Br. Med. Bull., *21*:153, 1965.

Gibson, T.: Cartilage grafts. *In* Seiffert, K. E., and Geissendorfer, R. (Eds.): Transplantation von Organen und Geweben. Stuttgart, Georg Thieme Verlag, 1967, p. 203.

Gibson, T.: Bone and cartilage transplantation. *In* Rapaport, F. F., and Dausset, J. (Eds.): Human Transplantation. New York, Grune and Stratton, 1968, p. 313.

Gibson, T., and Davis, W. B.: The fate of preserved bovine cartilage grafts in man. Br. J. Plast. Surg., *6*:4, 1953.

Gibson, T., and Davis, W. B.: Some further observations on the use of preserved animal cartilage. Br. J. Plast. Surg., *8*:85, 1956.

Gibson, T., and Davis, W. B.: The distortion of autogenous cartilage grafts: Its cause and prevention. Br. J. Plast. Surg., *10*:257, 1958.

Gibson, T., and Davis, W. B.: A bank of living homograft cartilage: A preliminary report. Trans. Int. Soc. of Plastic Surgeons, 2nd Congress, London. Edinburgh, Livingstone, 1960, p. 452.

Gibson, T., Davis, W. B., and Curran, R. C.: The long-term survival of cartilage homografts in man. Br. J. Plast. Surg., *11*:177, 1958.

Gibson, T., Davis, W. B., and Gillies, H. D.: The encapsulation of preserved cartilage grafts with prolonged survival. Br. J. Plast. Surg., *12*:22, 1959.

Gillies, H. D.: Plastic Surgery of the Face, Based on Selected Cases of War Injuries of the Face, Including Burns. London, Oxford University Press, 1920.

Gillies, H. D., and Millard, D. R.: The Principles and Art of Plastic Surgery. London, Butterworths, 1957.

Greeley, P. (1944): Quoted by Peer (1955).

Hagerty, R. F., Calhoon, T. B., Lee, W. H., and Cuttino, J. T.: Human cartilage grafts stored in air. Surg. Gynecol. Obstet., *110*:433, 1960.

Kenedi, R. M., Gibson, T., and Abrahams, M.: Mechanical characteristics of skin and cartilage. Hum. Factors, *5*:525, 1963.

Kluzak, R., Titlbach, M., and Zastava, V.: L'Autoresorp-tion de la greffe: (A propos des heterotransplantations de cartilage hyalin). Ann. Chir. Plast., *8*:169, 1963.

Krüger, E.: Absorption of human rib cartilage grafts transplanted to rabbits after preservation by different methods. Br. J. Plast. Surg., *17*:254, 1964.

Leopold, G.: Experimentelle Untersuchungen über die Aetiologie der Geschwulste. Virchows Arch., *85*:283, 1881.

Loewi, G., and Muir, H.: The antigenicity of chondromucoprotein. Immunology, *9*:119, 1965.

Medawar, P. B.: Immunity to homologous grafted skin. III. The fate of skin homografts transplanted to the brain, to subcutaneous tissue and to the anterior chamber of the eye. Br. J. Exp. Pathol., *29*:58, 1948.

Mikhelson, N. M.: Homogenous cartilage in maxillofacial surgery. Acta Chir. Plast. (Praha), *4*:3, 1962.

Millard, D. R., Jr.: Eyelid repairs with a chondromucosal graft. Plast. Reconstr. Surg., *30*:367, 1962.

Millard, D. R., Jr.: Corrective rhinoplasty. *In* Gibson, T. (Ed.): Modern Trends in Plastic Surgery. Vol. 2. London, Butterworths, 1966, p. 300.

Mühlbauer, W. D., Schmidt-Tintemann, U., and Glaser, M.: Long-term behaviour of preserved homologous rib cartilage in the correction of saddle nose deformity. Br. J. Plast. Surg., *24*:325, 1971.

Mustardé, J. C.: Repair and reconstruction in the orbital region. Edinburgh, E & S Livingstone, 1969.

North, J. F.: The use of preserved bovine cartilage in plastic surgery. Plast. Reconstr. Surg., *11*:261, 1953.

Peacock, E. E., Weeks, P. M., and Petty, J. M.: Some studies on the antigenicity of cartilage. Ann. N.Y. Acad. Sci., *87*:175, 1960.

Peer, L. A.: Fate of autogenous septal cartilage after transplantation in human tissue. Arch. Otolaryngol., *34*:697, 1941.

Peer, L. A.: Diced cartilage grafts. Arch. Otolaryngol., *38*:156, 1943.

Peer, L. A.: Transplantation of Tissues. Vol. 1. Baltimore, Williams & Wilkins Company, 1955.

Peer, L. A.: Sex chromatin study to determine the survival of cartilage homografts. Transplant. Bull., *5*:404, 1958.

Rasi, H. B.: The fate of preserved human cartilage. Plast. Reconstr. Surg., *24*:24, 1959.

Rasi, H. B.: Follow-up clinic. Plast. Reconstr. Surg., *49*:83, 1972.

Smith, A. U.: Survival of frozen chondrocytes isolated from cartilage of adult animals. Nature (Lond.), *205*:782, 1965.

Straith, C. L., and Slaughter, W. B.: Grafts of preserved cartilage in restoration of facial contour. J.A.M.A., *116*:2008, 1941.

Szabon, J.: Unsere Erfahrungen mit Septumknorpelimplantationen in post-traumatischen Fallen. Otolaryngol. Pol., *16*:1a, 1962.

Thomas, L.: Reversible collapse of rabbit ears after intravenous papain and prevention of recovery by cortisone. J. Exp. Med., *104*:245, 1956.

Weaver, J. M., Algire, G. H., and Prehn, R. T.: The growth of cells in vivo in diffusion chambers. II. The role of cells in the destruction of homografts in mice. J. Natl. Cancer Inst., *15*:1737, 1955.

Woodruff, M. F. A.: Cellular and humoral factors in the immunity to skin homografts: Experiments with a porous membrane. Ann. N.Y. Acad. Sci., *64*:1014, 1957.

CHAPTER 13

TRANSPLANTATION OF BONE

J. J. LONGACRE, M.D., PH.D.,
JOHN MARQUIS CONVERSE, M.D.,
AND DAVID M. KNIZE, M.D.

Bone is a dynamic living substance which shows marked structural alterations in response to injury, changes of stress, and vascular, endocrine, genetic, and nutritional influences. It is one of the few human organs that can undergo regeneration rather than repair with formation of scar tissue. Bone is a specialized form of connective tissue which provides support and protection for the vital and delicate organs of the body and also allows for locomotion. It is characterized by the presence of cells (*osteocytes*) that occupy cavities (*lacunae*). Long, branching processes from these cells lie in fine canals (*canaliculi*), which course through a hard, dense matrix consisting of collagenous fibers embedded in an amorphous ground substance (*cement*) impregnated with calcium phosphate complexes (Fig. 13–1). The primary structural unit of bone is the *osteon* (Fig. 13–2), laid down in laminated layers around central blood vessels in the haversian canal.

According to its origin, bone may be divided into *chondral* and *mesenchymal* forms. Growth of any long bone, a chondral bone, is occasioned by cartilaginous growth of the epiphysis, which is gradually replaced by new bone from the diaphysis. Membranous bone is formed by the replacement of a membrane of preexisting condensed mesenchyma. The regenerative powers of bone are limited except in the very young.

Every bone contains two types of tissue:

The outer layer is *compact cortical bone*, the surface of which is penetrated by canals (Volkmann's canals) which carry blood vessels that anastomose with those of the haversian canals (Fig. 13–3). Blood from the haversian canals supplies the osteocytes through the canaliculi. The osteons of the long bones are

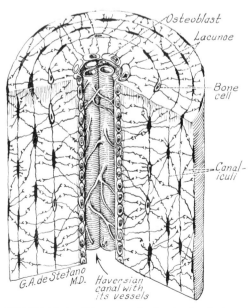

FIGURE 13–1. Diagrammatic sketch of a single osteon of the haversian system.

313

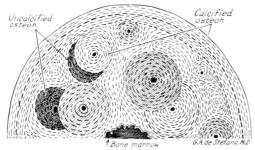

FIGURE 13-2. Cross section of compact bone as seen by microradiography. Note that the osteons are oriented in the longitudinal axis of the long bone. The dark masses represent recent uncalcified osteons. The light masses represent older calcified osteons.

oriented in the general direction of the longitudinal axis (see Fig. 13–2). Cortical bone is covered with periosteum, which has two layers of cells. The cells of the outer layer resemble fibrocytes, while those of the deeper (cambium) layer resting on the cortical bone surface are plump and round. The latter layer contains the blood vessels, and its cells differentiate into osteoblasts, which add new bone to the cortical surface (Fig. 13–3, *A*).

The inner layer is *coarse cancellous bone* (Fig. 13–3, *B*), open and trabeculated but similar in structure to compact bone. It differs in that complete osteons are present only in the thickened trabeculae, which branch out to

form the framework surrounding the marrow-filled spaces. The surfaces of the trabeculae are covered with resting osteoblasts.

OSTEOGENESIS

Bone tissue is in a continuous flux throughout life, and its osteocytes have a limited life span. Portions of bone with osteocytes nearing the end of their life span must be removed and replaced by new bone with young and vital osteocytes. Regenerative activity is the result of the interplay of multinucleated cells (*osteoclasts*), which erode the old bone, and large, single, nucleated cells (*osteoblasts*), which lay down the osteogenic fibers. According to Bourne (1972), a great amount of extracellular phosphatase appears on the fibrous matrix aggregate, and it is in these areas that the osteoid tissue begins to form. Following the formation of the new bone, phosphatase activity is lost, to return to the osteocyte only under certain conditions (necrosis or tumor formation). In mature bone the phosphatase reaction appears to be restricted to the periosteum (osteoblasts, capillaries, and fibers), the endosteum (including that of the haversian canals), and the more superficially placed osteocytes. As the osteocytes become more deeply em-

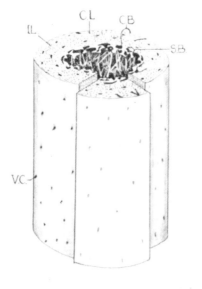

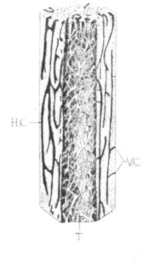

FIGURE 13-3. *A*, A diagrammatic sketch of compact cortical bone of the human tibia. C.L., circumferential lamellae. I.L., interstitial lamellae. C.B., compact bone. S. B., spongy bone. V.C., Volkmann's canal. *B*, Wedge of compact bone removed as demonstrated in Figure 13–1, looking into the marrow side. Note the direction of the osteons of the long bone oriented in a longitudinal axis. H.C., haversian canal. V.C., Volkmann's canal. T., trabeculae.

A

B

bedded and thus older, they become more and more enzymatically inactive until they finally become negative. According to Ham and Gordon (1952), in addition to the periosteum and endosteum, the bone marrow is a descendant of the original anlage of the "periosteal bud." It is this undifferentiated "mother cell" in the bone marrow that retains the potential to form osteogenic cells.

Because bone is a dense substance which cannot grow by interstitial expansion, growth of mature bone is accomplished by apposition of new bone on its surface areas. Although subperiosteal or subendosteal deposition is necessary to increase the diameter of a bone, growth does not occur simply by an evenly distributed apposition onto all surfaces; rather, the regulatory mechanism called *remodeling* occurs, which involves the simultaneous processes of bone deposition and resorption in selective areas. For example, the midportion of a long bone grows in diameter by subperiosteal deposition, while the endosteal surface is proportionally removed by resorption. However, with growth of the mandible or the metaphysis of a long bone, the remodeling process may require deposition of new bone on the endosteal surface, while the subperiosteal surface undergoes resorption. Much of this complex mechanism of remodeling has been clarified by Enlow (1963).

During the period of skeletal growth the formation of new bone outweighs resorption. In the healthy adult both processes are in balance. In the aged, regenerative apposition lags behind resorption, thus leading to senile osteoporosis. The presence of resting or reversal lines in a section of bone permits the reconstruction of a history of that area in much the same manner as a geologist reconstructs the past from the study of the rock strata of a region. The biophysical investigations of bone by Engström, Amprino, and Finean (1946, 1950, 1953, 1955) and Holmstrand (1957) allow the study of the differentiation of the newly laid down bone from the old, the degree of calcification, and the orientation of the inorganic hydroxyapatite crystals along with the orientation of collagen fibrils embedded in or resting on the bone. The collagen fibrils in a lamella are arranged in bundles which encircle the canal in continuous spirals, resulting in a trellislike arrangement. This arrangement imparts maximal structural strength to the tissue; it gives a characteristic appearance when viewed in polarized light. The inorganic crystals of hydroxyapatite are deposited in this highly ordered matrix of collagen and ground substances. The crystals are aligned with their long axes parallel to the longitudinal axis of the fibril. The distribution of these crystals can be studied by microradiography and their direction determined by microdiffraction.

In order to resist mechanical strain in the most efficient manner, the trabeculae of the cancellous bone are oriented along the lines of maximum stress. It is thought by some that the size and orientation of these trabeculae can change in response to altered mechanical demands. This concept of the functional adaptation of bone was first advocated by Wolff (1892). To date no adequate explanation of the mechanism has been presented. The work of Holmstrand (1957) has challenged Wolff's law by showing that the direction of the vessels growing into a compact bone graft in rabbits accounts for the orientation of the bone crystallites in the new osteons of the graft, and that mechanical forces in spite of previous assertions do not influence the ultrastructural organization of the substituting bone. In 1960 Holmstrand, Longacre and DeStefano were able to confirm this finding further in the study of a series of split rib autografts and allografts used to reconstruct skull defects in seventeen Macaca rhesus monkeys. The "healing-in" time of these grafts varied from two weeks to two years. Microdiffraction studies again showed that the structure of the original split rib graft and the placement of it either sagittally or transversely in the skull defect are the deciding factors in the ultrastructure of the new substituting bone in the graft. The following is a summary of the findings in these experiments:

1. Vascularization of the graft is brought about by vessels originating from the host skull bone and entering the graft primarily at its ends and extending along the old haversian systems of the graft. This has been observed by microangiography as early as two weeks following implantation (Fig. 13–4).

2. Demineralization of the graft is the main activity during the first six months. This is followed by replacement of the old haversian systems by new osteons that are only slightly mineralized. These follow the original pattern of the original osteons of the graft.

3. During the first six months postoperatively, the vascularization and demineralization in the autografts take place sooner than in the fresh allografts (Fig. 13–5), but after an interval of two years there is little discernible difference.

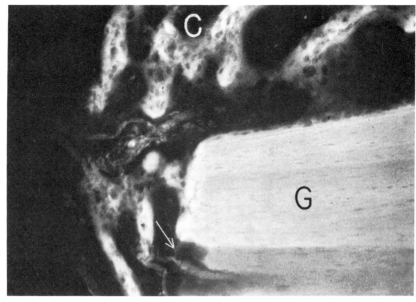

FIGURE 13–4. Microradiogram of an 80-micron thick sagittal section of a split rib graft (the rib is sectioned lengthwise) two weeks after surgery. Callus structures are seen at C. Notice the large lacunae of the osteocytes in the callus in comparison with the finer lacunae seen in the graft at G. The arrow points to a contrast-filled vessel which enters an old haversian system in the graft. Notice the demineralization occurring around this vessel. Recorded with Cu K alpha radiation at 27 kv. Primary magnification × 80.

4. Studies by microradiography and in polarized light disclose the fate of the graft after a "healing-in" period of 16 months. Both autografts (Fig. 13–6) and allografts (Fig. 13–7) retain their original orientation and their morphologic characteristics.

5. The osseous union between adjacent rib grafts and between rib grafts and skull results in a structure which in many respects resembles the normal calvarium after the final formation of an inner and outer table (see Fig. 13–6). The direction of the osteons in this newly laid down bone corresponds to the direction of the osteons of the donor site.

6. The fibrous union (Fig. 13–8) between adjacent rib grafts and between rib grafts and skull has the morphologic characteristics of a normal cranial suture (Fig. 13–9).

7. Microdiffraction studies prove that the ultrastructural organization of the inorganic hydroxyapatite crystals depends on the direction of the osteons of the original graft (see Figs. 13–7 and 13–10).

The Role of the Ground Substance

The ground substance consists of less than 5 per cent of the matrix. In attempting to assign a specific role to the ground substance in cal-cification, two properties stand out as important. One is that its state of aggregation is probably that of a gel in which the mucopolysaccharides are combined with a protein moiety as a mucoprotein. The anionic groups of this mucoprotein are free and reactive (Schubert and Hammerman, 1956), and this accounts for the large cation-binding capacity of the ground substance. In vivo the rapid depolymerization of the mucopolysaccharide protein complexes and the subsequent decrease in their cation-binding properties may lead to release of free cations, including calcium. This increase in calcium ion concentration may end in the initiation of calcification.

Rather than beginning by the process of simple precipitation, calcification is thought to begin with crystal nucleation followed by crystal growth, with the collagen portion of the matrix as the nucleation site. Anderson's (1969, 1970) and Matsuzawa and Anderson's (1971) electron microscopic observations of endochondral calcification appear to have located vesicles containing the earliest recognized deposits of hydroxyapatite. This work holds promise for clarifying the mechanism of calcification.

The mineralization of bone is a vital process that demands exquisite homeostatic control mechanisms. Though the blood and tissue fluids

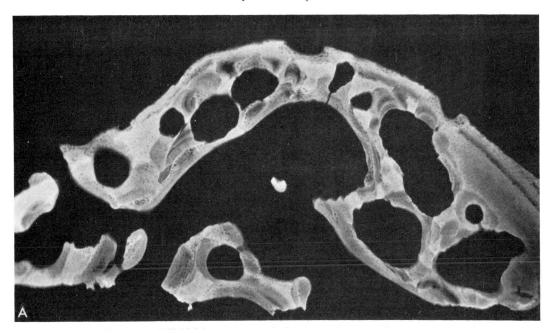

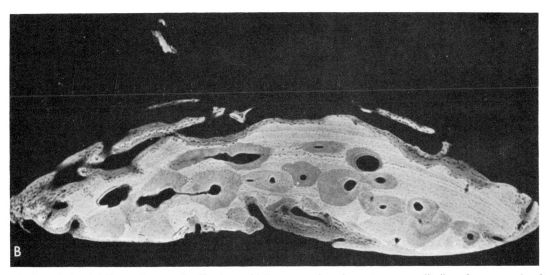

FIGURE 13–5. *A,* Microradiogram of a 90-micron thick cross section of an autogenous split rib graft seven weeks after surgery. Notice the large resorption cavities inside the graft, giving it the appearance of spongy bone. *B,* Microradiogram of an 80-micron thick cross section of a split rib allograft seven weeks after surgery. This graft was grafted in the same animal as the autogenous graft in *A.* Microradiograms in *A* and *B* recorded with Cu K alpha radiation at 27 kv. Primary magnification for *A* and *B* × 20.

contain calcium and phosphate ions, hydroxy-apatite crystal formation does not occur in any collagenous tissue other than bone, cartilage, or tooth except in ectopic bone formation. According to Glimcher (1960), the control of this specificity is apparently placed in the detailed intramolecular structure of the collagen macromolecules, their linear polymers, and their lateral aggregation patterns.

EXPERIMENTAL BONE TRANSPLANTATION: A HISTORICAL REVIEW

In order to appreciate the significance of recent contributions, a short historical review is indicated. Though Van Meekren (1668) reported an attempt to repair a cranial defect in a Russian soldier with a dog's skull bone, the failure of

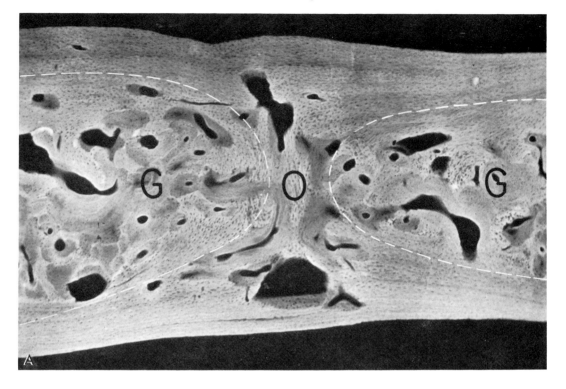

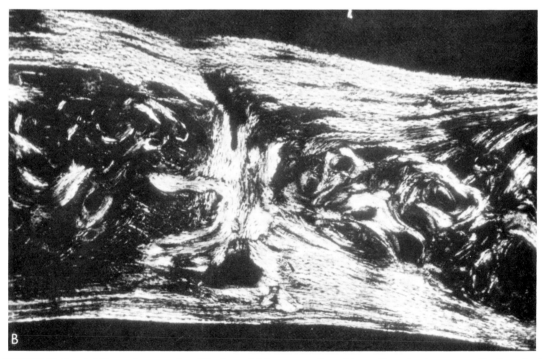

FIGURE 13–6. *A,* Microradiogram of an 80-micron thick cross section of two adjacent autogenous split rib grafts 16 months after surgery. Inner and outer tables of calvarium have reformed. The dotted lines indicate the approximate original size of the rib grafts in cross section. O is the osseous union between the ribs. Some resorption cavities are seen between the outer and inner tables. Many haversian systems with a low mineralization are indicative of the rebuilding activities inside the "reconstructed" calvarium. Registered with Cu K alpha radiation at 27 kv. Primary magnification × 20. *B,* The same specimen as in *A* but seen in polarized light. The birefringent collagen bundles in the outer and the inner tables are oriented transversely in the picture and parallel with the skull roof, whereas the collagen in the haversian osteons inside the "regenerated" ribs is oriented perpendicular to the plane of the picture. Primary magnification × 20.

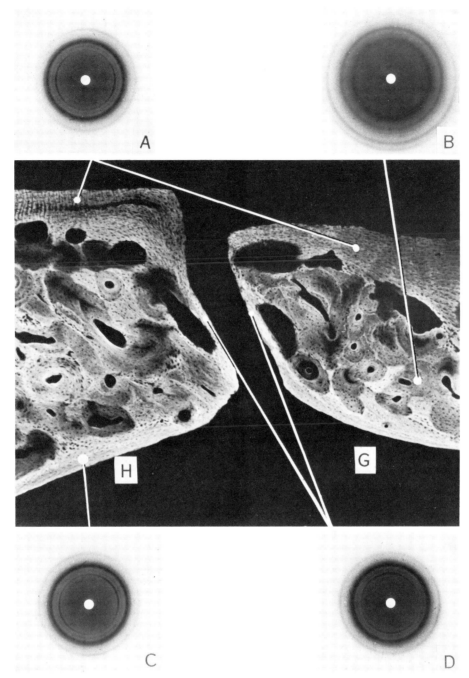

FIGURE 13–7. Microradiogram of an 80-micron thick cross section of a split rib allograft at 16 months after surgery. The letters G and H refer to the rib graft and the host skull bone, respectively. The white lines point out the sites where the microdiffraction examinations were recorded. All diffractograms, *A* to *D*, show the typical pattern of hydroxyapatite. Diffractogram *A* gives the orientation of the bone crystallites in the outer table of the host skull bone and of the graft. It is parallel to the plane of the picture and parallel to the skull roof; this is indicated by the position in the diffractogram of the arcs constituting the 002 reflection. The same orientation was obtained for the bone crystallites in the inner table of the host skull bone, as is indicated by diffractogram *C*. On the other hand, the orientation of the bone crystallites in the new haversian osteons in the graft is perpendicular to the plane of the picture, as shown by diffractogram *B* (this orientation is indicated by the absence of the 002 reflection). Diffractogram *D* recorded from bone adjacent to the fibrous union between the host bone and the graft shows that the orientation of the bone crystallites is parallel to that of the collagen fibers in the fibrous union (compare Figure 13–8). Microradiogram and diffractograms recorded with Cu K alpha radiation at 27 kv. Primary magnification × 20.

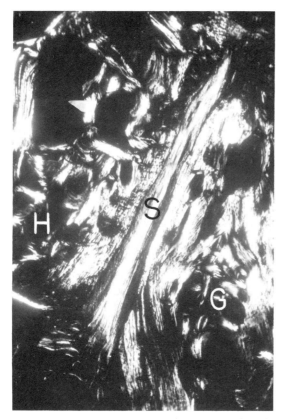

FIGURE 13–8. An 80-micron thick cross section of a split rib allograft with a healing-in time of 16 months. H, G, and S, respectively, refer to the host skull bone, the rib graft, and the fibrous union between the two. Notice in this picture the similarity between the orientation of the collagen in the fibrous union and the orientation of the collagen in the cranial suture seen in Figure 13–9. Polarized light; primary magnification × 50.

this heterogenous graft did not become evident inasmuch as Van Meekren was forced to remove the bone graft or else suffer excommunication. The real interest in the grafting of bone followed the publication in 1867 of the fundamental experimental work of Ollier. Inspired by Claude Bernard, his work emphasized the importance of the periosteum in osseous regeneration. In 1878 Macewen reconstructed an extensive defect of the humerus in a child in three stages with bone fragments (allografts) of wedges removed from the curved exterior tibial crests of three other children. However, the defect in this case was produced by the removal of a large sequestrum for chronic osteomyelitis. In 1912 Macewen reported the repair of a defect of the mandible with strips of autogenous rib.

Phemister (1914) showed that osteogenesis in experimental animals occurs from both the periosteum and the endosteum and that the bone cells and fibrous content of the haversian canals participate but to a lesser extent. Moreover, he noted that a bone graft split longitudinally showed marked callus formation along the entire length of the medullary canal. He also showed that if a bone graft devoid of periosteum was cut into small pieces, more callus was formed. He thought that this finding was due to the fact that more bone cells survive because of the increase in surface area, the increase in facilities for nutrition, and the factor of greater functional irritation. As a result considerable callus is formed about each piece, and the pieces fuse and rapidly restore the continuity of the shaft. It is of interest that, though he noted this, he did not change his conclusions except to advise the use of chips at the ends of the grafts. It was Phemister (1914) who emphasized that the fate of transplanted bone depended upon perfect hemostasis, perfect asepsis, and perfect coaptation of parts.

Gallie and Robertson in 1918 proved that the periosteum alone cannot be depended upon for osteogenesis but that its importance lies in the preservation of the blood supply to the recipient bone ends and that undue stripping of the periosteum is to be avoided. Their experiments emphasized the superiority of the autogenous cancellous transplant over the compact cortical graft. They pointed out that the grafts should be porous so that osteoblasts may obtain the necessary supply of tissue fluid nitrients to permit their maximum survival until revascularization can occur. They also suggested that small pieces of bone should be packed about the graft so as to increase the number of surviving osteoblasts. Their work also indicated the part that function plays in the ultimate survival and hypertrophy of bone grafts, thus reemphasizing the observations of Roux (1895) that bone obeys the laws of functional adaptation: "There is a distinct relation between the form, size and structure of a tissue or organ and the function it has to perform and a change in any of these factors results in corresponding changes in the other."

Much experimental investigation followed. The following are some of the landmarks: Keith (1919) felt that the osteoblasts were a specialized type of bone-forming cells which seemed to conduct the work of bone building as if they had been given the training of expert and unerring engineers. Likewise, Cartier (1951) expressed the view that the osteoblasts

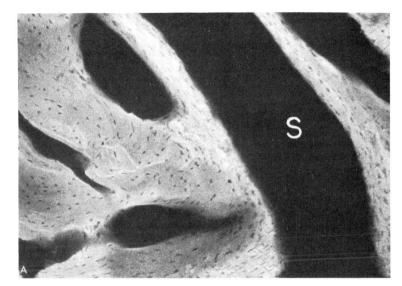

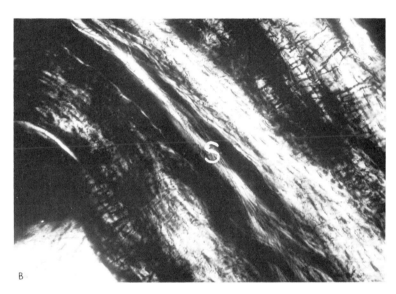

FIGURE 13–9. *A,* Microradiogram of a 90-micron thick cross section of a normal calvarium in an adult rhesus monkey. S refers to the cranial suture, which does not contain any mineral salts and therefore appears dark in the microradiogram. Recorded with Cu K alpha radiation at 27 kv. *B,* From the same specimen as is seen in *A* but photographed in polarized light. S indicates collagen inside the cranial suture. The collagen is oriented in the longitudinal extension of the suture and is parallel with the plane of the picture. Primary magnification for *A* and *B* × 80.

preside over the formation and life of osseous tissue. This is entirely contrary to the view of Leriche and Policard, who in 1926 regarded these cells as "banal reactionary fibroblasts." They denied them any special function and claimed that they were degenerated fibroblasts trapped in the spread of bone matrix. An opposing view was held by Bourne (1956), who presented evidence that the osteoblast is responsible for the secretion of the fibrous protein (collagen) and alkaline phosphatase and that the osteoblast may also contain hexose-phosphate and mucopolysaccharides. It seems clear that the osteoblast is the essential cell for bone formation, but the necessity of its continued presence within lacunae in the bone as

an osteocyte is open to question. The bone of higher orders of teleosts is acellular and without lacunae or canaliculi, yet it has the histologic, chemical, and physical properties of human bone (Moss and Frielich, 1963; Simmons, Simmons and Marshall, 1970). Moss (1961) believed that acellular bone is formed by osteoblasts which recede before becoming trapped as osteocytes. The function of the osteocyte in human bone is still not clear.

The origin of the osteoblast has been attributed to the multipotential cell, the local fibroblast cell (Anderson, 1961), and cells of vascular origin. There is now evidence to support the latter possibility. The earliest evidence of osteogenic activity in a bone

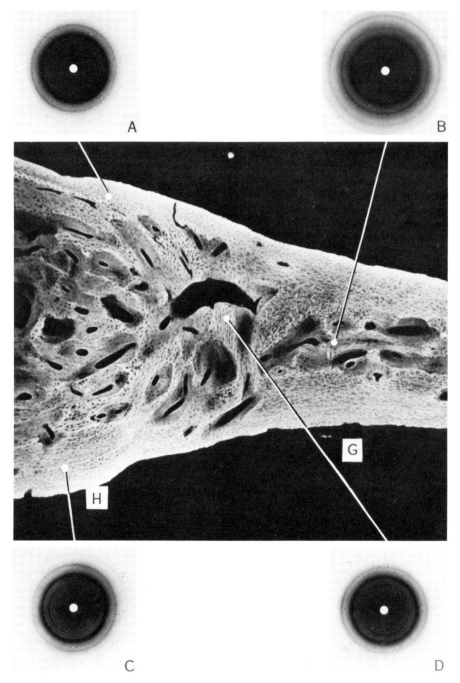

FIGURE 13–10. Microradiogram of an 85-micron thick cross section of an allograft 16 months after surgery. Letters H and G refer to the host bone and the rib graft, respectively. Diffractogram *D* was recorded from the osseous union between the graft and host bone and shows that the orientation of the bone crystallites is perpendicular to the skull roof and parallel to the plane of the picture; therefore it is the same as the orientation of the collagen fibers in a fibrous union between a graft and skull bone. For explanation of the diffractograms *A, B,* and *C* reference is made to Figure 13–7. Microradiogram and the diffractograms were recorded with Cu K alpha radiation at 27 kv. Primary magnification × 20.

transplant is the observation of a faint ring of calcification about vessels penetrating the graft. Makin's (1964) convincing study using tritiated thymidine–labeled cells suggests that the endothelial or perivascular adventitial cell can assume the function of the osteoblast. Trueta (1963) further supported the vascular origin of osteogenetic cells with his micro-photographic studies.

In 1930 Ham pointed out that the osteogenic

cell has a dual potential: whether it forms bone or cartilage depends primarily on the environment in which it differentiates. If the vascularity is good, bone will be produced. As the cells outrun their blood supply, cartilage will be formed first. In this case the new bone will be formed by a process similar to that on the diaphyseal side of the epiphyseal plate. Ham's theory has been more recently supported by Bassett, Hurley and Stinchfield (1962), who observed that low oxygen tension induced the formation of cartilage in skeletal tissue culture. Later Hall (1969) found that pressure is a much more potent stimulus to cartilage formation than low oxygen tension in tissue culture studies.

Living bone stimulated by direct current forms new bone about the cathode (Becker, Bassett and Bachman, 1964), and there is bony resorption about the anode (Friedenberg and Kohanim, 1968). These findings suggest that electronegativity stimulates the osteoblasts, and electropositivity stimulates the osteoclast.

Recent evidence indicates that calcitonin (Knize, 1973) and growth hormone (Knize, Gershberg and Ballantyne, 1973) stimulate the activity of the osteoblast, or at least inhibit osteoclastic activity, in bone transplants. These mechanical, chemical, and hormonal factors probably act through the osteogenetic cell, possibly by affecting its genetic machinery.

THE IMMUNE RESPONSE TO BONE ALLOGRAFTS AND XENOGRAFTS

For a number of years following World War II there was a certain amount of enthusiasm for the use of preserved bovine bone implants (xenografts). Several years of careful follow-up revealed such a high percentage of failures and absorption that the technique fell into disfavor. A second wave of enthusiasm for the use of lyophilized calf bone implants has developed in the United States. Careful and unbiased followers are now reporting a high percentage of absorptions and failures. Carefully controlled experimental work at Oxford by Stringa (1957) showed that the fresh living autograft was quickly vascularized, while there was delayed vascularization and a high rate of complications when allografts were used. However, in a xenograft there was an immediate walling off of the foreign body by the tissues of the host. The xenograft was never incorporated or vascularized, and eventually the chances of extrusion were comparable to those for other foreign bodies.

Studies of the antigen-antibody reaction demonstrate that in the case of the bone allograft the main antigens are associated with the nucleated marrow cells, while in the xenograft the matrix and the serum proteins are antigenic.

According to Enneking (1962), bone tissue antigens are not different from other tissues. They stimulate cellular antibodies and hemoagglutinins, which in turn destroy the proliferating transplanted cells and remaining matrix. However, bone is antigenic for only a limited time, and the intensity and effectiveness of the immune response vary considerably. These factors combined may lead to temporary immunoparalysis.

The success of a graft depends upon its early vascularization. Holmstrand (1957) demonstrated that new blood vessels from the bed enter the haversian systems of the bone graft as early as the second week.

Burwell (1962) has shown that primary fresh allografts are less well vascularized than autogenous bone and that substances were carried directly to the lymph nodes draining the area and produced a proliferative response of the lymphocytes within three days. However, when "second set grafts" were then introduced into the host, the reaction was much more rapid and violent, with marked lymphoid hyperplasia and enlargement of the regional nodes. The large and medium lymphoid cells quickly destroyed all exposed cells of the graft, and there was no new bone formation.

Graft antigenicity has been diminished by freezing (with or without radiation), by freeze drying, and by methods which extract the soluble antigens. These basic studies help to explain why certain preserved, nonviable bone allografts and processed xenografts are occasionally successful in orthotopic sites, where large numbers of host osteogenic cells are available, as in spinal fusion.

In an attempt to reduce the immune response to the xenograft, cobalt irradiation has been used to sterilize the bone. Short-term observations of these implants showed that there was less reaction on the part of the host. Long-term studies, however, showed that 95 per cent of the implant remained after 20 months and that there was no creeping substitution, as was noted along fresh allografts. Bassett, Hurley and Stinchfield (1962) concluded that further clinical use was not indicated.

While the work by Burwell (1968) confirmed the existence of intrinsic osteogenic inductors, it is increasingly apparent that cells of the graft (particularly those on its surface) may survive and form bone shortly after transplantation. For this reason fresh, autogenous, cancellous bone continues to be the best material to aid osteogenesis in the recipient region. On the other hand, a preserved allograft and processed (deantigenetic) xenograft, when employed for mechanical support, seem to perform as well as a cortical autograft.

The state of cell variability is involved not only in the function of a bone graft but also in the semantics of bone grafting. Viable bone transplants should be considered as grafts, while nonviable ones (allografts and xenografts) must be classified as implants, since their behavior is similar to that of metallic or alloplastic implants. A graft must be defined as anything inserted which becomes an integral part of the host. Finally it is not sufficient to have merely a stimulus for bone formation. It is necessary to have a good vascular bed, for in the absence of a proper nutritional and physical milieu, the osteocytes may not synthesize the organic precursors of an osseous matrix.

It is thus strongly suggested that fresh bone autograft remain the graft of choice, followed by the graft of freeze-dried bone, which is far less desirable. The long-term results with all forms of grafted anorganic bone leave much to be desired.

Using the accelerated rejection of a skin allograft as a test to demonstrate the immune response to a previously implanted fresh bone allograft, according to the technique of Chalmers (1959), Brooks and coworkers (1963) investigated the immune response to various types of bone implants. These included fresh allografts; frozen allografts; frozen, irradiated allografts; freeze-dried allografts; frozen, dried, and irradiated allografts; deproteinized, nonautoclaved allografts; deproteinized, frozen allografts and decalcified allografts. The various transplants were placed, in a first stage, into the lateral thigh muscles of the anesthetized C57 mouse. The bone allografts were all removed from C3H donors. After a three-week delay, to allow the C57 mouse recipient to become sensitized to the C3H bone allograft, a full thickness graft from another C3H donor was transplanted to the C57 recipient of the allografts. Both C57 and C3H mice were isogenic strains. The accelerated rejection of the skin allograft was used as a test to demonstrate that the recipient had undergone an immune response to the implanted bone. As judged from the accelerated rejection of the skin allograft, fresh bone allografts have

antigens in common with skin. Freezing and freeze-drying the bone allograft seemed to inactivate the antigens. Decalcification, deproteinization, and deproteinization and freezing of the bone allografts seemed to leave intact a sufficient quantity of common antigens with skin to produce an acceleration of the skin allograft rejection.

It should be noted that in this experimental series, virtually all of the calcium had been removed, but the organic matrix which remained seemed to retain antigenic properties. It was also interesting that freezing and drying from the frozen state altered the antigens and provoked a lesser response to the challenge by the skin allografts.

CLINICAL ASPECTS OF BONE TRANSPLANTATION

The manner in which bone behaves as a transplant depends first upon its original structure.

Compact Cortical Bone Autograft

Some of the osteoblasts of an autogenous transplant may survive and give rise to new bone when the transplant is adequately supplied by tissue fluids. Studies using supravital dye, which is incorporated into areas of bone where osteogenic activity is in progress at the time of the dye injection, suggest that osteogenesis occurs in an autograft within the first week after transplantation (Fig. 13–11). This early osteogenic activity is thought to be that of the surviving transplanted osteoblasts. The callus tissue from the bed spreads over the transplant and fixes it. The haversian canals are slowly invaded by the blood vessels and osteogenic cells from the host. Two processes occur simultaneously—absorption and new formation. The transplant comes to consist of an interwoven mixture of dead and new bone.

Cancellous Bone Autograft

The open trabeculae of the cancellous graft permit the survival of the maximal number of osteoblasts, and hence this graft will become incorporated more quickly and more completely. Gordon and Ham (1950) transplanted cancellous bone chips to muscle and found that only those close to capillaries of living muscle survived. They, in turn, proliferated and gave

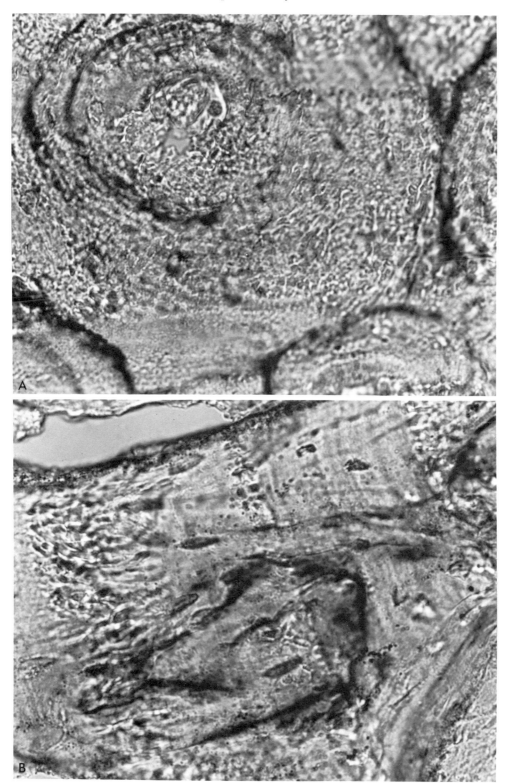

FIGURE 13–11. *A*, Section of bone in situ, with supravital dye marker of lead sulfate which indicates areas of new bone formation at the time of dye injection. Note outline of haversian systems. × 400. *B*, Section of a bone transplant labeled by the supravital dye which was injected on the seventh day post grafting. This suggests that transplanted osteogenic cells survive and continue to function in new bone formation. × 500.

rise to new trabeculae which grew toward the capillaries. Ham and Gordon (1952) found that they had to freeze and thaw these bone grafts three successive times in order to destroy this growth potential. From this they concluded that new bone comes from the osteogenic cell and that it is not produced by fibroblasts induced by "ergastoplasm" released from the bone; they presumed that the osteoblasts survive in cancellous bone fragments following transplantation.

For all practical purposes the surgeon should depend on the osteoblasts living on the surface of the bone graft and its many trabeculae and on the undifferentiated cells of the bone marrow for osteogenesis. Such bone induction as usually occurs in fractures and in association with bone transplants depends on these osteogenic cells' growing abundantly.

Practical Applications

Despite the experimental observations just mentioned, the proper clinical application did not follow for some years. Under the persuasive influence of Murphy (1913) and Albee (1915) in America and Groves (1917) in England, bone grafts were handled more as a cabinet maker would saw and fit his wood, rather than as a surgeon should handle living tissue. Little thought was given to the fact that the heat generated by the elaborate motor-driven saws would destroy the osteoblasts not only on the cut edges of the bone graft but also on the edges of the defect in the bone. Likewise, the use of cortical bone to produce the rigidity which these workers regarded as so essential also added to their difficulties. The concept finally arose that bone seldom, if ever, survives in its entirety and slowly undergoes "creeping substitution" from the host bone. Thus Orell of Stockholm (1937), thinking of the bone graft as a calcium bridge, reasoned that the removal of all organic substances should provide an "os purum." The use of this material, though successful in obliterating a bone cavity, failed to produce fusion either in an ununited fracture or in the arthrodesis of a joint. In short, more was needed for osteogenesis than the availability of calcium salts from a so-called bridge.

The observations of Mowlem (1952) have shown that the more trabeculae of the cancellous bone graft that are opened so that serum may enter and early vascular penetration occur, the higher will be the percentage of bone cells that survive. This is reflected by

evidence of cellular activity along the surfaces of the exposed trabeculae. The surviving osteoblasts cover the remaining trabeculae with a new layer of osteoid substance, and in time new bone will invade and replace the inner portion of the trabeculae where the osteocytes have failed to survive. Long before this occurs, the cancellous grafts will have fused with the recipient bone ends, and the muscular forces will provide the guiding force for the laying down and shaping of new bone. According to Mowlem, "The method should be directed to the creation of circumstances under which the maximum cellular survival is insured under conditions which will make the subsequent activity of the cells most effective. No longer is a bone graft that inorganic bridge which is to be completely resorbed and slowly replaced. Instead it is only the scaffold to carry these cells which can rapidly envelop it with new bone and incorporate it in the new repair."

This idea is not opposed to well documented work showing that most of a cortical graft is absorbed and replaced not only from the recipient bone bed but also from islands surviving in the graft. Bone is a living tissue, serving the function of support and designed to resist stress and strain. Its reactions must be the function of its cells. If their survival is ensured, its transplantation is satisfactory. If, in its new position, it serves the function of resisting stress and providing support, then it will persist and will be modified in shape and structure for the demands made upon it.

Clinical Use of Bone Grafts

In man the end result depends on the age of the patient, the condition of the graft and recipient bed, and the sterility of the wound. However, it has been shown that fresh autogenous grafts will survive in spite of a complicating infection. This is not true if the autograft has been boiled or refrigerated or if an allograft from a bone bank has been added. It will then be necessary to remove the bone if there is a draining sinus. The banked or boiled bone frequently is absorbed.

Tibial Bone Grafts. Prior to World War I and for many years after, the tibia was used as a source of osteoperiosteal grafts of cortical and cancellous bone. The approach is made along the anteromedial surface of the tibia through an incision parallel to the tibial crest. The osteoperiosteal grafts may be removed by cutting the periosteum with a knife and then removing shavings of cortex and periosteum with a chisel or gouge (Fig. 13–12). In order to fill a defect numerous grafts must be superimposed, and the contour is rather irregular. The fact that these grafts are thin accounts for the excellent osteogenic properties of this type of graft. If the amount of bone removed is small, there is little residual defect. If, however, the amount removed is large, for example, following the removal of a corticocancellous graft, a bone defect is produced that not only is disfiguring but also is the cause of a great deal of pain and frequently of secondary fracture.

The graft is kept moist with saline and then is carved using an osteotome, chisel, rongeur, or paring knife. Following this, it is carefully wedged into the defect and is usually fixed with wire or metallic screws.

Iliac Bone Autograft. Over the past three decades the ilium has become a favorite source of bone grafts. The ilium is composed almost entirely of cortical bone with an abundant supply of cancellous bone and is of variable thickness surrounded by two thin plates of cortex. The fact that the iliac crest is so accessible makes

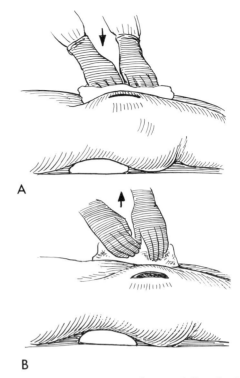

FIGURE 13–13. Exposure of crest of ilium for bone graft. *A*, Patient's hip is elevated by a sandbag to make the iliac crest prominent. The assistant presses a gauze pad against the skin just below the crest of the ilium and retracts the skin over the crest. *B*, Skin incision lies lateral to the crest of the ilium.

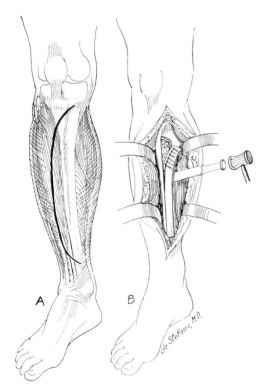

FIGURE 13–12. *A*, Incision for removal of tibial graft. *B*, Removal of graft.

the removal of the graft relatively simple, and the secondary defect is usually covered. However, the morbidity that follows the removal of this graft (in terms of bleeding, ileus, pain, and limping due to muscular spasm) is great in relation to the amount of bone removed.

One of the thicker (1.3 to 1.7 cm) areas of the iliac crest is the anterior third between the anterior superior iliac spine and the tubercle of the crest. Posterior to this area the crest and ala become thinner until the posterior iliac spine is reached; this thicker region provides an additional source of bone.

TECHNIQUE. The incision extends through the skin and periosteum to the crest of the ilium. Just before the incision, the skin is retracted by the assistant in order that the incision will lie lateral and below the crest instead of over the crest (Fig. 13–13). The periosteum is then reflected and raised with a periosteal elevator (Fig. 13–14, *A*). A part of the crest, the full thickness of the crest (Fig. 13–14, *B*), or the inner table is exposed (Fig. 13–14, *C*), depending on the amount and shape

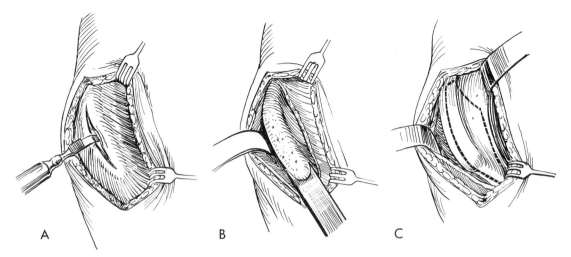

FIGURE 13-14. Removal of bone from the ilium. *A*, The periosteum has been incised and is being raised by an elevator. *B*, Resection of bone from the crest. *C*, Resection of bone from the inner table.

of the bone graft required. The periosteum covering the outer surface of the ala is also raised if the full thickness of the ala is required (Fig. 13-14, *B*). The inner table of the ilium and adherent cancellous bone are resected when a wider surface of bone is required; the periosteum is further elevated, raising the iliacus muscle with the periosteum and thus exposing a portion of the iliac fossa. By vertical sectioning of a portion of the crest and horizontal splitting of the crest between the vertical cuts, a section of the inner cortical table, with its underlying cancellous bone, may be separated and removed from the outer table (Fig. 13-14, *C*). The inner surface of the ilium is exposed rather than the lateral aspect, for the periosteum is raised with greater ease over the smooth medial surface, which is roofed over the iliacus muscle. The lateral aspect of the bone is uneven in the adult, serving as the area of insertion for the gluteal muscles.

In the adult, when cancellous bone alone is needed an osteotomy is made over the central portion of the iliac crest, and a wedge of cancellous bone is resected (Fig. 13-15); the outer and inner tables of the ilium are then fractured toward each other with heavy forceps in order to eliminate the resulting dead space between them. This technique does not disturb the continuity of the crest and leaves no visible deformity.

The technique advocated by Robertson and Baron (1946) can be employed when a large amount of cancellous bone is required; in this technique, the bone is sectioned below the crest of the ilium, reflecting the crest upward

and preserving the origin of the abdominal muscles (Fig. 13-16). Cancellous bone is removed from the center of the bone after separation of the cortical surfaces, and the crest is then replaced in its original position; cancellous chips can be removed with a gouge.

Patients experience more discomfort and difficulty in early ambulation when the full thickness of the ala is removed than when the outer table of the ilium is preserved. This inconvenience may be the result either of the extensive stripping of the lateral surface of the ilium to obtain wide exposure or of the weakening of the attachments of the gluteal musculature, the fascia lata, and the tensor of the fascia lata. The result is the so-called "gluteus gait," a persistent type of dragging limp. When the wound is being closed, care should be exercised to obtain a strong repair of the fascia lata, if divided, and an accurate apposition of the edges of the periosteum from which the abdominal and gluteal muscles arise.

Although it is occasionally necessary to remove all or part of the anterior superior iliac spine, this is likely to be attended by a definite morbidity and is better avoided. The outer edge of the crest gives attachment to the fascia lata and origin to the tensor fascia lata. Failure of good repair and sound healing of these may result in disturbances of gait, as already noted, or a "clicking" sound when the patient walks, produced by the fascia slipping suddenly over the greater trochanter instead of gliding smoothly over it.

The lateral cutaneous nerve of the thigh, in its pelvic location, takes a retroperitoneal course

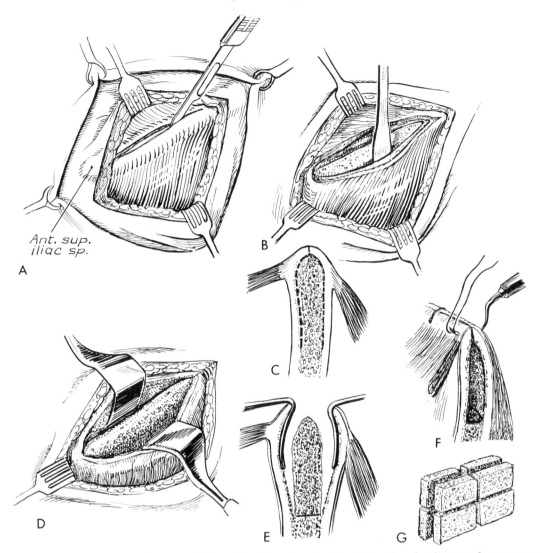

FIGURE 13–15. A technique for removal of cancellous bone from the ilium. *A*, Incision of periosteum after exposure of the crest. *B*, Separation of cortex with osteotome. *C*, Cross section showing lines of separation of inner and outer cortex from cancellous bone. *D*, Exposure of cancellous bone. *E*, Cross section showing exposure. *F*, Reunion of inner and outer cortex by stainless steel wire suture (after Tessier). *G*, Blocks and lamellae of cancellous bone obtained.

on the deep surface of the iliacus muscle. It leaves the pelvis by a variable route, usually just deep to the attachment of the inguinal ligament to the anterior and superior iliac spine, but sometimes through the ligament or even across the spine itself (Ghent, 1961). The nerve is thus easily damaged in this region, producing paresthesia and hypesthesia, which may be permanent over the lateral aspect of the thigh.

Interference with the attachment of the inguinal ligament or removal of massive grafts of the full thickness of the ilium may lead to the formation of hernias (Oldfield, 1945; Reid, 1968).

Cancellous bone bleeds readily, and hematoma formation is common, particularly if the inner table of the bone has been exposed, for a dead space remains between the bone and the detached iliacus muscle. Gelfoam soaked in thrombin solution or bone wax may be rubbed into the bleeding cancellous bone; hemorrhage from a spurting vessel is arrested by crushing the bone around the vessel. If the full thickness of the ala is removed, the dead space can be eliminated by suturing the iliacus muscle to the glutei, as advised by Dingman (1950). When relatively small bone grafts are resected from the iliac crest, a pressure dressing will collapse the dead space and prevent hematoma. It is our

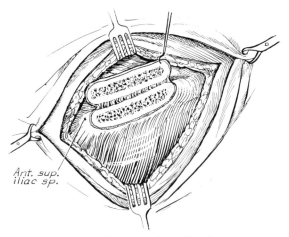

Ant. sup. iliac sp.

FIGURE 13–16. The crest of the ilium has been separated, remaining attached to the abdominal musculature. The cancellous bone is exposed.

practice, after exposure of the inner table, to leave a drain with continuous suction to evacuate the accumulated blood. The drain is placed in such a way that it may be removed without displacing the entire dressing. Early ambulation reduces the period of discomfort and disability.

The button-hole incision for cancellous chips. When cancellous chips are required to enhance the osteogenic processes along a line of osteotomy or to provide additional contour restoration, a short incision is made immediately behind the anterosuperior spine. Cancellous bone is abundant in this area and is resected without submitting the patient to a major operation.

THE ILIUM AS A SOURCE OF BONE GRAFTS IN CHILDREN. Bone grafts, either in the form of corticocancellous grafts or cancellous chips, are in general use for a number of reconstructive procedures. In infants, Breine and Johanson (1966) found that the tibia yields sufficient material for alveolar grafts in the cleft palate deformity. Knowledge of the various dimensions of the ilium in a child will allow the surgeon to obtain a surprising amount of corticocancellous and cancellous bone (Crockford and Converse, 1972). Moreover, it is possible to secure such bone through a subepiphyseal lateral approach, without in any way disturbing the integrity of the epiphyses of the crest—a disadvantage of the previously described techniques (Crenshaw, 1963).

Applied anatomy. At birth, the crest of the ilium is composed of a thick cap of primary cartilage which forms the rim and superior part of the ala, and which sits on the ossifying part of the body of the bone (Fig. 13–17, *A*). By the age of 9 years, this layer is but 1 cm in height. It is not until puberty that one or two secondary centers appear in it; they unite at 20 to 25 years of age (Brash, 1951).

Before puberty and the adolescent growth spurt, there is little difference between the pelvic bones of the sexes (Tanner, 1962). Thereafter, the characteristic changes of shape, angulation, and thickness occur, the female bone remaining thinner than that of the male (Bryce, 1915).

In the adult, because of the firm attachment of the gluteal muscles and the resultant irregularities of the surface, it can be difficult to strip cleanly the periosteum from the lateral surface of the bone. The crest and medial surface of the ilium are more easily exposed. In children this problem does not arise because the surface of the bone is smooth, and the firm attachment of the periosteum to the epiphyseal line is readily appreciated (this attachment marks the superior limit of the dissection). Thus the growing edge of the crest of the ilium, together with the attached abdominal muscles, may be left intact.

To illustrate the proportions of the ilium, a small adult female pelvis was studied, transilluminated, and sectioned. Further information was obtained from observations made in 26 infants, children, and young adolescents in the course of bone graft removals. Figure 13–18 shows, by transillumination, that the bone in the center of the iliac fossa is the thinnest part and may even be defective. This thin area lies posterior to a radius drawn through the tubercle of the crest—an easily identifiable landmark (Fig. 13–19, marker line 2). As the tubercle also indicates the posterior limit of the thickest part of the crest, it is the bone between the tubercle and the anterior superior iliac spine which forms the best source of grafts.

Measurements of fresh adult cadavers show that, for an "average" pelvis, the thickness of the crest 2 cm posterior to the anterior superior iliac spine is 1.5 cm; this increases to 1.7 cm through the tubercle. However, along a radius taken through the first point (Fig. 13–19, marker line 1), the thinnest area is 0.9 cm; an equivalent figure in the line of the tubercle is 0.5 cm. As can be readily appreciated from Figure 13–19, cut 3, the bone becomes progressively thinner posterior to the tubercle, until the region of the sacroiliac articulation is reached. These dimensions in childhood will be proportionately less. In the 9 year old, the

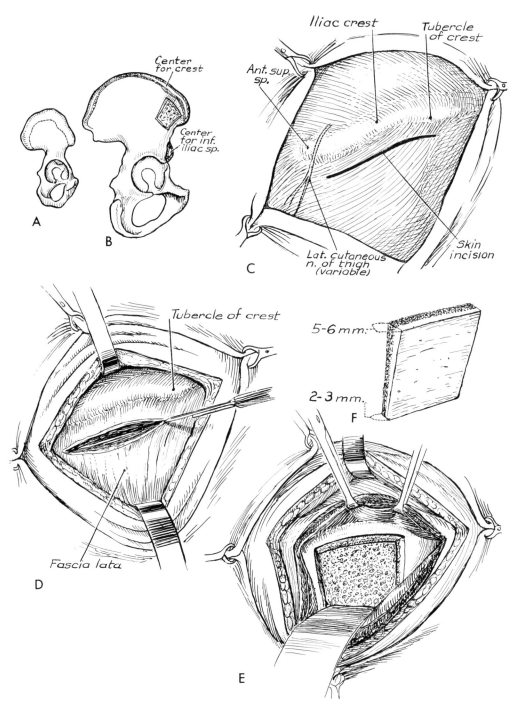

FIGURE 13–17. The ilium as a donor site for bone grafts in children. *A,* At birth about two-thirds of the ilium is ossified. The width of the cartilaginous epiphyseal crest is indicated by the dotted line. *B,* The ilium at birth. The growth centers for the iliac crest and the anteroinferior spine are indicated, as well as the site of bone graft removal. *C,* The site of the skin incision. *D,* The fascia lata and muscles are incised down to bone. *E,* The bone graft has been removed; the inner table is spared. *F,* The thickness of the bone graft removed in a 12 year old child. (From Crockford, D. A., and Converse, J. M.: The ilium as a source of bone grafts in children. Plast. Reconstr. Surg., *50*:270, 1972. Copyright 1972, The Williams & Wilkins Company, Baltimore.)

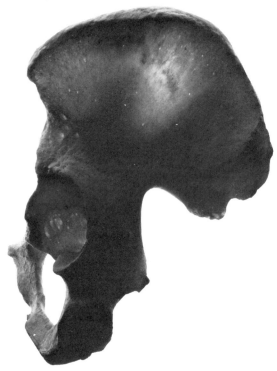

FIGURE 13–18. Transillumination shows that the thinnest part of the bone is in the center of the iliac fossa. (From Crockford, D. A., and Converse, J. M.: The ilium as a source of bone grafts in children. Plast. Reconstr. Surg., *50*:270, 1972. Copyright 1972, The Williams & Wilkins Company, Baltimore.)

thickest part of the crest is between 0.8 and 1.0 cm.

When a child is operated on, the immediate region of the anterior superior iliac spine should remain inviolate, owing to its important ligamentous and muscular attachments.

The two important structures disturbed by this operation are the *fascia lata,* which is attached along the line of the crest, and the *tensor fascia lata* muscle, which originates in the anterior quarter of the lateral edge of the crest. The normal locking of the knee joint in extension is dependent on the perfect function of these two structures.

Technique. Before draping, the pelvis is rotated 30 to 40 degrees away from the surgeon on sand bags. It is also advisable to place a sand bag under the ipsilateral shoulder to prevent excessive spinal rotation. The skin is then prepared and draped in the usual fashion, leaving the anterior superior iliac spine and the anterior half of the crest exposed.

Following retraction of the skin medially by an assistant (to ensure that the final position of the scar is well clear of the iliac crest), the incision is made in the line of the crest, starting

1 to 2 cm posterior to the anterior superior iliac spine and extending posteriorly as far as necessary. The wound is deepened through the superficial fascia to the *fascia lata,* and hemostasis is secured (Fig. 13–17, *C, D*). Then, with a clean knife, a firm incision is made through the *fascia lata* and the underlying muscle straight down onto the bone; the line of this incision should lie about 2 cm below the curve of the crest (Fig. 13–17, *C, D*). The bone is then exposed by subperiosteal dissection; care is taken superiorly not to disrupt the firm attachment of the periosteum to the epiphyseal line.

When hemostasis has been obtained, the corticocancellous graft or grafts required may be marked out with the corner of an osteotome, keeping at least 1 to 1.5 cm posterior to the anterior superior iliac spine and the anterior edge of the ilium. Then, using a curved-on-the-flat osteotome of the required width, the grafts may be removed (Fig. 13–17, *E, F*). With care, such an instrument will stay in the plane of the medulla. When sufficient graft has been obtained, a large curette or gouge may be used to harvest the cancellous bone lying between the two tables of the anterior (so far untouched) part of the ilium.

Bleeding should be controlled, but it is usually impossible to prevent bony surface oozing. This makes it imperative to close the wound around a suction drain. The wound should be closed in layers—*fascia lata* and muscle, Scarpa's fascia, and skin. It is rarely possible to make a comprehensive repair of the periosteum, but it cannot be too strongly emphasized that if the *tensor fascia lata* muscle and the *fascia lata* are not thoroughly repaired, an abnormal gait may result. Patients so affected walk with a limp, the affected leg swinging lateral to the normal straight line of advance (Casson, 1971).

The postoperative care of the wound presents no unusual problems. We have found that children can walk unaided with little discomfort after the removal of the drain 48 to 72 hours later.

The area below the posterior superior iliac spine was employed in a number of patients as a source of bone grafts for craniofacial surgery. Bone grafts could be removed from this site without repositioning the patient during the course of the operation and without leading to difficulties in the postoperative care of the donor site.

Complications. A number of complications may follow the removal of bone from the ilium.

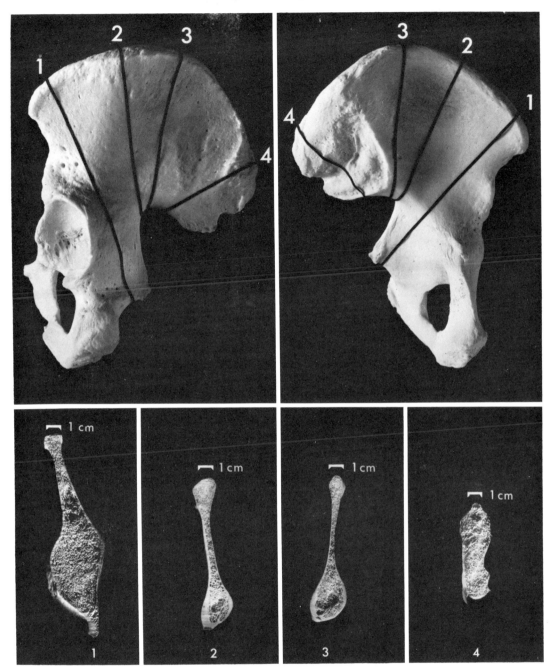

FIGURE 13–19. The same specimen as that in Figure 13–18. In the two top photographs, the black marker tapes show the lines of section. In the lower photographs, the cross-sectional appearance of the bone is shown — at the lines of section, looking anteriorly at each. *Cut 1,* Through the crest 2 cm posterior to the anterior superior iliac spine. *Cut 2,* Through the tubercle of the crest. *Cut 3,* Through the thinnest part of the crest. *Cut 4,* Through the posterior superior iliac spine. These photographs are all of the same scale. (From Crockford, D. A., and Converse, J. M.: The ilium as a source of bone grafts in children. Plast. Reconstr. Surg., *50:*270, 1972. Copyright 1972, The Williams & Wilkins Company, Baltimore.)

The steps necessary to reduce the incidence of most of these have already been mentioned.

Reports of herniation of abdominal contents through the scar, mentioned earlier, refer to adults in whom the abdominal muscles were dissected from their attachment to the iliac crest, and large full-thickness bone grafts were taken. With the subepiphyseal lateral approach, herniation is extremely unlikely because the medial table should remain intact. Even if it is removed, its periosteum should remain to form new bone. Moreover, any full thickness defect will be small and will be well protected from intra-abdominal pressure by the overlying iliacus muscle.

Grafts of Adjacent Bone

Following the original experimental work of Ollier (1867), osteoperiosteal grafts from the lamina and dorsal spines have been used with great success in spinal fusion. Since the work of Albee (1915) and Groves (1917), ununited fractures of the long bones have been fused by removing a section of bone at the site of the malunion and reversing it so that the fracture site is bridged in part by normal bone. In 1890 Mueller used a flap of scalp, to which was attached a portion of the outer table of the skull, to repair an adjacent cranial defect. More recently the outer table has been removed and used as a free graft to repair smaller defects of the skull.

Greater Trochanter and Olecranon Process Grafts

When only a small volume of autologous bone is needed, as is often the requirement for many hand surgical procedures, convenient, easily harvestable areas are the greater trochanter and the olecranon process. The olecranon process is especially convenient, since it can be included in the same surgical field as the hand.

An incision over the proximal end of the olecranon process is made down through periosteum. A periosteal elevator is used to expose a 1-cm square area of bone. A 4-mm osteotome is effective to transect the cortex, permitting the removal of a 1 × 1 cm section of cortical bone. Through this opening, cancellous bone can be removed with a curette. If the cortical bone is not needed, it can be replaced over the opening.

The greater trochanter is approached through a 3- to 4-cm vertical incision directly over this bony landmark. Fascia lata and tendinous insertions are split longitudinally, and with the wound retracted, periosteum is raised from the surface of the greater trochanter. An osteotome is used to remove a 1- to 2-cm square section of cortical bone, permitting access to the

abundant supply of cancellous bone available in the greater trochanter, which can be removed with a curette. If the cortical bone is not required, it can be used to cover the defect. The wound is closed in layers. Drains have not been necessary.

Unlike bone removal from the iliac crest, postoperative morbidity from using either the greater trochanter or the olecranon process is low. In the case of the trochanter, the patient may ambulate early with minimal discomfort.

Rib Grafts

Macewen in 1912 was among the first to utilize the rib in the repair of a mandibular defect. In 1915 Kappis employed full thickness rib with periosteum to cover a dural and cranial defect. The rib graft fell into disfavor principally because of the way in which it was utilized. When a whole rib is inserted, the only possible vascular penetration is through the cut ends of the graft and several Volkmann's canals. Otherwise, the rib presents only dense cortical bone on its surfaces with little chance of survival. The early work of Brown of Australia (1917) and Ballin of America (1921), both of whom suggested splitting the rib, leaving the inner portion of the rib to maintain an intact thoracic wall, made little impression. In 1928 Brown presented a ten-year "postal card" follow-up of his split rib cases, including

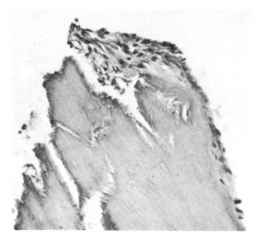

FIGURE 13–20. Split rib graft removed one week following insertion into cranial defect. Note absence of cells in the lacunae. Also note that there are living osteoblasts still present along the surface of the trabeculae.

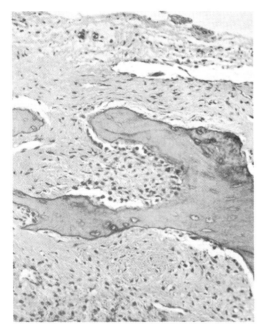

FIGURE 13-21. Two-week specimen shows rapid ingrowth of granulation tissue between the trabeculae. Note the absorption of bone with beginning formation of Howship's spaces in certain areas. In other areas there are living osteoblasts, and some have already surrounded themselves with osteoid tissue.

the roentgenograms of one patient. In 1937 Fagarasanu split the rib in order to gain more substance.

Until 1955, no one indicated the fact that rib bone differed from other bone in its osteogenic properties, in its adaptability to fit many defects, and in its extraordinary power to

regenerate repeatedly and thus provide a constant source of fresh autogenous bone to repair even the largest defects. Histologic studies were then made on numerous cases (Longacre and deStefano, 1957). At one week (Fig. 13-20) the osteocytes are absent from the lacunae, but there are living osteoblasts still present along the surface of some of the trabeculae. It is our impression that many of these "marginal" surviving cells are separated from the early specimen during the course of decalcification and preparation so that only a few remain. At two weeks (Fig. 13-21) there is rapid ingrowth of granulation tissue between the trabeculae and beginning regeneration. There are many areas of resorption of bone with beginning formation of Howship's spaces. In other areas there are living osteoblasts, and some have already surrounded themselves with osteoid substance (osteocytes). The five-week specimen (Fig. 13-22) reveals continuing absorption along with the increase in the vascularity of the granulation tissue between the trabeculae. There is now active regeneration of new bone along the surfaces of most of the trabeculae. This process is most active in the neighborhood of blood vessels with the beginning of osteon formation. The six-month specimen (Fig. 13-23) shows the split rib grafts attached to the skull by a layer of fibrous tissue, and between the two there is an area of newly formed bone with some areas not yet calcified. There is osteoid substance around some rather large (young) osteocytes. The remaining portion of the graft reveals reversal lines and a few areas of absorption, but for the

FIGURE 13-22. Five-week specimen shows continuing absorption along with increase in vascularity of the granulation tissue between the trabeculae. There is now active regeneration of new bone all along the surface of the trabeculae. This process is most active in the neighborhood of blood vessels.

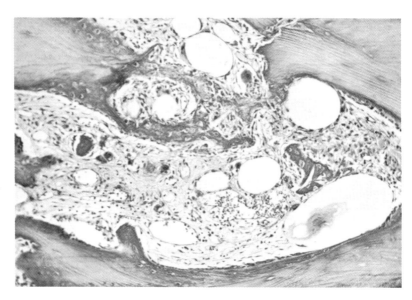

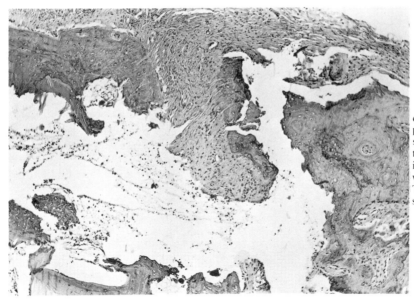

FIGURE 13–23. Six-month biopsy shows rib graft attached to portion of the skull. They are separated by a layer of fibrous tissue, and between the two there is an area of newly formed bone with some areas not yet calcified. There is osteoid substance around some rather large osteoblasts.

most part the split rib graft is replaced with new bone. The studies at the end of one year (Fig. 13–24) show the graft and host skull to be joined by a band of tissue resembling a cranial suture. Whether this suture would close in time cannot be stated, but there is new bone formation by metaplasia from stroma along the line at a slow rate (that is, by the same mechan-

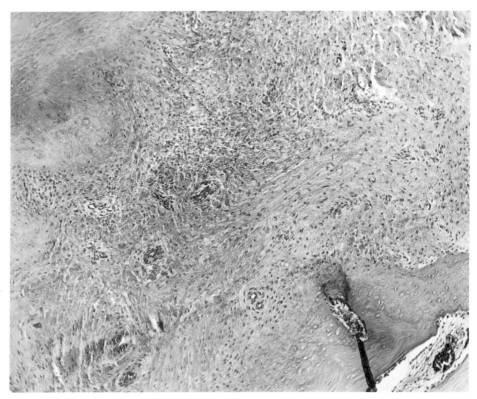

FIGURE 13–24. One-year specimen shows the graft and host bone to be joined by a band of tissue resembling a cranial suture. Note that new bone is being formed by metaplasia from stroma along the line at a slow rate (namely by the same mechanism as membrane bone formation).

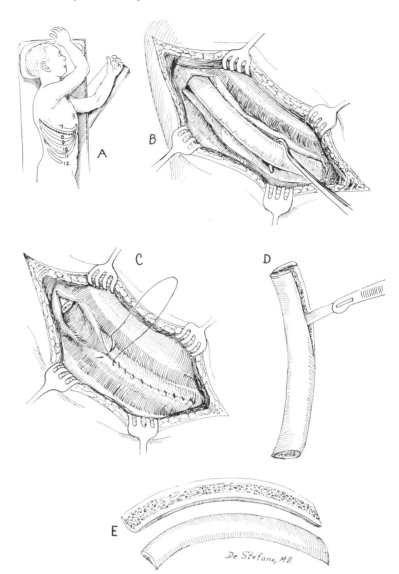

FIGURE 13–25. *A, B,* Removal of a full length of rib by the subperiosteal technique. The Doyen elevator is used to free the periosteum of the rib bed. *C,* Closing the periosteal bed with a running chromic catgut suture. *D, E,* Technique of splitting the rib utilizing the Beaver knife.

ism as membrane bone formation). These findings on transplanted human bone thus confirm the work of Mowlem.

Technique of Obtaining the Split Rib Graft. If only a small portion of bone is required, an incision is made directly over the seventh rib anteriorly. If the defect is very extensive, the utilization of the posterolateral thoracoplasty approach over the seventh rib will open up a fascial plane for dissection, through which three to four full length ribs may be removed at one sitting. Care should be taken that only alternate ribs are removed and that each rib bed is closed with a running suture.

Under intratracheal anesthesia the incision is made parallel to the seventh rib from the angle of the scapula to the anterior axillary line, cutting through the latissimus dorsi and raising the lower edge of the trapezius (Fig. 13–25, *A*). The fibers of the serratus anterior are split anteriorly. On elevating the scapula, a fascial plane is opened which allows access to the full extent from the second to the tenth ribs. The periosteum is incised and carefully elevated (Fig. 13–25, *B*). Following the removal of each rib, the periosteum is carefully closed with a running suture of catgut, the muscle is closed in layers with figure-of-eight sutures of chromic catgut, and the skin is

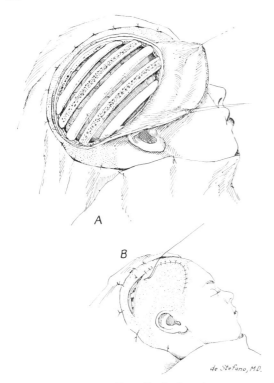

A

B

de Stefano, M.D.

FIGURE 13–26. *A,* The split ribs have been contoured to fit snugly against the host skull in the reconstruction of cranial defects. *B,* The split rib grafts are secured into position within the defect under the replaced scalp flap.

sutured with silk or nylon (Fig. 13–25, *C*). With careful technique, perforation of the pleura should seldom occur. Should it be punctured, careful closure of the wound under positive pressure following the introduction of a catheter with a water seal is required. After the lung has expanded fully, the catheter may be removed. The ribs are split lengthwise using a Beaver blade, opening up the cancellous portion and at the same time preserving the cortex as a scaffold (Fig. 13–25, *D, E*). The split rib graft may now be bent and contoured to fit almost any defect (Fig. 13–26, *A*). In placing the grafts, the authors have purposely avoided the use of any foreign material to maintain fixation except where absolutely necessary (Fig. 13–26, *B*).

REFERENCES

Albee, F. H.: Bone Graft Surgery. Philadelphia, W. B. Saunders Company, 1915.

Anderson, H. C.: Electron microscopic studies of induced cartilage development and calcification. J. Cell Biol., *35*:81, 1961.

Anderson, H. C.: Vesicles associated with calcification in the matrix of epiphyseal cartilage. J. Cell Biol., *41*:59, 1969.

Anderson, H. C., and Matsuzawa, T.: Membranous particles in calcifying cartilage matrix. N.Y. Acad. Sci., *32*:619, 1970.

Ballin, M.: A method of cranioplasty. Surg. Gynecol. Obstet., *33*:79, 1921.

Bassett, C. A. L., Hurley, L. A., and Stinchfield, F. E.: The fate of long-term anorganic bone implants. Transplant. Bull., *29*:51, 1962.

Becker, R. O., Bassett, C. A. L., and Bachman, C. H.: Bioelectric Factors Controlling Bone Structure. *In* Frost, H. (Ed.): Bone Biodynamics. Boston, Little, Brown & Company, 1964, pp. 209–232.

Bourne, G. H.: Biochemistry and Physiology of Bone. Vol. I. New York, Academic Press, 1956.

Bourne, G. H.: Biochemistry and Physiology of Bone. Vol. II. New York, Academic Press, 1972, pp. 75–120.

Brash, J. C.: Cunningham's Textbook of Anatomy. 9th Ed. London, Oxford Medical Publications, 1951.

Breine, U., and Johanson, B.: The tibia as donor area for bone graft in infants. Acta Chir. Scand., *131*:230, 1966.

Brooks, D. B., Heiple, K. G., Herndon, C. H., and Powell, A. E.: Immunological factors in homogenous bone transplantation. 4. The effect of various methods of preparation and irradiation on antigenicity. J. Bone Joint Surg., *45*:1617, 1963.

Brown, R. C.: The repair of skull defects. Med. J. Aust., *11*:409, 1917.

Brown, R. C.: Cranioplasty by split-rib method. J. Coll. Surg. Australasia, 1928.

Bryce, T. H.: Quain's Anatomy. 11th Ed. Vol. 14, Part 1. London, Longmans, Green and Company, 1915, p. 177.

Burwell, R. G.: Studies in the transplantation of bones. IV. The immune responses of lymph nodes draining second-set homografts of fresh cancellous bone. J. Bone Joint Surg., *44-B*:688, 1962.

Burwell, R. G.: Studies in the transplantation of bone. Treated composite homografts of cancellous bone: An analysis of inductive mechanisms. J. Bone Joint Surg., *48-B*:532, 1968.

Cartier, P.: Biochimie de l'ossification. Le rôle de l'acide adenosine triphosphorique dans la mineralisation du cartilage ossifiable. J. Physiol. (Paris), *43*:677, 1951.

Casson, P. R.: Personal communication, 1971.

Chalmers, J.: Transplantation immunity in bone homografting. J. Bone Joint Surg., *41*:160, 1959.

Crenshaw, A. H.: Campbell's Operative Orthopedics, 4th Ed. St. Louis, Mo., C. V. Mosby Company, 1963, p. 57.

Crockford, D. A., and Converse, J. M.: The ilium as a source of bone grafts in children. Plast. Reconstr. Surg., *50*:270, 1972.

Dingman, R. O.: The use of iliac bone in the repair of facial and cranial defects. Plast. Reconstr. Surg., *3*:24, 1950.

Engström, A.: Quantitative micro- and histochemical elementary analysis. Acta Radiol., Suppl. 63, 1946.

Engström, A.: The dection of small difference in cellular mass by historadiography and a new equipment for microradiography. Exper. Cell Res. (Suppl.), *3*:117, 1955.

Engström, A., and Amprino, R.: X-ray diffraction and X-ray absorption studies of immobilized bones. Experientia, 6:267, 1950.

Engström, A., and Finean, J. B.: Low-angle X-ray diffraction of bone. Nature (Lond.), *171*:564, 1953.

Enlow, D. H.: Principles of Bone Remodeling. Springfield, Ill., Charles C Thomas, Publisher, 1963.

Enneking, W. F.: Immunologic aspects of bone transplantation. South. Med. J., *55*:894, 1962.

Fagarasanu, I.: Procédé de cranioplastie par des greffons costaux redoublés: Procédé du "grillage protecteur." Tech. Chir. (Paris), *29*:57, 1937.

Friedenberg, Z., and Kohanim, M.: The effect of direct current on bone. Surg. Gynecol. Obstet., *126*:97, 1968.

Gallie, W. E., and Robertson, D. E.: The transplantation of bone. J.A.M.A., *70*:1134, 1918.

Ghent, W. R.: Further studies on meralgia paraesthetica. Can. Med. Assoc. J., *85*:871, 1961.

Glimcher, M. J.: Specificity of the Molecular Structure of Organic Matrices in Mineralization. *In* Sognnaes, R. F. (Ed.): Calcification in Biological Systems. Washington, D.C., American Association for the Advancement of Science, 1960, pp. 421–487.

Gordon, S., and Ham, A. W.: Essays in Surgery. Toronto, University of Toronto Press, 1950, p. 296.

Groves, E. W. H.: Bone transplantation. B. J. Surg., *5*:185, 1917.

Hall, B. K.: Hypoxia and differentiation of cartilage and bone from common germinal cells *in vitro*. Life Sci., *8*(Part II):553, 1969.

Ham, A. W.: A histological study of the early phases of bone repair. J. Bone Joint Surg., *12*:827, 1930.

Ham, A. W., and Gordon, S.: The origin of bone that forms in association with cancellous chips transplanted into muscle. Br. J. Plast. Surg., *5*:154, 1952.

Holmstrand, K.: Biophysical investigations of bone transplants and bone implants; an experimental study. Acta Orthop. Scand., Suppl. 26, 1957.

Holmstrand, K., Longacre, J. J., and deStefano, G. A.: Biophysical studies of split-rib grafts in the repair of defects of the cranium. Plast. Reconstr. Surg., *26*:3, 1960.

Kappis, A.: Zur Deckung von Schadeldefekten. Zentralb. Chir., *42*:897, 1915.

Keith, A.: Bone growth and bone repair. Br. J. Surg., *5*:685, 1917; *6*:19, 1918–1919; *6*:160, 1918–1919.

Knize, D. M.: The influence of periosteum and calcitonin on onlay bone graft survival. A roentgenographic study. Plast. Reconstr. Surg., *53*:190, 1974.

Knize, D. M.: Gershberg, H., Ballantyne, D. L., and Converse, J. M.: Hormonal enhancement of autologous onlay bone grafts. Surg. Forum, *24*:511, 1973.

Leriche, R., and Policard, A.: Some fundamental principles of the pathology of bone. Surg. Gynecol. Obstet., *43*:308, 1926.

Longacre, J. J., and deStefano, G. A.: Further observations of the behavior of autogenous split-rib grafts in reconstruction of extensive defects of the cranium and face. Plast. Reconstr. Surg., *20*:281, 1957.

Macewen, W.: The Growth of Bone. Observation on Osteogenesis. An Experimental Inquiry into the Development and Reproduction of Diaphyseal Bone. Glasgow, James Maclehose and Sons, 1912.

Makin, H. J.: Osteogenesis in the subchondral bone of rabbits. J. Bone Joint Surg., *46-A*:1252, 1964.

Matsuzawa, T., and Anderson, C. H.: Phosphatases of epiphyseal cartilage studied by electron microscopic cytochemical methods. J. Histochem. Cytochem., *19*:801, 1971.

Moss, M. L.: Studies of the acellular bone of teleost fish. Acta Anat., *46*:343, 1961.

Moss, M. L., and Frielich, M.: Studies of the acellular bone of teleost fish. Acta Anat., *55*:1, 1963.

Mowlem, R.: Editorial. Br. J. Plast. Surg., *4*:231, 1952.

Mueller, W.: Zur Frage der temporaren Schadelresektion an stelle der Trepanation. Zentralb. Chir., *17*:65, 1890.

Murphy, J. B.: Osteoplasty. Surg. Gynecol. Obstet., *16*:493, 1913.

Oldfield, M. C.: Iliac hernia after bone grafting. Lancet, *1*:810, 1945.

Ollier, L.: Traité expérimental et clinique de la régénération des os et de la production artificelle du tissu osseux. Paris, P. Masson et fils, 1867.

Orell, S.: Surgical bone grafting with "os purum," "os novum" and "boiled bone." J. Bone Joint Surg., *19*:873, 1937.

Phemister, D. B.: The fate of transplanted bone and regeneration of its various constituents. Surg. Gynecol. Obstet., *19*:303, 1914.

Reid, R. L.: Hernia through an iliac bone-graft donor site. Case report. J. Bone Joint Surg., *50-A*:757, 1968.

Robertson, I. M., and Baron, J. N.: A method of treatment of chronic infective osteitis. J. Bone Joint Surg., *28*:19, 1946.

Roux, W.: Gesammelte Abhandlungen. Leipzig, I. W. Engelmann, 1895.

Schubert, M., and Hammerman, D.: Metachromasia: Chemical theory and histochemical use. J. Histochem. Cytochem., *4*:158, 1956.

Simmons, D. J., Simmons, N. B., and Marshall, J. H.: The uptake of calcium-45 in the acellular-boned toadfish. Calcif. Tissue Res., *5*:206, 1970.

Stringa, G.: Studies in the vascularization of bone grafts. J. Bone Joint Surg., *39-B*:3955, 1957.

Tanner, J. M.: Growth at Adolescence. 2nd Ed. Oxford, Blackwell Scientific Publications, 1962, p. 45.

Trueta, J.: The role of the vessels in osteogenesis. J. Bone Joint Surg., *45-B*:402, 1963.

Van Meekren, J.: Observationes Medicochirurgicae. Amsterdam, Henrici and T. Bloom, 1682.

Wolff, J.: Das Gesetz der Transformation der Knochen. Berlin, A. Hirschwald, 1892.

CHAPTER 14

PRINCIPLES AND TECHNIQUES OF MICROVASCULAR SURGERY

B. M. O'BRIEN, F.R.C.S., F.R.A.C.S.,
AND J. W. HAYHURST, M.D.

The application of microsurgical techniques permits the achievement of surgical goals that are not possible with conventional techniques. Two major advantages are offered. First, the lighting and high magnification of modern microscopes allow the surgeon to see small structures that he has never been able to see adequately before. Second, fine microinstrumentation and microsutures enable repair of the small structures with a precision not previously possible.

Early plastic surgeons founded a specialty by virtue of their appreciation for tissue techniques and their ability to operate with great precision. To their centimeter-conscious peers, plastic surgery became the "surgery of millimeters." Microsurgery heralds the dawn of a new age in surgery, the "surgery of microns." The contrast between "millimetric" and "micron surgery" can be demonstrated by a series of illustrations (Figs. 14–1 to 14–4).

HISTORY

The compound microscope was invented in 1590 by Zacharias Janssen. It found early medical use in microbiology, histology, and pathology. The microscope proved to be an invaluable aid for surgery on the small structures of the ear during the 1920's, and despite the fact that the foundations for vascular surgery were well established early in this century (Guthrie, 1912), for some unexplained reason the seemingly obvious application of the microscope to small vessel surgery was not made until almost 50 years later.

Paré used ligatures on vessels as early as 1564. However, 200 years elapsed before Hallowell performed the first repair of a vessel in 1759 by transfixing the vessel edges with metal pins, each of which was tied with a thread (Guthrie, 1912). In 1889 Jassinovski used fine interrupted silk sutures for the repair of human vascular lacerations (Hershey and Calnan, 1967). He suggested that the vascular sutures should not penetrate the intima of the vessel.

The actual anastomosis of the entire circumference of an artery was reported by Briau on canine carotid arteries in 1896 (Hershey and Calnan, 1967). Carrel (1902) contributed the triangulation method of vessel repair. After the turn of the century, Carrel and Guthrie did extensive work on vascular repairs and tissue replantation, laying the ground work for

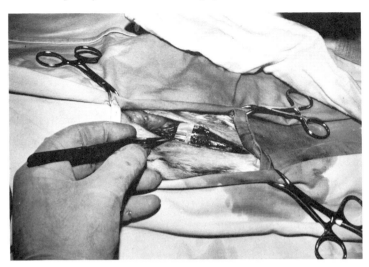

FIGURE 14–1. Surgeon's naked-eye view from 24 inches.

modern-day vascular surgery and transplantation surgery. Guthrie later published a book on blood vessel surgery which remains pertinent (Guthrie, 1912).

In 1948 Shumacher and Lowenberg reported high patency rates with anastomoses of canine arteries as small as 3.2 mm in diameter. In comparing the various methods of suturing vessels, they reaffirmed that simple interrupted sutures gave the highest patency rates. Their successful repairs stimulated the interest of other surgeons to study anastomosis techniques in smaller vessels.

Seidenberg, Hurwitt, and Carton (1958) were the first investigators to make a concerted effort to repair vessels in the microvascular range (1.5 to 3 mm). Unfortunately, they were hampered by the unavailability of small sutures and they failed to take advantage of magnification for their repairs.

The introduction of the microscope as an aid to microvascular repairs was a major advance which heralded the arrival of modern-day microvascular surgery. Jacobson and Suarez (1960), using the microscope at up to 25 × magnification, reported a 100 per cent patency rate following the anastomosis of 26 vessels which were 1.6 to 3.2 mm in diameter. After this epoch-making report, many surgeons quickly realized that trained hands were capable of a greater surgical precision than the previously unaided eye could perceive. This report provided considerable stimulus to the study of microvascular surgery.

In 1962 Chase and Schwartz reported their studies of approximately 800 small arterial

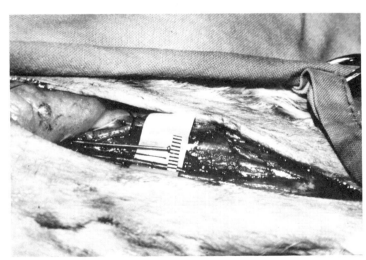

FIGURE 14–2. View with 2× magnification (loupe) from 9 inches.

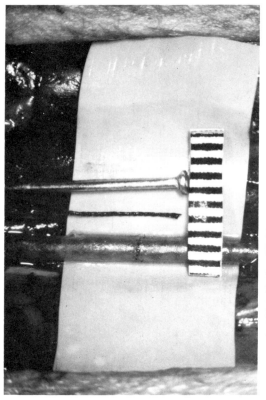

FIGURE 14–3. The lowest power through the microscope (6×); millimeter rule is on the right.

ioned to progressively smaller dimensions (Buncke and McLean, 1971; Acland, 1972a).

With the use of improved sutures and an increasing experience in microvascular surgery, O'Brien and his coworkers were able to report an 81 per cent patency rate in 58 rabbits' arteries averaging approximately 1 mm in diameter (O'Brien and coworkers, 1970a). Systemic heparin was used, and the vessels were examined at various intervals up to six weeks postoperatively.

With the development of more refined surgical techniques and improved sutures, Hayhurst and O'Brien (1975) have reported a 98 per cent long-term patency rate following anastomosis of 50 rabbits' arteries averaging 0.9 mm in diameter and a 92 per cent patency rate for a group of 25 veins averaging 1.1 mm in diameter (Table 14–1). This study emphasized the critical importance of technique and demonstrated that high patency rates can be achieved without anticoagulation (Table 14–2). It was further determined that, for the evaluation of true patency rates in vessels 1 mm in

anastomoses. They emphasized atraumatic technique, the importance of continued practice in the laboratory, and the value of a good assistant. Adequate microvascular sutures were not yet available, but even with 7–0 silk they were able to report satisfactory patency rates following the anastomoses of canine brachial arteries (1.2 to 1.7 mm) (Chase and Schwartz, 1962, 1963).

Further advances in the techniques of microvascular repair were closely associated with the improvement in available suture materials. In 1965 Buncke and Schulz described a needle which was prepared by plating metal onto the end of a small nylon thread. Though the needles were rather soft and malleable, these sutures were superior to anything previously available and enabled the authors to achieve limited success in the replantation of rabbits' ears and monkeys' digits (Buncke and Schulz, 1965, 1966). A smaller, improved suture based on the same principle was later described by O'Brien, Henderson, and Crock (1970b) and by O'Brien and Hayhurst (1973b). The more conventional machined needles were also fash-

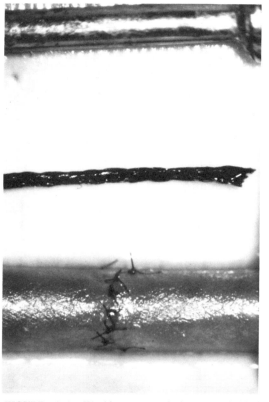

FIGURE 14–4. Working power of 20×. Household pin above, 4–0 silk, and rabbits femoral artery below (repaired with sutures 19 microns in diameter)

TABLE 14–1. *Patency Rates*

VESSELS	IMMEDIATE PATENCY	LONG-TERM PATENCY (DAYS)
50 arteries	100%	98% (3–41)
50 veins	98%	80% (3–41)
25 veins	100%	92% (7–13)

diameter, the examination should be made during the second postoperative week.

INSTRUMENTATION

Instruments. Only a few simple instruments are required for microsurgery (Fig. 14–5). Nontoothed forceps should be of good quality and resistant to staining and rusting. The tips should be fine, smooth, and uniform with the jaws meeting at the ends of the forceps. Forceps that are not uniform, have sharp edges, and do not meet at the tips are unsatisfactory. Numbers 2 and 5 jeweler's forceps (Dumont, Switzerland) are generally satisfactory (see Fig. 14–5). Occasionally it is helpful to modify the tips with a fine carborundum stone or emery paper. The attachment of rounded handles to these forceps may be an aid in holding the forceps (Lendvay, 1973b).

Scissors should be spring-operated with delicate, sharp blades. Most handheld microsurgery instruments should be approximately 15 cm in length. A Westcott scissors with the tips of the blades slightly rounded is useful for dissection of the adventitia. Both straight and slightly curved blades are useful.

Spring-loaded needle holders should also be approximately 15 cm in length and should rest in the first web space between the thumb and index finger. The needle holder is held as one holds a pencil and is rolled between the index, middle finger, and thumb during the motion of inserting sutures. Consequently, needle holders with a rounded handle are preferred. The jaws of most ophthalmology needle holders are too large for the smaller microsurgery needles. The jaws do not grasp the small needles well, and the sutures tend to slide off the shoulders of these instruments during tying. Microsurgery needle holders should have thin jaws with very narrow shoulders capable of grasping and tying a suture only a few microns in diameter. A gentle curve to the jaws is preferred

by most microsurgeons. A needle holder without the locking device is essential, because the movement of the locking and unlocking maneuver can be traumatic to the vessels being repaired. A needle holder incorporating these qualities is shown in Figure 14–6 (O'Brien and Hayhurst, 1973).

A lacrimal duct syringe with a blunt tip is useful for irrigation of the microvascular field. A blunt No. 25 gauge needle and small Silastic tubing attached to a 5-ml syringe are aids in the irrigation of the ends of the vessels (see Fig. 14–5).

Small strips of thin plastic are useful for fashioning a cuff around the anastomosis just after its completion. This "cuffing" technique allows the use of fewer sutures than would otherwise be necessary for an arterial anastomosis (McLean and Buncke, 1973) (see Fig. 14–24). Ordinary household kitchen Saran-Wrap or Glad Wrap is suitable for this purpose, and small strips can be gas-sterilized

TABLE 14–2. *Surgeon's Subjective Estimation of—*

1. Technical adequacy of venous anastomosis (A).
2. Degree of spasm (S) of vein.
3. Amount of blood (B) coming in contact with external surface of the vein.

    1. = Excellent or minimal.
    2. = Good or mild.
    3. = Fair or moderate.
    4. = Poor or considerable.

ANASTOMOSIS	NUMBER OF VEINS	NUMBER OCCLUDED	% OCCLUDED
A1	1	0	0
A2	39	7	17.9
A3	8	2	25.0
A4	2	1	50.0
SPASM			
S1	7	1	13.8
S2	35	7	20.0
S3	8	2	25.0
S4	0	0	0
BLOOD			
B1	0	0	0
B2	36	7	19.4
B3	11	3	27.3
B4	3	0	0

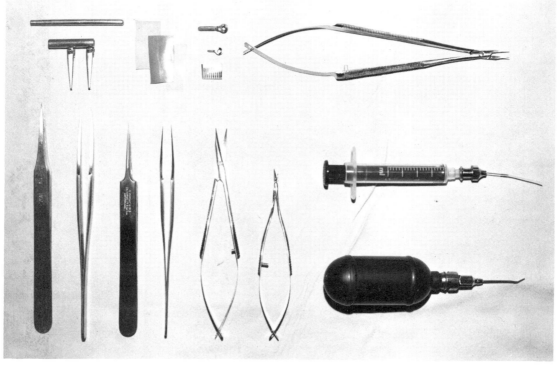

FIGURE 14-5. A standard set of microvascular instruments. Top row, left to right: microvascular clamp, yellow and green background material and Saran Wrap, Scoville clamps and millimeter rule, micro needle holder. Bottom row, left to right: jeweler's forceps (numbers two and five), Westcott scissors, Vanass scissors, 5-ml syringe with 29-gauge needle and Silastic tubing for irrigation, lacrimal duct syringe.

prior to the operative procedure. Other varieties of cellophane and thicker plastics are not suitable for this purpose because of frequent bleeding after their removal.

A background material of a color which suits the surgeon is useful in performing small anastomoses (see Fig. 14–5). It provides a color contrast against which a fine suture is more easily seen, and it complements the photography of these small vessels. Many soft plastics or ordinary toy balloons can be used as background materials. A millimeter rule should be included in the photograph for easy comparison of the sizes of different vessels.

Microvascular Clamps. A number of microvascular clamps are commercially available (Fig. 14–7). The Henderson-O'Brien double microvascular clamp is adjustable by means of a small key and screw mechanism (Henderson, O'Brien and Parel, 1970). The amount of pressure at the tips of the clamp can be varied manually, a feature which enables the surgeon to use the same clamp for small or large vessels. It should be applied while observing through the microscope, as it is relatively easy to crush the

intima of the vessel with only a slightly overzealous application of the screw mechanism. The clamp will also separate into two parts, so that each may be applied to different vessels which are then brought together as the two clamps are joined, although this feature is seldom required. Serrations on the jaws of the clamp are intended to prevent slippage of the vessel, but these are inefficient and the vessel may slip from the clamp if it is not applied snugly enough. The jaws of the microvascular clamp can be brought into approximation and the clamp introduced into small surgical fields. This clamp has had extensive experimental and clinical use.

The second microvascular clamp (see Fig. 14–7) was developed by Acland (Spingler and Tritt, Germany). A small wire rectangle surrounds the jaws of the clamp and incorporates a suture-holding device which is helpful for microsurgeons working alone. However, the wire encircling the jaws of the clamps necessitates the dissection of a longer length of vessel than would otherwise be necessary and prevents the insertion of the clamp into small spaces, a requirement which is frequently

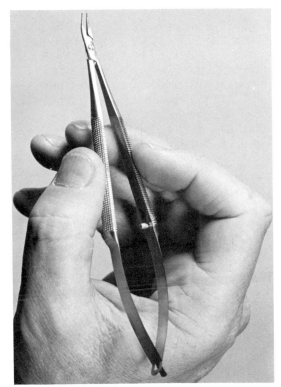

FIGURE 14-6. A microvascular needle holder (G. Ginch Company, Australia). (From O'Brien, B. M., and Hayhurst, J. W.: Metallized microsutures and a new micro needle holder. Plast. Reconstr. Surg., *52*:673, 1973.)

necessary in digital replantations and other clinical situations. The nonadjustability of the jaws in the original model has been overcome by producing an adjustable version of the clamp, which is shown in the illustration. The closing pressure of the jaws is fixed at approximately 30 to 50 g, depending upon the size of the clamp. This is appropriate for most smaller vessels but inadequate for some larger vessels. The jaws of this clamp also offer little resistance to longitudinal slippage of the vessel. This is the least expensive of the microvascular clamps and is very suitable for the experimental situation in which the surgeon is working alone and is restricted by a limited budget. There are three sizes, the largest of which is the most useful for the majority of clinical cases.

Two vascular clips essentially similar to Heifetz clips (see Fig. 14–7) have been incorporated onto a sliding bar which permits their approximation and use as a microvascular clamp. The closing pressure of the microvascular clamps is said to be 80 g at a point 2 mm from the tips (Tamai, 1974). Because of the two opposing biconvex surfaces presented to the vessels, most of the pressure is concentrated along a narrow line and can cause considerable endothelial damage.

Single clamps of the various types are also available (see Fig. 14–7). Tamai has ingeniously suggested the use of two Scoville clamps and a No. 19 gauge needle to fashion a workable double microvascular clamp (Tamai and associates, 1972). The Scoville clamps, though variable in their closing pressure, are often much too strong to apply to smaller vessels without causing significant damage.

Dopplers. Dopplers are instruments which can frequently detect blood flow in vessels beneath the skin. Several types are equipped with microprobes capable of detecting vessels 1 mm in diameter or smaller. These instruments are used by some surgeons for mapping out the course of vessels in proposed microvascular flaps and can be used as an adjunct in monitoring blood flow in microvascular flaps, replanted digits, or major extremities. The novice should be cautioned that these instruments are to be used only as an *aid* in the management of patients. The experienced microsurgeon, using all his clinical senses, remains the most reliable instrument for monitoring a microvascular repair.

Bipolar Coagulation. The bipolar coagulator is an invaluable aid in coagulating small branches during dissection. It conducts current between the tips of the forceps and when used carefully can safely coagulate small branches near the main vessel. The tips should be as

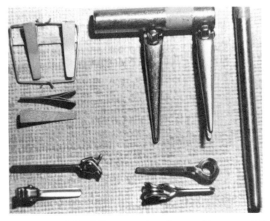

FIGURE 14-7. Microvascular clamps. Top row, left: Acland adjustable clamp and two single Acland clamps; right: Henderson-O'Brien clamp with key. Bottom row, left: two Heifetz clamps; right: two Scoville clamps.

small as a jeweler's forceps and of superior quality. The power source for the bipolar coagulator must be capable of small increments of current and is preferably one that is designed specifically for this purpose. Some neurosurgical instruments have micro tips available which can be used for microsurgery. One instrument which is designed for microsurgery is the MET Bipolar Coagulator.* The use of the standard type of conduction coagulator may be disastrous in microvascular surgery, because the current may extend up a small branch on to the parent vessel, causing its coagulation and destruction.

Microscopes. A good microscope is invaluable for microsurgery. The ideal microscope should have strong lighting with magnifications of approximately 6 to 40 power. A foot-operated switch should control changes in magnification and focus, with the capacity to move the microscope horizontally in two planes. The head of the microscope should tilt in all planes to provide ready access for all clinical situations. The assistant's binocular system should view the same operating field as the surgeon, and the assistant should be able to sit at any point 90 to 180 degrees from the surgeon. The microscope should be capable of mounting both a still *and* a movie or television camera at the *same* time. The lighting of the microscope should be sufficient for good photomicrography or, as an alternative, have a photolight attachment.

*F. L. Fisher, Vertiebsgruppe MET, Postfach 529, Guntramstrasse 14, 7800 Freiburg, Germany.

There are no microscopes presently available which incorporate all of these requirements. The Zeiss OP-Mi7-PH combines most of the features necessary for a good microsurgical microscope. A disadvantage is that at present it cannot accommodate two cameras at the same time. There are numerous other microscopes available which incorporate some of the qualities of the ideal microscope.

Sutures. The proper suture size for a microvascular repair depends upon the size and consistency of the vessel to be anastomosed. The ideal needle for microsutures should be the same size as the suture material itself. Unfortunately, this is not yet possible. The size of the needle remains the critical factor in microsutures (Fig. 14–8).

The U.S.P. terminology used by most suture companies is unsatisfactory for microsutures. For example, nonabsorbable sutures 18 to 38 microns in diameter may all be designated 9–0 (Buren and Ryan, 1974), whereas most 10–0 microsutures also fall within this same range. A different size range is allowed for absorbable sutures under the U.S.P. system.

The authors believe that all sutures should give the diameter of the needle and the suture material in microns, the arc length of the needle in millimeters, and the curve of the needle in eighths of a circle. This could be coded with a system similar to that used by Spingler and Tritt. For example, 7 ST 43–18 would be a 70μ needle by Spingler and Tritt with a 4-mm cord length and a $^3/_8$ circle with an 18μ thread, and a 7 E 43–22 would be a

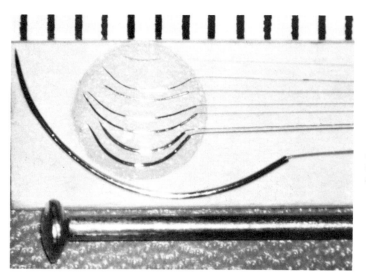

FIGURE 14–8. Microsutures. From top to bottom: 3 MF 21–12, 5 St. 43–18, 7 MF 32–19, 7 D G 43–18, 10 D G 43–18, 13 E 33–22, 14 DG 33–35. The large needle is a 6–0 Ethilon cardiovascular suture. For size comparison a household pin is shown below and a millimeter rule at the top.

70μ needle by Ethicon with a 4-mm cord length and a ⅜ circle on a 22μ thread.

For vessels 0.5 to 1.0 mm in diameter, a needle 60 to 80 microns in diameter with a nylon thread of approximately 20 microns in diameter is satisfactory. There are now several sutures of this size which are commercially available.

The needle of the metallized microsuture (MicroFine*, Australia) is 70 microns in diameter with a monofilament nylon thread of 19 microns (7 MF 32–19). The needle is 3 mm in length with a ⅖ circle (Figs. 14–8 and 14–9). The needle is produced by plating the end of the nylon suture material with metal.

---

*MicroFine, 5 Cedar Court, Glen Waverley, Melbourne, Australia.

Each needle is sharpened by hand under the microscope. The needle is attached to a small tab of adhesive plastic on a small strip of yellow cardboard with a 7.5 cm length of nylon. The suture on the cardboard can be introduced into the microscopic field, where the surgeon removes it from its holder under microscopic vision. The suture is admirably suited for the repair of small tubular structures below 1 mm in diameter and has the advantage of a very firm suture-needle junction. The newer versions of this suture have overcome previous difficulties with roughness on the external surface and malleability of the needle. The short 7.5-cm length of the suture material accelerates the repair of small vessels but is used up rapidly for larger vessels or in experimental applications.

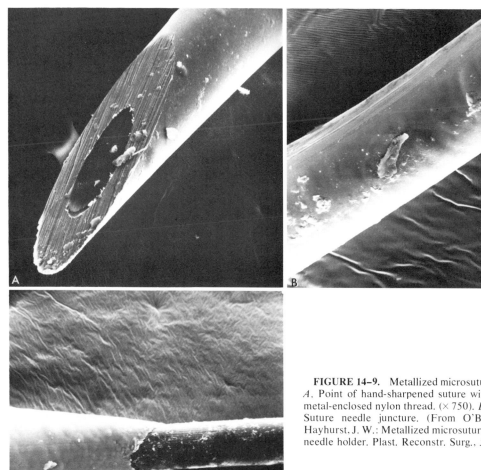

FIGURE 14–9. Metallized microsuture. (7 MF 32–19). *A*, Point of hand-sharpened suture with exposed end of metal-enclosed nylon thread. (× 750). *B*, Needle body. *C*, Suture needle juncture. (From O'Brien, B. M., and Hayhurst, J. W.: Metallized microsutures and a new micro needle holder. Plast. Reconstr. Surg., *52*:673, 1973.)

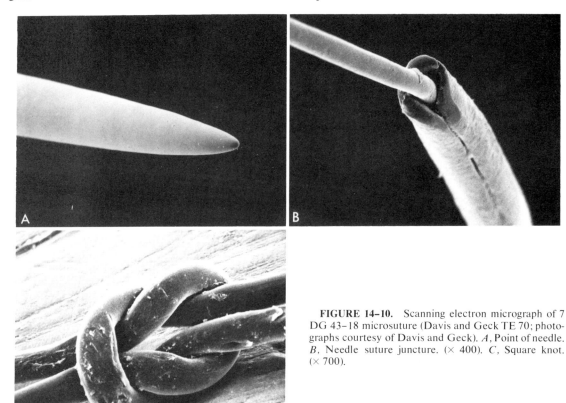

FIGURE 14–10. Scanning electron micrograph of 7 DG 43–18 microsuture (Davis and Geck TE 70; photographs courtesy of Davis and Geck). *A,* Point of needle. *B,* Needle suture juncture. (× 400). *C,* Square knot. (× 700).

The needle shown in Figures 14–10 and 14–11 is a 70μ ³⁄₈ circle needle with a cord length of 4 mm. These finely machined needles are also sharpened by hand under magnification. This needle is produced in Germany (Spingler and Tritt) and marketed by three separate companies, each with its own nylon suture material. The sutures are: 7 ST 43–18 (Spingler and Tritt 7 V 43, 10–0); 7 E 43–22 (Ethicon, BV–6, 10–0); and 7 DG 43–18 (Davis and Geck, TE 70, 10–0) (see Figs. 14–10 and 14–11). All of these sutures are suitable for the repair of vessels in the range of 0.5 to 1 mm in diameter.

For the anastomosis of vessels 1 to 3 mm in diameter, a needle 100 to 130 microns in diameter is easier to handle and yet is not too large for satisfactory microvascular repairs. The 10 DG 43–22 (Davis and Geck TE 100 with a 22-micron suture [10–0]) and the 10 ST 43–25 (Spingler and Tritt 10 V 43 with a 25-micron suture [10–0]) use the same excellent needle. The 13 E 33–22 (Ethicon BV–5 needle with a 22-micron suture [10–0]) is also a suitable suture (see Fig. 14–8).

For vessels above 3 mm in diameter, the microsurgeon can use needles of 100 to 130 microns in diameter, or he may wish to use a slightly larger needle, such as the 14 DG 33–35 (Davis and Geck TE 143, 9–0). The surgeon would seldom require suture materials or needles larger than this for microvascular repairs.

PATHOPHYSIOLOGY OF MICROVASCULAR OCCLUSIONS

In order to appreciate how and why a microvascular anastomosis may become occluded, an understanding of the *mechanisms* of thrombus and clot formation is essential. The tendency for a microvascular anastomosis to become occluded may be affected by (1) the coagulability of the blood, (2) changes in the vessel wall, and (3) disturbances of blood flow. It has been over 100 years since Virchow outlined the three variables operating in the pathogenesis of thrombosis (Samuels and Webster,

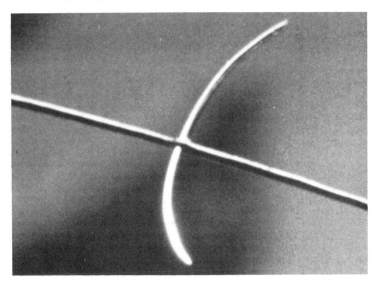

FIGURE 14–11. Needle of 7 E 43–22 microsuture through human hair (Ethicon BV6; photograph courtesy of Ethicon).

1952). Early and late microvascular occlusions and each of the above variables will be discussed, particularly as they relate to microvascular occlusions.

Platelets. Platelets usually have an ovoid or discoid shape, but when they come in contact with a thrombogenic substance they become more rounded, form pseudopods, and become "sticky" (Mustard and Packham, 1970). Simple contact with collagen, microfibrils, cell walls, sutures, or any number of substances is sufficient to cause "stickiness" and adherence of the platelets to a thrombogenic surface (Spaet and Gaynor, 1970; MacMillan and Kim, 1970). The irreversibly stimulated platelets then undergo a "release reaction," with disintegration and release of the contents of their storage granules into the surrounding medium. The storage granules contain ADP, serotonin, and histamine, all of which may cause additional platelets to form pseudopods and undergo a potentially reversible form of aggregation (Mustard and Packham, 1970). Stimulation by ADP appears to be the usual mechanism of secondary platelet aggregation. This phenomenon requires the presence of calcium and is reversible. In the absence of further stimulation and in the presence of magnesium, ADP-stimulated platelets rapidly deaggregate (Mustard and Packham, 1970). Epinephrine, norepinephrine, and thrombin also stimulate platelet aggregation.

Early Occlusion. The sequence of events which follows a vascular injury can, with the aid of a microscope, be observed through the translucent vessel wall (Spaet and Gaynor, 1970; Zucker, 1972; Acland, 1972b; Honour, Pickering and Sheppard, 1973). Within a few seconds platelets can be seen adhering to the site of injury. The platelets soon become covered with additional platelets to form a thrombus, which is whitish in color. The thrombus may grow to completely occlude the blood flow of the vessel; alternatively it may grow and stabilize, then begin to decrease in size with embolism of the platelets from the parent thrombus. In experimental lesions in microvessels, the thrombus usually reaches maximum size in about 10 minutes. Subsequently, it begins to decrease in size within 20 minutes of the initial injury (Didisheim, 1968; Spaet and Gaynor, 1970; Acland, 1972b). Histologic examination of the thrombus reveals that it is composed primarily of platelets. Some of the platelets have become irreversibly altered, and others are in a progressively less severe and reversible state of alteration. Those platelets on the outer perimeter of the thrombus which are less severely stimulated may revert to their normal state as deaggregation takes place. Following the disappearance of the outer layers of adhering platelets, a residual, nonthrombogenic amorphous material from the disintegrated platelets can be seen coating the original thrombogenic area (Spaet and Gaynor, 1970). Therefore, at least in the experimental situation, if the vessel does not become occluded by the initial platelet thrombus formation during the first 10 to 20 minutes of blood flow, the thrombus decreases in size, and threat of early occlusion is diminished (Didisheim, 1968; Acland, 1972b).

Late Occlusion. Although the first 20 minutes after a microvascular repair appears to be the critical period for occlusion from the initial platelet thrombus, later occlusion may also occur. In a study of microvascular repairs of femoral arteries in rabbits, it was found that occlusion most often occurred during the first 48 postoperative hours. The risk of occlusion decreases rapidly, with few vessels becoming occluded after 72 hours (Ketchum and coworkers, 1974). This finding fits well with the clinical experience of other investigators who have lost most of their digital replants because of venous occlusion, usually on the second or third postoperative day (Kleinert and coworkers; 1976; Lendvay, 1973a). When an arterial occlusion occurs, it is usually an earlier phenomenon.

The causes of microvascular occlusions in the later postoperative period are not well understood. The events which occur after the initial thrombus has grown to its maximum size and then shrunk to leave a residual amorphous coating over the sutures and exposed tissues at the site of the anastomosis are largely unknown. Particularly at venous anastomotic sites, fibrin strands can be found forming a meshwork in the outer platelet layers of the thrombus (Mustard and Packham, 1970). Although pure fibrin itself is not thought to be thrombogenic, fibrin breakdown products and thrombin in the anastomosis area cause platelet aggregation and the release of additional platelet constituents, including platelet factors 3 and 4, which further facilitate blood coagulation (Mustard and Packham, 1970; Zucker, 1972). Therefore, the slow growth of a thrombus may occur by the alternate layering of platelets and fibrin, with each further stimulating the production of the other.

Late venous occlusions may also result from the gradual growth of a thrombus at the venous anastomotic site secondary to the trapping of sensitized and activated platelets and coagulants. The sensitized platelets and activated procoagulants originate from the arterial anastomotic site and other sites of vessel injury between the arterial and venous repairs. This will be discussed in greater detail later in the chapter.

Infection may play a role in some late microvascular occlusions, although the authors feel this is rarely a major factor. In a study of the factors influencing patency rates, the authors found no correlation between occluded vessels and infected operative sites (Hayhurst and O'Brien, 1975; Hayhurst, 1976a). *Staphylococcus aureus* and *Streptococcus faecalis* have been cultured from both patent and occluded microvessels with little apparent correlation to occlusions (Elcock and Fredrickson, 1972). The authors do not feel that *minor* infections have adversely affected the outcome of free microvascular flaps or digital replants clinically, but a more severe infection may have caused the demise of at least one major extremity replantation.

Edema in the postoperative period can most definitely cause pressure on the microvascular replant with a reduction in blood flow and can lead to microvascular occlusion.

Coagulability of the Blood. A number of rather impressive changes in blood coagulation have been noted during surgery and in the immediate postoperative period. These changes have been implicated in the formation of postoperative venous thrombosis. It has been shown that at least 50 per cent of these thrombi may develop during the actual surgical procedure (Flanc, Kakkar and Clarke, 1968). These same changes in the coagulability of blood may be a factor in intraoperative and postoperative microvascular occlusions.

During and after surgery, there is an increase in platelet adhesiveness, Factor VIII activity, and fibrinogen, and there is a decrease in plasminogen and spontaneous fibrinolytic activity (Sharnoff and coworkers, 1960; Ham and Slack, 1967, 1968; Ygge, 1970; J. R. O'Brien and coworkers, 1974). Even in minor surgical procedures, such as herniorrhaphies, there is often a considerable increase in platelet adhesiveness, with a peak usually at 48 hours postoperatively. Operation may also increase the response of platelets to thrombin. This finding, together with a reported decrease in the postoperative heparin thrombin clotting time, has been suggested as a reason why small doses of heparin are useful in preventing postoperative venous thrombosis (J. R. O'Brien and coworkers, 1974).

Minute doses of heparin (as small as 1 to 10 I.U. per kg body weight) reduce the increased platelet adhesiveness seen after major and minor surgical procedures. Even these extremely low doses of heparin decrease platelet adhesiveness to preoperative levels or below, and the therapeutic effect lasts for more than one hour. The low doses of heparin have no effect on normal platelet adhesiveness, as seen in the preoperative period (Ham and Slack, 1967, 1968).

Changes in the Vessel Wall. Microvessels and capillaries are normally lined with a layer of nonthrombogenic endothelial cells. Immediately beneath the endothelial cells is the extremely thrombogenic "subendothelium," consisting of occasional collagen fibrils, numerous noncollagenous microfibrils (embedded in the internal elastic lamina), the vascular basement membrane, and elastin (Stemerman and Spaet, 1972; Spaet, Gaynor and Stemerman, 1974). These components are listed in the order of their reactivity with platelets, collagen being very reactive and elastin being almost nonthrombogenic. Cell wall material and cell contents also stimulate the aggregation of platelets (MacMillan and Kim, 1970; Mustard and Packham, 1970).

It is known that endothelial cells are replaced only a few times during the life of an animal (Spaet and Gaynor, 1970). This is in marked contrast to other "surfaces" of the body which are exposed to friction and stress, i.e., the bronchi, the gut, and the urinary tract. In these tissues, the lining cells have a rapid turnover, and each lining cell is required to endure stress for only a short time. Periodic interaction of normal endothelial cells with platelets may be necessary to add additional healthy cellular and membrane material to the endothelial cells. This enables them to withstand the constant friction of blood flow while maintaining the proper "pore" size between the endothelial cells necessary for normal capillary permeability. In various thrombocytopenic states, the absence of regular "renewal" of the endothelial cells by an adequate number of platelets would explain the increased capillary permeability and fragility which is seen in these cases.

The edema which is noted during in vitro perfusion of organs has been considerably reduced when a platelet-rich medium is used as a perfusate (Gimbrone and coworkers, 1969). This finding may well be the result of platelets covering or plugging any endothelial ulcerations or defects and of endothelial support via regular interactions with platelets (Majno and Palade, 1961; Tranzer and Bumgartner, 1967; Wojcik and coworkers, 1969). Platelets may perform a similar function in preserving the capillary integrity of microvascular replants.

In addition to their ability to form a hemostatic plug, platelets may have at least three other functions: first, the ability to recognize any foreign thrombogenic material in the bloodstream and to cover it with a layer of platelets to form an amorphous, nonthrombogenic coating over the surface; second, to plug any abnormally large gaps between endothelial cells to maintain normal vascular permeability; and third, to interact with endothelial cells to assist in maintaining normal vascular integrity.

Microvascular repairs result in a number of thrombogenic factors at the anastomotic site. Sutures are particularly thrombogenic. Almost any foreign material, including sutures, may cause primary aggregation of platelets. Exposed to flowing blood, sutures soon become covered with layers of platelets forming a thrombus. The outer platelets revert to normal and deaggregate, and the deeper platelets disintegrate to leave a residual, protective, amorphous, nonthrombogenic coating onto which *normal* platelets do not adhere (Spaet and Gaynor, 1970). In addition to providing a foreign body for platelet adherence, sutures may also cause other thrombogenic changes in the vessel wall. It has been shown that a small incision in a vessel results in a larger thrombus formation if it is closed with a single small suture than if the incision is left open and allowed to seal itself (Acland, 1973). Other thrombogenic materials include the partially exposed ends of the vessels, the subendothelium with its collagen fibrils and microfibrils, exposed cell walls, and the contents of cells, including ADP, epinephrine, and serotonin (MacMillan and Kim, 1970; Spaet and Gaynor, 1970; Stemerman and Spaet, 1972).

Damage to the vessel wall may result from trauma, ischemia, chemicals, electrical current, extremes of temperature, and desiccation. The amount of injury necessary to produce a platelet thrombus is unknown. Preparation for a microvascular anastomosis, including dissection of the adventitia, gentle clamping of the vessel, and touching and gentle stroking of the intima, does not seem to result in the formation of a significant amount of thrombus in veins, at least when observed after ten minutes of venous flow (Acland, 1973). However, the longterm effect of these maneuvers and their effects on arteries should also be determined. The authors have certainly found that the injudicious application of a microvascular clamp or a firm pinch with a jeweler's forceps can lead to complete thrombosis of a microvessel, particularly an artery.

Unrecognized trauma to microvessels is felt

to be the primary reason for the generally poor results obtained in the replantation of avulsed digits and extremities. The stretching of the vessels prior to their breaking may result in tears and separation of the intima at a considerable distance from the actual site of transection of the vessel. With the separation of the intima, the subendothelial structures become exposed and provide a thrombogenic site which may lead to occlusion of the vessel.

The effect of ischemia on vessels is a significant factor in the failure of many microvascular replants. In a study of digital replantation in monkeys after prolonged storage of the digit, it was noted that there were vascular changes and early disintegration of the vessels after overnight storage at 4°C (Hayhurst and coworkers, 1974). The effects of various periods of ischemia on the endothelium of microvessels and capillaries have not been well delineated, but one could certainly speculate that with varying periods of ischemia there is a variable degree of endothelial cell damage, detachment, and desquamation with resultant exposure of small areas of thrombogenic subendothelium. Endothelial ulcerations may result in the formation of small platelet thrombi which grow and embolize sensitized platelets. Small platelet thrombi alone can cause additional tissue damage (Mustard and Packham, 1970). The clumps of sensitized platelets, or individually sensitized platelets, are then inflicted on the venous anastomotic site. This may be an important factor in the greater frequency of venous occlusions seen in many digital replantations (Lendvay, 1973; Kleinert and coworkers, 1976).

Chemicals. Contrast media in various concentrations, as used for angiograms, have been shown to cause considerable changes in the microcirculation. The changes begin first in the venules and include endothelial damage and the formation of thrombi on the vessel walls (Brånemark and coworkers, 1969). All contrast media studied showed some vascular and tissue damage. The changes were reversible to some extent by rapidly perfusing the vessels with a washing solution after the angiograms. Routine angiograms may cause damage to the microvessels and capillary circulation of the microvascular replant. The authors have personally had to cancel one attempted microvascular flap to the lower extremity because of inadequate flow of blood from an anterior tibial vessel which had previously been demonstrated by angiograms to be patent. The suspicion was that angiography had adversely af-

fected the vessel. Vascular changes following an arteriogram performed to confirm the patency of microvascular anastomoses have also been suggested as a possible cause of failure in at least one free flap (Kaplan, Buncke and Murray, 1973). Unless such angiograms can definitely be shown to offer possible benefit to the patient, they should be avoided.

Chemicals or drugs which are relatively well tolerated in the normal circulation may become toxic when infused into the vasculature of an ischemic part or when placed in contact with the microvessels of an ischemic part.

There have been few studies on the effects of chemicals on the microcirculation, and any substance which has not been proved innocuous should be regarded as potentially toxic to the microcirculation. There is some suggestion that substances such as procaine may indeed be toxic under these circumstances (Mehl, Paul and Shorey, 1964).

Chlorpromazine is a vasodilator which has been used in microvascular surgery (Buncke and Blackfield, 1963; Lendvay, 1973a). Topical application of chlorpromazine to surgically injured vessels has been found to increase greatly the amount of thrombus formed (Acland, 1975).

Electrical Current. The internal surface of vessels carries a negative charge, as do the formed elements of the blood, including platelets (Sawyer and Srinivasan, 1967). When a positive electrode at 300 millivolts or greater is applied to a small vessel, the negatively charged platelets form a platelet thrombus on the interior of the vessel within a few seconds, followed by varying degrees of vessel damage (Honour, Pickering and Sheppard, 1973; Sawyer and Srinivasan, 1967). A negative current has also been used in the prevention of thrombosis in metal conduits (Schwartz and Richardson, 1961). *Thrombosis* has also been produced experimentally beneath a negative electrode (Didisheim, 1968). In this study a constant *current* of 200 milliamperes was maintained at an unstated voltage for two minutes, following which the largest thrombosis was noted beneath the *negative* electrode. The explanation for these differences may lie in the pH changes which could occur beneath the electrodes. In the latter study, the pH beneath the negative electrode was noted to rise to 10 to 11, and beneath the positive electrode the pH dropped to 1 to 2.

Changes in Temperature. The small vessels of skin may respond readily to cold or heat with vasoconstriction or vasodilatation, respectively. It has been suggested that a stream of warm saline directed against a microvessel in constriction is a satisfactory means of breaking the vasoconstriction (Horn, 1969). However, the authors have not found that this method offers any great advantage over the more simple procedure of just leaving the vessel alone for a few minutes. In a study of the effects of temperature of the operative field on the degree of vasoconstriction of vessels, the authors found that controlling the temperature of the operative field at 38 to 39°C with a radiant energy source did not significantly alter the amount of vasoconstriction present in either the arteries or veins (Hayhurst and O'Brien, unpublished work). The resistance of ischemic tissue, such as in an amputated part, to changes in temperature is not known, but it is possible that this tissue may be less tolerant of the extremes of temperature than normal tissue. At least one amputated digit was thought to have been lost as a result of tissue freezing

while it was packed in ice for transport to a replantation center (Lendvay, 1973a).

Arteries Versus Veins.   The patency rates in most well-controlled series are better for arterial repairs than for venous repairs (Hayhurst and O'Brien, 1975). However, the reported patency rates vary considerably from author to author, with some authors reporting higher patency rates for their venous repairs than the arterial repairs of other authors (Table 14–3).

The excellence of microvascular technique is the single most important factor in determining patency rates. Veins are technically more difficult to repair because of their flimsy wall structure, and this has been suggested as the primary reason for the lower patency rates in microvenous repairs (Hayhurst, 1976a). In a histopathologic study of microvascular repairs, the most common accompaniment of venous occlusion was the inaccurate apposition of the vein edges (Baxter and coworkers, 1972). In

TABLE 14–3.   *Summary of Previously Published Series of Experimental Microvascular Repairs*

AUTHORS	SIZE OF VESSELS (mm/diameter)	TIME OF PATENCY DETERMINATION	PATENCY RATE (%)	NUMBER OF VESSELS	ANTI-COAGULATION	ANIMAL
Arteries						
Ts'ui et al., 1966	3.1–5.0	1–32 days	100	5	No	Dog
Ts'ui et al., 1966	3.1–3.1	1–32 days	86	24	No	Dog
Ts'ui et al., 1966	1.1–2.1	1–32 days	81	43	No	Dog
Hattori et al., 1970	1.1–1.2	7 days	35	51	No	Dog
Ts'ui et al., 1966	0.74 1.0	1–32 days	41	6	No	Dog
Hattori et al., 1970	1.0	7 days	32	38	No	Dog
Hattori et al., 1970	0.8–0.9	7 days	7	45	No	Dog
Ts'ui et al., 1966	0.3–1.0 (0.67 av)	1–32 days	73	22	Systemic acenocoumarol	Dog
O'Brien et al., 1970a	0.8–1.0	1–16 weeks	81	58	Systemic heparin	Rabbit
Tamai et al., 1972	1.0	3 months	95	20	No	Dog
Kolar et al., 1973	0.8–1.2	1 week	31	26	No	Rabbit
Kolar et al., 1973	0.8–1.2	1 week	46	26	Systemic acenocoumarol	Rabbit
Ketchum et al., 1974	0.5–1.5	0–7 days	55	42	No	Rabbit
Ketchum et al., 1974	0.5–1.5	0–7 days	86	48	Pluronic F–68	Rabbit
Hayhurst et al., 1975	0.9	3–41 days	98	50	No	Rabbit
Acland, 1972	0.49	1 hour (8 days)	30 (90)	20 –	No –	Rat
Acland, 1972	0.49	1 hour (8 days	90 (95)	20	5% Magnesium sulfate	Rat
Veins						
Ts'ui et al., 1966	1.5–3.5	17 weeks	88	17	No	Dog
O'Brien et al., 1970a	1.1	1–16 weeks	90	90	Systemic heparin	Rabbit
Hayhurst et al., 1975	1.2	1–43 days	80	50	No	Rabbit
Hayhurst et al., 1975	1.1	7–14 days	92	25	No	Rabbit
Tamai et al., 1972	1.0	16 weeks	90	20	No	Dog

this study it was also demonstrated that venous repairs heal much more slowly than arterial repairs, with re-endothelization of veins sometimes beginning as long as three weeks postoperatively, whereas arterial repairs usually begin to show re-endothelization at the end of one week. In addition, it was demonstrated that rather massive areas of vein wall necrosis were commonly seen at the anastomotic site. In contrast to the case in arteries, this finding seldom led to occlusion of the venous anastomosis.

The difference in flow rates between arteries and veins may be implicated as a cause for the lower patency rates at the venous anastomotic site. Any platelet thrombi which are formed at an arterial anastomotic site may be swept away by the rapidly flowing arterial blood, whereas the lower flow rates at the venous anastomotic site do not provide this "scouring effect" (Spaet and Gaynor, 1970). Indeed, there seems to be an architectural difference between the arterial and venous thrombi, the arterial thrombus being composed almost entirely of platelets and a few fibrin strands, usually on the surface of the platelet thrombus. However, the venous thrombus is composed of a more heterogeneous population, with numerous entrapped erythrocytes and leukocytes within a more coarse fibrin network enclosing a platelet mass (Didisheim, 1968).

There are also qualitative differences in venous and arterial blood. In microvascular replants, the brief contact of platelets and procoagulants with the arterial anastomotic site may produce only a mild stimulus of the platelets, which increases their stickiness but may be insufficient to cause their aggregation at the anastomotic site. The procoagulants may not have been adequately stimulated to form fibrin at the arterial anastomotic site. The sensitized platelets and activated procoagulants then pass through the capillaries and approach the venous anastomotic site at a much slower rate of flow. Traumatic ischemic endothelial ulcerations also provide a nidus for platelet thrombus formation from which platelet emboli may originate and pass into the venous circuit. Thus, the venous anastomotic site is exposed to numbers of "sticky" platelets that would be more likely to adhere to the thrombogenic substances at the venous anastomotic site.

Disturbances of Blood Flow.   Disturbances of flow alone may be adequate to cause the deposition of platelets onto a vessel wall (Didisheim, 1968). Spontaneous thrombi on normal

mouse aortas have been seen to be laid down with a curved form, suggesting that the aggregates had formed in vortices (Jørgensen, Haerem and Moe, 1973). Irregularities of the vessel surface which upset the normal laminar flow of blood may result in a "trapped vortex" (Fig. 14–12, *A*) (Leonard, 1972). Portions of the blood in the trapped vortex travel in a continuous circle, effectively isolated from the circulation. Blood cells which are traumatized by the turbulence in the vortex can liberate ADP, which will further stimulate platelets and precipitate their aggregation (Jørgensen and coworkers, 1973). Platelets and procoagulants in the blood may be stimulated by the build-up of thrombogenic factors which are trapped in the vortex. Under the influence of ADP or thrombin, platelets may adhere to what appear to be normal endothelial cells. Sites which have been shown to be prone to platelet accumulation are the areas lateral to the ostia of the intercostal arteries. That this is an influence of flow configuration is suggested by the fact that the same platelet patterns are deposited in similar areas in siliconized flow chambers of the same configuration (Jørgensen and coworkers, 1973). Other sites of increased turbulence occur at sharp vessel curves and at the site of a smaller proximal vessel discharging into a larger distal vessel (Fig. 14–12, *B*) (Fox and Hugh, 1966). The authors have also observed, in two separate clinical situations, that small arteries which originate from larger arteries at a right angle (Fig. 14–12, *C*) are not satisfactory for donor arteries because of their propensity to become occluded. This finding may be due to the flow characteristics around the origins of such vessels with the production of sensitized platelets and activated procoagulants.

MICROVASCULAR REPAIR

Proficiency with microvascular anastomoses can and should be attained and maintained in the laboratory. Microvascular surgeons are fortunate in that they can become proficient at performing microvascular repairs before doing their first anastomosis in a human. A microvascular surgeon should be able to achieve patency rates of well over 90 per cent on experimental repairs of 1-mm vessels prior to undertaking clinical anastomoses. There is a moderate amount of physical skill required in attaining this degree of proficiency. However, once attained, it is somewhat more easily

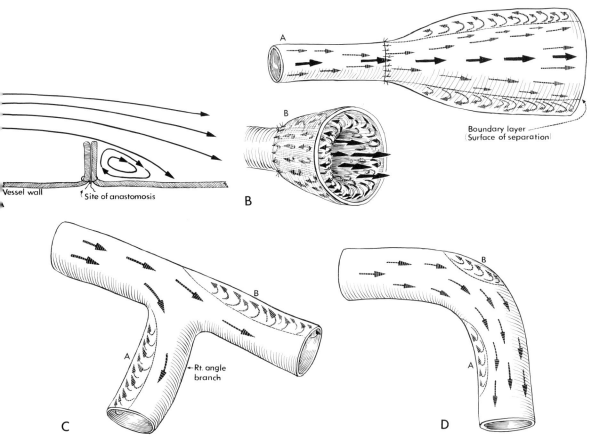

FIGURE 14–12. *A*, Trapped vortex. The recirculation of blood in the trapped vortex results in repeated stimulation of the blood elements, allowing the build-up of stimulated procoagulants. (Adapted from Leonard, E. F.: The role of flow in thrombogenesis. Bull. N.Y. Acad. Med., *48*:273, 1972.) *B*, Fast flowing blood entering a larger vessel creates areas of turbulence. Larger vessels should be avoided on the downstream side of an arterial anastomosis. *C*, Maximum turbulence near a right angle branch occurs at areas A and B. An anastomosis should not be placed near a vessel bifurcation. *D*, A sharp bend in a vessel causes turbulence at points A and B. This should be avoided, particularly at a position proximal to an anastomosis. *(B, C,* and *D* adapted from Fox, J. A., and Hugh, A. E.: Localization of atheroma: A theory based on boundary layer separation. Br. Heart J., *28*:388, 1966.)

maintained with regular exercise of the skill. The ability to achieve excellence in laboratory microvascular repairs is the basis upon which the surgeon can begin to build his clinical experience and judgment.

Position and Preparation. Most standard operating tables are not satisfactory for microvascular surgery because of their instability. A stainless steel table approximately 24 inches wide with four strong, rubber-covered legs is more suitable. The height of the table should allow the surgeon to sit comfortably while observing through the microscope. The hands, forearms, and elbows should rest comfortably on a firm support at right angles to the vessel to be anastomosed. This support should be roughly at the same height as the microvascular anastomosis and should extend to a point as near the anastomosis as possible. Folded

sheets or wooden blocks can be used to provide such forearm and hand rests. Mechanical hand rests which attach to the table offer excellent support and may occasionally prove useful, particularly for areas on the head and neck, but usually are not necessary. It is much easier to concentrate on the anastomosis if the chair height allows observation through the microscope without undue strain. The height requires frequent changing, and chairs that are readily adjustable by the surgeon are preferable.

Exposure. As with most surgery, time spent in obtaining adequate exposure is never wasted. When a surgeon finds himself struggling with a microvascular anastomosis, it is all too frequently because of poor exposure. While in a comfortable position, the surgeon should have an unobstructed view of the vessels to be repaired. Skin edges and projections of subcutaneous tissue which obstruct the surgeon's clear access to the microvascular anastomosis are retracted. This is done with self-retaining retractors and traction sutures which leave the assistant's hands free to provide adequate assistance.

Principles of Microvascular Technique

The essential technical requisites of successful microvascular anastomoses are: (1) gentle handling of tissues; (2) adequate debridement; (3) similar size of vessels; (4) proper vessel stance; (5) correct suture tension; (6) appropriate suture spacing; and (7) recheck of anastomoses.

Gentle Handling of Tissues. In microvascular surgery, the necessity for gentle handling of tissues must be carried to the extreme. Every effort is made to avoid grasping the ends of the vessels to be anastomosed. They should instead be handled by grasping small bits of loose adventitia on the external surface or by external manipulation with forceps or polished manipulators. Small veins can tolerate variable amounts of manipulation, including stretching and pinching, but they do not readily withstand the crush of a firm grasp by a forceps or clamp (Acland, 1973).

Adequate Debridement. Microvascular repairs should be performed only on normal undamaged vessels. The recipient vessels are frequently in an area of trauma, and occasionally the donor vessels may be subjected to trauma, as in digital or major extremity replantation. All vessels are carefully inspected under the high power of the microscope for signs of damage which would indicate the need for further debridement. Any vessel which contains a clot should be resected. The interior of the vessel is irrigated and inspected for signs

of retained fibrin deposits on the intimal wall. Such fibrin deposits serve as a nidus for platelet thrombus formation, and their presence is an indication for further debridement of the vessel.

The interior of the vessel is also observed for signs of intimal tears or intimal "ruffling," findings which are commonly seen proximal and distal to the site of avulsion injuries. These signs call for additional debridement until no more damage can be seen. This may require the resection of several centimeters of vessel. The generally poor results obtained in the replantation of avulsed digits and extremities can usually be attributed to an inadequate debridement of vessels proximal and distal to the site of amputation.

Hydrostatic pressure has been used to detect small intimal tears by saline leakage from the vessel (Ts'ui and associates, 1966). However, this maneuver can be traumatic to the vessel and is usually not necessary.

After adequate debridement there should be a *strong* pulsatile flow of blood from the recipient artery. If a catheter is necessary to obtain flow, this suggests proximal vascular damage, and these vessels should be avoided as recipient vessels in microvascular surgery. These catheters have been shown to strip the endothelium, exposing the very thrombogenic subendothelium (Sawyer and coworkers, 1973). Failure to obtain full pulsatile arterial flow is a strong indication of the possible failure of any microvascular surgery relying on such flow.

Similar Size of Vessels. Vessels with a discrepancy in size of up to 50 per cent of their diameters can usually be anastomosed satisfactorily (Fig. 14–13). When the size discrepancy is much greater, an interposing vein graft, each end of which more readily approximates the size of these vessels, gives better results (Fig. 14–14).

Some surgeons find it helpful to divide the

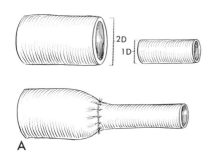

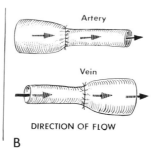

FIGURE 14–13. *A*, Vessels of one diameter size difference can be satisfactorily anastomosed without difficulty. *B*, The larger vessel should be on the upstream side for arteries and on the downstream side for veins.

A   B

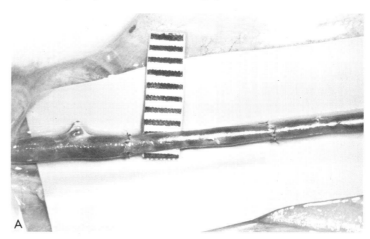

FIGURE 14–14. Vein grafts may be used to (*A*) join vessels of greatly dissimilar diameter or (*B*) bridge gaps in arteries or veins.

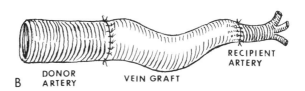

smaller vessel obliquely when suturing vessels of a dissimilar size. The use of an end-to-side repair is an alternative technique.

Proper Vessel Stance. On several occasions, when a small, sharply angled branch of a larger vessel has been used for a microvascular anastomosis or the anastomosis has been placed near a major branch, the outcome has been poor. It is our feeling that vascular configurations which contribute to turbulence at or just above the anastomosis predispose the anastomosis to occlusion (see Fig. 14–12, *A* to *D*). This is probably due to the formation of trapped vortices and other forms of turbulence which initiate platelet reaction and the stimulation of blood procoagulants (Leonard, 1972; Jørgensen, Haerem and Moe, 1973). In general, small end branches which emerge from a larger vessel at a right angle are not satisfactory donor vessels when the microvascular anastomosis has to be placed near the branch.

For the same reasons, any kinking or twisting of the vessel upstream from the repair predisposes the anastomosis to occlusion. Such situations are best avoided by adjusting donor and recipient vessels or interposed vein grafts to the proper length, with minimal tension, but without an excess of vessel which would cause twisting or kinking. In addition, care is exercised in replacing vessels beneath skin closures or other tissues to avoid kinking or twisting of the anastomosis at the time of closure.

Suture Tension. Proper suture tension is extremely important. This is particularly true for microarterial repairs and slightly less so for microvenous repairs. Sutures which are tied too tightly cause small tears in the wall and exposure of the subendothelium, cell walls, and cell contents, all of which cause platelet reaction, aggregation, and disintegration, leading to thrombus formation (MacMillan and Kim, 1970; Spaet and Gaynor, 1970). Sutures which are tied too tightly also cause damage to the media of the arterial wall. If at least one-third of the media does not survive, re-endothelization does not occur, and occlusion of the anastomotic site invariably follows (Baxter and coworkers, 1972; Spaet, Gaynor and Stemerman, 1974).

To ensure that the arterial sutures have not been tied too tightly, a small "suture circle" should remain visible through the translucent arterial wall at the end of three ties (Hayhurst, 1976a) (see Fig. 14–19). The diameter of this "suture circle" should be roughly equal to the thickness of the arterial wall, and its persistence after the suture has been tied indicates that the encompassed portions of the arterial wall have not been strangulated.

Excessive suture tension and resultant wall necrosis should also be avoided in venous repairs, but this is not as critical for veins because large areas of vein wall necrosis are often seen at or near the venous anastomotic site without causing occlusion. Re-endothelization of such veins also occurs relatively late, sometimes as late as three to four weeks postoperatively (Baxter and coworkers, 1972).

Appropriate Suture Spacing. The correct spacing of sutures is critical to the performance of a successful anastomosis. Suture spacing depends upon the size of the vessels, the consistency of the vessel wall, the size of the suture used, and the pressure of the system, i.e., arterial or venous. The philosophy of suture spacing is different for microarterial and microvenous repairs.

ARTERIAL REPAIR. The media is the key to a satisfactory microarterial anastomosis. Each suture which passes through the vessel wall causes significant damage and disturbs the normal physiology of the vessel. A suture which is placed through the full thickness of the arterial wall causes less damage than oblique sutures which pass through a longer portion of the media in an attempt to avoid piercing the intima.

In general, the larger the vessel, the further apart the sutures can be placed. This is primarily because of the more substantial consistency of the larger vessel wall. However, some large veins have a thin wall consistency which will require more closely spaced sutures than the same size artery with a thicker wall. In addition, the smaller the suture size, the more closely the sutures must be placed.

The pressure of the vascular system which is being repaired also affects the suture spacing. An artery of the same size and *consistency* will require a relatively greater number of sutures than would a similar size vein, because of the tendency of the higher pressure of the arterial system to cause leakage at the anastomotic site.

Each suture causes damage to the vascular wall and contributes to the potential for the occlusion of the anastomosis. With this in mind, it would seem wise to use as few sutures as possible to avoid disruption of the normal vascular physiology and damage to the vessel. On the other hand, failure to place an adequate number of sutures in an arterial repair will result in prolonged bleeding from the anastomosis. Therefore, the goal in spacing arterial sutures should be to achieve an ultimately leak-free anastomosis with as few sutures as possible. This usually involves about eight to ten 7 MF 32-18 sutures for a 1-mm artery. The "cuffing" technique allows the use of fewer arterial sutures than would otherwise be necessary (McLean and Buncke, 1973). A microsurgical arterial repair is illustrated in Figures 14-15 to 14-23. A small strip of thin plastic is used to form a "cuff" around the arterial anastomosis, which is left in place for about five minutes following the repair (Fig. 14-24). After release of the clamps, patency of the anastomosis can be confirmed by "stripping" a segment of the vessel "downstream" and then allowing the empty segment to be filled (Figs. 14-25 and 14-26).

VENOUS REPAIR. A different philosophy must be used in spacing sutures in a venous repair. If the same procedure were followed for venous repairs as for arterial repairs, one would attempt to repair the vein with a minimal number of sutures. One can use as few as four to six sutures for a 1-mm venous repair,

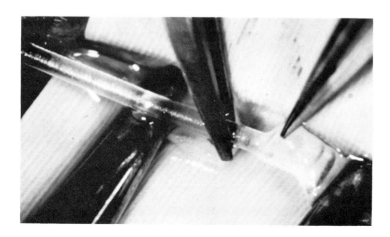

FIGURE 14-15. Irrigation of the ends of the artery with normal saline.

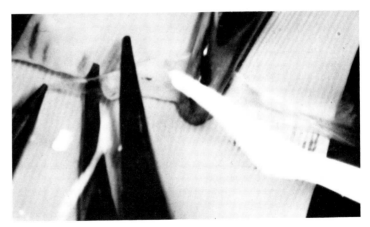

FIGURE 14–16. Trimming the loose adventitia only near the end of the vessel.

but this is not good technique, even though the anastomosis will generally be leak-free in a matter of a few minutes. In this low pressure system, the gaps between the widely spaced sutures rapidly become filled with platelet thrombi and clots. These occluding plugs narrow the effective lumen of the anastomosis and predispose it to occlusion.

Improvement in the patency rates of venous repairs has been obtained by a more careful attention to the end-to-end approximation of the veins and by the addition of a few sutures to each anastomosis (Hayhurst and O'Brien, 1975). The goal in spacing sutures for a venous anastomosis should be to achieve an accurate edge-to-edge approximation of the vessel ends. There should be no hesitation in using an adequate number of sutures to accomplish this, e.g., eight to ten sutures for most 1-mm veins. The fear of suture crowding and the avoidance

of suture tension are of secondary importance for venous repairs, contrary to the case in arteries. The "cuffing" technique has also not been of help in venous anastomoses because it tends to narrow the anastomotic site in this low pressure system. The technique of microsurgical venous anastomosis is illustrated in Figures 14–27 through 14–31.

Recheck of Anastomoses. All anastomoses are rechecked prior to final skin closure. If an occlusion occurs, an evaluation of the possible cause of occlusion and a specific correction should be made. It will be found that most occlusions during the operative period are due to technically faulty microvascular repairs. It is inadequate to dislodge the occluding plug from the anastomosis in the hope that it will remain open. This treatment of a thrombosis is frequently rewarded by reocclusion of the vessel

Text continued on page 364.

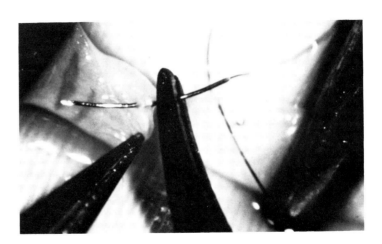

FIGURE 14–17. Full-thickness bites are taken. Note the needle visible through the vessel end.

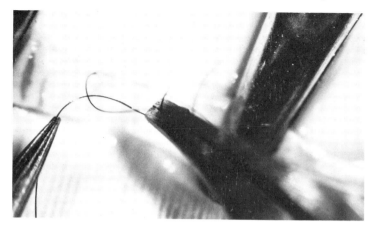

FIGURE 14-18. Ties are made with the forceps and needle holder. There is no need to change the position of the hands.

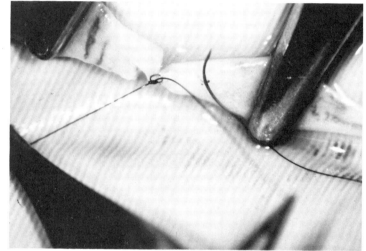

FIGURE 14-19. Be sure the "suture circle" is still present after three square knots. The "feel" of the suture is not a reliable index of tension.

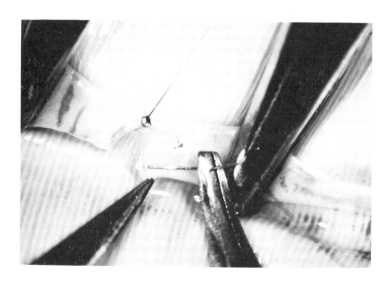

FIGURE 14-20. The assistant provides countertraction as the second suture is placed 120° from the first. Note grasping of the adventitia instead of the vessel edge.

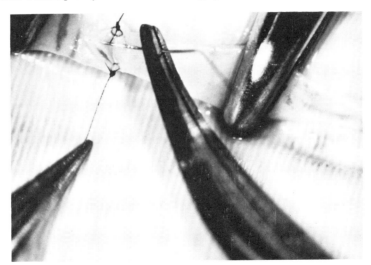

FIGURE 14–21. Slight tension on the stay sutures provides adequate counter-traction for needle placement.

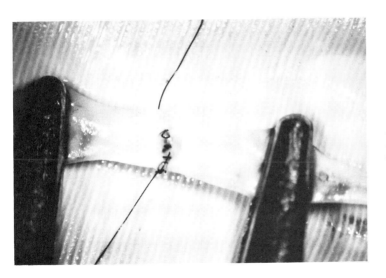

FIGURE 14–22. After completion of the front of the anastomosis, the micro-vascular clamp is rotated 180° to expose the remainder of the vessel for repair.

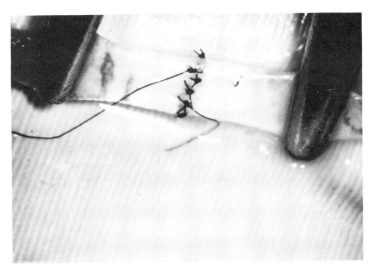

FIGURE 14–23. The completed anas-tomosis, showing the two original stay sutures ready to be cut.

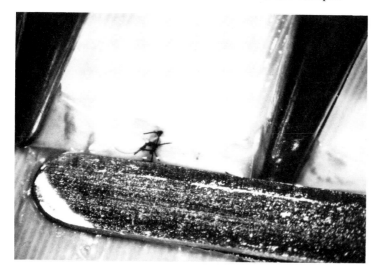

FIGURE 14-24. The anastomosis "cuffed" with Saran Wrap.

FIGURE 14-25. Beginning patency check as blood is stripped from a small segment of the vessel "downstream" from the anastomosis. Apply the forceps *gently* to avoid crushing the vessel wall.

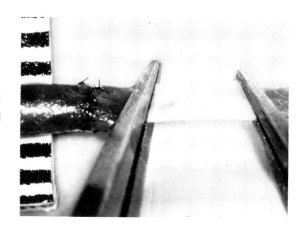

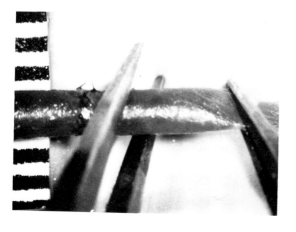

FIGURE 14-26. Release of the forceps near the repair allows blood to flow through the anastomosis and fill the empty distal segment.

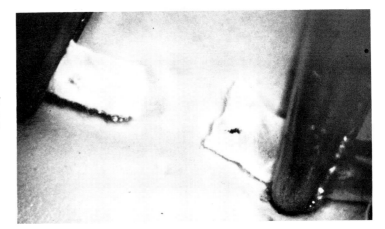

FIGURE 14–27. Vein under pool of saline prior to repair. Note bubbles on the vein and the shadow beneath the vein.

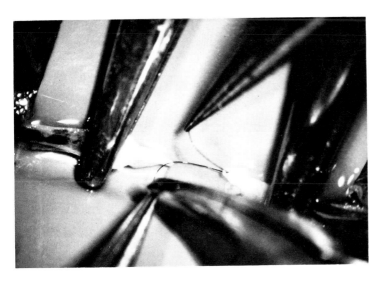

FIGURE 14–28. Although the suture is inserted while the vein is immersed under saline, fluid is removed to facilitate tying of the suture. Note collapse of the vein ends by the surface tension of the fluid. The assistant applies tension by holding the end of the suture.

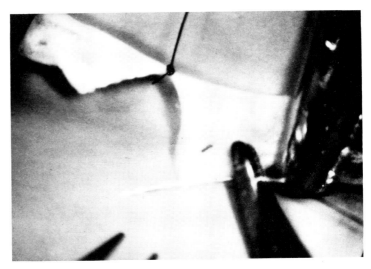

FIGURE 14–29. The second suture being placed 180° from the first.

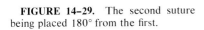

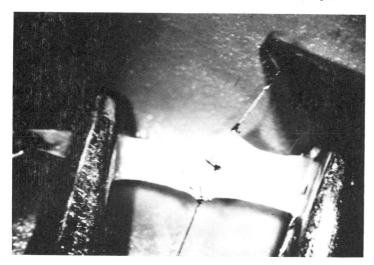

FIGURE 14-30. With the stay sutures in place, it may be possible to place the remainder of the sutures in a "dry" field.

at a less opportune time. Any faulty repair must be resected and a better anastomosis accomplished.

Number of Vessels Repaired

Most microvascular replants will survive if at least one artery and vein of approximately 1 mm in diameter remain patent. This has been demonstrated either experimentally or clinically for digital replants, microvascular free flaps, and penile replantations (O'Brien and coworkers, 1973a,b; Hayhurst, 1976b; Hayhurst and coworkers, 1976b; Horton and coworkers, 1976). Although one artery and one vein are usually sufficient to provide an adequate circulation for full survival of a microvascular replant, the repair of one additional artery and two or more veins greatly improves the

statistical chance that at least one artery and one vein will remain open.

If one assumes that the repair of the arteries and veins of a microvascular replant are independent events (they are not entirely independent) and not dependent upon each other, the following statistical analyses are valid (Table 14-4) (Hayhurst, 1976b). From the table one can see that if a microsurgeon is capable of only an 80 per cent patency rate for arteries and veins and if he repairs only a single artery and vein, the statistical likelihood that both the artery and the vein will remain open is only 64 per cent. If the microsurgeon is capable of a 90 per cent patency for both arteries and veins, the statistical chance of the the artery and vein remaining open is 81 per cent. On the other hand, if the microsurgeon repairs two arteries and two veins, the repair of this one additional artery and vein increases the chances of at

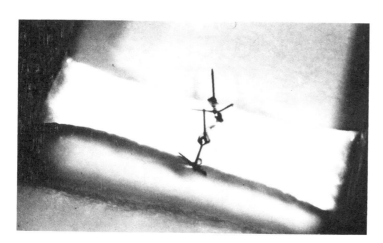

FIGURE 14-31. Completed venous repair.

TABLE 14-4. *Relationship of the Percentage Likelihood That at Least one Artery and one Vein Will Both Remain Open to the Number of Arteries and Veins Repaired and the Known Patency Rates of the Surgeon*

NO. OF VESSELS REPAIRED		PATENCY RATES	
Arteries	*Veins*	80%*	90%*
1	1	64%	81%
1	2	78.4%	89%
2	2	92.1%	98%
2	3	95.2%	98.9%

*Surgeon's known patency rates.

least one artery and vein remaining patent to 92 per cent for a surgeon capable of an 80 per cent patency rate and to 98 per cent for a surgeon capable of a 90 per cent patency rate.

This is particularly applicable to digital replantation when two arteries and two or more veins are readily available for repair. In such instances, the repair of one additional artery and one or two additional veins greatly increases the statistical likelihood that adequate circulation will be achieved.

ANTICOAGULATION

It has been shown that technically satisfactory anastomoses in vessels approximately 1 mm in diameter do not require anticoagulation for high patency rates (Hayhurst and O'Brien, 1975; Hayhurst, Mladick and Adamson, 1976b). Experimentally the authors have had excellent results with the repair of 1-mm vessels for the replantation of microvascular flaps and the penis without the use of any sort of anticoagulation (Hayhurst and coworkers, 1976b; Horton and coworkers, 1976).

However, several experimental studies on patency rates in normal vessels have shown an increased patency rate with the use of anticoagulants such as heparin, acenocoumarin, and Pluronic F-68 (Elcock and Fredrickson, 1972; Kolář, Wieberdink and Reneman, 1973; Ketchum and coworkers, 1974). Clinical microsurgeons have almost universally felt the need to use some form of anticoagulation during the care of their free flaps and digital replants (O'Brien and coworkers, 1973a,b; Lendvay, 1973a; Buncke, 1974; Harii, Ohmori and Ohmori, 1974; Hayhurst, 1976b; Hayhurst, Mladick and Adamson, 1976b).

It is thus clear that the role of anticoagulation in microvascular surgery is at present uncertain. It would appear that, if normal vessels are adequately repaired, anticoagulation is not necessary to achieve high patency rates or reliable microvascular replants. However, in microvascular repairs which are inadequate, in vessels which have suffered a significant amount of damage, and in certain other clinical situations, the judicious use of anticoagulants may improve patency rates and the survival of microvascular replants.

The surgeon should not be tempted to rely upon the supposedly magical properties of the anticoagulant which is presently in vogue to forge a patent vessel from a poorly executed anastomosis. If a surgeon performs an inadequate anastomosis, he should recognize this early, assess the cause of the inadequacy, make the proper adjustments, and revise the anastomosis rather than turning quickly to some form of anticoagulation therapy. Whether or not some anticoagulants can improve the patency rates in a series of poorly executed anastomoses is a question that has not yet been adequately answered.

Topical Anticoagulants

When applied topically, magnesium sulfate is a vasodilator and is thought to be an antithrombogenic agent. Its use in small experimental vessels has been described by Acland (1972b), who believes that if a thrombus can be prevented from forming for the first 20 to 30 minutes following a microvascular repair, there is no additional thrombus formation. In a series of rat arteries approximately 0.5 mm in diameter, he demonstrated a 30 per cent patency in the controls and a 90 per cent patency in the magnesium sulfate–treated group. Didisheim (1968) had previously pointed out the great importance of the diameter of small vessels and its influence on patency.

Dipyridamole (Persantin) is frequently used because of its antithrombogenic action orally, and its action as a vasodilator. However, a less well known property of dipyridamole is its ability to cause vasodilatation when applied topically to a microvessel. The authors have observed this action in the laboratory but have not studied it extensively (Hayhurst and O'Brien, unpublished work).

A heparinized saline solution is commonly used for irrigation of vessels in the operative field during microvascular repairs. The use of a heparinized saline irrigant has not been shown to improve patency rates (Elcock and Fredrickson, 1972). One secondary benefit of the use of heparinized saline for an irrigation solution is that it makes the microvascular field somewhat less "sticky" than if saline alone is used. Heparinized Ringer's lactate solution may be preferable, as some evidence has become available that saline may be injurious to endothelium.

Systemic Anticoagulants

Heparin

MODE OF ACTION. Heparin is a heterogeneous polysaccharide with a molecular weight of approximately 6000 to 20,000; it is primarily derived from animal sources, usually the lungs, liver, or gut. Its primary action is on blood coagulation, and it inhibits the conversion of prothrombin to thrombin by its inhibition of thromboplastin and thromboplastin generation. It also inhibits Factors V, IX, and XI. It requires approximately 30 to 40 times as much heparin to inhibit the action of thrombin already formed than it does to prevent the formation of thrombin (Goodman and Gilman, 1970).

It is only when it is given in extremely high doses that heparin affects platelet response to collagen and ADP (Mustard and Packham, 1970). However, heparin has been shown to reduce platelet adhesiveness in vitro but not to prevent platelet adherence to the site of injury of the vessel wall (Salzman, 1965; Negus, Pinto and Slack, 1971). Some investigators believe that heparin given in the usual anticoagulant doses has little or no effect on platelet function (Mustard and Packham, 1970). Heparin is said to inhibit the aggregation of platelets by thrombin but not by ADP (Goodman and Gilman, 1970).

Following even minor surgery, such as a herniorrhaphy, there is often a marked increase in platelet adhesiveness which peaks at about 48 hours postoperatively (Ham and Slack, 1967). Minute heparin dosages from 1 to 10 I.U. per kg have been shown to reduce increased postoperative platelet adhesiveness within ten minutes of injection; the effect lasts more than one hour (Negus, Pinto and Slack, 1971). However, the small doses of heparin had no effect on normal preoperative levels of platelet adhesiveness.

EXPERIMENTAL STUDIES. In a randomized controlled series of microvascular anastomoses

in femoral arteries (rabbit) averaging approximately 1 mm in diameter, a 55 per cent patency was obtained for 42 controls and a 57 per cent patency for 42 heparin-treated rabbits, indicating no significant difference in the patency rates for normal vessels (Ketchum and coworkers, 1974). In another study of somewhat smaller mesenteric arteries in rats, heparin had a minimal beneficial effect in preventing a thrombus caused by a direct current (Didisheim, 1968). However, following endothelial damage of canine femoral arteries, heparin-treated animals showed an increased patency rate over controls (Haimov and Danese, 1973). In a double-blind study of a series of 2-mm rabbit neck veins using the Nakayama ring pin, patency rates were increased from 46 per cent for a series of eight controls to 94 per cent for a series of 16 experimental animals (Elcock and Fredrickson, 1972).

In experimental studies on digital replantation in monkeys after a prolonged period of ischemia, heparin was of benefit in maintaining a viable digit (Hayhurst and coworkers, 1974). In these limited studies, the authors did not determine whether the beneficial effect was secondary to pharmacologic action on the veins, arteries, or both.

In studies on rat veins, deposits of fibrin have been noted on endothelial cells, with platelets adhering to the fibrin strands (Spaet and Gaynor, 1970). It has been suggested that in some cases fibrin deposition may precede and even initiate a platelet thrombus. By its action in preventing fibrin formation, heparin could be of benefit in preventing this type of thrombosis.

Heparin has also been shown to have an affinity for endothelial intercellular cement, as demonstrated by toluidine blue, a specific stain for heparin (Samuels and Webster, 1952). In this study heparin was felt to prevent the aggregation of platelets on intercellular cement and injured endothelium.

The limited experimental studies currently available suggest that there is little objective evidence to indicate the benefit of heparin in preventing the occlusion of technically satisfactory microvascular repairs in normal *arteries* of approximately 1 mm in diameter. Some studies seem to suggest that there is possibly some benefit in the use of heparin in preventing the occlusion of small veins, and possibly *damaged* arteries.

CLINICAL STUDIES. Several studies have recently demonstrated the benefit of low doses of heparin in reducing postoperative venous thrombosis (Kakkar and coworkers, 1971). The reduction of the postoperative increase in platelet adhesiveness may account for the effectiveness of heparin.

In the management of digital replantation, many different anticoagulant regimens are used, but the single anticoagulant that is common to all is heparin (O'Brien and coworkers, 1973b; Lendvay, 1973b; Kleinert and coworkers, 1976; Hayhurst, 1976b). It should be noted that many successful microvascular free flaps, requiring the anastomosis of the same size vessels, have been accomplished without the use of heparin (Harii, Ohmori and Ohmori, 1974; O'Brien and coworkers, 1974; Hayhurst, Mladick and Adamson, 1976b). Although it has not been our experience, some authors feel that venous occlusions are the most common causes of digital replantation failure (Lendvay, 1973a; Kleinert and coworkers, 1975). Heparin may be most beneficial in preventing venous thrombosis in vessels which have been subjected to considerable ischemic damage. It may also be helpful in preventing the occlusion of arteries and veins which have suffered considerable ischemic, chemical or traumatic damage. For satisfactory microvascular repairs in normal arteries, it should not be expected that heparin will improve patency rates.

Coumarin

MODE OF ACTION. The coumarin anticoagulants interfere with blood coagulation by preventing vitamin K synthesis which is necessary for the production of prothrombin. Coumarin derivatives also inhibit Factors VII, IX, and X and are thought to interfere with platelet adhesiveness and clumping, although a direct effect has not been demonstrated in vitro (Goodman and Gilman, 1970; Murphy and Mustard, 1960).

EXPERIMENTAL STUDIES. Ts'ui and associates (1966) reported a 41 per cent patency rate for 17 control vessels averaging 0.77 mm in diameter and a 73 per cent patency rate for a series of 22 experimental vessels averaging 0.67 mm. In the experimental dogs, the prothrombin time was maintained at approximately 40 to 60 per cent during the entire period of observation, which ranged from 1 to 32 days (Ts'ui and associates, 1966). It was not stated whether the vessels were arteries, veins, or a mixture of both.

The effect of acenocoumarin on microvascular repairs of rabbit femoral arteries averaging 0.8 to 1.2 mm in diameter was studied by Kolář, Wieberdink, and Reneman (1973). They reported a 31 per cent patency rate for 26 controls. In the experimental group, there were only eight animals which were felt to have been adequately anticoagulated throughout the ten-day period of observation, and in this group there was a 70 per cent patency rate. However, in the five animals which were not felt to be adequately anticoagulated, the patency rate was only 20 per cent. This gave an overall patency rate of 46 per cent for this group of 26 experimental animals. The fact that in those animals which were *inadequately* anticoagulated with acenocoumarin the patency rates were lower than the controls is of interest in that Didisheim (1968) also showed a deleterious effect of coumarin on the patency rate of small mesenteric arteries in rats (100 to 325 μ in diameter).

CLINICAL APPLICATIONS. At least one group of replantation surgeons has treated its digital replants by initiating anticoagulation with heparin during the operative or early postoperative period and then converting the patient to anticoagulation with coumarin anticoagulants (Kleinert and coworkers, 1976). However, the results of their recently reported series are somewhat lower than those of other investigators for complete and incomplete amputations (O'Brien and coworkers, 1973b; Lendvay, 1973a; Hayhurst, 1976b). The authors know of no uses of coumarin anticoagulants for microvascular free flaps or other clinical microvascular replants.

Aspirin

MODE OF ACTION. Aspirin was introduced by Dreser in 1899 (Goodman and Gilman, 1970). It is a commonly used drug with many complex and poorly understood pharmacologic properties. It has been shown to inhibit collagen- and thrombin-induced platelet aggregation; it does not influence platelet aggregation induced by ADP (Evans, Packham and Nishizawa, 1968; Mustard and Packham, 1970). It also inhibits the "release reaction" of platelets (Mustard and Packham, 1970).

EXPERIMENTAL STUDIES. In a double-blind study performed on 2-mm rabbit veins, the postanastomosis patency rates were 66.6 per cent for the controls and 46.6 per cent for aspirin-treated animals. The Nakayama ring pin was used for the repair, but the number of animals and the dosages of aspirin were not given (Elcock and Fredrickson, 1972).

The authors have done 20 vein-to-vein grafts in the rabbit. The grafts averaged approximately 2.5 cm in length and 1.5 mm in diameter and were repaired with 19μ metallized microsutures. A 50 per cent patency rate was obtained in ten controls examined at one week postoperatively. In ten experimental animals that received a single dose of 5000 U. of heparin immediately after surgery and 600 mg of aspirin and 100 mg of dipyridamole by mouth daily for one week, a 50 per cent patency rate was observed in the experimental group (Hayhurst and O'Brien, unpublished work).

In canine peripheral arteries of unstated size, two injuries were induced either by endarterectomy or instillation of 0.1N H_2SO_4. After two days, 29 per cent of the chemically injured and 43 per cent of the endarterectomized segments were occluded. In dogs treated with 600 mg per day of aspirin, the occlusion rate was reduced to 2 per cent and 17 per cent, respectively. In the same study, treatment with 200 mg per day of dipyridamole had no effect (Weiss, Danese and Voleti, 1970).

In 20 endarterectomized canine femoral arteries, a daily dose of 0.75 mg per kg of aspirin initiated before surgery increased the patency rate to 95 per cent versus 0 per cent for 20 controls. In the same study, dogs treated with Pluronic F–68 had a 0 per cent patency rate, those with dipyridamole a 20 per cent rate, and those with dextran 70 a 95 per cent patency rate (Justice, Papavangelou and Edwards, 1974).

CLINICAL STUDIES. In a double-blind study, daily dosages of 600 mg of aspirin begun preoperatively failed to reduce the incidence of postoperative venous thrombosis (J. R. O'Brien, 1973). However, in another controlled study, 600 mg of aspirin given every six hours was found to be as effective as Warfarin and dextran 40 in reducing the incidence of postoperative venous thrombosis to 10 to 12 per cent (versus 34 per cent for the controls). In the same study, dipyridamole was not found to be effective (Salzman, Harris and DeSanctis, 1971).

In patients with prosthetic heart valves, 400 mg of dipyridamole per day was sufficient to prevent platelet consumption, and the addition of 600 mg of aspirin per day to the regimen reduced the required dosage of dipyridamole from 400 mg to 100 mg. Thus, it would appear that in humans aspirin potentiates the effect of dipyridamole on platelets (Harker and Slichter, 1970).

The authors have used aspirin in the dosage of 1 g per day in conjunction with 100 mg of dipyridamole (daily oral dosage for both digital replants and microvascular flaps). It is felt that this regimen potentiates the effects of dipyridamole on platelets and inhibits both collagen- and thrombin-induced platelet aggregation.

Dipyridamole. Dipyridamole (Persantin) can be given either orally or parenterally and is known to inhibit ADP-induced platelet aggregation and the release reaction of platelets. It also enhances platelet disaggregation (Emmons and coworkers, 1965; Mustard and Packham, 1970). It is a vasodilator and is thought to act as a relaxant of smooth muscles (Goodman and Gilman, 1970). It has also been observed in our laboratory that dipyridamole has rapid action as a vasodilator when applied topically to small vessels. In at least one clinical study, there were no significant changes in platelet function tests with daily (400 mg) dose of dipyridamole (Harker and Slichter, 1970).

EXPERIMENTAL STUDIES. Dipyridamole demonstrated a marked inhibition of electrically induced thrombi in small rat arteries (100 to 325 microns in diameter) when compared with results in controls and experimental groups treated with heparin and warfarin (Didisheim, 1968). It is not known whether the beneficial effect is the result of the vasodilatory properties of dipyridamole or its ability to inhibit platelet aggregation.

In dog femoral arteries which had been stripped of endothelium, a daily dose of 3 mg of dipyridamole per 5 kg body weight was noted to increase patency from 0 per cent in 20 controls to 20 per cent in 20 experimental animals treated with dipyridamole. In the same experiment, both dextran 70– and aspirin-treated animals had a 95 per cent patency rate following anastomoses of 20 experimental vessels (Justice, Papavangelou and Edwards, 1974).

CLINICAL APPLICATIONS. In patients with prosthetic heart valves, dipyridamole has been shown to prevent platelet consumption (Harker and Slichter, 1970). In this study it was also shown that when the drug is combined with aspirin, the dosage necessary to prevent complete consumption of platelets could be reduced to one-fourth the usual dose. It has been suggested that dipyridamole is primarily useful in the prevention of platelet thrombi (Sullivan, Harken and Gorlin, 1971). Dipyridamole combined with aspirin, heparin, and low molecular weight dextran has been extensively used in digital replantations (O'Brien and coworkers, 1973b; Hayhurst, 1976b; Hayhurst, Adamson and Mladick, 1976a). It has also been used in combination with aspirin and low molecular weight dextran without heparin in several microvascular flaps (Hayhurst and coworkers, 1976a). In a study of experimental digital replantations in monkeys after prolonged ischemia, aspirin and Persantin were not felt to be effective in preventing loss of the digit when used alone. However, when they were combined with heparin, there was a significant improvement in survival rates (Hayhurst and coworkers, 1974). Problems with hypertension were not noted in any of the clinical cases.

Dipyridamole may be useful in preventing platelet consumption and aggregation by virtue of its action on ADP-induced platelet aggregation and the prevention of the release reaction. Its use may be especially helpful when it is combined with aspirin, an agent which also inhibits collagen-induced platelet aggregation and apparently potentiates the action of dipyridamole.

Dextran. Dextran is a mixture of branched polysaccharides with glucose units in the main chain and a molecular weight which may approach 40 million (Goodman and Gilman, 1970). Dextran has been used clinically both as dextran 40 (average molecular weight 40,000) and dextran 70 (average molecular weight 70,000). Approximately 20 per cent of the molecules of dextran 40 have a molecular weight greater than 50,000, which is above the renal threshold. Thus, repeated administration of dextran 40 will eventually lead to a build-up of dextran molecules which are above the renal threshold and will thus have to be metabolized. The higher molecular weight fractions of dextran are thought to be the active components which cause both a decrease in platelet adhesiveness and a defect in the release reaction of platelets and in platelet aggregation (Clagett and Salzman, 1974; Salzman, Harris and DeSanctis, 1971). Dextran is thought to form a coating of platelets by reacting with the plasma proteins necessary for platelet aggregation. Dextran also improves the microcirculation by preventing sludging, an effect which may be secondary to hemodilution.

EXPERIMENTAL STUDIES. In a study of the effect of low molecular weight dextran on the patency of canine arteries averaging 1.1 mm in diameter, a 72 per cent postanastomosis patency rate was obtained for controls, and a 50 per cent patency rate was obtained for experimental vessels in animals which had received 500 ml of 10 per cent low molecular weight dextran intravenously over a period of 12

hours following the completion of the anastomosis (Ts'ui and associates, 1966).

In canine carotid or femoral arteries approximately 3.5 mm in diameter, a thrombogenic lesion was created by a 2-cm linear arteriotomy and intimectomy. There was only a 16.7 per cent patency rate for 24 controls and a 6.7 per cent patency rate for 16 dogs given 500 ml of low molecular weight dextran started 30 minutes *before* surgery and continued for 24 hours. However, there was a 95 per cent patency rate for 20 dogs in which the dextran was started immediately *after* surgery and which were otherwise treated in the same way. The poorer results in those dogs given dextran preoperatively was thought to be due to excessive bleeding from the operative site, which required continuous application of pressure as well as reclamping and resuturing of the arteriotomy for hemostasis (Winfrey and Foster, 1964). In another study using canine femoral arteries which had been stripped of their endothelium over a short segment, the administration of dextran 70 in a dose of 1 per cent per kilogram body weight begun immediately after surgery increased the patency rates from 0 per cent for 20 controls to 95 per cent for 20 experimental vessels (Justice, Papavangelou and Edwards, 1974).

CLINICAL APPLICATIONS. In a study of thromboembolic complications following hip arthroplasty, dextran 40 was found to be as effective as warfarin and aspirin in preventing venous thrombosis (12 to 14 per cent) and was found to be better than dipyridamole (26 per cent), and its effectiveness was found to be greater than in the controls (39 per cent) (Salzman, Harris and DeSanctis, 1971). Dextran 70 has also been shown to reduce postoperative clinical and postmortem thrombi in patients undergoing major general surgical procedures by roughly 50 per cent when the drug is administered during surgery and a second dose is given approximately 24 hours postoperatively. This dose achieved a level of approximately 0.4 mg per 100 ml for approximately 72 hours postoperatively (Stadil, 1970). Dextran 40 has also been shown to prevent thrombus formation following crush injury, electrical burn, and endothelial stripping caused by a Fogarty catheter (Sawyer and coworkers, 1973).

Pluronic F–68. Pluronic F–68 is a nonionic surfactant, composed of hydrophilic and hydrophobic groups with a molecular weight of approximately 8000. It is not absorbed when given by mouth and is not metabolized; it is excreted by the kidneys within 90 minutes of administration. It is said to decrease platelet adhesiveness and to improve microcirculation by decreasing blood viscosity without hemodilution. It also inhibits Factor VIII and Hageman factor (Ketchum and coworkers, 1974).

EXPERIMENTAL STUDIES. In a well-controlled study on rabbit femoral arteries averaging 0.8 to 1.2 mm in diameter, patency rates were increased from 55 per cent of 42 control repairs to 86 per cent of 48 repairs in which the Pluronic F–68 was given immediately before the microvascular repair (Ketchum and coworkers, 1974). In 20 repairs in which administration of the Pluronic F–68 was delayed for approximately one hour after the repair, the patency rates were only 60 per cent and were not significantly different from those of the controls.

In canine femoral arteries which had been stripped of a portion of their endothelium, there were no patent vessels in 20 controls, and in 12 experimental animals which were given Pluronic F–68 there were also no patent vessels. The Pluronic F–68 was begun one hour before surgery and continued postoperatively until a total dose of 2.0 to 12.0 g had been given. In the same study, both dextran 70 and aspirin gave a 95 per cent postanastomosis patency rate (Justice, Papavangelou and Edwards, 1974).

POSTOPERATIVE CARE

An uncomplicated microvascular replant requires a minimum of postoperative care. Mild elevation and frequent monitoring of the vascular status of the replant are the elements of good postoperative care. A light dressing is all that is required, with care being taken to avoid constricting bandages over the venous outflow tract. However, experimental studies have shown that microvascular flaps can tolerate pressure dressings (Hayhurst and coworkers, 1976b).

Capillary Refill Time. The capillary refill time is the single most important index of the adequacy of a microvascular replant's circulation. To observe capillary refill time, the gloved finger is used to exert gentle pressure on the skin of the replant sufficient to blanch an area of the skin approximately 1 cm in diameter. The time required for the color to return to the blanched area is known as the capillary refill time. The capillary refill time is probably a reflection of the total amount of blood in the capillary bed and the tone of that bed. This can be influenced by the rate of arterial inflow into the capillary bed or the rate of venous outflow from the capillary bed or both. The fact that capillary refill time is not an indicator of blood flow can be occasionally confirmed when a totally detached microvascular flap is seen to have a reasonably rapid capillary refill time, if both the artery and the vein have been occluded prior to separation of the flap. However, at present, the capillary refill time, when correlated with other clinical parameters, remains the best method of monitoring the circulatory status of a microvascular flap.

Color of the Microvascular Replant. The color of an adequately revascularized microvascular replant approaches that of the normal part in vivo. Free flaps, in fact, may appear remarkably pale in comparison to the more conventional flaps. The pale appearance of these flaps may at times be misleading, particularly to those accustomed to the appearance of standard skin flaps. With very early or mild venous congestion, the flaps frequently have a deceptively healthy-appearing color. Replanted digits have a normal color when adequately revascularized.

In general, the color of a microvascular replant should be relatively normal, and any change from that color warrants investigation. Nurses, in particular, seem to vary widely in their sensitivity to the color changes of microvascular replants, and their observations should not be relied upon too heavily. Unfortunately, the skin pigmentation of patients varies considerably, as does the color of the replants. For this same reason, color changes in darkly pigmented patients are frequently of little or no help.

Temperature of the Microvascular Replant. The surface temperature of a microvascular replant is dependent upon many factors, including the body temperature of the patient, ambient temperature, humidity, type of bandage, and circulatory status of the patient. The surface temperature of microvascular free flaps can be misleading. The warmth of a flap is usually reassuring, but flaps have been seen to succumb while maintaining their warmth, presumably by conduction from deeper lying structures. At the same time, flaps with a perfectly adequate circulation may be cool to the touch. In general, the temperature of a well-vascularized free flap approaches that of normal adjacent skin.

The temperature of replanted digits is a somewhat more reliable index of the total blood flow in the digit. As the digit is an end organ, it receives much of its warmth from the blood circulating from the body. The total blood flow in the hand and fingers correlates with the temperature of the finger. The normal temperature of a finger under standard conditions is approximately 86° F. Any interruption of blood flow to the digit is followed rapidly by a drop in temperature of the avascular part. A temperature sensing device for the finger with a reference point correlated with body temperature could thus prove useful in monitoring replanted digits. This would be particularly useful in patients with deeply pigmented skin, in whom capillary refill time and color are of little value in following the circulation of the replanted digit.

Venous Congestion. In the earliest stages of venous congestion, the color of the microvascular replant may be little changed, or it may have a deceptively healthy-appearing pink color. However, the brisk capillary refill time is a warning signal, and as the capillary refill time becomes even shorter, the color of the flap usually becomes progressively more pink, subsequently red, then purple, and finally a dusky blue. The pulp of a congested digit also has an increased tissue turgor and a feeling of "fullness."

At the first sign of venous congestion, the replant is inspected for constricting bandages, tight sutures, or hematomas. If there is any doubt, the suspect sutures should be removed and the wound probed for accumulations of blood. Additional elevation of the part may be of some value and should be tried. As a last resort, moderately vigorous massage of the replant in the vicinity of the microvascular anastomoses may occasionally dislodge a loosely adherent thrombus and improve the venous outflow. Incisions in the distal pulp are not advocated.

If the patient is receiving anticoagulants, the state of anticoagulation should be confirmed. If it is low or if doses have been missed, the reinstitution of heparin therapy should be accomplished at once. If the patient is not receiving anticoagulant therapy, anticoagulation is not begun except in the possible rare case in which difficulties develop after the first postoperative week and a decision not to reoperate has been made. The usual procedure is to return the patient to surgery if adjunctive measures do not improve or stabilize the vascular status within one or two hours and the decision whether or not to use anticoagulants is made at the time of reoperation.

Arterial Occlusion. The first sign of arterial insufficiency is generally a slowed capillary refill time. The slowing of the capillary refill time becomes more marked as the vascular inflow becomes progressively impaired. The color of the replant suffering from arterial insufficiency may vary from a pure white in extreme cases to the more usual light dusky blue appearance or a more dark blue-white mottled appearance. The temperature of the replant is usually distinctly cool. Arterial insufficiency may result in a somewhat empty feel, described by some surgeons as a "waxy" feel. This is particularly noticeable in digital replantations.

If a replant shows signs of arterial insufficiency, it should be inspected for constricting bandages, tight sutures, and hematoma formation, although these factors seldom are a source of arterial insufficiency. More frequently, a change of position by lowering the replant to heart level or slightly below may be of some value, particularly if the part has previously been excessively elevated. Massage of the replant near the anastomosis may also be tried; the maneuver is seldom of help and involves some risk to the microvascular anastomosis. The treatment of arterial insufficiency by adjunctive measures is less often successful than the treatment of venous congestion; early surgical intervention is usually the best course.

If the patient is on anticoagulant therapy, the level of anticoagulation should be evaluated, and if it is inadequate, it should be corrected at once. If the patient has not been on anticoagulant therapy, immediate reoperation is usually the best course, the decision whether or not to anticoagulate being made at the time of reoperation.

Reoperation. If reoperation is necessary, the anastomosis can usually be approached by reopening the skin near the microvascular anastomosis. All anastomoses are inspected and tested for patency. In most cases, if reoperation has been prompt, either the venous or arterial anastomosis will be found to be completely or partially occluded. In cases in which reoperation has been delayed for a considerable period of time, occlusions of both the arterial and venous sides may be found.

The vessels are inspected for excessive tension, kinking or other adverse positions, such as a sharp bend close to the anastomotic site, sources of external pressure, and poorly executed anastomoses. Unless an external cause of the occlusion can be determined and readily corrected, the anastomosis should be entirely resected and a new anastomosis or vein graft performed under ideal conditions. At the time of resection of the anastomosis, adequate forward flow of blood should be seen from the proximal artery. The vessels should be carefully inspected for signs of occult vascular damage not previously noted. If the latter is detected, further debridement should be performed. The surgeon should recall the principles of microvascular repairs and, if any serious departures from these principles have occurred, the surgeon should make every effort to correct these deficiencies.

If performed early, a reoperation usually has a good chance of success particularly in the early days postoperatively. If efforts to revascularize the replant are unsuccessful after several days of previous viability, the replanted part should not be removed unless it is definitely necrotic. In determining the viability of a replant that is in dire straits, the surgeon should not be too hasty to condemn a cool dark blue replant without capillary refill which remains soft and moist to the touch. If time permits, if there are no signs of infection, and if there are no other contraindications, the part may be left in situ, and the surgeon will occasionally be surprised by a gradual return of color to the entire part as it regains circulation. Recent experimental evidence suggests that microvascular flaps replaced in situ may survive without their axial vessels by the end of, and perhaps earlier than, the eighth postoperative day (Sharzer and O'Brien, 1974). A delay of two to three days is usually sufficient to allow for the resurrection of such jeopardized parts.

MICROVASCULAR FREE FLAPS

History

In 1893 Dunham described the transfer of a skin flap to the cheek of a man, followed later by a dissection of the vessels to the flap and a burying of the pedicle beneath the skin, i.e., a two-stage island flap procedure. Monks (1898) performed a one-stage transfer of an island of skin from the forehead to the lower eyelid,

with the circulation based only on the tunneled subcutaneous pedicle. Such island flaps soon found ready acceptance in reconstructive surgery. The goal of the immediate transfer of flaps to distant sites then awaited only the development of microvascular surgery.

It was 65 years later when transfer of the first experimental microvascular flaps was performed (Goldwyn, Lamb and White, 1963). Although there was survival of only three of five free microvascular flaps for only 48 hours, the feasibility of the survival of relatively large skin flaps on a single small artery and vein was proved.

The first successful free flaps made use of a small vascular cuff from the femoral artery and vein to transfer canine groin flaps without the need for microvascular anastomoses (Krizek and coworkers, 1965). Finally, Strauch and Murray (1967) were able to transfer skin flaps using microvascular anastomoses to maintain their viability. They achieved an overall survival rate of 61 per cent for the transfer of 33 groin flaps in rats. Fujino, Harashina, and Mikato (1972), using a microvascular stapler for the vascular anastomoses, achieved a 58 per cent survival rate following the transfer of 12 groin flaps in dogs. Pigs have also been used as models for the transfer of microvascular flaps, and an 80 per cent survival rate (groin flaps) using somewhat larger vessels was reported (Daniel and Williams, 1973). O'Brien and Shanmugan (1973) achieved a 100 per cent survival of 27 groin flaps in rabbits with the use of microvascular anastomoses on vessels approximately 1 mm in diameter. Hayhurst, Mladick and Adamson (1976b) have recently reported a 100 per cent survival of ten canine microvascular groin flaps following the anastomosis of a single 1-mm artery and vein for each flap without the use of any anticoagulants (Fig. 14–32).

The first attempted microvascular flap in humans was reported by Kaplan, Buncke, and Murray (1973). A groin flap was transferred to an intraoral defect and was reported to have survived 3½ weeks before being extruded.

The first successful microvascular free flap in man was performed by Harii and Ohmori in September, 1972 (Harii, Ohmori and Ohmori, 1974). A few months later, workers from O'Brien's laboratory in Melbourne, Australia, performed the microvascular anastomoses which made possible two separate successful microvascular flaps involving the transfer of groin flaps to the legs of two young men (O'Brien and coworkers, 1973a; Daniel and

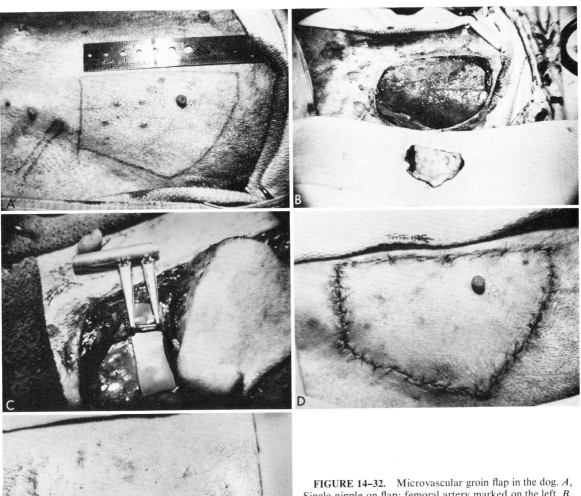

FIGURE 14–32. Microvascular groin flap in the dog. *A*, Single nipple on flap; femoral artery marked on the left. *B*, Flap totally detached. *C*, Repair of single artery and vein. *D*, Immediately after replacement of the flap. *E*, Six weeks postoperatively.

Taylor, 1973). The first successful microvascular flap in the United States was done in November, 1973 (Fig. 14–33) (Hayhurst and coworkers, 1976b).

Indications

It is axiomatic that a flap should not be used if a skin graft will suffice. A good general rule is to use the simplest procedure that will provide adequate coverage of the defect. The surgeon should not overlook the use of a skin graft or local skin flap, techniques which are much simpler, require less time, and involve less risk to the patient. Only when he has satisfied himself that the simpler procedure will not suffice should a surgeon entertain thoughts of a distant flap.

Each surgeon will develop his own indications for the use of microvascular flaps. These indications will be greatly influenced by past training experience and current technical skills. As a surgeon gains facility with the use of

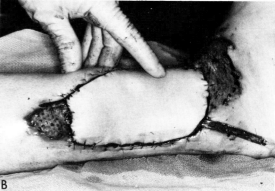

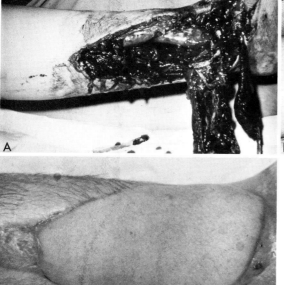

FIGURE 14–33. Microvascular free flap. *A,* Compound fracture of tibia with loss of skin and 10 cm segment of fibula in a 13 year old boy. *B,* Use of capillary refill time to evaluate the circulatory status of the microvascular flap at the end of surgery. *C,* Close-up view of healed flap.

microvascular flaps, his indications will likely expand.

Advantages

Microvascular Flaps Require Only a One-Stage Procedure. Cross-leg flaps and distant skin flaps require two or three or more procedures.

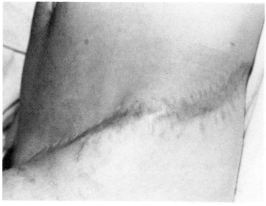

FIGURE 14–34. Healed scar following removal of a large groin flap. The donor defect had been closed primarily.

The Avoidance of Extremes of Immobilization. Distant flaps often require immobilization of one or more extremities in a flexed position for a considerable period of time. These positions may be particularly deleterious in older patients or in patients with concomitant fractures of the pelvis or lower extremities. Free microvascular flaps require only mild elevation and little or no immobilization.

Cosmetically Acceptable Donor Sites. Microvascular flaps can be taken from inconspicuous areas, such as the groin or the dorsum of the foot. These donor sites are easily concealed by even brief conventional clothing and are usually cosmetically more acceptable to the patient than the multiple scars associated with distant flaps or even some local flaps (Fig. 14–34).

Vascularity of the Flap. The microvascular free flap with its unique vasculature has a circulation which is *more* than adequate for its own needs and can provide additional blood supply to the recipient area. Distant flaps of the conventional type can provide a vascular input to the recipient area only so long as they remain attached to their donor pedicles. Once detached from the pedicles, these flaps are parasitic on the surrounding tissues, their vascularity being dependent upon such vessels as can grow through the surrounding circumferential scar.

Reliability. Even the earliest published series of free flaps demonstrate that these procedures are more reliable than most multi-staged distant flap transfers (O'Brien and co-workers, 1974; Harii and coworkers, 1974; Hayhurst and coworkers, 1976b).

Flexibility. The ability to perform one-stage transfers of skin flaps from a variety of distant donor sites greatly increases the options available to a reconstructive surgeon. Potential donor sites include the groin, deltopectoral area, dorsum of the foot, scalp, forehead, and various skin-muscle areas; the size, texture, and color of the donor flap can be varied to a degree not previously possible.

Disadvantages

Longer Operating Time. In the present state of the art, most microvascular flaps require approximately four to six hours of operative time. When one considers the operative times for the two or three or more operations necessary for a distant skin flap, the difference in total time is not great. As surgeons gain more experience with microvascular flaps, one may anticipate that the operative times will be reduced significantly.

Sacrifice of a Recipient Vessel. In the head and neck the blood supply is such that the sacrifice of almost any recipient microvessel (1 to 3 mm in diameter) is entirely safe. Likewise the trunk is generously supplied with multiple small vessels in such a way that the loss of any single microvessel is normally tolerated quite well. The distal areas of the extremities are sites which frequently require flap coverage, and it is fortunate that the dual arterial supply to the hand and foot is such that the loss of either major artery is usually tolerated without consequence.

Preoperative Evaluation

When evaluating the merits of a microvascular flap coverage for a particular defect, consider-

ation should be given to both the recipient site and the donor area.

Recipient Site. When presented with an acute wound which will eventually require a flap, the reconstructive surgeon should not overlook the possibility of primary free flap coverage. Though it would be injudicious to attempt primary microvascular flap coverage in many wounds, it would be equally unfortunate to miss an opportunity for an appropriate one-stage repair. Many wounds *will* be optimal at the first operation, and primary coverage with a well-vascularized flap may offer the best chance of maximal tissue salvage.

However, a more conservative approach (and often the correct one) is to prepare the wound for secondary coverage. For acute traumatic wounds, this requires thorough debridement, good wound care, and the prevention of sepsis and tissue desiccation. Temporary allograft or autograft coverage is often helpful. In chronic wounds a thorough debridement of all necrotic tissue is necessary. A well-vascularized microvascular free flap is resistant to infection and can perform a considerable amount of biological debridement; nevertheless, every effort should be made to debride as much necrotic and infected tissue as possible.

Recipient vessels of an appropriate size (usually 1 to 3 mm in diameter) must be available for the defect. Large defects, particularly on the extremities, often have interrupted the course of an appropriate recipient vessel, the free end of which can be found in the edge of the defect. Otherwise, a long vascular pedicle, either on the microvascular flap itself, from adjacent vessels, or a combination of both, can be employed. The placement of arterial and venous repairs on different sides of the flap may be helpful. When covering areas of irradiation damage, a long vascular pedicle is frequently imperative to avoid the use of irradiated vessels.

In the head and neck area, there is an abundance of small vessels and there is usually little difficulty in locating one or more recipient vessels. The anterior trunk is likewise criss-crossed with a number of appropriate sized vessels, such as the intercostal, epigastric, and internal mammary vessels. In the extremities the use of *one* of the major vessels to the foot or the hand is usually safe, provided the other major vessel is normal.

The unnecessary use of angiography on recipient or donor vessels should be avoided because of the potential for damage to the endothelium. A clinical evaluation, including evaluation of the pulses, usually provides an adequate circulatory survey. If an angiogram is felt to be necessary, the microvascular flap should preferably be delayed for several weeks to allow for endothelial repair. Dopplers may be an aid to locating and following the course of the smaller vessels.

A consideration for innervation of the flap may be beneficial, particularly when the recipient site is on the hand or foot. The lateral cutaneous branches of the lower intercostal nerves, particularly the eleventh and twelfth nerves, supply the lateral segments of most groin flaps. These nerves can be dissected out to the lateral margin of the groin flap and utilized for innervation of the flap. Most free flap donor sites possess a discrete nerve supply. The first web space of the foot and the dorsum of the foot appear especially favorable.

Donor Site. The microvascular surgeon is fortunate in being able to select microvascular free flaps from several donor areas, each with different qualities. Up to the present time, most microvascular free flaps have been chosen from areas known to have an axial pattern vascular supply, such as the forehead, deltopectoral region, chest wall, groin, dorsum of the foot, and toe (O'Brien and coworkers, 1974; Harii and coworkers, 1974; Morrison, 1974; Hayhurst and coworkers, 1976b; Hayhurst, unpublished work). Additional potential donor areas include the inner aspect of the arm, and the penis and scrotum. In most other areas of the body, the skin is supplied by small branches of larger muscular arteries that emerge from the muscles at various points to provide the major blood supply to only a small region of the skin (see Chapter 6). In the future it may be feasible to use these smaller vessels for small grafts either by direct anastomosis or by using the larger parent muscular arteries for repair.

Compound skin-muscle microvascular flaps have been used for reconstruction of the pharynx in dogs (Schecter, Biller and Ogura, 1969).* Large skin-muscle compound micro-

---

*The first successful compound skin-muscle microvascular flaps were reported by Harii (1973), using the gracilis muscle and its overlying skin to correct severe facial contour defects. The gracilis possesses upper, intermediate, and lower supply vessels. The upper group is the dominant one and is associated with the nerve. The gracilis has been transferred with microvascular anastomosis (O'Brien, 1976).

vascular flaps based on the rectus femoris and latissimus dorsi muscles have been suggested as suitable for microvascular transfers in humans (McCraw, 1974; Seijo, 1975). The use of the larger vessels of compound microvascular flaps should greatly extend the number of potential donor sites and provide larger vessels on which to perform the microvascular repairs.

GROIN FLAP. The details of the anatomy of the groin flap have been described (Smith and coworkers, 1972) (see also Chapter 6). The axial vessels are the superficial circumflex iliac artery and vein which originate from the femoral artery and saphenous vein, respectively. The origin of the artery is usually approximately 2 cm below the inguinal ligament from which it courses laterally parallel to the inguinal ligament. In a large number of cadaver and clinical dissections, the authors have not seen any cases in which these vessels were not of a sufficient size for microvascular repairs. Though the artery is often small, there have been no losses of the distal ends of the microvascular flaps, even when the latter were of large dimensions (20 × 24 cm). A groin flap 31 × 22 cm has been transferred to the shoulder region with a marginal loss of only 2 cm. The maximum length and width of a free groin flap should approximate the maximum size tolerated as a pedicle flap, and perhaps may even be made somewhat larger owing to the medial extension which is possible for a microvascular flap (Fig. 14–35).

The distal end of a free groin flap may be thinned considerably, just as in a pedicle groin flap. Thinning of the proximal end of the flap can be done but should be accomplished with caution to avoid damage to the axial vessels. The excessive thickness of the groin flap in obese patients may be a contraindication to its use in some recipient sites. These thick flaps are usually difficult to inset and may require thinning as a secondary procedure. The use of a small, triangular, medial extension of the flap is an aid to final closure over the proximal end of the flap and the axial vessels (Fig. 14–35). This is frequently the site of a "dog-ear" following closure of a conventionally designed flap.

With flexion of the leg, it is quite easy to close primarily most groin flap donor sites. The groin has been primarily closed after removing a 20 × 24 cm groin flap (see Fig. 14–34). The resultant scar in the groin is easily concealed by even brief clothing. The sartorius muscle may be transferred across the femoral vessels to provide extra protection. Larger donor defects can be closed with a skin graft.

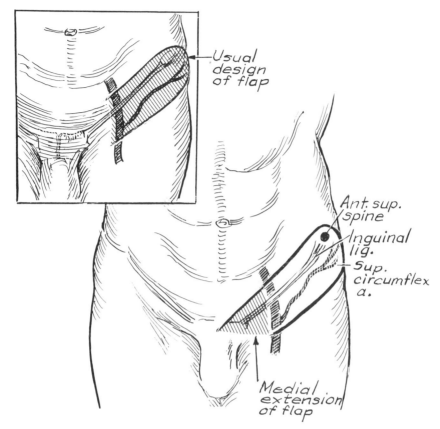

FIGURE 14–35. Medial extension of the groin flap when used as a microvascular flap (see Chapter 6 for the anatomy of this area).

DELTOPECTORAL FLAP. The anatomy of the free deltopectoral flap is similar to that of the deltopectoral flap originally described by Bakamjian (1965). The details of the flap are discussed in Chapters 6 and 63. Of the two major arteries supplying the flap, the perforating branch of the second intercostal artery is usually the larger and the one most used for a microvascular flap transfer (Harii, Ohmori and Ohmori, 1974). If a very large flap is used, the incorporation and use of the perforating branch of the first intercostal artery and its accompanying vein should give an improved vascular supply.

The size of vessels in the base of the deltopectoral flap usually varies from 0.8 to 2.5 mm in diameter, with the veins being slightly larger than the arteries. These vessels are of a suitable size for microvascular repairs. If smaller vessels are found, they can be dissected back to the internal mammary artery, and a section of the latter taken to provide a larger vessel which is more amenable to microvascular repairs.

In the usual patient, the deltopectoral flap is thinner than a groin flap of the same size. The color match for facial defects is better than with the groin flap but is still not ideal. In most patients, excepting some hirsute males, the deltopectoral area contains less hair than the groin.

For small to moderate sized free deltopectoral flaps, the donor site can be closed primarily. This may be surprising to those accustomed to the use of the standard deltopectoral flap. Primary closure is often possible because the total size required for a microvascular flap is smaller than that of a traditional (pedicle) deltopectoral flap; the latter is usually made somewhat larger than needed to allow for subsequent shrinkage or loss. The absence of the pedicle base also allows undermining which facilitates primary closure. When primary closure of the free deltopectoral flap donor site is possible, the resultant scar is usually much less obtrusive than if a skin graft is necessary.

DORSALIS PEDIS FLAP. The dorsalis pedis

free flap was first described by O'Brien and Shanmugan (1973) and by McCraw (1974), and the details of the anatomy of this flap are described in Chapter 86. The primary arterial supply is via the anterior tibial artery, which also has two venae comitantes which are of a suitable size for microvascular repairs. The vascular pedicle of this flap can be dissected from the lower leg to a length of at least 10 to 15 cm. If additional venous drainage is required, the saphenous vein may be included with the flap.

Even in obese patients, this flap usually is surprisingly thin. Because of this characteristic and because of the similarity in texture to the skin of the hand, this flap may well be the most useful for coverage of the hand. The presence of the superficial peroneal and the musculocutaneous nerves may also provide an opportunity for reinnervation of the flap.

The size of the flap is limited by the size of the dorsum of the foot but can often be as large as 10 × 10 cm. The flap donor area accepts a skin graft readily, and the final cosmetic and functional result has generally been excellent (McCraw, 1975).

Operative Technique

Two operative teams are preferable, one working at the donor site and the second at the recipient site. Each team should be familiar with the principles of microvascular surgery.

An initial step should be to confirm the suitability of the recipient vessels. At present, most microvascular flaps are satisfactorily transferred with vessels of less than 3 mm in diameter. Vessels smaller than 0.5 mm in diameter cannot, at present, be repaired with sufficient reliability to warrant the clinical transfer of flaps based on these small vessels alone.

A single 1-mm artery and vein can provide sufficient blood flow to support the survival of a microvascular flap several hundred square centimeters in size. However, a decreased venous resistance and increased total blood flow may be obtained with the repair of two or more veins. The repair of a greater number of vessels can also increase the reliability of microvascular free flaps.

In defects which are large enough to require a sizable flap, the course of the vessels, which are of suitable size for use as recipient vessels, is frequently interrupted. This is particularly true for the lower leg, forearm, and head and neck region. In acute wounds, the pulsating artery may be identified at the edge of the defect. In more chronic wounds, it is usually necessary to dissect the vessels only a few centimeters before finding a normal vessel with adequate blood flow. Although most microvascular anastomoses are resistant to minor infections, a microvascular anastomosis in an infected field should be avoided. This problem can sometimes be overcome with a long vascular pedicle, as can be developed in a free dorsalis pedis flap. Vessels in an irradiated area should also be avoided in microvascular repairs because of the frequent abnormalities seen in these vessels.

Normal, brisk, pulsatile arterial flow *must* be demonstrated in the recipient vessels as an initial maneuver. Failure to achieve normal flow should exclude the use of a microvascular free flap because of the associated high risk of failure of the flap. The necessity of using an arterial catheter to obtain good flow also suggests proximal vascular damage and indicates a high risk of subsequent arterial occlusion.

The vascular pedicle is usually placed on the proximal side of the defect. However, this is not necessary and any location of the flap vessels which will establish adequate circulation is satisfactory. The arterial and venous repairs can be situated on different sides of the flap.

Preparation of the Defect. Following confirmation of satisfactory recipient and donor vessels, the recipient defect is prepared. All necrotic tissue should be excised and hemostasis obtained. Any obviously infected or necrotic bone should be removed. One should remember that X-ray studies suggesting osteomyelitis and the superficial appearance of a bone may be misleading. The authors have observed several such cases which healed without incident following coverage with a healthy microvascular flap. The same finding has been noted following coverage of open infected joints with healthy free flaps.

If the original defect has been covered by a skin graft, often only a portion of the original defect requires resurfacing by a microvascular free flap.

Raising the Flap. The location, size, number, and general course of the flap vessels should be confirmed prior to raising the flap. This is best done by surgical exploration; according to some surgeons a Doppler instrument facilitates the tracing of the course of the axial vessels. Angiograms are often unreliable and can cause damage to the microcirculation

(Brånemark, Jacobsson and Sorensen, 1969). If the location and course of the vessels in the base of the flap are verified prior to raising the flap, changes in the alignment of the flap can be made to provide better ce tralization of the axial vessels.

The flap should be tailored to fit the defect and to allow for normal skin tension. A template taken from the recipient defect is useful in planning. Microvascular free flaps tolerate a normal or slightly greater than normal skin tension without ill effects. Groin flaps and deltopectoral flaps are normally subjected to considerable stretch in vivo during movement of the limbs, and this normal elasticity can be used to fit the flap to a particular defect. Temporal flaps, scalp flaps, and dorsalis pedis flaps are somewhat less elastic. The determination of the location of the axial vessels in the base of the flap aids the subsequent raising of the flap by helping to prevent inadvertent division of the flap vessels. Some microsurgeons prefer to raise microvascular flaps from distal to proximal, identifying the deeper artery and then making a medial incision to isolate the venous drainage of the flap (Harii, Ohmori and Ohmori, 1974).

Flap Care. Following isolation of the axial vessels and preparation of a suitably long vascular pedicle, if the recipient defect and recipient vessels are not yet prepared, the flap should be left attached to the axial vessels to reduce total ischemia time to a minimum.

It is only after the recipient defect is fully prepared and the recipient vessels are ready for anastomosis that the flap vessels should be divided. Prior to division of the flap vessels, they should be tagged with a suture to prevent their retraction and loss in the soft tissues. The proximal side of the axial vessels should be ligated and the vessels divided. The ends of the flap vessels should be left open and the flap drained of blood. Perfusion of the flap should *not* be done.

The flap should be transferred immediately to the recipient defect and preparations made for the microvascular anastomoses. The flap should be kept moist and protected from contamination.

Microvascular Technique. The principles of microvascular technique as discussed in the previous section should be carefully followed.

Insetting the Flap. The flap may be loosely inset prior to the microvascular repairs if this facilitates the anastomoses. The insetting of the flap should be completed with a good approximation of the skin edges. There is no need to leave excessive or redundant tissue, and a well-tailored flap is desirable. A small suction drain is often employed (see Fig. 14–33, *B*).

Postoperative Management. The suture line is protected from contamination for the first 12 to 24 hours, and thereafter the flap may be left uncovered if there is no drainage. The major portion of the flap is usually left exposed to facilitate frequent observation of the circulatory status. Drains are removed after 24 hours or as soon thereafter as possible. In the early postoperative period, most microvascular flaps will show some edema, which is minimized by elevation. Excessive elevation can impair arterial inflow and should be avoided.

Anticoagulants are not needed for uncomplicated microvascular flaps (O'Brien and co-workers, 1974; Harii, Ohmori and Ohmori, 1974; Hayhurst, Mladick and Adamson, 1976b).

Monitoring of the circulatory status of the flap is usually practiced at hourly intervals for the first 72 hours and every four hours thereafter. The color and temperature of the flap and the capillary refill time should be assessed. Any changes should be investigated as discussed in the previous section.

If the flap heals per primum, it should be able to survive without its axial vessels by the end of eight days or less (Sharzer and O'Brien, unpublished results). After this period of time, a microvascular flap can be treated essentially as any other type of new flap.

Clinical examples of microvascular free flaps can be found in Chapters 27, 34, and 86.

MICROVASCULAR FREE BONE GRAFTS

A microvascular free bone graft is one which is totally detached from the body and reattached by microvascular anastomoses to maintain osseous viability. On the other hand, a free bone graft does not have an intact blood supply; with inadequate revascularization many of the bone cells die, resulting in considerable resorption of the graft (see Chapter 13).

The feasibility of the replacement of a canine radius with a microvascular rib graft has been demonstrated (Fig. 14–36) (Hayhurst,

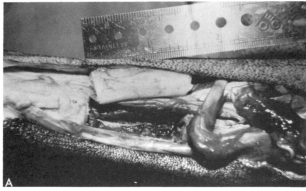

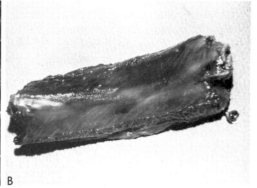

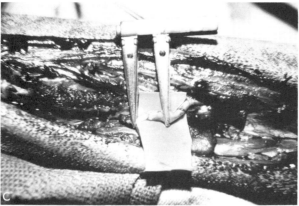

FIGURE 14–36. Microvascular bone graft to canine radius. *A*, Segment of radius removed. *B*, Rib with vascular clip on vessels. *C*, Microvascular anastomosis of intercostal vessel.

unpublished work). The patency of the microvascular anastomoses was shown by angiography, and remodeling of the rib in the shape of a normal radius was observed (Fig. 14–36, *E, F*).

Microvascular rib grafts have also been used to reconstruct canine mandibular defects (McCullough and Fredrickson, 1973; Ostrup and Fredrickson, 1974). In one study there was an 80 per cent bony union for ten experimental rib grafts transplanted to the mandible; bony union was not observed in six control grafts in which no microvascular anastomoses were done (Ostrup and Fredrickson, 1974).

McKee (1975) began in 1970 the clinical use of the sixth or seventh ribs supplied by the internal mammary vessels for grafting defects of the mandible. In addition to the intercostal vessels, additional smaller branches of the internal mammary vessels to the soft tissues surrounding the rib were also incorporated. Through an anterior approach, the cartilage is removed subperichondrially, and an adequate length of rib is removed together with surrounding muscles to preserve the intercostal vessels. The internal mammary vessels on their long pedicles are anastomosed to neck vessels of the opposite side, usually the facial vessels.

Bilateral neck dissections may present difficulties, as often no satisfactory recipient veins can be found. The large amount of soft tissue removed with the rib has the secondary advantage of filling neck defects following a block dissection. The technique has been performed by McKee in 11 patients with nine survivals, the two failures representing bone extrusions early in the postoperative period. He found that only six weeks of immobilization was required, as opposed to the three months required with a nonvascularized rib bone graft.

McKee has also transferred vascularized rib bone grafts for nonunion of the tibia, splitting these ribs longitudinally in order to expose more cancellous bone to the tibial segments and anastomosing the internal mammary vessels to the tibial vessels. Long-term evaluation of these patients is awaited.

O'Brien, Sykes, and Donahoe (1974, unpublished work) have suggested the use of the contralateral posterior eighth and ninth ribs as an alternative source of microvascular free rib grafts. The incision is placed directly over the

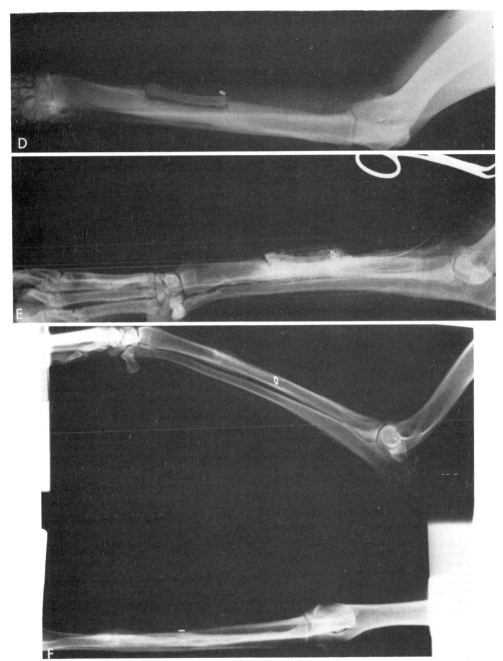

FIGURE 14–36 *Continued.* *D,* Radiograph immediately postoperatively. Note the metallic ring at the anastomotic site. *E,* Angiogram demonstrating patency of the artery two weeks postoperatively. *F,* Long-term healing with remodeling of the radius.

middle of the selected rib and follows the line of that rib commencing 1 to 2 cm from the posterior midline. The ninth rib has less serratus posterior inferior and less latissimus dorsi. The latissimus dorsi is divided over the middle of the rib along the line of the rib, and a plane is dissected under the latissimus dorsi to expose the interspace above and below the rib. The intercostal muscles are divided above, avoiding the pleura, and medially some of the serratus posterior inferior is also sectioned. For exposure of the interspace below, the intercostal muscles are divided close to the upper border of the lower rib, commencing laterally to avoid the intercostal vessels which can be identified on the undersurface of the intercostal musculature adjacent to the rib.

The portion of serratus posterior inferior that has been doubly divided is discarded, and the lateral border of the erector spinae can be defined, mobilized, and retracted medially. In this manner a plane is opened under the erector spinae as far medially as the vertebral spines. This maneuver permits division of any remaining medial fibers of the intercostal muscles and easier identification of the intercostal nerve and vessels. The nerve and vessels pass directly medially, with the rib curving superiorly away.

The pleura is dissected carefully from the rib, commencing superiorly and laterally. As the dissection proceeds inferomedially, the nerve and vessels are mobilized from the pleura. The rib is sectioned as far medially as possible, the limiting factor being the erector spinae muscle. In this way the safety of the vessels is enhanced because of their divergence from the rib, and the desired curve of the mandible is matched. The required length of rib is measured and divided laterally with the accompanying nerve, vessels, and intercostal muscles. It is possible to resect rib and vessels without taking the intercostal nerve, particularly if only a short length of rib is required. The distance separating the nerve varies, but the nerve is included if any risk to vessels might arise otherwise.

The specimen is raised and with blunt dissection the pleura is mobilized as far medially as the side of the vertebral body. The medial end of the nerve is divided. Mobilization of the artery is continued (Fig. 14–37) using a head light, and the distal end of the rib is checked

for bleeding. The artery is ligated to provide maximum length and flexibility at the recipient site.

Microvascular Fibula Bone Grafts

Independently, Ueba (1973, unpublished work) and O'Brien (1973, unpublished work) considered the use of the fibula as a donor bone graft utilizing the midshaft nutrient vessels supplied by the peroneal vessels (Fig. 14–38, *A*).

Exposure. The common peroneal nerve is palpated around the neck of the fibula. A long curvilinear incision is made just below and behind the nerve between the subcutaneous portion of the fibula and the tendocalcaneus. The soleus and peroneus longus are identified inferiorly, and the deep fascia is incised to open a plane between the soleus and flexor hallucis longus. The lateral border of the fibula is freed from its deep fascial attachment inferiorly and the soleus attachment superiorly. The soleus is reflected medially (superiorly some branches of the peroneal vessels may have to be divided as they lie under the deep surface of soleus) to expose the flexor hallucis belly which is reflected laterally (Fig. 14–38, *B*).

The following structures are located: (1) the posterior tibial nerve and vessels; (2) the peroneal vessels—proximally before entering the flexor hallucis longus; and (3) the origin of the nutrient artery from the peroneal artery.

If it is planned to remove the bulk of the flexor hallucis longus with the bone, the lower end of the muscle may be divided. If not, the

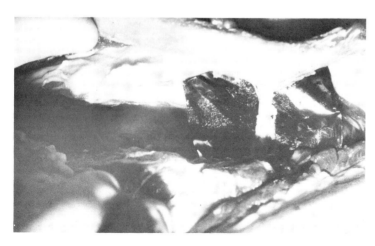

FIGURE 14–37. A cadaver dissection of the ninth left posterior rib (upper) with posterior intercostal vessels displayed in a vertical position.

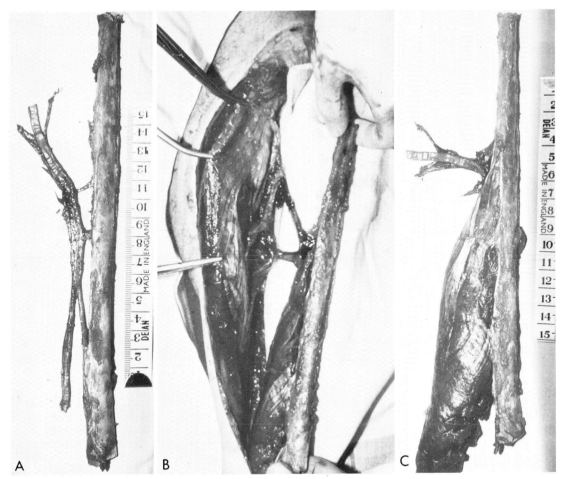

FIGURE 14–38. *A*, Fibula (flexor hallucis longus removed) demonstrating three nutrient vessels arising from the peroneal vessels. The middle nutrient vessels are the largest. *B*, Fibula with flexor hallucis longus attached. Branches of the peroneal artery are shown entering the undersurface of the retracted soleus muscle. *C*, Fibula with the attached flexor hallucis longus and with the nutrient vessels arising from the peroneal vessels.

peroneal artery is carefully dissected into the flexor hallucis muscle; this is necessary if the bone graft is to be relatively short. The peroneal muscles are dissected sharply from the lateral border of the fibula, preserving the periosteum. The bone above and below is sectioned by passing a Gigli saw around the bone, avoiding the peroneal artery and common peroneal nerve above, and the anterior tibial vessels both above and below.

Pulling the fibula posteriorly, the extensor digitorum longus and the extensor hallucis tendons are dissected off the anterior surface of the fibula, and the interosseous membrane is divided close to the fibula without damaging the periosteum. This maneuver frees the bone, leaving it attached by the tibialis posterior. The fibula is rotated forward, and, keeping the line of the peroneal artery under vision, the tibialis

posterior is divided as close to the fibula as possible. With the fibula attached only by vessels, the excess bulk of flexor hallucis can be removed and the bone shortened to the exact length required. The fibula ends are checked for bleeding, and then the peroneal vessels are ligated above and below (Fig. 14–38, *C*). The wound is closed with suction drainage.

Clinical Experiences. In December 1973, Ueba transplanted the contralateral fibula on the peroneal vessels to correct a deficiency of one-third of the right ulna of an 11 year old boy following resection for neurofibromatosis. The peroneal vessels were sutured to the ulnar artery and to a subcutaneous vein. Delayed union occurred at the proximal end and nonunion at the distal end, though radiologically the bone was vascularized without absorption or sclerosis. The possibility of neurofibromatosis in the distal radial fragment could not be excluded.

The fibula was employed as a donor bone in two cases of traumatic tibial deficiency of the opposite leg; the peroneal vessels were sutured to the tibial vessels (Taylor and coworkers, 1975). Infection destroyed the bone graft in the first case and the leg was amputated. Good union was obtained in the second case and the graft has hypertrophied. The use of the fibula for spinal defects has been demonstrated by O'Brien, Sykes and Crock (1975) following resection of the eleventh and twelfth thoracic vertebrae for a severe congenital kyphosis. A 6-cm fibular bone graft was used to bridge the gap, and the peroneal vessels were sutured to a posterior intercostal branch of the aorta and to a tributary of the azygous vein.

Microvascular bone grafts with an intact vasculature and well-vascularized periosteum would seem to offer the potential for a greater resistance to infection and more rapid vascularization of the bone cells than free bone grafts.

PENILE REPLANTATION

Traumatic amputation of the penis is fortunately not a common event (see Chapter 98). The relatively protected position of the penis and the fact that it is usually covered by clothing serve to decrease the number of inadvertent traumatic injuries to this area. Those accidents which do result in an isolated amputation of the penis are unusual and are frequently associated with avulsion of the loose clothing and the genitalia.

The majority of penile amputations are intentional, the result of self-mutilation or an act of vengeance. In some areas, amputation of the penis is a form of punishment for infidelity, often accomplished while the hapless victim is in a state of sleep or drunkenness.

Attempts at replantation of a completely amputated penis with conventional surgical techniques have met with consistent failure; even the most successful attempts have resulted in survival of only a portion of the penis (Best, Angelo and Milligan, 1962; McRoberts, Chapman and Ansell, 1968; Mendez and coworkers, 1972). However, even a small strip of skin can provide a marginal circulation that may be adequate for eventual survival of the penis (Mendez, Kiely and Morrow, 1972; Schulman, 1973).

Experimentally, the repair of one dorsal artery and vein is sufficient to support complete survival of the canine penis (Fig. 14–39) (Horton and coworkers, 1976). However, maximal healing and minimal swelling were achieved with the repair of two dorsal arteries, two dorsal veins, and an additional skin vein. Repair of the urethra and corpora, either alone, with repair of a single artery, or with additional use of the "pocket principle," failed to provide adequate circulation in the penis.

A proposal has been made for a protocol to be followed in the microsurgical replantation of the human penis (Horton and coworkers, 1976). The profuse bleeding which is to be anticipated should be controlled with pressure, avoiding the use of hemostats. The penis should be initially cooled in a crushed-ice solution, and cooling with sterile ice should be continued during surgery until full circulation of the penis is restored. Total primary microsurgical reconstruction of the penis is advocated. Repair should include the urethra, one deep penile artery within the corpora, a dorsal artery of the penis, a superficial and deep dorsal vein, the dorsal nerves, and the skin. If possible, all vessels exceeding 0.5 mm in diameter should be repaired. It is likely that up to six hours of normothermic and 24 hours of hypothermic (0° to 4° C) ischemia time would not preclude a successful replantation (Hayhurst, O'Brien, Ishida and Baxter, 1974). Perfusion of the amputated penis should not be done. Mild elevation and use of an indwelling bladder catheter are suggested. Anticoagulation should be withheld for at least 12 to 24 hours following surgery.

MICROLYMPHATIC SURGERY

Lymphaticovenous end-to-side communications have been observed under normal conditions (Rusznyak, Foldi and Szabo, 1967; Calnan and coworkers, 1967) and in abnormal circumstances (Neyazaki and coworkers, 1965; Threefoot and Kossoner, 1966; Pentecost and coworkers, 1966; Burn and coworkers, 1966; Ohara and Taneichi, 1973). Laine and Howard (1963) performed experimental end-to-side lymphaticovenous anastomoses to canine femoral veins over a temporary polyethylene splint which was subsequently removed through a lateral venotomy. A patency of 40 per cent was reported during a follow-up period ranging from three

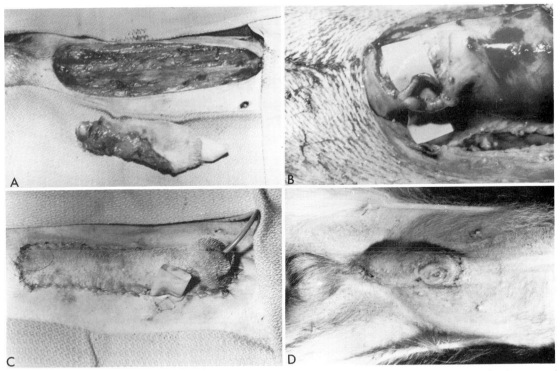

FIGURE 14–39. Experimental replantation of the penis in the dog. *A*, Penis totally detached. *B*, Repair of artery and vein. *C*, Appearance immediately after replantation. *D*, Appearance six weeks postoperatively.

weeks to three months. In a second series of 15 anastomoses, a "shirt tail" form of union, as used in ureterovesical anastomoses, with only one suture yielded a patency rate of 20 per cent after three months. The patency was observed by direct anastomosis and cannulation. It was noted that there was nearly always some stenosis at or near the anastomosis. Emphasis since that time has been placed on the anastomosis of transected lymph nodes to veins because of the technical difficulties associated with lymphaticovenous union. Niebulowicz and Olszewski (1968) and Politowski, Bartkowski, and Dynowski (1969) claimed clinical improvement in patients with secondary lymphedema using lymphonodovenous communications. Firica, Ray, and Murat (1969) demonstrated experimental evidence of lymphovenous flow. Rivero, Calnan, Reis, and Mercurius Taylor (1967) obtained 100 per cent patency at one month in dogs, but all of the anastomoses were stenosed by fibrous tissue at three months (Calnan and coworkers, 1967). However, these latter observations were made in dogs without established secondary lymphedema.

Calderon, Robert, and Johnson (1967) im-

planted lymphatics into veins and also performed direct end-to-end lymphaticovenous anastomoses but could not demonstrate the flow of lymph through these junctions.

Clinical trials of direct lymphaticovenous anastomoses have been few. Cockett and Goodwin (1962), Milstillis and Skyring (1966), and Sedláček (1969) have performed anastomoses for the treatment of chyluria, intestinal lymphangiectasia, and elephantiasis with reasonably successful clinical results. However, in these conditions the anastomoses had been performed on dilated lymph vessels, considerably larger than normal lymphatics.

Yamada (1969) succeeded in anastomosing lymph vessels to veins at the ankles of dogs with microvascular techniques utilizing a polyethylene catheter as a temporary internal splint. All of the branches entering the saphenous vein between it and the nearest venous valve were divided to protect the anastomosis, thus decreasing the venous pressure and avoiding backflow across the anastomosis.

Personal Experiences. In 1969 a number of lymphaticovenous anastomoses were attempted on the femoral vessels of dogs joining the lymphatic obliquely to the femoral vein using four or five metallized nylon microsutures. However, the primary patency was inconsistent; subsequently, a microsurgery technique was evolved joining the lymphatic end-to-end to a similar sized branch of the femoral vein over a Silastic splint, which was removed through the wall of the femoral vein after completion of the anastomosis. Angiography, re-exploration, and histopathologic examination were used to monitor the status of the anastomoses. Most of the anastomoses were blocked within 24 hours; hence, postoperative Calciparine (Australia) (700 mg per kg) was used subcutaneously twice daily for seven days in the remaining group of 15 dogs. Some improvement in patency rates was achieved in a follow-up period extending to 18 days.

An improved technique in adult greyhound dogs was developed, anastomosing femoral lymphatics to small neighboring veins away from the arterial pulsation (Gilbert and co-workers, 1975). The diameter of the veins and lymphatic vessels ranged from 0.3 to 1.2 mm. The vein was occluded with a soft clamp and the vein segment irrigated with heparinized saline (1000 units per 100 ml). The lymphaticovenous anastomoses were performed without tension with 19 μ metallized nylon sutures (7 MF 32–19) (O'Brien and Hayhurst, 1973). The lymphatic flow was not interrupted, and after the first few sutures, the lymph helped to distend the vein. Repair is easier when the sutures are passed through the vein walls first. Immediate patency of all anastomoses was obtained (Fig. 14–40). The surrounding lymphatics were divided and ligated. It was possible by raising venous pressure to demonstrate venous backflow across the anastomosis. Conversely, clearing the anastomosis with lymph by squeezing the limb to elevate the lymphatic pressure could also be demonstrated.

In assessing results, lymphangiography was not found to be reliable, and the best evidence of patency was obtained by surgical explora-

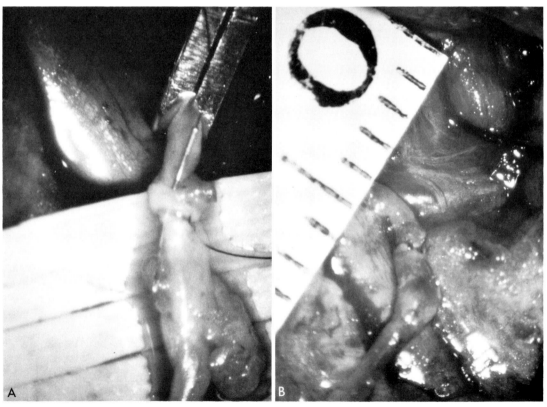

FIGURE 14–40. *A*, A lymphaticovenous anastomosis, accomplished using a 7 MF 32–19 metallized nylon microsuture and suturing from the vein (clamped) to the lymphatic. The diameter of the vessels is approximately 0.5 mm. *B*, The completed lymphaticovenous anastomosis. The lymphatic vessel runs across the main vein and joins its small tributary.

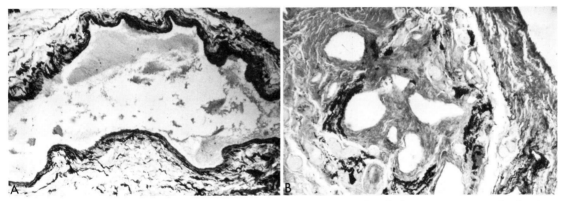

FIGURE 14-41. *A,* Transverse section of the lymphatic side of a patent lymphaticovenous anastomosis, showing a mural thrombus which is most prominent in the upper aspect of the photograph. Fibrinous coagulum is present within the lumen. Gomori's aldehyde fuchsin stain; section taken five weeks after anastomosis, × 100. *B,* Transverse section of the anastomotic site, showing a thrombosed anastomosis in which there is recanalization. The channels in the central region are of moderate dimension, while those in the adventitia are more recently formed proliferating capillaries. Gomori's aldehyde fuchsin stain; section taken six weeks after anastomosis, × 105.

tion with the injection of patent blue dye into the paw. Occlusion, distal emptying, and release also demonstrated distal to proximal flow.

Results. Results in the nonlymphedematous models revealed a patency rate at one week of 78 per cent (14 of 18). Between six and eight weeks, the patency rate was 73 per cent (24 of 33), and at six months 83 per cent (10 of 12). In a second series the thoracic duct was ligated, and at one month 63.6 per cent (7 of 11) were patent.

On histologic study, in the patent anastomoses a thin, circumferential, luminal thrombus was present in continuity with the fibrinous coagulum between the tissue gaps and the suture track (Fig. 14-41, *A*). The prime determining factor in the success of the anastomosis was achievement of correct apposition of the vessel edges without distortion, and this was dependent upon the number and placement of sutures, as well as the tension applied when they were tied. When an occlusion occurred, it stemmed in every case from the venous component. Lymph has very little coagulation potential. It was noted that where tissue disruption was greatest, the luminal thrombus was most prominent (Fig. 14-41, *B*). Further experiments are now being carried out utilizing lymphaticovenous anastomoses in dogs with experimental obstructive lymphedema established by the method described by Clodius and Wirth (1974). There is a difference of pressure within the peripheral veins and the lymphatics, the lymphatic pressure being higher than the vein during active mus-

cular contraction (Yamada, 1969). In obstructive lymphedema, the pressure gradient between the lymphatics and the veins might be higher.

Clinical Experience. Experimental microlymphaticovenous work appears to find its main clinical application in the treatment of secondary obstructive lymphedema, as primary lymphedema usually has few lymphatic vessels and little evidence of obstruction (see Chapter 87). In secondary lymphedema, microsurgical treatment ideally should be instituted before the peripheral lymphatics have been substantially destroyed by increasing pressure and repeated infections. In six cases of secondary obstructive lymphedema in the upper limb treated by microvascular surgery, two to seven lymphaticovenous anastomoses, usually at the elbow and/or the middle of the medial aspect of the upper arm level, have been performed with encouraging early results (O'Brien, 1976).

There has been significant reduction of limb volume with less swelling in the hand and forearm and, to a lesser extent, in the upper arm. The isolation of the lymphatics after injection of patent blue dye into the web space on the dorsum of the hand has been tedious. However, all sizable lymphatics demonstrable by preoperative lymphangiogram have been located, and usually there is a vein of similar diameter in the vicinity. In most cases it is thought that there is a valve in the vein proximal to the main vein in the area.

The preoperative lymphangiograms have caused some exacerbation of the lymphedema. The arm is elevated for approximately one month before operation until the arm volume is constant, and a compression pump is applied regularly. Postoperative elevation and compression are continued for one week following surgery, but no anticoagulant therapy is employed.

Obstructive lymphedema of both short and long duration has been treated. It has been noted that the earlier the patient is seen with the edema, the greater should be the chance of anastomosing a larger number of lymphatics to veins. However, no known method is yet available for detecting those cases which will develop obstructive lymphedema, nor is there any reliable technique of estimating lymphatic clearance, such as by radioactive methods.

A reduction in volume of 25 per cent of the limb has been observed at one month, but some of this improvement has been lost with ambulation and dependency. Elevation at night assisted with pump compression and the wearing of an elastic stockinette are required postoperatively, but these supportive measures were not used in some of the early cases. The patients have not tolerated warm weather well. Greater comfort and increased softness of the limbs have been evident, and, with more consistent, conservative, supportive measures, it is possible that permanent improvement may be obtained, particularly as it may take some time for the lymphaticovenous communication to function adequately. However, in view of the latent nature of obstructive lymphedema, observation over a period of years is indicated. The microsurgical methods are equally applicable to the upper and lower limbs and to localized cases of obstructive lymphedema following trauma.

REFERENCES

Acland, R.: A new needle for microvascular surgery. Surgery, *17*:130, 1972a.

Acland, R.: Prevention of thrombosis in microvascular surgery by the use of magnesium sulphate. Br. J. Plast. Surg., *25*:292, 1972b.

Acland, R.: Thrombus formation in microvascular surgery: An experimental study of the effects of surgical trauma. Surgery, *73*:766, 1973.

Acland, R.: Personal communication, 1975.

Bakamjian, V. Y.: A two stage method for pharyngoesophageal reconstruction with a primary pectoral skin flap. Plast. Reconstr. Surg., *36*:173, 1965.

Baxter, T. J., O'Brien, M., Henderson, P. N., and Bennett, R. C.: The histopathology of small vessels following microvascular repair. Br. J. Surg., *59*:617, 1972.

Best, J. W., Angelo, J. J., and Milligan, B.: Complete traumatic amputation of the penis. J. Urol., *87*:134, 1962.

Brånemark, P. I., Jacobsson, B., and Sorensen, S. E.: Microvascular effects of topically applied contrast media. Acta Radiol. [Diagn.] (Stockh.), *8*:547, 1969.

Buncke, H. J., Jr.: Personal communication, 1974.

Buncke, H. J., Jr., and Blackfield, H. M.: The vasoplegic effects of chlorpromazine. Plast. Reconstr. Surg., *31*:353, 1963.

Buncke, H. J., Jr., and McLean, D. H.: The advantage of a straight needle in microsurgery. Plast. Reconstr. Surg., *47*:602, 1971.

Buncke, H. J., Jr., and Schulz, W. P.: Experimental digital amputation and reimplantation. Plast. Reconstr. Surg., *36*:62, 1965.

Buncke, H. J., Jr., and Schulz, W. P.: Total ear reimplantation in the rabbit utilizing micro-miniature vascular anastomoses. Br. J. Plast. Surg., *19*:15, 1966.

Buren, E. A., and Ryan, R. F.: Standardization of measurements in medicine by conversion to the metric system. Plast. Reconstr. Surg., *54*:459, 1974.

Burn, J. L., Rivero, O. R., Pentecost, B. L., and Calnan, J. S.: Lymphographic appearances following lymphatic destruction in the dog. Br. J. Surg., *53*:634, 1966.

Calderon, G., Robert, B., and Johnson, L. L.: Experimental approach to the surgical creation of lymphaticovenous communications. Surgery, *61*:122, 1967.

Calnan, J. S., Reis, N. D., Rivero, O. R., Copenhagen, H. J., and Mercurius Taylor, L.: Natural history of lymph node to vein anastomosis. Br. J. Plast. Surg., *20*:134, 1967.

Carrel, A.: La technique opératoire des anastomoses vasculaires et la transplantation des viscères. Lyon Médical, *98*:859, 1902.

Chase, M. D., and Schwartz, S. I.: Consistent patency of 1.5 millimeter arterial anastomoses. Surg. Forum, *13*:220, 1962.

Chase, M. D., and Schwartz, S. I.: Suture anastomosis of small arteries. Surg. Gynecol. Obstet., *117*:44, 1963.

Clagett, G. P., and Salzman, E. W.: Prevention of venous thromboembolism in surgical patients. New Engl. J. Med., *290*:93, 1974.

Clodius, L., and Wirth, W.: A new experimental model for chronic lymphoedema of the extremities (with clinical considerations). Chir. Plast. (Berl.), *2*:115, 1974.

Cockett, A. T. K., and Goodwin, W. K.: Chyluria: Attempted surgical treatment by lymphatic-venous anastomosis. J. Urol., *88*:566, 1962.

Daniel, R. K., and Taylor, G. I.: Distant transfer of an island flap by microvascular anastomoses. Plast. Reconstr. Surg., *52*:111, 1973.

Daniel, R. K., and Williams, H. B.: The free transfer of skin flaps by microvascular anastomoses. Plast. Reconstr. Surg., *52*:16, 1973.

Didisheim, P.: Inhibition by dipyridamole of arterial thrombosis in rats. Thromb. Diath. Haemorrh., *20*:257, 1968.

Dunham, T.: A method for obtaining a skin flap from the scalp and a permanent buried vascular pedicle for covering defects of the face. Ann. Surg., *17*:677, 1893.

Elcock, H. W., and Fredrickson, J. M.: The effect of heparin on thrombosis at microvenous anastomotic sites. Arch. Otolaryngol., *95*:68, 1972.

Emmons, P. R., Harrison, M. J. G., Honour, A. J., and Mitchell, J. R. A.: Effect of dipyridamole on human platelet behavior. Lancet, *11*:693, 1965.

Evans, G., Packham, M. A., and Nishizawa, E. E.: The effect of acetylsalicylic acid on platelet function. J. Exp. Med., *128*:877, 1968.

Firica, A., Ray, A., and Murat, J.: Les anastomoses lymphoveineuses étude expérimentale. Lyon Chir., *65*:384, 1969.

Flanc, C., Kakkar, V. V., and Clarke, M. B.: The detection of venous thrombosis of the legs "using ^{125}I-labelled" fibrogen. Br. J. Surg., *55*:742, 1968.

Fox, J. A., and Hugh, A. E.: Localization of atheroma: A theory based on boundary layer separation. Br. Heart J., *28*:388, 1966.

Fujino, T., Harashina, T., and Mikato, A.: Autogenous en bloc transplantation of the mammary gland in dogs using microsurgical technique. Plast. Reconstr. Surg., *50*:376, 1972.

Gilbert, A., O'Brien, B. M., Vorrath, J. W., Sykes, P. J., and Baxter, T. J.: Lymphatico-venous anastomosis by microvascular technique. Br. J. Plast. Surg., *29*:355, 1976.

Gimbrone, M. A., Aster, R. H., Cotran, R. S., Corkery, J., Jandl, J. H., and Folkman, J.: Preservation of vascular integrity in organs perfused in vitro with a platelet rich medium. Nature, *222*:33, 1969.

Goldwyn, R. M., Lamb, D. L., and White, W. L.: An experimental study of large island flaps in dogs. Plast. Reconstr. Surg., *31*:528, 1963.

Goodman, L. S., and Gilman, A.: The pharmacological Basis of Therapeutics. 4th Ed. London, MacMillan & Company, 1970.

Guthrie, C. C.: Blood vessel surgery and its applications, 1912. Reprinted by University of Pittsburgh Press, 1959.

Haimov, M., and Danese, C.: Prevention of acute experimental arterial thrombosis by refibrination. Vasc. Surg., *7*:206, 1973.

Ham, J. M., and Slack, W. W.: Platelet adhesiveness after operation. Br. J. Surg., *54*:385, 1967.

Ham, J. M., and Slack, W. W.: Platelet adhesiveness after operation. Br. J. Surg., *54*:385, 1967.

Ham, J. M., and Slack, W. W.: The effect of small doses of heparin on platelet adhesiveness and lipoprotein-lipase activity before and after operation. Br. J. Surg., *55*:227, 1968.

Harii, K.: Personal Communication, 1973 and 1976.

Harii, K., Ohmori, K, and Ohmori, S.: Free deltopectoral skin flaps. Br. J. Plast. Surg., *27*:231, 1974.

Harker, L. A., and Slichter, S. J.: Studies of platelet and fibrinogen kinetics in patients with prosthetic heart valve. New Engl. J. Med., *283*:1302, 1970.

Hattori, H., Killen, D. A., and Green, I. W.: Influences of suture materials and technique on patency of anastomosed arteries of less than 1.5 mm in diameter. Am. Surg., *36*:352, 1970.

Hayhurst, J. W.: Factors influencing patency rates. *In* Symposium on Microsurgery. St. Louis, Mo., C. V. Mosby Company, 1976a.

Hayhurst, J. W.: Complications of digital replantation. *In* Symposium on Microsurgery. St. Louis, Mo., C. V. Mosby Company, 1976b.

Hayhurst, J. W., and O'Brien, B. M.: An experimental study of microvascular technique, patency rates, and related factors. Br. J. Plast. Surg., *28*:123, 1975.

Hayhurst, J. W., O'Brien, B. M., Ishida, H., and Baxter, T. J.: Experimental digital replantation after prolonged cooling. Hand, *6*:134, 1974.

Hayhurst, J. W., Adamson, J. E., and Mladick, R. A.: A reliable method of digital replantation. 1976a (in preparation).

Hayhurst, J. W., Mladick, R. A., and Adamson, J. E.: Experimental and clinical microvascular flaps. 1976b (in preparation).

Henderson, P. N., O'Brien, B. M., and Parel, J. M.: An adjustable double microvascular clamp. Med. J. Aust., *1*:715, 1970.

Hershey, F. B., and Calnan, C. H.: Atlas of Vascular Surgery. St. Louis, Mo., C. V. Mosby Company, 1967.

Honour, A. J., Pickering, G. W., and Sheppard, B. L.: The fate of mural thrombi produced by injury in the ear artery of the rabbit. Br. J. Exp. Pathol., *54*:608, 1973.

Horn, J. S.: The reattachment of severed extremities. *In* Recent Advances in Orthopaedics. Baltimore, The Williams & Wilkins Company, 1969, p. 49.

Horton, C. E., Devine, C., Morgan, R. G., and Hayhurst, J. W.: Replantation of the penis. An experimental study in dogs. 1976 (in preparation).

Jacobson, J. H., and Suarez, E. L.: Microsurgery in anastomosis of small vessels. Surg. Forum, *11*:243, 1960.

Jørgensen, L., Haerem, J. W., and Moe, N.: Platelet thrombosis and non-traumatic intimal injury in mouse aorta. Thromb. Diath. Haemorrh., *29*:470, 1973.

Justice, C., Papavangelou, E., and Edwards, W. S.: Prevention of thrombosis with agents which reduce platelet adhesiveness. Am. Surg., *40*:186, 1974.

Kakkar, V. V., Nicolaides, A. N., Field, E. S., and Flute, P. T.: Low doses of heparin in prevention of deep-vein thrombosis. Lancet, *2*:669, 1971.

Kaplan, E. N., Buncke, H. J., and Murray, D. E.: Distant transfer of cutaneous island flaps in humans by microvascular anastomoses. Plast. Reconstr. Surg., *52*:301, 1973.

Ketchum, L. D., Wennen, W. W., Masters, F. W., and Robinson, D. W.: Experimental use of Pluronic F68 in microvascular surgery. Plast. Reconstr. Surg., *53*:288, 1974.

Kleinert, H. E., Kutz, J. E., Atasoy, E., Neale, H. W., and Serefin, D.: Replantation of non-viable digits: 10 years' experience. J. Bone Joint Surg., 1976 (in press).

Kolář, L., Wieberdink, J., and Reneman, R. S.: Anticoagulation in microvascular surgery. Curr. Surg. Res., *5*:52, 1973.

Krizek, T. J., Taraburo, T., Desprez, J. A., and Kiehn, C. L.: Experimental transplantation of composite grafts by microsurgical anastomosis. Plast. Reconstr. Surg., *36*:538, 1965.

Laine, J. B., and Howard, J. M.: Experimental lymphatico-venous anastomosis. Surg. Forum, *14*:111, 1963.

Lendvay, P. G.: Replacement of the amputated digit. Br. J. Plast. Surg., *26*:398, 1973a.

Lendvay, P. G.: Personal communication, 1973b.

Leonard, E. F.: The role of flow in thrombogenesis. Bull. N.Y. Acad. Med., *48*:273, 1972.

MacMillan, D. C., and Kim, A. K.: A comparative study of platelet aggregation in man and laboratory animals. Thromb. Diath. Haemorrh., *24*:385, 1970.

Majno, G., and Palade, G. E.: Studies on inflammation. I. The effect of histamine and serotonin on vascular permeability: An electron microscopic study. J. Biophys. Biochem. Cytol., *11*:571, 1961.

McCraw, J.: Personal communication, 1974.

McCraw, J. B., and Furlow, L. T.: The dorsalis pedis arterialized flap. Plast. Reconstr. Surg., *55*:177, 1975.

McCullough, D. W., and Frederickson, J. M.: Neovascularized rib grafts to reconstruct mandibular defects. Can. J. Otolaryngol., *2*:96, 1973.

McKee, D.: Microvascular panel. Pan Pacific Surgical Association: Thirteenth Congress, Honolulu, 1975.

McLean, D. H., and Buncke, H. J.: Use of the Saran-Wrap cuff in microsurgical arterial repairs. Plast. Reconstr. Surg., *51*:624, 1973.

McRoberts, J. W., Chapman, W. G., and Ansell, J. S.: Primary anastomosis of the traumatically amputated penis: Case report and summary of the literature. J. Urol., *100*:751, 1968.

Mehl, R. L., Paul, H. A., and Shorey, W. D.: Patency of the microcirculation in the traumatically amputated limb—A comparison of common perfusates. J. Trauma. 4:495, 1964.

Mendez, R., Kiely, W. F., and Morrow, J. W.: Self-emasculation. J. Urol., 107:981, 1972.

Mistillis, P., and Skyring, A. P.: Intestinal lymphangiectasia—Therapeutic effect of lymph-venous anastomosis. Am. J. Med., 40:634, 1966.

Monks, G. H.: The restoration of a lower eyelid by a new method. Boston Med. Surg. J., 139:385, 1898.

Morrison, W. A.: Personal communication, 1974.

Murakami, M., Odake, K., Takase, M., and Yoshino, K.: Potentiating effects of adenosing on other inhibitors of platelet aggregation. Thromb. Diath. Haemorrh., 26:252, 1972.

Murphy, E. A., and Mustard, J. F.: Dicumarol therapy: Some effects of platelets and their relationship to clotting tests. Circ. Res., 8:1187, 1960.

Mustard, J. F., and Packham, M. A.: Thromboembolism. Circulation, 42:1, 1970.

Negus, D., Pinto, D. J., and Slack, W. W.: Effect of small doses of heparin on platelet adhesiveness and lipoprotein lipose activity before and after surgery. Lancet, 1:1202, 1971.

Neyazaki, T., Kupic, E. A., Marshall, W. H., and Abram, H. L.: Collateral lymphovenous anastomosis after experimental destruction of the thoracic duct. Radiology, 85:423, 1965.

Niebulowicz, J., and Olszewski, W.: Surgical lymphaticovenous shunts in patients with secondary lymphoedema. Br. J. Surg., 55:6:440, 1968.

O'Brien, B. M.: A modified triploscope. Br. J. Plast. Surg., 26:301, 1973.

O'Brien, B. M.: Microvascular Reconstructive Surgery. Edinburgh, Churchill Livingstone, 1976.

O'Brien, B. M.: Personal Communication, 1976.

O'Brien, B. M., and Hayhurst, J. W.: Metallized microsutures and a new micro needle holder. Plast. Reconstr. Surg., 52:673, 1973.

O'Brien, B. M., and Shanmugan, M.: Experimental transfer of composite free flaps with microvascular anastomoses. Aust. N.Z. J. Surg., 43:285, 1973.

O'Brien, B. M., Henderson, P. N., Bennett, R. C., and Crock, G. W.: Microvascular surgical technique. Med. J. Aust., 1:722, 1970a.

O'Brien, B. M., Henderson, P. N., and Crock, G. W.: Metallized microsutures. Med. J. Aust., 1:717, 1970b.

O'Brien, B. M., MacLeod, A. M., Hayhurst, J. W., and Morrison, W. A.: Successful transfer of a large island flap from the groin to the foot by microvascular anastomosis. Plast. Reconstr. Surg., 52:271, 1973a.

O'Brien, B. M., MacLeod, A. M., Miller, G. D. H., Newing, R. K., Hayhurst, J. W., and Morrison, W. A.: Clinical replantation of digits. Plast. Reconstr. Surg., 52:490, 1973b.

O'Brien, B. M., Morrison, W. A., Ishida, H., MacLeod, A. M., and Gilbert, A.: Free flap transfers with microvascular anastomoses. Br. J. Plast. Surg., 27:220, 1974.

O'Brien, J. R.: Aspirin in the prevention of thrombosis. Am. Heart J., 86:711, 1973.

O'Brien, B. M., Sykes, P. J., and Crock, H. V.: New methods in the treatment of spinal kyphosis including microvascular bone graft. 1975 (in preparation).

O'Brien, J. R., Tulevski, V. G., Etherington, M., Madgwick, T., Alkjaersig, N., and Fletcher, A.: Platelet function studies before and after operation and the effect of postoperative thrombosis. J. Lab. Clin. Med., 82:342, 1974.

Ohara, I., and Taneichi, N.: Lymphaticovenous anasto-

mosis in a case with primary lymphoedema tarda. Angiology, 24:668, 1973.

Ostrup, L. T., and Fredrickson, J. M.: Distant transfer of a free living bone graft by microvascular anastomosis. Plast. Reconstr. Surg., 54:274, 1974.

Pentecost, B. L., Burn, J. I., Davies, A., and Calnan, J. S.: A quantitative study of lymphovenous communications in the dog. Br. J. Surg., 53:630, 1966.

Politowski, M., Bartkowski, S., and Dunowski, J.: Treatment of lymphedema of the limbs by lymphatic-venous fistula. Surgery, 66:639, 1969.

Rivero, O. R., Calnan, J. S., Reis, N. D., and Mercurius Taylor, L.: Experimental peripheral lymphovenous communication. Br. J. Plast. Surg., 20:124, 1967.

Rusznyak, I., Foldi, M., and Szabo, G.: Lymphatics and Lymph Circulation. London, Pergamon Press, 1967.

Salzman, E. W.: The limitations of heparin therapy after arterial reconstruction. Surgery, 57:131, 1965.

Salzman, E. W., Harris, W. H., and De Sanctis, R. W.: Reduction in venous thromboembolism by agents affecting platelet function. New Engl. J. Med., 284:1287, 1971.

Samuels, P. B., and Webster, D. R.: The role of venous endothelium in the inception of thrombosis. Ann. Surg., 136:422, 1952.

Sawyer, P. N., and Srinivasan, S.: Studies on the biophysics of intravascular thrombosis. Am. J. Surg., 114:42, 1967.

Sawyer, P. N., Stanczewski, B., Pomerance, A., Lucas, T., Stover, G., and Srinivasan, S.: Utility of anticoagulant drugs in vascular thrombosis: Electron microscope and biophysical study. Surgery, 74:263, 1973.

Schecter, G. L., Biller, H. F., and Ogura, J. H.: Revascularized skin flaps: A new concept in transfer of skin flaps. Laryngoscope, 79:1647, 1969.

Schulman, M. L.: Reanastomosis of the amputated penis. J. Urol., 109:432, 1973.

Schwartz, S. J., and Richardson, J. W.: Prevention of thrombosis with the use of a negative electric current. Surg. Forum, 12:46, 1961.

Sedlácek, J.: Lymphovenous shunt as supplementary treatment of elephantiasis of lower limbs. Acta Chir. Plast. (Praha), 11:157, 1969.

Seidenberg, B., Hurwitt, E. S., and Carton, C. A.: The technique of anastomosing small arteries. Surg. Gynecol. Obstet., 106:743, 1958.

Seijo, M.: Personal communication, 1975.

Serafin, D.: Personal communication, 1974.

Sharnoff, J. G., Bagg, J. F., Breen, S. R., Rogliano, A. G., Walsh, A. R., and Scardino, V.: The possible indication of postoperative thrombo-embolism by platelet counts and blood coagulation studies in the patient undergoing extensive surgery. Surg. Gynecol. Obstet., 111:469, 1960.

Sharzer, L., and O'Brien, B. MC.: Unpublished work. 1974.

Shumaker, H. B., and Lowenberg, R. I.: Experimental studies in vascular repair. Surgery, 24:79, 1948.

Smith, P. J., Foley, B., McGregor, I. A., and Jackson, I. T.: The anatomical basis of the groin flap. Plast. Reconstr. Surg., 49:41, 1972.

Spaet, T. H., and Gaynor, E.: Vascular endothelial damage and thrombosis. Adv. Cardiol., 4:47, 1970.

Spaet, T. H., Gaynor, E., and Stemerman, M. B.: Thrombosis, atherosclerosis and endothelium. Am. Heart J., 87:661, 1974.

Stadil, F.: Prevention of venous thrombosis. Lancet, 2:50, 1970.

Stemerman, M. B., and Spaet, T. H.: The subendothelium and thrombogenesis. Bull. N.Y. Acad. Med., 48:289, 1972.

Strauch, B., and Murray, D. E.: Transfer of composite graft with immediate suture anastomosis of its vascular pedicle measuring less than 1 mm in external diameter using microsurgical technique. Plast. Reconstr. Surg., *40*:325, 1967.

Sullivan, J. M., Harken, D. E., and Gorlin, R.: Pharmacologic control of thromboembolic complications of cardiac-valve replacement. New Engl. J. Med., *284*:1391, 1971.

Tamai, S.: Personal communication, 1974.

Tamai, S., Sarauchin, N., Hori, Y., Tatsumi, Y., and Okuda, H.: Microvascular surgery in orthopaedics and traumatology. J. Bone Joint Surg., *54B*:637, 1972.

Taylor, G. I., Miller, G. D. H., and Ham, F. J.: The free vascularized bone graft. Plast. Reconstr. Surg., *5*:533, 1975.

Threefoot, S. A., and Kossoner, H. T.: Lymphaticovenous communication in man. Arch. Intern. Med., *117*:213, 1966.

Tranzer, J. P., and Bumgartner, H. R.: Filling gaps in the vascular endothelium with blood platelets. Nature, *216*:1126, 1967.

Ts'ui, C., Feng, Y. H., Tange, C. Y., Li, C. M., Yu, Y. C., Ch'en, C. C., Shih, Y. F., Wang, W. H., Chiang, L. P.,

Ch'iu, H. P., Ma, S. H., Lin, T. L., and Ch'en, C.: Microvascular anastomosis and transplantation: Experimental studies and clinical application. Chinese Med. J., *85*:610, 1966.

Ueba, Y.: Personal communication, 1974.

Weiss, H. J., Danese, C. A., and Voleti, C. D.: Prevention of experimentally induced arterial thrombosis by aspirin. Fed. Proc., *29*:381, 1970.

Winfrey, E. W., III, and Foster, J. H.: Low molecular weight dextran in small artery surgery: Antithrombogenic effect. Arch. Surg., *88*:82, 1964.

Wojcik, J. D., Van Horn, D. L., Webber, A. J., and Johnson, S. A.: Mechanism whereby platelets support the endothelium. Transfusion, *9*:324, 1969.

Yamada, Y.: The study on lymphatic venous anastomosis in lymphoedema. Nagoya J. Med. Sci., *32*:1, 1969.

Ygge, J.: Changes in blood coagulation and fibrinolysis during the postoperative period. Am. J. Surg., *119*:225, 1970.

Zucker, M. B.: Platelet function. *In* Williams, W. J., Beutler, E., Erslev, A. J., and Rundler, R. W. (Eds.): Hematology. New York, McGraw-Hill Book Company, 1972.

CHAPTER 15

INORGANIC IMPLANTS

Thomas D. Rees, M.D.,
Richard P. Jobe, M.D.,
and Donald L. Ballantyne, Jr., Ph.D.

Nearly all humans have received an inorganic implant during their life spans: an infant may receive minute particles of silicone preservative from the injection tract of a hypodermic syringe; the cavities of an adolescent's teeth may contain dental fillings; and the adult's laceration or surgical wound has been sutured. Silk suture material is probably the most natural as well as the earliest foreign substance used in surgery. It is a protein substance of very high strength and specificity. Human reaction to silk is a good example of early inflammatory response followed by fibrosis; occasional allergic reaction signifies its protein nature.

The development of inorganic materials for surgical application has produced significant changes in the scope and procedures of operations in all surgical specialties; plastic surgery in particular is a beneficiary of these devices.

It has been traditionally stated that the ideal tissue substitute is fresh autogenous tissue. In the view of the contemporary plastic surgeon, however, there are situations in which such a transplant is not the ideal solution to the patient's problem. Among the most important disadvantages of autogenous tissue grafts are: (1) restricted availability of donor tissue; (2) replacement of the graft on the host bed by scar; (3) graft absorption and shrinkage, as with bone or cartilage onlay grafts; and (4) infection. Hence, there is an obvious demand for inorganic implants.

The polymer chemists and metallurgists have developed significant tools for the plastic surgeon. Metals and polymer plastics have been altered by structural and compositional changes in an effort to create a chemical and physical composition that is relatively resistant to immunologic attack. The extreme versatility of contemporary implantable surgical prosthetic devices and the rapidity with which technology is now advancing suggest that in the 1970's we are on the threshold of an era of biologically acceptable inorganic implant materials.

IMPLANT MATERIALS

Silk, cotton, and catgut suture material, while still widely used, induce more reaction in tissue than the more recently introduced metallic and synthetic substances. Dacron, polyethylene, nylon, polypropylene, and steel are more modern substitutes which achieve the same objective of approximation of tissues without creating the inflammatory reaction of the more natural substances.

Similarly, nylon, Dacron, Mylar, Teflon, polypropylene, and various acrylic resins are used as carefully fabricated prostheses. Each synthetic material with its peculiar physical characteristics and usefulness evokes a slightly different biological response.

Among the metals currently acceptable for implantation are gold, stainless steel, tantalum, titanium, and vitallium. Stainless steel wire is the material of choice for direct fixation of fractures of the facial bones because of its low tissue reactivity, high strength, and resistance to corrosion. In addition, it is used in the manufacture of many successful prostheses and fixation devices. In order for a metallic implant to remain in the tissues with relatively little reaction, the chemical and physical structure of the metal must be resistant to changes in the tissue environment resulting from the presence of a foreign body within living tissue.

The selection of the metallic substance from which the prosthesis is to be fabricated is a complex metallurgical problem and primarily concerns the strength that is required of the prosthesis. In the development of metallic prostheses, design plans must include the avoidance of fracture of the implant as a result of stress either within the implant or at the point of attachment to the adjacent bony structure.

Observations by Nilles and Lapitsky (1973) have indicated that if the surface of a metallic implant which is in contact with bone has pores greater than 150 microns but less than 1 mm in size, there is an opportunity for the bone to infiltrate the surface and establish a solid fixation between the metal and the bone. Haversian canals do not develop in pores less than 150 microns in size. Consequently, the adherence and resistance to shear is not as likely. The same observations have been made in the interface between porous ceramic materials and bone (Hentrich and coworkers, 1971).

Synthetic Implants

While metallic prostheses have been used primarily in surgical procedures, synthetic plastics have been of particular interest to the plastic surgeon.

The synthetic plastics have been the focus of extensive experimental and clinical research, though the criteria for such investigations are still somewhat ill-defined. In general, in addition to being more malleable, pliable plastics may be carved and shaped and, in all respects, are easier for the surgeon to handle than comparable metals. Exceptions to this generalization are some of the hard solid plastics, such as methylmethacrylate, polypropylene, and polyethylene, which are very hard and must be prefabricated to fit the defect. The softer plastics, silicone and Dacron, have achieved wide acceptance as implants at the present time because of their exceedingly low biological activity and their ease in fabrication.

Adhesives and Glues

The α-cyanoacrylate adhesives were originally compounded in Germany in the early 1900's. In 1952, Eastman* introduced its industrial cyanoacrylate adhesive monomer 910, methyl α-cyanoacrylate, which was first used as a tissue adhesive in about 1959. In the body, this ultimately degraded into formaldehyde and alpha-cyanoacetate—both toxic products which are metabolized and disposed of by way of the excretory systems. The rapidity with which methyl α-cyanoacrylate breaks down, however, apparently produces sufficiently high concentrations of toxic metabolites to cause a rather marked inflammatory response (Cameron and coworkers, 1965). To remedy this problem, Leonard and associates (1966) developed higher homologous monomers of alpha-cyanoacrylate which degrade more slowly, thus preventing the aggregation of significant concentrations of toxic metabolites at any given time. It should be noted that the lower monomer, methyl α-cyanoacrylate, forms weaker bonds than the higher monomers, suggesting that the intense inflammatory response has an adverse effect on the resulting bond to the tissues (Houston and coworkers, 1969).

Although there are many reports of the isolated application of these glues, investigators and clinicians have yet to find wide surgical application for these compounds other than for the fixation of orthopedic appliances. The compound N-butyl cyanoacrylate was used in Vietnam as an effective hemostatic agent coating the lacerated liver. Limited use has also been found for these substances in blood vessel anastomoses, wound closure, and the application of skin grafts (Souther, Levitsky and Roberts, 1971). However, they are mainly of interest as the first example of a useful exogenous polymer group that can be disposed of by the body when their usefulness has ended.

The Silicones

The silicones, in particular, are in wide industrial and medical use because of their many physical forms. They are available as sponges, meshes, gels, liquids of various viscosities, and elastomers (rubbers) of varying degrees of hardness and elasticity. Even the hardest of sil-

---

*Eastman Corporation.

icone rubbers can be carved at the operating table by the surgeon and sculptured to fill a defect or to provide a nearly exact contour restoration. Furthermore, following implantation, silicone implants retain their resiliency, an important attribute in reconstructive surgery. The use of silicones in plastic surgery was recently reviewed by Braley (1973).

Silicone is a general term for the organopolysiloxanes, a class of polymers consisting of chains of basic units made up of silicone, oxygen, and organic radicals of the formula $CH_3-Si-O-CH_3$, and its proper chemical name is dimethylpolysiloxane. It is manufactured for medical purposes in many physical forms, including liquids, foams, resins, sponges, and rubbers.

Special mention should be made of room temperature vulcanizing silicone (RTV), which forms a soft rubbery mass immediately after the polymer and catalyst are mixed. It vulcanizes in the tissues at either room or tissue temperature. This vulcanizing fluid, though only investigated briefly, is available for surgical applications and in this form can be used to augment a predesigned implant at the operating table. Mixtures of the polymer and catalyst can be packed into spaces as a tissue filling for immediate fabrication of tissue augmentation materials, and the substance has been experimentally injected through large-bore needles as well. The uses of this form of silicone are still being evaluated.

The more solid form of silicone, commonly known as silicone rubber, is widely used in surgery as an implant material because of its low tissue reaction, absence of toxicity, and nonallergenic properties. These properties have been well documented in many laboratory and clinical studies, dating from early reports by Brown and his group in 1953 and 1954 and by Marzoni, Upchurch and Lambert, (1959), and have recently been summarized by Speirs and Blocksma (1963), Zarem (1968), and Braley (1973). Clinically, it is used for shunts in the treatment of hydrocephalus and for pacemakers and heart valves in cardiovascular surgery; in plastic surgery it has been employed for contour restoration in facial and breast reconstruction. It has also been used to fashion artificial joints (Swanson, 1972) and as a prosthesis for tendon sheath reconstruction (Nicolle, 1969)

Body Response to Silicone Implants. Body response to silicone implants—whether sponges, semisolids, such as gels, or solids

(rubber)—is similar and has been well documented. Initially there is a mild inflammatory reaction consisting of round cell infiltration, which gives way to the formation of a pseudosheath generated by collagen formation; occasional giant cells are seen in the sheaths. Such pseudosheaths are generally delicate and thin, causing little untoward effect in the host organism except when subjected to excessive motion, as well as to low grade latent or late infection; in both situations the sheath can thicken and become hypertrophic. Contraction of such a pseudosheath capsule is ordinarily of no consequence around a firm prosthesis, such as a chin or nose implant; however, it can be troublesome in mammary augmentation because of excessive firmness and distortion around the softer gel or inflatable prostheses. The adverse reactions of the pseudosheath have been histologically documented by Thompson (1973) and are being evaluated by Williams, Aston and Rees (1975) and others because of the extensive use of breast prostheses. Electron microscopic studies of the cellular nature of the pseudosheaths, particularly in view of the recent findings of the myofibroblast by Gabbiani, Ryan and Majno (1971), suggest a similar process in the contraction of the typical silicone pseudosheath. Recent studies of the mammary implant pseudosheath are described in Chapter 89. The erosive action of a solid silicone implant in juxtaposition to bone is discussed later in this chapter. In general, silicone implants have proved successful for implantation in plastic surgery because of their high degree of biocompatibility. Since silicone fluid is also available for contour restoration by injection and is currently under investigation, the histologic, immunologic, and toxicologic effects of this physical state of silicone will be detailed in this chapter.

It is well to remember that an apparently innocuous membrane can develop thickening and late contracture months or even years after implantation. When infection is introduced, an accelerated inflammatory response leads to increased fibrosis and cellular reaction. Such infections are thought to be bloodborne from a primary site, such as the pharynx or genitourinary system.

Injectable Silicone Fluid. Dimethylpolysiloxane fluid, popularly known as injectable liquid silicone, has been investigated in laboratory animals and in humans as a soft tissue substitute. Because of its clinical misuse, particularly in mammary augmentation, it has acquired an unfavorable reputation which it does not deserve.

Early experimental work was conducted with the Dow-Corning 200 Fluid, which was replaced by a purified form of the fluid known as 360 Medical Fluid. However, its current designation is the highly purified Medical Grade Fluid MDX 44011, prepared in several standard viscosities and expressed in centistokes, the centistoke viscosity of water being equal to one. Most of the animal and human research was done with silicone fluid of 350 centistokes.

Those who have been using injectable liquid silicone under controlled circumstances consider it to be an advantageous "fat substitute" in restoring soft tissue contour in such deformities as hemifacial atrophy (Fig. 15–1) and lipodystrophy (see Chapter 53). Since the volume can be absolutely controlled, this material seems to be superior to biological grafts in the treatment of many such defects. Laboratory and clinical experiences with the use of liquid prostheses have been summarized by Rees, Ashley, and Delgado (1973), Rees (1973), and Ashley, Thompson, and Henderson (1973).

Tissue Response to Silicone Implantation and Injection. If an implant is relatively free of toxicity, the tissue response to it is primarily a local reaction at the intersurface between the implant and the surrounding tissues. In the absence of other surgical trauma, hemorrhage, or infection, the initial reaction to the implant is formation of a granulation tissue layer, not unlike that which occurs in any wound. In this situation, the implant separates the two edges of the surgical wound, and the granulation tissue establishes an interface with the plastic or metal rather than with the opposite side of the wound. The granulation tissue then converts, as eventually does all granulation tissue, to fibrous tissue. The amount of granulation tissue produced will be in direct response to the amount of irritation caused by the physical presence of the prosthesis, the amount of motion between the adjacent tissue and the prosthesis, and the amount of initial trauma. The amount of fibrosis, in turn, will reflect the amount of granulation tissue, the amount of motion, the amount of physical irritation, and the toxicity of the implant.

In the uncomplicated implant, a thin, fibrous capsule will form in a reasonably short time.

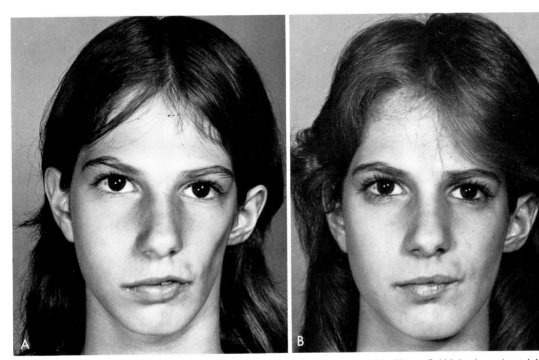

FIGURE 15–1. Patient with hemifacial atrophy before and after treatment with silicone fluid injections. A total dose of 20 ml was used.

Thicker fibrous capsules generally appear around implants which elicit a greater degree of local inflammatory response or in patients biologically inclined to excess fibroplasia. In such patients, a thick capsule will form even with an implant which usually induces minimal local inflammatory response. Similarly, a fibrous capsule forms around the silicone cysts after injection (Fig. 15–2).

In general, tissue response to liquid silicone is not unlike, if not identical to, that found around gel or solid forms of silicone, and both processes can therefore be considered one and the same.

If the initial acute cellular response is considerable, the chances of secondary infection, wound breakdown, or slough and the need for ultimate removal of the implant are increased.

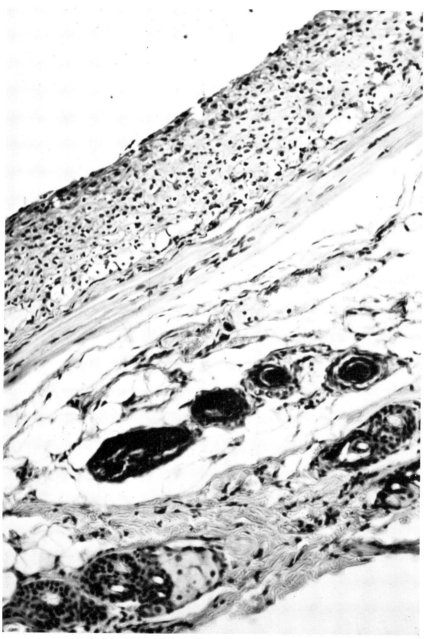

FIGURE 15–2. Appearance of a typical fibrous capsule formed around a silicone cyst (upper left hand corner). The initial inflammatory response is mild and gives way to a thin, fibrous capsule formation similar to that which forms around all silicone implants. × 3.5.

However, if the initial inflammatory reaction is minimal, the likelihood of such complications is reduced, and the chances of a successful implant increase. The initial inflammatory reaction can, however, be influenced by factors not related to the nature of the implant.

For several decades the clinical application of silicone fluid as an injectable tissue prosthesis took precedence over responsible and controlled experiments in animals. To remedy this, a series of experiments were initiated in 1963 at the Institute of Reconstructive Plastic Surgery, New York University Medical Center, at the Division of Plastic Surgery, University of California at Los Angeles, and elsewhere to evaluate the local tissue effects and possible carcinogenic properties of dimethylpolysiloxane (silicone) fluid in animal recipients. For most of the laboratory studies, injectable silicone fluid of 350 centistokes was used. Collectively, more than 1000 animals, including mice, rats, guinea pigs, rabbits, dogs, monkeys, and subhuman primates, have been used in silicone fluid investigations; mice and rats were the most commonly used animals. Monkeys, apes, and baboons in smaller numbers were also studied. Current emphasis is on primate studies.

From these data, including the work of Grasso, Golberg, and Fairweather (1964), Winer, Sternberg, Lehman, and Ashley (1964), and Andrews (1966), certain conclusions are emerging about the local and systemic responses to liquid silicone in various animal species. The following summary of research observations is derived mostly from a review by Rees, Ballantyne, and Hawthorne (1970).

LOCAL TISSUE RESPONSE. The preliminary study in humans and rats indicated that subcutaneous injection of silicone fluid was well tolerated by tissues (Rees and coworkers, 1965). The absence of measurable tissue response to the subcutaneous injection of silicone has been a constant observation in all animal species tested. Specific differences in the gross or microscopic appearance depend on the site, volume, and procedure of administration. The injected material apparently diminishes in volume after a single administration of a large dose (Ballantyne, Rees and Seidman, 1965). This phenomenon of shrinkage also results when large volumes are injected into potential spaces where the fluid can disseminate, such as the suprapannicular, subpannicular, intramuscular, intraperitoneal, and subcutaneous spaces.

The gross appearance of subcutaneous injection sites shows multiple cysts resembling a honeycomb (Ballantyne and coworkers, 1965). There is infinite variety in the size of the honeycomb compartments. The multilocular cystic area eventually becomes localized by a pale, white, glistening capsule, the thickness of which varies with the number of injections and the total volume deposited.

The early microscopic local response to single or multiple injections is a mild inflammatory one, characterized by a round cell infiltration. The inflammatory phase usually subsides within six months (Symmers, 1968). When massive doses are given, a fine, membranous capsule forms around the injected material and divides it into delicate, thin-walled, spherical or ellipsoid spaces (Ballantyne and coworkers, 1965); the lining of these cysts consists of flattened endothelium-like cells of connective tissue. Moderate fibrosis persists around the cysts six months after the injections. Occasional giant cells are seen. There is an absence of significant chronic inflammatory response.

Varying degrees of a mild, chronic, inflammatory reaction are seen if the injection is delivered intradermally. In the interstices between the cyst walls, the collagen content of the dermal fibrous tissue appears increased, and there is some disruption of dermal and subdermal architecture; also present are a moderate number of histiocytes, a few lymphocytes, and an occasional giant cell. Evidence of phagocytosis can be assumed from the presence of large round cells with nuclei flattened against the cell walls, creating an appearance similar to fat cells (Rees and coworkers, 1965; Ballantyne and coworkers, 1965).

REACTION OF ADIPOSE TISSUE. As illustrated in Figure 15–3, when large doses of silicone are given subcutaneously, adipose tissue is transformed into cysts of varying sizes and shapes at the local injection sites (Ballantyne and coworkers, 1965). The fat cells surrounding the cysts appear shrunken and show varying degrees of atrophy, with small intracellular vacuoles present. Their nuclei are prominent and thin, and a "ground-glass" appearance is occasionally seen.

When massive subcutaneous (Ballantyne and coworkers, 1965) and/or intraperitoneal doses (Rees and coworkers, 1967; Ben-Hur and coworkers, 1967) of the injectant are given, irregular foci of atrophy of omental and mesenteric fat are observed. These adipose tissue changes in animals suggest the possibility of a specific lipodystrophy-like effect in the fatty cells, but whether there is an affinity of

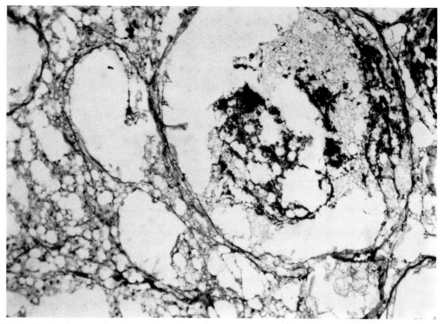

FIGURE 15-3. Photomicrograph of a section of a subcutaneous nodule of a treated rat showing a varying degree of atrophy and a focus of calcification. × 100. (From Ballantyne, D. L., Jr., Rees, T. D., and Seidman, I.: Silicone fluids: Response to massive subcutaneous injection of dimethylpolysiloxane fluid in animals. Plast. Reconstr. Surg., *36*:330, 1965.)

silicone fluid for fat is not clear. Other studies are indicated to determine the possible effect of silicone fluid on cholesterol metabolism and its role in cardiovascular disease.

VISCERAL AND SYSTEMIC DISTRIBUTION. Silicone fluid has been shown to be phagocytized in rodents (Ballantyne and coworkers, 1965; Ben-Hur and coworkers, 1967; Rees and coworkers, 1967; Hawthorne and coworkers, 1970) and is probably absorbed by other mechanisms. After intraperitoneal injection or massive subcutaneous doses, vacuoles can be found throughout the reticuloendothelial system—in the regional lymph nodes, liver, spleen, kidneys, adrenals, and elsewhere. These vacuoles are assumed to be composed of silicone fluid until proved otherwise.

Accumulations of such vacuoles can be seen in the corticomedullary junction of the adrenal glands (Fig. 15-4) of mice approximately 14 weeks after intraperitoneal injection (Ben-Hur and coworkers, 1967). Because this area is rich in reticuloendothelial cells, it is a common site of drug accumulation.

Systemic distribution and deposition of silicone fluid seem governed by the following variables: (1) the route of administration, (2) the amount given, and (3) the time interval after injection.

HEMATOLOGIC EFFECTS. In 1966, An-

drews made a small incision at the injection site in a patient and collected blood samples from exuded bloody fluid, presumably mixed with silicone. From such evidence of clear cytoplasmic vacuoles in several neutrophils and mononuclear cells, the author concluded that the leukocytes could phagocytize silicone fluid.

Similarly, it has been reported that subcutaneous and/or intraperitoneal deposits of silicone fluid are subject to a certain degree of local phagocytosis (Ballantyne and coworkers, 1965; Rees and coworkers, 1965; Andrews, 1966; Rees and coworkers, 1967; Brody and Frey, 1968; Nosanchuk, 1968), as well as systemic deposition in the reticuloendothelial system (Andrews, 1966; Ben-Hur and coworkers, 1967; Rees and coworkers, 1967). These observations suggest that injected silicone may be collected by the mobile phagocytic cells and ultimately stored in distant organs. These transitory findings occurred several weeks after injection and persisted for a few weeks. Vacuoles were identified in tissue leukocytes and some monocytes. Vacuolization of erythrocytes (Fig. 15-5) in the peripheral blood smears of rats has also been found by Hawthorne, Ballantyne, Rees, and Seidman (1970). However, the investigators were unable to duplicate this finding in other animal species.

These findings suggest that the injection of

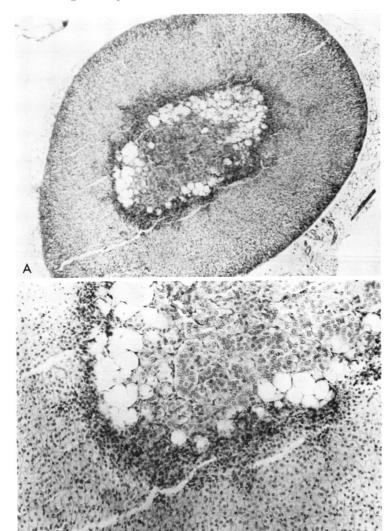

FIGURE 15–4. Adrenal. *A*, Numerous histiocytes at the cortico-medullary junction of the adrenal gland. *B*, The clear cytoplasm presumably represents silicone fluid that has been phagocytized. Higher power, × 10. (From Rees, T. D., Ballantyne, D. L., Jr., Seidman, I., and Hawthorne, G. A.: Visceral response to subcutaneous and intraperitoneal injections of silicone in mice. Plast. Reconstr. Surg., *39*:402, 1967.)

very large doses of silicone fluid may have some effect on the hematopoietic system. Hawthorne and associates (1970), using a large number of rats, found that silicone deposits in the peritoneal cavity and organs seem to have no effect on the total and differential leukocyte counts, hemoglobin levels, and hematocrit readings when compared with the controls.

After subcutaneous administration of silicone fluid into guinea pigs, Nosanchuk (1968) failed to detect evidence of antibody reaction.

EFFECTS ON THE VASCULAR SYSTEM. An evaluation of the effects of silicone fluid on the viability and revascularization of full-thickness suprapannicular skin autografts in rats was reported by Rees, Ballantyne, Hawthorne, and Seidman (1968).

Injection of 6 to 8 ml of silicone fluid around

and beneath autografts does not adversely affect the vascularization or viability of the transplants. No alteration in the morphology of grafted skin or in the blood vessels is indicated in histologic sections.

In a microscopic study in guinea pigs, Thompson (1973) showed the formation of a pseudosheath around an implanted silicone block within eight days after insertion. An independent blood supply and some nerve fibers were demonstrated in the pseudosheaths; removal of the silicone implant was followed by rapid capsule resolution, and the latter was complete by two weeks.

According to Folkman and his associates (1964, 1966), silicone rubber sheets possess certain unusual qualities related to metabolic processes. Gases, such as oxygen and carbon

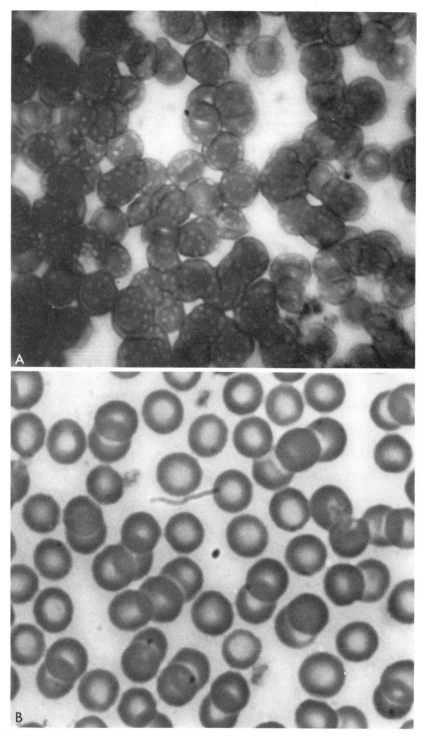

FIGURE 15–5. *A*, Blood smear from rat injected with silicone fluid nine months previously. Note the vacuoles. × 970. *B*, Blood smear from control rat. × 970. (From Hawthorne, G. A., Ballantyne, D. L., Jr., Rees, T. D., and Seidman, I.: Hematological effects of dimethylpolysiloxane fluid in rats. J. Reticuloendothel. Soc., 7:587, 1970.)

dioxide, and certain metabolites, particularly those of a fat-soluble nature, pass through silicone rubber sheets *in solution*—even though silicone sheeting is not considered to be a semipermeable membrane. It may be assumed that silicone fluid possesses similar qualities, which explains why the liquid is apparently innocuous to the vascularization and survival of a skin graft.

Technique and Complications of Injection Therapy. Complications following the injection of silicone fluid are usually the result of excessive dosage, the addition of adulterants such as lipids, improper injection technique, or poor site selection.

Correct injection techniques in regard to site, dosage, frequency of injections, and actual needle technique are most important and have been emphasized by Ashley and coworkers (1967) and by Rees (1973). Injections are spaced at weekly intervals or longer, and the volume of injectant is kept at appropriately low levels. Small contour defects, minor depressions, and the like should receive no more than 0.5 ml per *subcutaneous* injection, while significant soft tissue atrophy, such as hemifacial atrophy, may receive as much as 2 to 3 ml at each injection, provided that this volume is deposited at multiple sites by continually moving the needle. Frequent aspirations are helpful to determine that the needle tip is not in a vascular lumen. Postinjection massage or vibration is an important maneuver to disperse the silicone fluid into the tissue planes as minute droplets and to prevent pooling of the material. The initial injections of a series should be particularly small in volume until a fibrous stroma is present. Subsequent injections are then appropriately increased in volume without fear of migration, since the fibrous scaffold retains the injected dose in situ.

Breast injections are considered unwise at this time since the massive doses required to achieve augmentation interfere significantly with normal gland architecture, and the systemic effects of such volumes in humans are unknown. Severe complications of such mammary injections have been reported by Ortiz-Monasterio and Trigos (1972), Delage, Shane, and Johnson (1973), and others. These complications are essentially the formation of mammary granulomas with multiple silicone cysts and often lymphatic blockage with involvement of the dermal lymphatics. Breast amputation or subcutaneous mastectomy has been necessary in many patients (Vinnik, 1974).

Such mammary granulomas clearly camouflage normal breast tissue, making breast examination difficult or impossible; however, no carcinogenic effect has been demonstrated.

The thin skin of the eyelid renders this a poor site for injections. Rees, Ballantyne, and Seidman (1971) demonstrated severe deformities of the lids after injections for wrinkle ablation. Such problems are difficult to treat, particularly since it is virtually impossible to aspirate or remove silicone fluid once it is injected unless the entire area is extirpated.

The wide use of adulterants in silicone fluid in many parts of the world undoubtedly accounts for many untoward results which have been reported or rumored. These adulterants are thought to be fatty acids, for the most part.

Infections are remarkably rare when medical grade fluid is used, and surgery (even skin grafting) heals uneventfully in heavily injected areas. A localized inflammatory reaction following injection therapy in facial atrophy rarely occurs, and when it does, it responds to intralesional steroid injections and antibiotics (Rees, 1975).

Accumulated experience (since 1962) by several investigators with silicone fluid injection therapy indicates that, when pure medical grade fluid is utilized in small, spaced, and controlled doses and in favorable deformities located in favorable sites, complications are rare.

The accumulated data on silicone fluid injection therapy are under review by the Federal Food and Drug Administration of the United States Government. Future use of the material in the United States will be determined by this review.

Silicone injection therapy has found its greatest use in the treatment of localized soft tissue loss from trauma, developmental defects, hemifacial atrophy, and lipodystrophy and in the treatment of some types of wrinkles. A ten-year study of the use of this technique in facial atrophy was reported by Rees, Ashley, and Delgado (1973).

Dacron and Teflon

In addition to the silicones, Dacron and Teflon are established as implant materials of choice for many prostheses such as vascular pellets, artificial vessels, and orbital floor implants.

These materials are not unlike silicone in the type and amount of tissue response they evoke upon implantation. These reactions were recently summarized by Rigdon (1974). Polymorphonuclear leukocytes emigrate to Dacron cloth, Dacron polyester, and Teflon fluorocarbon fibers after subcutaneous implantation in mice, rats, and rabbits. Such leukocytic infiltration persists for varying periods of time, depending upon the species, and is thought by Rigdon to be an electrical phenomenon in which electronegative leukocytes emigrate to a positively charged plastic. Plasma proteins may become adsorptive onto a positively charged plastic surface.

Proliferation of fibroblasts and mononuclear cells begins around these plastics with the decrease in emigration and destruction of leukocytes similar to any inflammatory response. The mononuclear cells are usually phagocytic and are thought to be macrophages. Subsequently, collagenization occurs, and in a manner similar to silicone, the Dacron and Teflon implants eventually become surrounded by fibroblasts, fibrosis, and collagenous tissue. Rigdon suggests that such studies with plastic materials provide excellent models for the study of acute inflammation.

In addition, Teflon is highly inert and is not unlike the "naturally healing process" noted in silicone implants by Speirs and Blocksma (1963). LaVeen and Barberio (1949) published a comprehensive report on tissue reaction to Teflon.

PROPLAST

A combination of two polymers, polytetrafluroethylene and pyrolytic graphite, has recently become available as a porous, low modular implant for many applications in skeletal augmentation and skeletal fixation. This material, developed at the Prosthetic Research Laboratory, Fondren Orthopedic Center, Methodist Hospital, Houston, Texas, is said to induce relatively little foreign body reaction. It is porous, with interconnecting pores of 100- to 500-micron orifice size. This pore size permits, as has been mentioned earlier in this chapter, the penetration of vessels, fibrous tissue, and eventually bone, providing early and permanent fixation of the implant at its site of implantation.

Proplast appears to represent a contemporary application of established principles of material selection, host reaction, and prosthetic configuration. As a result of this concept, its use in plastic surgical, orthopedic, and oto-

logic procedures seems promising (Homsy, Kent and Hinds, 1973; Homsy, 1973; Janeke, Komorn and Cohn, 1974; Janeke and Shea, 1975; Freeman, Anderson and Homsy, 1973). The material can be shaped before or after heat sterilization. It should not be sterilized in gases or chemical substances, as such materials cannot easily be removed from the porous structure. It is relatively easy to shape with sharp instruments; it should not be compressed, lest one collapse the porous structure. The ultimate structure of Proplast suggests its use primarily as a solid tissue substitute. Success with this implant requires diligent attention to the rules of implant surgery, adequate asepsis, soft tissue cover, and gentle handling of tissues.

SOFT SILICONE IMPLANTS IN RABBITS

Lilla, Vistnes and Jobe (1974) studied the response in rabbits to several soft implants bearing similarities to currently used soft silicone- or saline-filled breast implants. The implants in rabbits were bare, backed with perforated silicone sheet, backed with Dacron mesh, or coated with a 2-mm shell of polyurethane foam of 250- to 800-micron pore diameter (Fig. 15–6). Observation in this study, in which the animals were sacrificed at 1, 6, 12, and 18 months, showed a typical reaction at the silicone implant surface as described earlier in this chapter. The content of the prosthesis did not alter the reaction in the tissue. The reaction was intensified and the capsule was thickened in the area adjacent to the perforated silicone, to a greater extent at the Dacron patch, and to the greatest extent in the polyurethane-coated prostheses. At 18 months the typical capsule around the smooth silicone was 150 to 200 microns thick; at the perforated sheet, 750 microns; at the Dacron patch as well as around the polyurethane implant, 1 mm (1000 microns). Contrary to expectations, capsules of implants with Dacron or perforated silicone sheets on one side were not thickened on the side opposite the fixation patch.

The Dacron-backed, and particularly the polyurethane-coated, prostheses were less mobile than the others. Mobility of the prosthesis was roughly in inverse proportion to the capsular reaction. One interesting phenomenon noted in the polyurethane-coated prosthesis was the formation of a "composite capsule"

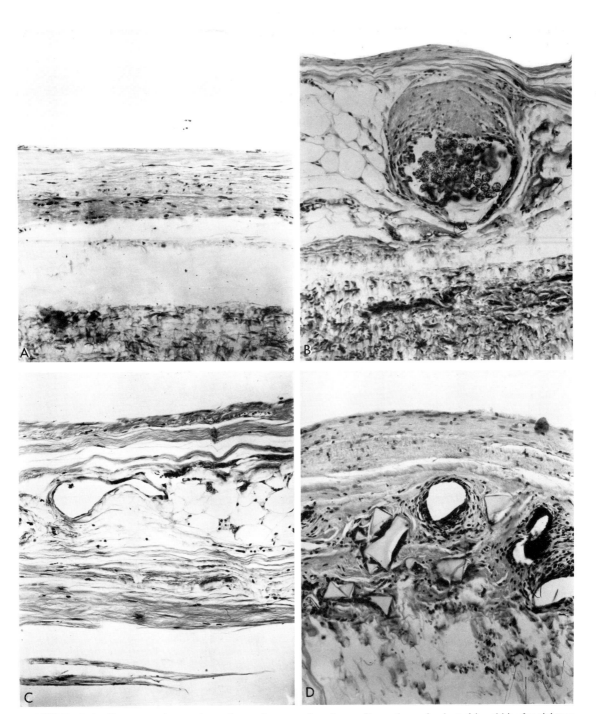

FIGURE 15–6. Representative sections of capsules around various soft prostheses implanted in rabbits for eighteen months (border of prosthesis at top). *A*, Plain silicone shell. *B*, Silicone shell with Dacron backing. Note foreign body reaction around fiber while capsule remains thin and relatively acellular. *C*, Silicone shell with perforated silicone backing at site of backing. *D*, Silicone shell covered with polyurethane foam. Note the polyurethane fragments in the external portion of the capsule which have apparently become separated from the silicone shell of the prosthesis. Between the relatively irregular capsular structure containing the polyurethane fragments and the silicone capsule there is a relatively orderly fibrous layer typical of the capsule around silicone alone. All photomicrographs approximately × 100. (From Lilla, J., Vistnes, L., and Jobe, R. P.: Long-term study of soft alloplastic prostheses in rabbits. Unpublished data, 1974.)

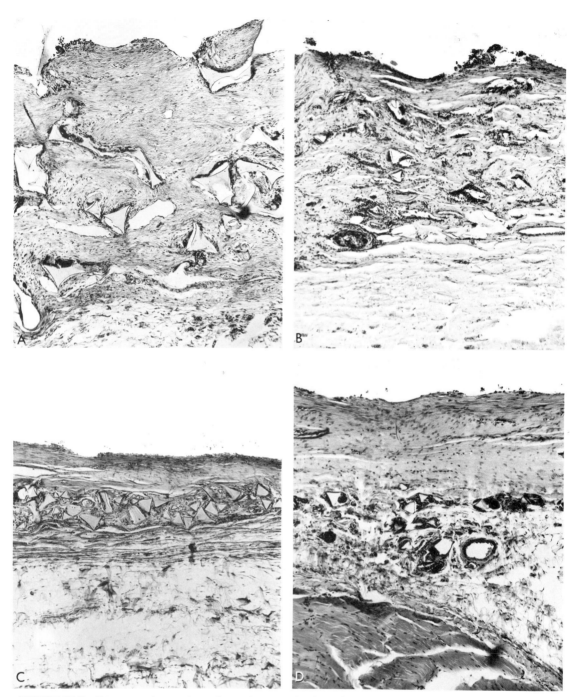

FIGURE 15–7. Representative sections of capsules around polyurethane covered soft silicone prostheses at various intervals after implantation (border of prosthesis at top). *A*, One month. *B*, Six months. *C*, Twelve months. *D*, Eighteen months. Note (1) the reduction of polyurethane fragment size as time progresses; (2) the compaction of polyurethane fragments; (3) the separation of polyurethane fragments from the silicone shell with interposition of relatively orderly fibrous tissue structure; and (4) the persistence of inflammatory cells throughout the period of study. (Lilla, Vistnes, and Jobe, 1974.)

(Fig. 15–7) at a point at which the polyurethane foam appears to separate itself from the underlying silicone shell. Why this occurs is not yet clear, but it may involve fragmentation due to motion and microtrauma, adhesive failure, and/or dissolution and weakening of the polyurethane. Peacock (1970) includes polyurethane in his list of slowly soluble plastics. This is further supported by the apparent reduction in polyurethane fragment size seen in the microscopic study of the specimens removed as time progresses from implantation. The inner section of the "composite capsule" resembles a typical orderly silicone capsule, while the section permeating the polyurethane foam has a more disorderly distribution of fibroblasts and collagen and more inflammatory reaction. Such separation of the silicone shell from the capsule has been noted clinically on removal of long-standing polyurethane-coated breast prostheses. This phenomenon appears to have no adverse effect, and this viewpoint is supported by the data in animals. Contracture of the polyurethane-infiltrated capsule does not appear to pose a clinical problem.

IMPLANTS OVER BONE

It has recently been observed that inorganic implants placed over osseous structures appear to recede into the bone (Figs. 15–8 and 15–9). Radiologic evidence of this phenomenon was first reported by Robinson and Shuken (1969). Subsequent studies by Jobe, Iverson, and Vistnes (1973), in which silicone implants were placed over and under the periosteum of the skulls of rabbits for periods of approximately 20 months, showed that the process intensified if there was an absence of natural fibrous tissue between the implant and the bone (Figs. 15–10 and 15–11). Osteosclerosis also occurred in the subjacent bone. Molding, which might be expected according to the principles of Wolfe's law (see Chapter 13), occurred even if an abundant amount of fibrous tissue was present between the surface of the implant and that of the bone. When there was no interposition of fibrous tissue, 12-mm hemispheres of firm silicone produced a depression of as much as 2 mm in the bone.

It has been observed by Spira (1973) that in humans the osseous changes occur in the first few months following implantation. The implant thereafter appears to establish a point of residence. Calcification of the capsule around the implant has also been noted. This phenomenon may influence the surgeon's choice of implants and their location.

In a retrospective cephalometric analysis of 85 patients who had undergone the insertion of silicone rubber implants for chin augmentation, over half of the patients showed some degree of bone absorption beneath the implant (Friedland, Coccaro and Converse, 1976). Bony absorption was less when the implant was placed over the hard bone of the lower part of the mandible rather than over the more superior alveolar bone. If absorption of the bone is only minimal, removal of an implant in an adequate position was not recommended.

Dacron has been attached to the flat undersurfaces of implants in an attempt to "fix" the implant to the underlying fascia or bone. Concurrent osteogenic response was evidenced by the fact that the bone invaded the Dacron and was found in the interface between the implant and the fibers of the Dacron mesh.

When they are properly used, there appears, however, to be no significant adverse response which would contraindicate the use of alloplastics in contact with bone.

THE EFFECT OF SURGICAL TECHNIQUE

The technique by which the implant is inserted contributes to the success or failure of the implant. A carefully executed surgical procedure with a minimum of trauma, directed toward achieving a clean, healed wound within a minimal period of time, is of utmost importance. Hemostasis should be as exact as possible to avoid hematoma formation around the implants, an occurrence that has been associated with the presence of thick encapsulation, especially in breast implants which feel unnaturally hard (Williams, 1972). Tissue handling should be exceptionally gentle to avoid areas of focal necrosis. Suture material that is buried with the implant should be carefully selected for its nonreactivity and should be as closely related chemically to the implant as possible.

The amount of fibrosis surrounding an implant is determined by several factors, including its composition, size, shape, and surface, as well as its form—that is, whether the implant is a solid, gel, fabric, mesh, or sponge with either open or closed pores. Impurities which might be introduced with the implant should also be

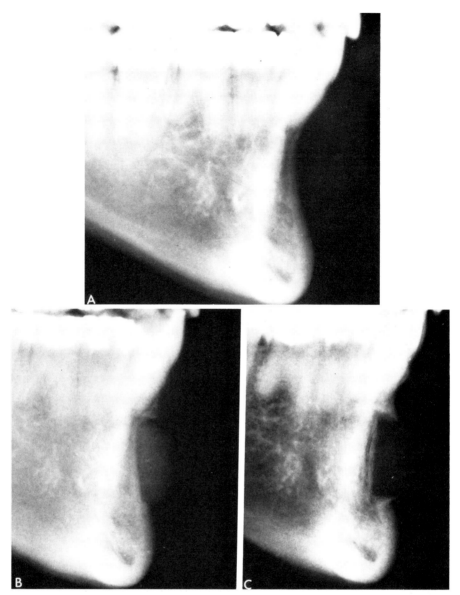

FIGURE 15–8.   Bone deformity beneath silicone elastomer chin implant. *A,* One month before chin augmentation at age 17 years. *B,* Two months after chin augmentation. Note erosion of bony surface. *C,* At age 23, 5½ years after chin augmentation, there has been extensive loss of bony surface with calcification around the implant. Presumably the position of the implant has been stable for some time. (The reproduction of the X-ray film has been printed to show the calcification extending forward into the capsule of the implant.) (From Jobe, R. P., Iverson, R., and Vistnes, L.: Bony formation beneath alloplastic implants. Plast. Reconstr. Surg., *51*:169, 1973.)

avoided. While many implants in themselves elicit only minimal tissue reaction, this response can be considerably intensified if preservative agents, debris, sebaceous material, or other impurities are not thoroughly removed from the implant before its insertion. The manufacturer's instructions for proper preparation of implantable prostheses should be strictly followed. Particular attention should be given to cleansing of the prosthesis when it is necessary before sterilization.

CHOICE OF PROSTHETIC MATERIAL

Occasionally the design of the implant includes substances which will specifically elicit more

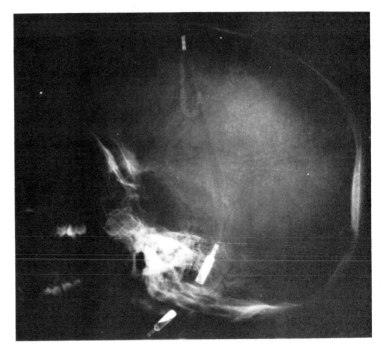

FIGURE 15–9. Bone deformity beneath a silicone elastomer ventriculovenous shunt is demonstrated in a 3 year old child who had the shunt in place (presumably over the periosteum) for two years. The groove of radiolucency shows its location. (Courtesy of Dr. R. P. Jobe.)

intense reactions in the tissue for a useful purpose. For example, Dacron or polyurethane is placed on a silicone implant for the purpose of increasing fibrosis and thereby improving fixation. Thus a response which is adverse in one circumstance can be effectively used to advantage in another.

Certain sponge implants are specifically designed to encourage collagen deposition. In these implants the fibrous capsule formed acts to fix the implant in its site. The interstices of Ivalon sponges, for example, may be completely filled with fibrous tissue, which can undergo calcification and eventually heterotopic ossification.

This type of reaction is desirable in specific reconstructive techniques, such as the implantation of Marlex mesh in the repair of abdominal and thoracic wall defects. The formation of fibrous tissue around metallic orthopedic implants is considered by many a prerequisite stage of callus formation, leading to firm bony union.

Nevertheless, the same fibrous reaction led to failure and early discouragement of the use of sponge implants for breast augmentation. Sponges of polyvinyl materials (Ivalon), popular in the early development of breast prostheses, caused such extensive fibrosis, with ossification within the interstices, that an unnatural hardness often resulted; Etheron

sponges had similar disadvantages. These poor results stimulated the search for a more suitable material with a solid or smooth surface for use in mammary augmentation. Silicone sponges of a fine cell variety are still being used for many reconstructive procedures and are preferred by many surgeons for chin augmentation. These fine-celled sponges are not invaded by fibrous tissue because of the small size of the cells and also, possibly, because of the fact that they are not true sponges. They are closed pore sponges and the cells do not intercommunicate.

BIOCOMPATIBILITY STUDIES

Biocompatibility of implant materials is now being studied, using more refined scientific techniques that are not adequately standardized as yet. The technique of implanting these substances in animals and examining the results with standard physical and chemical tests is both expensive and time-consuming. To remedy this situation, Homsy (1970) developed a technique for assaying biocompatibility in vitro using tissue culture techniques. The polymer is incubated in a pseudoextracellular fluid, a fluid that is used for tissue culture, and growth inhibition occurs in direct proportion to

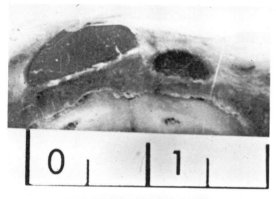

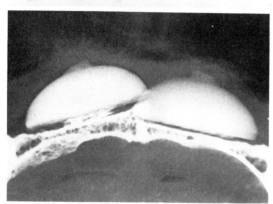

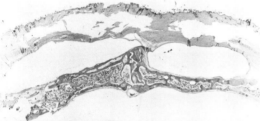

FIGURE 15–10. Twenty months after two 12-mm solid silicone hemispheres were placed on the skull of a rabbit. The three views of the same 24-mm transverse section removed from the rabbit's head show brain at the bottom and skin at the top. The implant on the left was placed above the periosteum and is without Dacron. The cut surface is more tangential in its contact with the prosthesis on the right; therefore, the latter appears smaller. Note the definite flattening and increased density of the bone contour beneath the implant, the loss of bone thickness beneath the right implant with downward displacement of the implant, and the calcification beneath the left implant (evoked by Dacron?).

Since most implants in plastic surgery are either solid or semisolid in nature and are not apt to elicit systemic responses, laboratory procedures for investigating the tissue reactivity of new material are directed toward histologic evaluation of the degree and extent of the inflammatory response at the site of implantation. An exception is the still experimental injection of dimethylpolysiloxane (silicone) fluid as a contour-restoring prosthesis. A study by Ballantyne, Rees, and Seidman (1965) has shown that this fluid can be sequestered by the reticuloendothelial system; consequently,

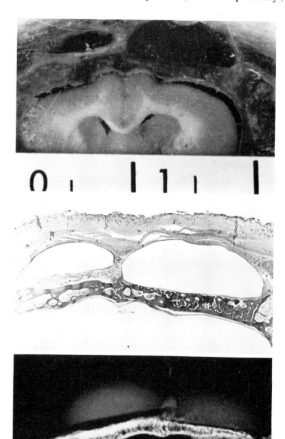

FIGURE 15–11. Another pair of implants placed on the skull of a rabbit. The implant on the left is above the periosteum and is with Dacron; the one on the right is on bone without Dacron. Note the osteosclerosis beneath the implant on the right and the marked fibrous response (evoked by Dacron?) around the left implant. Compare the differences in quality and quantity of the reactions to those seen in Figure 15–10).

the inflammatory response elicited by the polymer under investigation. If this type of technology is used, it can be expected that improved preliminary evaluation of new polymeric substances can be achieved before embarking on expensive animal implantation studies.

systemic distribution can be achieved throughout the body when massive doses are used. However, such a systemic effect is exceedingly rare or absent following usual doses.

THE QUESTION OF MALIGNANCY

Oppenheimer and his associates (1948, 1952, 1953, 1961) have conducted extensive studies on the development of sarcomas and occasional malignant tumors in rodent recipients of various foreign implants. After the publication of their original animal findings in 1948, considerable concern arose over the possibility of similar tumors developing in humans who have received implantable materials. Manufacturers and researchers have conducted frequent surveys on this subject. Extensive studies of this question, particularly in relation to breast implantation, have been done more or less continuously over the past few years. Although a breast malignancy has developed over implants, there has been no evidence to date to suggest that the implant played a direct etiologic role in the development of the tumor. The case of a malignancy occurring in the presence of alloplastic implants was reported by Herrman, Kanhouwa, Kelley and Burns (1971). In this report a woven Teflon graft, inserted to repair a laceration of the left superficial femoral artery, had been in place in the thigh of a 31 year old man for $10\frac{1}{2}$ years when a tumor developed, surrounding but not invading the artery, the vein, and the graft. The only other case of malignancy following insertion of a prosthetic implant in humans was reported by McDougall (1956), who found a Ewing's sarcoma of the humerus 30 years after implantation of a bone plate.

According to Rees (1973), the question of a granuloma-like response to the injection of silicone or silicone mixtures has been raised by several investigators. Sternberg and his associates (1964) described two cases of "tumors" in apes injected with silicone mixtures. This was followed by a subsequent report (Winer and coworkers, 1964) of three patients who developed benign tumors after receiving large volumes of silicone mixtures by injection into their breasts.

However, the patients were apparently injected not with pure medical grade silicone fluid but with mixtures to which had been added various adulterants, such as "1 per cent animal and vegetable fatty acids of unknown types."

Ben-Hur and Neuman (1963) reported development of "malignant epithelial tumors" in two out of 36 mice injected with 3 ml of silicone fluid. However, their slides were reviewed by Grasso, Golberg, and Fairweather (1964), who believed the growths to be adenomas of the mammary gland, a common tumor in mice.

Karfik and Šmahel (1968) reported what they considered to be a subcutaneous silicone granuloma in a 29 year old Arab woman who had been injected for glabellar wrinkles. Histologic sections of the granuloma demonstrated multiple cystic formations with cellular elements composed of lymphocytes and histiocytes, as well as multiple small "pseudocysts" lined by a fibrous capsule containing macrophages and giant cells. The exact chemical composition of the substance used was not known.

Since this time, reports of granulomatous lesions following injections of silicone fluid mixtures into the breasts have been made by Symmers (1968), Ortiz-Monasterio and Trigos (1972), and Delage, Shane and Johnson (1973). Symmers reported three such cases of breast lesions after injection of compounds presumably containing silicone fluid. According to his paper, it is not clear exactly what mixture was injected. The histologic picture of the breast biopsies did, however, correspond to that described by previous authors and was highly suggestive of granuloma. In one of the patients, unusual histiocytes were identified in regional lymph nodes. It is known that after massive and rapid administration, silicone fluid can be found in the lymphatics (Rees and coworkers, 1967). It is worth noting that the amount of any material necessary to effect augmentation of the breast constitutes an unusually high dose. It is certainly not improbable that such high doses can instigate the formation of granulomas.

There is some confusion over the propriety of the term "siliconoma." Ben-Hur and Neuman (1965) coined the term on the basis of finding a collection of macrophages, presumably containing ingested silicone fluid, which were clumped together in one of a series of 60 mice. The word suggests a tumor or neoplasm composed of silicone or silicone-containing cells. A collection of macrophages does not, however, constitute a tumor. The Greek suffix "-oma" is properly added only to words derived from Greek roots denoting a tumor or neoplasm. According to this definition, a siliconoma would be interpreted at least as a "proliferation of cells containing silicone." However, no one has yet convincingly shown that the injection of silicone fluid mixtures has produced a proliferating neoplasm. One cannot deny, however, that an intense local inflammatory reaction can be incited by the local injection of adulterated silicone fluid; occasionally a granuloma-like response may occur following the local misuse, either by technique or by dosage, of medical grade silicone fluid. At present, it seems fair to conclude that a cause and effect relationship has not been established.

THE FUTURE

On the horizon there are materials currently little used in plastic surgery that have distinct promise. Elemental carbon in its many forms offers a multitude of prospective uses (Bensen, 1971). The "swelling implant," polyglyceryl-methacrylate, (Refojo, 1971), is under study for ocular applications and may find a number of roles in plastic surgery since it can be inserted and can be expected to enlarge to a predictable size. The porous ceramics (Hentrich and coworkers, 1971), which are invaded by fibrous tissue in bone and replaced by the same in time as the naturally occurring elemental constituents of the ceramic are metabolized, offer possibilities to the plastic surgeon as a technological assist in the augmentation of bony structures requiring mass but little strength.

ATTEMPTS TO ACHIEVE ORDER

The first surgical implant materials were those originally used for larger industrial purposes. Only recently have new materials been designed for the specific needs of the medical market.

At the present time systems of quality control, environmental testing, and structural durability do not exist. There is no agreement about how materials and devices should be tested and standardized against chemical, physical, mechanical, and biological criteria. Hegyeli (1971), in a review of this problem, has suggested a systematic approach focused in three areas: (1) matching the engineering properties of the materials and devices with those of the corresponding human tissue; (2) defining the aspects of the implant materials which might have an effect on the biological system; and (3) defining those properties of the implant which might be altered by the environment.

Public agencies are assuming the surveillance of these aspects of medical care.

Professional societies have an obligation to define the criteria for responsible implantable product development and use. An established agency of the American industrial culture, the American Society for Testing and Materials, at the encouragement of the American Association of Orthopedic Surgeons, embarked in 1962 upon this task with the formation of the Committee F-4 on Surgical Implants. Following established patterns that have proved effective in other fields, the American Society for Testing and Materials brings together specialists in industry, medicine, and government with the intent of obtaining viable voluntary consensus standards for materials, products, systems, and services. A subcommittee of the Committee F-4 on Plastic and Reconstructive Surgery exists and will, hopefully, with the support of the societies of plastic surgeons, play a contributing and influential role.

REFERENCES*

Andrews, J. M.: Cellular behavior to injected silicone fluid: A preliminary report. Plast. Reconstr. Surg., *38*:581, 1966.

Ashley, F. L., Braley, S., Rees, T. D., Goulian, D., and Ballantyne, D. L., Jr.: The present status of silicone fluid in soft tissue augmentation. Plast. Reconstr. Surg., *39*:411, 1967.

Ashley, F. L., Thompson, D. P., and Henderson, T.: Augmentation of surface contour by subcutaneous injections of silicone fluid. Plast. Reconstr. Surg., *51*:8, 1973.

Ballantyne, D. L., Jr., Rees, T. D., and Seidman, I.: Silicone fluids: Response to massive subcutaneous injection of dimethylpolysiloxane fluid in animals. Plast. Reconstr. Surg., *36*:330, 1965.

Ben-Hur, N., and Neuman, Z.: Malignant tumor formation following subcutaneous injection of silicone fluid in white mice. Isr. Med. J., *22*:15, 1963.

Ben-Hur, N., and Neuman, Z.: Siliconoma—another cutaneous reaction to silicone fluid. Plast. Reconstr. Surg., *36*:629, 1965.

Ben-Hur, N., Ballantyne, D. L., Jr., Rees, T. D., and Seidman, I.: Local and systemic effects of dimethylpolysiloxane fluid in mice. Plast. Reconstr. Surg., *39*:423, 1967.

Bensen, J.: Elemental carbon as a biomedical material. J. Biomed. Mater. Res., *2*:41, 1971.

Braley, S.: The use of silicone in plastic surgery—A retrospective view. Plast. Reconstr. Surg., *51*:3, 1973.

*The authors are grateful to Dr. D. Ousterhaut for suggesting valuable references.

Brody, G. L., and Frey, C. F.: Peritoneal response to silicone fluid. Arch. Surg., 6:237, 1968.

Brown, J. B., Fryer, M. P., and Randall, P.: Silicones in plastic surgery. Plast. Reconstr. Surg., 12:374, 1953.

Brown, J. B., Fryer, M. P., and Lu, M.: Polyvinyl and silicone compounds as subcutaneous prosthesis. A.M.A. Arch. Surg., 68:744, 1954.

Cameron, J. L., Woodward, S. C., Pulaski, E. J., Sleeman, H. K., Brandes, G., Kulkarni, R. K., and Leonard, F.: Degradation of cyanoacrylate tissue adhesive. I. Surgery, 58:424, 1965.

Delage, C., Shane, J. J., and Johnson, F. B.: Mammary silicone granuloma. Arch. Dermatol., 108:104, 1973.

Folkman, J., and Long, D. M.: The use of silicone rubber as a carrier for prolonged drug therapy. J. Surg. Res., 4:139, 1964.

Folkman, J., Long, D. M., and Rosenbaum, R.: Silicone rubber: A new diffusion property useful for general anesthesia. Science, 154:148, 1966.

Freeman, B. S., Anderson, M. S., and Homsy, C. A.: Bony Fixation of a New Implant Material, presented to the American Association of Plastic Surgeons, New York, June, 1973.

Friedland, J. A., Coccaro, P. J., and Converse, J. M.: Retrospective cephalometric analysis of mandibular bone absorption under silicone rubber chin implants. Plast. Reconstr. Surg., 57:144, 1976.

Gabbiani, G., Ryan, G. B., and Majno, G.: Presence of modified fibroblasts in granulation tissue and their possible role in wound contraction. Experientia, 27:549, 1971.

Grasso, P., Golberg, L., and Fairweather, F. A.: Injection of silicones in mice. Lancet, 2:96, 1964.

Hawthorne, G. A., Ballantyne, D. L., Jr., Rees, T. D., and Seidman, I.: Hematological effects of dimethylpolysiloxane fluid in rats. J. Reticuloendothel. Soc., 7:587, 1970.

Hegyeli, R. J.: Limitations of current techniques for the evaluation of bio hazards and bio compatibility of new candidate materials. J. Biomed. Mater. Res., 1:1, 1971.

Hentrich, R. L., Graves, G. A., Stein, H. F., and Bajpa, P. K.: An evaluation of inert and resorbible ceramics for future clinical orthopedic applications. J. Biomed. Mater. Res., 5:25, 1971.

Herrman, J. B., Kanhouwa, S., Kelley, R. J., and Burns, W. A.: Fibrosarcoma of the thigh associated with a prosthetic vascular graft. New Engl. J. Med., 284:91, 1971.

Homsy, C. A.: Biocompatibility in the selection of materials for implantations. J. Biomed. Mater. Res., 4:341, 1970.

Homsy, C. A.: Implant stabilization—Chemical and biochemical consideration. Orthop. Clin. North Am., 4:295, 1973.

Homsy, C. A., Kent, J. N., and Hinds, E. C.: Materials for oral implantation—Biological and functional criteria. J. Am. Dent. Assoc., 86:817, 1973.

Houston, S., Hodge, J. W., Ousterhout, D. K., and Leonard, F.: Effect of alphacyanoacrylates on wound healing. J. Biomed. Mater. Res., 3:281, 1969.

Janeke, J. B., and Shea, J. J.: Self-stabilizing total ossicular replacement prosthesis in tympanoplasty. Laryngoscope, 85:1550, 1975.

Janeke, J. B., Komorn, R. M., and Cohn, A. M.: Proplast in cavity obliteration and soft tissue augmentation. Arch. Otolaryngol., 100:24, 1974.

Jobe, R. P., Iverson, R., and Vistnes, L.: Bony formation beneath alloplastic implants. Plast. Reconstr. Surg., 51:169, 1973.

Karfik, V., and Smahel, J.: Subcutaneous silicone granuloma. Acta Chir. Plast. (Praha), 10:328, 1968.

LaVeen, H. G., and Barberio, J. R.: Tissue reaction to plastics used in surgery with special reference to Teflon. Ann. Surg., 129:74, 1949.

Leonard, F., Kulkarni, R. K., Brandes, G., Nelson, J., and Cameron, J. L.: Synthesis and degradation of poly alkyl alphacyanoacrylates. J. Appl. Polym. Sci., 10:259, 1966.

Lilla, J., Vistnes, L., and Jobe, R. P.: Long-term study of soft alloplastic prostheses in rabbits. Unpublished data, 1974.

McDougall, A.: Malignant tumor at site of bone plating. J. Bone Joint Surg., 388:709, 1956.

Majno, G., Gabbiani, G., Hirschel, B. J., Ryan, G. B., and Statkov, P. R.: Contraction of granulation tissue in vitro: similarity to smooth muscle. Science, 173:548, 1971.

Marzoni, F. A., Upchurch, S. E., and Lambert, C. J.: An experimental study of silicone as a soft tissue substitute. Plast. Reconstr. Surg., 24:600, 1959.

Nicolle, F. V.: A silastic tendon prosthesis as an adjunct to flexor tendon grafting: An experimental and clinical evaluation. Br. J. Plast. Surg., 22:224, 1969.

Nilles, J. L., and Lapitsky, M.: Biomechanical investigations of bone-porous carbon and porous metal interfaces. J. Biomed. Mater. Res., 7:63, 1973.

Nosanchuk, J. S.: Injected dimethylpolysiloxane fluid: A study of the antibody and histologic response. Plast. Reconstr. Surg., 42:562, 1968.

Oppenheimer, B. S., Oppenheimer, E. T., and Stout, A. P.: Sarcomas induced in rats by implanting cellophane. Proc. Soc. Exp. Biol. Med., 67:33, 1948.

Oppenheimer, B. S., Oppenheimer, E. T., and Stout, A. P.: Sarcomas induced in rodents by embedding various plastic films. Proc. Soc. Exp. Biol. Med., 79:366, 1952.

Oppenheimer, B. S., Oppenheimer, E. T., Stout, A. P., et al.: Malignant tumors resulting from embedding plastics in rodents. Science, 118:305, 1953.

Oppenheimer, E. T., Willhite, M., Danishefsky, I., and Stout, A. P.: Observations on the effects of powdered polymer in the carcinogenic process. Cancer Res., 21:132, 1961.

Ortiz-Monasterio, F., and Trigos, I.: Management of patients with complications from injections of foreign materials into the breasts. Plast. Reconstr. Surg., 50:42, 1972.

Peacock, E. E., Jr., and Van Winkle, W., Jr.: Surgery and Biology of Wound Repair. Philadelphia, W. B. Saunders Company, 1970.

Rees, T. D.: Silicone injection therapy. In Rees, T. D., and Wood-Smith, D. (Eds.): Cosmetic Facial Surgery. Philadelphia, W. B. Saunders Company, 1973, pp. 232–267.

Rees, T. D.: Unpublished data, 1975.

Rees, T. D., Platt, J. M., and Ballantyne, D. L., Jr.: An investigation of cutaneous response to dimethylpolysiloxane (silicone liquid) in animals and humans—A preliminary report. Plast. Reconstr. Surg., 35:131, 1965.

Rees, T. D., Ballantyne, D. L., Jr., Seidman, I., and Hawthorne, G. A.: Visceral response to subcutaneous and intraperitoneal injections of silicone in mice. Plast. Reconstr. Surg., 39:402, 1967.

Rees, T. D., Ballantyne, D. L., Jr., Hawthorne, G. A., and Seidman, I.: The effects of dimethylpolysiloxane fluid on rat skin autografts. Plast. Reconstr. Surg., 41:153, 1968.

Rees, T. D., Ballantyne, D. L., Jr., and Hawthorne, G. A.: Silicone fluid research: A follow-up summary. Plast. Reconstr. Surg., 46:50, 1970.

Rees, T. D., Ballantyne, D. L., Jr., and Seidman, I.: Eyelid deformities caused by the injection of silicone fluid. Br. J. Plast. Surg., 24:125, 1971.

Rees, T. D., Ashley, F. L., and Delgado, J. P.: Silicone fluid injections for facial atrophy. Plast. Reconstr. Surg., *52*:118, 1973.

Refojo, M. F.: The swelling implant. J. Biomed. Mater. Res., *1*:179, 1971.

Rigdon, R. H.: Inflammation associated with Dacron and Teflon: An experimental study in mice, rats and rabbits. Tex. Rep. Biol. Med., *32*:2, 1974.

Robinson, M., and Shuken, R.: Bone resorption under plastic chin implants. J. Oral Surg., *127*:116, 1969.

Souther, S. G., Levitsky, S., and Roberts, W. C.: Bucrylate tissue adhesive for microvascular anastomosis. Arch. Surg., *103*:496, 1971.

Speirs, A. C., and Blocksma, R.: New implantable silicone rubbers: An experimental evaluation of tissue response. Plast. Reconstr. Surg., *31*:166, 1963.

Spira, M.: Published comments on bone deformation paper by Jobe, Iverson and Vistnes. Plast. Reconstr. Surg., *51*:174, 1973.

Sternberg, T. H., Ashley, F. L., Winer, L., and Lehman, R.: Gewebereaktionen auf injizierte flussige Siliciumver bindungen. Hautartz, *15*:281, 1964.

Swanson, A. B.: Flexible implant resection arthroplasty. Hand, *4*:119, 1972.

Symmers, W. S.: Silicone mastitis in "topless" waitresses and some other varieties of foreign body-mastitis. Br. Med. J., *3*:19, 1968.

Thompson, H. G.: The fate of the pseudosheath pocket around silicone implants. Plast. Reconstr. Surg., *51*:667, 1973.

Vinnik, C.: Personal communication, 1974.

Williams, C. W., Aston, S. J., and Rees, T. D.: The effect of hematoma on thickness of pseudosheaths around silicone implants. Plast. Reconstr. Surg, *56*:2; 194, 1975.

Williams, J. E.: Experiences with a large series of silastic breast implants. Plast. Reconstr. Surg., *49*:253, 1972.

Winer, L., Sternberg, T. H., Lehman, R., and Ashley, F. L.: Tissue reactions to injected silicone liquids. Arch. Dermatol., *90*:588, 1964.

Zarem, H. A.: Silastic implants in plastic surgery. Surg. Clin. North Am., *48*:129, 1968.

ADDITIONAL REFERENCES

Cahoon, J. R., and Paxton, H. W.: A metallurgical survey of current orthopedic implants. J. Biomed. Mater. Res., *4*:223, 1970.

Dunn, H. K., King, R., Andrade, J. D., Jr., and DeVries, K. L.: Polyester textile bioadhesion to muscle and bone. J. Biomed. Mater. Res., *7*:109, 1973.

Hahn, H., and Palich, W.: Preliminary evaluation of porous metal surface titanium for orthopedic implants. J. Biomed. Mater. Res., *4*:571, 1970.

Hulbert, S. F., Cooke, F. W., Klawitter, J. J., Leonard, R. B., Sauer, B. W., Mowle, D. D., and Skinner, N. B.: Materials and design considerations for the attachment of prostheses into the musculoskeletal system. J. Biomed. Mater. Res., *4*:1, 1973.

Jones, L., and Liberman, B. A., Jr.: Interaction of bones to various metals. Arch. Surg., *32*:990, 1936.

Kulkarni, R. K., Moore, E. G., Hegyelli, A. F., and Leonard, F.: Biodegradable poly (lactic acid) polymers. J. Biomed. Mater. Res., *5*:169, 1971.

Laing, T., Ferguson, R. B., Jr., and Hodge, E. S.: Tissue reaction in rabbit muscle exposed to metallic implants. J. Biomed. Mater. Res., *1*:135, 1967.

Zierold, A. A.: Reaction of bone to various metals. Arch. Surg., *9*:365, 1924.

CHAPTER 16

SCARS AND KELOIDS

GEORGE F. CRIKELAIR, M.D.,
DAVID M. C. JU, M.D.,
AND BARD COSMAN, M.D.

A scar, or cicatrix, may be defined as the new tissue that is formed in the healing of a wound (Dorland, 1974). Human soft tissue healing is basically nonregenerative. That which is destroyed is not restored but replaced by a less well-differentiated tissue—scar—which contracts and draws the remaining normal parts together (Van Den Brenk, 1956). A scar is the inescapable result of the healing process.

Despite the inevitability of the process of scar formation, there exists in the population, both lay and medical, the strange belief that a plastic surgeon can make an incision and leave no visible scar and that he can in fact do away with previously existing scars. The simple facts of wound healing make this physically impossible. There is, of course, little question that a patient suffering a laceration or incision wants it to heal without leaving a visible scar and that the surgeon suturing a laceration or making an operative incision never wants to produce anything but an invisible scar. This wished-for result is often spoken of in medical circles as the "fine hairline scar."

In considering the realities of scars, the discussion will be divided under five headings:
1. Basic observations on cutaneous scars.
2. The physical basis of scar contraction.
3. Skin sutures and skin suture marks.
4. Keloids and hypertrophic scars.
5. Scar revision and its complications.

BASIC OBSERVATIONS ON CUTANEOUS SCARS

Every incision incites an inflammatory process which ends without fail with the formation of a scar. A "good scar" is one which is no more than a fine line, level and even with the surrounding surface; it is the same color as the surrounding skin and causes no contracture, pull, or distortion of the surrounding structures. Accurate photographs of scars are difficult to obtain because minor variations in the features mentioned are apt to be "burned out" by the lighting needed for obtaining the picture. Flat lighting will make a scar invisible; intense cross lighting may accentuate it if it has variations in height or depth.

Some areas of the body rather consistently heal with less noticeable scars than others. For example, incisions in the eyelids usually leave fine, almost invisible scars. The forehead, palms and soles, penis and scrotum, and all mucous membranes generally share this happy result. Other areas are not so kind to the surgeon or the patient. Scars over the lower portion of the nose often become depressed. Scars about the chin, sternal area, shoulders, and upper back are apt to spread, as are incisions on the lower extremities. This all too frequently happens despite proper attention to

413

the best surgical precepts. Certain conditions such as lymphedema also predispose to unsightly scars.

The idea is frequently presented that children "heal" better than adults and that therefore scarring will be less and the resultant scar less noticeable. It is perhaps true that children develop tensile strength in a sutured wound more rapidly than do adults, but in the process the scars are usually redder and maintain this color longer than comparable scars in elderly patients. This results in poorer looking scars for longer periods of time. Generally, if a surgeon wants to get the best cosmetic result from an incision in the least possible time, he should choose a patient closer to the age of 90 than 9 years.

Tincture of time is perhaps the best, the kindest, the least expensive, and the easiest medication for any scar, provided, of course, there is not too much tissue loss and no anatomical malalignment. Patients with facial scars following automobile injuries are excellent examples of this process. Seen a few weeks after repair by whatever technique, the scars and surrounding facial skin may be red, indurated, uneven, and bumpy. Seen six to 12 months later, what may have looked like a problem necessi-

tating several operations may so improve spontaneously that little further need be done to improve the condition (Fig. 16–1).

Only when a scar is soft and white has the healing process completely subsided. The time for this varies from person to person. Some scars never develop redness and induration; others may require one to two years for these conditions to subside. A covering make-up is of great help to both patient and doctor while awaiting the settling of a scar (Thorne, 1966).

Massage, pressure, the application of ointments and grease, and X-ray therapy have been suggested to hasten the process of scar resolution. There seems to be no benefit from massage other than giving the patient something to do while time passes and the scars improve spontaneously. The use of pressure per se, continued over long time periods and combined with immobilization, may be of real value, as in the case of skin grafts to the anterior neck (Cronin, 1961; Lintilnac and associates, 1966; Fujimori and coworkers, 1968). Applying this technique to a simple incised wound seems unwarranted in most instances. The use of pressure in the treatment of burn scars is discussed in Chapter 33. The addition of creams and greases falls into the same

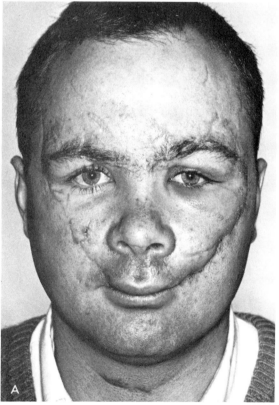 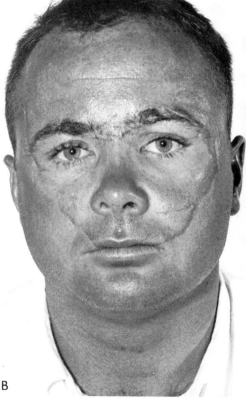

FIGURE 16–1. Patient one month (*A*) and seven months (*B*) after windshield laceration. No surgery was performed in the interval. The initial apparent need for major scar revision has been much reduced.

category, except that by their use the patient is more fully occupied during the waiting period. X-ray therapy may hasten the scar resolution process slightly, but the wisdom of using radiation for a benign, self-limited process is questionable. Despite better understanding of radiation therapy and its more judicious application, the late hazard of radiation in the form of radiation change in the skin remains. Deeper structures may also be affected. There may be interference with osseous development. And the possibility of malignancy in the thyroid gland following irradiation therapy of benign lesions in the neck is well known (Hanford, Quimby and Frantz, 1962).

If the anatomical arrangement of the surrounding tissues is distorted at the time of the original suturing, obviously no improvement in alignment will come with the passage of time, although the scar itself may improve. Proper alignment of structures therefore is always necessary and should be attended to without waiting for too much time to pass. Excessive skin loss is comparable to the contraction of a scar and usually distorts the surrounding structures. Such problems can improve only to a degree with the passage of time but usually will benefit from the addition of tissue in the form of skin grafts or flaps.

Chronic unstable scars may give rise to cancer. Interest in this problem dates from the classic publication of Marjolin (1828). Celsus in the first century noted the development of cancer in burn scars. The reported cases of cancer in burn scars have been mainly squamous cell in type and have developed in large, deep, burn scars that were slow to heal (Bowers and Young, 1960; Arons and associates, 1965). Chronic osteomyelitis may also give rise to malignant changes if draining sinuses have been present for many years. Any fistula of a chronic nature appears to have the same malignant potential.

Treves and Pack (1930) considered the avascular scar tissue around Marjolin's ulcer as a barrier against metastases. Furtell and Myers (1972) suggested that the circumferential scar prevented the growth of lymphatics, thus placing the carcinoma in an immunologically privileged site. Arons, Lynch, Lewis and Blocker (1965), in a reassessment of their clinical data, and Bostwick, Pendergrast and Vasconez (1976) have obtained clinical evidence negating this concept. The latter authors have observed recurrence of the malignancy and regional lymph node metastases within 6 months after radical excision of the carcinoma and repair of the wound.

With more extensive skin grafting of burns and better surgical treatment and reconstruction for osteomyelitis and other causes of tracts and fistulas, fewer of these cases will be observed in the future.

The possibility of a fibrosarcoma developing in a scar is very rare but should be mentioned (Fleming and Rezek, 1941; Kanaar and Oort, 1969). We have seen a patient who 13 years postoperatively developed "lumps" in an appendectomy scar. Repeated excisions followed with a pathologic diagnosis initially of fibroma and later of fibrosarcoma (Ju, 1966).

A discussion of scars is incomplete without reference to the vast amount of work being done in the biochemistry and histochemistry of wound healing (Edwards and Dunphy, 1958; Levenson and coworkers, 1966; Peacock and Van Winkle, 1970). However, at the present time, despite advances in our knowledge of wound healing, despite advances in surgical techniques, despite the achievements of biochemistry and histochemistry, scars remain unpredictable in behavior. With the best understanding and technique of trained surgeons, some scars will spread, some will hypertrophy, and others will form keloids. Both practical and theoretical considerations therefore make it unwise for the operating surgeon to promise a patient that the result of an operative incision or a traumatic wound will be "a fine hairline scar."

THE PHYSICAL BASIS OF SCAR CONTRACTION

The healing of a wound by *first intention* is divided into three phases: first, there is a transient lag phase, second, a short phase of fibroplasia, and third, a gradual and ill defined phase of contraction of the scar (see Chapter 3). During the first two days—the lag phase—a fibrinous network studded with leukocytes and red blood cells binds the wound edges together. From the third to the fifth day, during the phase of fibroplasia, fibroblasts start to proliferate in the fibrinous network, and new capillaries are formed. The strength of the wound increases rapidly, and the epithelial cells proliferate to cover the narrow gap between the edges of the incised wound. In normal instances the tensile strength of the wound is great enough at the end of the first week to hold the wound edges together without benefit of the sutures (Findley and Howes, 1950). At this stage a scar usually appears reddish in color and feels somewhat firm in consistency. The contraction phase follows, and gradually the new blood vessels become obliterated, the young fibroblasts mature, and the scar contracts (Dunphy, 1963; Van Winkle, 1967). After a varying period of months, the resolution process is completed and the scar becomes soft and pliable, slightly shiny, and whitish in color. The fibrous tissue in the wound that heals by first intention is rather small in amount. Usually it is represented by a thin sheet of scar tissue extending through the dermis to the depths of the incision.

If there is a gross physical gap between the wound edges to be filled by the formation of granulation tissue, healing is said to be by *second intention*. The duration of healing depends upon the dimension of the wound, the presence or absence of infection, the mobility of the adjacent structures, the general condition of the patient, plus other local and general factors. While the depths of the wound are being filled with granulation tissue, epithelization occurs on the surface peripherally. At the same time obliteration of the blood vessels and deposition of collagen fibers in the granulation tissue take place. Usually wound contraction occurs simultaneously with the epithelial proliferation from the margin of the wound. This contraction of the wound is to be distinguished from the later scar contraction. All wounds show the phenomenon of size decrease. It is still a moot point as to precisely which structures in the wound or about it generate the forces required for this alteration. The phenomenon has been systematically investigated and varying interpretations offered (Billingham and Russell, 1956; Van Den Brenk, 1956; Watts, 1960; Ramirez and coworkers, 1969). The weight of evidence now available suggests that it is the fibroblasts within the healing wound, i.e., in the granulation tissue, that actually contract, thereby exerting the necessary force (Peacock and Van Winkle, 1970). Gabbiani, Ryan and Majno (1971) identified a cell in contracting wounds which they called the myofibroblast because on electron microscopic examination it possessed ultrastructural characteristics of a fibroblast and a smooth muscle cell.

Eventually the young granulation tissue in the wound is completely covered by new epithelium, and the initial stages of healing by second intention are completed. Since there is more scar tissue in this kind of wound, additional contraction of the scar is to be expected later. The scar of a wound newly healed by second intention appears as an area or mass of dense, indurated, reddish fibrous tissue which usually takes much longer to resolve. Not infrequently these heavy scars, when in an area of frequent trauma, are unstable and tend to break down. Ulcers may occur, the cycle of healing by second intention is repeated, and more scar is formed.

The young fibroblasts in a scar, whether arising from the healing by first intention or second intention, are, in the first six months, rather vulnerable to physical irritation. The resolution process can be delayed or caused to revert to active proliferation of fibroblasts with increase in vascularization, by intermittent change of tension in the scarred area. Constant steady tension in a scar is probably not so potent a stimulant as are changing stresses in the stimulation of the proliferative process of the fibroblasts in a new scar (Altemeier and Stevenson, 1960). This is well illustrated by a scar which runs longitudinally across the transverse creases of the neck (Fig. 16–2). The scar may appear to be fine and linear in the first two weeks of the healing process. As soon as the immobilization is removed and the patient starts to use the muscles of the head and neck, the scar invariably starts to thicken and eventually to contract. Flexion and extension of the neck constantly change the tension in the scar, and proliferation of fibroblasts is stimulated. The fibrous tissue, consisting chiefly of collagenous fibers and less elastic than the normal tissue, is also less pliable and resilient. Forceful exercise may produce microscopic tears

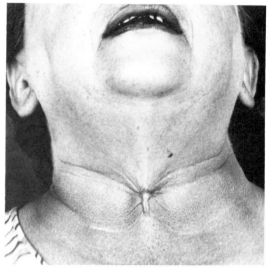

FIGURE 16–2. The contraction forces at the upper and lower ends of a vertical scar distort the normal transverse skin creases. (Courtesy of Dr. J. P. Webster.)

and induce microscopic bleeding which may become organized to form more scar with further increase in the thickness and rigidity of the scar tissue. These events, postulated by Skoog (1948), lead to a vicious circle and scar contracture occurs.

Factors Affecting Scar Contraction. The physical factors that affect the extent of scar contraction are the initial amount of scar tissue formed in the wound healing process; the position of the scar in relation to the skin tension lines on the surface of the body; the position of the scar in relation to joints; and the shape of the scar.

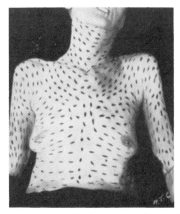

FIGURE 16–3. Langer's lines on a cadaver. (From Cox, H. T.: The cleavage lines of skin. Br. J. Surg., *29*:234, 1941.)

1. THE AMOUNT OF SCAR. The amount of scar formation varies according to whether the wound heals by first intention or by second intention. However, even in the former case great variations in scar formation are observed. The presence or absence of hematoma and devitalized tissue and the method of wound closure and dressings are factors accounting for the variation. The hematoma is usually replaced by fibrous tissue, as is tissue necrosed by a ligature. Foreign bodies are usually surrounded by dense fibrous tissue and foreign body giant cells. Moreover, in a wound healed by second intention, in addition to the depth or dimension of the initial gap, the presence or absence of infection and the duration of the open wound play a role in determining the amount of eventual scarring. A third degree burn of considerable area without the benefit of skin graft usually requires weeks or months to heal. The granulation tissue is excessive, and the collagen fibers are thick and dense.

The age and sex of the patient as well as the site of the injury are also factors. The initial fibroblastic activity may be greater in children and pregnant women; thin, elderly patients do not usually manifest similar activity. There is great variation in the amount of scar formation in different individuals, and this same variation may be found in varying anatomical areas in the same person. In extreme examples of individual or site variation, scar formation may be so intensified as to resemble a benign tumor growth, i.e., a keloid is formed.

2. THE TENSION LINES OF THE SURFACE OF SKIN (LANGER'S LINES). In 1861 Langer noted that puncture holes in human cadavers had a tendency to spread open in a definite direction that corresponded to a certain general pattern. He was able to map these lines, which were subsequently called Langer's lines (Fig. 16–3). Since a cadaver has no muscle activity,

the cause for this spreading must be entirely physical. The physical phenomenon, however, arises out of the living organism's adaptation to function. Langer's lines in general correspond to the tension lines of the skin. Since the skin is constantly pulled and stretched by muscular activities and joint motions, it is advantageous from an architectural viewpoint for the collagen fibers and the elastic fibers in the skin to be arranged in a special way to facilitate these changes (Cox, 1941). The fibrous network is thus arranged more or less in an accordion plait fashion. An accordion moves to and fro in a longitudinal direction without changing its transverse dimension greatly. The general direction of the majority of the transverse fibers of the skin is perpendicular to the underlying muscle (Rubin, 1948; Kraissl, 1949). This is nature's economy in architecture: the contracting muscles do not have to pull against the general direction of the tension of the dermal fibers of the skin, and the skin maintains its tension during muscular activity (see Chapter 1). A scar parallel to these skin lines is not subject to tension by muscle pull; it will resolve earlier and remain fine and delicate. On the contrary, a linear scar perpendicular to the skin tension lines is parallel to the long axis of the underlying muscles. During the contraction and relaxation of the muscles, these scars are alternately pulled and relaxed. Fibroblastic activity is constantly stimulated, and the scars have a tendency to hypertrophy. An L-shaped scar usually will have one limb of the L thicker and more hypertrophic than the other, since it is physically impossible to place both limbs of the L parallel to Langer's lines. In such an incision on the neck, for example, the vertical portion parallels the sternocleidomastoid muscle and the transverse one parallels the skin crease; the vertical scar usually is much thicker and more unsightly than the transverse one.

3. THE POSITION OF THE SCAR IN RELATION TO THE JOINT. The greatest tension changes in the skin occur in the vicinity of joints. A scar across a joint is constantly subjected to stress and pull, particularly in the area of hinge joints such as the fingers and elbows. The changes in skin tension are different at the different axes of the joint. There is considerable change of skin tension along the longitudinal axis of the joint but little or no change in the transverse axis. During each joint motion, the change of tension on the flexor surfaces is the reverse of that on the extensor surfaces. When a joint is flexed, the flexor surface is relaxed and tension reduced, while the extensor surface is stretched and tension increased; when the joint is extended the reverse process occurs. Whether the joint is extended or flexed, the effect of the motion is to produce a positive tension surface and a negative tension surface at the same time. From a mathematical viewpoint, there must be a plane of zero tension between the flexor and extensor surfaces. Clinically, this plane is midway between the extensor and flexor surfaces; this is the neutral zone. Any incision across the joint in this midlateral plane is not subject to

the dynamics of joint activity, and scars in this plane will remain static. The midlateral incision is thus used safely in the exploration of fingers, knees, and elbows, while scars in the middle of the extensor or flexor surfaces usually produce contractures (Fig. 16–4).

Such contractures can be corrected by a Z-plasty (Davis and Kitlowski, 1939; Furnas, 1968). The scar is partially or totally excised at first, the Z incisions are made, and two triangular flaps are transposed to a reversed Z position (see Chapter 1). The longitudinal scar is thus converted into three segments; the midportion of the scar is made to become more or less parallel to the transverse axis of the joint and therefore not subject to change of tension during joint motion. The two lateral limbs of the Z are placed away from the center of the longitudinal axis and therefore closer to the neutral zone or the midlateral plane of the joint. A Z-plasty also lengthens and inserts additional normal skin along the longitudinal axis of the joint where the change of tension is greater during motion. This gives more normal elasticity during motion (Fig. 16–5).

4. THE SHAPE OF A SCAR. A semicircular scar made on any part of the body is apt to contract and produce the deformity called "trapdoor effect." The tissue within the semicircle becomes puffy and raised (Fig. 16–6). This has been explained on the basis of lymphatic or venous obstruction. However, the

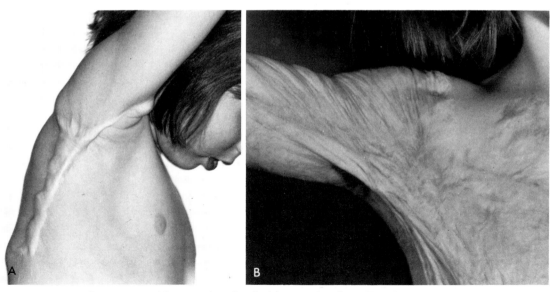

FIGURE 16–4. Contracture and hypertrophy of an incision crossing the axillary flexion crease (*A*) and an elevated contracture band without hypertrophy (*B*) of a burn scar involving the anterior axillary line.

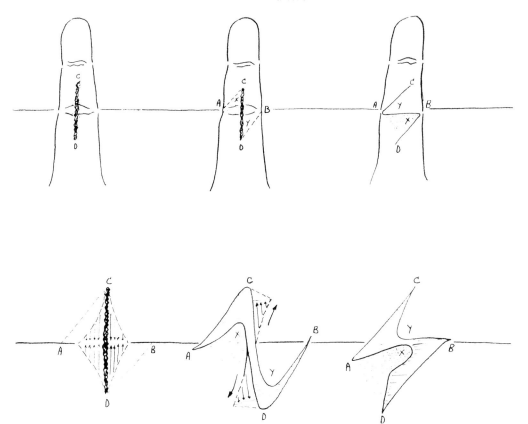

FIGURE 16–5. Correction of cross-joint scar by Z-plasty. CD is converted to CA–AB–BD. As soon as the incisions AC and DB are made, the triangular flaps X and Y tend to transpose themselves to the desired position because of the inherent contraction forces in the scar. This is a phenomenon first noted by Davis and Kitlowski (1939).

condition will occur in any semicircular incision whether its base is situated away from or toward the general direction of the lymphatic or venous drainage. In addition, the trapdoor effect occurs weeks or months after a wound is healed. Lymphatic or venous obstruction, therefore, cannot be substantially responsible for this phenomenon, and another explanation must be sought.

When a linear scar undergoes contraction, the contracting force is distributed graphically in a triangular fashion (Ju, 1951). The force of contraction of a straight scar being equal on both sides, the influence of the contracting force is greatest at the area closest to the scar and is gradually reduced away from the scar (Fig. 16–7). In a semicircular scar there is a concentration of this contracting force and convergence of the forces of contraction; this causes the wrinkling and raises the level of the

tissue within the semicircle. The trapdoor effect is the result (Fig. 16–8).

A circumferential scar of a limb or finger usually produces severe contracture, and quite often causes interference with venous return and lymphatic drainage (Stevenson, 1946). This effect is particularly notable in the congenital circular bands of children. The circular scar, since it is a continuous ring, has no intervening normal skin to offer the normal elasticity for the excursion of vascular pulsation or muscular contraction. The rate of growth of the extremity is affected. In addition to this, a circular scar is a combination of two semicircles, so that a double trapdoor effect is present in the ring. Any attempt that is made to relieve the constricting scar by mere excision of the ring and resuturing the skin and soft tissues along the circle does not basically change the scar pattern, and the constriction will recur.

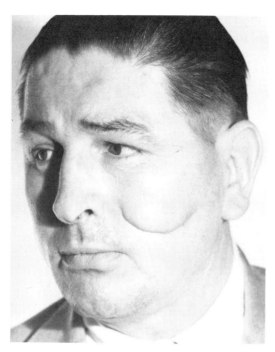

FIGURE 16-6. Trapdoor scar of the cheek.

SKIN SUTURE MARKS

At the termination of most operative procedures, the surgeon sutures the cut skin edges. It is his aim to place each stitch in the skin properly, to have it do its work well, and to remove it, leaving no mark. Any mark that a suture may leave is nothing less than scar tissue and manifests all the histologic features of incisional scars (Gillman and Penn, 1956; Ordman and Gillman, 1966).

Gillies (1943) in discussing suturing said: "How tight to tie is a matter of experience and lies between that adequate to bring the edges closely opposed and that that cuts through by causing tissue necrosis. Err on the loose side. Stitch marks are indisputable evidence of a stitch that has caused a local pressure necrosis and its accompanying infection."

Webster (1949) has stated: "Buried sutures take the burden of tension from the skin sutures and allow the early removal of the latter so that they leave no scars. Constriction of the skin by sutures causes necrosis, and necrosis means scarring and deformity. The more loosely the skin sutures can be tied, in conformance with good approximation of the cut surfaces, and the earlier they are removed, the smaller will be their permanent mark on the skin."

Such scars are benefited by Z-plasties, since these increase the dimension of the scar, change its direction, and also break the ring by inserting normal elastic skin into the circumference of the circle (Fig. 16-9).

To avoid suture marks many measures have been advanced and many suture techniques ad-

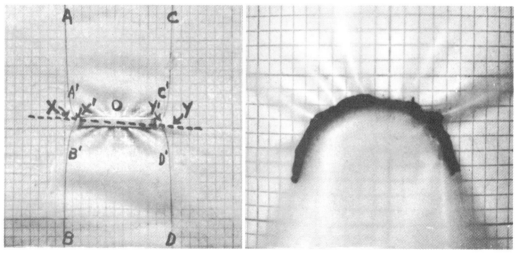

FIG. 16-7   FIG. 16-8

FIGURE 16-7. Experimental study of scar contraction. A rubber band is glued under tension onto an elastic membrane. Contraction of the rubber band pulls straight lines AXB to A'X'B' and CYD to C'Y'D'. Note also the wrinkles above and below the rubber band X'OY'. The forces of contraction can be graphically represented by triangle A'X'B' and triangle C'Y'D'.

FIGURE 16-8. Experimental production of trapdoor effect. A semicircular rubber band under tension is glued onto the elastic membrane. The membrane within the semicircle becomes raised and "puffy."

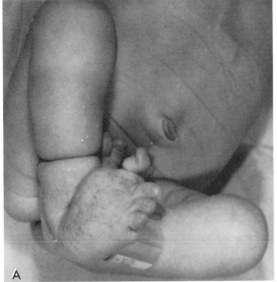

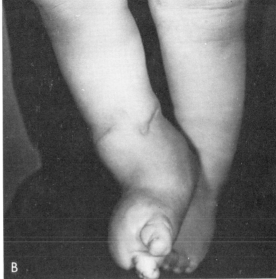

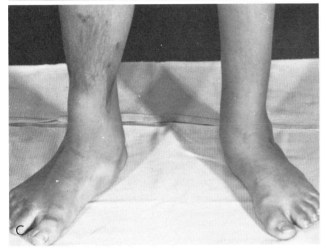

FIGURE 16–9. Congenital constricting band of the right ankle before (*A*) and three months after (*B*) two Z-plasties. Distal swelling is regressing. Result 12 years later (*C*) shows relatively normal appearing foot.

vised. The epithelial stitch (Halsted, 1924), the vertical mattress or end-on vertical mattress suture (Davis, 1919), and subcuticular sutures have been advocated. The use of very closely spaced sutures, the addition of tape support for the wound edge after early suture removal (Straatsma, 1947), the use of collodion strips for closure and for later support (Uchida and Uchida, 1961), the closure of the wound by suturing only strips of adhesive fastened on the skin parallel to the cut edges (Gosis, 1939; Radcliffe, 1943), and very early removal of sutures have been among these approaches. The use of tape closure alone was reviewed by Golden (1960) in his presentation of a new surgical tape.

Of the many causes offered for suture marks, tension is the most frequently mentioned. The tension may be a direct result of the surgical technique. A well-healed rotation flap employed to close a decubitus ulcer is illustrated in Figure 16–10. The right half of the incision was closed by the surgeon and the left half by his assistant. The same needles and sutures were used by both, and all sutures were removed at the same time. However, one-half of the scar has prominent suture marks and the other has none. This suggests that control of skin suture marks can be at the proximal rather than at the distal end of the needle holder. In addition to initial tension, the edema that develops in a wound in the first 48 hours further tightens tight sutures (Howes, 1940). However, the factor of tension as well

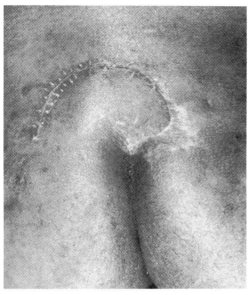

FIGURE 16–10. Excision of sacral decubitus ulcer closed by a rotation flap. Note the suture marks in the left half of the incision.

scars in some patients may also lead to keloids at the site of skin sutures (Fig. 16–11).

2. STITCH ABSCESS. Owing to the activity of bacteria—usually low grade skin contaminants—an abscess may occur around the exits of the sutures from the skin. In some instances this is associated with the necrosis caused by the tension of the tied suture. The suture behaves as a foreign body, and only after its removal will the inflammation subside. When the infection is controlled, repair begins. If the cavity is small, it becomes filled first with granulation tissue, then scar. The size of the suture mark secondary to a stitch abscess depends on the size of the abscess.

3. SKIN TYPE. Suture marks do not seem to occur as commonly in some areas of the body as in others. This parallels the formation of scars as mentioned earlier. The skin of the eyelids seldom shows suture marks, and the marks seem to be less common on the palms of the hands and the soles of the feet. The skin of the back, the chest, the upper arms, and the lower extremities by comparison, is more likely to show suture marks. The same is true of the skin of the lower third of the nose and the cheeks adjacent to the nasal alae as compared to the rest of the face. It may be that the presence of secondary skin appendages, sweat glands, sebaceous glands, and hair follicles, or rather the type of these structures present in a

as the other possible factors warrant further comment, since these points apply to the formation of scars in general.

Possible Factors in the Formation of Suture Marks

1. KELOID TENDENCY. The inherent "something" that causes keloids and keloidal

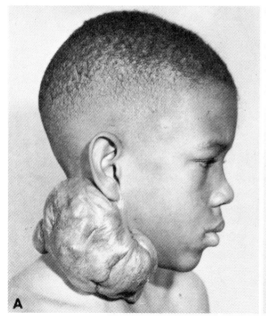

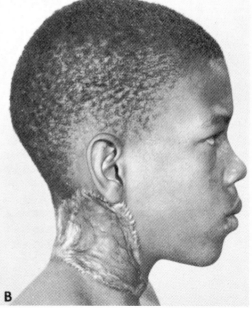

FIGURE 16–11. A large keloid of the neck excised and grafted. Note the marks of the sutures at the edge of the split-thickness skin graft.

given area, is a contributing factor to the formation of suture marks.

4. SUTURE MATERIAL. There are many reports on the effects of suture materials, absorbable and nonabsorbable, and the relative merits of the various nonabsorbable sutures—silk, cotton, linen, wire, nylon, and other synthetics. As a result of these studies, there is general agreement that nonabsorbable sutures are preferable for skin closure, but the type of nonabsorbable material may perhaps always remain a matter of personal preference. Localio, Casale, and Hinton (1943) observed little difference among wounds sutured with various nonabsorbable sutures.

5. TENSION. Intrinsic tension depends on the tightness of the suture in relation to the tissue mass it encompasses (Fig. 16–12). This is the tension referred to by most authorities. If the suture is too tight, local pressure gives rise to ischemia and to tissue necrosis with subsequent scar formation and visible suture marks. These marks may be punctate or actually linear. The edema of the encompassed tissue increases the effective tightness of the suture. Tension may also be affected by the suture size in that the heavier the suture material, the easier it is to apply excessive tension. A 6–0 suture has a limited tensile strength in itself as compared to a 2–0 suture and therefore can exert only a certain amount of tension before breaking. This does not imply that a smaller suture will not cause tissue necrosis and suture marks; it is only a comparison between the possible abuse of small and large sutures.

The mass of the tissue included in a skin suture may also make a difference. The greater the bulk of tissue or the farther from the cut skin edge the suture is placed, the greater the force needed to approximate the edges. Also, there is then a greater bulk of tissue which may become edematous after the suture has been placed.

Extrinsic tension pertains to the tensions applied to the cut surfaces themselves. Inasmuch as the sutures, while in place, are sustaining the approximation of the cut edges, the force applied against the cut surfaces is transmitted through the sutures to the tissues encompassed (Fig. 16–12). These tensions are influenced by the direction of the incision in relation to the normal skin tension lines and by the tensions on the edges being approximated. The latter are partly dependent on the size of the gap to be sutured and the looseness of the cut edges. Thus, undermining has been advised to relieve tension. Movement of a sutured incision that runs at right angles to the skin tension lines will exert forces away from the center. Rest and immobilization while the sutures are in place may help to eliminate these extrinsic tension forces and exert an influence on the prevention of suture marks.

Control of Factors Causing Suture Marks. With the exception of tension, these factors are variables not always controllable by the surgeon. Keloid formation is inherent in a given individual. Stitch abscesses may reflect an error in skin preparation or operative technique or may arise from too much tension. They can occur even in the most guarded situations. The type of skin sutured will depend on the anatomical location, and little can be done to change this. The type of suture material certainly can be altered, but clinically there is as yet insufficient evidence for stating that one type is more likely to cause suture marks than another type.

The variable factors under control of the surgeon are the size of the suture needle, the size of the suture, and the number of days the sutures are left in place. These factors were investigated (Crikelair, 1958), using transverse thoracoabdominal incisions in white male patients. With varying combinations of needles and sutures the wounds were sutured, and the sutures were removed at varying intervals. Regardless of the size of the needle or the size of the suture, the severe marks in all instances were caused by the sutures which were left in place 14 days. Those removed at or before seven days left no appreciable permanent mark. The marks made by the 14-day sutures were all about the same size. Most of the

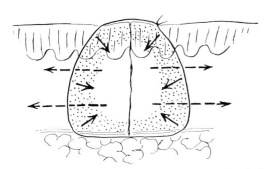

FIGURE 16–12. If the suture is tied too tightly, the intrinsic tension is toward the center, and ischemia and necrosis occur in the encompassed tissue, as shown by the stippled area. If extrinsic tension tends to distract the wound edges, the force is away from the center, but the adversely affected tissue area is the same.

marks were round; a few were slightly more linear.

In some instances fewer sutures were used, and they were placed at a greater distance from the cut surfaces and from each other. This resulted in tension and some bunching of the cut edges. Sutures removed early, despite the initial bunching of the cut edges and the slight reaction about points of exit of the sutures from the skin, left practically no visible marks.

In plastic surgery, small instruments, sutures, and suture needles are generally used. This is in part due to the delicacy of the work. However, on occasion larger needles and sutures may be helpful. Where needed they may be employed, since neither the size of the suture nor the size of the suture needle appears to be a cause of suture marks. In general, if sutures are properly placed without tension and the other causes of suture marks are reasonably eliminated, those sutures left in beyond seven days are more likely to cause suture marks. If sutures are placed under tension, removal within seven days may avoid suture marks. Usually sutures tied without tension, with the wound immobilized, can be left until the seventh day at least without causing suture marks. By this time enough tensile strength has developed in the wound so that it can maintain itself, although some support to the wound with adhesive tape is advisable for a longer period of time. Obviously, these are not "all or none" laws but aids in thinking and planning in our surgery where fine scars and the absence of suture marks are so important.

KELOIDS

The most carefully planned and executed plastic surgical procedure is from time to time defeated by keloid formation. In the surgical treatment of patients with painful, pruritic, unsightly keloids the best efforts of the plastic surgeon are, in a substantial proportion of cases, insufficient to prevent recurrence. Keloid formation is a problem with elements common to the investigation of wound healing and the study of neoplasia. The suffering of the individuals affected and the fundamental importance of the subject challenge the inadequacy of our present knowledge (Fig. 16–13).

Characteristics of Keloids. A keloid is an abnormal fibrous proliferation localized in the dermis and characterized by elevation, extension laterally into the surrounding normal tissue, continued, albeit intermittent, growth, absence of significant regression, and a profound tendency to recur after excision. Symptoms of pruritus and pain are present at some time in most lesions. Ulceration is rarer; small areas of infection with draining sinus tracts, skin bridges, and pockets are somewhat more common. Early in development or during periods of active growth, the lesions tend to be tense, reddish, or violaceous in hue with moderate vascularization, and small blood vessels are visible beneath the skin surface. Later in development and during quiescent periods, the keloid is less tense and vascularized but remains elevated and firmer than normal tissue. The lesions have a definite predilection for the upper half of the body, with the head, neck, chest, shoulder, and arm being the most common sites (Cosman and associates, 1961; Crockett, 1964). Within this area there is a centripetal distribution, with the midline of the body—the head, neck, and chest—having the greatest density of lesions. The sternal region is the most common site of keloids arising from inapparent trauma. However, abdominal scars are also frequent sites of keloid formation, especially in the umbilical and pubic extensions. In general, keloids tend to grow along rather than across skin lines, whatever the initial orientation of the lesion.

While many keloids are clinically unmistakable, it must be emphasized that some of their clinical characteristics are shared by hypertrophic scars. The hypertrophic scar is elevated, vascular, reddish, tense, pruritic, and painful, and early in its course it shows signs of growth. Such scars may recur after excision, especially if those local factors, such as tension or shape, initially responsible for the excessive scar formation are not altered in the revision. The distinctive signs of a keloid—the lack of regression with time, the tendency to recurrence, and the extension into normal tissue laterally—are events in time that immediate clinical observation cannot establish. It is therefore not possible clinically to differentiate a hypertrophic scar from a keloid in every instance.

Pathology. Pathologically, the keloid is a poorly circumscribed, dense connective tissue mass located in the dermis. This dermal location appears significant in that submucosal keloids are rare or nonexistent. Our experience includes no keloids occurring primarily be-

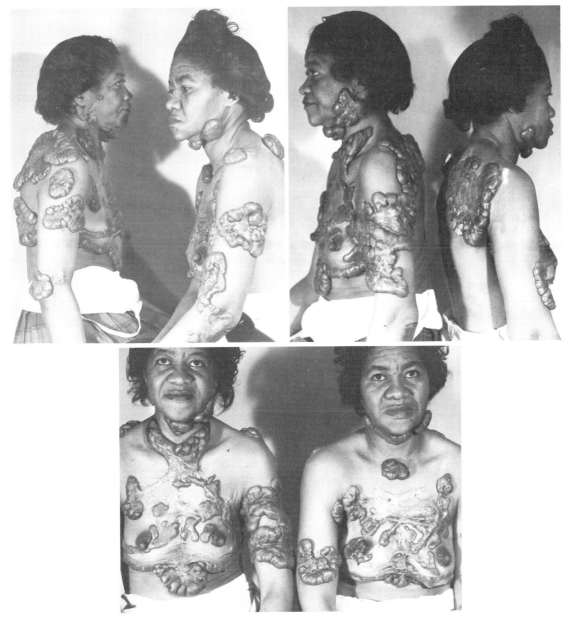

FIGURE 16–13. Severe keloid formation in identical twins. Note similar locations of the keloids in each despite different initiating traumas. Their mother and maternal grandmother also had keloids.

neath mucosa, and the few reports in the literature do not sustain critical examination (Sedgewick, 1861; De Beurmann and Gougerot, 1906; Mook, 1924; Schmidt, 1934; Strand, 1945). The specialized skins of the eyelids, areola, and penis, which have thin, highly modified dermal layers, are also relatively free of keloid formation, although rare cases have been described (Parsons, 1966).

The stratified epithelial layer overlying the dermal lesion is flattened and often thinned. Rete pegs as well as dermal papillae may be absent, and epithelial appendages are either reduced in number or are absent. Elastic fibrils also are usually absent. Characteristically there are abnormally broad, swollen, eosinophilic, interlacing, glassy-appearing collagen fibers forming the mass of the lesion (Fig. 16–14). The margin between the lesion and the surrounding tissue has been the object of much

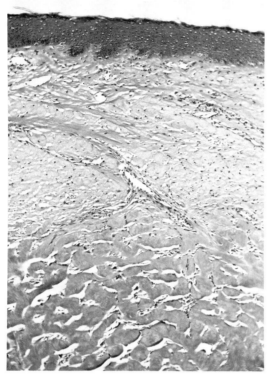

FIGURE 16–14. Photomicrograph of a keloid lesion with characteristic broad, eosinophilic, glassy, hyalin-like collagen fibers and a poorly defined border of more normal connective tissue between it and the flattened overlying epithelium, which lacks rete pegs and accessory skin structures. × 110.

study and varying interpretation. Some view the keloid as extending into surrounding tissue by expansion and describe the margin as discrete and formed of compressed but normal scar tissue (Heidingsfeld, 1909). Other interpretations suggest a progressive transformation of surrounding scar into the characteristic keloid morphology (Sylven, 1945). Various estimates of mast cell frequency and activity around the keloid lesion have also been offered (Sylven, 1945; Robinson and Hamilton, 1953).

The exact point of origin of a keloid remains obscure. It has been suggested that the lesions form in the adventitia of blood vessels and the branching spread of the keloid is a consequence (Crocker, 1886; Unna, 1896). The connective tissue of the corium (Geschickter and Lewis, 1935) and the fibrous envelopes of sweat glands and hair follicles (Heidingsfeld, 1909) have also been mentioned. Small bundles of abnormal collagen fibers have been noted in the dermis in early keloid lesions (Gaulin and Lattes, 1960). Normal scar fiber morphology, however, seemed to shade imper-

ceptibly into that of keloid, according to other authors (Mancini and Quaife, 1962). The appearance of the fibroblasts on routine histologic section of keloids is unremarkable. Mitotic activity is not marked in early keloids and is very rare in mature lesions. Anderson (1888) and Horton (1953) have reported cancer developing in keloids, but in the first instance the lesion appears to have been a fibrosarcoma from onset, and in the second, the tumor was a basal cell carcinoma in the skin of an irradiated keloid. Only a single authentic case of sarcomatous degeneration in a keloid has been reported (Biemans, 1963).

Historically, keloids were first described by Alibert in 1806. He termed them cancer-like—"les cancroïdes." In 1816 he introduced the name "chéloïde," referring both to the clawlike extension of the lesions and to their tendency to grow laterally into normal tissue, thus moving sideward like crabs. In 1825 he entitled the chapter of his dermatologic text, "Les Cancroïdes ou Kéloides," using the latter word for the first time in the form in which it was later taken up by English, American, and German authors.

While Alibert's description was classic, no definitive histologic correlation was established. This problem became increasingly difficult as clinical subdivisions multiplied. Thus, a distinction was drawn between "true" or spontaneous keloids and "false" ones, those arising from known trauma. Further, Addison (1854) described as "true keloids" the lesions of what we now know as morphea or scleroderma and called Alibert's lesions "false." Additional confusion arose with the practice of dividing the lesions as to anatomical location, physical configuration, and precise nature of the initiating trauma.

In the course of time these clinical distinctions have been critically reviewed and dropped. It has been recognized that an initiating trauma, however minor, can usually be found for any keloid and that keloids of whatever etiology have profound similarities in clinical behavior. However, the early attempts to find pathologic distinctions to fit the clinical ones engendered the impression that the pathologist's difficulty in distinguishing keloids from scars was so great as to preclude his help in diagnosis and prognosis.

This last point of view is distinctly counter to our experience (Cosman and associates, 1961). On review of our surgical treatment of 340 keloids, or lesions termed so clinically, we found a striking correlation between the pathologic diagnosis and the clinical results of treatment. Our pathology laboratory employed the single criterion of the presence of the characteristic broad, eosinophilic, hyalin-like collagen fibers in diagnosing a keloid. Lesions so diagnosed had a 47 per cent recurrence rate, as compared to only 17 per cent in lesions with the pathologic diagnosis of scar or "doubtful." We have therefore come to view the pathologic examination as most significant in resolving the clinical uncertainty in the diagnosis and prognosis of hypertrophic scars and keloids (Blackburn and Cosman, 1966).

Incidence. The absence of pathologic confirmation of clinical impressions clouds most studies of the keloid problem. Thus the actual incidence of keloids in any large population group remains undetermined. In samples in the Swiss population, Naeglie (1931) reported a clinical incidence of 4.5 per cent in children and 13.3 per cent in adults. It was reported that 3.4 per cent of the children on the island of Aruba had keloids (Bernstein, 1964). These figures seem higher than our experience suggests. While keloids are certainly more frequent in Negroes than in white persons, the relatively asymptomatic nature of many keloids and the unwillingness of most individuals to lose time seeking treatment for minor problems must be kept in mind in evaluating figures for relative incidences in the two races. This point was made by Matas (1896) in his monograph in which, on the basis of ten cases seen over a ten-year period and corrected for hospital admission rates, he reached the now widely quoted ratio of nine Negroes with keloids to each white person. In similar fashion ratios ranging from 6:1 to 18.7:1 have been calculated (Geschickter and Lewis, 1935). The inherent limitations of these studies as well as our own prevent a statistically significant statement.

Etiology. Many etiologic factors have been held responsible for keloid formation. The heavy scars following the healing of draining tuberculous lymph nodes and syphilitic lesions led to an early association with these lesions. No present evidence, however, supports this concept.

Because of the greater incidence of treated keloids in women and because of the apparent peak of case incidence noted in the immediate postpubertal years, the possibility of female hormone influence on keloid formation has been advanced. However, it is in both this sex and this age group that treatment for cosmetic blemishes is most likely to be sought. Further, the practice of ear piercing may contribute to early female cases (Cosman and Wolff, 1974). In our series the treated lesions were preponderantly in women, but no peak incidence was noted when the time of onset of the lesions was considered rather than the age when treatment was begun. In addition, the median age of onset was about 22 years, and was the same in both sexes. Laboratory evidence of high estrogenic content in keloid tissue (Geschickter and Lewis, 1935) has not been confirmed. Cutaneous keloid lesions have not been produced by high estrogen administration in laboratory animals (Vargas, 1943). Hormonal influence has been cited by Jacobsson (1948) and Edgerton, Hanrahan, and Davis (1951), who observed instances of the growth of keloids during pregnancy.

The hyperthyroid state has been linked with keloid tendency by Justus (1919), but no major series including our own bears out this association. No confirmation exists for the suggestion of an abnormality in parathyroid function in keloid patients (Pautrier and Zorn, 1931). Similar lack of confirmation exists for Marshall and Rosenthal's (1943) concept of local or general accumulations of tissue fluids resulting in "herniations of the integument," i.e. keloids. The same authors also claimed that inspissated blood was the cause of keloids. The notion of mucopolysaccharide-induced plasma clots and consequent vascular and lymphatic stasis advanced by Barnard, Garnes, and Oppenheim (1961) is also speculative. That some factor in the serum of keloid patients accelerates fibroblast proliferation was suggested by Robinson, Corbett, and Hamilton (1952, 1953) but later denied. An autoimmunologic etiology has been suggested by Chytilova, Kulhanek, and Horn (1959) but remains conjectural.

Race and heredity seem more important in keloid susceptibility than any other general factors known. The prevalence of keloids in Negroes is a matter of general agreement. The view of Bohrod (1937) that sexual selection in African Negro tribes practicing scarification favored development of the racial characteristic of heavy scarring has been widely, if tacitly, accepted though without ethnographic confirmation. In addition, it must be noted that earth and pigment are regularly introduced into these scarification wounds, and the amount of these materials tends to regulate the bulk of the scars which lack the spreading characteristics of keloids (Lacassagne and Rousset, 1931; Lespinne, 1931).

The literature on family groups with keloids in several generations has been well summarized by Bloom (1956) and by Goeminne (1968). However, few of our patients gave such histories, and in other large series a similar paucity of positive family histories has been noted. That this may represent a deficiency in history-taking is possible, or it may be that hereditary influence is not strong in the usual patient with keloids. It is certainly true that some of our patients with severest involvement have had positive family histories (see Fig. 16–13).

Local factors appear to play a significant part in the problem because many individuals with keloids have other scars whose behavior and appearance is normal. Importance has been attached to the tension on the wound, the wound's orientation relative to skin lines, the presence or absence of infection, and the achievement of primary healing. A most significant contribution concerned with local factors in keloid formation was that of Glücksman (1951). In the examination of hypertrophic scars and keloids, he frequently found foreign body reactions with hair and endogenous keratinized material. Based on this, the suggestion was advanced that lanugo caught up in wounds was the factor of prime importance in hypertrophic scarring (Mowlem, 1951). The failure to distinguish between scars and keloids and the absence of clinical follow-up weaken this argument. Few others have noted so high an incidence of foreign body reaction, and slow disappearance of deliberately buried dermal elements has been well demonstrated (Thompson, 1960). Another intriguing observation of local influence is that of Calnan and Copenhagen (1967), who autotransplanted the skin of histologically diagnosed excised keloids. Keloids recurred at the excision sites but did not occur at the skin recipient locations. This supports the safety of the use of the keloidal skin as a graft when this is technically feasible (Cosman and coworkers, 1961; Sugawara and Hashimoto, 1967).

Of great interest insofar as local alterations are concerned is the report by Conway, Gillette, and Findley (1959) and Conway, Gillette, Smith, and Findley (1960) of an "abnormal" fibroblast in tissue cultures of keloids. This finding, which could make the cellular study of keloids possible, has not yet been verified. Another technique applied to keloid material is that of paper chromatography (Woringer and Zimmer, 1958). No marked alteration from normal connective tissue was noted, but increase in tissue water in keloids and some qualitative differences in peptides and in amino acids was observed. Quantitative electrolyte differences between keloids, scars, and normal skin have been investigated, with calcium reported to be present in greater amounts in keloids than in normal scar or skin (Psillakis and associates, 1971). Some histochemical studies have not revealed profound differences between scars and keloids (Kurnatovski and Pruszcynski, 1968). On the other hand, significant findings have been reported by others. Acid phosphatase activity in keloid nodules in the reticular layer was found to be increased tenfold over that in normal connective tissue (Im and Hoopes, 1971). Glucose-6-phosphate dehydrogenase levels have been reported to be markedly elevated in both keloids and hypertrophic scars as compared to normal scar. Of possible diagnostic importance is the further observation that alanine transaminase activity in keloid epithelium is twice the normal, whereas it is not increased in epithelium overlying hypertrophic scars (Hoopes, Su and Im, 1971). More recently, keloid proline hydroxylase activity has been reported to be thrice that of hypertrophic scars, while collagenase activity was only twice as great (Ketchum, Cohen and Masters, 1974). Additional work remains to be done in these areas of investigation.

Results of Treatment. Unfortunately, the clinical study of the keloid problem and evaluation of therapy have been handicapped by a surprising lack of documentation of the long-term course of treated and untreated lesions. The necessity for long periods of follow-up has been demonstrated in our material by the finding of a median period from excision to recurrence of 12.9 months. Many factors previously thought to influence the results of excision proved of no importance in our experience. Thus, prognosis did not vary significantly with any one anatomical location if the pathologic diagnosis was keloid. The race of the patient did not influence the result of excision. The same proved true so far as the size of the lesion, the preoperative duration, or the nature of initiating trauma was concerned. While what was clinically termed a "burn keloid" proved to be a hypertrophic scar pathologically somewhat more frequently than was true of the other clinically diagnosed keloid lesions, the prognosis of a burn-induced keloid was no better than that of any other keloid lesion. Surprisingly too, the presence of another keloid or nonkeloid scar in an individual who had one lesion surgically excised proved of no help in the prognosis of the excision result. The pathologic diagnosis of the excised lesion was the significant factor. A slightly poorer success rate, however, was noted in those individuals with multiple other keloids. Patients whose major complaints were pruritus, pain, or recent growth of lesion had higher recurrence rates than patients without these symptoms and signs. The lower success rate in all these groups, however, did not seem great enough to contraindicate an attempt at treatment. The same was true in our group of recurrent lesions. Reoperation was attended by about the same rate of success as in lesions never treated before. There was no correlation between completeness of local excision and lesion recurrence, nor, in retrospect, was there any way of distinguishing the recurring from the nonrecurring member of excised pairs of earlobe keloids (Cosman and Wolff, 1972, 1974).

The limited success of any therapy was as well known to Alibert (1806) as to all who have subsequently treated keloids. Excision alone without adjuvant treatment has had no specific advocates. Excision and skin grafting has been reported favorably (Goldman, 1901; Krieger, 1958), but our results do not support the claims for the special efficacy of this method. In addition, those of our patients with keloids treated in this way showed a 46 per cent incidence of keloid formation in the donor sites. Our attempts to use the skin surface of the keloid as a graft for the excision site have not, as yet, shown any special success and occasionally have been technically difficult. Others have reported more favorably on this technique (Sugawara and Hashimoto, 1967). The effectiveness of intrakeloidal excision, as well as claims for special suture or nonsuture methods, has yet to be investigated systematically.

Method of Treatment. The combination of therapies used most widely in the past is excision and postoperative X-ray therapy. De Beurmann and Gougerot (1906), Freund (1913), and Wickham and Degrais (1913) were early proponents of this method. The original use of preoperative X-ray therapy in addition to postoperative X-ray was claimed by Gillies (Levitt and Gillies, 1942).

In our series, dose schedules of 800 R in four parts pre- and postoperatively, using varying factors of kilovoltage and filtration, were the rule, although a substantial number of patients received no X-ray therapy at all. Review of our results demonstrated that histopathologic diagnosis was far more significant than the administration or the lack of X-ray therapy in achieving eradication of the keloid. However, those lesions that received some irradiation did slightly better than those that received none. There appeared to be no advantage to the combination of preoperative and postoperative treatment as compared to early postoperative X-ray therapy alone. In the group of irradiated lesions, our observations do suggest that irradiation was most efficacious if given within the period of two weeks following excision. This time factor is supported by other studies, and there are indications that high doses of X-ray therapy (1000 to 1500 R) are needed if the treatment is to be most meaningful (Arnold and Grauer, 1958; Van Den Brenk and Minty, 1960). Postexcisional irradiation by iridium 192 in a plastic tube implanted at the time of wound closure has been reported, but there is no reason to believe this technique will be better than more conventional modes of radiotherapy (Caronni, 1967).

Large series using X-ray or radium therapy alone or in combination have been presented. Since the pathologic diagnosis of the treated lesions was not verified, it is difficult to assess the results. Where detailed figures are available, as in Jacobsson's series (1948), the suggestion is strong that the successfully treated lesions were hypertrophic scars and not keloids. The success rates with those lesions that appear to have been keloids are strikingly similar to those we have achieved, as well as to those achieved by others. It must be emphasized, however, that X-ray therapy, in common with a wide variety of other agents, including vitamin E (Edgerton, Hanrahan and Davis, 1951), vitamin K (Mienicki and Kossakowska, 1963), and ultrasonic energy (Kuitert and coworkers, 1955), seems able temporarily at least to alleviate symptoms of pain and pruritus. In the present state of our knowledge, the use of roentgen therapy in this way and with adequate shielding cannot be condemned.

Enzyme therapy using hyaluronidase alone and in combination with other substances (Cornbleet, 1954) has enjoyed a brief vogue but has proved unsatisfactory in most hands. Other abandoned enzymatic agents have included fibrinolysin, pepsin, turtle bile, and Kutapressin. The oral use of tetrahydroxyquinone has had less than the originally promised success (Kelly and Pinkus, 1958; Sheard, 1961; Kelly, 1963). Application of nitrogen mustard–like agents either locally or intralesionally has had some proponents (Fischl, 1965; Ehlers and Knoth, 1966).

Of greater significance has been the development of local and systemic hormone therapy employing ACTH and adrenal steroid derivatives introduced by Conway and Stark in 1951. Asboe-Hansen (1956) favorably reported the use of hydrocortisone injected locally, and the use of local ointment on the open wound and on the healing wound later was reported by Feller (1959). Reports such as those of Whitehill (1954) on the prophylactic use of hydrocortisone ointment on abdominal wounds and the work of Mancini, Stringa, and Canepa (1960) suggested that very early or very prolonged treatment was useful.

Highly favorable reports of the intralesional use of triamcinolone acetonide have appeared, but the number of pathologically proven cases treated remains small (Maguire, 1965; Griffith, 1966; Ketchum and coworkers, 1966; Minkowitz, 1967). Nevertheless, it is clear that steroids are valuable agents in keloid therapy. While no one agent has been demonstrated to be clearly superior to all others, triamcinolone acetonide has been the most widely used. The consensus favors the use of suspensions rather than soluble forms (Barra, Mouly and Dufourmentel, 1973). Injection of steroid locally by needle or by pressure jet apparatus alone or accompanied by local anesthetic or hyaluronidase is the most usual mode of administration (Vallis, 1967; Griffith, Monroe and McKinney, 1970; Ketchum and coworkers, 1971). Three therapeutic regimens may be distinguished: intralesional injection alone; excision and intraoperative wound margin injection; excision, wound injection, and postoperative injection as well. The experience of the authors with intralesional injection alone has been less favorable than that reported by others (Ketchum and coworkers, 1971) in so far as control of lesion growth is concerned; relief of the symptoms of pruritus and pain seems to be comparable to that achieved by X-ray therapy under the same circumstances. In young patients and over areas of bone growth or endocrine gland location, it may be wiser to avoid the use of X-ray. Steroids are the therapy of choice if excision has been ruled out because of the size and position of the keloid or by patient choice. There has been less evaluation of excision combined with wound injection than of the regimen of excision, wound injection, and postoperative injection. The latter is the more commonly chosen course (Griffith and coworkers, 1970; Ketchum and coworkers, 1974). Most authorities report injecting steroid post-

operatively one or more times starting at a variable time within the first three postoperative weeks. Maximum doses have been suggested for single lesions (Ketchum and coworkers, 1974), but it is not truly known what the limits of therapy should be either in terms of single treatments or in terms of multiple injections. At present, the authors are evaluating a program of excision, intraoperative injection, and postoperative injection, with institution of the latter at the first, second, and third weeks after excision. Further three-week courses are given if scar pruritus increases steadily and/or if scar hypertrophy appears to be recurring. For all such studies, however, strict control and adequate follow-up and definitive pathologic diagnosis are required if the results are to be significant.

Hypertrophic scars were treated by compression by Dupuytren (1832), and Fujimori, Hiramoto, and Ofuji (1968) advocated compression treatment of hypertrophic scars of the lower extremity. Custom-made elasticized conforming masks (Jobst) have reduced the degree of hypertrophic scar formation following facial burns (Larson and associates, 1973). The technique is discussed in detail in Chapter 33.

SCAR REVISION

A scar has three components—line, contour, and color. Each of these elements contributes in varying degree to the overall defect. The relative importance of each, subjectively for the patient and objectively so far as the surgeon is concerned, helps to determine the appropriate operative procedure, as well as the extent to which surgical intervention is either feasible or desirable.

The line of a scar though "fine" may be distinctly visible on the face and may subtly alter appearance. Its linear form "catches the eye." Or the scar may be prominent because it passes through malaligned normal structures. A scar line may be noticeable because it is wide or spread (Fig. 16–15). Of some interest is the fact that this latter type of scar is called "hypertrophic" by English authors (Mowlem, 1951), whereas we reserve this term for an enlarged, elevated scar.

The scar contour, or the scar's effect on the contour of surrounding tissue, may be the significant feature. The scar may be depressed (Fig. 16–16) and so be noticeable. Elevation or hypertrophy may be the complaint (Fig. 16–17). Contracted scars are often elevated (Fig.

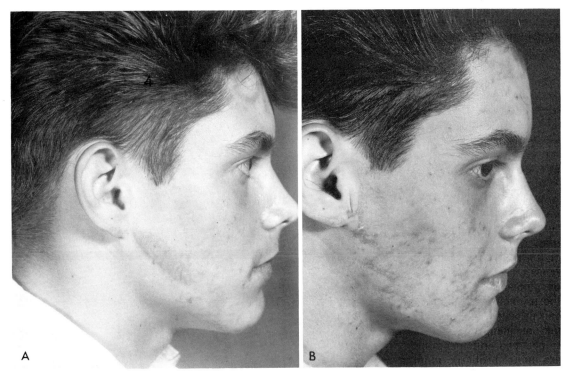

FIGURE 16–15. Spread scar (*A*) crossing the skin lines. Eleven months after revision (*B*) accomplished by step excision with least spread of the scar elements placed in the skin lines.

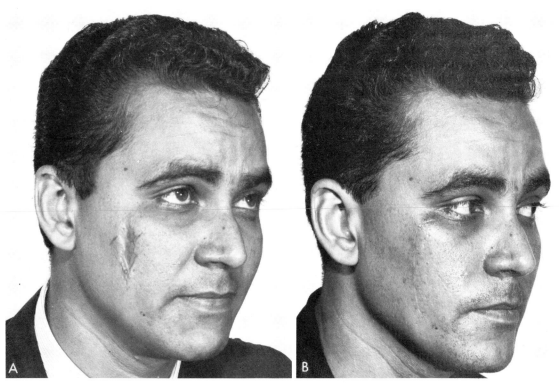

FIGURE 16–16. Depressed scar (*A*) treated by excision of scar skin, wide undermining, and direct advancement of the wound margins over the residual dermal scar (*B*) with the closure in the appropriate skin lines.

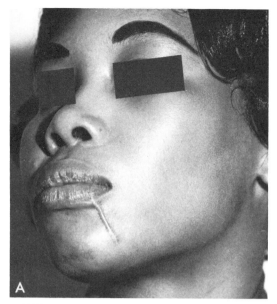

FIGURE 16–17. Hypertrophic scar producing slight deformity of the lip. Note that the hypertrophy extends up to but not within the vermilion.

16–18). They may displace mobile linear structures such as the eyebrows or they may distort lips or eyelids. The contour alteration may take the form of the trapdoor effect (Figs. 16–6 and 16–19).

The scar may be obtrusive because of a color difference as compared to the surround-ing area. A red childhood scar, a depigmented scar in dark skin, and a darkly pigmented scar in a lighter skin area (Fig. 16–20) are examples of this. The color difference may be consequent upon the presence of retained foreign bodies—a traumatic tattoo (Crawford, 1953).

In selecting scars for treatment, attention must be paid not only to the features of the defect as seen objectively but also to the element of the defect most disturbing to the patient. A scar line is the inevitable result of any surgical excision. If, for instance, the patient is a woman belonging to an ethnic group for whom any facial scar has the implication of discovered adultery, the substitution of a multiple Z-plasty line for the previous scar will hardly prove satisfactory. The complete scar erasure the patient desires cannot be achieved (Crikelair and Cosman, 1964).

In understanding a scar defect from the patient's point of view, however, it is sometimes unexpectedly revealing to view the scar as the patient himself sees it, that is, through a mirror. A scar that seems insignificant when seen by the examiner in a three dimensional view may have a quite different aspect in the two dimensional reflector. In some cases of minimal defects which the mirror magnifies, it may become necessary to convince the patient that others see a three dimensional view and not the mirror's image.

The timing of scar treatment also bears a

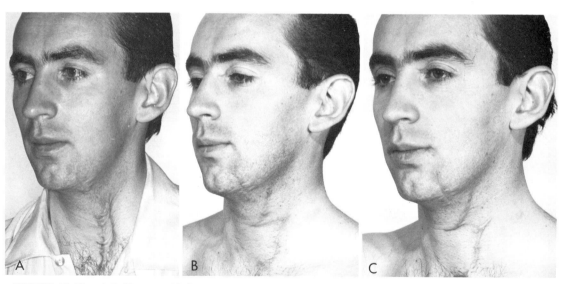

FIGURE 16–18. *A, B,* Hypertrophied scar contracture corrected by excision and Z-plasty. *C,* Recurrent hypertrophy of portions of the scar eight months following operation.

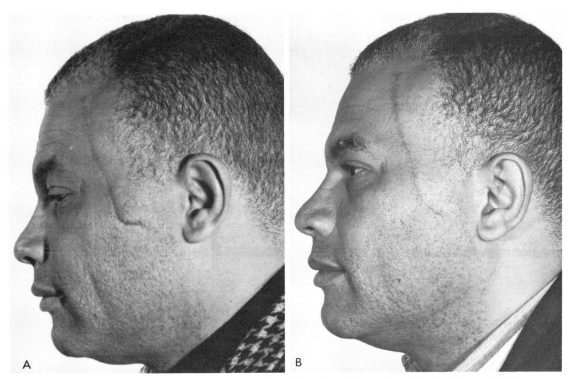

FIGURE 16–19. Trapdoor scar of cheek (*A*) treated by elliptical excision and straight line closure. (*B*) Appearance ten months later.

relation to the nature of the predominating element of the defect. Linear defects associated with malalignment are entitled to early repair, since no spontaneous improvement in the basic problem can be anticipated. Similarly, a spread scar does not show a tendency to become thinner with the passage of time, although other of its elements, such as color, may improve. On

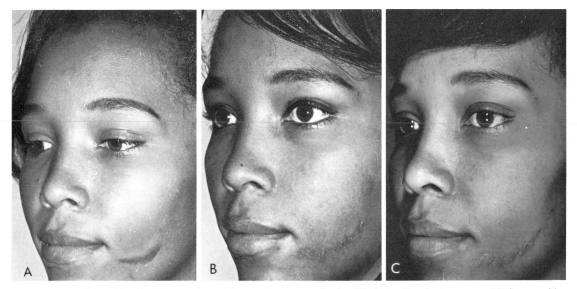

FIGURE 16–20. *A*, Darkly pigmented spread scar; *B*, one month after W-plasty. Result at one year (*C*) is marred by slight hypertrophy of scar and artificiality of zigzag line on face.

the other hand, early scar depression may become ameliorated, and hypertrophic scars will flatten. Contracted scars producing distortion are deserving of early repair. Trapdoor scars will not show significant improvement once the effect becomes apparent. Color contrasts, however, may be expected to improve with time, and delay in repair is justified. As mentioned earlier, toned cosmetics are of value during this period (Thorne, 1966).

The methods of scar excision are legion, yet in essence limited. Basically one can simply excise a scar and close the wound, or one can excise and replace the area. Within these categories, however, several subgroups may be distinguished for the sake of discussion, although the distinctions are somewhat artificial.

Simple excision and closure is useful in instances of depressed scars of limited width and in cases of spread scars of similarly limited dimension. However, the scar so treated must already be in proper skin lines, else it becomes necessary to redirect the scar line and the ex-

cision becomes complex. Further, the undermining to achieve closure without tension, a vital part of successful revisional surgery, requires the mobilization of deeper layers in the wound. The layered closure of the wound then introduces an element of tissue replacement into the "simple excision."

Multiple partial excisions of wide defects have been advocated by Morestin (1915), Davis (1919), and Sistrunk (1927). More recent advocates of this approach include Vilain (1965) and Webster (1969). Wide undermining for closure, repeated procedures, and the necessary limitation of these measures to areas of soft tissue redundancy make the method of infrequent application in routine scar revision.

Split-thickness excision is useful in some instances and may take two forms. The scar may be denuded of epithelium and a portion of dermis, leaving the bulk of the dermal and subcutaneous scar in place. The surrounding skin and subcutaneous tissue is undermined and advanced over the remaining scar (see Fig. 16–16).

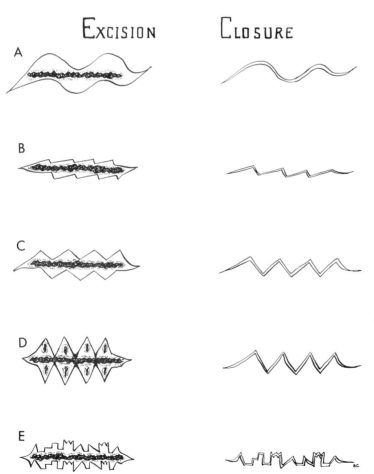

Excision   Closure

A

B

C

D

E

FIGURE 16–21. *A,* Multiple curve excision. Note the large amount of normal tissue to be excised in order that significant alteration of scar direction be achieved. *B,* Step excision. *C,* W-plasty. *D,* Diamond excision including suture marks. In closure the upper and lower lines of triangles are shifted on each other, and the result, after modification of the ends of the excision, is similar to *C. E,* Geometric broken line closure employing small triangular, rectangular, and square flaps.

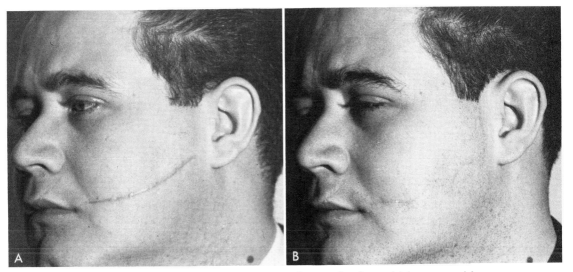

FIGURE 16-22. *A,* Long scar of cheek; *B,* five months after multiple curve excision.

Shallow, depressed scars may be treated by this method introduced by Poulard (1918). The safety of burying dermal grafts has been demonstrated (Thompson, 1960), and, in any case, scar tissue in general lacks or is deficient in accessory skin structures likely to produce cysts. The latter, however, appear to be a definite problem if any substantial amount of epithelium is buried (Reid, 1952).

Split-thickness scar excision can also be combined with dermis grafting and/or skin grafting over the partially excised area. This technique was proposed for the treatment of unstable scars by Hynes (1957) (see Chapters 6 and 33). This method has been used for broad scars of irregular contour and pigmentation (Serafini, 1962). The cosmetic limitations of the procedure preclude its general applicability (Pigott, 1968).

The most useful methods of surgical treatment of scars in our practice may be classified as complex excisions. In the case of a scar crossing skin lines, multiple Z-plasties may be used to redirect portions of the scar into proper lines. For the same reason this method is useful in instances where a scar has spread as a result of skin tension directed across it transversely (see Fig. 16-15). The Z-plasty, of course, has its most striking application in the correction of elevated scar contractures (see Fig. 16-18).

An effect somewhat similar to that of the Z-plasty in redirecting portions of a long scar lying across skin lines, but without the inter-position of tissue, can be achieved by excising the scar in a predetermined pattern of multiple interlocking curves (Figs. 16-21 and 16-22). This method is essentially analogous to that of interlocking steps, that called "W-plasty" by Borges (1959), and that of interdigitating diamonds advocated by Penn (1960) for the removal of suture mark scars. The curving scar is somewhat more natural in final appearance than that of these other methods. It suffers from the objection that to be effective in redirecting the scar line the curves must be large ones, and the amount of tissue sacrificed in the initial excision is greater; the possibility of a trapdoor effect in the curves also exists. The geometric broken line closure of Webster (1969), which employs small triangular, rectangular, and square flaps in irregular sequence, also seeks to gain the advantage of the Z-plasty in scar line redirection while avoiding its disadvantageous artificial look (Fig. 16-22).

Another form of complex excision is required in the case of trapdoor scars. Here the effect of the curved scar's contracting forces can be broken by multiple Z-plasties or by step excisions. A more certain means, however, is the staged excision of the borders of the trapdoor in noncontinuous, simple, elliptical excisions. This alters the trapdoor to a triangular or to a rectangular flap (see Fig. 16-19).

The treatment of scars with minor degrees of depression has already been mentioned. However, deep subcutaneous tissue losses beneath scars can be replaced by dermis-fat grafts, or, rarely, dermis-fat flaps may be needed. We have also employed rolled or folded dermis grafts for the same purpose in depressed scars. The use of muscle flaps and of bone or cartilage grafts in depressed scars appropriately located for their employment has also proved useful. The use of foreign materials, such as Silastic, in either solid or injectable form is discussed in Chapter 15. Replacement of scarred areas by skin grafts or by local or distant flaps with and without skin grafts is beyond the scope of this chapter. Such replacement techniques are more appropriate to the treatment of broad areas of tissue loss than to the isolated scars under discussion here.

Scars which are significantly elevated are best excised. Minor degrees of elevation are very frequent, however. This is especially true in the multiple tiny trapdoor scars often seen after windshield glass injuries. Shaving or dermabrasion (see Chapter 17) is very useful in these cases. Indeed, this technique often has a role in scar revisions being carried out primarily by other means. It is also of importance in treating traumatic tattoos (Crawford, 1953).

As to the actual mechanics of wound closure and the nature of suture materials, as has already been indicated, there is little that should be stated dogmatically. These details will perhaps always remain a matter of preference for each surgeon.

Complications of Scar Revision

Scar revision procedures are subject to all of the usual operative complications as well as to some special problems. Prime among the general complications are those of hemorrhage and postoperative hematoma formation. Such bleeding is, in the ordinary instance, not life-endangering, involving as it does small, superficial vessels of the skin and subcutaneous tissue. However, if the revision is being carried out within scar tissue, the oozing may often be most annoying and may complicate the operative result. Hemostasis is difficult to achieve in scarred tissue whose tiny vessels surrounded with scar do not retract, close, and clot but remain open and bleeding. Clamping and tying may be technically difficult; precise and meticulous electrocautery may be useful in some instances. Pressure on the wound for a brief period while it is covered with gauze soaked in epinephrine-containing solution may also be helpful. In spite of the natural disinclination to leave a drain site in a wound being revised, the use of a small rubber band drain removed early in the postoperative period (24 to 48 hours) may be the wisest course of management for even a small wound whose hemostasis remains uncertain.

Another general operative complication shared by scar revisions is that of infection. Several factors add to the normal potential for such an event. Not infrequently, the wound being revised has been acutely or chronically infected prior to its healing, albeit it has been healed for quite some time. The clinical impression that bacteria may reside in an area long after overt clinical signs of infection have subsided is a strong one. Reoperation in such a region may "light up" the inflammation. Further, the scarred area may have healed with many retained foreign bodies. Their presence further decreases the already reduced ability of scar tissue to sustain contamination without developing infection.

Wound dehiscence, early or late, is a complication of some scar revisions, especially those being done as stages in serial excisions of scarred area. Such wounds are of necessity being closed under some tension. Indeed, except in revision by replacement, most scar revisions must overcome the fact that tissue is being removed. Wide undermining, Z-plasties, and other local flaps are useful in avoiding such tense wound closures. Buttressing the wound closure by suturing the advanced wound margin to a residual sheet of scar dermis is, on occasion, a useful maneuver (Engdahl, 1968) (Fig. 16–23). Tape support and dressing immobilization are important aids.

Despite such techniques, upon removing the sutures, many a surgeon will still undergo the embarrassment of seeing the scar revision wound separate. Inaccuracies in suturing skin and dermal edges of differing thicknesses may lead to a "step" at the wound edge closure, an in-turning of epithelium which prevents dermal contact and so reduces the early development of wound tensile strength. A 1- to 2-mm edge undermining at the time of closure can permit easier coaptation of such unequal edges and also serve to allow more dermis-to-dermis apposition of the two edges (Fig. 16–23). Tape or collodion applied immediately upon suture removal is another means to avoid this complication (Uchida and Uchida, 1961).

In an occasional patient the complication of "suture allergy" occurs. Usually the problem occurs following the use of subcutaneous or subcuticular catgut. A red, swollen, tender

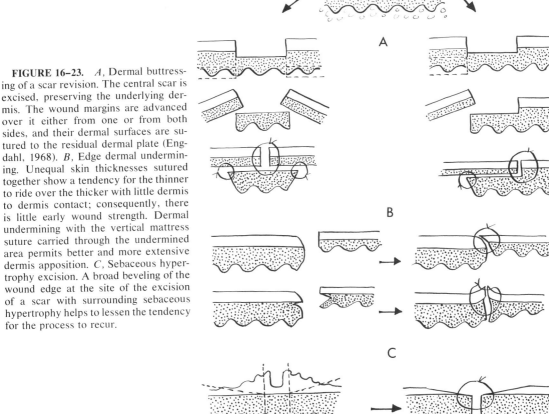

FIGURE 16–23. *A*, Dermal buttressing of a scar revision. The central scar is excised, preserving the underlying dermis. The wound margins are advanced over it either from one or from both sides, and their dermal surfaces are sutured to the residual dermal plate (Engdahl, 1968). *B*, Edge dermal undermining. Unequal skin thicknesses sutured together show a tendency for the thinner to ride over the thicker with little dermis to dermis contact; consequently, there is little early wound strength. Dermal undermining with the vertical mattress suture carried through the undermined area permits better and more extensive dermis apposition. *C*, Sebaceous hypertrophy excision. A broad beveling of the wound edge at the site of the excision of a scar with surrounding sebaceous hypertrophy helps to lessen the tendency for the process to recur.

wound is exposed on the first dressing. Subsequently, the wound may drain from several spots, and catgut sutures can be extracted from beneath the draining points. It is not possible to predict which patients will show this reaction to catgut. Milder forms with foreign body reactions around the buried suture material probably account for the occasional scar revision which, appearing satisfactory externally, is nevertheless complicated by the persistence of multiple firm nodules within the scar. Despite these occasional untoward reactions, catgut remains very useful for subcutaneous and subcuticular closure, since the technical difficulty of using monofilamentous nylon sutures subcutaneously, the discomfort of wire sutures beneath the skin, and the well-known tendency of silk sutures to be extruded make the use of such nonabsorbable materials less than completely desirable.

Sebaceous hypertrophy is another complication of scar revisions. This problem is most often seen in the revision of facial scars in patients with seborrhea and more generally in the revision of scars of the nasal tip. It is often said that scars of the tip of the nose tend to be "depressed." One can observe, however, that in many instances it is not the scar that is depressed, but rather there is such hypertrophy of the sebaceous glands adjacent to the scar that it appears as a valley between hills. The difficulty of overcoming this tendency of the incision to stimulate the sebaceous apparatus on the incision margins makes shaving or dermabrasion the preferred treatment of scars of this region. When excision and approximation become necessary, the beveling of the wound edges prior to their suture may sometimes be useful (Fig. 16–23, *C*).

Epithelial tunnels may complicate surgery, particularly in two areas. The thin eyelid skin appears to heal around sutures passed through it, so that in a very few days an epithelial lined tract remains to fill up with epithelial debris, forming a bump where each suture had been. While this process probably occurs to some degree in all sutured wounds (Gillman and Penn, 1956; Ordman and Gillman, 1966), the eyelid tracts do not disappear as do most others. The tracts must be unroofed, and occasionally a strip will have to be re-excised. The tip of the nose also exhibits this phenomenon in a slightly different form. An occasional suture hole becomes the permanent opening for deeper lying sebaceous glands to discharge through. Unfortunately, the use of such techniques as tape closure is especially difficult on the nasal tip, precisely because of the sebaceous activity of the area and the consequent difficulty of securing the tape.

An otherwise well-healed scar revision is sometimes marred by the development of firm, pearly white cysts along the scar line. These are milia and result from trapping of lanugo hair follicles in the scar tissue and beneath the epithelium. Usually small and self-limited in growth, they may reach a size of 2 to 3 mm. They are best treated by incising their thin overlying epithelium with a No. 11 blade, then extruding the tiny cyst and its lining.

Another troublesome form of adnexal structure trapping is that which may occur after scar revisions in the beard area. Especially in the revision of burn scars of this area, hair follicles caught up in the scar may grow in disoriented fashion, piercing or reentering the epithelium at odd angles and leading to frequent small foreign body reactions and folliculitis. It may be necessary to excise an entire area and resurface it with a skin graft in order to overcome this annoyance. The reverse of this problem is the more usual complication resulting from scar revisions in hair-bearing areas—that is, the almost inevitable loss of hair follicles on either side of the incision. Such a hair loss in the eyebrow or in the beard area may be narrowed but rarely eliminated, despite the most atraumatic technique.

Lastly we return full circle to the initiating problems of scar spread, of scar hypertrophy, and of keloid formation. These adverse results are more properly failures of scar revision rather than complications. It is true that striking and memorable successes in scar revision can be achieved. However, maximal effort all too frequently achieves minimal result. It is to be emphasized that all objective reviews of scar revision surgery demonstrate the difficulty of the field and the frequent failure of the actual result to satisfy either the hope of the surgeon or the expectation of the patient.

REFERENCES

Addison, T.: On the keloid of Alibert and on true keloid. Med.-Chir. Trans., *37*:27, 1854.

Alibert, J. L. M.: Description des maladies de la peau observées à l'hôpital Saint-Louis et exposition des meilleures méthodes suivies pour leur traitement. Barrols l'aîné et fils, Paris, 1806, p. 113.

Alibert, J. L. M.: Quelques recherches sur la chéloïde. Mém. Soc. Médicale d'Emulation, 1817, p. 744.

Alibert, J. L. M.: Description des maladies de la peau observées à l'hôpital Saint-Louis et exposition des meilleures méthodes suivies pour leur traitement. Auguste Whalen, Bruxelles, Tome Second, 1825, p. 37.

Altemeier, W. A., and Stevenson, J. M.: Physiology of Wound Healing. *In* Davis, L. (Ed.): Christopher's Textbook of Surgery. 7th Ed. Philadelphia, W. B. Saunders Company, 1960, p. 28.

Anderson, W.: Cheloid of abdomen assuming malignant characters. Lancet, *1*:1025, 1888.

Arnold, H. L., and Grauer, F. H.: Keloids: Etiology, and management by excision and intensive prophylactic radiation. A.M.A. Arch. Dermatol., *80*:772, 1959.

Arons, M. S., Lynch, J. B., Lewis, S. R., and Blocker, T. G., Jr.: Scar tissue carcinoma. Part I. A clinical study with special reference to burn scar carcinoma. Ann. Surg., *161*:170, 1965.

Asboe-Hansen, G., Brodthogen, H., and Zachariae, L.: Treatment of keloids with topical injections of hydrocortisone acetate. Arch. Dermatol. Syph., *73*:162, 1956.

Barnard, R. D., Garnes, A. L., and Oppenheim, A.: Hemagglutinative vaso-occlusion in the pathodynamics of keloid. Am. J. Surg., *101*:192, 1961.

Barra, J., Mouly, R., and Dufourmentel, C.: Traitement des chéloides et des cicatrices chéloidiennes par injection locales de corticoides. Ann. Chir. Plast., *18*:59, 1973.

Bernstein, H.: Treatment of keloids by steroids with biochemical tests for diagnosis and prognosis. Angiology, *15*:253, 1964.

Biemans, R. G. M.: A rare case of sarcomatous degeneration of a cheloid. Arch. Chir. Neerl., *15*:175, 1963.

Billingham, R. E., and Russell, P. S.: Studies on wound healing, with special reference to the phenomenon of contracture in experimental wounds in rabbits' skin. Ann. Surg., *144*:961, 1956.

Blackburn, W. R., and Cosman, B.: Histologic basis of keloid and hypertrophic scar differentiation: Clinicopathologic correlation. Arch. Pathol., *82*:65, 1966.

Bloom, D.: Heredity of keloids. N.Y. State J. Med., *56*:511, 1956.

Bohrod, M. G.: Keloids and sexual selection. Arch. Dermatol. Syph., *36*:19, 1937.

Borges, A.: La W-plástia en el tratamiento de las cicatrices. Rev. Latino-Am. Cirurg. Plast., *4*:10, 1959.

Bostwick, J., Pendergrast, W. J., Jr., and Vasconez, L. O.: Marjolin's ulcer: An immunologically privileged tumor? Plast. Reconstr. Surg., *57*:66, 1976.

Bowers, R. F., and Young, J. M.: Carcinoma arising in scars, osteomyelitis, and fistulae. Arch. Surg., *80*:564, 1960.

Calnan, J. S., and Copenhagen, H. J.: Autotransplantation of keloid in man. Br. J. Surg., *54*:330, 1967.

Caronni, E. P.: Asportazione chirurgica e terapia radiante immediata (Iridio 192) nel trattamento dei cheloidi. Nota preliminare. Chir. Ital., *19*:874, 1967.

Chytilova, M., Kulhanek, V., and Horn, V.: Experimental production of keloids after immunization with autologous skin. Acta Chir. Plast., *1*:72, 1959.

Conway, H., and Stark, R. B.: ACTH in plastic surgery. Plast. Reconstr. Surg., *8*:354, 1951.

Conway, H., Gillette, R. W., and Findley, A.: Observations on the behavior of human keloids in vitro. Plast. Reconstr. Surg., *24*:229, 1959.

Conway, H., Gillette, R. W., Smith, J. W., and Findley, A.: Differential diagnosis of keloids and hypertrophic scars by tissue culture technique with notes on therapy of keloids by surgical excision and Decadron. Plast. Reconstr. Surg., *25*:117, 1960.

Cornbleet, T.: Treatment of keloids with hyaluronidase. J.A.M.A., *154*:1161, 1954.

Cosman, B., and Wolff, M.: Correlation of keloid recurrence with completeness of local excision. Plast. Reconstr. Surg., *50*:163, 1972.

Cosman, B., and Wolff, M.: Bilateral earlobe keloids. Plast. Reconstr. Surg., *53*:540, 1974.

Cosman, B., Crikelair, G. F., Ju, D. M. C., Gaulin, J. C., and Lattes, R.: The surgical treatment of keloids. Plast. Reconstr. Surg., *27*:335, 1961.

Cox, H. T.: The cleavage lines of skin. Br. J. Surg., *29*:234, 1941.

Crawford, B. S.: Pigmented scars. Br. Med. J., *1*:969, 1953.

Crikelair, G. F.: Skin suture marks. Am. J. Surg., *96*:631, 1958.

Crikelair, G. F.: Surgical approach to facial scarring. J.A.M.A., *172*:160, 1960.

Crikelair, G. F., and Cosman, B.: Facial scars in Puerto Rican women. Plast. Reconstr. Surg., *33*:556, 1964.

Crocker, H. R.: The anatomy of keloid in an early stage. Br. Med. J., *2*:544, 1886.

Crockett, D. J.: Regional keloid susceptibility. Br. J. Plast. Surg., *17*:245, 1964.

Cronin, T. D.: The use of a molded splint to prevent contracture after split skin grafting on the neck. Plast. Reconstr. Surg., *27*:7, 1961.

Davis, J. S.: Plastic Surgery. Its Principles and Practice. Philadelphia, P. Blakiston's Son & Co., 1919, p. 26.

Davis, J. S., and Kitlowski, E. A.: The theory and practical use of the Z-incision for the relief of scar contractures. Ann. Surg., *109*:1001, 1939.

De Beurmann, L., and Gougerot, H.: Chéloïdes des muqueuses. Ann. Dermatol. Syph., 7:151, 1906.

DeBeurmann, L., Noire, H., and Gougerot, H.: Traitement des chéloïdes par l'ablation suivie de la radiothérapie. Bull. Soc. Fr. Dermatol. Syphiligr., *1*:414, 1906.

Dorland's Illustrated Medical Dictionary. 25th Ed. Philadelphia, W. B. Saunders Company, 1974.

Dunphy, J. E.: The fibroblast — A ubiquitous ally for the surgeon. New Engl. J. Med., *268*:1367, 1963.

Dupuytren, G.: Leçons Orales de Clinique Chirurgicale. Vol. 1. Paris, G. Balliére, 1832–34.

Edgerton, M. T., Jr., Hanrahan, E. M., and Davis, W. B.: Use of vitamin E in the treatment of keloids. Plast. Reconstr. Surg., *8*:224, 1951.

Edwards, L. C., and Dunphy, J. E.: Wound healing, I and II. New Engl. J. Med., *259*:224, 275, 1958.

Ehlers, G., and Knoth, W.: Oligo-N-methylmorpholinium-propylenoxyd, ein neus Mittel zur Behandlung von Keloiden und Verwandten Krankheitszustanden. Dermatol. Wochenschr., *152*:625, 1966.

Engdahl, E.: Strengthening of scars with a buried dermal sheet. Scand. J. Plast. Surg., *2*:109, 1968.

Feller, H.: Zur Therapie der Keloide. Munch. Med. Wochenschr., *101*:1894, 1959.

Findley, C. W., Jr., and Howes, E. L.: Effect of edema on tensile strength of incised wounds. Surg. Gynecol. Obstet., *90*:666, 1950.

Fischl, R. A.: Keloids: A new treatment. Three case reports. J. Mt. Sinai Hosp., *32*:65, 1965.

Fleming, R. M., and Rezek, P. R.: Sarcoma developing in an old burn scar. Am. J. Surg., *54*:457, 1941.

Fox, H.: Observations on skin diseases in the Negro. J. Cutan. Dis., *26*:67, 109, 1908.

Freund, L.: Die Strahlenbehandlung der Fehlerhaften Narben und Keloide. Wien. Med. Wochenschr., *63*:2355, 1913.

Fujimori, R., Hiramoto, M., and Ofuji, S.: Sponge fixation method for treatment of early scars. Plast. Reconstr. Surg., *42*:322, 1968.

Furnas, D. W.: The four fundamental functions of the Z-plasty. Arch. Surg., *96*:458, 1968.

Furtell, J. W., and Myers, G. H.: The burn scar as an immunologically privileged site. Surg. Forum, *23*:129, 1972.

Gabbiani, G., Ryan, G. B., and Majno, G.: Presence of modified fibroblasts in granulation tissue and their possible role in wound contraction. Experientia, *27*:549, 1971.

Gaulin, J. C., and Lattes, R.: Personal communication, 1960.

Geschickter, C. F., and Lewis, D.: Tumors of connective tissue. Am. J. Cancer, *25*:630, 1935.

Gillies, H.: Technique of good suturing. Clin. J., *72*:223, 1943.

Gillman, T., and Penn, J.: Studies on the repair of cutaneous wounds. M. Proc. Johannesburg, (Suppl.) 2:1, 121, 150, 1956.

Glücksman, A.: Local factors in the histogenesis of hypertrophic scars. Br. J. Plast. Surg., *4*:88, 1951.

Goeminne, L.: A new probably X-linked inherited syndrome: Congenital muscular torticollis, multiple keloids, cryptorchidism and renal dysplasia. Acta Genet. Med. Gemellol. (Roma), *17*:439, 1968.

Golden, T.: Non-irritating, multipurpose surgical adhesive tape. Am. J. Surg., *100*:789, 1960.

Goldman, E.: Zur Pathogenese und Therapie des Keloids. Beit. Z. Klin. Chir., *31*:581, 1901.

Gosis, M.: Painless rendering closure of superficial wounds. Am. J. Surg., *44*:400, 1939.

Griffith, B. H.: The treatment of keloids with triamcinolone acetonide. Plast. Reconstr. Surg., *38*:202, 1966.

Griffith, B. H., Monroe, C. W., and McKinney, P.: A follow-up study on the treatment of keloids with triamcinolone acetonide. Plast. Reconstr. Surg., *46*:145, 1970.

Halsted, W. S.: Surgical Papers. Vol. I. Baltimore, Johns Hopkins Press, 1924, p. 36.

Hanford, J. M., Quimby, E. H., and Frantz, V. K.: Cancer arising many years after radiation therapy. J.A.M.A., *181*:404, 1962.

Heidingsfeld, M. L.: Keloid: A comparative histologic study. J.A.M.A., *53*:1276, 1909.

Hoopes, J. E., Su, C. T., and Im, M. J. C.: Enzyme activities in hypertrophic scars and keloids. Plast. Reconstr. Surg., *47*:132, 1971.

Horton, C. E., Crawford, J., and Oakey, R. S.: Malignant change in keloids. Plast. Reconstr. Surg., *12*:86, 1953.

Howes, E. L.: A renaissance of suture technique needed. Ann. Surg., *48*:548, 1940.

Hynes, W.: The treatment of scars by shaving and skin graft. Br. J. Plast. Surg., *10*:1, 1957.

Im, M. J. C., and Hoopes, J. E.: Alpha-naphthyl acid phosphatase activity in normal human skin and keloids. J. Invest. Dermatol., *57*:184, 1971.

Jacobsson, F.: The treatment of keloids at Radium-hemmet 1921–1941. Acta Radiol., *29*:251, 1948.

Ju, D. M. C.: The physical basis of scar contracture. Plast. Reconstr. Surg., *7*:343, 1951.

Ju, D. M. C.: Fibrosarcoma arising in surgical scars. Plast. Reconstr. Surg., *38*:429, 1966.

Justus, J.: Beobachtungen und Experimente zur Ätiologie des Keloides. Arch. Dermatol. Syph., *127*:274, 1919.

Kanaar, P., and Oort, J.: Fibrosarcomas developing in scar-tissue. Dermatologica, *138*:312, 1969.

Kelly, E. W., Jr.: The effects of tetrahydroxy quinone on connective tissue. J. Chronic Dis., *16*:335, 1963.

Kelly, E. W., Jr., and Pinkus, H.: Oral treatment of keloids. Arch. Dermatol., *78*:348, 1958.

Ketchum, L. D., Smith, J., Robinson, D. W., and Masters, F. W.: The treatment of hypertrophic scar, keloid and scar contracture by triamcinolone acetonide. Plast. Reconstr. Surg., *38*:209, 1966.

Ketchum, L. D., Robinson, D. W., and Masters, F. W.: Follow-up on treatment of hypertrophic scars and keloids with triamcinolone. Plast. Reconstr. Surg., *48*:256, 1971.

Ketchum, L. D., Cohen, I. K., and Masters, F. W.: Hypertrophic scars and keloids. A collective review. Plast. Reconstr. Surg., *53*:140, 1974.

Kraissl, C. J., and Conway, H.: Excision of small tumors of the skin of the face with special reference to the wrinkle line. Surgery, *25*:592, 1949.

Krieger, K.: Der Spalthautlappen bei Keloid behandlung. Chirurg., *29*:219, 1958.

Kuitert, J. H., Davis, M. J., Brittis, A. L., and Aldes, J. H.: Control of keloid growth with ultrasonic energy. Am. J. Phys. Med., *34*:408, 1955.

Kurnatovski, A., and Pruszcynski, G.: The histoenzymological pattern of the keloids and hypertrophic scars. Acta Chir. Plast., *10*:232, 1968.

Lacassagne, J., and Rousset, J.: Tatouages et chéloïdes. Bull. Soc. Fr. Dermatol. Syphiligr., *38*:919, 1931.

Langer, K.: Zur Anatomie und Physiologie der Haut. Sitzungsb. Acad. Wissensch., *45*:223, 1861.

Larson, D. L., Abston, S., Dobrkowsky, M., Huang, T., Evans, E. V., and Lewis, S.: The Prevention and Correction of Burn Scar Contracture and Hypertrophy. Galveston, Texas, Shriner's Burn Institute, Galveston Unit, 1973.

Lespinne, V.: Tatouages en relief et chéloïdes chez le Nègre du Congo. Bull. Soc. Fr. Dermatol. Syphiligr., *38*:927, 1931.

Levenson, S. M., Stein, J. M., and Grossblatt, N. (Eds.): Wound Healing: Proceedings of a Workshop. Natl. Acad. Sci.–Natl. Res. Council, Washington, D.C., 1966.

Levitt, W. M., and Gillies, H.: Radiotherapy in the prophylaxis and treatment of keloids. Lancet, *1*:440, 1942.

Lintilnac, J. P., Cochain, J. P., Sablayroles, D., and Tichadou, M.: Rôle de la compression élastique continue prolongée dans la prévention des cicatrices rétractiles et hypertrophiques. Maroc Med., *45*:253, 1966.

Localio, S. A., Casale, W., and Hinton, J. W.: Wound healing: Experimental and statistical study. Surg. Gynecol. Obstet., *77*:481, 1943.

Maguire, H. C.: Treatment of keloids with triamcinolone acetonide injected intralesionally. J.A.M.A., *192*:325, 1965.

Mancini, R. E., and Quaife, J. V.: Histogenesis of experimentally produced keloids. J. Invest. Dermatol., *38*:143, 1962.

Mancini, R. E., Stringa, S. G., and Canepa, L.: The action of ACTH, cortisone and prednisone on the connective tissue of normal and sclerodermic human skin. J. Invest. Dermatol., *34*:393, 1960.

Marjolin, J. N.: Dictionnaire de Médecine; Article sur l'ulcère verruqueux, *21*:31, 1828. Chez Béchet Jeune, Paris.

Marshall, W., and Rosenthal, S.: Pathogenesis and experimental therapy of keloids and similar neoplasms in relation to tissue fluid disturbances. Am. J. Surg., *62*:348, 1943.

Matas, R.: The surgical peculiarities of the Negro. Trans. Am. Surg. Assoc., *14*:483, 1896.

Mienicki, M., and Kossakowska, H.: Recherches sur le taux de la vitamine K et plus particulièrement l'influence thérapeutique exercée par celle-ci dans le traitement de chéloïdes. Ann. Dermatol. Syphiligr. (Paris), *90*:389, 1963.

Minkowitz, F.: Regression of massive keloid following partial excision and post-operative intralesional administration of triamcinolone. Br. J. Plast. Surg., *20*:432, 1967.

Mook, W. H.: Keloid of the tongue. Arch. Dermatol. Syph., *10*:304, 1924.

Morestin, H.: La réduction graduelle des difformités tégumentaires. Bull. Mém. Soc. Chir. Paris, *41*:1233, 1915.

Mowlem, R.: Hypertrophic scars. Br. J. Plast. Surg., *4*:113, 1951.

Naeglie, T.: Recherches statistiques expérimentales et biologiques sur les chéloïdes. Bull. Soc. Fr. Dermatol. Syphiligr., *38*:905, 1931.

Ordman, L. J., and Gillman, T.: Studies in the healing of cutaneous wounds. II. The healing of epidermal, appendageal, and dermal injuries inflicted by suture needles and by the suture material in the skin of pigs. Arch. Surg., *93*:883, 1966.

Parsons, R. W.: A case of keloid of the penis. Plast. Reconstr. Surg., *37*:431, 1966.

Pautrier, L. M., and Zorn, R.: Calcémie: Teneur en calcium de la peau dans les chéloïdes et les acnés chéloïdiennes. Bull. Soc. Fr. Dermatol. Syphiligr., *38*:953, 1931.

Peacock, E. E., Jr., and Van Winkle, W., Jr.: Surgery and Biology of Wound Repair. Philadelphia, W. B. Saunders Company, 1970.

Penn, J.: The removal of "cross-hatch" scars. Plast. Reconstr. Surg., *25*:73, 1960.

Pigott, R. W.: A review of 50 cases of skin scarring treated by shave and split skin graft. Br. J. Plast. Surg., *21*:180, 1968.

Poulard, A.: Traitement des cicatrices faciales. Presse Méd., *26*:221, 1918.

Psillakis, J. M., De Jorge, F. B., Sucena, R. C., Mariani, U., and Spina, V.: Water and electrolyte content of normal skin, scars and keloid. Plast. Reconstr. Surg., *47*:272, 1971.

Radcliffe, W.: A simple method of wound closure. Practitioner, *150*:122, 1943.

Ramirez, A. T., Soroff, H. S., Schwartz, M. S., Mooty, J., Pearson, E., and Raben, M. S.: Experimental wound healing in man. Surg. Gynecol. Obstet., *128*:283, 1969.

Reid, D. A. C.: Experience in burying live scars. Br. J. Plast. Surg., *4*:235, 1952.

Robinson, D. W., and Hamilton, T. R.: Investigation into the role of heparin in proliferative tissue reactions. Surgery, *34*:470, 1953.

Robinson, D. W., Corbett, E., and Hamilton, T. R.: Some observations on connective tissue growth and tissue culture in relation to keloid formation: A preliminary report. Surg. Forum, 1952, p. 505.

Rubin, L. R.: Langer's lines and facial scars. Plast. Reconstr. Surg., *3*:147, 1948.

Schmidt, W.: Über ein Keloid der Zungenspitze bei einem Trompetenblässer. Dermatol. Wochenschr., *99*:1341, 1934.

Sedgewick, W.: Miscellaneous specimens including malformations of external parts, diseases of skin, diphtheria, etc. Trans. Pathol. Soc. London, *12*:234, 1861.

Serafini, G.: Treatment of burn scars of the face by dermabrasion and skin grafts. Br. J. Plast. Surg., *15*:308, 1962.

Sheard, C.: Keloids. Arch. Dermatol., *83*:873, 1961.

Sistrunk, W. E.: Contribution to plastic surgery. Removal of scars by stages, etc. Ann. Surg., *85*:185, 1927.

Skoog, T.: Dupuytren's contraction with special reference to etiology and improved surgical treatment in epileptics. Acta Chir. Scand., Suppl. 139, 1948.

Stevenson, T. W.: Release of circular constricting scars by Z-flaps. Plast. Reconstr. Surg., *1*:39, 1946.

Straatsma, C. R.: Surgical technique helpful in obtaining fine scars. Plast. Reconstr. Surg., *2*:21, 1947.

Strand, S.: On keloids and their treatment. Acta Radiol., *26*:397, 1945.

Sugawara, M., and Hashimoto, K.: A surgical treatment method for keloid; "Kurinuki" or hollowing-out method. Jap. J. Plast. Reconstr. Surg., *10*:313, 1967.

Sylven, B.: Ester sulphuric acids of high molecular weight and mast cells in mesenchymal tumors. Acta Radiol. (Suppl.), 1945, p. 57.

Thompson, N.: The subcutaneous dermis graft. Plast. Reconstr. Surg., *26*:1, 1960.

Thorne, N.: Camouflage of blemishes and scars. Br. J. Clin. Pract., *20*:593, 1966.

Treves, N., and Pack, G. T.: The development of cancer in burn scars. Surg. Gynecol. Obstet., *51*:749, 1930.

Uchida, K., and Uchida, J. I.: Evaluation of collodium treatment in operative scars. Br. J. Plast. Surg., *14*:325, 1961.

Unna, P. G.: The Histopathology of the Diseases of the Skin. Edinburgh, W. F. Clay, 1896, p. 841.

Vallis, C. P.: Intralesional injection of keloids and hypertrophic scars with the Dermo-Jet. Plast. Reconstr. Surg., *40*:255, 1967.

Van Den Brenk, H. A. S.: Studies in restorative growth processes in mammalian wound healing. Br. J. Surg., *43*:525, 1956.

Van Den Brenk, H. A. S., and Minty, C. J.: Radiation in the management of keloids and hypertrophic scars. Br. J. Surg., *47*:595, 1960.

Van Winkle, W.: The fibroblast in wound healing. Surg. Gynecol. Obstet., *124*:369, 1967.

Vargas, L., Jr.: Attempt to induce formation of fibroids with estrogens in the castrated female rhesus monkey. Bull. Johns Hopkins Hosp., *73*:23, 1943.

Vilain, R.: L'excision itérative partielle des lésions cutanées: A propos de 38 observations. Presse Méd., *73*:2307, 1965.

Watts, G. T.: Wound shape and tissue tension in healing. Br. J. Surg., *42*:555, 1960.

Webster, J. P.: Plastic surgery: General principles. *In* Christopher, F. (Ed.): Textbook of Surgery. 5th Ed. Philadelphia, W. B. Saunders Company, 1949, p. 1403.

Webster, R. C.: Cosmetic concepts in scar camouflaging—Serial excision and broken line techniques. Trans. Am. Acad. Ophthalmol. Otolaryngol., *73*:256, 1969.

Whitehill, J. L.: Prophylaxis of surgical keloids. Arizona Med., *11*:399, 1954.

Wickham, L., and Degrais, P.: Die Vervendung des Radiums bei der Behandlung, der Haut-Epitheliome, der Angiome und der Keloide. Handbuch des Radium-Biologie und Therapie. Wiesbaden, J. F. Bergmann, 1913, p. 402.

Woringer, F., and Zimmer, J.: Untersuchungen über das Keloidgewebe. Hautarzt, *9*:341, 1958.

CHAPTER 17

SURGICAL AND CHEMICAL PLANING OF THE SKIN

ROSS M. CAMPBELL, M.D.

Dermabrasion or Surgical Planing

Surgical planing, also known as dermabrasion, consists of the removal of the epidermis and as much of the superficial dermal layer as is necessary and the preservation of the epidermal adnexa in sufficient quantity to allow for spontaneous re-epithelization with minimal or no scarring.

The purpose of surgical abrasion is the smoothing of irregularities and discolorations on the surface of the skin resulting from traumatic scars, the scars and pits of acne, smallpox, or chickenpox, benign tumors, lentigines, commercial tattoos, and so forth. Surgical abrasion is also employed in overgrafting of grafts or flaps in order to increase the thickness or to improve the color of the transplanted skin (see Chapter 6).

HISTORICAL SURVEY

Scarification was reported by Rossignol in 1881. In this procedure numerous small superifical skin incisions were made in the hope that the entire skin surface would heal with a more nearly homogeneous appearance. Acupuncture or puncturing of the skin with fine needles was used for centuries as a form of therapy for neuralgic pain or the release of tissue fluid. It was also ingeniously used to de-

posit pigment permanently in the dermis to produce human picture galleries and subsequently to deposit other pigments to mask the earlier ones and thus obliterate evidence of former indiscretion or folly. McDowell (1974) has given a succinct summary of "tattoo erasing." Variot in 1888 described such a form of tattooing. It has been employed in its more modern form by Conway (1953) and other authors to mask colored lesions of the facial skin, such as nevus flammeus and other types of hemangioma.

Kromayer (1905) was probably the first to introduce mechanical methods of planing or leveling the skin in the treatment of various dermatologic lesions. At first he used cylindrical knives; later, dental burs in various shapes and sizes driven by electric engines were used on skin initially sprayed with ethyl chloride. He reported the effects of these treatments, commencing in 1905 and continuing until 1923. That he was an astute observer is shown by the significant statement credited to him that if the planing were not carried below the papillary layer of the dermis there would be healing without scarring. This statement was confirmed by the studies of Bishop (1945).

Janson in 1935 described the use of the wire brush technique in the treatment of tattoos.

The modern revival of the abrasive therapy of skin lesions should be ascribed to Iverson, whose report in 1947 described the use of sandpaper manually applied to traumatic tattooed lesions. In 1950 McEvitt described a similar method for the treatment of acne pits. There was a quick resurgence of interest by other plastic surgeons, with subsequent improvements in the manual sandpaper technique and later in the form of motor-driven cylinders of sandpaper, Carborundum, and other abrasive materials.

Kurtin in 1953 described his procedure employing a rapidly revolving wire brush and an ethyl chloride spray for anesthesia, hardening of the skin surface, and a bloodless field. He also emphasized the use of a blower for quicker freezing.

The toxic and explosive ethyl chloride has been superseded by the commercial refrigerant solution Freon; motors have been modified; the cutting instruments and aftercare of the patient have changed, but the principles of mechanically abrading or planing the skin to the appropriate level have remained essentially unchanged over the years. If it has yielded less than its promise, it is not because of an unrecognized inadequacy in the method, but rather because many of its proponents were overenthusiastic in the beginning or were insufficiently trained in its use and limitations. As now performed within its recognized limitations and with a proper selection of cases, it is a valued weapon in the plastic surgeon's therapeutic arsenal.

HEALING OF ABRADED AREAS

The successful employment of dermabrasion rests wholly on the inherent ability of the skin to reconstitute a new epidermal layer from the cutaneous adnexa made up of the pilosebaceous apparatus and the sweat glands. It follows logically, therefore, that the areas of the body where these components are in the greatest number and at the greatest depth should respond most favorably to planing or abrasion. Conversely, scarred or irradiated areas or body regions (the eyelids, the skin of the lower anterior neck, the inner aspect of the arm, and the volar aspect of the forearm) which are deficient in sebaceous glands, hair follicles, or sweat glands may not only fail to heal satisfactorily after even superficial planing but also in some instances heal with disfiguring scars. The face, with the exception of the eyelid, consists not only of thick skin but also of skin co-

piously endowed with epithelial adnexa. It is therefore a more favorable site for dermabrasion than any other area of the body. The skin of the back, which is approximately the same thickness as that of the face, i.e., about 4 mm exclusive of subcutaneous fat (Luikart, Ayres, and Wilson, 1959), is deficient in these necessary components in many individuals and does not always respond favorably. The base of the neck and the suprasternal and sternal areas are also susceptible to hypertrophic scarring. The areas to be abraded must be selected with discretion and with a knowledge of anatomical and histologic variations.

To be successful, planing must be extended below the level of the epidermis into varying depths of the dermis. Judgment and training dictate the depth to which the abrasion should be extended.

Healing of abraded areas is similar to that of donor areas of split-thickness grafts (see Chapter 6). An immediate outpouring of serum forms a coagulum extending across the abraded surface, in which necrotic cells and other debris are entrapped. There is immediate activity in the adnexal cells subjacent to those adnexal cells exposed by the planing. The exposed cells become necrotic, but those below assume certain of the attributes of squamous epithelium. According to Eisen, Holyoke, and Lobitz (1955) they appear to crowd the degenerating cells above them outward onto the surface of the wound. Marginal epithelial cells migrate from the edges of the abraded areas. In three days new epidermal cells are seen growing across the surface and extending out from the adnexal components. The findings of Luikart, Ayres, and Wilson (1959) of tonguelike projections of prickle cells from the pilosebaceous units at the three-day period are similar to the findings of Eisen, Holyoke, and Lobitz.

By the fifth day the epidermis is completely regenerated; it is thinner and lacks rete pegs but shows developing hair follicles and sebaceous glands. Not only do these elements contribute to the epidermal resurfacing, but in addition they are on their way toward resuming their functional activity.

The period required for complete epidermal regeneration varies from five to seven days on the face to ten days on the back, and it precedes dermal regeneration. At three days a cell-free area under the new epidermis is noted; there is no connection between the new epidermis and the dermal bed in this area. By five days some dermal regeneration is occurring, and by seven days a loose attachment of the dermis to the new epidermis can be observed. Because of the absence or the loose nature of the attachment in the first week, it would appear wise to avoid early dressing changes or injury.

In the newly regenerated dermis, many young fibroblasts are seen lying with their long axes in a horizontal plane, together with many new capillaries. A considerable amount of collagen is being laid down at the two-week period, appearing first in the form of a reticulum which is colored black by a special stain, in contrast with mature collagen in the lower depths, which stains brownish red. According to Luikart, Ayres, and Wilson, the new collagen shows a horizontal striated pattern that persists for at least four years after the abrasion. They feel the new collagen is responsible for the filling out of the skin which gives the youthful, rounded appearance frequently seen after facial abrasion.

An additional factor contributing to the filling out of the skin is intradermal edema. As it subsides and there is progressive restratification of the newly regenerated epidermis, the abraded area becomes slightly slacker and loses some of its smooth texture to the disappointment of the patient and surgeon. A general tightening of the abraded area can be attributed to the *inter-island contraction phenomenon* described by Converse and Robb-Smith in 1944. This phenomenon, observed in healing donor areas of skin grafts, is caused by the progressive approximation of the new islands of epithelium in the contracting, healing dermal wound. Inter-island contraction is responsible for a reduction in the surface area of the dermal wound and a tendency to constrict and collapse the deep pits of acne scars. It is this contraction that produces the shiny, smooth skin observed over the dorsum of the hand following the healing of a burn which penetrates the dermis and destroys the adnexal structures.

For the first month there is little evidence of *pigment formation* in the basal layers of the epidermis. By the end of one month, some return in the form of fine pigment granules can be noted on microscopic section. Murray (1958) noted in blacks that the first return of pigment after a month was seen around the pores of the skin, giving a polka dot appearance to the area. There was a gradual coalescence through spreading of the pigmented areas until the entire area was repigmented, although somewhat irregularly. Microscopic section of the basal layer showed uneven but marked hypertrophy with, as stated previously, diffuse, fine pigment granules gradually becoming more profuse and larger. He felt that it was the considerable hypertrophy of the basal layer that contributed to the darkening of the skin in the abraded areas, with lightening of color occurring at a later date as the hypertrophy subsided. Pigmentation is not a problem in the black patient alone, but appears with unhappy frequency in Caucasians as well. When the newly abraded areas are exposed to sunlight, the problem of hyperpigmentation is intensified. It may last from 3 to 18 months, or occasionally remain as a permanent stigma. Johnson (1960) considered hyperpigmentation one of the most serious adverse reactions. He utilized certain measures recommended to him by Fitzpatrick to counteract this development. The treatment consists of (1) the use of a broad-spectrum, sun-protective ointment, (2) the administration of 2 g of ascorbic acid daily by mouth to inhibit melanin formation and (3) 25 mg of cortisone daily to inhibit the pituitary melanocyte-stimulating hormone. Small (1956) has recommended the use of 4 per cent Benoquin. On the other hand Baker and coworkers (1974), while acknowledging the occurrence of occasional hyperpigmentation, have shown that the quantity of melanin granules in the basal epidermal layer is markedly diminished and remains so in the majority of cases. However, they were reporting the results of histologic studies done on chemically peeled skin, which resulted, most writers have felt, in a situation akin to dermabrasion.

Milia are small cysts arising from the epithelial cells of the hair follicles, sebaceous gland ducts, and sweat ducts which were separated at the time of the surgical abrasion, became isolated, but continued to function in the dermis. These appear within a month of operation but can be demonstrated even up to six months after surgery.

By the end of six months, the epidermis is of normal thickness, but the papillary ridges remain smaller than normal. In the average person there is a normal amount of epidermal pigment. The blood vessels may still be engorged, but the adnexa appear normal.

At the end of ten months the elastic fibers in the regenerated dermal tissue are almost nonexistent. There is nearly normal vascularity; the rete ridges are essentially normal in appearance; the epidermis is of the usual thickness; the adnexal appendages are functioning satisfactorily; but there is a decrease in the overall thickness of the epidermal-dermal complex due to incomplete regeneration of the full thickness of the dermis. The final result is a net decrease in the thickness of the dermis. It is for this reason that a planed area never fully recovers to the level of the surrounding unplaned skin unless the planing has been so superficial that only the epidermal layers have been removed, in which case the regeneration of the epidermis to its full thickness will restore it to the level of the surrounding untreated areas. This factor is of importance in treating the pits of acne and also in planing the tissue around depressed scars down to the level of the scar.

EQUIPMENT

Having employed this treatment since 1948, the author has used nearly all of the methods that have been advocated, beginning with manually applied hardware store sandpaper wrapped around a roll of gauze bandage and progressing through the more sophisticated developments, including the Snyderman metallic hand abrader, low and high speed wire brushes, burs, steel cutting wheels, and diamond fraises. The author is currently utilizing the Stryker dermabrader developed by Iverson (1957), a device which uses special emery paper cylinders available in three sizes. By the use of a Jacobs chuck with the Stryker apparatus, the range of its usefulness is greatly extended. The same instrument with adaptations can be used with the wire brush or, if desired, a dental bur or three sizes of cone-shaped carborundum attachments can be utilized for fine abarasion in close quarters, such as the nasolabial angle. The Hall Air Drill is also adapted to dermabrasion.

The Stryker instrument is employed with a choice of three cylinders in varying sizes and a medium grit emery paper or carborundum. The large cylinder with a protector shield is useful for planing large areas rapidly. The smaller sizes have their own appropriate fields of usefulness, and they are most valuable for work in critical areas—for example, close to the eyes, the alae of the nose, and the ears.

An additional benefit is that there is little or no tendency to gouge the skin, a problem frequently encountered with the wire brush. The foot pedal rheostat provides a wide range of speeds.

Opponents of grit paper often refer to the dangers of the formation of granulomas. However, if any particles of silica remain on the wound surface after flush irrigations with saline, they are enmeshed in the coagulum that forms and are removed when it separates.

OPERATIVE PROCEDURE

All patients undergoing extensive planing, e.g., the entire face, are preferably treated in a hospital operating room and not in the office. Office treatment should be confined to areas of small extent.

Preoperative preparation consists of washing the part to be treated with pHisoHex for several days before surgery. This has a beneficial effect on any active acne or folliculitis lesions that may be present by reducing skin surface bacterial counts.

Whether to employ general or local anesthesia is often a matter of personal choice. When the patient is given a relatively light anesthesia by a qualified anesthesiologist, the risk is minimal and it makes the task of abrading much easier for both patient and surgeon. If local anesthesia is used, the patient should receive adequate preoperative sedation, and the skin should be infiltrated with 1 per cent procaine-epinephrine solution to secure anesthesia and partial hemostasis. It is unnecessary to balloon the tissues.

It is helpful to mark the bottoms of the pockmarks or pits with surgical ink and to make an outline in ink of the general extent of the area to be treated. A slightly subdued light coming in from the side when applying the marks is recommended, since a bright direct overhead light tends to obliterate the unevenness of the surface and some minor areas might be overlooked.

Gauze packs are placed intraorally beneath the cheeks to provide a slightly stretched, firm surface so that the skin is taut. The abrader is moved slowly back and forth and in a circular manner across the surface, abrading through epidermis down to the desired level in the dermis, counterchecked by the dye previously applied to the depths of the pits.

As the operator approaches the inked outline of the area under treatment, the pressure and depth should be reduced gradually so that the edges of the treated areas are feathered or beveled out instead of ending abruptly. Unless beveling is performed, a sharp line of demarcation between the treated and untreated sections will remain and may eventually require revision.

At this point a word of caution should be given about all abrading instruments; the pressure of application must always be moderated when treating skin that overlies superficial bony prominences. This is one reason for avoiding Freon freezing. The yielding quality of unfrozen skin is easily overcome by stretching and conveys a proper sense of feel to the operator, allowing more discriminating applications of pressure and avoiding the excessive removal of skin layers.

Capillary bleeding is a natural response to planing the unfrozen skin but is seldom a cause of delay. The assistant drops or sprays saline slowly on the part being treated, thus aiding the clearing of blood from the field and allowing easier removal of the detritus. When an area has been completed, the surface is copiously irrigated to flush away all by-products of planing, and a cold pack of saline containing a small amount of epinephrine will control the bleeding and protect the treated part while work is progressing elsewhere.

At the conclusion of the operation there is generally a slight serous ooze from the treated surfaces. If one chooses, a layer of xeroform gauze or Telfa may be applied, followed by fluffed gauze and a pressure dressing. This is kept in place 24 to 48 hours; the dressing is then removed down to the innermost layer, which is not touched until it is ready to separate spontaneously approximately one week later. The postoperative pressure dressing contributes to the comfort of the patient and also minimizes the amount of ooze.

An alternate method is the application of a thick paste of thrombin, obtained by mixing thrombin powder with a small amount of saline. This is applied liberally to the abraded parts. Such a mixture controls bleeding and serous ooze and, when dry, forms an excellent protective eschar. Drying of the paste may be hastened by using a hairdryer to blow dry, warm air over the abraded area.

The operator should protect his eyes throughout the dermabrasion using a pair of safety goggles or a bronchoscopy shield.

POSTOPERATIVE CARE

When bulky dressings have been left in place eight or nine days postoperatively, as recommended by some authors, the patients have generally been more distressed, especially in warm weather. Perspiration and blood under the dressing make an obnoxious mixture with a strong odor and form an ideal culture medium. Pyocyaneous with its own particular odor is a frequent invader, increasing the general messiness and discomfort.

If the exposure method is employed, no ointments of any kind are used initially, but there is no objection to the application of Neosporin, bacitracin, or ordinary cold cream in the late stages of healing (five or six days) when the ointment may aid in the removal of the coagulum, not all of which separates at the same time, owing to variations in the depth of planing. The application of an ointment also relieves the patient of the discomfort associated with the tight coagulum.

The patient may be discharged the day following surgery. Many elect to remain in the hospital because of their appearance.

The coagulum should never be removed forcibly. To do so is to tear away some of the delicate new epithelium and delay healing. The young, pink epithelium is protected by the application of such preparations as cold cream, cocoa butter, or lanolin.

In two weeks the average patient can use make-up, at first lightly, then as desired.

Patients are advised to avoid exposure to direct or reflected sunlight. Even skyshine (as occurs under a shade tree) has been estimated to contain as high as 50 per cent of the ultraviolet rays of direct sunshine. Patients should be warned against going outdoors unless they have first applied a good quality sun-screening cream to the treated parts. Even the most effective creams available will screen out only about 85 to 90 per cent of the ultraviolet and infrared rays. The cream must be reapplied frequently and should be used for two to three months postoperatively.

If hyperpigmentation occurs, it regresses spontaneously in 3 to 18 months in most patients. Hypopigmentation is less commonly encountered, and it usually regresses spontaneously. It can be masked easily in female patients by the application of colored cosmetic bases.

Additional planing, if required, may be done at intervals of three months.

INDICATIONS FOR SURGICAL PLANING

Acne Scars and Pockmarks. An abrasion extending to a moderate depth will yield marked improvement in the case of shallow acne, chickenpox, or smallpox scars. When the lesions are deeper, a second or even a third planing may be indicated and can be done safely, although there is a lesser percentage of improvement at each subsequent procedure.

Scars. Scars, whether traumatic or surgical, can respond favorably to dermabrasion (Fig. 17–1). Both elevated and depressed linear scars may be abraded with good to excellent results, particularly in the former (Figs. 17–2 and 17–3). The puckered scar also responds satisfactorily, and this has proved to be an eminently satisfactory method for treatment in the type of suture line in which one side is higher than the other. The technique is also helpful in adjusting the level of junction of a skin graft to the level of the edge of the recipient site.

In all cases, however, the regenerative epithelial elements must be present. When the scar is wider than 0.5 cm, it is more effective to excise and suture either alone or in combination with abrasion. When the latter method is chosen, the surface of the scar and the surrounding skin is abraded, the pale white, deeper surface of the scar is exposed and excised, and the defect is closed (Fig. 17–4, *B*). As re-epithelization occurs, the site of the scar may be nearly obliterated, thus yielding a result generally free of suture marks (McAndrew, 1959).

The straddling technique (Fig. 17–4) assures the planing and equalization of the skin surface level of the scar and surrounding skin; it must be emphasized that, in depressed scars, it is important to reduce the projection of the normal surrounding skin to the level of the base of the scar.

Burn Scars. Burn scars lacking adnexal components are generally unsuited to this form of treatment unless they are small in area. They are better treated by the method of Webster (1954) and of Hynes (1956, 1957, 1959) of abrasion and overgrafting of the affected area when total excision down to the subcutaneous tissue is not feasible for functional or cosmetic reasons (see Chapter 6). This involves shaving the skin with a blade or abrading the scar (Fig. 17–5). Surgical abrasion is as precise as shaving the skin with a blade, is more easily controlled, gives a more uniformly smooth underface, and is rapid. If one desires to fit the graft exactly rather than chance some ridging at the beveled edges, the perimeter of the defect is incised vertically to a controlled depth. This technique was employed in the patient shown in Figure 17–6. A similar principle can be used to treat chronic radiodermatitis, nonhairy pigmented moles (the hairy types pierce the graft), and other types of scarring.

In dermal overgrafting as described by Webster, Peterson, and Stein (1958), when a scarred area or a thinly grafted site is susceptible to slight trauma and breakdown, successive skin grafts may be applied to the dermabraded surfaces of either a preexisting scar or a previously transplanted skin graft to build up a tough, well-cushioned, protective covering.

Dermabrasion may also be utilized to increase the area of vascular contact by abrading the epidermis when implanting tube skin flaps or composite grafts.

Tattoos. Amateur and traumatic tattoos are benefited considerably by this treatment because of the diffuse distribution of the tattoo pigments or particles in all layers of the skin, unlike the professional tattoo in which most of the pigment is deposited deep in the dermis. A great deal, if not all, of the material can be removed quite safely without impairing epithelial regeneration (Fig. 17–7). Sometimes the uncovering of the upper layers will reveal fairly gross deposits, which can then be removed by forceps or curettement. When healing occurs, it is generally fairly rapid, and scarring and residual tattooing may be minimal. Dermabrasion may be repeated several times.

At present our preference for treatment of the professional tattoo is dermabrasion and/or excision by either scalpel or dermatome, followed by a skin graft cut to a non-revealing shape (e.g., if the tattoo is a heart, the author does not make the skin graft heart-shaped). Small linear or oval tattoos can be excised and closed primarily. The author does not feel that salabrasion, as proposed by Manchester (1974), is superior to the above technique.

Pigmented Nevi. Pigmented nevi may respond well to abrasion. Among the types that do so are lightly pigmented lesions with the pigment confined to the basal epithelial layers. Iverson (1953), Wynn-Williams (1959), Epstein (1962), and Cronin (1953) reported satisfactory results with light abrasion, although recurrences were frequent, especially in the lentigines and chloasma. Iverson felt that the explanation of so-called recurrence might lie in inadequate abrasion, with patches of pigment being overlooked in the course of the procedure. Recurrences undoubtedly occur and have been reported by Mopper and Mercantini (1960).

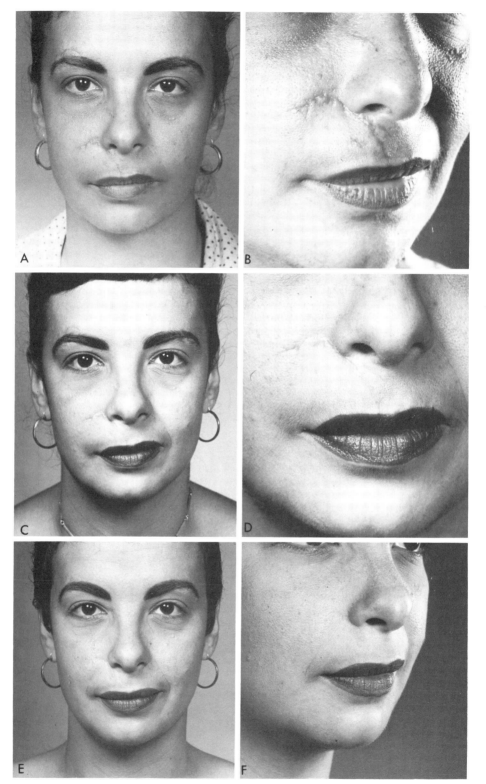

FIGURE 17–1.   Facial scars treated by excision and dermabrasion. *A, B,* Preoperative condition. *C, D,* Interim appearance after excision combined with dermabrasion. *E, F,* Final result after a third conservative abrasion treatment.

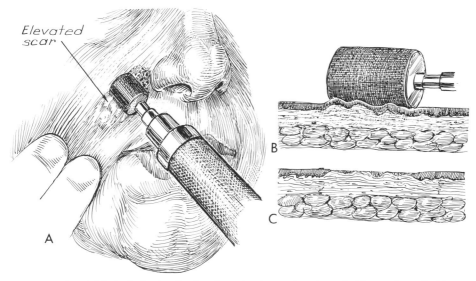

FIGURE 17–2. *A, B, C,* Method of using Stryker dermabrader to plane irregularities as shown in Figure 17–1.

The deeply pigmented nevus is less amenable to dermabrasion because of the danger of mechanical stimulation of metaplasia (a biopsy before operation is advisable) and because of a potential heavy scar resulting from the excessive depth of planing necessary for eradication of the lesion.

Hemangiomas. Hemangiomas, unless extremely superficial, are not successfully treated by abrasion. Bernard (1958) attempted to treat port-wine stains by dermabrasion, which removed a small superficial area of the stain, followed immediately by the application of a pigment for the purpose of tattooing and lightening the color of the part. The color "take" was inconstant, and the technique has not found clinical acceptance.

Keratotic Lesions. Keratotic lesions of small or large size, senile or seborrheic in nature but nonmalignant by preoperative biopsy,

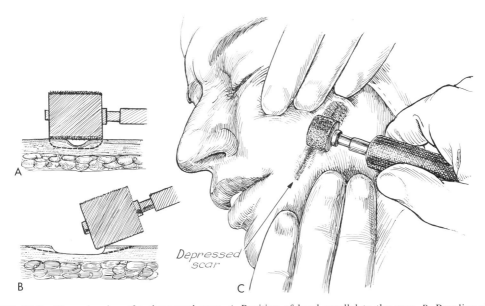

FIGURE 17–3. Dermabrasion of a depressed scar. *A,* Position of head parallel to the scar. *B,* Beveling of edges. *C,* Direction of dermabrasion.

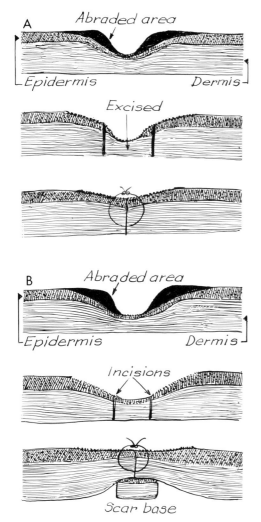

FIGURE 17–4. Straddling technique. A wide area on either side of the depressed shallow scar is abraded. *A,* Straddling technique of abrasion combined with excision and closure. *B,* Deeply depressed scar abraded and margins closed over the scar base.

can be safely and quickly removed by dermabrasion. The cosmetic result is excellent and extensive, and disfiguring surgery may be avoided. Pickrell, Matton, Huger, and Pound (1962) have performed abrasion in this type of lesion with excellent results. They found it especially satisfactory in large lesions of the scalp where surgical removal would result in an extensive hairless, skin-grafted area.

The use of dermabrasion as a prophylactic or therapeutic measure in the treatment of patients with senile or actinic precancerous skin lesions has been advocated by dermatologists, including Epstein (1962), Burks (1959), and Luikart, Ayres, and Wilson (1959). The planed skin with its new layers of collagen appears younger than the unplaned adjacent skin,

where long years of exposure to sun have resulted in marked collagen degeneration. When the entire face is planed, the whole appearance is more youthful, the skin becoming pinker and plumper. The so-called "rejuvenation of the skin" is said to retard the onset of premalignant change by several years (Epstein, 1962). The author's preference is chemical peeling of old actinic, leathery, and weathered skin.

Epitheliomas. Epitheliomas comprising basal cell, squamous cell, intradermal and basal cell, plus radiodermatitis were dermabraded by Pegum and coworkers (1959) and reported as being "clear" or successfully treated when they were assessed an indeterminate time after treatment by two dermatologists. Nevertheless, it is not recommended that malignancies be treated by this method, despite the fact that it has been claimed that ablation is complete and seeding and spreading of the tumor does not occur.

Rhinophyma. Rhinophyma is best treated by excising slices of the grossly thickened and irregular nasal skin; dermabrasion can assist in the treatment by further smoothing the remaining tissue (see Chapter 29). This method can also be employed in treating thick nasal skin of the type that prevents adequate draping of the skin over an altered nasal framework following rhinoplasty. The result can be very satisfactory in such cases. An extra benefit is the reduction of the oiliness of the nasal skin owing to the abrading away of many of the sebaceous glands. Ortiz-Monasterio and associates (1974) recommended simultaneous dermabrasion and rhinoplasty as treatment for the thick-skinned nose.

Fine Wrinkles. Fine wrinkles of the type not benefitted by facial surgery are frequently present on the upper and lower lips in older persons, and also in the outer canthal and glabellar regions. A medium light abrasion can be helpful in reducing their prominence. The abrasion must not be carried down onto the neck or to the eyelids. If it is, the danger of gross scarring and deformity occurring must be borne in mind. The author, however, prefers chemical peeling.

Limitations. The surgeon who employs dermabrasion most successfully will be the one who uses judgment in the selection and rejection of cases.

Although it has been claimed by some that almost any area of the body can be dermabraded, it is the author's experience that the

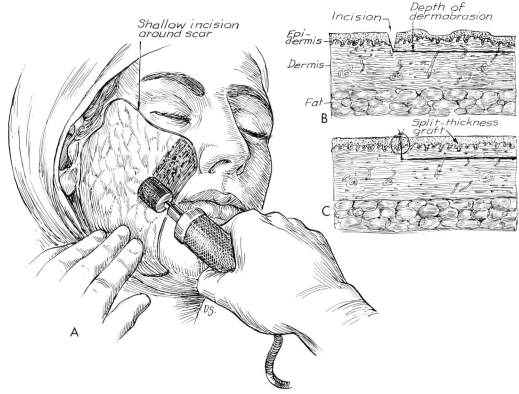

FIGURE 17–5. Technique of dermabrasion and overgrafting. *A,* Shallow incision around periphery of burn scar and abrasion down to the desired level. *B,* Depth of dermabrasion on cross section. *C,* Split-thickness skin graft in place.

face and scalp respond best to the treatment and heal fastest with minimal untoward healing reaction. The back and hands fare less well, while the chest, the forearms, especially the flexor surfaces, the inner upper arm, and the lower legs and feet do most poorly. The penalty of abrading too deeply is slow healing and excessive scarring.

To employ this method in a lesion such as a keloid or a wide hypertrophic scar, in both of which instances the affected part is deficient in adnexa, is manifestly an error in judgment. Healing of such an abraded area will be slow and will result, therefore, in the formation of a scar equally as thick or unsightly as the one treated.

It is likewise an error to attempt to treat pathologic conditions that extend below the dermis, since in order to encompass their ablation, the epithelial adnexa would have to be sacrificed. This accounts in part for the imperfect results obtained in acne scars of the so-called "icepick" type, in which the scar defect is columnar with steep vertical walls and a scarred base which enters the subdermis. For these, surgical excision and approximation,

perhaps in association with dermabrasion, as recommended by Iverson (1953) and McAndrew (1959), are preferable.

Cystic acne occupies a peculiar position in the literature on this subject. During abrasion, the cystic spaces are opened and their contents discharged. Wynn-Williams (1959) felt that as many of these spaces as possible should be marsupialized by superficial abrasion, while Luikart, Ayres, and Wilson (1959) held a completely opposing view, stating emphatically that if such cysts are so opened, a scar, frequently hypertrophic, will result. Both groups agree with Burks (1956), however, that acute acne lesions of lesser extent may be benefited by surgical abrasion.

In the case of large cysts, it is our practice to excise and close surgically, leveling the area of surrounding skin by planing.

Contraindications. Many of these have been discussed in the preceding sections on limitations and indications. It is sufficient to mention that pigmentation of skin, whether in the black or the brunette Caucasian, occupies

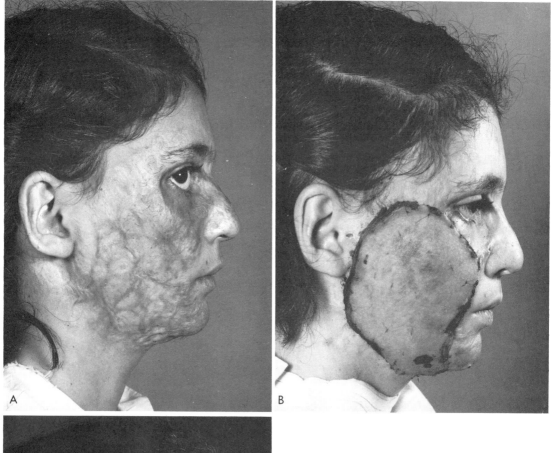

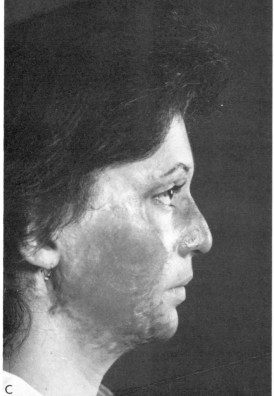

FIGURE 17–6. Treatment of burn scar by dermabrasion and overgrafting. *A*, Burn scar of cheek. *B*, split-thickness skin graft applied to the abraded area. *C*, Final result of overgrafting.

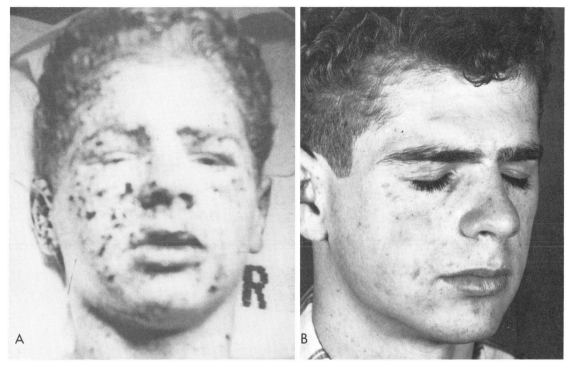

FIGURE 17–7. *A*, Widespread traumatic (gunpowder explosion) tattooing of face treated by scrubbing, abrading, and curettement. *B*, After an additional abrasion treatment. Note that some marks are likely to be permanent because of deep deposition of pigment. Further excision combined with abrasion is indicated.

a position high on this list. Postoperative hyperpigmentation has been described by Murray (1958) and Maneksha (1960), the latter reporting on dermabrasion of 150 cases of smallpox scarring in Indian patients. Maneksha felt that there were two explantations for the hyperpigmentation that developed in his patients; the first being that the abrasion may have been carried too deeply into the dermis, and the second that freezing of the skin contributed to the development of excessive pigment.

Wide scars, keloids, artistic tattoos, and deep burn scars are not benefited by dermabrasion.

MALIGNANCIES. Treatment of malignant skin lesion by this method has had some enthusiastic support (Burks, 1956; Pegum, 1959; Luikart, Ayres, and Wilson, 1959), but a surgeon *cannot* accept this as a definitive form of therapy for such lesions. One would be more inclined to believe that it could act as a mechanical metastasizer, particularly since Dorsey (1960) reported a case of widely disseminated flat warts on a face following planing of four wart scars caused by treatment with trichloroacetic acid.

RADIODERMATITIS. Abrasion by itself is of little value in this condition because of the paucity, if not complete absence, of the necessary regenerative epithelial elements. It may be useful in combination with skin overgrafting, as has been described in Chapter 6.

PSYCHOLOGIC CONTRAINDICATIONS. Psychologically unbalanced patients or those with psychoses are generally not accepted for abrasion therapy.

Criminals are also listed by Burks (1958) as unacceptable. He has reported some experimental work on the successful obliteration of fingerprints by the planing method and makes the startling statement that all fingerprint records and identification could be made obsolete and ineffective by this form of treatment.

COMPLICATIONS OF SURGICAL PLANING

If proper selection of patients has been combined with the appropriate skill and care in the execution of the procedure, serious complications are relatively infrequent. There are, however, fairly frequent complications of an annoying but generally temporary nature.

Edema and Erythema. Edema and erythema are natural responses on the part of the organism to trauma. Edema may last three to six weeks but rarely persists longer. Erythema, which initially occurs in every case, may persist for quite a long time beyond the normal period of involution. This has been attributed by various authors to excessive freezing of the skin, early exposure to sun or weather, or early resumption of topical therapy for active acne. The faint blush of the skin may be an attractive feature in some, or it may mar the appearance if the color is too ruddy. There appears to be no adequate therapy to correct this condition so that prevention is most important.

Milia. These are common sequelae occurring in about half of the patients some two to six weeks after planing. While most clear spontaneously, occasionally one must resort to incision and expression of the contents by pressure.

Incomplete Treatment. Inadequate planing of the affected areas may result in incomplete removal of the lesion. This type of complication is largely induced by unfamiliarity with the technique but occasionally is a result of laudable conservatism. The extensively pitted face calls for two or three treatments to achieve the desired improvement. Some patients will never be completely satisfied, their subjective desires exceeding the objective potential.

Linear Scarring. Linear scarring is occasionally seen where there has been an inadvertent gouging of tissue, particularly when the wire brush has been used. Deeper planing of the adjacent skin will not correct the defect that was left. Reapproximation of the edges by several fine sutures is the best method of treatment. With re-epithelization of the abraded skin on either side, new epithelium may grow over the suture line, reducing the scar to a minimum.

Hypertrophic Scarring. Hypertrophic scarring results when the abrasion is extended too deeply, causing delayed healing, or when the abrasion, even though superficial, has been done in an unfavorable area, such as the base of the neck.

Infection. Infection is extremely rare, occurring principally in those patients in whom dressings have been in place for some days. Severe cellulitis has not been observed.

Ridging. Marginal ridging or demarcation is occasionally encountered where beveling at the junction of treated and untreated areas has not been performed. It requires a light blending of the deeper abraded area with the surrounding skin by progressively abrading more superficially at the margins.

Chemical Planing

There are many synonymous terms for chemical planing: chemosurgery, chemabrasion, chemical face peeling, chemical face-lifting, and other terms limited only by semantic ingenuity. They all refer to the application of a cauterant to the skin for the purpose of causing a superficial destruction of the epidermis and upper layers of the dermis. After healing, the treated area has new epithelium and a somewhat more youthful appearance.

The application of caustic substances to the skin has been practiced for many years. Until quite recently it was in the hands of laymen incapable of exercising medical judgment. While there can be no doubt that some patients have achieved some measure of improvement, many others have been permanently disfigured and several have died as a result of inexpert administration.

CHEMICAL AGENTS AND TOXICOLOGY

Phenol. Phenol, a keratocoagulant, has been perhaps the most frequently used agent. It has been combined with other substances to form a solution of variable penetrability and coverage. Buffer agents have been used in combination with phenol (Combes, Sperber, and Reisch, 1960) which enable ready neutralization by the simple addition of water. Their formula is listed as follows: sodium salicylate, 0.3 g; powdered citric acid, 0.3 g; glycerin, 4.0 ml; water, 1.0 ml; anhydrous (99.5 per cent) phenol crystals, 30 g (Reisch, 1962).

Baker (1962) listed a somewhat different formula: phenol U.S.P., 3 ml; distilled water, 2 ml; croton oil, 2 drops; liquid soap, 8 drops. When it is compounded, there is approximately 5.5 ml of solution, of which perhaps only one-half is used in a total face application. A variation of slight degree is the formula used by Rees and Wood-Smith (1973), who recommend a freshly made solution compounded as follows: phenol 88 per cent U.S.P., 3 ml; croton oil, 3 drops; septisol soap, 8 drops; distilled water, 2 ml. This volume is sufficient for full face application.

Litton (1962) used a similar formula with some variations. It is as follows:

1. Phenol crystals diluted to 50 per cent with (2) and (3).
2. Glycerin.
3. Distilled water.
4. Croton oil. This is used to enhance skin irritation and thus penetration.

Baker and Litton recommend the use of a 50 per cent solution and occasionally a slightly stronger concentration, and both add croton oil in minute amounts for its irritant action, which appears to enhance the action of the phenol. Ayres (1962b) appears to have used full strength phenol in his trial of this substance, and for this reason his objections to its use appear to be less valid than if he had used dilutions in the 85 to 90 per cent range.

TOXICITY. The toxic effect following the absorption of phenol through the skin has been widely discussed, particularly that on the kidney, liver, medullary centers, and myocardium. Vasomotor collapse, convulsion, respiratory failure, and ultimate death can occur if prompt treatment with intravenous stimulants is not instituted (Aronsohn, 1972). Litton has drawn up a chart showing the systemic reaction to phenol (Fig. 17–8). Deichmann and Witherup (1944) reported the survival of a man who ingested an unknown quantity of phenol and whose blood level reached 23 mg per 100 ml.

In Litton's series the highest recorded figure was 0.68 mg per 100 ml one hour after administration of a 50 per cent solution to the entire face using a maximum of 3 ml of the solution. Baker reported no significant blood level or urinary changes in a personal series of 40 patients. Combes, Sperber, and Reisch (1960) have done intensive studies for longer than the 24-hour period criticized by Ayres as being insufficient in reporting blood levels and toxic results; they found no untoward effects or elevations to significantly dangerous levels, using 88 to 90 per cent phenol concentrations.

Ayres, in his own work, using full strength phenol found blood levels reaching as high as 50 mg per 100 ml when large areas of skin (8 × 19 cm) were treated at intervals of two to three days; transient urinary signs consisted largely of granular casts and albuminuria. In one of his patients albuminuria and positive urinary tests for phenol persisted for several months following treatment. It appears, however, that the concentration of phenol in his series is excessive when it is applied over rather large areas at too close intervals, a situation which is hardly likely in the usual clinical application of this substance. Dilution increases absorption because it slows down keratocoagulation, thus enabling a longer absorption time. The freshness of the solution has no influence on either its activity or its absorption. The author prefers to discard the preparation when it turns color. It is not denied that there is potential danger in the use of phenol, not only to the patient but also to the operator who inhales the phenol fumes.

SYSTEMIC REACTION TO PHENOL

(PHENOL-SKIN-BLOOD STREAM)

- FREE PHENOL AND CONJUGATED WITH {GLYCURONIC ACID, SULFURIC ACID} EXCRETED BY KIDNEYS.

or

- DETOXIFIED BY OXIDATION TO {HYDROQUINONE, PYROCATECHIN}

SIGNS AND SYMPTOMS OF PHENOL POISONING:

- CENTRAL DEPRESSION, FALL IN BLOOD PRESSURE, HEADACHE, NAUSEA.

- CAN HAVE TOXIC EFFECT ON MYOCARDIUM.

FIGURE 17–8. Toxic effect of phenol.

Trichloroacetic Acid. This substance, when used in full strength, has an extremely destructive action. It is used by Ayres as the cauterant of choice, mainly in dilutions of 25 to 50 per cent with occasional applications of 75 per cent to full strength. While thus achieving a destructive effect comparable to that obtained from phenol, he feels that he obtains a greater margin of safety from the systemic standpoint, since there is no evidence of a nephrotoxic effect from this agent. Wolfort, Dalton, and Hoopes (1972), employing a 50 per cent solution of tricholoracetic acid neutralized after 5 minutes by a benzalkonium chloride sponge, reported satisfactory results in 38 patients. They felt that there is no systemic toxicity; the depth of penetration is more easily controlled (benzalkonium chloride), and a chemical wound is left open, allowing for close observation. However, Aronsohn (1972) felt that its action is too unpredictable and more apt to generate scarring.

Salabrasion. This technique, as practiced by Manchester (1974) for tattoo removal, combines a chemical and a mechanical action. The results are, in the author's opinion, not as satisfactory as those of other methods. The technique awaits additional clinical trials.

MODE OF ACTION

The cauterants act in a way similar to surgical dermabrasion: they destroy the entire epidermis and the upper portion of the dermis by chemical coagulation rather than by mechanical removal. The coagulated portion of the skin remains in place, while new epidermal cells, derived from the adnexa of the skin, resurface the epidermis in five to seven days; dermal regeneration occurs in two to three weeks.

According to Ayres (1960), the depth of penetration of phenol is from 0.3 to 0.4 mm, the depth being controlled to some extent by the pressure of application. Thus there is penetration to the papillary layer of the dermis with little or no involvement of the reticular layer. Healing progresses in a fashion similar to that seen in dermabrasion or the healing of a skin graft donor site.

The effects of the treatment are explained as follows: The destruction of the epidermis results in the removal of roughened, withered, pigmented skin, which is replaced by young, fresh, pink epidermis. Because of the overall inter-island contraction (Converse and Robb-Smith, 1944), there is a diffuse tightening of the epidermal layer. There may also be a slight coarsening of texture of the skin if the application has been too heavy and the penetration too deep, giving it an appearance similar to that seen following the healing of a deep second degree burn. The firmness and elastic quality of the new skin are the result of the thickened papillary layer of the dermis, with its plumper, horizontally oriented collagen fibers. The increased vascularity yields an appearance not only of firmness but also of fresh, slightly pink, and thus more youthful skin.

However, there is at present real argument as to the presence of increased elastin in the dermis, although the discussions pro and con wax and wane. Baker and associates (1974) feel that there is an increase in "elastotic" material, demonstrated by means of Verhoeff's stain for elastin. They show some impressive photomicrographs containing untreated and treated contiguous areas after 15 years (Fig. 17–9). Their claim is disputed by Bhangoo (1974), who feels that Verhoeff's stain is unreliable for proving the presence of elastin and who quotes Litton (1962), Spira and co-workers (1970), Gillman and coworkers (1955), Gillman and Penn (1956), and Turnbridge (1964) in support of his view.

Litton, in a personal communication (1974), acknowledged that there may be considerable truth in Bhangoo's statement.

Other reported histologic changes occurring in human skin following chemical peeling are homogenization of the architecture of the dermal collagen and diminution in the quantity of melanin granules in the basal layer of the epidermis (Baker and associates, 1974). The latter finding is probably responsible for the bleaching of skin following chemical peeling.

TECHNIQUE

The patients should usually be admitted to the hospital for treatment. The exceptions to this routine are patients who are having only small areas treated; these can be handled in the office. When a full-face treatment is given, the experience is uncomfortable and traumatizing, both physically and psychologically. The post-treatment appearance is frightening and only a small percentage of patients are willing to face either strangers or members of their own family in such a state.

Chemical peeling is neither painless nor

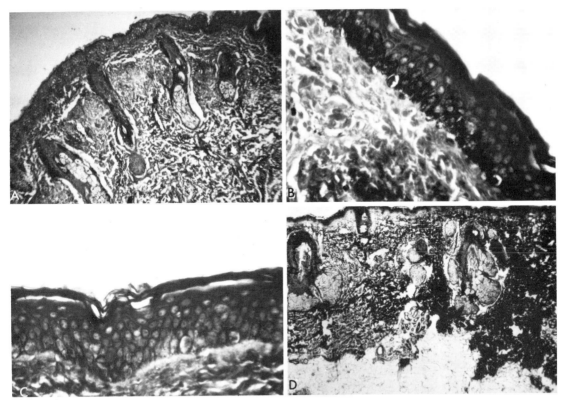

FIGURE 17–9. Histologic changes following chemical peel. *A,* Low power view showing breakdown in collagen in a lamellar distribution. *B,* Fontana stain of normal skin. Note densely pigmented basal layer of epidermis. *C,* Fontana stain 24 months after chemical peel. Note decrease in melanin cells in basal layer. *D,* Elastin stain showing junction between nontreated and treated skin. Note collection of "elastotic" material. (Courtesy of Dr. T. J. Baker.)

quick. The risk of losing the patient's confidence is great when one de-emphasizes the nature of the procedure.

Another reason for having a patient admitted to a hospital is to obtain a complete medical evaluation, especially regarding the kidneys and liver. If kidney damage has been revealed by the history or laboratory studies, chemical peeling should not be undertaken, regardless of the fact that, to date, all of the evidence seems to indicate that the small amounts of phenol used are harmless.

If corrective surgery on the eyelids and face is planned because of excessively redundant skin, the surgical procedure should be performed, and at that time only one area of the face should be treated by chemical application, namely the forehead or perioral region, with the remainder of the face and eyelids being treated after an interval of at least 8 to 12 weeks. Litton, Fournier and Capinpin, (1973) cautioned against combined facialplasty and chemical peeling at the same procedure.

When the chemical treatment alone is undertaken, the entire face, including both upper and lower eyelids, may be treated at one session, although Litton and others prefer a two-stage procedure. A more uniform treated surface is obtained than when secondary treatment is required, since it is difficult to match a treated with an untreated area. Edema of the eyelids does occur and may occlude the lids, but it has not constituted a serious obstacle.

Preoperative Sedation. General anesthesia is unnecessary, and all patients treated so far have appeared to do well with a compound medication consisting of an analgesic and a tranquilizer given about one-half hour before treatment. It may be necessary to repeat or reinforce the medication through an intravenous route during the procedure.

The treatment can be done at the patient's bedside or preferably in the operating room under a suitable light and with assistance.

Choice of Chemical. The phenol compound

recommended by Baker and Litton has been used extensively by the author. The solution thus made up is approximately 50 per cent phenol, and the proportions may be altered so as to lower or increase this percentage as the situation dictates.

It cannot be stressed too often that dilution increases skin absorption and thus potentiates toxicity.

The writer is not in a position to comment on the efficaciousness of trichloroacetic acid or salicylic acid, not having used them in his practice.

Procedure. The patient's face is cleaned thoroughly with pHisoHex, following which it is dried and the parts then further cleaned of oily residue by sponges containing ether. Care is taken to avoid the eyes and as far as possible to prevent the patient from inhaling the ether vapor. Excessive hair should be removed before the patient reaches the operating room. The face and whatever additional parts are to be treated are draped in routine fashion.

The freshly prepared solution is applied in an orderly fashion using cottontipped applicators. For finer work around the eyelids and the palpebral margins, cotton-tipped round toothpicks can be used. No applicator should be flooded with the solution. A good practice is to dip a number of applicators in the solution and then transfer them, with the tips down, into a sterile medicine glass. In this way an excess of solution runs off, and the remainder can be lightly blotted when the applicator is picked up for use.

In general, it is wise to adopt a regular order of treatment. The forehead extending upward into the hairline and downward into the eyebrow line may be treated first; next the application is extended to the temporal hairline. The solution is applied with even brush strokes on and into the skin, criss-crossing where necessary to secure complete coverage and making certain that the solution penetrates into all crevices and furrows. Where lines are especially heavy, additional force of application will exert some effect on the depth of penetration. The treated area quickly assumes a frosty white color accompanied by a sensation of burning pain which lasts several minutes and then as a general rule disappears.

With the skin under slight tension, strips of waterproof adhesive tape are applied, care being exercised to make sure that no wrinkling occurs beneath the tape. It may be advisable to apply these first strips in an edge-to-edge, end-to-end fashion, rather than in the overlapping manner which may be used for the second layer of tape. The taping is extended to the hairline and the eyebrows. Following the application of the tape, there will be a recurrence of the burning sensation, and some pain may be experienced by the patient. If the patient becomes unduly restless, it is wise to stop and reassure her.

After the forehead unit is taped, the second major area to be treated comprises both the eyelids and nose. The application is extended to within 2 to 3 mm of the palpebral margins using a wrung-out toothpick applicator. The application should be extended out over the entire nose, including the alae and the margins of the vestibules, in order that no areas show any sharp lines of demarcation between treated and untreated skin. The larger applicators are used for these regions, and in this second phase one can complete the entire middle third of the face. The upper lip should be stretched lightly and the solution rubbed in briskly, extending down to the vermilion border. One must never stop above the border, as this line will show in the final result. If the solution runs onto the vermilion, no permanent damage results. Once again the entire treated area is taped, and the actual application of the chemical solution is interrupted.

The remaining lower third of the face including the cheeks is then treated in a similar fashion, the treatment stopping below the mandible in an area that is not normally conspicuous. By the time the taping of this last area is completed, the oral aperture will have been reduced to a small opening which is incapable of being opened widely because of the splinting effect of the tape. This is beneficial because it prevents undue movement and loosening of the tape.

It should be again stressed that no creasing of skin is permissible; unless the skin in such areas as the outer canthus, the upper lip, the eyelids, and the forehead is stretched gently as the tape is being applied, there is a strong tendency for the reinforcement of wrinkles in these regions rather than their elimination.

Postoperative Care. With the treatment completed, the patient is kept on a liquid diet and warned against excessive efforts to talk or to be active. Considerable discomfort is felt over the next two days, and this should be controlled by adequate amounts of Demerol or some other analgesic. Hypnotics should be prescribed for bedtime. Most patients are slightly more comfortable if the head of the bed is elevated.

Forty-eight hours later the patient is again sedated and the adhesive tape mask is removed. Without adequate sedation this can be an extremely painful procedure, and the surgeon should stop frequently to give the patient a few moments of relief. As the tape is removed, the skin will show tiny punctate areas of hemorrhage, some serous weeping, and a deep red blush in general. Some swelling will be present. Removal of the tape takes with it the necrotic epidermis and dermis.

Thymol iodide powder is then dusted over the entire treated area including, lightly, the eyelids. The patient's appearance at this time is ghostlike. Further applications of the powder are made every three to four hours, and by the following day the color changes to a dark brown and the texture to that of a hard crust.

When the restraining effect of the tape is released, considerable edema of the tissues, to the point of a moon face, can be anticipated, and the patient should be warned that this may occur.

The crust is left in place until about the fourth day after tape removal, when the entire area can be liberally covered with petrolatum or cold cream. Twelve to 24 hours after this application, most if not all of the crust can be peeled away, showing bright, pink epidermis in most regions, with a few scattered areas still not healed. If the crust is adherent, it should not be removed forcibly.

Following the removal of the tape, there will be some persistent edema which gradually subsides during the next three to four weeks; it is not usually sufficient to cause the patient embarrassment. The new epidermis should be protected by light application of a thin lubricant such as cold cream. At the end of two weeks the patient is allowed to apply cosmetics lightly, and at the end of three weeks she can use her normal make-up.

Gentle cleansing of the face with a mild soap and water is permissible 12 to 14 days postoperatively.

There must be no exposure to actinic rays to avoid hyperpigmentation. This rule should be enforced as soon as the patient leaves the hospital or as soon as the crust is removed. If there is any risk of exposure to sun, a sunscreening cream should be applied frequently to all of the treated parts.

If the patient has been treated in the hospital, there is no reason why she should not go home after the tape mask has been removed. Most patients prefer to avoid public exposure, however, and some even elect to remain in the hospital.

RESULTS

For the first eight to ten weeks following treatment, the skin blush is fairly pronounced. It may be camouflaged by the application of cosmetics. This interval is also the time when the good results of therapy are at their height owing to the generalized edema. Few if any wrinkles are seen, and the patients are generally delighted at the "miraculous" results. It is at this time that one must warn them that there is still some swelling in the face and that some wrinkles or lines, while not as pronounced as before treatment, may later become visible. If the patient has not been warned that this can happen, she will be dejected later.

Milia may appear four to eight weeks following treatment, and they are handled in the same fashion as after dermabrasion.

Hyperpigmentation may occur despite the use of sun screen preparations and may persist for many months. A good rule to follow might be to use this treatment only in the early winter months when the hazard of exposure to excessive sunlight is minimal. In part, the pigmentation may be due to carelessness on the part of the patient, who feels that one application of the protective cream suffices for an entire day, not realizing that perspiration will dilute the effectiveness of the screening agent. Baker and Gordon (1971) noted that even reflected light, such as that received when driving an automobile for a lengthy period, has caused irregular pigmentation on the side of the face that was exposed. All practitioners seem to agree that patients must avoid direct sunlight for at least three to six months after chemical peel.

If the solution has been applied in an even fashion over the whole face, there should be no marked discrepancy between the various areas of treatment. Sometimes, however, treatment has been uneven, and this occasionally reflects itself in patchy, irregular discoloration. These areas of irregularity can usually be corrected by a second treatment, which may be administered in 8 to 12 weeks. The second treatment will also help reduce some of the residual lines remaining after the first application of the chemical.

Hypopigmentation, if it occurs, is generally

of a temporary nature, and the patient should be reassured as to the return of color, which may require 9 to 18 months; occasionally, repigmentation does not occur.

Occasional white streaking may be seen in some areas of the face, and it is generally the result of a solution that has been applied too lightly. If this occurs and is of a limited nature, it may be aided by a local application to the affected area.

Hypertrophic scarring and *scar contractures* are seen occasionally, but seldom or not at all when the treatment is administered by a skilled plastic surgeon. Spira and associates (1974) refer to it as being more apt to occur if a perioral peel has been combined with a face lift.

Nevi darkening may occur. Previously existing nevi on a peeled face frequently become much darker. Patients should be warned of this in advance, and surgical excision of the nevi should be performed either before (one to two weeks) or after the procedure.

Telangiectases appear more prominent because of the bleaching effect of the peel solution. If this occurs, electrocoagulation may be of some help; a whiter scar occasionally results (Spira and associates, 1974).

Pore prominence is generally enhanced. This is possibly due to phenol running down into the pores, thus increasing the possibility of greater systemic absorption and allowing deeper penetration than is desirable (Aronsohn, 1972).

A demarcation line is unavoidable. The treated area is always lighter than the untreated, especially in dark-complexioned individuals. It is minimal in light-skinned people but still can be detected. Feathering of the edges of the treated area helps, as does restricting the limits of the peel to a part one to two inches beyond the jaw line. Litton does chemical planing of the neck on occasion, but most practitioners, including the author, have been reluctant to try it or have had unsatisfactory results when they have tried it; thus neck peels should be avoided as a general rule.

In general, the results can be said to be satisfactory, and the technique has become widely accepted by plastic surgeons.

INDICATIONS

Chemical peeling is not a substitute for corrective surgery, although it may well supplement it. The patient with a deep nasolabial line, heavy vertical or horizontal furrows in the forehead region, excessive skin in the eyelids,

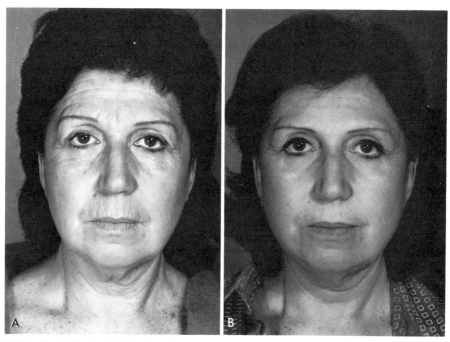

FIGURE 17–10. Perioral and glabellar chemical peeling used in conjunction with a facial and eyelidplasty. *A*, Preoperative view. *B*, Postoperative view. (Courtesy of Dr. Cary L. Guy.)

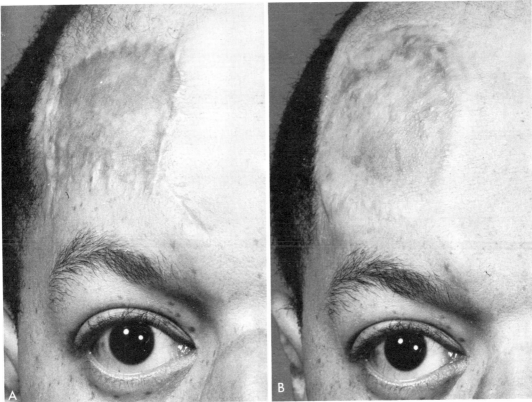

FIGURE 17–11. Chemical planing of the line of junction of a skin graft and the recipient site edge. *A*, Donor area of a scalping flap for subtotal reconstruction of the nose. Note the uneven junction line of the skin graft with the surrounding tissue. *B*, Smoothing effect following chemical planing.

and heavy jowls with redundancy of skin in the neck cannot possibly secure the desired amount of improvement by chemosurgery alone. Residual fine lines in the periorbital region and perioral region, particularly the upper lip, shallow forehead lines, and fine checkering of the skin respond best to this form of treatment (Fig. 17–10).

It can be used as the sole form of treatment in combination with surgery in patients with a greater degree of skin laxity.

It is a useful office procedure for the treatment of minor degrees of scar irregularity (Fig. 17–11) and has been successful in reducing multiple small elevations or puckering resulting from healing after certain types of burns.

Sternal keloids, which respond in a notoriously poor fashion to nearly every form of surgery, have been flattened in several instances by repeated application of a phenol solution. In such cases the chemical is applied solely within the boundaries of the keloid. It is sometimes useful to test the effect of the chem-ical on a small area of keloid before treating the whole lesion.

The lines of separation between dermabraded and untreated skin, which are frequently quite sharp, can be skillfully brushed out or blended by the application of the chemical solution.

Sun-irradiated and damaged skin responds to chemical peeling in much the same way as it does to dermabrasion insofar as improving the condition of the skin and reducing its susceptibility to malignant change is concerned.

Contraindications. In general, the contraindications are the same as for dermabrasion, and areas of the body that are either deficient in or devoid of the epithelial elements should be avoided.

Dark-skinned individuals and particularly blacks, while not completely excluded, should be approached with considerable caution for the reasons previously discussed in the section of this chapter devoted to dermabrasion.

Patients with poor nutritional status or diabetes in whom healing is likely to be prolonged, should, as a general rule, be eliminated as candidates.

REFERENCES

Aronsohn, R. B.: Complications of chemosurgery. Eye Ear Nose Throat Mon., *51*:19, 1972.

Ayres, S.: Dermal changes following application of chemical cauterants to aging skin (superficial chemosurgery). Arch. Dermatol., *82*:578, 1960.

Ayres, S.: Superficial Chemosurgery. *In* Epstein, E. (Ed.): Skin Surgery. 2nd Ed. Philadelphia, Lea & Febiger, 1962a.

Ayres, S., III: Superficial chemosurgery in treating aging skin. Arch. Dermatol., *85*:385, 1962b.

Baker, T. J.: Chemical face peeling and rhytidectomy. A combined approach for face rejuvenation. Plast. Reconstr. Surg., *29*:199, 1962.

Baker, T. J., and Gordon, H. L.: Chemical face peeling and dermabrasion. Surg. Clin. North Am., *51*:387, 1971.

Baker, T. J., Gordon, H. L., Mosienko, P., and Seckinger, D. L.: Long-term histological study of skin after chemical face peeling. Plast. Reconstr. Surg., *53*:522, 1974.

Bernard, F. D.: Dermabrasion tattooing, a preliminary report. Plast. Reconstr. Surg., *22*:267, 1958.

Bhangoo, K. S.: Histological changes following chemical face peeling. Plast. Reconstr. Surg., *54*:599, 1974.

Bishop, G. H.: Regeneration after experimental removal of skin in man. Am. J. Anat., *76*:153, 1945.

Burks, J. W.: Wire Brush Surgery. Springfield, Ill., Charles C Thomas, 1956.

Burks, J. W.: Wire brush planing—an office procedure. Postgrad. Med., *20*:652, 1956.

Burks, J. W.: The effect of dermabrasion on fingerprints. A.M.A. Arch. Dermatol., *77*:8, 1958.

Burks, J. W.: Prophylactic planing of the aged patient for cancer of the skin. J. Louisana Med. Soc., *111*:169, 1959.

Combes, F. C., Sperber, P. A., and Reisch, M.: Dermal defects: Treatment by a chemical agent. N.Y. Physicians & Am. Med., *55*:36, 1960.

Converse, J. M., and Robb-Smith, A. H. T.: The healing of surface cutaneous wounds: Its analogy with the healing of superficial burns. Ann. Surg., *120*:873, 1944.

Conway, H.: Tattooing of nevus flammeus for permanent camouflage. J.A.M.A., *152*:666, 1953.

Cronin, T. D.: Extensive pigmented nevi in hair-bearing areas: Removal of pigmented layer while preserving the hair follicles. Plast. Reconstr. Surg., *11*:94, 1953.

Deichmann, W., and Witherup, S.: Phenol studies. VI. The acute and comparative toxicity of phenol and *o*-, *m*- and *p*-cresols for experimental animals. J. Pharmacol. Exp. Therap., *80*:233, 1944.

Dorsey, C.: Dissemination of flat warts by wire brush surgery. Arch. Dermatol., *82*:262, 1960.

Eisen, A. Z., Holyoke, J. B., and Lobitz, W. C.: Responses of superficial portion of human pilosebaceous apparatus to control injury. J. Invest. Dermatol., *25*:145, 1955.

Epstein, E.: Skin Surgery. 2nd Ed. Chapter 14, Dermabrasion. Philadelphia, Lea & Febiger, 1962.

Gillman, T., and Penn, J.: Studies on the repair of cutaneous wounds. Med. Proc., *2*:121, 1956.

Gillman, T., Penn, J., Branks, D., and Roux, M.: A re-examination of certain aspects of the histogenesis of the healing of cutaneous wounds. A preliminary report. Br. J. Surg., *43*:141, 1955.

Hynes, W.: The treatment of pigmented moles by shaving and skin graft. Br. J. Plast. Surg., *9*:47, 1956.

Hynes, W.: The treatment of scars by shaving and skin graft. Br. J. Plast. Surg., *10*:1, 1957.

Hynes, W.: "Shaving" in plastic surgery with special reference to the treatment of chronic radiodermatitis. Br. J. Plast. Surg., *12*:43, 1959.

Iverson, P. C.: Surgical removal of traumatic tattoos. Plast. Reconstr. Surg., *2*:427, 1947.

Iverson, P. C.: Further developments in the treatment of skin lesions by surgical abrasion. Plast. Reconstr. Surg., *12*:27, 1953.

Iverson, P. C.: Dermal abrasion. Am. J. Nursing, *57*:860, 1957.

Janson, P.: Eine einfache Methode der Entfernung von Tatauierungen. Dermatol. Wochenschr., *101*:894, 1935.

Johnson, H. M.: Headache and risks of dermabrasion. A.M.A. Arch. Dermatol., *81*:26, 1960.

Kromayer, E.: Rotationinstrumente: Ein neues technisches Verfahren in der dermatologischen Kleinchirurgie. Chir. Dermatol. Ztschr., Berlin, *12*:26, 1905.

Kromayer, E.: Die Behandlung der kosmetischen Hautleiden unter besonderer Berüchsichtigung der physikalischen Heilmethoden und der narbenlosen Operationsweisen. Leipzig, Georg Thieme, 1923, p. 15.

Kurtin, A.: Corrective surgical planing of skin; new technique for treatment of acne scars and other skin defects. A.M.A. Arch. Dermatol. Syph., *68*:389, 1953.

Litton, C.: Chemical face lifting. Plast. Reconstr. Surg., *29*:371, 1962.

Litton, C.: Personal communication, 1974.

Litton, C., Fournier, P., and Capinpin, A.: A survey of chemical peeling of the face. Plast. Reconstr. Surg., *51*:645, 1973.

Luikart, R., Ayres, S., and Wilson, J. W.: Surgical skin planing. N.Y. State J. Med., *59*:3413, 1959.

McAndrew, J. J.: Removal of linear scars. A.M.A. Arch. Dermatol., *80*:227, 1959.

McDowell, F.: Tattoo erasing. Plast. Reconstr. Surg., *53*:580, 1974.

McEvitt, W. G.: Treatment of acne pits by abrasion with sandpaper. J.A.M.A., *142*:647, 1950.

Manchester, G. H.: The removal of commercial tattoos by abrasion with table salt. Plast. Reconstr. Surg., *53*:517, 1974.

Maneksha, R. J.: Dermoabrasion therapy for scars. Experience of 150 cases of smallpox scars. Plast. Reconstr. Surg., *25*:615, 1960.

Mopper, C., and Mercantini, E. S.: The inadequacy of dermabrasion in therapy of nevi. Can. Med. Assoc. J., *83*:1015, 1960.

Murray, R. D.: Abrasive surgery in Negroes. Plast. Reconstr. Surg., *21*:42, 1958.

Ortiz-Monasterio, F., Lopez-Mas, J., and Araico, J.: Rhinoplasty in the thick-skinned nose. Br. J. Plast. Surg., *27*:19, 1974.

Pegum, J. S., Ridley, C. M., Russell, B., Thorne, B., and Morrison, S. L.: Dermabrasion: An appraisal. Br. J. Dermatol., *71*:371, 1959.

Pickrell, K., Matton, G., Huger, W., and Pound, E.: Dermabrasion of extensive keratotic lesions of the forehead and scalp. Plast. Reconstr. Surg., *30*:32, 1962.

Rees, T. D., and Wood-Smith, D.: Cosmetic Facial Surgery. Philadelphia, W. B. Saunders Company, 1973.

Reisch, M.: Personal communication, 1962.

Rossignol, M.: Des scarifications dans les maladies de la peau. Arch. Belges Méd., *20*:298, 1881.

Small, A. A.: Kurtin's surgical planing procedure: A review of experiences with special reference to post-acne scarring. Can. Med. Assoc. J., *75*:279, 1956.

Spira, M., Dahl, G., Freeman, R., Gerow, F. J., and Hardy, S. B.: Chemosurgery—A histological study. Plast. Reconstr. Surg., *45*:247, 1970.

Spira, M., Gerow, F. J., and Hardy, S. B.: Complications of chemical face peeling. Plast. Reconstr. Surg., *54*:397, 1974.

Turnbridge, R. E.: Aging of connective tissues. *In* Rock, A., and Champion, R. H. (Eds.): Progress in Biological Sciences in Relation to Dermatology. London, Cambridge University Press, 1964, pp. 67–75.

Variot, M. G.: Nouveau procédé de destruction des tatouages. C. R. Soc. Biol., *40*:636, 1888.

Webster, G. V.: Report at the Annual Convention of the American Society of Plastic and Reconstructive Surgeons, Hollywood. Florida, October, 1954.

Webster, G. V., Peterson, R. A., and Stein, H.: Dermal overgrafting of the leg. J. Bone Joint Surg., *40-A*:796, 1958.

Wolfort, F. S., Dalton, W. E., and Hoopes, J. E.: Chemical peel with trichloroacetic acid. Br. J. Plast. Surg., *25*:333, 1972.

Wynn-Williams, D.: Dermabrasion. Br. J. Plast. Surg., *12*:170, 1959.

CHAPTER 18

THERMAL BURNS

JOHN B. LYNCH, M.D.,
AND TRUMAN G. BLOCKER, JR., M.D.

Electrical Burns
*John Marquis Converse, M.D.,
and Donald Wood-Smith, F.R.C.S.E.*

INTRODUCTION

There are estimated to be approximately 2,000,000 burns that occur annually in the United States. Approximately one-half of these are limited and require only first aid treatment for the relief of pain. An estimated 250,000 are more severe and require bed rest or home treatment. Each year 70,000 burn patients are hospitalized in the United States, and 12,000 of them die. Although large burn services continue to report mortality rates in excess of 20 per cent, the National Safety Council Bulletin indicates that progress is being made with regard to prevention of fatalities from fires and other burns. Since 1910 the mortality rate per 100,000 from burns has dropped from 9 to 4.

Trends in present-day burn therapy are toward: (1) standardization and simplification of care for the average patient with lesions involving 20 to 80 per cent of the body surface; and (2) treatment of complications due to loss of critical amounts of skin, unusual depth of burn, involvement of critical areas such as the hands, face, or eyes, respiratory tract injury, fluid and electrolyte abnormalities, concomitant disease or trauma, and infection. Certainly in the past 25 years, burn treatment has achieved a measure of status in surgery, whereas it was once a relatively neglected field.

HISTORICAL ASPECTS

The most important early discussion of burns in the English language was by John Kentish, who in 1797 published a monograph entitled "An Essay on Burns." In this essay he advocated exposure therapy in the early stages of the burn, but later he preferred the use of occlusive dressings. James Earle (1799), in a series of publications which appeared at about the same time, discussed many aspects of burn treatment, including the use of ice for treatment of the initial pain. Few changes were made in therapy throughout the nineteenth century, except for the use of the continuous baths of Hebra at the Allgemeines Krankenhaus in Vienna. Although this type of therapy never gained popularity in the United States, it was enthusiastically reported by Emanuel Friend in the Journal of the American Medical Association in 1895.

Standard textbooks and medical journals at the end of the nineteenth century indicate that there was little or no emphasis on burn physiology and supportive therapy but that a wide variety of local nostrums were in vogue. The latter included carron oil, carbolic acid, bichloride of mercury, lead carbinate, zinc oxide ointment, gum arabic, lard, collodion, silver nitrate, castor oil, Ichthyol, and a wide variety of other concoctions. The first modern discussion of burn therapy was published by Sneve (1905) in a remarkable article entitled "The Treatment of Burns and Skin Grafting." This paper, which advocated exposure therapy, was followed by a prize-winning essay in 1906 by Oppenheimer, who advocated picric acid therapy. Picric acid therapy was used intermittently for many years following this publication.

Between 1909 and 1915 reports on the open air treatment of burns appeared under the authorship of Neathery (1909), St. John (1910), Hermann (1915), and Haas (1915). With the advent of World War I Barthe de Sandfort (1914) introduced paraffin wax or Ambrine in the treatment of acute extensive burns, a method which rapidly became popular and widely used.

In 1925 Davidson published his paper on "Tannic Acid in the Treatment of Burns," and as a consequence the exposure technique rapidly declined in popularity. In addition to tannic acid, topical agents in wide use at this time included silver nitrate, saline packs and baths, and gentian violet. In 1941 the era of antibiotic topical agents was introduced with the preliminary reports on the topical use of sulfanilamide. In 1942 Allen and Koch encouraged the use of pressure dressings, and in the same year the National Research Council manual officially abandoned tannic acid and other types of chemical eschar agents for local burn wound care.

It was not until Wallace's article of 1949 that exposure treatment of burns was revived in the literature. Blocker (1950) and Pulaski (1950) observed Wallace's techniques in Edinburgh and reintroduced them for clinical trial in the United States.

Since 1950, increased understanding of fluid and electrolyte therapy, improved methods of combating shock, and better understanding of the metabolic, nutritional, hematologic, and psychologic aspects of burn care have been recognized. Since 1950 voluminous international papers have appeared on all aspects of burn care. In addition, several national and international burn meetings have been held in recent years, and specialized institutes for the treatment of burns have been developed in many countries. A comprehensive review of the historical aspects of burn treatment appears in the first edition of this book, and it is recommended for the reader desiring more historical information.

ETIOLOGY

The cause of burns varies from one part of the world to another, depending on local customs with respect to the use of fire. Burns occur frequently in India because of the small, open cooking stoves in common use; molten metal burns occur frequently in certain specialized industrial areas; and the custom of setting a child on a hot brick for the purpose of toilet training is practiced in some parts of South America. Of the 70,000 burns which require hospitalization in the United States annually, approximately 50 per cent occur in the home; of these home accidents, at least two-thirds are preventable. The cause of burns in 1000 consecutive patients is illustrated in Table 18–1. The majority of patients receive injuries from direct contact with flash or flames. Flammable clothing, the use of open fires for heating, the use of gasoline and kerosene for cleaning purposes or to start fires, carlessness with cigarettes, and small children playing with matches have accounted for the majority of accidents in the home. In some instances, alcoholism and epilepsy are etiologic factors.

When the causes of these accidents are reviewed, it is apparent that certain legislative requirements could significantly reduce the frequency of burn injuries. Certain clothing, such as women's and children's sleepwear, which tends to be caught up in the draft of any open fire, should be given flame retardant treatment. Additional building code requirements should prohibit the use of open floor furnace heaters and prevent the installation of open gas heaters at or near floor level, where the draft can ignite clothing.

Home safety programs in the past have emphasized maintaining and checking electrical wiring and avoiding the storage of oily rags, cloths, or paper in closets where ignition can occur. By far the greatest danger results from the inadequate or improper storage of gasoline and the use of gasoline for starting fires, burning leaves, and so forth.

CLASSIFICATION AND DIAGNOSIS OF BURNS

Although the diagnosis of a burn does not pose a problem, the evaluation of the magnitude of

TABLE 18–1. *Cause of Burn in 1000 Consecutive Patients*

Flame and flash burns	77.1%
Scalds	13.0%
Contact burns	5.1%
Electrical burns	3.0%
Chemical burns	1.4%

TABLE 18–2. *Factors Which Determine the Severity of a Burn Injury in an Individual Patient*

1. Extent of body surface burned
2. Depth of the burn
3. Age of the patient
4. Causative agent
5. Fractures or associated injuries
6. Concomitant illness, such as preexisting cardio-vascular, renal, or metabolic disease
7. Obesity or alcoholism
8. Burns sustained in a closed space with inhalation of smoke, carbon monoxide, and noxious fumes

injury is more difficult. The important factors contributing to the severity of injuries are listed in Table 18–2.

Extent of Body Surface Burned

The first factor to consider in determining the severity of the injury in an individual patient is the extent of body surface involvement. An approximation of surface area involvement can be rapidly made by application of the "rule of nines" (Fig. 18–1). In adults, approximately 9 per cent is allowed for the head and neck, 9 per cent for each upper extremity, 18 per cent for the anterior thorax and abdomen, 18 per cent for the back and buttocks, and 18 per cent for each lower extremity. In children, a relatively greater amount is allowed for the head and trunk, and less for the lower extremities. Although the "rule of nines" is useful for an initial estimate of the body surface involved, a more accurate determination is desirable. For this purpose a body surface chart, such as that illustrated in Figure 18–2, is preferred.

Depth of Burn

The depth of the burn is largely dependent upon the temperature of the burning agent and the duration of contact. Burns are usually classified as *first degree, second degree,* or *third degree,* depending on the depth of tissue destruction.* As illustrated in Figure 18–3, a first degree burn is one which involves only the epidermis. It is characterized by erythema; the classic ex-

ample is a sunburn. A second degree burn is one which destroys the epithelium and a variable portion of the dermis. In the absence of infection, second degree burns will heal spontaneously in two to four weeks by regeneration of the epithelial surface from the epithelium persisting in the base of hair shafts and skin glands. A third degree burn is one in which the entire thickness of skin including epithelium and dermis is completely destroyed. Unless third degree lesions are extremely small, spontaneous regeneration does not occur, and skin grafting is required. The term *"fourth degree,"* indicating involvement of underlying muscles, tendons, nerves, bones, or blood vessels, is not commonly employed in the burn literature, but it is still included in many tables of classification.

The diagnostic points which are helpful in differentiating the depth of the burn are listed in Table 18–3.

Determination of the depth of the burn at the time of initial examination is often difficult. The wound will vary in appearance, depending upon the cause of the burning agent, the time elapsed since injury, and prior therapy that the patient may have received. In general, a first degree burn is characterized by only a red,

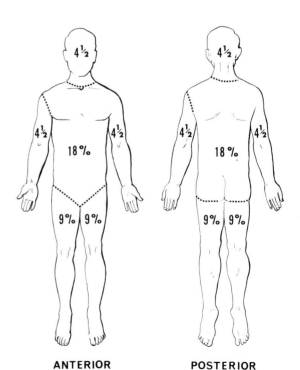

ANTERIOR   **POSTERIOR**

FIGURE 18–1. "Rule of Nines" used to determine the percentage of body surface area burned.

---

*Dupuytren (1832) classified burns in six degrees; the classification in three degrees is that of Boyer (1814).

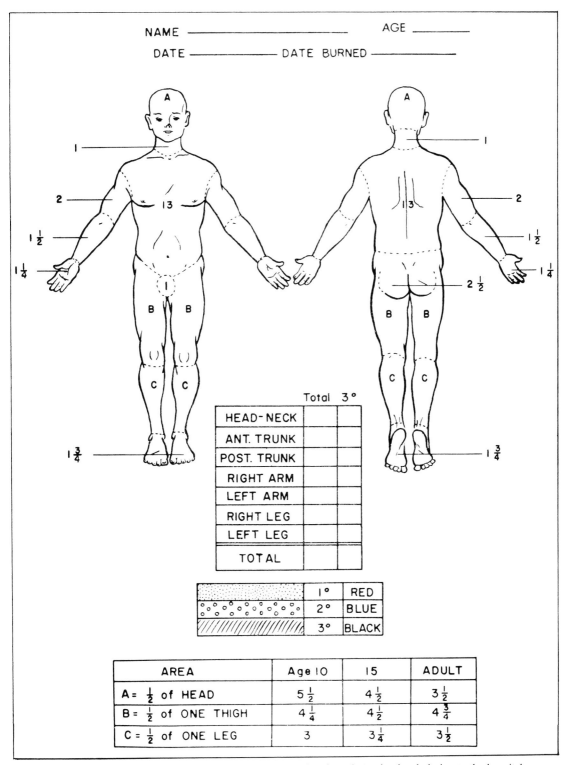

FIGURE 18–2. Body surface chart. This can be completed on the patient's admission to the hospital.

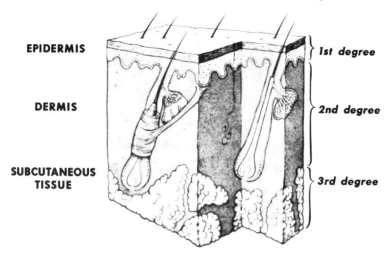

EPIDERMIS

DERMIS

SUBCUTANEOUS TISSUE

1st degree

2nd degree

3rd degree

FIGURE 18-3. Classification of burns according to the depth of injury.

warm, inflamed surface. A second degree burn is usually pink or red with the presence of considerable blisters which may have broken, resulting in a weeping surface. Third degree wounds can vary from pale to white to brown to frankly charred; the appearance of coagulated vessels in a waxy appearing skin is pathognomonic of a third degree burn. In general, second degree burns tend to retain sensitivity to pin prick, but several hours after injury, when considerable tissue edema has developed, sensation may be considerably blunted. In contradistinction, third degree burns usually rapidly lose sensitivity to pin prick stimulation, although deep pressure sensation is retained. Over the years, many experimental techniques utilizing dyes, radioisotopes and thermography have been devised and reported for the differentiation of second and third degree wounds. However, these are not used as a routine clinical measure.

One of the most helpful methods in determining the depth of the burn is knowledge of the causative agent. In general, direct contact with flame or ignition of clothing will usually produce a third degree burn wound. By contrast, a patient who is exposed to a sudden flash or explosion, but whose clothes do not ignite, will usually receive second degree burns of the exposed portions of the body such as the face and hands. In scald injuries the depth is variable, but frequently hot liquids, such as those from an overturned pot, splashed on the body will produce a second degree burn (Fig. 18-4). On the other hand, immersion of the body into heated liquids can produce not only third degree burns but also extremely deep subcutaneous tissue destruction from the "parboiling" effect.

Contact burns which result from touching hot objects usually produce localized injuries whose depth is related to the temperature of

TABLE 18-3. *Determination of the Depth of the Burn*

	FIRST DEGREE	SECOND DEGREE	THIRD DEGREE
Color	Pink or red	Pink, red, or mottled red or white	White, brown, or charred
Presence of blisters	Absent	Present with a weeping surface if blisters are broken	Usually absent
Sensation to pin prick	Present	Present	Absent
Surface of the wound	Uniform	Frequently elevated above normal skin	Frequently depressed below surrounding normal unburned skin
Dye and isotope tests	First, second, and third degree variable, depending on the material and technique utilized		
Time	Heals	Heals	Produces granulating wounds

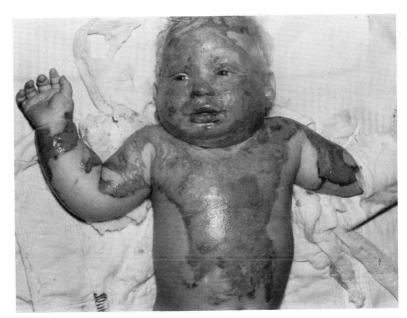

FIGURE 18–4. Predominantly second degree burn resulting from a scald injury.

the burning object and the duration of exposure. Electrical burns are usually deceiving and are almost invariably much deeper and more extensive than indicated on initial examination. Relatively innocuous electrical lesions at the time of initial examination can produce a remarkable amount of tissue destruction when reexamined after a few days (Fig. 18–5). Lynch, Wisner and Lewis (1971a) have reviewed a large group of electrical injuries and found that if the patient does not succumb from acute electrocution and survives to be admitted to the hospital, the mortality rate is low. However, the frequency of amputations of digits or extremities is quite high, occurring in 30 per cent of patients.

Although it may be impossible during the first few days to determine accurately the depth of a burn in a given area, it is usually possible to ascertain if the burn is predominantly second or third degree. In some instances, however, the most experienced observer may be unable to determine with accuracy the exact depth of burn in a given area, and the true depth becomes apparent with the passage of time. The second degree burn in the absence of infection or other complications will heal spontaneously, and the third degree burn will produce a granulating surface necessitating skin grafting. The differentiation of second and third degree burns is more difficult since the advent of effective topical therapy. Prior to the use of topical agents, wounds that initially appeared to be third de-

gree would usually progress to granulating wounds requiring skin grafts. Now similar wounds often heal, apparently as a result of prevention of conversion of deep second degree to third degree burns by bacterial infection. Consequently, the present tendency is to overestimate the depth of injury at the time of initial evaluation.

Age of the Patient

The age of the patient is the third most important factor in estimating the severity of injury. Burns are tolerated extremely poorly by indi-

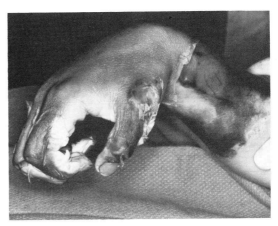

FIGURE 18–5. Extensive electrical burn of the hand.

viduals at the extremes of life, and the mortality rate in infants under the age of 12 months and in individuals past the age of 65 is quite high, even in the presence of limited burns. In general, the mortality rate is quite low for individuals under the age of 50 who sustain burns of 30 per cent of the body surface or less. As the extent of burn increases beyond 30 per cent of the body surface, the mortality rate rises in all age groups, and as the age increases above 50, the mortality rate rises, even in burns of less than 30 per cent. For example, a 30 per cent third degree burn in a 60 year old individual will result in significant mortality, while a younger person with the same lesion may be expected to recover, without unusual complications, in the majority of cases. The mortality rates published in a number of studies of burn patients show considerable varia- tion according to the type of service involved, but a general reference for mortality is illustrated in Tables 18–4 and 18–5 for males and females, respectively.

If large numbers of small localized burns are seen, burn deaths may fall below 10 per cent of the total number of patients treated. In burn centers in which the more severely burned patients, particularly elderly patients and those with lesions of more than 50 per cent burn surface area, are selectively sent from a large referral area, the most recent figures for hospitalized patients fall within the 20 to 30 per cent mortality range. The rise in mortality rate reported from the Galveston Burn Center over recent years is illustrated in Table 18–6. It will be noted from Table 18–6 that the percentage of patients admitted with larger burns has risen proportionately with the mortality rate.

TABLE 18–4.   *Predicted Mortality in Males (%)**

AGE OF PATIENTS IN YEARS	PER CENT OF BODY SURFACE BURNED									
	10	20	30	40	50	60	70	80	90	100
2	0	5	17	40	63	80	92	98	100	100
4	0	5	16	39	63	79	92	98		
8	0	4	14	37	60	78	91	97		
12	0	4	13	36	59	77	91	97		
16	0	3	13	35	59	77	90	97		
20	0	3	13	35	59	77	90	97		
24	0	4	14	37	60	78	91	97		
28	0	4	15	38	62	78	92	97		
32	0	5	17	40	63	80	92	98		
36	1	6	19	44	66	81	94	98		
40	1	7	22	47	69	84	94	98		
44	2	9	27	52	71	87	92	99		
48	3	11	32	56	75	89	96	99		
52	4	15	39	62	79	92	97	100		
56	6	20	45	67	83	94	98			
60	9	27	53	72	87	96	99			
64	13	36	59	77	91	97	100			
68	19	45	67	83	94	98				
72	29	54	73	88	96	99				
76	40	63	80	92	98	100				
80	51	71	86	95	99					
84	61	78	92	97	100					
88	71	86	95	99						
90	75	89	97	99						

*Galveston Mortality Table (Males). (Modified from McCoy, J. A., Micks, D. W., and Lynch, J. B.: Discriminant function probability model for predicting survival in burned patients. J.A.M.A., *203*:644, 1968. Copyright © 1968, The American Medical Association.)

TABLE 18–5.   *Predicted Mortality in Females (%)**

	PER CENT OF BODY SURFACE BURNED									
AGE OF PATIENTS IN YEARS	10	20	30	40	50	60	70	80	90	100
2	0	5	17	40	64	80	93	98	100	100
4	0	5	16	39	63	79	93	98		
8	0	4	14	38	61	78	91	97		
12	0	4	14	36	60	77	91	97		
16	0	4	13	36	59	77	90	97		
20	0	4	14	36	59	77	90	97		
24	0	4	14	37	60	78	91	97		
28	0	4	15	39	62	79	92	97		
32	0	5	17	40	64	80	92	98		
36	1	6	19	45	66	81	94	98		
40	1	7	22	48	69	84	94	98		
44	2	9	27	52	72	87	95	99		
48	3	12	33	56	75	89	97	99		
52	4	15	39	62	79	92	97	100		
56	6	20	46	67	83	94	98			
60	9	27	53	72	87	96	99			
64	14	36	60	77	91	97	100			
68	20	45	67	83	94	98				
72	29	57	74	88	96	99				
76	40	63	80	92	98	100				
80	51	71	87	95	99					
84	62	79	92	98	100					
88	71	86	95	99						
90	75	89	97	99						

*Galveston Mortality Table (Females). (Modified from McCoy, J. A., Micks, D. W., and Lynch, J. B.: Discriminant function probability model for predicting survival in burned patients. J.A.M.A., *203*:644, 1968. Copyright © 1968, The American Medical Association.)

Associated Injury or Concurrent Disease

In addition to the extent and depth of the burn and the age of the patient, other factors involved in determining the severity of the injury include any fractures or associated injuries sustained at the time of burning. It is becoming more common to encounter patients involved in automobile accidents and other forms of trauma in which associated injuries are quite frequent. Particular attention should be paid to blast effects on the lung in individuals involved in explosions.

Any illness that the patient had prior to the time of burning may complicate an otherwise smaller burn. For example, patients with preexisting renal or cardiovascular disease tolerate burning poorly. Metabolic disorders such as diabetes, obesity, and alcoholism increase the magnitude of severity in burn injuries. It is also important to keep in mind that the patient sustaining facial burns or the patient who has sustained his burn in a closed space may have pulmonary complications resulting from a burn involving only a limited percentage of the body surface.

TABLE 18–6.   *Comparison of Extent of Burn and Mortality*

YEAR	PATIENTS WITH GREATER THAN 20% BURNS	MORTALITY
1958–62	45%	17.0%
1963–64	52%	23.4%
1965–66	63%	26.4%
1968–69	64%	28.5%

TABLE 18–7. *Classification of Burns*

CRITICAL BURNS
  Second degree burns of over 30% of body surface
    area
  Third degree burns of face, hands, feet, or over 10%
    of body surface area
  Burns complicated by:
    1. Respiratory tract injury
    2. Major soft tissue injury
    3. Fractures
  Electrical injuries

MODERATE BURNS
  Second degree burns of 15 to 30% of body surface
  Third degree burns of less than 10% (except hands,
    face, feet, and genitalia)

MINOR BURNS
  Second degree of less than 15%
  Third degree of less than 2%

With the above facts in mind it is possible to categorize burns according to the severity of injury. A workable classification for the disposition of burn patients is illustrated in Table 18–7.

In general, hospitalization is required for second degree burns involving 15 per cent or more of the body surface and for third degree burns involving 10 per cent of the body surface or critical areas such as the face, hands, genitalia, or lower extremity.

MORBIDITY

Prognosis is dependent upon the extent, depth, and location of the burn injury and upon the development of complications. First degree and superficial second degree burns below 20 per cent will usually heal spontaneously in a period of 7 to 14 days, although alterations in pigmentation may persist for weeks or even months. Deep second degree burns, if not converted to full thickness skin loss or unduly complicated by infection, may be expected to heal in three to six weeks, depending upon the amount of surface involvement and, in particular, upon the extent of lower extremity lesions, which usually heal slowly (Fig. 18–6). Recovery is often characterized by permanent changes in the character and color of the skin in accordance with the amount of destruction of dermal elements.

The time required for healing of third degree burns is affected by the number of skin grafting procedures required, by both local and systemic complications, and by the type of early care. Small areas of 5 to 10 per cent full thickness skin loss require nearly twice as long to heal as larger (30 to 40 per cent) second degree burns. Unless early excision can be practiced in selected cases of localized third degree burns, an average of three to four weeks usually elapses from the time of injury until the first grafting procedure in patients admitted immediately following burning. Patients with less than 20 per cent burns ordinarily require only one or two grafting procedures and will be ready for discharge approximately six weeks after the injury. For burns involving between 20 and 50 per cent of the body surface, 8 to 12 weeks of hospitalization are usually required, and over 50 per cent of the body surface requires three to four months or longer,

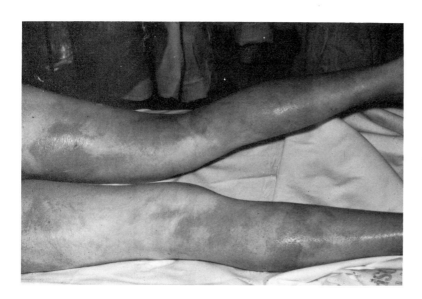

FIGURE 18–6. Second degree burns of the lower extremities.

according to the individual characteristics of the patient's injury.

Spontaneous healing in third degree lesions of appreciable size (5 per cent of the body surface) occurs only with cicatrization and contractures. Recognition of this fact and encouragement of routine early skin grafting represent perhaps the greatest single advance in burn therapy in our time, although the improvement in general supportive measures cannot be minimized.

PATHOPHYSIOLOGY

Systemic Response

Although there is a tendency for the uninformed to consider a burn as a superficial skin problem, the stress associated with the burn injury is severe and at times can involve virtually every organ system in the body. The most striking immediate systemic effects following burning are related to the hemodynamic changes that occur. Immediately after burning there is altered capillary permeability, so that water, sodium, chloride, and protein escape from the vascular compartments into the burn wound. This creates the "obligatory" burn edema, which is characterized by extensive swelling about the face and neck following burns in this area.

As a result of excessive fluid, electrolyte, and protein shift in burn edema, there is resulting hypovolemia and hemoconcentration, conditions which require intensive fluid replacement therapy. Extravasation of fluid into the burn wound continues for 24 to 48 hours, although the major shift has occurred after 18 hours. The shift in fluids following a severe burn is due to (1) the stress mechanism, especially the elaboration of the mineralocorticoids, which results in retention of sodium, chloride, and water and excretion of potassium; (2) alteration of capillary permeability, which allows egress of electrolytes and protein from the vascular compartment; and (3) variation in osmotic effects.

Salt is lost from the vascular system in relatively greater amounts than water; water in relatively greater amounts than protein; albumin in relatively greater amounts than the globulin fraction; and plasma in relatively greater amounts than red cell mass. Because of the greater loss of water and electrolytes from the vascular compartment, some degree of concentration of plasma proteins and red blood cells is produced as the circulating blood volume decreases. Compensatory attraction of fluids from unburned areas thus occurs from increased intravascular osmolarity. The loss of fluid from the vascular compartment results in hemoconcentration with the characteristic early elevation in the hemoglobin concentration and hematocrit. The total water content of the body increases during the edema period, paralleling the increase in the extracellular space in response to fluid therapy, and in the presence of reduced urinary output. Insensible water loss varies considerably from one patient to another but may affect the fluid balance considerably.

Although the immediate hemodynamic changes are the most obvious and the most dramatic aspects of a burn, the systemic response to a burn injury is by no means limited to these changes. An abbreviated outline of the pathophysiologic changes associated with burn injury is as follows:

ACUTE PHASE

1. Clinical Shock
   a. Increased capillary permeability
   b. Decreased cardiac output, circulating blood volume, and liver blood flow
   c. Transient rise in blood pressure with peripheral vasoconstriction followed by lowered blood pressure (not as severe as in hemorrhagic shock)
   d. Plasma volume reduction; hemoconcentration with elevation of hematocrit
   e. Tissue anoxia: specific organ and general metabolic disturbances following decreased blood flow
   f. Depression of the central nervous system
   g. Accelerated nitrogen excretion
   h. Endocrine response (pituitary, adrenocortical, adrenal medullary, thyroid, renal, etc.)
2. External Loss of Plasma
   a. Decreased plasma volume
   b. Loss of protein and electrolytes
3. Loss of Circulating Red Cells
   a. Relative and absolute decrease in circulating red cells
   b. Trapping in dilated capillaries
   c. Destruction in burned area
   d. Hemolysis from increased fragility
   e. The sludge phenomenon
   f. Masked anemia from hemoconcentration
4. Burn Edema
   a. Severe localized swelling in areas of injury
   b. Fluid shifts between undamaged and affected tissues
   c. Sequestration of sodium and protein in edema fluid
   d. High blood potassium from redistribution of electrolytes and destroyed tissue cells and erythrocytes
   e. Physiologic alterations in pulmonary, renal, and cardiac function

SUBACUTE PHASE

1. Diuresis
   a. Subsidence of edema
   b. Increased urinary output
   c. Mobilization of sodium
   d. Potential pulmonary edema
2. Clinical Anemia
   a. Hypochromia and microcytosis following initial hemolysis
   b. Need for increased protein and iron for red cell regeneration
   c. Continued loss of red cells during dressings and at surgery
   d. Expansion of capillary bed in granulating areas
   e. Increased red cell fragility
   f. Elevated COHb levels initially
3. Accelerated Metabolic Rate
   a. Increased cellular and biochemical activity
   b. Increase from acceleration of vaporizational water loss through burn wound
4. Nitrogen Disequilibrium
   a. Increased nitrogen catabolism
      (1) Tissue catabolism
      (2) Loss of muscle protein from disuse atrophy
      (3) Poor oral intake secondary to anorexia
      (4) Loss of protein through granulating wounds
   b. Normal or accelerated nitrogen anabolism
      (1) Increased need for acclerated metabolism and tissue repair
      (2) Primary response to trauma in specific organs
   c. Qualitative and quantitative changes in plasma protein components affecting immune response
5. Disordered Fat Metabolism
6. Abnormal Vitamin Metabolism
   a. Increased requirements for vitamin C, thiamine, riboflavin, etc.
   b. Deficient intake because of poor appetite
7. Impairment of Hepatic Function
   a. Evidence of damage on standard tests and biopsy
   b. Disturbance of carbohydrate and protein metabolism
   c. Increased liver storage of fat
8. Bone and Joint Changes
   a. Intra-articular and skeletal disturbances in calcification
   b. Stimulation to skeletal growth in children
9. Endocrine Disturbances
   a. Possible adrenal exhaustion
   b. Depression of gonad function
   c. Curling's ulcer
   d. Other endocrine dysfunction
10. Electrolyte and Chemical Imbalance
    a. Increased need for potassium and calcium for the healing process
    b. Loss of sodium, potassium, and calcium through granulating tissue
    c. Deficient intake
11. Circulatory Derangements
    a. Low blood volume
    b. Low osmotic pressure
    c. Tendency toward thrombotic phenomena
    d. Diminished cardiac reserve
    e. Complications from preexisting cardiovascular and renal disease
12. Loss of Function of the Skin as an Organ
    a. Temperature regulation and insulation
    b. Excretion of water and chloride
    c. Mechanical protection against chemical and physical trauma

   d. Storage of salt and glucose
   e. Sensory link between central nervous system and external environment
   f. Protection against invasion by pathogenic organisms

From the above outline the magnitude of the sytemic response which *may* be elicited in various patients can be appreciated. No further discussion is required of the first item, *clinical shock*, which is appreciated by all clinicians caring for seriously injured patients. External loss of plasma, with decreased plasma volume and loss of protein and electrolytes, has been alluded to in the introduction to this section. The external loss of plasma occurs chiefly in second and third degree "weeping" burns, and many workers, Fox and his associates (1960) in particular, believe that profound differences exist in response to therapy in scald burns as opposed to flame burns. The amount of fluid lost from the surface of the burn wound has been variously estimated, as outlined in Table 18–8, from which it will be noted that an average figure of 4000 ml per square meter of burn per day is a realistic figure. Water loss is an important factor because evaporation of each 1000 ml of water requires the expenditure of 567 kilocalories.

Loss of Circulating Red Cells. The loss of circulating red blood cells has been the subject of considerable discussion. Regardless of internal fluid or electrolyte shifts, the red blood cell is the major oxygen-carrying component of the blood, since only insignificant amounts of oxygen are dissolved in the plasma. At the time of burn injury, the red blood cells located in the immediate burn wound are destroyed, together with the epithelial and dermal cells. In addition to the outright destruction of red blood cells, the slowing of flow in the microcirculation, which was first reported by Knisely (1962) in his description of the sludge phenomenon, renders much of the remaining circulating red blood cell mass ineffective.

TABLE 18–8. *Surface Water Loss from the Burn Wound*

AUTHOR	GRAMS OF WATER LOSS/ SQUARE METER BURNED/DAY
Roe and Kinney (1964)	1000 to 4000
Moncrief and Mason (1964)	3360 to 7200
Moyer and Fallon (1963)	5008 to 7440

The absolute quantity of red blood cell destruction has been studied by Salzburg and Evans (1950), Davies (1960), Topley, Moe, and Jackson (1957), and Muir (1961). Despite the technical difficulties associated with the absolute determination of red blood cell destruction, it is probable that the extent of loss of red blood cells as a direct result of the injury varies from 5 to 40 per cent, depending on the extent and depth of the burn, and probably averages 15 per cent of the red blood cell mass. Moore (1959), having obtained similar results in his studies, advocated the administration of 1 to 2 units of packed red blood cells during the first 24 to 48 hours following a burn injury. Levin and Blocker (1958) have demonstrated that the red blood cell survival time is markedly decreased following thermal injury.

The results of the above studies have resulted in concern for replacement of the red blood cell mass, with the effect that many patients have been overtransfused with whole blood, often to their detriment. Many studies are currently available to demonstrate that even those with major burns, in the absence of preexisting anemia or acute hemolytic episode, can be adequately resuscitated without the use of whole blood transfusions during the first 48 hours.

Metabolic Changes. After the first 72 hours following the burn have elapsed, if initial fluid therapy and general supportive measures have been adequate, a period of homeostasis ensues. This is characterized by some subsidence of edema, increased urinary output, and mobilization of sodium. However, with these changes the potential of pulmonary edema exists. With the mobilization of fluid back into the vascular system, the early hemoconcentration is corrected, and the actual anemia present resulting from red blood cell destruction is manifested by a hypochromic microcytic anemia. Associated with this period of stress there is an accelerated metabolic rate with an increase of both catabolism and anabolism.

Increased oxidation of fat in response to trauma is one factor in the marked weight loss that may occur in severely burned patients. The fundamental mechanism involved is not completely understood, but the weight loss represented by fat oxidation may, after severe trauma, total two to four times that of starvation alone (Moore, 1959).

Protein imbalance is one of the most spectacular sequelae of thermal trauma. Under normal conditions there exists a state of equilibrium between the rates of protein synthesis and breakdown. In severely burned patients, catabolism is greatly accelerated, and studies with radioactive compounds by Blocker and his associates (1954, 1955, 1962) indicate that a state of equilibrium is not attained until late in convalescence. However, in the severely burned patient, the rates of anabolism are either normal or accelerated, although in the latter case to a much less degree than catabolism.

In addition to the primary alteration in protein equilibrium that is initiated by the burn, poor oral intake secondary to anorexia, loss of muscle from disuse atrophy, and external losses through granulations and raw surfaces all contribute to the negative nitrogen balance. These summations of anabolic and catabolic processes, represented by graphs of nitrogen intake and excretion, show, in chronologic sequence, (1) initial positive balance, (2) greatly accelerated nitrogen excretion with persistent negative balance until wound coverage can be obtained or sufficiently large amounts of protein can be administered to offset the urinary losses, and (3) gradual return to positive balance with healing of the burn wounds.

Musculoskeletal Changes. One of the most interesting and unexpected findings in burn patients is the bone and joint changes. Most of the alterations of the musculoskeletal system in patients with severe burns occur sometime after the acute injury and do not represent the direct result of thermal injury. Although several authors have reported skeletal abnormalities in association with burn patients, the most extensive studies have been conducted by Evans (1973), and his classification of the musculoskeletal changes is shown in Table 18–9.

Evans (1966) has shown that many of the above listed deformities can be prevented and has outlined the orthopedic correction of these deformities when they occur.

Endocrine Changes. The endocrine changes that occur in association with burns are widespread and include depression of gonad function with a decrease in libido, cessation of menstruation, abnormal hair growth, and the development of signs of cortisone excess late in the convalescent period, such as the moon face and "buffalo hump." Stimualtion of skeletal growth in children and young adults is a common phenomenon in both males and females immediately following skin coverage and healing. The acute endocrine changes and the electrolyte abnormalities secondary to mineralocorticoids have been referred to earlier.

Determination of blood and urinary levels of

TABLE 18–9. *Evans' Classification of Musculoskeletal Changes in Burns*

1. Alterations limited to bone
   A. Osteoporosis
   B. Periosteal new bone formation
   C. Irregular ossification
   D. Diaphyseal exostosis
   E. Acromutilation of fingers
   F. Pathologic fractures
   G. Osteomyelitis
   H. Necrosis and tangential sequestration
2. Alterations involving pericapsular structures
   A. Pericapsular calcification
   B. Heterotopic para-articular ossification
   C. Osteophytes
3. Alterations involving the joint proper
   A. Septic arthritis
   B. Spontaneous dissolution
   C. Ankylosis
   D. Dislocation
4. Alterations secondary to soft tissue contracture
   A. Muscle contracture
   B. Malposition of joints
   C. Scoliosis
5. Abnormalities of growth
6. Nonviability of extremity leading to amputation

corticosteroids has been performed, and correlations have been noted between the severity of the burn and laboratory data by a number of workers, including Hume and Haynes (1961), Hardy (1958), and Feller (1962). Examples of extremely low excretion patterns were observed and were considered as an extremely unfavorable prognostic sign.

At the present time the consensus of opinion is that *steroid replacement therapy is not required during the acute phase of burn management* except for the acute management of certain pulmonary complications which will be discussed later. The possible role of ACTH as one factor in the production of the typical Curling's ulcer has been discussed, and ACTH has also been implicated in the "pseudodiabetes" of stress. According to Gardner (1953), however, the movement of potassium from the intracellular to the extracellular compartment interferes with glycogen deposition and thus produces a typical diabetic glucose tolerance curve with the attendant glycosuria. Although thyroid activity may be increased during the early phases of a burn, the thyroid gland has not been directly implicated in the pathologic changes frequently associated with burns.

No discussion of burn pathophysiology would be complete without mention of the possibility of a burn toxin. The possibility of heat-denatured protein complexes being absorbed and producing untoward effects has been stud-

ied in many parts of the world for many years. The effects of bacteria and sepsis are difficult to control experimentally in human studies. Despite the mass of experimental and clinical studies performed, there is no evidence at the present time of any "toxic" antigenic substances caused by the burn or elaborated by burn patients which are of significant clinical importance.

Excellent discussions of the physiologic derangements that occur in response to severe thermal trauma are to be found in the reports of Allgöwer and Siegrist (1957), Sevitt (1957), Levenson and Lund (1957), Hardy (1958), Moore (1959), Artz and Moncrief (1969), and Dolecek (1969).

IMMEDIATE HOSPITAL CARE

With the above pathophysiologic alterations in mind, it is apparent that, when treatment of an acute burn is instituted, a well-organized and coordinated approach is essential to assure that all required treatment is administered in an orderly fashion and in proper sequence. It is imperative that unnecessary handling or movement be eliminated, since this is poorly tolerated by the burned patients. Far too often patients are transferred from stretcher to bed to stretcher to X-ray table to stretcher to bed. In the absence of associated injuries, it is important to avoid delay in initiating treatment for the purpose of obtaining diagnostic studies which can usually be obtained with portable equipment at the bedside. Moreover, such studies can be safely delayed for a few hours until initial resuscitation measures are underway. Adequate assistance should be initially obtained, and all attendants involved in the direct care of the patient should wear masks and gloves. An orderly method of treatment is required in order to assure that the patient's urgent needs are corrected before the more obvious but less urgent ones are treated. The following outline is suggested as a workable guide in the institution of immediate treatment for burn patients:

1. General evelution of the patient
2. Establishment and maintenace of an adequate airway
3. Emergency sedation, if required
4. Fluid replacement therapy to combat shock
5. Insertion of an indwelling catheter to monitor urinary output

6. Prophylaxis against tetanus
7. Evaluation for antibiotic therapy
8. Nutritional requirements
9. General supportive measures
10. Initiation of burn wound care

General Evaluation

A rapid preliminary evaluation should be immediately performed to assess the magnitude of injury and to establish the priority of treatment. This can usually be obtained in a short period of time, and treatment should be initiated prior to the recording of a detailed history and the physical examination. The patient's clothing should be removed and all burned areas inspected for estimation of the extent and depth of the burn. While this is being accomplished, a history, including the cause of the burn, time elapsed since the burn, and the therapeutic measures which may have been initially instituted, should be obtained. Information concerning the patient's age, drug allergy (particularly to antibiotics and anesthetic agents), status of tetanus immunization, and use of medications (particularly insulin, digitalis, diphenylhydantoin, sedatives, narcotics, reserpine, or steroids) is important.

A complete preliminary examination must be performed to detect any associated disease which may influence subsequent burn therapy. It should be remembered that photographs constitute an important part of the record, and arrangements should be made for photographs at a convenient time during the initial treatment plan for the patient. The majority of the history and preliminary evaluation can be obtained while the patient is being undressed, placed in bed, and evaluated. As much of the history as possible should be obtained from the patient. If the patient is unable to give a history, information should be obtained from any family member or ambulance attendants who accompany the patient.

Establishment and Maintenance of an Adequate Airway

A mechanically clear airway and free respiratory exchange must be assured at the outset. The head, neck, and pharynx must be examined for evidence of mandibular fractures or other injuries; aspiration of the nasopharynx to remove any mucus or foreign material should be performed if the patient is unconscious. The oral and nasal mucous membranes must be inspected for evidence of injury, such as hyperemia, and direct burning effect, such as singeing of the nasal hair and presence of soot and particulate matter. Relatively minor initial physical findings may herald the onset of serious pulmonary complications.

In burns involving the face and neck, considerable edema can be anticipated within 24 to 48 hours. For this reason, prophylactic tracheotomy has been frequently employed in the past. The performance of a tracheotomy necessitates increased vigilance on the part of the nursing staff, and the tracheostomy cannula itself can be a source of mechanical irritation to the trachea and cause other complications. For that reason, *tracheotomy is not routinely performed,* and if transient respiratory difficulty develops during the first few days of treatment, the insertion of an indwelling nasotracheal tube is preferable. These tubes can usually be safely left in place for five to seven days with a lesser incidence of complications than when tracheotomy is performed. In some instances endotracheal tubes have been left in place without ill effects for periods exceeding seven days. If a cuffed endotracheal tube is used, the cuff should be made of soft material to avoid pressure on the trachea, and periodic deflation of the cuff is indicated. Tracheostomy should be reserved for the occasional patient with associated chest injuries or significant pulmonary complications.

Most patients benefit from a humidified atmosphere for the first 48 to 72 hours following an acute burn. This is particularly true if there are burns of the face and neck region. Humidified oxygen through a nebulizer is part of the initial treatment. It should be noted that, of the commercially available nebulizers, the ultrasonic machines are by far the most effective. However, excessive wetness of the lung can be produced in some patients, and for this reason the use of ultrasonic nebulizers in burn patients is *not* routinely recommended.

At the time of initial examination, the patient is often noted to have dusky or cyanotic mucous membranes and nailbeds, even in the presence of an elevated hemoglobin concentration and hematocrit. When one remembers the circulatory derangements which occur following burn injury and the associated destruction of red blood cell mass, it is not surprising that some decrease in arterial oxygen saturation is noted even in the absence of overt pulmonary complications. The administration of humidified oxygen by a nebulizer while the circulatory derangements are being corrected with fluid therapy is a worthwhile adjunctive measure. It must also be kept in mind that *undue restlessness on the part of the patient is often a manifestation of hypoxia.*

Emergency Sedation

Most patients immediately after a burn not only are in some pain from the injury but also have suffered considerable anxiety as a result of being involved in an accident. For immediate sedation, full therapeutic doses of a narcotic, such as morphine sulphate (10 to 15 mg for adults and 1 mg/year of age for children) or Demerol (meperidine hydrochloride), are recommended. Because of the uncertain status of the circulatory system, the narcotic should be slowly administered intravenously in order to assure absorption. A calm and reassuring attitude on the part of the physician and attendants is equally important to allay the patient's anxiety and apprehension.

Because a third degree burn destroys the majority of the sensory endings in the area, burn patients may be reasonably comfortable except during dressing changes, turning or manipulating of the patient, or other procedures. For this reason, regular narcotic administration should be limited to the first 24 to 48 hours. Following that period, milder analgesics such as codeine or nonnarcotic analgesics can be substituted, especially during dressing changes.

Fluid Replacement Therapy for Burn Shock

Immediately following burning there is alteration of capillary permeability in the burn area, which results in a rapid extravasation of fluid from the vascular compartment to the extracellular space. Following this extensive fluid shift, there is hypovolemia with hemoconcentration, which leads to decreased venous return, decreased cardiac output, decreased renal blood flow, decreased glomerular filtration, and oliguria. These changes occur at a slower rate than after acute hemorrhage, and, as a result, compensatory mechanisms tend to maintain the blood pressure and pulse rate at a relatively normal level during the early phase. There may be significant hypovolemia with inadequate renal blood flow and impending renal complications, even in the presence of relatively normal blood pressure or pulse. At the same time the extravasation of fluid from the vascular to extracellular space is occurring, there is a release of potassium from cells that are destroyed in the area of the burn wound and a shift of sodium into the intracellular space. Thus serum potassium levels tend to be elevated at a time when urinary output is compromised. These internal fluid electrolyte derangements are of significant magnitude and require intensive fluid replacement therapy.

As a rule, *adults with 20 per cent burns and children with 15 per cent burns* require administration of intravenous fluids for treatment of actual or impending shock. In some instances, particularly with electrical burns, patients with lesions of lesser extent will require immediate shock therapy.

At the time of institution of intravenous therapy, blood should be drawn for a complete blood count and hematocrit and for baseline blood chemistry studies. These include serum sodium, potassium, carbon dioxide, chlorides, and protein with A-G ratio. In addition, the blood urea nitrogen and blood sugar should be determined in older individuals, and blood type and cross matching should be performed, although blood is not usually required during the first 48 hours of burn therapy. Other blood tests are ordered, if indicated by the history and physical, and arterial blood gases must be monitored if any complication is present.

Since the severe burn requires not only immediate fluid resuscitation but also continuous intravenous therapy, it is wise at the time of admission to evaluate the venous portals available for therapy. In many instances superficial veins are not available because they lie in the area of the burn or in an adjacent region in which edema is or will become a problem. It is therefore wise to insert initially a small plastic catheter into a peripheral vein of the lower or upper extremity, bearing in mind the possibility of local thrombophlebitis which may render that particular site unsuitable for future fluid administration. The saphenous vein at the ankle or the cephalic vein at the wrist or shoulder are the most commonly employed. Cannulation of the subclavian vein by a physician experienced in the method is a reliable technique in the massively burned patient. A polyethylene catheter of No. 16 or 18 caliber should be inserted and fixed securely. It may be utilized for a period of five to seven days, after which time a new site should be utilized to minimize cannulation complications if further fluid therapy is required. It must be emphasized that it is not wise to attempt fluid replacement through a simple needle inserted into a vein. As edema progresses and hypovolemia becomes more acute, it becomes technically more difficult to recannulate a vein as required.

Estimation of Fluid Requirement. The primary requirement of fluid therapy is the restoration of circulating blood volume. For this purpose, normal saline, Ringer's lactate, colloids, blood, albumin, and various synthetic materials have been employed in the past. Experience with large numbers of burn patients has resulted in the development of several formulas for burn fluid replacement, as illustrated in Table 18–10.

Although adequate fluid resuscitation can be accomplished by a variety of methods, as illustrated above, the Brooke Army modification of the Evans formula has proved to be quite workable as a guide for initial fluid estimates. It must be emphasized that all of the treatment regimens outlined above are for the purpose of preliminary planning to estimate the patient's fluid requirement. *They are not formulas to be followed rigidly*, and the subsequent clinical course of the patient, including urinary output, response to initial therapy, and onset of complications, will determine the amount and type of subsequent fluids which must be administered.

The Brooke formula allows 1.5 ml of electrolyte-containing solution and 0.5 ml of colloid per kilogram of body weight times the percentage of body surface burn. An additional adult average requirement of 2000 ml of dextrose in water should be kept in mind to replace insensible fluid loss. Fluid requirement for burns of more than 50 per cent should never exceed that calculated for 50 per cent burns. This is based on the fact that the fluid requirement parallels the extent of burn fairly closely up to 50 per cent. Above 50 per cent the fluid requirements are variable, and all patients with burns of more than 50 per cent should be initially calculated as 50 per cent burns. As a general rule, smaller amounts of colloid are required in second degree burns than in third degree burns. Furthermore, patients in whom fluid therapy is instituted very early following a burn will require less fluid replacement for adequate resuscitation than patients in whom institution of therapy is delayed for some hours. It must be reemphasized that these formulas are simply estimates of what the patient is likely to require and must not be rigidly followed.

The fluid alterations associated with a burn occur more rapidly immediately after the injury and proceed at a progressively slower rate thereafter. As a result fluid replacement therapy must be concentrated in the early postburn period. The commonly employed rule is to administer one-half of the first 24-hour fluid requirement in the first eight hours following the burn (*not* eight hours following admission to the hospital), one-quarter of the first 24-hour requirement in the second eight hours following burn, and the last quarter in the third eight hours following burn. In general, the intravenous replacement therapy required for the second 24 hours will be approximately one-half of that required during the first 24 hours, but it is variable, depending on fluid intake, nausea, vomiting, extent and depth of the burn, and other individual factors.

The priority for replacement of fluids is as follows:
1. Electrolyte-containing solutions (sodium)
2. Colloid- or protein-containing solutions
3. Free water

There is a tendency for inexperienced physicians to start intravenous fluid therapy with electrolyte-free glucose solutions. The disadvantage of electrolyte-free solutions is that they dilute the serum sodium and accentuate the electrolyte problems. Free water without electrolytes should only be administered after adequate replacement therapy with electrolytes and/or colloids has resulted in stable vital signs and adequate urinary output for several hours. Despite the inclusion of water for insensible loss in many of the formulas listed above, it should be used with caution, if at all. A more physiologic method of administering water is

TABLE 18–10. *Representative Types of Replacement Fluid Formulae*

FORMULA	COLLOID	ELECTROLYTE SOL.	H_2O
Evans formula	1 ml/kg/%	1 ml/kg/%	2000 ml
Brooke formula	0.5 ml/kg/%	1.5 ml/kg/%	2000 ml
Massachusetts General Hospital formula	125 ml plasma/%	15 ml/%	2000 ml
Parkland Hospital formula	—	4 ml/kg/%	—

to administer glucose solutions in 0.2 N saline, since the inclusion of some sodium is important for renal function, and glucose solutions in free water should not be used in burn patients at all during the first few days.

Choice of Replacement Fluids. The choice of fluids for replacement therapy depends upon the etiology of the burn, the depth and extent of the injury, the availability of commercial solutions in the individual hospital, and the preference of the surgeon. There is a large variety of commercially available electrolyte solutions. Over the years, sodium chloride has been undoubtedly the most widely used. However, it contains 155 milliequivalents of chloride, which is considerably higher than the normal serum level and tends to increase the acidosis that occurs following burns. A more physiologic solution, such as lactated Ringer's solution, does not have this disadvantage. Although exogenous potassium administration is contraindicated during the early shock phase, the 4 mEq/L present in Ringer's solution is acceptable except in infants or in patients with inadequate urinary output.

Of the various colloid solutions available for replacement, virus-free plasma, whole blood, and dextrans are the ones which have been most widely used. Serum albumin and other synthetic substitutes have been occasionally used in various centers but are not widely used at the present time. Although burn patients can be adequately resuscitated during the first 48 hours without the administration of colloid (Baxter and Shires, 1968) the major *potential* advantages derived from the use of plasma as a colloid fluid are: (1) a tendency for a smaller total fluid replacement requirement with less possibility for circulatory overload with pulmonary edema; (2) the replacement of some albumin can minimize the marked hypoalbuminemia which may occur; and (3) the administration of the immunoglobulins present in plasma can potentially enhance the host's resistance to infection. Baxter (1973) has presented conclusive evidence that the fluid shift in burn patients occurs more rapidly than had been previously appreciated. Baxter has also demonstrated that the decreased cardiac output and many of the circulatory derangements can be corrected by rapid infusion of electrolyte solution without colloid, using 4 milliliters per kilogram per per cent burn as a guide. However, an occasional patient, usually an infant or an elderly patient, may require addition of colloid for adequate maintenance of urinary output and stable vital signs. The increased volume infused rapidly also increases the possibility of requiring prophylactic administration of digitalis. When digitalization is required, it should be slowly administered intravenously in divided doses, and great care should be exercised since the usual digitalizing dose for a healthy patient may result in an increased frequency of arrhythmia in the burn patient due to increased myocardial sensitivity. For these reasons, one should employ a regimen of three-fourths lactated Ringer's solution and one-fourth plasma during the initial 24 to 48 hours; the plasma should be virus-free. The National Research Council has warned of the hazard of hepatitis with plasma administration, and plasma is not usually available. Plasminate is recommended unless group-specific individual units of plasma are available.

There has been a complete reversal of practice in recent years in the use of whole blood during the acute resuscitative phase. In the early fifties, whole blood was utilized as the primary fluid replacement therapy in many burn centers, including that of the authors. Fox, Lasker, and Winfield (1960), Wilson and Stirman (1960), Fogelman and Wilson (1960), and others believe that whole blood is harmful during the acute phase. Their publications, together with those by Quinby and Cope (1952) on blood viscosity and by Markley and coworkers (1961) and Markley and Kefalides (1962) (the Lima project), who have studied the efficacy of saline versus plasma versus dextrose, have influenced considerably the current trends in fluid administration. Moreover, the pattern of mortality in burns has not changed considerably during the past 20 years irrespective of the type or amount of fluid therapy during the first 48 hours.

The amount of acute red cell destruction at the time of burn varies according to the type of burn and the extent and depth of the burn, and it can vary from 5 to 40 per cent of the red cell mass. An average figure is probably closer to 10 to 15 per cent of the total red cell mass during the first several hours following burning. Many regimes of whole blood replacement have been utilized in various centers. At the present time, the most prevalent practice is to type and cross match patients for whole blood at the time of admission, but in the absence of a preexisting anemia or other specific complication, whole blood replacement therapy is deferred until after the first 72 hours, since adequate resuscitation and oxygen transport can be accomplished otherwise. On most burn services it is very uncommon for the burn patient to receive any whole blood replacement therapy during the first 72 hours.

Insertion of an Indwelling Catheter

From this discussion, it is apparent that the various formulas available for estimating the initial fluid requirements are only for preliminary planning, and the amount and type of fluid administration are determined by the patient's clinical response. The most important parameter of the adequacy of fluid therapy is the urinary output. For this reason, a Foley catheter should be inserted into the bladder immediately upon the patient's admission and simultaneously with the insertion of an indwelling venous catheter for fluid administration. At the time of initial catheterization, the quantity and character of the urine present in the bladder should be noted, and the time since the patient was burned, and last voided, should be recorded. If the patient has a large burn, has been admitted more than one hour following injury, and has not had any prior therapy, it is not uncommon, upon initial catheterization, to obtain a few milliliters of blood-tinged or frankly bloody urine. At the time of injury the red cell destruction can be a source of free hemoglobin, and muscle injury can also release myoglobin. These substances can impart a blood-tinged color to the urine and may precipitate in the renal tubules with resulting obstruction.

A useful guide for determining adequate urinary output in burned patients has been modified from Wolferth and Peskin (1959) and is illustrated in Table 18–11.

The blood pressure and pulse are unreliable guides to the adequacy of fluid replacement therapy during the early burn shock period. The single most reliable indicator is the urinary output, which should be maintained between 30 and 50 ml per hour in an adult. If the urine output falls below this level, the rate of fluid therapy administration should be increased. Moreover, if the urinary output exceeds 75 ml per hour, the patient should be reevaluated to ascertain that the extent of the burn has not been overestimated, and the rate of fluid administration may be cautiously decreased.

TABLE 18–11. *Adequate Urinary Output According to Age*

0 to 1 year	8 to 20 ml/hr
1 to 4 years	20 to 25 ml/hr
4 to 10 years	25 to 30 ml/hr
10 years plus	30 to 50 ml/hr

Central Venous Pressure. Monitoring central venous pressure is not required for the vast majority of burns. The average patient with a 30 to 50 per cent burn who was in good health prior to injury, who has been admitted within a reasonable time after the burn, and in whom adequate initial fluid resuscitation is instituted can ordinarily be followed successfully without central venous pressure measurements. On the other hand, with patients who have failed to respond adequately to an appropriate immediate treatment regimen or in whom pulmonary or cardiac abnormalities exist, the monitoring of central venous pressure can be an important adjunct. For the purpose of monitoring central venous pressure, a polyethylene catheter is usually placed in the external jugular or subclavian vein and passed into the intrathoracic vena cava. The length of tubing required to place the tip of the catheter at or near the right atrium is estimated. The antecubital, basilic, or cephalic veins may also be utilized, but the increased length makes the estimation of the tip location more difficult. The catheter is connected through a three-way stop cock to a manometer which is positioned at the same height as the right atrium. The positioning of the catheter, the subsequent positioning of the manometer, and the respiration of the patient at the time the reading is made can all contribute to technical errors in the central venous pressure reading.

A central venous pressure reading of 7 cm of water or below indicates inadequate venous return and suggests that fluid therapy is inadequate. If this is confirmed by decreased urinary output and other clinical signs of hypovolemia, fluid therapy should be intensified. If the central venous pressure reading is from 7 to 15 cm of water and is corroborated by adequate urinary output and satisfactory clinical signs, the infusion of intravenous therapy should be continued. When the central venous pressure rises above 15 cm of water, great caution should be exercised, as the possibility of pulmonary edema exists and there may be a need for digitalization.

Renal Failure. An occasional patient is seen in whom there is scanty urine output during the initial period of fluid administration or in whom urinary output becomes markedly reduced during the course of fluid therapy. The possibility of renal failure (acute tubular necrosis) is always raised and must be differentiated from inadequate urinary output resulting from inadequate fluid replacement therapy. In general, acute tubular necrosis is rarely encountered during the first 48 hours of burn treatment if the patient has been admitted within a reasonable period of time after the burn (up to three hours) and if initial resuscitative measures have been adequate. The overwhelming majority of instances in which urinary output is or becomes inadequate are related to insufficient fluid replacement therapy. Nevertheless, the differentiation between these two clinical situations is mandatory because the therapy is diametrically opposed. To differentiate the two, the following points are helpful: (1) urinary output tends to be scanty to almost absent in true renal failure and somewhat higher in inadequate fluid replacement therapy; (2) specific gravity of the urine will tend to be in the range of 1.015 to 1.020 in early renal failure and will usually exceed 1.025 in inadequate fluid replacement therapy; (3) differential between serum and urinary osmolarity and urinary sodium excretion studies may be helpful in establishing the diagnosis; and (4) response to a fluid load is a useful test.

At the bedside the urinary specific gravity and the response to a fluid test are the most important diagnostic aids. In general, no patient should be considered to have acute tubular necrosis until it has been demonstrated that he has failed to respond to a fluid test load. It must also be remembered that a plugged catheter or other mechanical problems can block urine excretion, and *total absence of urinary output is almost always related to a mechanical obstruction of the drainage system* rather than acute tubular necrosis or inadequate fluid replacement.

For a fluid test load, the administration of 1000 ml of lactated Ringer's solution over a 30- to 45-minute period is suggested. A slight, transient, or absent response will be noted in acute tubular necrosis, while some evidence of diuresis with increased urinary output usually occurs in the patient with inadequate fluid therapy unless his fluid deficit is extremely large. If there is an increased urine output suggesting inadequate fluid therapy, the rate of administration should be increased and the judicious use of an osmotic diuretic will be helpful in maintaining adequate glomerular filtration and minimizing renal tubular precipitates. The use of obligatory osmotic agents should be reserved for the occasional patient experiencing low renal output as a result of inadequate

fluid replacement therapy, and the administration should be limited in time and amount to tide the patient over the transient episode.

The use of mannitol for a fluid test load is often advocated but is not recommended for the burn patient. If mannitol is infused into a patient who has, in fact, acute tubular necrosis, the excretion of the material cannot be accomplished; it is poorly metabolized and remains in the vascular compartment, where it tends to potentiate the possibility of pulmonary edema because of its osmotic properties.

Tetanus Prophylaxis

The possibility of tetanus is ever present in the burn patient because of necrotic tissue which cannot be immediately eliminated. In patients who have been adequately immunized prior to burn, the use of a tetanus toxoid booster is all that is required. In the presence of a complete primary series of tetanus toxoid immunizations, a booster of tetanus toxoid is adequate if a previous booster has been given within the prior six years. In patients who have had a basic immunization but have not had a booster dose within six years of the time of injury, a booster dose of toxoid is probably all that is required; however, the presence of large amounts of necrotic tissue under anaerobic conditions makes the use of supplementary passive immunity desirable. Passive immunity has been accomplished in the past with tetanus antitoxin prepared from horse serum. The sensitivity problems are well known and, although skin testing will minimize the possibility of an immediate anaphylactic type of reaction, the skin test does not give any indication related to delayed sensitivity, such as urticaria and hives, which constitute the characteristic serum sickness seen seven to ten days following administration. It should also be pointed out that the skin test is not reliable in the presence of shock, and if tetanus antitoxin prepared from horse serum is to be utilized, the skin test should be delayed for 24 to 48 hours until adequate circulation has been restored.

With the advent of human immune globulin (human tetanus antitoxin), an effective material for passive immunization against tetanus is available and should replace the equine or bovine antitoxin. Administration of 500 units of human immune globulin is recommended for patients at the time of admission who have not been previously immunized or who have not received a booster within the previous six years. This should be repeated every two weeks for the period of time that necrotic tissue is present in the wound in patients requiring passive immunization.

Antibiotic Therapy

At the time of admission to the hospital, a baseline culture of the burn wound should be obtained from representative areas, and this should be repeated at regular intervals (at least weekly and more often if the patient's course indicates) throughout the course of treatment. The burn wound is never sterile, and persistence of bacteria in the depth of the wound can be routinely anticipated. The initial cultures usually show a wide variety of organisms, but as time progresses the predominant burn wound flora consists of Staphylococcus, Pseudonomas, Proteus, and other coliform organisms. The intact burn eschar may act as a satisfactory wound dressing for the immediate postburn period, while the eschar is intact. Invasive infection or septicemia is unlikely for the first 72 hours except with beta-hemolytic Streptococcus. Most strains of this organism have remained sensitve to penicillin over the years. It is therefore recommended that procaine penicillin (600,000 units) be administered twice daily for the first five days, after which time antibiotic therapy should be administered on the basis of clinical indication and should be guided by culture and sensitivity reports. In the event of penicillin allergy or in the presence of respiratory tract injury or other associated infections, broad-spectrum antibiotics may be initially indicated in a limited number of patients.

Evaluation of the effect of early administration of systemic antibiotics on mortality is difficult because of the present tendency for patients with fatal burns to succumb later in the course of burn treatment than they did in previous years. Monasterio and coworkers (1962), in a study of 100 burn patients with lesions of more than 20 per cent of the body surface area, found that morbidity and mortality in patients treated without the use of antibiotics were comparable to those obtained in a similar group of 100 patients previously treated with antibiotics. Some decrease in the percentage of graft takes in the patients not treated with antibiotics was also noted. Haynes (1959), Haynes, Jones and Gibson (1960), and others have noted that discontinuance of routine prophylactic penicillin therapy

results in an increase in incidence of hemolytic streptococcal infections, and the majority of burn centers prescribe some type of prophylactic systemic antibiotic treatment for the control of the virulent and invasive organism. With the advent in recent years of numerous topical chemotherapeutic agents, the importance of prophylactic antibiotic therapy for Streptococcus is unclear. The use of procaine penicillin for the first five days is still recommended at the present time, with avoidance of broad-spectrum antibiotics unless pulmonary injury or other complications are present.

Nutritional Requirements

All patients with extensive burns should be given nothing by mouth for the first several hours after being burned. Following a severe burn, intense thirst is usually present. If patients are allowed unlimited access to water, large amounts may be consumed with resulting hyponatremia, which may be sufficiently severe to produce cerebral edema and convulsions. Frequently, there will be an associated paralytic ileus with gastric and abdominal distention and associated nausea and vomiting. The administration of oral fluids during this period increases the gastric distention and the possibility of vomiting with aspiration. If distention and vomiting occur in the absence of oral feeding, an indwelling nasogastric tube should be inserted and connected to suction to produce decompression. Placing a cool, moist cloth between the patient's lips is of some value in minimizing the thirst. The practice of administering ice chips or water is extremely hazardous, because the volume ingested can produce acute gastric distention and compound the electrolyte abnormalities.

After 24 hours, some oral intake may be permitted in major burns if there is no evidence of abdominal distention, nausea, and vomiting, and if peristalsis is present. It is preferable to begin oral intake with limited amounts, at frequent intervals, of milk or other fluids. The initial administration of 1 to 2 ounces per hour is recommended. If this is tolerated for 24 hours, a clear liquid diet is prescribed. A soft diet may be ordered when tolerated by the patient, usually on the third or fourth day. By the end of the first week, it is desirable to increase gradually the feedings to a high protein, high caloric diet in an attempt to maintain an intake of 50 to 80 calories per kilogram of body weight with 2 to 4 grams of protein per kilogram. Such a large intake usually requires supplementary protein feeding between meals and at night, and often requires the insertion of a nasogastric feeding tube to provide the desired calories and proteins.

Larson (1970) has demonstrated that a major portion of the desired protein and calorie intake can be accomplished by administering milk orally or through an indwelling nasogastric tube. The advantages of milk appear to be twofold: (1) the osmolarity of milk is more nearly that of intestinal contents and tends to prevent the explosive diarrhea which can occur when protein hydrolysates and other protein compounds with high osmolarity are administered; and (2) the early and sustained administration of milk may decrease the frequency with which clinically apparent stress ulcers are encountered.

In addition to the caloric and protein requirements, B complex vitamins should be provided in at least twice the usual daily requirements, and 1000 mg of ascorbic acid should also be adminstered daily. Vitamin administration should continue until all wounds are healed and the patient is well into the convalescent period. Later in the course of the burn, iron is recommended for hematopoiesis. Studies with other trace metals are in progress at the moment, with zinc receiving considerable attention. Although low serum zinc levels can be measured in burned patients, and many experimental reports related to the role of zinc in wound healing are appearing, the results available at this time are inconclusive, and routine zinc administration cannot be advocated as helpful in the average burn patient.

General Supportive Measures

In addition to the specific items mentioned above, any seriously ill, hospitalized patient will require certain supportive measures related to his age, prior medical condition, and progress during the course of burn therapy. In addition to the usual general supportive measures, there are some items of specific importance to burn patients.

Positioning and Exercise. The patient should be positioned in bed with the head of the bed elevated, especially for burns of the upper portion of the body. Elevation of the head of the bed tends to minimize the head and neck edema and at the same time makes the patient more comfortable. Attention should be given to positioning burned extremities and

other joint surfaces to minimize the possibility of contractures. It should be remembered that the position of comfort is usually the position of contracture. As a result, efforts should be made to maintain joints such as the elbows, wrists, knees, and hips in extension or only moderate flexion to avoid the development of severe flexion contractures.

Since bed rest is required initially for patients with burns of the lower half of the body, these patients must be encouraged to exercise actively various muscle groups. In fact, active physiotherapy should be started shortly after admission to the hospital to put all joints through a functional range of motion several times during the day. Exercise not only preserves mobility of joints but also tends to preserve muscle tone. The use of foot boards to prevent plantar flexion of the feet is important, and if the patients are to be nursed in the prone position, the use of a double mattress in order to allow the feet to hang free is recommended.

HAND BURNS

A special note of caution is urged with respect to hand burns. In general, all burns of the hands and forearms should be elevated for the first four to five days following burning in order to minimize the edema and subsequent fibrosis which can result from the swelling. Compression dressings are often desirable but should be limited to the first 48 to 72 hours when swelling is most acute and patients are generally least able to cooperate with the physician and therapist. Following this time the maintenance of the hand in a functional position with the use of a fitted splint is recommended. The hand should not be left in the splint as a full time measure but should be removed from the splint several times during the day in order to encourage the patient to participate in active and passive exercise of all finger joints. The proper functional position for acute burned hands consists of opposition of the thumb, neutral or dorsiflexion of the wrist, acute flexion of the MP joints, and slight, if any, flexion of the proximal and distal interphalangeal joints. This position will minimize the tendency for the hand to assume the typical postburn deformity, which occurs in the improperly managed hand: adduction of the thumb, straight or hyperextension of the metacarpal phalangeal joints, and flexion of the interphalangeal joints. If this is combined with a flexion contracture of the wrist, the problem of rehabilitation of the hand is compounded. The management of burns of the upper extremity is discussed in Chapter 81.

Anemia. Following the initial red cell destruction, there is continued hemolysis as a result of increased red cell fragility. Combined with this is the blood loss at the time of dressing changes from the open wounds and the requirement for blood replacement during surgery. Although blood transfusions are usually not required during the first 48 to 72 hours of burn care, periodic transfusions are necessary to maintain the hemoglobin at about 12 g per 100 ml and to replace blood lost during dressing and operative procedures. Blocker and coworkers (1960b) have reported that, even with the most conservative methods of management after the acute phase of a burn, an average of 1 ml of blood per day has been required for each 1 per cent of body surface involvement in order to maintain the hemoglobin at 12 g or more.

In addition to the usual anticipated blood loss, occasional hemolytic destruction of red cells can occur acutely, and the reason is usually not apparent. The acute hemolysis of red cells can result in considerable release of hemoglobin with associated renal complications and may necessitate early transfusions.

Therapeutic administration of virus-free plasma at intervals is of some limited value in patients referred late with extreme emaciation and hypoproteinemia. The administered protein is of value in elevating the albumin levels and in providing immunoglobulins. There are adequate clinical studies available to indicate that the serum albumin levels must be kept above 3.0 g per 100 ml for satisfactory healing, and the inability of the patient to maintain an albumin level of 3.0 despite therapeutic measures is a poor prognostic sign. The administration of gamma globulin as an adjunctive measure to massive antibiotic therapy in the treatment of septicemia has been reported and may be of limited value.

ACTH and Cortisone. Although a number of years ago both ACTH and cortisone were believed to be of value in the shock phase of extensive burns, subsequent clinical trials have proved disappointing, and both have been abandoned for routine use. An exception should be made in patients who have recently received some type of steroid therapy. Moncrief (1962) has suggested that hydrocortisone might be employed in a severe burn as transient therapy in the absence of resuscitative fluids, and Moore (1959) has recommended its use in patients with "hypermature" granulation tissue in whom repeated skin graft failures have occurred. Although a number of workers have extensively studied the steroid levels in blood and urine, Haynes (1959) has indicated that there are no clear-cut indications for ACTH and cortisone therapy, even in patients with low serum and urinary levels who fail to respond to the standard ACTH tests. Artz and Moncrief (1969) have reviewed the available data regarding adrenal cortical response and concluded that adrenal cortical insufficiency can occur in burns but is not common. They suggest that, when one suspects adrenal cortical insufficiency in a burn patient who is not doing well, an immediate eosinophil count and plasma and urine sodium and chloride determinations should be done. In the face of documented adrenal cortical insufficiency, the administration of ACTH or hydrocortisone does not necessarily correct the condition.

It would appear, therefore, that there is no evidence to support the use of ACTH or cortisone in the management of the average patient, even with extensive burns.

Psychologic Aspects. The burned patient necessarily goes through a difficult psychologic adjustment. Initially there is the fear of death, followed by the fear of disability and physical disfigurement. The burned patient who is subjected to repeated painful experiences may become demoralized. Attention to the psychologic needs of the patient and calm reassurance during the course of therapy are essential. It is important to emphasize the progress made toward recovery and to minimize the psychologic problems. It is not uncommon for patients to enter a period of depression during the early convalescence, at the time when they are preparing to leave the hospital and reenter their community, as they realize that they may be scarred or disfigured and not in the same condition that they were prior to injury.

Lewis and coworkers (1963) made a study of the reaction of patients to severe burns by developing and validating rating scales of ward behavior, taking into account the patient's basic personality type and his adjustment following injury. Six empirical catagories were developed as follows:

1. Well-adjusted group
2. Overly compliant—submissive group (inadequate character)
3. Complaining—demanding group (rebellious-aggressive personality)

4. Uncooperative — obstructive group (rebellious-aggressive personality)

5. Passive — helpless group (passive-dependent personality)

6. Unresponsive group (depressive reaction)

The findings indicated that approximately 30 per cent of the patients fell within the well-adjusted group and 45 per cent within the passive-helpless catagory with respect to their hospital adjustment. The passive-helpless patients showed greater interest in the details of their nursing and medical care than did the well-adjusted patients, who had a greater degree of understanding of the aims and goals of treatment and generally responded to the therapy in a manner superior to the other groups. It would appear that the success of the patient's adjustment to his injury depends more on his preburn personality than on any other single factor. In extreme cases the assistance of psychiatric counseling may be necessary.

Acute psychotic episodes are most commonly encountered in burn patients as a toxic manifestation in relation to generalized sepsis or as a result of withdrawal of the patient from alcohol or drugs, especially narcotics and barbiturates.

Many of the unexplained acute psychotic episodes which are occasionally encountered in burn patients are apparently due to absorption of hexachlorophene if this compound is used in soaps for tubbing or cleansing burn wounds. Larson (1968) has demonstrated that abnormally high serum levels of hexachlorophene can be obtained in burn patients and correlated with otherwise unexplained CNS symptoms. Larson has been able to reproduce these same symptoms under experimental laboratory conditions. For that reason, hexachlorophene-containing compounds should not be used for cleansing large open wounds or for repeated washing in the Hubbard tank.

Other General Measures. Obviously the patient must be examined daily or more often and appropriate measures instituted as indicated. The importance of maintaining an optimal nutritional intake cannot be overemphasized. The use of proper positioning and splinting to minimize functional contractures and the active and passive exercise of joints under the supervision of a physical therapist are mandatory from the beginning of burn treatment. Small doses of sedatives such as barbiturates may be helpful during the course of therapy, and occasional patients may benefit from the administration of tranquilizing agents or muscle relaxants. Although small amounts of tranquilizing agents may be helpful in occasional adult patients, one should not use them as a routine measure. It should be emphasized that some of these drugs (such as diazepam) can produce a degree of mental confusion which is undesirable in burn patients. The use of phenothiazine prior to tubbing or dressings is particularly helpful in children.

Local Wound Management

Although immediate attention to the burn wound is mandatory, it should not take precedence over the initial fluid therapy, respiratory evaluation, and other more urgent requirements. The majority of flash and flame burns actually require no cleansing, although adherent clothing, dirt, or other foreign material should be removed by gentle rinsing with bland soap and warm water. Breaking of blisters is unnecessary during the first few hours and may actually contribute to an increased fluid loss. Chemical burns should be treated with copius irrigations of water for dilution for several hours.

Complete examination of the burn wound should encompass a careful oral-pharyngeal evaluation for any evidence of singeing of hair or hyperemia, which may herald subsequent pulmonary problems.

Decompression of Circumferential Burn Scars. Circumferential burns of the extremities must be inspected carefully for evidence of circulatory impairment. The thick, leathery eschar of a circumferential third degree burn is unyielding and, as the internal fluid shifts occur, can result in sufficient rise of pressure to produce ischemia of the extremity. This is usually manifested by a distal extremity which is cool, pale, or cyanotic, and distal pulses may be absent (Fig. 18–7). If there is a circumferential constricting eschar of an extremity, it should be decompressed with a vertical incision extending from the uninvolved skin above to the uninvolved skin below. Since third degree burns are relatively insensitive, these incisions can often be performed on the ward without anesthesia. However, care should be taken to minimize additional bacterial contamination. All attendants should be wearing caps, gowns, and masks, and if decompression is contemplated, the proposed incision lines should be painted with an iodine solution and gloves and sterile instruments should be utilized. The incision should be made sufficiently deep into the

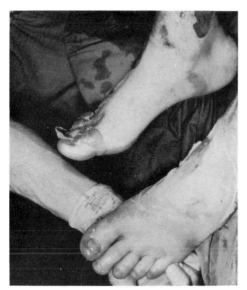

FIGURE 18–7. Pale, cyanotic appearance of the feet in a circumferential third degree burn of the lower extremities. Distal pulses could not be palpated.

(4) maintaining the interphalangeal joints straight. This is best accomplished by the use of a splint during the first two to three days of acute burn treatment; thereafter the hand is removed from the splint several times during the day for both active and passive exercising, and the splint is then replaced to prevent or minimize the deformity when active exercise programs are not being conducted and during sleep.

If the lower extremities are burned, they should also be elevated and can be managed by exposure unless the wound is limited to one or both lower extermities, where dressings may facilitate nursing care, particularly in children and in elderly patients. For circumferential wounds of the trunk, the use of circa-electric beds or Stryker frames for turning the patient in order to avoid maceration of the dependent wound surface is desirable.

TOPICAL AGENTS

In the introduction to this chapter, a wide variety of topical agents, escharotics, and other applications were mentioned for historical purposes. In addition to the "healing" compounds, numerous enzymatic debriding agents, analgesic compounds, and conventional antibiotics (penicillin, sulfanilamide, etc.) have been tried in past years and have proved to be of such limited value that their use could not be recommended.

Despite disappointment with earlier attempts at enzymatic debridement of the eschar, interest has continued, since early chemical removal of the eschar to facilitate early grafting would be beneficial for the burn patient. Levine and coworkers (1973) have reported effective experimental debridement of third degree burn eschar in animals using bromelain, an enzyme derived from pineapple. Since the report of McConn and coworkers (1964) on a neutral proteinase of high specific activity obtained from *Bacillus subtilis*, considerable clinical interest has been expressed in this compound, and many different authors have reported beneficial effects from the use of this enzyme. Pennisi, Capozzi and Friedman (1973), Krizek and Robson (1974), and others have reported that this enzyme, when applied to burn wounds, is effective in accomplishing early debridement of the necrotic eschar. Application of this agent requires that it be kept continuously moist, and it should be applied to a limited area of the body,

subcutaneous tissue to release the pressure, but ordinarily it is not necessary to deepen the incision to or through the underlying deep muscle fascia (Fig. 18–8). If the circulation to the hands and fingers is compromised, adequate decompression will require incisions on both sides of the fingers connected to incisions in the hand to ensure adequate decompression of the distal phalanges.

Exposure therapy or compression dressings can be utilized according to the surgeon's preference and in accordance with other proposed topical wound medication. In general, hand burns are best managed by incorporating them into a dressing that includes a splint to maintain the hand in the desired position and allows for elevation, support, and compression for the first 48 to 72 hours. The desired position for the acutely burned hand is not the classic position of function. As mentioned earlier, the burned hand deformity that results from ignoring the position of the hand during the course of burn treatment is characterized by flexion of the wrist, adduction of the thumb, hyperextension of the metacarpal phalangeal joints, and flexion of the interphalangeal joints. The initial positioning of the hand should be aimed at preventing this deformity and should consist of (1) maintaining the wrist in neutral or slight extension, (2) maintaining the thumb in opposition toward the fingers, (3) maintaining the metacarpal phalangeal joints flexed 75° to 80°, and

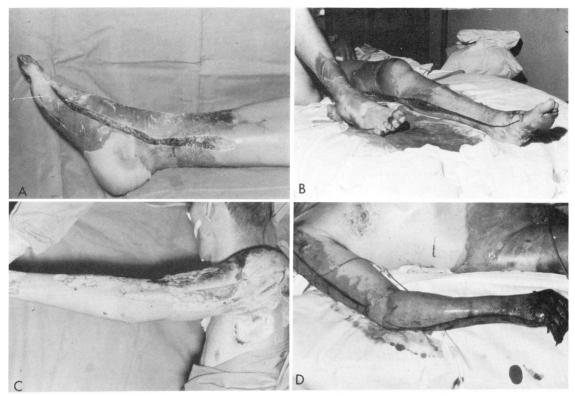

FIGURE 18–8. Decompression incisions for circumferential full-thickness burns of the extremities.

not exceeding 10 per cent of the body surface at one time. It should be instituted two to five days after burning, when the patient's general condition has stabilized, and becomes less effective late in the course of the burn, when a stable, leathery eschar has existed for several days. In addition to being inactivated by drying, the enzyme is also inactivated by heavy metals, such as silver.

The basic problem in the topical use of antibacterial or other compounds is related to the fact that most of these agents do not penetrate the dead eschar sufficiently to produce a significant therapeutic effect at the interface between the living and devitalized tissue. Systemic antibiotic and other agents administered parenterally are also not effectively carried into this interface because of the absence of adequate circulation in this area. As a result, burn wound sepsis has historically been the major complication of burn therapy and has resulted in invasive infection and septicemia; it is also the largest single cause of burn mortality.

Since 1965, a number of topical agents which have the capability of permeating the eschar with sufficient antibacterial activity to control burn wound sepsis have been utilized. Included among the compounds in current use are:

1. Silver nitrate, 0.5 per cent solution
2. Sulfamylon acetate, 10 per cent
3. Silver sulfadiazine
4. Neosporin
5. Other compounds

Silver Nitrate. Although 10 per cent silver nitrate had been advocated as a topical burn wound preparation at the turn of the century, the use of this compound gained widespread

TABLE 18–12. *Advantages of 0.5% Silver Nitrate Solution*

1. Bacteriostatic property
2. Patients seem less toxic
3. Burn wounds cleaner with less odor
4. Elimination of dressing procedures in the operating room under anesthesia
5. Prevention of conversion of second degree to third degree wounds by infection
6. Joint mobility maintained with wet dressings

TABLE 18–13. *Disadvantages of 0.5%*
Silver Nitrate Solution

1. Delays eschar separation by two or three weeks
2. Dilutional hyponatremia
3. Adverse effect on donor sites and dermatomes
4. Expense of the dressings required, although the nitrate itself is inexpensive
5. Difficulty in judging depth of burn and evaluating burn wound after applying silver nitrate
6. Deep black staining of the entire environment

popularity as a 0.5 per cent solution following the clinical studies of Moyer and coworkers (1965). Monafo (1967) has reported reduction in the number of bacteria present in the burn wound and in the incidence of septicemia. The advantages and disadvantages of silver nitrate are summarized in Tables 18–12 and 18–13.

The recommended procedure for application of silver nitrate is to apply bulky, coarse mesh gauze to the surface of the wound saturated with silver nitrate in 0.5 per cent solution. The bulky, coarse mesh gauze is held in place with 6-inch kerlix and covered with stockinet. The inner dressings are continuously moistened with 0.5 per cent silver nitrate to prevent drying. Dressings are changed either every 12 hours or daily. If the inner dressings are allowed to dry by evaporation of moisture, the silver nitrate concentration is increased, and increased concentrations are caustic to open wounds.

The use of the hypotonic solution adjacent to the burn wound can result in a severe dilutional hyponatremia with convulsions. This complication is rarely encountered because it can be anticipated and supplementary sodium administered if silver nitrate dressings are being employed. The wounds do, in fact, remain clean with a healthy color, and the frequent repeated dressing changes are an effective method of wound debridement.

The separation of the eschar is delayed by two to three weeks if silver nitrate soaks are utilized; in addition, the silver nitrate effect on the potential donor areas makes removal of skin grafts more difficult, and mechanical problems are encountered with the dermatome. The evaluation of the subeschar area for microabscesses is much more difficult if the eschar has been treated with silver nitrate, and application of skin grafts to partially debrided wounds can be troublesome if some silver nitrate–treated eschar is still present.

The most apparent disadvantage to the use of 0.5 per cent silver nitrate solution is the deep black staining of hospital linen, floors, and equipment, as well as the clothing of attendants and personnel, which requires special care in cleansing (Fig. 18–9).

Silver nitrate enjoyed a tremendous surge of popularity, and although it is still used in some burn centers, such as the Shriner's Burn Institute in Boston, it is not as widely used in the United States as it was a few years ago. In the

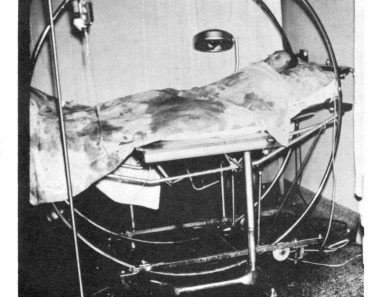

FIGURE 18–9. Dark staining of bedclothes, a major problem associated with the use of silver nitrate dressings.

TABLE 18–14.   *Advantages of Sulfamylon*

1. Bacteriostatic property
2. Penetrates the eschar well
3. Easy to apply
4. Nonstaining
5. Low toxicity

authors' experience with 100 consecutive patients treated with silver nitrate at the University of Texas (Dominguez and associates, 1967), there was a decrease in mortality of patients with 40 to 60 per cent body surface burns.

Sulfamylon. Ten per cent Sulfamylon cream has been widely used in burn centers in the United States since its introduction by Lindberg and associates (1965). This is an old compound that had been used in Germany many years ago. The initial clinical trials in burn patients in this country demonstrated an antibacterial activity when the substance was applied to the burn wound; these trials were performed with Sulfamylon hydrochloride, which had a tendency to produce metabolic acidosis which could be a troublesome complication, particularly in children. Sulfamylon is currently marketed as the acetate salt, which has minimized the electrolyte abnormalities. The advantages and disadvantages of the compound are listed in Tables 18–14 and 18–15.

Sulfamylon is applied as a 10 per cent cream directly on the open wound, using a gloved hand or tongue blade, to a depth of approximately 1/2 cm. No covering is necessary, but turning the patient in bed results in smearing of the cream onto the bed clothes, so frequent reapplication may be necessary during the early course of the burn. Application twice a day is recommended to ensure an adequate covering of Sulfamylon over the burn wound. Much of the problem associated with displacement of Sulfamylon from the burn wound can be obviated and nursing care can be facilitated by impregnating the Sulfamylon in a single

TABLE 18–15.   *Disadvantages of Sulfamylon*

1. Acidosis (more marked with the hydrochloride than with the acetate salt)
2. Painful at the time of application
3. Sensitivity reaction (in 15 per cent of patients)
4. Delays eschar separation
5. Carbonic anhydrase inhibitor
6. Retards epithelial regeneration

layer of fine mesh gauze, which is applied to the burn wounds twice a day and which may be covered with one or two layers of loose dressing to maintain the compound in position on burned extremities. This limited dressing does not produce a warm, moist wound environment, which can promote maceration and bacterial proliferation, as seen in conventional occlusive dressings. The changing of the fine mesh gauze twice a day also facilitates wound debridement, with small sloughing portions of the eschar being removed at the time of each dressing change. The burn wound must be completely cleansed on a daily basis for inspection and reapplication of the Sulfamylon. This is best accomplished in the Hubbard tank, where active and passive exercising is performed under the supervision of the physical therapy staff. During the first few days when the patient's general condition will not tolerate his being moved to the Hubbard tank, the Sulfamylon is removed daily by gentle cleansing in bed.

Sulfamylon acetate exerts a bacteriostatic effect on the burn wound by virtue of its ability to penetrate the eschar. Although the burn wound is not sterilized, the proliferation of bacteria is controlled to the point that the incidence of burn wound sepsis and secondary infectious complications is reduced. Sulfamylon is easy to apply and has the distinct advantage over silver nitrate that it is nonstaining and does not obscure evaluation of the wound or interefere with donor sites.

The disadvantages of Sulfamylon have been well documented by numerous studies. The acidosis originally produced with the Sulfamylon hydrochloride was troublesome but could easily be controlled by anticipating its occurrence and using appropriate electrolyte therapy. The incidence of acidosis has been decreased with the use of Sulfamylon acetate. Application of the compound is painful; the patient experiences a burning sensation which usually subsides within a period of 30 minutes. In some patients the pain on application can be severe, and can require narcotic sedation. In an occasional patient the pain may be so severe that discontinuance of the Sulfamylon therapy is indicated. Sensitivity reactions manifested primarily by a genrealized skin rash occur during the course of treatment in 10 to 15 per cent of patients. This usually subsides spontaneously with the discontinuation of Sulfamylon, and in some patients Sulfamylon has been reinstituted following previous sensitivity reaction. However, this should be done with caution and only if burn wound sepsis is a significant problem.

Sulfamylon, in common with all topical antibacterial compounds which have any bacteriostatic effect, reduces bacterial autolysis of the eschar, which results in delayed eschar separation and prolongs the hospital treatment time prior to the first grafting. The delayed eschar separation makes it mandatory to remove mechanically with forceps and scissors any adherent eschar which does not spontaneously separate during the first four to five weeks. The removal of eschar can be performed at the time of daily soaking in the Hubbard tank but should be extremely conservative and meticulous to prevent the production of bleeding wounds. Only superficial, partially separated eschar should be removed by this method.

Another characteristic of Sulfamylon is its carbonic anhydrase inhibition. This interferes with the effectiveness of the renal tubular buffering mechanism and causes a respiratory compensation with elevation of the respiratory rate, which may approach 40 to 50 per minute. Although the respiratory compensation may maintain the blood pH in normal range, the rapid respiratory rate can be exhausting in a seriously ill patient. Artz and Moncrief (1969) recommended that, when the respiratory rate increases regardless of whether or not the patient's blood studies show an acidosis, Sulfamylon acetate should be discontinued for two or three days until the reaction subsides.

In an occasional patient with deep second degree burns, separation of the eschar occurs uneventfully, but re-epithelialization of the burn wound is inordinately prolonged with the continued use of Sulfamylon acetate. For this reason the authors have frequently discontinued the use of Sulfamylon after the eschar has separated and the resulting wound surface is a clean second degree wound in an attempt to facilitate the spontaneous healing of the area. Experimental studies by Scapicchio, Constable and Opity (1968), Wisner and coworkers (1970), and Bellinger and Conway (1970) have shown that regeneration of epithelium on experimental wounds is retarded by Sulfamylon, and the same phenomenon has been observed in patients.

In addition to the disadvantages of Sulfamylon listed above, Maurer and coworkers (1970) have reported a patient with agranulocytosis resulting from the use of Sulfamylon. This must be rare, as Sulfamylon has been used in various centers on thousands of patients with no other complications of this type reported.

Silver Sulfadiazine. Fox and coworkers (1969) reported experimental studies showing that silver sulfadiazine is an effective bacteriostatic agent in experimental animal burns. Subsequent clinical trials have demonstrated that silver sulfadiazine appears to be comparable in bacteriostatic effect to Sulfamylon. The advantages and disadvantages of silver sulfadiazine are listed in Tables 18–16 and 18–17.

An examination of these tables shows that silver sulfadiazine is comparable to Sulfamylon in bacteriostatic effect, but patient acceptance is much higher since silver sulfadiazine is less painful on application. Furthermore, it does not have the carbonic anhydrase inhibiting capacity and is extremely low in toxicity. As a result, silver sulfadiazine is currently a widely utilized and effective topical chemotherapeutic agent.

Other Topical Agents. Stone (1967) has reported his experience with the use of gentamicin as a topical wound agent. Since that time the FDA has withdrawn approval of this agent for topical use, and Stone and Bush (1973) are currently using Neosporin ointment with occlusive dressings. Georgiade and coworkers (1967) have reported preliminary results using furazolium chloride. Other topical agents are currently under experimental and clinical evaluation, and new ones will undoubtedly appear in the future.

PREGRAFTING PHASE OF WOUND MANAGEMENT

The time required for conservative preparation of a third degree burn wound for grafting will average three to six weeks, depending on the location and extent of the burn and on the topical medication utilized. The importance of evaluating circumferential third degree wounds of an extremity for a constricting effect has previously been emphasized. The burn wound itself requires no specific therapy for the first few days. The intact eschar serves as a satisfactory wound covering, and invasive infection

TABLE 18–16. *Advantages of Silver Sulfadiazine*

1. Bacteriostatic property
2. Penetrates the eschar well
3. Easy to apply
4. Nonstaining
5. Low toxicity
6. Less painful on application than Sulfamylon

TABLE 18–17. *Disadvantages of Silver Sulfadiazine*

1. Delays eschar separation

is unlikely in the immediate postburn period. The management of burn shock and general supportive measures take precedence over definitive wound management during this period.

Between seven and ten days post burn, the intact eschar begins to show necrosis and liquefaction, and some method of cleansing and debridement is necessary. The most widely used technique is to rely primarily on daily bathing in the Hubbard tank for mechanical wound cleansing. Upon return from the Hubbard tank, each patient should have any loose or shredding eschar removed, and Sulfamylon or silver sulfadiazine should be applied to the wound. The topical ointment may be held in place by one or two layers of gauze on the extremities. The repeated removal of the gauze and tubbing will effectively remove the major portion of the eschar during the first few weeks of burn therapy. An occasional patient may require surgical debridement in the operating room under anesthesia to complete the removal of the eschar and to prepare the burn wound for grafting. It must be emphasized that the daily removal of the limited bandages and daily Hubbard tank cleansing is a method aimed at maintaining meticulous mechanical wound cleanliness; the use of any of the topical agents is not a substitute for the continuation of sound surgical principles.

Because all of the effective topical chemotherapeutic agents retard bacterial autolysis of the eschar and tend to delay the time for initial grafting, other methods have been evaluated for hastening eschar removal. Richards and Feller (1973) have reported that grid escharotomy is helpful in early removal of the eschar, while it decreases the probability of wound infection and sepsis. The escharotomy is performed with an electrocautery by cutting through the eschar, but not into deeper tissues, in a grid fashion to divide the eschar into 1-inch squares and to increase the peripheral surface area available for debriding. This type of escharotomy is performed not for relief of pressure, as in circumferential third degree burns, but rather for early eschar removal. A more widely utilized method of eschar removal is tangential excision, as reported by Janzekovic (1970), Jackson and Stone (1972), and others. This technique is performed two to five days post burn and utilizes a dermatome or skin graft knife to remove repeated parallel slices of the burn eschar until a bleeding surface is obtained; the latter is covered immediately with skin grafts. Jackson and Stone have reported earlier wound closure by this method without increased mortality. The application of grafts is essential following the tangential excision, since the excision alone offers no advantage.

Another method currently being evaluated for removal of the eschar is use of the carbon dioxide laser. In experimental animals Levine and coworkers (1974a) have reported laser debridement of third degree burns. With this technique there was a decreased blood loss, no evidence of toxicity, and satisfactory skin graft take. Link and coworkers (1974), utilizing a carbon dioxide laser, have presented a series of experimental studies with encouraging results. Levine and coworkers (1974b) have compared laser excision, scalpel excision, electrosurgical excision, and tangential excision of third degree burns and feel that, although the laser may be a helpful adjunct in selected cases, it does not represent a panacea at the present time.

Occlusive Dressings. Since Allen and Koch (1942) emphasized the use of pressure dressings, this method has been widely utilized in burn patients. The use of bulky occlusive dressings for large burn wounds is not in common use at the present time and, in general, other methods are preferable. The use of bulky compression dressings produces a warm, moist environment, which is optimal for bacterial proliferation. This wound environment not only produces maceration and increases the probability of infection of the wound but also can produce maceration of the adjacent uninvolved skin. Wound complications and abscesses which are not readily apparent until the time of dressing change can also develop. Even in air conditioned hospital environments, the use of bulky compression dressings can result in hyperpyrexia, with the associated increased metabolic demand, which is so detrimental for burned patients. The dressing materials themselves are expensive, and the changing of the dressings is usually painful, requiring sedation or anesthesia. Furthermore, the use of bulky dressings limits motion, a desirable function in all burn patients. For these reasons, bulky compression dressings have largely been supplanted by other forms of therapy, and at the present time dressings are limited to occasional patients with small burns, such as elderly patients or children with limited burns of one extremity, in whom nursing care can be greatly facilitated with the application of a bandage. The use of a compression bandage to maintain burned hands in a functional position as a temporary measure during the first two or three days of burn care is also useful. Otherwise, dressings should be limited to minor burns being treated on an outpatient basis, when wound covering for prevention of further contamination is desirable.

Exposure Therapy. Another technique for management of the burn wound for the past 25 years has been the use of exposure therapy. This is an effective method, and the rationale of this form of treatment is to leave the wound exposed in order that the surface coagulant may form a firm, intact eschar. The coagulum and eschar should ideally be cool and dry in order to minimize bacterial proliferation. Epidermal regeneration occurs spontaneously under second degree burn eschars, and separation of the eschar occurs two to six weeks after the burn. The proliferation of bacteria beneath a third degree eschar results in autolysis and liquefaction of the burn eschar. At this time regular mechanical cleansing and conservative debridement are required to eliminate the eschar and prepare the wound for grafting. During this period the wound surface is continually available for observation and inspection to detect abscesses or other wound complications.

Simple exposure therapy is most often utilized for limited second degree burns, such as those that occur on the face and hands following exposure to a flash. Otherwise, exposure therapy is supplemented by the application of one of the chemotherapeutic topical agents mentioned above.

Excision of the Burn Wound. The burn wound is the only example in surgery in which the basic principle of early surgical debridement of all necrotic tissue is routinely violated. Excision of severe extensive burns is a major surgical procedure associated with significant blood loss and operative mortality. Massive excision has been tried in many centers in the past and has been reported by MacMillan (1958), Jackson and coworkers (1960), and others. However, no improvement in mortality has been demonstrated. The use of serial excision of a small portion of the burn wound at repeated intervals to minimize the magnitude of the surgical procedure was evalu-

ated by Cramer, McCormack, and Carroll (1962), and some patients were salvaged who otherwise would have probably succumbed. Nevertheless, at the present time surgical excision of extensive burns (over 20 per cent) is not often employed.

Burke and associates (1974) have reported a sophisticated experimental approach to staged excision of massive burns with allograft coverage in patients immunosuppressed by drugs to prolong the survival of allografts until the limited autograft donor areas can be used for resurfacing. With this highly technical approach and its many associated problems, these workers have reported survival of patients who certainly would not have survived by any conventional approach.

On the other hand, in limited burns, surgical excision of the burned tissue followed by skin grafting, either at the same time or after an interval of 24 or 48 hours to obtain hemostasis, is a satisfactory method of therapy. This method is particularly applicable over the dorsum of the hand, where early wound coverage and functional restoration are important. Many examples are seen, such as the laundry worker who catches one hand on a steam press and produces a well-demarcated, localized third degree burn of limited extent; in such a situation, surgical excision with skin grafting is the optimum treatment. Surgical excision and grafting should usually be limited to burns that involve 15 per cent of the body surface or less and to burns that are clearly third degree, in which spontaneous healing cannot be anticipated (Fig. 18–10).

An alternative technique is that of tangential excision, as discussed previously.

GRAFTING PROCEDURES

Three to five weeks following burning, the third degree wounds will usually be ready for grafting. Wounds are clinically ready for grafting when the eschar has separated and the granulating bed is free of necrotic tissue and active infection. At this stage granulation tissue, characterized by a thin, flat red surface will be present, and grafts should be applied as soon as possible because open granulations, as time elapses, tend to proliferate, become boggy and edematous, and bleed easily. Skin grafts do not take as well in this hypermature stage. In extensive burns it may not be possible to cover the entire wound at one surgical procedure. It is seldom possible to graft more than

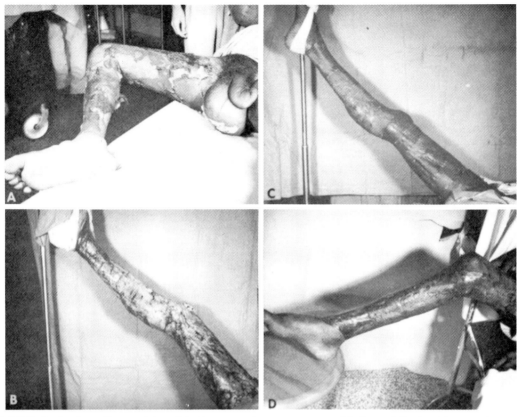

FIGURE 18-10. Immediate excision of the burn wound. *A*, Appearance eight hours following injury. *B*, Appearance following excision of the burned tissue down to the deep fascia. *C*, Appearance 48 hours later, after delayed split-thickness skin grafting. *D*, Appearance three months after skin grafting.

20 to 30 per cent of the body surface at one operation. In extensive burns the first procedure should ordinarily be done as soon as a suitable wound is ready, provided that the patient's general condition is satisfactory.

The first priority for wound coverage should be given to the face, the hands, and the flexion joint surfaces. It is not necessary to wait until all burned areas are ready for grafting before applying the initial skin coverage. No specific preparation of the burn wound is required in the majority of patients, although application of continuous wet dressings for 24 hours may be helpful in locally infected wounds. If grafting has been delayed beyond the optimum time and the granulation tissue has become hypertrophic, thick, boggy, and edematous, some surgeons have advocated scraping of the excessive granulation tissue prior to the time of grafting. If the burn wound is large, this can result in a significant amount of blood loss. The vascularization of grafts will not necessarily be improved and may actually be hampered by the formation of multiple, small subgraft

hematomas if grafting is performed at the same operation. The hypertrophic granulation tissue can usually be flattened and made more optimum for grafting by the application of a firm compression bandage for 24 hours prior to grafting.

Anesthesia Considerations

A burn graft is a major surgical procedure, and the patient should be taken to the operating room with an empty stomach and with appropriate premedication. Since many of these patients are seriously ill, premedication should be minimal, consistent with adequate sedation for smooth induction. Endotracheal intubation will be required in the majority of patients, particularly if the patient is to be turned from one position to another. An adequate amount of blood should be typed and cross matched for infusion at the time of surgery to replace the blood loss and to correct any deficiency of red blood cell mass which may exist at the time.

The surgical procedure should be performed expeditiously in order to minimize the length of anesthesia time. An adequate intravenous portal must be established prior to induction for the administration of medication and blood transfusions. In the seriously ill patients electrocardiographs and temperature monitoring should be routinely employed. A drop in body temperature is usually encountered during burn grafting procedures. In selected, critically ill patients, additional monitoring of the central venous pressure may be desirable.

In children, *ketamine hydrochloride* has been the subject of extensive clinical investigation in many surgical centers. It is a dissociative agent which can be administered either intramuscularly or intravenously. The duration of a single injection is limited to a few minutes, but with repeated injections patients can be maintained for a period of 1 to 1½ hours without difficulty. Because of the dissociative character of this compound, the patients do not require intubation, and postoperative nausea and vomiting are infrequently encountered. The patients are actually awake, can move spontaneously, and may respond to questions. Despite the conscious attitude of the patient, pain perception is eliminated, and the removal of skin grafts, debridement of wounds, and other usually painful procedures can be accomplished. Because of distressing hallucinatory episodes which may occur in adults, it is preferable to confine its use to the pediatric age group.

Donor Sites

The donor sites in order of preference are the upper thighs, abdomen, back, chest, upper arms, buttocks, legs, and dorsum of the feet. The lower thighs, legs, and feet are avoided if early ambulation is anticipated. The patient's age, sex, percentage of surface involvement, and burn distribution will affect the selection of donor sites in an individual patient. In limited burns it is desirable to select the donor sites on the same surface of the body as the burn wound in order to facilitate postoperative positioning and nursing.

The donor areas should be carefully prepped with a surgical soap, and surgical drapes should be utilized to isolate the donor area from the contaminated burn wounds as much as possible. Obviously in very extensive burns this is not always possible, and in some instances it is necessary to remove skin grafts from areas immediately adjacent to open burn wounds. Even when this is performed, the frequency of infection in donor sites should be low if meticulous attention to wound care is observed.

For removal of skin grafts the Brown electric or air-driven dermatome, the Padgett or Reese dermatomes, or the variety of freehand knives can be utilized. For extensive burns the authors prefer to use the Brown air-driven dermatome because considerable amounts of skin can be removed in large sheets within a minimum amount of time (Fig. 18–11). The thickness of the grafts removed will vary according to the location and extent of the burn wound and the character of the wound at the time of grafting. In relatively localized burn wounds with an optimal granulating surface, removal of skin grafts with the Brown dermatome set at 16 to 18/1000th of an inch* is rec-

---

*1 inch = 2.540 cm metric.

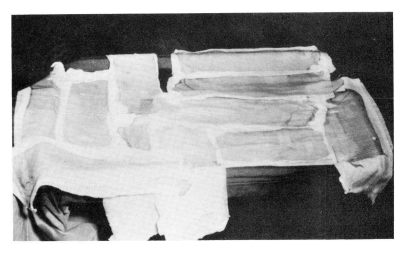

FIGURE 18–11. Large sheets of split-thickness skin removed by the Brown air-driven dermatome.

ommended in adults. In more extensive burn wounds or in suboptimal wound conditions, setting the dermatome at 10 to 15/1000th of an inch produces a thinner graft with an improved chance of graft survival. If a second crop of grafts must be harvested from the same donor area within two to three weeks, thinner grafts (8 to 10/1000th of an inch) are recommended; this thickness is usually more appropriate for small children.

As the sheets of skin are removed with the Brown dermatome, they are passed to the assisting nurse who spreads them out on saline-soaked gauze sponges with the raw surface exposed. The nurse keeps the grafts moist with saline during the few minutes required for removal of additional grafts and preparation for application of the grafts to the burned surface.

Many devices have been described over the years for expansion of skin grafts to allow a limited donor area to cover a much larger recipient area. Of those in current use, the mesh dermatome (Tanner, Vandeput and Olley, 1964) is the most widespread. This device produces a series of perforations in the graft of a geometrical design that allows expansion of the skin graft to many times its original size. The coverage of additional area is at the expense of leaving multiple small raw areas between the transplanted grafts. Although these grafts take well and are effective in covering large raw wounds, the healed surface presents a cobblestone effect which is cosmetically not as acceptable as the effect presented by large sheets of graft. Excessive scarring with increased contracture formation is at least a theoretical possibility. For that reason, mesh grafting is best reserved for patients with large open wounds and limited donor areas. In general, the mesh should not be expanded more than three to one, although current instruments allow considerably more expansion. In general, the authors agree with DiVincenti, Curreri and Pruitt (1969), who emphasized that mesh grafts should be restricted to broad, flat, and immobile burn wound surfaces. Meshing is specifically contraindicated on the face, hands, forearms, flexion and joint areas, and, in adult patients, below the knee.

Following the removal of skin grafts, the donor area presents a raw, denuded, bleeding surface. The surface can be managed by the application of a variety of agents, including Gelfoam powder, Congo red, and fine mesh gauze impregnated with a variety of compounds. Our own preference is to cover the donor area with a single layer of fine mesh gauze soaked in glycerine and to cover the fine mesh gauze wtih moist, warm, bulky pads while the skin grafts are being applied. When the patient is ready to leave the operating room, the bulky saline-soaked pad is removed, leaving the single layer of glycerine-impregnated gauze exposed. The use of heat lamps continuously for a few hours, and intermittently for the next four to five days, will result in drying of the serum and coagulum within the fine mesh gauze. Once the coagulum has dried to a brown crust, the possibility of infection is minimized, and the gauze is left in place while spontaneous epidermal regeneration takes place beneath it. After a few days, the edges tend to curl and are trimmed away with scissors to avoid their catching onto bed clothing. After a period of five to seven days when the coagulum in the donor site is dry, tubbing of the patient is acceptable. Upon removal of the patient from the tub, the donor site is simply blotted dry. With this technique, infection in the donor site is uncommon.

Application of Skin Grafts

An effort should be made to use large pieces of skin in contradistinction to "postage stamps" or thin strips with intervening raw areas. The use of mesh expanded grafts should also be limited, as mentioned above, although Neale (1974) has reported the use of meshed grafts without expansion to provide drainage. Optimum wound healing is obtained by complete coverage of the burn wound with large sheets of skin, which results in the best cosmetic effect and minimizes the chance of subsequent contracture of the grafts and functional deformities.

If the burn wounds are limited to one surface of the body where it is possible by positioning to leave the area exposed, the grafts are spread out on the granulating surface and trimmed to fit the defect. Trimming must be sufficiently accurate to prevent the skin grafts from overlapping the normal skin edges, where the proliferation of skin bacteria will result in a thin margin of peripheral skin loss. If the wound can be positioned for exposure, no sutures or dressings are required, as the skin grafts rapidly become adherent to the underlying wound (Figs. 18–12 and 18–13). The liberal use of Steristrips is helpful in securing the

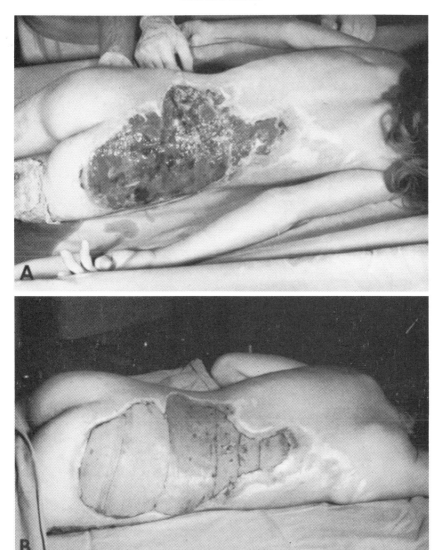

FIGURE 18–12. Skin grafting of the burn wound. *A,* Appearance of mature granulation tissue prior to skin grafting. *B,* Ten days following "lay on" application of skin grafts without scraping of the granulations and without the use of sutures.

graft in position until it becomes adherent. These can be applied rapidly and without the bleeding associated with suturing.

"Pie-crusting" is not recommended, since improved graft vascularization is obtained with the "rolling" technique described below. The exposed grafts are available for inspection, and any small seroma, hematoma, or purulent collection can be promptly evacuated. The use of lamps continuously for several hours and intermittently for the first four or five days is helpful in keeping the grafted surface dry and facilitating the maturation of the skin grafts. The nursing personnel are trained to inspect the

grafts and, at hourly intervals for the first 24 hours, to use cotton-tipped applicators to express small collections of serum from beneath the grafts. Small collections of serum and small localized hematomas can be effectively evacuated from beneath the grafts with enhancement of the percentage of skin graft vascularization. After the first 24 hours, the rolling technique is continued at less frequent intervals four or five times during the day until the grafts are stabilized (five to seven days) (Fig. 18–14).

In circumferential wounds of an extremity, it is not possible to position the patient for ex-

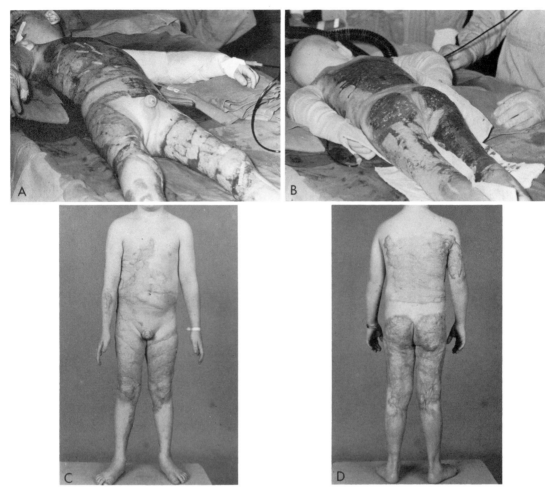

FIGURE 18-13.   Skin grafting of extensive burn wounds. *A,* Skin grafts are applied and secured by Steristrips on the anterior surface of the trunk and lower extremities. *B,* Posterior burn wounds. *C, D,* Appearance after several grafting procedures.

posure of the entire wound. A suitable alternative method is the use of dressings to stabilize the grafts and to prevent their being dislodged by contact with the bed clothes.

In circumferential wounds of the extremities, the grafts should be placed transversely around the circumference of the extremity, not laid in a vertical fashion, for optimum cosmetic and functional results. After completion of the application of skin grafts, the use of a firm compression dressing to stabilize the grafts is satisfactory, and sutures or other stabilizing devices are usually not required. The use of Steristrips at the time of application of the grafts is often helpful in maintaining them in position until dressings can be applied. After application of the grafts to a lower extremity, the grafts are covered with a single layer of glycerine-impregnated gauze, which should be placed transversely. The single layer of gauze is reinforced with several layers of saline-saturated gauze sponges placed transversely. Bulky padding is placed over this layer, and the entire dressing is secured with a kerlix and an ace bandage. The technique is particularly effective for wounds limited to one or both of the lower extremities. After the dressings are in place, the patient is returned to his room and the lower extremities are elevated on pillows. In the absence of unusual pain, temperature elevation, or oozing from the bandage, all of which would indicate a wound complication, the dressings are ordinarily left in place for about five days, and the first dressing change is often performed under some analgesia. At this time the dressings can be reapplied for an additional four or five days prior to commencing therapy in the Hubbard tank.

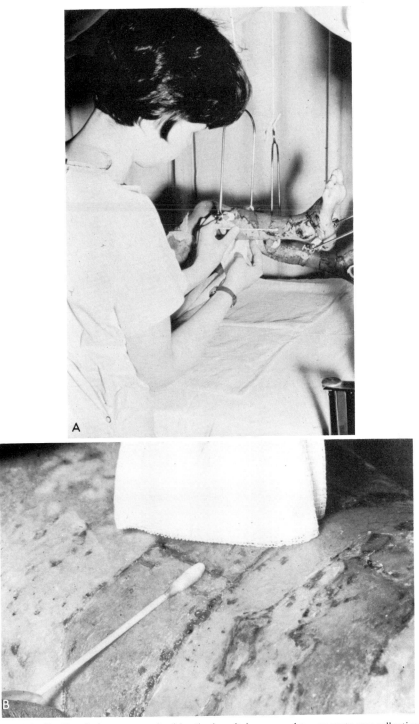

FIGURE 18–14. "Rolling" technique as practiced by the hospital personnel to evacuate any collections from beneath the skin grafts.

Skeletal Traction

Although exposure of skin grafts when the patient can be positioned for exposure and the use of circumferential dressings to immobilize skin grafts are accepted procedures, certain limitations to these techniques exist. These limitations are related to certain anatomical sites where exposure or compression dressings are difficult to apply and maintain in the proper position. This problem is most evident in circumferential burn wounds of the trunk and extremities, and in burn wounds that extend over the flanks or over certain flexion areas, such as the axilla (Fig. 18–15). For this reason, skeletal traction in selected patients, as described by Evans, Larson, and Yates (1968), has been used by the authors for some years. By this technique, it is often possible to position patients for optimum placement and postoperative management of grafts. At the same time

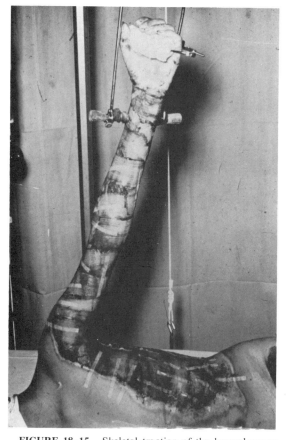

FIGURE 18–15. Skeletal traction of the burned upper extremity. The skin grafts of the arm, axilla, and trunk are secured by Steristrips. Skeletal traction permits the use of the exposure method and the joints are maintained in optimum position.

the joints are maintained in optimum position for the prevention of contractures (Fig. 18–16). The technique is particularly useful for circumferential grafting of an extremity without the use of sutures or compression dressings. This permits the wound to be exposed for evacuation of any small seromas, hematomas, or localized areas of purulent material.

The technique not only allows positioning of joints in the optimum position for minimizing contracture but also can be used for gradual stretching of any flexion deformities which may be present (Fig. 18–17). Gentle, steady traction over a period of three to seven days is effective in correcting flexion contractures of the elbows, hips, and knees which can occur in patients who have been allowed to maintain their joints in flexed positions for extended periods. In addition, the weights can be removed from the traction daily and the joints exercised through an active and passive range of motion.

The use of skeletal traction is ordinarily limited to the time of grafting and the immediate postgrafting period. At the time when all wounds are ready for grafting, the patient is taken to the operating room, and under anesthesia surgical preparation of the burn wounds and donor areas is performed. The donor areas are appropriately draped, and the skin grafts are removed. After removal of the skin grafts and application of fine mesh gauze to the donor areas, Steinmann pins are placed in the appropriate position after additional preparation of the skin by wiping with an iodine-containing solution. The patient is placed in balanced suspension or skeletal traction, as indicated by the location of the wounds, to obtain the desired postoperative position. At this point the skin grafts are placed on the open wound. Although no sutures or dressings are required to maintain the grafts in position, the use of Steristrips is often helpful in maintaining the grafts in the desired position until adherence to the underlying wound has occurred.

The most commonly utilized points for placement of the Steinmann pins are through the distal radius approximately 2 inches proximal to the wrist joint for upper extremity suspension, and through the proximal tibia and calcaneus for suspension of the lower extremity. The usual smooth Steinmann pins are satisfactory for the short-term immobilization required in the majority of patients. Frequently, however, threaded Steinmann pins are utilized to avoid slippage of the extremity on the pin in the adult, especially when more extended use

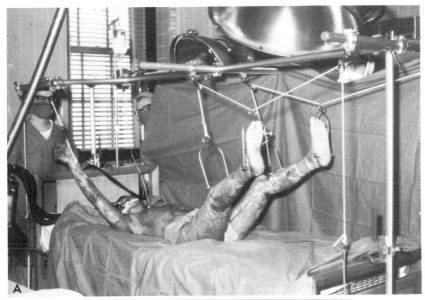

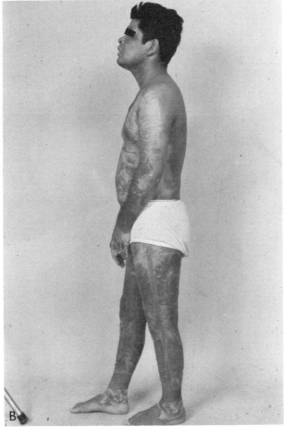

FIGURE 18–16. *A*, Skeletal traction of an upper and both lower extremities in an extensively burned patient. *B*, Appearance after resurfacing of burn wounds.

of skeletal traction is anticipated. The use of power drills and equipment is essential for placing pins through multiple large bones. Skeletal traction is ordinarily required for only ten days to two weeks following the application of grafts, until they are sufficiently vascularized that the skeletal traction and Steinmann pins can be removed and the patient returned to the

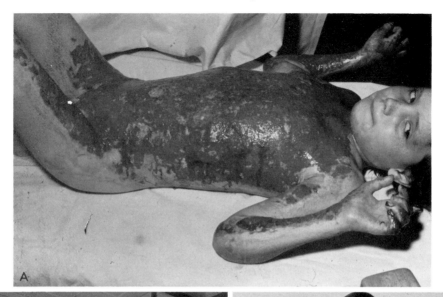

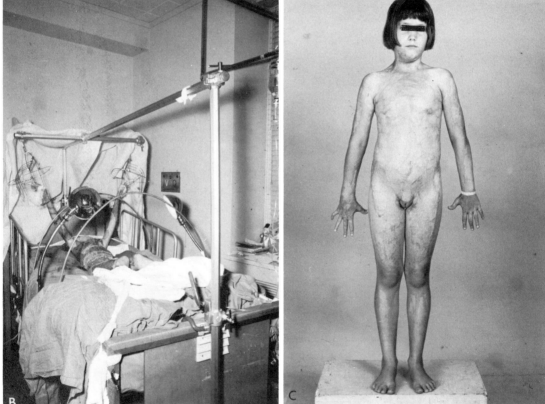

FIGURE 18–17. *A*, Flexion deformities following burn injury. *B*, Skeletal traction was employed to facilitate skin grafting and to correct flexion deformities by gradual stretching. *C*, Appearance after healing of wounds.

Hubbard tank. However, pins have frequently been left in extremities for periods of three to six weeks without any increase in the frequency of complications. It should be noted that the patients can be removed from a trac-

tion apparatus and placed in the Hubbard tank with the pins still present in the extremities when desired. The point of exit of the pin through the skin is meticulously cleaned several times during the day and following cleansing is swabbed with alcohol. Pins have been placed through bones using the skin immediately adjacent to the burn wound or in some instances through granulating surfaces. Although this technique has been used on hundreds of extremities, major complications have not been encountered. Minor pin tract infections develop from time to time, but these have responded to removal of the pin without development of osteomyelitis. Although Constable (1969) has reported one patient who developed a sequestrum of the radius associated with the use of Steinmann pins, major complications of this type are extremely rare.

The hand is a specialized area that lends itself to the use of skeletal traction at the time of grafting. The use of a pin through the distal radius can be combined with a pin through the proximal portion of the metacarpals of the index and long finger to maintain the wrist in dorsiflexion. When pins are placed through the metacarpals, the index and long fingers should be used, since these are fixed to the metacarpals. The proximal portion of these bones should be used in order to avoid impaling the cross communications of the extensor tendons, which occur more distally. A metallic frame developed at the Shriner's Burn Institute in Galveston in collaboration with the Orthopedic Service allows for the attachment of rubber bands to additional pins placed through the fingertips for positioning of the fingers (Fig. 18–18). At the time of grafting, this appliance is placed on the hand and the hand is positioned with the wrist neutral or in mild dorsiflexion. The metacarpal phalangeal joints are flexed to avoid shortening of the collateral ligaments during the postoperative period and to allow application of skin grafts to minimize the possibility of contracture.

Although skeletal traction can be employed prior to grafting for the correction of any flexion deformities that may be present, the use of this technique is usually limited to the grafting phase. Skeletal traction is ordinarily applied at the time of the skin graft and is left in place for ten days to two weeks postoperatively, at which time the pins and traction devices are removed.

Allografts

Allograft skin has been used as a temporary method of wound coverage for many years. It is particularly useful in the occasional large burn, in which the wound area is ready for grafting but exceeds the area of available donor sites. Under these circumstances the application of allografts will provide temporary wound coverage which seals the wound and minimizes fluid, electrolyte, and protein loss through the burn wound. The survival of allograft skin is variable in the burn patient but usually averages from ten days to three weeks. Rappaport and associates (1964) reported prolonged survival of allografts in burn patients. The rejection phenomenon is characterized by a gradual spotty dissolution of the skin, with shredding and sloughing of the allograft, leaving a wound that is not optimum for the application of autografts for a period of several days. For this reason if additional donor sites become available, it is desirable to remove the allografts at three to five days and replace them with autografts. Since additional donor sites may not be readily available, it is not unusual to allow the allografts to proceed to full rejection while donor areas are healing in preparation for removal of additional crops of skin autografts.

The use of allografts in this manner will provide temporary wound coverage which is often helpful in extensive burns or in patients who are anemic or hypoproteinemic or who have other complications. The use of skin allografts to provide temporary coverage in the large burn in which adequate donor sites are not available for autografting is the most frequent indication for allografts and the most useful method for employing them.

The use of allografts as a biological dressing has been described by Zaroff and associates (1966) and Silverstein and Pruitt (1973). The usual regime is to remove the allograft prior to take and to reapply additional allografts as a biological dressing. The serial application of allografts is a useful way to determine when the wound is ready for acceptance of autografts. The use of allografts in this fashion as a biological dressing is of some help in the preparation of wounds for grafting, but the limited availability of allograft skin in most hospitals limits its use.

Storage of allograft skin can be accomplished for a few days without any requirement for expensive or unusual equipment. Skin grafts can be removed and simply wrapped in sterile gauze sponges soaked with saline and an antibiotic, such as penicillin or 0.25 per cent neomycin solution. The skin grafts wrapped in moistened sponges can be placed in sterile jars and refrigerated in ordinary refrigerators without freezing. When stored in this manner, the grafts retain their viability and are useful for a period of seven to ten days on the average.

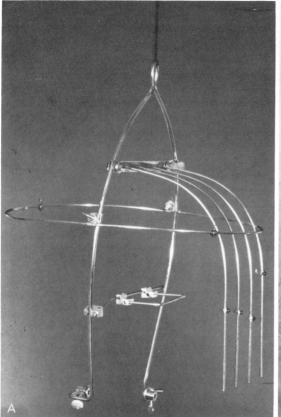

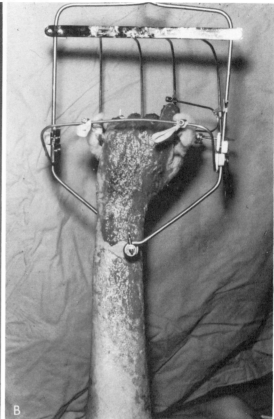

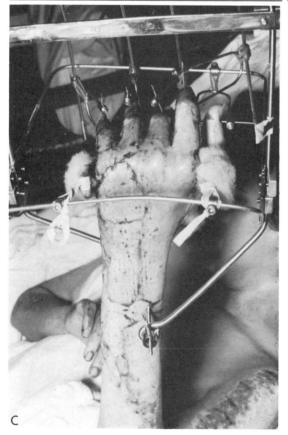

FIGURE 18–18.   Skeletal traction for a hand burn. *A*, Design of metallic frame. *B*, Skeletal traction in place prior to skin grafting. *C*, Close-up view following the application of split-thickness skin grafts.

After this time, although some cells remain viable, the grafts become friable and are usually not satisfactory.

Skin allografts and the storage of skin grafts are discussed in Chapter 6.

Xenografts

Because of the limited availability of allografts in many hospitals, trials have been conducted with various xenograft materials. At the present time, the one in use in several burn centers is pig xenograft, as popularized by Bromberg, Song and Mohn (1965). Pig skin can be removed under sterile conditions using the same dermatomes used for clinical practice. When applied to granulating wounds, the pig skin will produce an effective wound coverage for a period of a few days. Porcine grafts appear to be as satisfactory for biological dressings as human allografts and have been used in many burn centers on large numbers of patients without apparent complications. Porcine grafts become adherent to the burn wound and often cannot be removed without producing bleeding, although "take" of the skin does not occur, as evidenced by lack of revascularization. Although porcine grafts appear to be clinically satisfactory and are in widespread use at the present time, it should be cautioned that the full immunologic impact of their use in human patients has not been extensively studied. Porcine xenografts are also discussed in Chapter 6.

Clinical and research studies have investigated the use, in addition to porcine grafts, of other materials as biological wound dresssings. These include lyophilized human allografts, collagen film, and bovine embryo skin. O'Neill (1973) has reported a comparison between xenograft and a polytetrafluoroethylene-polyurethane laminate and suggests that this prosthesis is useful as a temporary wound dressing with characteristics at least equal to, and in some respects superior to, those of pig skin. Although the development of a nonantigenic biological wound dressing is desirable, none of the materials available to date is ideal, and in general all are of limited usefulness.

POSTGRAFTING PHASE

Following the application of skin grafts, the general management of the burn patient is similar to that of other postoperative patients. General supportive measures, pulmonary toilet, intravenous fluid replacement, transfusions, and pain medication may be required. For the first few days following the application of skin grafts, patients are usually placed on penicillin or other antibiotics until the skin grafts have stabilized. If the grafts are exposed, meticulous wound attention, consisting of frequent inspection and elimination of blisters or hematomas by expressing them with cotton-tipped applicators, is indicated. Ordinary "goose neck" lamps to minimize hypothermia and to promote drying of burn wounds and donor sites are routinely utilized. If skeletal traction is employed, the points of exit of pins through the skin must be meticulously cleansed several times during the day and swabbed with alcohol. In the absence of complications, the skin grafts will become stable over the ensuing days. During this time it is important to maintain adequate nutritional intake with vitamin supplements, particularly ascorbic acid in doses of 1000 mg per day, and to encourage the patient to exercise all joints that are not immobilized as a temporary measure.

After approximately seven to ten days, the grafts are usually sufficiently stable that the patient can be placed in the Hubbard tank daily for cleansing and exercise. The donor sites can be safely soaked at this time without the fear of infection. If there are no grafts or donor sites below the waist, ambulation is encouraged. If there is lower extremity involvement, ambulation must be delayed until three weeks after the grafts have been healed, and elastic supportive dressings should be used until complete restoration of circulatory equilibrium has been established in the skin transplants. This usually requires the use of elastic support for several weeks as a minimum, and in many older patients the elastic supports are worn permanently.

In order to expedite the treatment of acute burn patients, the following treatment outline is suggested as a checklist:

1. General evaluation
   a. History
      Patient's age
      Type of burn and circumstances
      Time of burn and time elapsed since injury
      Prior treatment
         Sedation
         I.V. therapy
         Status of tetanus immunization
      Allergies to medication such as penicillin, etc.
      Current medications such as steroids, digitalis, or insulin

History of peptic ulcer, cardiac disease, etc.
Symptoms since burn
Mental status
Urinary output
Vomiting
b. Physical examination
Extent of burn ("rule of nines")
Estimate of depth of burn
Temperature, pulse, respiration, blood pressure, if unburned areas available
Mental status
Check for constricting circumferential wounds
Check nasal and oral mucous membranes for hyperemia, soot, singed hair, etc.
Chest — rales or rhonchi
Abdomen — distention, bowel sounds
Skeletal — fractures or associated injuries
Weight on admission
2. Establish and maintain an adequate airway
a. Check for facial fractures if unconscious
b. Remove any foreign material in pharynx
c. Evaluate for endotracheal tube or tracheostomy
d. O_2 via nebulizer for humidity
e. Elevate head of bed for burns of upper half of body
3. Immediate sedation
a. Morphine sulfate, 10 mg, or Demerol, 75 mg, in adults
b. Give slowly I.V. — not I.M. or subcutaneously
c. Exhibit a calm confident attitude
4. Institute fluid therapy by cutdown or intracath
a. Brooke formula fluid estimate
1.5 ml lactated Ringer's solution + 0.5 ml plasminate × kg body wt. × % body surface burned in first 24 hours
Estimate 1/2 of this amount to be given in first 8 hours post burn — 1/4 next 8 hours — 1/4 next 8 hours
b. Maintain urine output, 30–50 ml/hour in adults
c. Avoid electrolyte-free solutions during early hours of treatment
d. Blood pressure and pulse not reliable guide to adequacy of fluid therapy
e. Insert central venous pressure catheter if complications develop
f. Consider rapid digitalization in selected patients
5. Draw blood for baseline determinations when fluid therapy is started
a. CBC
b. Urinalysis
c. Serum electrolytes
d. Blood urea nitrogen
e. Total serum proteins with A/G rates
f. Serum bilirubin
g. Blood sugar
h. Arterial blood gases if complications present
i. Repeat (a) through (e) in 12 hours, then daily for 3 days, then twice weekly
6. Insert Foley catheter
a. Record amount and character of initial bladder urine
b. Measure hourly urine output (bedside specific gravity may be useful)
c. Adjust rate of fluid administration to maintain 30–50 ml/hr output
d. Irrigate with commercial GU irrigant every 6 hours
e. Remove catheter as early as possible when condition stable (3 to 7 days)
7. Tetanus toxoid, 0.5 ml if previously immunized, 500

units human immune globulin if not previously immunized
8. Procaine penicillin, 600,00 units b.i.d., I.M. if not sensitive, × 5 days
9. NPO initially with *no* ice chips, sips of water, etc.
a. Institute nasogastric suction for distention and/or vomiting
b. After 12–24 hours, if no distention and peristalsis present, start milk, 100–250 ml/hr
c. 2–3 days — soft diet
d. 3–7 days — high caloric, high protein diet
e. 50–80 cal/kg/day
f. 2–4 g protein/kg/day
10. Chest X-ray on admission (portable technique frequently required); obtain early photographs; electrocardiogram for electrical burns and all patients over 40
11. Wound care
a. Gentle cleansing for removal of dirt and debris with bland soap and water
b. Copious irrigation for chemical burns for 24 hours
c. Decompression incisions if required
d. Splint and elevate burns of hands; elevate burned lower extremities
e. Bed rest with head elevated until shock period is over
f. Alternating air mattress when at bed rest
g. Turn, cough, deep breath every 2 hours
h. Topical agents applied
12. Medications
a. Analgesics and sedatives as needed
b. Aspirin for temperature over 101° F
c. Multivitamin preparation daily
d. Ascorbic acid, 1000 mg daily
e. Antacids and antispasmodics for epigastric pain or distress
f. Laxative p.r.n.
g. Steroids not required
h. Avoid tranquilizers except on specific indication
13. General
a. Wound cultures on admission and twice per week
b. Draw blood cultures for sudden change in temperature or level of consciousness
c. Record detailed history, physical examination, and burn diagrams
d. Place patient on critical list
e. Evaluate need for special duty nurses
f. Consultations as required

COMPLICATIONS

Shock Phase

During the shock phase the chief complications are as follows:

1. Inadequate initial fluid treatment with prolonged shock leading to renal shutdown. This may result as a consequence of prolonged transporatation without fluid therapy or inadequate ventilation in head and neck burns, or may be associated with concomitant fractures

or other injuries resulting in liberation of large amounts of myoglobin and hemoglobin.

2. Electrolyte derangement and acidosis during treatment. Because of the possibility of hyperkalemia during the early hours post burn due to the liberation of potassium from destroyed cells and the intracellular shift of sodium for potassium, the exogenous administration of potassium-containing solution should be avoided, particularly in children or in patients with inadequate urine output. Electrolyte abnormalities and acidosis can be accentuated by certain of the topical agents currently in widespread use, as mentioned earlier.

3. Water intoxication or hyponatremia from overtreatment with electrolyte-free solutions orally or intravenously, with resulting disorientation, irrational behavior, and convulsions. Many of these symptoms can also be produced by the absorption of hexachlorophene if this solution is used for repeated cleansing of large open burn wounds.

4. Associated fractures and other injuries. Concomitant fractures, head injuries, soft tissue lacerations, and other injuries should be given precedence over specific therapy of the burn wound.

Respiratory Tract Complications

Immediately following a burn, particularly if the injury is sustained in a closed space, there is the possibility of inhalation of smoke, carbon monoxide, and fumes and the possibility of direct thermal injury to the upper respiratory tract. This is manifest by singeing of the nasal hair, hyperemia of the oral and pharyngeal mucosa, and the presence of soot or other foreign material in the upper airway. There may be associated hoarseness, respiratory distress, poor breath sounds, cyanosis, or restlessness on physical examination. The chest X-ray is usually normal early after the burn injury unless there are associated injuries. It should be pointed out that, although carbon monoxide may be a cause of death in patients trapped in a burning building, when the patient is removed from the immediate area, the carbon monoxide is cleared from the bloodstream in a matter of several hours and apparently leaves no sequelae.

The initial effects of the thermal trauma are complicated by the progressive edema which develops over the next two or three days. During this time the use of humidified oxygen, frequent position change of the patient, en-couragement of coughing, and forced breathing are essential. If airway impairment from the progressive edema is evident, the use of an endotracheal tube for a few days is preferable to a tracheostomy. Because the possibility of pulmonary edema is real during the fluid resuscitative phase, digitalization is frequently employed, particularly in burns of more than 40 per cent of body surface in adult patients.

The respiratory tract sequelae of thermal injury have been recognized for many years. At the present time there is an increasing number of patients seen who develop respiratory problems after a latent period of two to five days, during which respiratory symptoms may have been minimal. The onset of respiratory difficulty during this time period is a significant pulmonary complication associated with a high mortality. The first symptom may be an increase in the respiratory rate, some increased difficulty with respiratory exchange, or the appearance of rales or wheezes. This is followed in a short time by the development of tenacious sputum containing debris and epithelial cells from the respiratory tract; mechanical obstruction of the minor bronchi with the development of atelectasis and emphysema can result. Cyanosis and disorientation may shortly follow, and the monitoring of arterial gas tensions and blood pH are mandatory in managing patients with this complication. The chest X-ray film may be initially normal but may show a more severe confluent consolidation as time progresses. The respiratory distress and cyanosis become more severe; inadequate respiratory exchange with hypoxia develops; spontaneous pneumothorax and right heart strain may develop; and pulmonary edema may ensue with a fatal outcome. This delayed form of pulmonary involvement demands vigorous therapy, but the response is often poor; the mortality rate is high.

Although the response to any form of therapy is poor, the following treatment modalities appear to have some value. Humidified oxygen should be administered via a nebulizer. The patient must be turned frequently and encouraged to cough for the purpose of clearing the airway and expelling the sputum containing debris and epithelial sloughs. Pounding on the chest wall has been reported as being of some assistance in freeing and expelling plugs of the obstructing materials. Although tracheal aspiration may temporarily remove secretions, the catheter is an additional source of bacterial contamination, even under the most ideal circumstances, and repeated suction further traumatizes the tracheal mucosa with a deleterious effect. Tracheostomy may be required to minimize dead space, to assist in expelling secretions, and to facilitate the administration of intermittent or continuous positive pressure respiration. The administration of steroids in pharmacologic doses (Solu-Medrol, 1 to 2 g) may be of value in reducing the bronchial constriction and inflammatory response. If utilized, it should be given early and limited to one administration in the majority of patients to minimize spread of the subsequent pneumonia. Occasionally a second or a third injection is given over 12 to 24 hours. Bronchial dilators may be used as well as the nebulizer to attempt to minimize bronchospasm. Bronchodilators should be used intermittently and infrequently. Antibiotics should be administered in large doses, using culture and sensitivity reports for selection of the most appropriate agent. Intravenous digitalization should be used early in the course of treatment.

Infection Complications

The most common and most serious complication of the burn is infection. From the burn wound there can usually be cultured at any given time the prevailing flora of the individual patient and of the hospital attendants and ward environment. Even without contamination from outside sources, organisms imbedded in the hair follicles and sweat glands survive the effects of the initial burn and serve as potential sources of localized and systemic infection.

With necrotic tissue serving as a nutrient medium for pathogens, there may occur in succession cellulitis, invasion of adjacent tissue with extending necrosis, lymphangitis, and finally septicemia. With the development of septicemia there may be associated metastatic abscesses to the lungs, liver, and other internal organs. Burn septicemia is rare during the first few days post burn, presumably because of the latent or incubation period required for bacterial proliferation. Order and coworkers (1965) have shown that, when the quantitative bacterial concentration of the burn wound is 10^5 organisms or less per gram of tissue, invasive infection and septicemia are uncommon. When the multiplication of bacteria results in a wound concentration in excess of 10^5 organisms per gram of tissue, invasive infection is likely. When the necrotic burned tissue has been removed from the wound and healthy granulation tissue develops, the likelihood of invasive infection is considerably decreased. Healthy granulation tissue not only serves as a mechanical barrier but also, as Eade (1958) has shown, contains phagocytic cells which rapidly eliminate organisms following wound coverage with skin grafts. Sterilization of the burn wound is not possible prior to the application of skin grafts. Consequently, the mainstay of therapy has been adherence to sound surgical principles with mechanical cleansing and debridement, although the use of the topical agents currently available is an effective adjunct to surgical principles.

The organisms producing wound infection vary from one patient to another. During the middle 1950's, staphylococcal organisms, frequently resistant to penicillin, were commonly the bacteria producing septicemia in at least 50 per cent of the patients. Since 1960 there has been a progressive rise in the frequency of Pseudomonas and other gram-negative organisms, with a concomitant decrease in the frequency with which staphylococcal organisms are involved. Pseudomonas has been particularly troublesome in many burn centers, and full-blown Pseudomonas septicemia is characterized by proliferation of vast numbers of organisms within the local tissue, a peripheral vasculitis, satellite necrotic infected areas in the surrounding unburned skin, and blood-borne abscesses of the lungs, brain, liver, and other internal organs. The development of full-blown Pseudomonas septicemia is refractory to treatment, and the mortality rate remains extremely high, despite the availability of a continually enlarging number of antibacterial agents.

The onset of septicemia may be insidious. Many burn patients commonly have a temperature of 99 to 101° F for the first several postburn days; the white blood cell count may normally range up to 15,000, depending upon the state of hemoconcentration and hydration. The onset of septicemia may be heralded by a rising and spiking temperature, with an increase in the white blood cell count above 15,000 and with a shift in the neutrophil components of the differential white blood cell count. This is usually accompanied by an increased respiratory rate, disorientation, restlessness, and signs of clinical deterioration. The course of gram-negative septicemia may be extremely rapid, with the development of a preterminal, endotoxic, shocklike syndrome characterized by hypothermia, leukopenia, progressive ileus, anuria, and death over a 24- to 72-hour period. Baines, Lynch and Lewis (1970) have indicated that the sudden appearance of immature neutrophils in significant numbers in the bloodstream may herald the onset of significant septicemia by a few hours or a few days. If other signs suggesting infection are present, there is sufficient justification to warrant antibiotic therapy.

The treatment of Pseudomonas infections, as well as septicemia caused by Aerobacter, Klebsiella, and other pathogens, is quite difficult. At the present time the drug which is most often effective against the Pseudomonas organism is gentamicin, although polymyxin, colistin sulfate, and a variety of other drugs are available. There are also efforts to develop suitable antisera against specific organisms. The use of sensitivity tests prior to employment of specific antibiotics is recommended in all cases of systemic infection. Moreover, wound cultures and sensitivity reports will usually give some indication of the offending organism during the time required for culturing specific organisms from the blood.

With the current use of effective topical antibacterial agents and with the development of septic complications while the patient is receiving systemic antiboitic therapy, the emergence of certain fungi and yeast as colonizers of the burn wound is being reported with increasing frequency (Bruck and associates, 1971). In addition, the development of bloodstream invasion with these organisms (particularly Candida) has also been reported. Viral agents such as Herpes can produce clinically difficult burn wound infectious complications, but this is uncommon. The evolution of these changing patterns of infection has been summarized by Lynch and associates (1971b).

Other bacteriologic complications in burn patients arise from ascending infection of the urinary tract in association with prolonged catheterization. Furuncles and secondary abscesses are occasionally seen in the burn patient; they not only constitute a hazard to surgery but also may serve as sources of systemic infection.

Superficial thrombophlebitis commonly occurs at the site of previous cutdowns for intravenous fluid therapy, and spread of the infection may occur along the course of the veins. Embolic phenomena from this source are uncommon.

Chondritis of the ear and the nose may develop in deep burns involving these areas because of the thin covering of skin over the cartilage. Local incision and drainage are usually inadequate in the case of the ear, and it is necessary to remove all affected cartilage. Management of the facial burn is also discussed in Chapter 33.

Septic arthritis is particularly prone to occur in deep burns of the hand, in which there is direct involvement of the phalanges and interphalangeal joints with joint destruction. On the other hand, exposure of the skull and long bones, such as the tibia, occurs frequently without the sequela of osteomyelitis

General and Metabolic Complications

One of the most significant complications associated with burns is the sudden occurrence of gastrointestinal bleeding, which may be massive and life-endangering. This usually involves multiple ulcerations of the gastric and intestinal mucosa and is commonly called Curling's ulcer. This complication can be found at autopsy in approximately one-third of burned patients and gives rise to clinically significant bleeding in approximately 10 per cent of patients. It characteristically does not occur during the first few days following burning but is a possibility from the fifth day through the third to fourth week of burn care. Although many patients may have prior symptoms suggestive of peptic ulcer disease, this is not a constant finding, and Curling's ulcer is seen in all age groups, including children. Sudden significant bleeding may be the first indication of this complication. In other patients there may be some premonitory symptoms, such as epigastric pain, distress, or cramping. At the earliest symptom antispasmodics and antacids should be immediately administered, and most patients with large burns are prophylactically treated with antacids from the time of admission. With the use of milk in amounts of 100 to 250 ml every hour as soon as oral feedings are tolerated, it is possible that the frequency with which clinically significant bleeding occurs may be decreased. Although Curling's ulceration is usually recognized by the onset of bleeding, perforation and other secondary intra-abdominal complications are possible. Treatment should be aimed at prevention by administration of antacids and antispasmodics. When bleeding is the first indication that ulceration is present, conservative measures consisting of sedation, blood transfusion, and/or gastric suction should be instituted. Conservative measures should be continued if at all possible, since emergency surgery is usually associated with mortality.

Other metabolic complications consist of hypoproteinemia, anemia, weight loss, and loss of muscle mass in relation to increased nitrogen catabolism and bed rest. Unless suitable nutritional care is given and early skin coverage can be obtained, the patient is prone to develop other sequelae.

Serious pulmonary, cardiac, and renal complications are generally related to preexisting disease, to infection, or to pathologic changes accompanying an overwhelming burn. Acute renal insufficiency is usually associated with inadequate fluid therapy, and occasionally hemodialysis is required in centers where such facilities are available. Impaired liver function has been demonstrated in severe burns by such workers as Stenbert and Hogeman (1962) and others. In addition, an occasional patient is seen with homologous serum hepatitis as a result of plasma and blood transfusion therapy.

Local Complications

In addition to the complications that have been mentioned, particular consideration must be given to certain special structures. These include the eye, burns of which fortunately occur only rarely except in accidents involving chemicals, and the eyelids, burns of which may cause ectropion, resulting in corneal ulceration or chronic conjunctivitis. When the area around the eye is burned, the eye must be carefully protected, particularly if the patients are to be nursed prone. The advent of a Pseudomonas ophthalmitis can result in total destruction of an eye in a matter of hours. At times, there is loss of portions of the nose, the cheek, the lips, and the ears, and in these cases extensive cosmetic deformities can be produced which may have profound socioeconomic implications. The subject is discussed further in Chapter 33.

Soft tissue contracture deformities in flexion creases and in joint areas, as well as hypertrophic scars and keloids, present problems in reconstructive surgery. Early skin grafting, physiotherapy, splinting, skeletal traction, and the avoidance of local infection minimize the more severe functional defects, which were once the rule in the majority of burned patients.

Neurologic complications due to poor positioning of the patient with secondary pressure on the peripheral nerves must be avoided. The majority of bone and joint alterations in which there is no direct thermal involvement may be prevented, as Evans (1966) has shown, by a supervised program of physical therapy with active and passive motion and isometric muscle tension exercises.

Unfortunately, decubitus ulcers can be a serious problem, particularly in elderly patients in whom early ambulation is difficult or impossible, and meticulous nursing care is essential to prevent the development of pressure sores.

As noted previously, the constricting effects of burn eschar occasionally result in distal gangrene unless prompt relaxation incisions can be done. In order to be effective, the escharotomies should be done as early as possible to avoid the prolonged tissue hypoxia which can result from a constricting burn eschar. In severe burns of the extremities, there may frequently be involvement of the deep structures with compromise of the circulation, particularly in electrical injuries, so that amputation may become a necessary and, in fact, life-saving procedure.

One complication of the local burn that has not been previously mentioned is the failure to form adequate granulation tissue to support skin grafts. This occurs most frequently in association with gram-negative septicemia, when characteristic spreading, black, necrotic patches are noted within the burn wound. In other patients it develops in the terminal phase of wound care when one or more grafting procedures may have been successfully accomplished, and only multiple, small, raw areas are present. These multiple, small areas may be extremely refractory to successful skin graft resurfacing for reasons which have not been adequately elucidated. The control of any minor local wound infection, together with optimum nutritional and vitamin intake, is imperative in the management of the occasional patient with refractory, scattered, small open areas.

CONVALESCENCE AND REHABILITATION

At the time of discharge from the hospital, most extensive burn patients may still have a few scattered unhealed areas present. These normally should not exceed 1 cm in greatest diameter. At the same time, the patient will have usually sustained considerable weight loss and will generally be weak from the prolonged hospitalization and trauma of multiple surgical procedures. If there are skin grafts or donor sites below the knee, ambulation must be delayed until these are well healed, and elastic support must be utilized for a minimum of several weeks. Although the blood count may not be entirely normal, major degrees of anemia should be corrected prior to release from the hospital. Most patients will be released from the hospital with instructions to maintain a high protein diet supplemented with multivitamins and ascorbic acid for a period of several weeks. After discharge from the hospital, most patients at home are allowed ambulation unless the lower extremities are a problem, as indicated above. The majority of patients rapidly regain their lost weight and their sense of well-being. During this time, maintenance of an active exercise program to regain range of joint motion is mandatory. In addition, splinting of certain burns, particularly about the hand, may be helpful in minimizing subsequent contracture.

The recently healed second degree burn wounds, skin grafts, and donor areas are quite fragile for a period of several weeks, and the development of small clear blisters, either spontaneously or after minimal trauma, is quite common. These blisters characteristically rupture, leaving a small granulating wound which slowly heals. With the passage of several weeks to several months, the circulatory stability of the skin recovers and, with additional maturation, spontaneous blistering ceases.

After healing of deep burns, either spontaneously in the case of second degree injury or following split-thickness skin grafts in third degree wounds, there is a characteristic hypertrophic healing phase. Clinically, this appears as a thick, elevated, indurated, hypertrophic scar that may be fiery red in color. At this time, some symptoms, such as itching, stinging, and minor discomfort, are usually present. These symptoms can be alleviated by regular application of bland lubricating ointments, which should be applied several times daily. However, in occasional patients the pruritus may be so intense that antipruritic medication is required. In some patients, the symptoms associated with hypertrophic scars can be minimized by local injection of steroid preparations if the burn scars are localized. It is necessary to recognize that this type of scarring is to be anticipated following most burns and usually does not represent an early stage of keloid formation. After several months, maturation of the scar tissue occurs, as evidenced by regression of the red color, softening and improved texture of the scars, and disappearance of the symptoms of itching and burning. The most effective method available at the present time for minimizing hypertrophic scar formation consists of continuous application of pressure over the recently healed skin grafts and scars. This can be accomplished by the use of ace bandages on the extremities or trunk or by the use of custom-made pressure suits (Jobst) which are designed to fit virtually all parts of the body. It must be emphaiszed that, to be effective, these must be used on a 24-hour basis and left off for only brief periods, such as when bathing (see Chapter 33).

The exact cause of postburn hypertrophic scarring is not fully understood but is probably related to a multiplicity of factors (Lynch, 1973). The biochemical reactions related to the production of collagen and the physicochemical reactions related to alignment of collagen in a healing burn are usually exaggerated in the postburn patient for reasons that are not fully understood. In addition to the chemical abnormalities, part of the hypertrophic scarring is apparently caused by a chronic inflammatory reaction. The bacterial counts that are invariably high on an open burn wound are rapidly eliminated by the application of skin grafts, and the number of recoverable bacteria under the graft drops to nearly zero after several hours. However, during reconstructive procedures performed during the thick hypertrophic scar phase, viable bacteria can be cultured from the depth of the scar tissue after a period of several weeks. It would seem, therefore, that some of the thick hypertrophic scar reaction is, in fact, caused by the persistence of bacteria that require several weeks for complete clearance. The effects of mechanical forces are not well understood, but it is well known that a thick, hypertrophic scar over a flexion joint crease subjected to continual tension will rarely complete the normal scar maturation process.

In burn scar reconstruction, it is wise to delay surgical procedures, if possible, until the major portion of the hypertrophic scar period has subsided. This usually requires 6 to 12 months, and the scars continue to mature in most instances for two years or more. Obviously, in severe functional deformities, such as ectropion of the eyelids, contractures about the mouth, or severe flexion contractures of the neck or fingers, earlier release may be required. However, the results are usually not as good as when performed later, and the rate of complications is higher during this period. The patient should be advised that when mandatory early release is undertaken during the hypertrophic scar phase, secondary revisions may be required. Burn reconstruction techniques are discussed in Chapters 33 and 34.

It is imperative during the posthospitalization period that patients be encouraged to assume as much responsibility for their own care as they safely can and that they continually be encouraged to resume their normal daily activities. In the case of workmen, they should be released to some form of gainful employment as soon as their condition permits. In addition, any reconstructive procedures should be timed and spaced so that the patient does not become totally dependent upon the hospital. The patient and his family must also realize that the more severe the original deformity, the more realistic should be the goals of reconstruction and, in general, the greater will be the permanent deformity.

ELECTRICAL BURNS*

Because of the almost universal exposure to electrical devices in the modern home, accidents associated with electrical burns are fairly common. Dale (1954) and Baldridge (1954), in discussing the physical aspects of electrical burns, mentioned two general types: arc and contact. In the arc burn the involved area is heated to a temperature of 2500 to 3000°C, with charring of the soft tissue. In the contact burn an electric current passes from the point of contact through the body to a "ground" exit, with burns occurring at both sites. Death may occur if the current travels through and disrupts vital cerebral and cardiac centers.

In the child the electrical burn occurs most commonly in the 9 month to 4 year old age group, with the peak incidence in the 1 and 2 year old age groups. The burn is commonly of the arc type secondary to contact with a live electric socket, the injury being confined to the immediate area of burn. A frequent type of burn in this age group is sustained by the child's placing a live electric socket in his mouth, the moisture of the mouth completing the electric circuit. Arc burns of the mouth result in a moderate to massive degree of microstomia.

If the child is wet or is touching a ground object (i.e., a radiator), the current may pass through the body, even resulting in electrocu-

tion. Although it is generally believed that voltages of 110 to 120 are not fatal, the authors know of one child who was electrocuted by contact with a live Christmas tree light socket and a radiator.

A point of major clinical importance in the electrical burn, in contradistinction to the more usual thermal burn, is that the severity of the electrical arc burn may not be apparent at the initial consultation. Examination of the site usually discloses a third degree burn with a central charred area and a pale gray elevation of the surrounding skin. However, pathologic examination will show an extensive coagulation necrosis extending for a considerable distance beyond the apparent limits of the wound. Microscopically, blood vessel walls are disrupted, sensory nerves widely destroyed, and the supporting tissues devitalized. Because of the extensive vascular involvement, there is an imprecise line of demarcation and a minimum of surrounding tissue reaction with slow spontaneous repair.

Deformities Associated with Electrical Burns. Burn lesions of the lips, alveolar processes, and tongue, structures which are commonly involved in "live socket" burns, follow a fairly constant pattern. The damage to the tongue is not usually severe, although the tip of the tongue may show considerable ulceration in the initial stages. Secondary involvement of the floor of the mouth may occur and result in some degree of scarring with lack of the normal motility of the tongue.

Slow sequestration of the alveolar processes and the teeth is common, but eruption of the permanent teeth after loss of the deciduous incisors is not usually affected. Lips generally suffer the most extensive damage, the lower lip being usually more severely injured than the upper. The burn involves the entire thickness of the lip, including the mucosa in the inner surface. The contraction during the slow healing phase results in severe deformities, especially when a large portion of the lip tissue has been lost. For details of the repair of these deformities, the reader is referred to Chapters 32 and 33.

The Treatment of Electrical Burns. The usual tendency in the treatment of an electrical burn is to underestimate the severity of the lesion in the early stages (Brown and Fryer, 1957; Muir, 1958; Bell, Poticha, and Mehn, 1962), and it is for this reason that the previously held view of Wells (1952) that early excision and grafting were the treatment of

---

*Contributed by John Marquis Converse, M.D., and Donald Wood-Smith, F.R.C.S.E.

choice in the majority of cases is not regarded as valid.

Unfortunately, many electric socket burns of the lips and cheeks in children are not seen early and they may involve areas which are not amenable to primary repair. When the burn involves the corner of the mouth, it is probably preferable, as advocated by Pitts, Pickrell, Quinn and Massengill (1969), to await the spontaneous separation of the eschar and healing and softening of the wound before undertaking the definitive repair of the resultant defect. It has been our experience that final reconstruction is best achieved not only after healing of the burn wound but also after a significant period during which the scars are allowed to soften. Children have a tendency to develop hypertrophic scarring, and reconstructive procedures done while the scars are hypertrophic often cause additional hypertrophic scarring. After a period of a year or more, the scars tend to flatten and soften, and the tendency for hypertrophic scarring has usually lessened.

In carefully selected cases, early excision and grafting may be done to advantage; however, it is often impossible to judge the extent of damage, and there is a possibility of either excessive resection of normal tissue or inadequate resection of irreversibly damaged tissue. These lesions should be treated conservatively until the full extent of the damage has become apparent, especially when amputation is contemplated.

REFERENCES

Allen, H. S., and Koch, S. L.: The treatment of patients with severe burns. Surg. Gynecol. Obstet., *74*:914, 1942.

Allgöwer, M., and Siegrist, J.: Verbrennungen. Berlin, Springer-Verlag, 1957.

Artz, C. P., and Moncrief, J. A.: The Treatment of Burns. 2nd. Ed. Philadelphia, W. B. Saunders Company, 1969.

Baines, J. W., Lynch, J. B., and Lewis, S. R.: The differential white cell count in burn septicemia. Presented at the annual meeting of the American Association of Plastic Surgeons, Colorado Springs, Colorado, 1970.

Baldridge, R. R.: Electric burns. New Engl. J. Med., *250*:46, 1954.

Barthe de Sandfort, E.: De la keritherapie. Nouvelle application thermale des paraffines. Bull. Acad. Med. Paris, *26*:249, 1914.

Baxter, C. R.: Response to initial fluid and electrolyte therapy of burn shock. Symposium on the Treatment of Burns. St. Louis, Mo., C. V. Mosby Company, 1973, p. 42.

Baxter, C. R., and Shires, T.: Physiological response to crystalloid resuscitation. Ann. N.Y. Acad. Sci., *150*:874, 1968.

Bell, J. L., Poticha, S. M., and Mehn, W. H.: Electrical injuries with special reference to the hand. Arch. Surg., *85*:852, 1962.

Bellinger, C. G., and Conway, H.: Effects of silver nitrate and Sulfamylon on epithelial regeneration. Plast. Reconstr. Surg., *56*:582, 1970.

Blocker, T. G., Jr.: An introduction to disaster problems. Symposium on Burns. National Research Council, National Academy of Sciences, Washington, D.C., 1950.

Blocker, T. G., Jr., Levin, W. C., Lewis, S. R., and Snyder, C. C.: The use of radioactive sulphur-labeled methionine in the study of protein catabolism in burn patients. Ann. Surg., *140*:519, 1954.

Blocker, T. G., Jr., Levin, W. C., Washburn, W. W., Nowinsky, W. W., Lewis, S. R., and Blocker, V.: Nutrition studies in the severely burned. Ann. Surg., *141*:589, 1955.

Blocker, T. G., Jr., Eade, G., Lewis, S. R., Jacobson, H. S., Grant, D. A., and Bennett, J. E.: Evaluation of a semi-open method in the management of severe burns after the acute phase. Texas State J. Med., *56*:402, 1960b.

Blocker, T. G., Jr., Lewis, S. R., Grant, D. A., Blocker, V., and Bennett, J. E.: Experiences in the management of the burn wound. Plast. Reconstr. Surg., *26*:579, 1960a.

Blocker, T. G., Jr., Washburn, W. W., Lewis, S. R., and Blocker, V.: A statistical study of 1000 burn patients admitted to the plastic sugery service at the University of Texas Medical Branch, 1950–59, J. Trauma, *1*:400, 1961.

Blocker, T. G., Jr., Lewis, S. R., Levin, W. C., Perry, J., and Blocker, V.: The problem of protein disequilibrium following severe thermal trauma. *In* Artz, C. P. (Ed.): Research in Burns. Washington, D.C., American Institute of Biological Sciences, Publ. No. 9, 1962.

Boyer, A.: Traité des Maladies Chirurgicales et des Opérations qui leur Conviennent. Vol. 1. Paris, L'Auterur et Migneret, 1814.

Bromberg, B. W., Song, I. C., and Mohn, M. P.: The use of pigskin as a temporary biological dressing. Plast. Reconstr. Surg., *36*:80, 1965.

Brown, J. B., and Fryer, M. P.: Reconstruction of electrical injuries, including cranial losses with preliminary report of cathode-ray burns. Ann. Surg., *146*:342, 1957.

Bruck, H. M., Nash, G., Foley, F. D., and Pruitt, B. A.: Opportunistic fungal infection of the burn wound with Phycomycetes or Aspergillus. Arch. Surg., *102*:476, 1971.

Burke, J. F., May, J. W., Albright, N., Quinby, W. C., and Russell, P. S.: Temporary skin transplantation and immunosuppression for extensive burns. New Engl. J. Med., *290*:269, 1974.

Constable, J. D.: Presented at the American College of Surgeons annual meeting. San Francisco, October, 1969.

Cramer, L. M., McCormack, R. M., and Carroll, D. B.: Progressive partial excision and early grafting in lethal burns. Plast. Reconstr. Surg., *30*:595, 1962.

Dale, R. H.: Electrical accidents (a discussion with illustrative case). Br. J. Plast. Surg., *7*:44, 1954.

Davidson, E. C.: Tannic acid in the treatment of burns. Surg. Gynecol. Obstet., *41*:202, 1925.

Davies, J. W. L.: A critical evaluation of red cell and plasma volume technique in patients with burns. J. Clin. Pathol., *13*:105, 1960.

DiVincenti, F. E., Curreri, P. W., and Pruitt, B. A.: Use of mesh skin autografts in the burned patient. Plast. Reconstr. Surg., *44*:464, 1969.

Dolecek, R.: Metabolic response of the burned organism. Springfield, Ill., Charles C Thomas, Publisher, 1969.

Dominguez, O., Baines, J. W., Lynch, J. B., and Lewis, S. R.: Treatment of burns with silver nitrate versus exposure method: Analysis of 200 patients. Plast. Reconstr. Surg., *40*:489, 1967.

Dupuytren, G.: Leçons Orales de Clinique Chirurgicale faites a l'Hotel Dieu de Paris. Vol. 1. Paris, G. Baillière, 1832–1834.

Eade, G. G.: The relationship between granulation tissue, bacteria, and skin grafts in burned patients. Plast. Reconstr. Surg., *22*:42, 1958.

Earle, J.: Means of lessening the effect of fire on the human body. London, C. Clark, 1799.

Early Care of Acute Soft Tissue Injuries. Edited by the Committee on Trauma, American College of Surgeons. Philadelphia, W. B. Saunders Company, 1960.

Evans, E. B.: Orthopaedic measures in the treatment of severe burns. J. Bone Joint Surg., *48A*:643, 1966.

Evans, E. B.: Bone and joint changes secondary to burns. *In* Lynch, J. B., and Lewis, S. R. (Eds.): Treatment of Burns. St. Louis, Mo., C. V. Mosby Company, 1973, p. 76.

Evans, E. B., Larson, D. L., and Yates, S.: Preservation and restoration of joint function in patients with severe burns. J.A.M.A., *204*:843, 1968.

Feller, I.: A second look at adrenal cortical function in burn stress. *In* Artz, C. P. (Ed.): Research in Burns. Washington, D. C., American Institute of Biological Sciences, Publ. No. 9, 1962.

Fogelman, M. J., and Wilson, B. J.: A different concept of volume replacement in traumatic hypovolemia. Am. J. Surg., *99*:694, 1960.

Fox, C. L., Jr., Lasker, S. E., and Winfield, J. M.: Relative lack of efficiency of fluid therapy. Am. J. Surg., *99*:690, 1960.

Fox, C. L., Rappole, B. W., and Stanford, W.: Control of Pseudomonas infection in burns by silver sulfadiazine. Surg. Gynecol. Obstet., *128*:1021, 1969.

Friend, E.: The treatment of extensive burns. J.A.M.A., *24*:41, 1895.

Gardner, L. I.: Experimental potassium depletion: Effect on carbohydrate metabolism and pH of muscle. Journal-Lancet, *73*:190, 1953.

Georgiade, N., Lucas, M., Georgaide, R., and Garrett, W.: The use of a new potent topical antibacterial agent for the control of infection in the burn wound. Plast. Reconstr. Surg., *39*:349, 1967.

Haas, S.: The treatment of burns in children. Am. J. Surg., *29*:61, 1915.

Hardy, J. D.: Pathophysiology in Surgery. Baltimore, Williams & Wilkins Company, 1958.

Haynes, B. W., Jr.: Thermal, chemical, and electrical injuries. *In* Ochsner, A., and DeBakey, M. E. (Eds.): Christopher's Minor Surgery. Philadelphia, W. B. Saunders Company, 1959.

Haynes, B. W., Jr., Jones, V., and Gibson, C. D., Jr.: A nine year study of coagulase-positive staphylococcus in a burn unit. Antibiot. Ann., *7*:728, 1959–60.

Hermann, C.: A note on the open method of treating burns. Am. J. Surg., *29*:61, 1915.

Hume, D., and Haynes, B. W., Jr.: Discussion in Conference on Burn Therapy. Medical College of Virginia, Virginia, 1961.

Jackson, D. M., and Stone, P. A.: Tangential excision and grafting of burns. The method and a report of 50 consecutive cases. Br. J. Plast. Surg., *25*:416, 1972.

Jackson, D., Topley, E., Carson, J. S., and Lowbury, E. J. L.: Primary excision and grafting of large burns. Ann. Surg., *152*:167, 1960.

Janzekovic, A.: A new concept in the early excision and immediate grafting of burns. J. Trauma, *10*:1103, 1970.

Kentish, J.: An Essay on Burns, Which Happen to Workmen in Mines. Edinburgh, G. G. and J. Robinson, 1797.

Knisely, M. H.: Postburn pathologic circulatory physiology. *In* Artz, C. P. (Ed.): Research in Burns. Washington, D. C., American Institute of Biological Sciences, Publ. No. 9, 1962.

Krizek, T. J., and Robson, M. C.: Clinical experience with Travase®, enzymatic debridement in the burned patient. Presented at annual meeting American Society of Plastic and Reconstructive Surgeons, Houston, Texas, October, 1974.

Larson, D. L.: Studies show hexachlorophene causes burn syndrome. Hospitals, *42*:63, 1968.

Larson, D. L.: Can Curling's ulcer incidence be modified in acute burns? Presented at Singleton Surgical Society Meeting, Galveston, Texas, 1970.

Levenson, S. M., and Lund, C. C.: Thermal Burns. Chicago, Year Book Medical Publishers, 1957.

Levin, W. C., and Blocker, T. G., Jr.: Studies in burn anemia. Annual Report, U.S. Army Contract, DA-49-007-MD-447, 1958.

Levine, N., Seifter, E., Connerton, C., and Levenson, S. M.: Debridement of experimental skin burns of pigs with bromelain, a pineapple-stem enzyme. Plast. Reconstr. Surg., *52*:413, 1973.

Levine, N., Ger, R., Stellar, S., and Levenson, S. M.: Use of a carbon dioxide laser for debridement of third degree burns. Ann. Surg., *179*:246, 1974a.

Levine, N. S., Peterson, H. D., Salisbury, R. E., and Pruitt, B. A.: Laser, scalpel, electrosurgical, and tangential excision of third degree burns. A preliminary report. Presented at the annual meeting of the American Society of Plastic and Reconstructive Surgeons, Houston, Texas, October, 1974b.

Lewis, S. R., Goolishian, H. A., Wolf, C. W., Lynch, J. B., and Blocker, T. G., Jr.: Psychological studies in burn patients. Plast. Reconstr. Surg., *31*:323, 1963.

Lindberg, R. B., Moncrief, J. A., Switzer, W. E., Order, S. E., and Mills, W.: The successful control of burn wound sepsis. J. Trauma, *5*:601, 1965.

Link, W. J., Zook, E. G., and Glover, J. L.: Plamsa scapel excision of burns: An experimental study. Presented at the annual meeting of the American Society of Plastic and Reconstructive Surgeons, Houston, Texas, October, 1974.

Lynch, J. B.: General principles of reconstruction following burns. *In* Lynch, J. B., and Lewis, S. R. (Eds.): Symposium on the Treatment of Burns. St. Louis, Mo., C. V. Mosby Company, 1973, p. 189.

Lynch, J. B., Wisner, H. K., and Lewis, S. R.: Management of electrical injuries. South. Med. J., *64*:97, 1971a.

Lynch, J. B., Kim, K., Larson, D. L., Doyle, J. E., and Lewis, S. R.: Changing patterns of mortality in burns. Plast. Reconstr. Surg., *48*:329, 1971b.

McConn, D., Tsuru, D., and Yasonobu, K. T.: *Bacillis subtilis* neutral proteinase: a zinc enzyme of high specific activity. J. Biol. Chem., *239*:3706, 1964.

MacMillan, B. G.: Early excision of more than twenty-five per cent of body surface in the extensively burned patients. Arch. Surg., *77*:369, 1958.

MacMillan, B. G., and Altemeier, W. A.: Massive excision of the extensive burn. *In* Artz, C. P. (Ed.): Research in Burns. Washington, D.C., American Institute of Biological Sciences, Publ. No. 9, 1962.

Markley, K., and Kefalides, N. A.: Further studies in the evaluation of saline solutions in the treatment of burn shock. *In* Artz, C. P. (Ed.): Research in Burns. Washington, D. C., American Institute of Biological Sciences, Publ. No. 9, 1962.

Markley, K., Bocanegra, M., Chiappori, M., Morales, G., and John, D.: The influence of fluid therapy upon water and electrolyte equilibria and upon the circulation during shock period in burned patients. Surgery, *49*:161, 1961.

Maurer, L. H., Andrews, P., Ruechert, F., and McIntyre,

O. R.: Lymphocyte transformation observed in Sulfamylon associated agranulocytosis. Plast. Reconstr. Surg., *46*:458, 1970.

Monafo, W. W.: Bacteriologic studies of burn wounds treated with silver nitrate solution. J. Trauma, *7*:99, 1967.

Monasterio, F., Rebeil, A. S., Barrera, G., Araico, J., Bosque, R. G., Escobosa, J. E., and Barreto, F. R.: Comparative study on the treatment of extensive burns with and without antibiotics. *In* Artz, C. P. (Ed.): Research in Burns. Washington, D. C., American Institute of Biological Sciences, Publ. No. 9, 1962.

Moncrief, J. A.: Discussion, Symposium on Burns. University of California School of Medicine, 1962.

Moncrief, J. A., and Mason, A. D., Jr.: Evaporative water loss in the burned patient. J. Trauma, *4*:180, 1964.

Moore, F. D.: Metabolic Care of the Surgical Patient. Philadelphia, W. B. Saunders Company, 1959.

Moyer, C. A., and Fallon, R. H.: Rates of insensible perspiration through normal, burned, tape-stripped and epidermally denuded living human skin. Ann. Surg., *158*: 915, 1963.

Moyer, C. A., Brentano, L., Bravens, D. L., Margraf, H. W., and Monafo, W. W.: Treatment of large human burns with 0.5 per cent silver nitrate solution. A.M.A. Arch. Surg., *90*:812, 1965.

Muir, I. F. K.: The treatment of electrical burns. Br. J. Plast. Surg., *10*:292, 1958.

Muir, I. F. K.: Red cell destruction in burns, with particular reference to the shock period. Br. J. Plast. Surg., *14*:273, 1961.

Neale, H. W.: Use of the non-expanded mesh graft. J. Trauma, *14*:247, 1974.

Neathery, E. J.: Treatment of extensive burns. Texas State J. Med., *4*:229, 1909.

O'Neill, J.: Comparison of xenograft and prosthesis for burn wound care. J. Pediatr. Surg., *8*:705, 1973.

Oppenheimer, L. S.: The treatment of burns. N.Y. Med. J., *84*:646, 1906.

Order, S. E., Mason, A. D., Walker, H. L., Lindberg, R. B., Switzer, W. E., and Moncrief, J. A.: The pathogenesis of second and third degree burns and conversion to full thickness injury. Surg. Gynecol. Obstet., *120*:983, 1965.

Pennisi, V. R., Capozzi, A., and Friedman, G.: Travase®, an effective enzyme for burn debridement. Plast. Reconstr. Surg., *51*:371, 1973.

Pickrell, K. L.: A new treatment of burns: Preliminary report. Bull. Johns Hopkins Hosp., *69*:217, 1941.

Pitts, W., Pickrell, K., Quinn, G., and Massengill, R.: Electrical burns of lips and mouth in infants and children. Plast. Reconstr. Surg., *44*:471, 1969.

Pulaski, E. J.: Exposure method. Symposium on Burns, National Research Council, National Academy of Sciences, Washington, D. C., 1950.

Quinby, W. C., Jr., and Cope, O.: Blood viscosity and the whole blood therapy of burns. Surgery, *32*:316, 1952.

Rappaport, F. T., Converse, J. M., Horn, L., Ballantyne, D. L., and Mulholland, J. H.: Altered reactivity to skin homografts in severe thermal injury. Ann. Surg., *159*:390, 1964.

Richards, K. E., and Feller, I.: Grid escharotomy for debriding burns. Surg. Gynecol. Obstet., *137*:843, 1973.

Roe, C. F., and Kinney, J. M.: Water and heat exchange in third degree burns. Surgery, *56*:212, 1964.

St. John, D.: The open air treatment of burns. Am. J. Surg., *24*:256, 1910.

Salzburg, A. M., and Evans, E. I.: Blood volumes in normal and burned dogs. Ann. Surg., *132*:746, 1950.

Scapicchio, A. P., Constable, J. D., and Opity, G.: Comparative effects of silver nitrate and Sulfamylon acetate on epidermal regeneration. Plast. Reconstr. Surg., *41*:319, 1968.

Sevitt, S.: Burns, Pathology and Therapeutic Applications. London, Butterworths and Company, Ltd., 1957.

Silverstein, P., and Pruitt, B.: Allograft coverage of the burn wound. *In* Lynch, J. B., and Lewis, S. R. (Eds.): Symposium on the Treatment of Burns. St. Louis, Mo., C. V. Mosby Company, 1973, p. 172.

Sneve, H.: The treatment of burns and skin grafting. J.A.M.A., *45*:1, 1905.

Stanford, W., Rappole, B. W., and Fox, C. L.: Clinical experience with silver sulfadiazine, a new topical agent for control of pseudomonas infections in burns. J. Trauma, *9*:377, 1969.

Stenbert, T., and Hogeman, K.-E.: Experimental and clinical investigations of liver function in burns. *In* Artz, C. P. (Ed.): Research in Burns. Washington, D. C., American Institute of Biological Sciences, Publ. No. 9, 1962.

Stone, H. H.: Use of gentamycin sulfate in burn therapy. J. Trauma, *7*:109, 1967.

Stone, H. H., and Bush, C. A.: Topical burn chemotherapy with antibiotic creams (Neosporin or gentamicin). *In* Lynch, J. B., and Lewis, S. R. (Eds.): Symposium on the Treatment of Burns. St. Louis, Mo., C. V. Mosby Company, 1973, p. 129.

Tanner, J. C., Vandeput, J., and Olley, J. F.: The mesh skin graft. Plast. Reconstr. Surg., *34*:287, 1964.

Topley, E., Moe, D., and Jackson, G.: The clinical control of red cell loss in burns. J. Clin. Pathol., *10*:1, 1957.

Wallace, A. B.: Treatment of burns; a return to basic principles. Br. J. Plast. Surg., *2*:232, 1949.

Wells, D. B.: Treatment of electric burns by immediate resection and skin graft. Ann. Surg., *90*:129, 1952.

Wilson, B. J., and Stirman, J. A.: Initial treatment of burns. J.A.M.A., *173*:509, 1960.

Wisner, H. K., Lynch, J. B., Larson, D. L., and Lewis, S. R.: Correction of retarded epidermal regeneration due to sulfamylon by administration of oral zinc. *In* Matter, P., Barclay, T. L., and Koníčková, Z. (Eds.): Research in Burns. Bern, Hans Huber Publishers, 1971, pp. 129–133.

Wolferth, C. C., Jr., and Peskin, G. W.: Fluid therapy in burns, trauma, and shock. Pediatr. Clin. North Am., *6*:169, 1959.

Zaroff, L. I., Mills, W., Puckett, J. W., Switzer, W. E., and Moncrief, J. A.: Multiple uses of viable cutaneous homografts in the burned patient. Surgery, *59*:3668, 1966.

CHAPTER 19

COLD INJURY

DAVID M. KNIZE, M.D.

Cold injury remains a perplexing surgical challenge. Few conditions in medical history have been so enveloped in confusion regarding the underlying pathologic process and the many methods of treatment, some of which have been contradictory and even detrimental. The basis for our present knowledge about cold injury is provided by centuries of recorded clinical observations augmented in recent years by experimental evidence which has begun to clarify the long-undefined pathogenesis. The wealth of older knowledge will be reviewed, and the more recent concepts derived from experimental evidence will be examined.

CLASSIFICATION OF COLD INJURIES

Because the course of any cold injury is characterized by unpredictability, a satisfactory means of classification, relating acute clinical findings and injury conditions to the ultimate tissue loss, has been difficult to develop. Nevertheless, the two traditionally used classification systems will be described.

Degrees of Injury

The acute physical findings after cold exposure and subsequent rewarming, together with the eventual depth of tissue necrosis, provide the basis for this retrospective classification system (Table 19–1).

First degree injury is characterized by skin erythema and edema localized in the injured area (Fig. 19–1). Gangrene and tissue loss do not occur; however, lingering causalgic pain frequently develops, indicating that some element of nerve injury has been produced.

Second degree injury consists of vesicle formation in addition to skin erythema and edema. Although the skin eventually sloughs superficially, deeper necrosis does not occur.

Third degree injury is typified by local edema and grayish blue discoloration. Gangrene of skin progressively becomes evident over several postinjury days. Areas of cold-injured skin which develop vesicles will usually undergo partial thickness necrosis. However, areas of skin without vesicle formation are usually associated with skin loss down to the subcutaneous level (Fig. 19–2).

Fourth degree injury is indicated by deep

TABLE 19–1. *Degrees of Injury Classification**

DEGREE	APPEARANCE	LOCAL EDEMA	VESICLES	GANGRENE	TISSUE LOSS
First	Erythema	+	–	–	–
Second	Erythema	+	+	–	Superficial skin
Third	± Cyanosis	+	±	Late (days)	Full thickness skin
Fourth	Cyanosis	–	–	Early (hours)	Skin + deep tissues

*Five characteristic states are based upon physical findings in the injured limb.

516

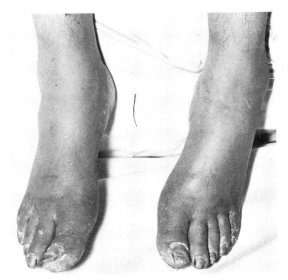

FIGURE 19-1. First degree injury; erythema and edema of foot present on admission. Although no loss of tissue subsequently developed, causalgic type pain persisted for several weeks. (Courtesy of University of Colorado Medical Center.)

cyanosis of the injured part without the development of vesiculation and local edema. Tissue is injured to a level into or below the subcutis (Fig. 19-3, *A, B*), and gangrene of the involved areas is evident within a few hours after injury (Fig. 19-3, *C*).

Since this classification system is found in the older cold injury literature and because its use will undoubtedly persist for years, the reader should be familiar with it. From the practical standpoint, one can attempt to distinguish only "superficial" (first or second degree) from "deep" (third or fourth degree) injury; this is sometimes difficult to do, even for the experienced clinician, since the initial physical appearance is often a deceptive indicator of the ultimate extent of injury. The four-degree system does have merit as a means of retrospective classification of a cold injury when the patient is discharged from the hospital.

Clinical State

In addition to physical findings, the following classification system includes the environmental conditions under which the cold insult occurred. Cold injuries are grouped into five categories, as listed below in order of increasing severity (Table 19-2).

Chilblains is a skin condition resulting from chronic intermittent exposure to the environmental conditions of high humidity and low ambient temperature without developing tissue freezing. It is characterized by discomfort in the involved limbs; the symptom usually resolves spontaneously, and no tissue is lost.

Immersion foot, also known as trench foot, results from exposure of wet feet to a temperature range of 32 to 50°F (1 to 10°C) for at least several hours and possibly extending to several days without actual tissue freezing. A large proportion of World War I cold injury casualties was due to immersion foot, which developed when infantry men under enemy fire stood in trenches for long periods with water or mud above their ankles. Symptoms include a tingling sensation or dull discomfort in the foot, followed by numbness. Immediately after exposure, the skin appears erythematous and eventually becomes pale. Occasionally, tissue loss can result, and prolonged disability is not uncommon.

Frostbite develops after exposure to temperatures at freezing levels or below, usually for more than one hour. Clinically tissues become frozen to variable depths, and this process can develop more rapidly when clothing is penetrated by environmental dampness. Except when exposure time is short, gangrene with tissue loss of varying severity occurs. In a clinical group of 140 patients, exposure to an ambient temperature of 20°F (−6.5°C) or below for a duration of one hour or more consistently resulted in tissue loss (Knize, Weatherly-White, Paton and Owens 1969b).

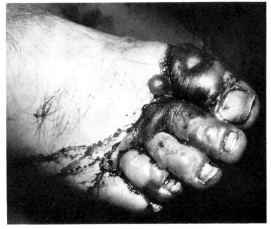

FIGURE 19-2. Third degree injury; slight cyanosis, edema, and vesiculation of foot present on admission. Full thickness skin was lost distal to vesicles on the toes. (Courtesy of University of Colorado Medical Center.)

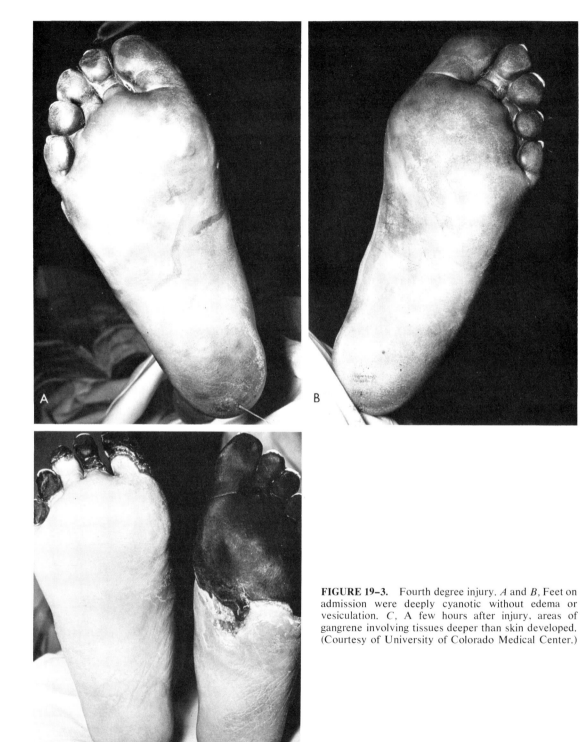

FIGURE 19-3.   Fourth degree injury. *A* and *B*, Feet on admission were deeply cyanotic without edema or vesiculation. *C*, A few hours after injury, areas of gangrene involving tissues deeper than skin developed. (Courtesy of University of Colorado Medical Center.)

TABLE 19–2.   *Clinical State Classification**

NONFREEZING	FREEZING	WITH OR WITHOUT FREEZING
Chilblains	Frostbite	Hypothermia
Immersion foot	High altitude frostbite	

*The five clinical states are subdivided to indicate the usual presence or absence of tissue freezing.

This critical ambient temperature is similar to that seen by Blair (1964) in Korean War casualties. The early symptoms are much like those of immersion foot: tingling or dull pain and eventual numbness in the involved parts. After tissue freezes, the limb appears waxy white and immobile, the skin is hard to palpation, and sensation is absent. When the injured areas have been thawed prior to the examination, immersion foot and frostbite are usually indistinguishable without a history of the nature of the exposure. This illustrates the value of a classification system incorporating the environmental conditions under which injury occurred, since the prognosis for tissue survival with immersion foot is better than that with frostbite.

High altitude frostbite, while not uncommonly seen, is a vicious form of cold injury. Classically it has been a hazard for aviators and mountaineers who were exposed to conditions of low atmospheric oxygen concentration and extreme cold enhanced by high wind velocities. The contribution of "wind chill" to cold by accelerating heat loss is well known (Molnar, 1958). Although the exposed skin of the face can be involved, the hands are more frequently affected. The distinctive clinical feature of high altitude frostbite is extensive loss of tissue, ranging from epithelial slough to gangrene and autoamputation (Fig. 19–4), occurring after exposure as brief as one minute under the above environmental conditions.

High altitude frostbite was first described by Davis, Scarff, Rogers, and Dickinson in 1943 following their clinical experience with treating aviators in World War II. Typically tissue freezing appears when an aviator removes a glove for a delicate instrument adjustment. In the *mild* form of injury, exposure for a few seconds produces numb, waxy white, hard and stiff fingers. Usually after thawing there is no blistering, gangrene, or other gross anatomical residua, but subsequent vasomotor instability is common. The *severe* form may at first appear clinically similar to the mild type, with the exception that vesicles may develop and the skin may take on a dull, ground-glass appearance; frequently, subungual hemorrhages are seen. Tissue loss results from the severe form.

Hypothermia, the most severe form of cold injury, occurs when protective clothing and body thermoregulatory mechanisms fail to retain body heat adequately. When the core (rectal or esophageal) temperature drops below 90°F (32°C), physiologic derangements become progressively more severe and are directly related to both the depth of the temperature drop and the exposure duration.

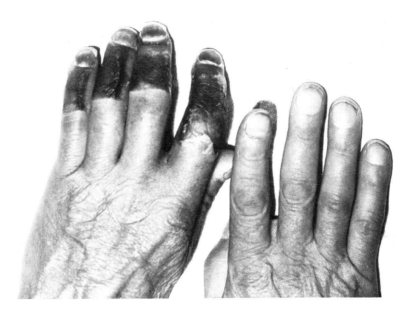

FIGURE 19–4. High altitude frostbite. Short exposure following removal of left glove resulted in loss of distal digits. (Courtesy of University of Colorado Medical Center.)

The latter is believed to be the more critical factor in producing the total insult (Zingg, 1967). Such changes include (1) a massive intravascular fluid shift producing hemoconcentration (Fruehan, 1960); (2) adrenal cortical and pituitary hypofunction (Hume, Egdahl and Nelson, 1956); (3) microvascular erythrocyte aggregation (Bigelow, Lindsay and Greenwood, 1950); and (4) whole blood viscosity increase (Alexander, 1947; Fukusumi and Adolph, 1970). Central nervous system changes, as manifested by abnormalities in the EEG, neurologic examination, and cerebrospinal fluid pressure, are probably related to body fluid shifts (Block, 1967).

Three phases of progressive hypothermia are clinically recognized:

1. At the rectal temperature of 90 to 98.4°F (32 to 37°C), thermoregulatory mechanisms act against continued chilling by shivering, increasing pulse rate and blood pressure, as well as constricting peripheral skin capillaries (Adolph, 1951).

2. At 75 to 90°F (24 to 32°C), the general body tissue metabolic rate is depressed, while pulse rate, blood pressure, and respiratory rate progressively decrease as body temperature falls. In this phase, near the rectal temperature range of 77 to 82.5°F (25 to 28°C) and below, cardiac arrhythmias frequently occur.

3. Lastly, when the core temperature is lower than 75°F (24°C), temperature regulatory centers cease to function, and heat is lost as from an inanimate object (Talbott, Consolazid and Pecora, 1941). A more detailed description of these physiologic and clinical changes can be found in the German literature (Alexander, 1947; Killian, 1949).

The lower limit of rectal temperature compatible with continued physical exercise is believed to be near 95°F (35°C) (Freeman and Pugh, 1969). With progressive hypothermia, the victim will collapse and eventually become unconscious when the rectal temperature drops to about 86°F (30°C). At such a level the skin is pale, dry, and cold with an almost corpselike appearance, and a variable degree of subcutaneous edema is present. Pupils react poorly to light, and tendon reflexes are delayed or sluggish. Peripheral pulses are usually absent, and respiratory effort may be so shallow as to be imperceptible. The victim often has the clinical appearance of death, even though an ECG (Fig. 19–5) could demonstrate the myocardial electrical activity characteristic of hypothermia with the well-described "J" waves (Osborn, 1953).

While the classification systems utilizing the

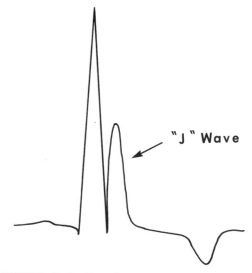

FIGURE 19–5. Hypothermia produces several nonspecific changes in the electrocardiogram, but the presence of a "J" (junctional) wave in most leads, similar to that shown here in lead II, is characteristic. The amplitude of the wave is variable.

"degrees of injury" or the "clinical state" attempt to aid the clinician with the problem of prognosis, neither system is practical for this purpose. Perhaps after the complex pathogenic factors involved in any type of cold injury are more clearly defined, it will be possible to identify those particular features of the acute phase which relate to final tissue damage. Formulation of a classification system as a useful tool for prognostication can only follow this development. Those recognized general clinical prognostic signs which can be observed after thawing a cold-injured area will be described later.

PREDISPOSING FACTORS

The development of a cold injury does not depend simply upon the depth of the ambient temperature and duration of exposure. Several other contributory conditions designated as "predisposing factors" will be described.

Insufficient Conservation of Body Heat

The degree of inadequacy of protective clothing varies with environmental conditions. Tight-fitting clothing may produce areas of constriction which can hinder blood circulation and lessen the extent of heat-retaining air insulation. Wet clothing transmits heat from the body into the environment, because water is a thermal conductor. For example, if the boots of a soldier walking in snow are penetrated by moisture through to the skin of the feet, there will exist a mechanism for accelerated heat loss from the feet. By the same principle, metal objects in contact with bare skin in a freezing environment produce loss of body heat.

Mental State

Clinical studies of military cold injuries during World War II (Whayne and DeBakey, 1958) and the Korean conflict (Orr and Fainer, 1952) showed a correlation between fatigue and apathy and the incidence of cold injury among combat troops. In such states or while under starvation, men often become indifferent to their personal hygiene and to the condition of their clothing. Cold injuries occur with high frequency among soldiers in retreat (Kinmouth, Rob and Simeone, 1962).

Among civilians, the most common factor contributing to cold injury has been impairment of judgment due to excessive alcohol consumption. Intoxicated patients and others whose consciousness, judgment, or self-protective instincts are depressed by psychosis or drug abuse often expose themselves to dangerous environmental hazards. In the Denver series (Knize, Weatherly-White and Paton, 1969b), alcohol intake or mental instability led directly to cold injury in 50 per cent of the patients. Once the injury had occurred, however, alcoholic intake probably did not significantly alter the course of events.

Previous Cold Injury

Based on clinical observations, an individual who has experienced a prior cold injury must be placed in a high risk category during subsequent exposure to low environmental temperatures (Whayne and DeBakey, 1958; Mills and Whaley, 1964). For reasons not yet determined, a cold injury in some way sensitizes an individual, with the result that subsequent cold exposure, even of a lesser degree, produces tissue damage more rapidly.

Mobility

Military studies have shown that long periods of physical immobility contribute to the extent of cold injury (Whayne and DeBakey, 1958). This has been observed in soldiers pinned down by prolonged enemy fire. Motion is necessary for the production of body heat and efficient circulation, especially with respect to endangered limbs.

Race and Climate

While civilian clinical studies are inadequate for statistical evaluation of factors such as race and previous climatic environmental conditions, military series from World War II (Whayne and DeBakey, 1958) and the Korean conflict (Orr and Fainer, 1952) suggest that dark-skinned soldiers under the same combat conditions are more susceptible to cold injury. Similarly, individuals from regions of warmer climates within the United States tend to be more susceptible (Whayne and DeBakey, 1958).

PATHOGENESIS

Important advances in understanding the mechanisms by which cold exposure inflicts damage to living tissues have taken place in recent years. Present knowledge suggests that tissue loss results either from *direct cellular injury* or a *basic microvascular insult* which progresses to local ischemia. The current evidence for the contribution of each of these two mechanisms of tissue damage to the total cold injury will be discussed.

Direct Cellular Injury

Direct cellular death can be produced under low temperature conditions in the following ways:

Cellular Dehydration. One of the early important studies investigating the critical temperature for tissue death was reported by Moran in 1929. He attributed tissue necrosis to dehydration of individual cells by the formation of extracellular ice crystals. According to Moran, the formation of the ice crystals progressively incorporated more extracellular water, producing an osmotic gradient which attracted water from the intracellular space. Supporting evidence was produced by Merryman (1956) in his study of "ice-crystal nucleation." Over subsequent years it has been confirmed that cellular dehydration can induce cellular death through the following mechanisms (Mazur, 1963, 1965): modification of protein structure by high electrolyte concentration, alteration of membrane lipids, alteration of cellular pH, and imbalance of chemical activity.

Mechanical Injury from Ice Crystal Formation. Whether the physical presence of ice crystals can disrupt the cell membrane by puncture or compression is now questioned. Although it has been experimentally shown that rapid freezing forms intracellular ice crystals which could mechanically disrupt the cell (Merryman, 1956), a freezing rate sufficiently fast to produce intracellular crystals is unlikely in the clinical cold injury (Merryman, 1970). The slow freezing rate observed clinically produces primarily extracellular ice crystals, which deform cells physically but do not actually disrupt cell membranes (Smith, 1961; Merryman, 1970). The mechanical injury theory is attractive, but it has little supporting evidence thus far.

Inactivation or Depression of Cellular Systems by Lowered Temperatures Above Freezing. Cellular structures after freezing injury have been studied under the electron microscope. Stowell and coworkers (1965) described alterations in the nucleus following freezing. In addition, they observed changes occurring in the *cytoplasmic structures,* notably mitochondria, endoplasmic reticulum, and Golgi bodies (Trump and coworkers, 1965). *Enzyme systems* are known to be affected by lowered temperatures. Shikama and Yamuzahi (1961) reported depression of ox catalase activity at 22°F (−6°C), with a maximum loss in activity at 11°F (−12°C). Markert (1963) showed structural alteration of lactic acid dehydrogenase after freezing and thawing.

The evidence cited leaves little doubt that direct cellular injury can occur with freezing. However, the contribution of this mechanism to the final tissue loss following a cold exposure injury is surprisingly small, as was shown by the following study: epidermal tissue subjected to a standard injury of freezing and thawing in vivo, which had consistently produced necrosis, survived as a full-thickness skin graft transplanted to an uninjured recipient site. In contrast, uninjured full-thickness skin did not survive transplantation to a recipient area pretreated with the same freezing injury (Weatherley-White, Sjostrom and Paton, 1964). Similarly it was shown by Kreyberg and Hanssen (1950) that frozen skin survived when transplanted to a subcutaneous pocket in normal intact tissue. It appears that the direct cell injury after cold insult is not an irreversible process and that some mechanism besides cellular injury alone must lead to tissue necrosis. Evidence suggests that this mechanism begins at the microvascular level.

Microvascular Insult

Microangiographic studies have shown microvascular failure after cold injury (Quintanella, Krusen and Essex, 1947; Bellman and Strombeck, 1960). Although capillary patency initially appeared normal in post-thawed tissue, blood flow rate was observed to decline within three minutes by Bellman and Adams-Ray (1956) and within five minutes by Quintanella, Krusen and Essex (1947).

Following cold insult to living tissue, Kulka (1956, 1964) found local vascular thromboses advancing from the capillary levels to larger vessels and resulting in ischemic death of progressively larger areas. Viable cells were observed histologically in cold-injured tissue for as long as eight days or until occlusion of the local vessels occurred. This work indicates that a major role is played by vascular insufficiency and that the direct injury to cellular structures and mechanisms may be reversible.

Considerable evidence has accumulated to support the microvascular insult theory of cold injury and to suggest that the starting point in the pathologic pathway is a primary alteration in the vascular endothelium. After experimentally damaging vessel walls using a microprobe technique, Zweifach (1961) observed platelet agglutination at the site of injury, a phenomenon confirmed by several other investigators (Allison, Smith and Wood, 1955; Majno, Schoefl and Palade, 1961; Maggio, 1965). As suggested by recent studies (Skjorten, 1968; Kattlove and Alexander, 1971), after a cold injury the platelet may play a more active role in this process than was formerly believed. A "platelet plug" develops within the injured vessel (Friedman, Lange and Weiner, 1947; Robb, 1963; Bergman, 1964; Deykin, 1974), and this partial occlusion reduces the blood flow rate. Erythrocytes then aggregate behind the plug and contribute bulk to the obstruction (Sandison, 1931; Lutz, 1951; Gelin, 1956; Bergentz, Eiken and Nilsson, 1961; Maggio, 1965). Subsequently, within this total cellular mass, fibrin clot formation occurs and blood flow ceases. The initial obstruction usually begins at the level of the capillary and the postcapillary venule, and the clot progresses in retrograde fashion into the arterial system.

Since erythrocyte bulk provides most of the obstructing mass, the factors affecting erythrocyte behavior deserve further comment. Emphasis on the role of erythrocyte aggregation in the pathologic process originated from a study (Kulka, 1964) showing that high molecular weight dextran, a compound known to produce erythrocyte aggregation, produced more severe tissue loss when administered intravenously after a cold injury. The recognized conditions which induce aggregation and have relevance to cold injury can best be considered under the following categories (Fig. 19–6).

1. *Plasma protein alterations* result when plasma proteins are lost from the intravascular space owing to increased vessel wall permeability after the initial endothelial cell injury. The plasma proteins first lost are the small molecules, such as albumin; only later do the larger molecules, such as fibrinogen and the globulins, leave the vessels. Thus, shortly after tissue injury, there is a relative local increase in the plasma concentration of the macromolecular plasma protein fractions, particularly fibrinogen and alpha$_2$-globulin (Gelin, 1956). A diminution in plasma albumin concentration or a real or relative increase in globulin or fibrinogen plasma concentration has been observed by Merrill and his coworkers (1966) to be associated with erythrocyte aggregation and increased blood viscosity. Experimentally produced cold injury has been shown to increase whole blood viscosity (Weatherley-White and coworkers, 1969), presumably in a manner similar to the above mechanisms.

2. *Elevated serum lipid concentrations* (Fig. 19–6) induce erythrocyte aggregation (Swank, 1951; Bergentz, Gelin and Rudenstam, 1960). The stress of cold exposure has been shown to mobilize serum triglycerides while inhibiting lipid storage in fat depots (Radomski, 1971). Following a cold injury, hemolysis of the erythrocytes agglutinating in the vessels has been observed (Quintanella, Krusen and Essex, 1947; Mundth, 1964), producing a local increase in serum lipid levels when phospholipids are released from disrupted cell membranes. This is similar to the cell disruption which occurs from hemolysis of erythrocytes circulating through a burned area, and in both cases erythrocyte lysis is produced by a yet unexplained alteration in the physical and chemical structure of the erythrocyte membrane (Lovelock, 1957).

3. *Hemodynamic alterations* (Fig. 19–6) in

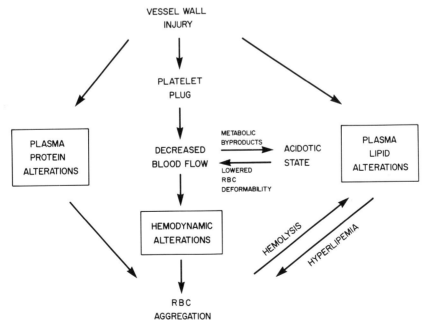

FIGURE 19–6. Theoretical schema of events following cold injury which lead to cessation of microvascular blood flow. (Modified from Knize, D. M., Weatherley-White, R. C. A., and Paton, B. C.: Use of antisludging agents in experimental cold injuries. Surg. Gynecol. Obstet., *129*:1019, 1969. By permission of Surgery, Gynecology & Obstetrics.)

whole blood develop simultaneously with decreased flow rates (Eiseman and Spencer, 1962); the pseudoplastic characteristics of whole blood at low shear rates result in erythrocyte aggregation. Furthermore, the erythrocyte, which is normally capable of being pressed into unnatural shapes for passage through the capillary bed, loses its deformability in the presence of acidosis. Following a cold injury, after the platelet plug forms and the local pH decreases, both these mechanisms would be expected to play a role in the complex processes leading to microvascular insufficiency.

TREATMENT

In view of the current understanding of the pathologic process, the most significant part of treating any cold injury should be an effort to prevent collapse of the microvascular circulatory system. Indeed, antisludging agents, low molecular weight dextran, and a nonionic surfactant (Pluronic F-68, manufactured by the Wyandotte Chemical Company) were shown experimentally to have a definite protective effect when administered intravenously after cold injury and thawing (Mundth, Long and Brown, 1964; Knize, Weatherly-White and Paton, 1969a). Clinical studies of this type, however, have not yet been performed; large numbers of patients are unavailable, and a control series would be almost impossible because of the lack of adequate criteria to determine the severity of injury and to predict expected tissue loss prior to starting treatment. Nevertheless, development of microvascular circulatory support will undoubtedly be the cornerstone in future cold injury treatment. Until that time, the knowledge and techniques now available must be utilized to the best advantage.

Primary Treatment

Typically, travel conditions from the site of injury make it difficult to transport the patient to a hospital for several hours after a cold injury; therefore, it is essential to provide appropriate first aid measures. Constricting or wet clothing should be removed from the injured parts, and these areas must be protected from further cold exposure with any available material. Since the part may be insensitive, care must be taken to avoid any trauma which could compound the injury.

Smoking should be prohibited, for nicotine causes vasoconstriction.

The patient should be transported in the prone or supine position whenever possible. However, if *survival* depends on the patient's walking, no attempt should be made to warm frozen feet until reaching a treatment facility where controlled therapeutic thawing can be achieved. This is important for optimal limb salvage, because once rewarmed, the patient's injured parts must no longer be allowed to remain in a dependent position or be further exposed to cold. Mills, Whaley and Fish (1961) have cautioned against the "freeze-thaw-freeze" injury produced when a thawed part is allowed to freeze again, for in such cases the cumulative insult to tissue is considerably more severe.

First aid at the site of injury for a *hypothermic* patient consists of providing an airway and prevention of further heat loss by placing the victim into a plastic bag which can then be placed within a sleeping bag or wrapped with blankets. Detection of cardiac arrest may be difficult, but should it occur during evacuation, external cardiac massage and mouth-to-mouth breathing must be administered until a hospital is reached.

Thawing

When the earliest suitable situation permits, and the rectal temperature is within normal range and the limb is still frozen, i.e., hard and inflexible, the affected part should be thawed *rapidly* by immersion in water warmed to between 104 and 108°F (40 to 42°C). The narrow temperature range for the water bath must be observed closely, because rewarming at lower temperatures has been found to be less beneficial for tissue survival (Fuhrman and Crimson, 1947); water temperatures above 108°F (42°C) may produce a burn injury and thereby compound the total insult (Mills, Whaley and Fish, 1961). If the rectal temperature is subnormal, special treatment measures (described below) should be observed.

Usually pain experienced with thawing is severe, and a parenteral analgesic such as morphine is recommended if no contraindications exist. The frozen extremities remain in the water bath until the skin becomes erythematous as far as the most distal parts of the cold-injured area; usually thawing requires less than 30 minutes. By this time, the previously frozen skin should be soft to palpation, but caution should be exercised not to massage the limb because of the danger of further tissue injury. All nonfreezing cold injuries should be rewarmed to normal body temperatures.

Upon completion of rewarming, the injured parts must be elevated and the patient taken promptly to a hospital. At this stage, certain physical changes develop in the thawed tissue, and these may serve as general prognostic signs for tissue survival (Table 19-3). Rapid return of skin warmth and sensation with the presence of an erythematous color is a favorable sign, while the persistence of cold, anesthetic, and pale skin is unfavorable. The presence of vesiculation is favorable, especially if the vesicles are large and contain clear fluid, but the absence of vesiculation or sanguineous vesicles is usually associated with the development of early gangrene. The absence of edema carries a poor prognosis.

Hospital Care for the Normothermic Patient

It is unusual for the patient to reach a hospital before thawing has been administered or has taken place spontaneously, but if the injured parts are still frozen or incompletely thawed, rapid thawing should be carried out immediately, provided the rectal temperature is within normal range (care of the hypothermic patient will be described subsequently). The injured parts should be gently washed with a bland soap and the patient put at bed rest with the parts elevated. Low molecular weight dextran should be given intravenously on a dosage program to be outlined. Antihistamines, steroids, vasodilators, and anticoagulants previously used have not proven consistently beneficial. A tetanus toxoid booster is given unless the last immunization has been received within the previous 12 months. If the status of

tetanus immunization is uncertain, human hyperimmune globulin should be administered in addition to the tetanus toxoid. Thousands of Napoleon's soldiers in the Russian campaign perished from tetanus as a complication of cold injury (Campbell, 1964). At present, there is no evidence that prophylactically administered antibiotics are of real benefit; therefore, antibiotics should be withheld until evidence of infection presents itself. Narcotics, after the initial thawing procedure, are usually not required in the uncomplicated case; sedatives or tranquilizers should be sufficient. A diet high in protein and caloric value is recommended.

Absolute bed rest is essential for foot injuries; slight elevation should be used for all injured parts until edema and vesiculation have subsided. Attempts to prevent edema by external pressure (Shumaker and coworkers, 1951) or the use of hyaluronidase (Pirozynski and Webster, 1952) have not been effective.

The injured parts should be left exposed to comfortably warm room air with a "cradle" device to prevent contact with the bed clothing. No topical medications or dressings are to be applied, with the exception of cotton padding between the toes or fingers to prevent maceration. During the bleb period involving several days after rewarming, sterile sheets and reverse isolation techniques should be used.

Whirlpool treatments at body temperature using a bland soap are recommended twice daily. Preferably attendants should wear masks, caps, gowns, and gloves. After bleb rupture and subsequent drying of the affected areas, sterile technique is no longer necessary. It is advisable to begin physical therapy at the earliest possible time to avoid joint flexion contractures. Regardless of the condition of the limb, even in the presence of large bullae, active motion of all involved joints including digits should start on the day of admission. Otherwise, as is often the case, the limb may be preserved even though useful joint function is never regained. Buerger's exercises are recommended for 20 minutes four times daily.

Antisludging Agents. Although no supportive clinical evidence is available, experimental studies show that antisludging agents provide a definite protective effect. The microvascular obstruction process begins shortly after thawing, and maximal beneficial effect would be expected if intravenous administration of the antisludging agent began during thawing. Unfortunately this circumstance would be only rarely possible, because in most instances the

TABLE 19-3. *Prognostic Signs*

FAVORABLE	UNFAVORABLE
Rapid return of skin warmth and sensation	Cold, anesthetic skin
Erythema of skin	Skin pallor
Vesicles with clear fluid	Vesicles absent or sanguinous
Edema	Absence of edema

injured part is thawed before the arrival of the patient at a treatment facility. Since vascular obstruction and the resulting ischemic necrosis progress slowly over several hours to days (Kulka, 1956), support of the remaining patent vasculature to prevent microvascular stasis would appear to be essential in order to salvage the more proximal marginally viable tissue. Therefore, at this time, it is suggested that low molecular weight dextran should be administered intravenously as soon as possible following the cold exposure. The dosage is 500 ml of the 10 per cent solution over an initial two to three hours, followed by 500 ml. slowly administered over each subsequent 12-hour period for five days. Pluronic F-68, a nonionic surfactant, has provided a protective effect superior to that of low molecular weight dextran (Knize, Weatherly-White and Paton, 1969a). However, it is not yet commercially available for this use.

Surgical Treatment. Active surgical treatment has no role in the acute care of a cold injury. Since it is usually impossible to determine tissue viability for several days, debridement should not be attempted; blebs must be left undisturbed. Incisions from premature debridement only invite further tissue loss, because the edematous tissue often has marginal blood supply and is highly susceptible to deep infections. If tendons or joints are exposed, additional functional loss can result. The most practical course is to utilize daily whirlpool treatments for gentle "physiologic debridement"; these will serve to elevate the eschar slowly as it becomes separated. Limited debridement of the loose eschar can then be done with safety. After a period of up to three or four months, dry gangrene should indicate a definite line of demarcation between viable and nonviable tissues; at this time, amputation can be performed. Often the amputation level is more distal than expected, as compared to the extent of the early dry eschar, because viable deep tissues underlying the eschar shell are re-epithelized. Although tissue salvage is worth the expenditure of time, situations must be individualized. Nursing home care is frequently satisfactory during the long period of waiting for the line of demarcation to become clear. In many cases, the patient can return home for much of this time.

Reconstructive plastic surgical procedures should not be considered before the final amputation. However, should any small granulating area become exposed, split-thickness skin grafts may be applied as indicated.

Two exceptions to the rule of "no incision" during the early treatment period are (1) ischemia from a constricting dry eschar, and (2) development of infection under the eschar. Decompressing incisions through the eschar should be made carefully in order to avoid injury to the underlying delicate, re-epithelizing tissues. To decompress digits and to facilitate digital joint motion for the daily physical therapy program, incisions just through the eschar along the transaxial line (Fig. 19–7) are satisfactory. This incision can be made unilaterally or on both sides of the digit when required. In the event of suppuration beneath the eschar, an escharectomy is required; however, the daily whirlpool treatments will usually prevent this complication. If wet gangrene and sepsis occur, early amputation should be performed.

Although some cold injuries in the superficial category recover totally, most deep category injuries have troublesome late sequelae, even in the face of apparent tissue preservation and good functional recovery. These sequelae include causalgic pain, hyperesthesia, sensory loss, hyperhidrosis, nail bed deformity, and various other forms of epidermal scarring. In cold-injured children, growth disturbances in digits secondary to epiphyseal damage is well documented (Schatzki, 1956; Hakstian, 1972; Tishler, 1972). Lumbar or cervical sympathectomy has shown definite benefit in the late phase for symptomatic relief of causalgic pain, hyperhidrosis, and vasospastic disorders and for improved healing of cutaneous ulcers persisting 6 to 12 months after injury.

Hospital Care for the Hypothermic Patient

Treatment for the hypothermic patient basically consists of rewarming the body of the victim by applying heat externally. The optimal

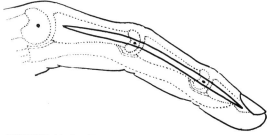

FIGURE 19–7. Transaxial line; position of digital decompression incision along line joining the dorsal-most end of each transverse volar digital crease. (Courtesy of Dr. R. W. Beasley.)

rate at which this treatment should be received has been the subject of debate for over 25 years. It was concluded from the Dachau experiments (Alexander, 1947) that rewarming should be accomplished rapidly by total body immersion in warm water. However, those subjects were rendered hypothermic rapidly over a very brief exposure period of one to two hours, and the physiologic derangements described on page 520 did not have sufficient time to become severe. Duguid, Simpson and Stowers (1961) reported that attempts to rapidly rewarm the accidental hypothermia patient with a longer duration of cold exposure met with unusually high mortality rates. Death during rewarming has been attributed to what has been termed "rewarming shock" (Zingg, 1967). This condition is initiated when the peripheral vessels dilate in response to the heat applied externally. With the blood volume contracted secondary to hemoconcentration, hypotension is produced as blood shunts into these dilated peripheral vessels. The shock state which can result becomes more severe because of the multiple preexisting physiologic derangements.

The following guidelines can be used in planning the treatment of a hypothermic patient:

Hypothermia and Prolonged Exposure to Cold. Without a reliable history it must be assumed that the patient has endured a lengthy period of cold exposure if he is unconscious or the rectal temperature is less than 93°F (34°C) when he is admitted to the hospital. This patient should be rewarmed slowly over 24 to 36 hours by wrapping him with blankets and monitoring closely in a warm room. This approach is based on the generally held belief that the physiologic derangements which develop with hypothermia of long duration must necessarily require several hours to return toward normal. The risk of rewarming shock should be lessened if externally applied heat is not used until the core temperature rises above the upper limit of the 77 to 82.5°F (25 to 28°C) range, in which cardiac arrhythmias and cardiac arrest frequently occur (Virtue, 1955).

Respiratory assistance with oxygen is important during rewarming. Hillman concluded in 1972 that the most critical defect in a hypothermic patient is hypoxemia from respiratory depression, and correction of this state should be commenced at the earliest possible time. Since intubation often aggravates cardiac arrhythmias in the face of hypothermia, it should be deferred until at least after the patient is well oxygenated by mask and the rectal temperature is above the high risk range (77 to 82.5°F or 25 to 28°C) for cardiac irritability. Because hypothermic lungs lose pulmonary compliance, care must be taken to avoid excessive inflation pressures. Hillman (1971) felt that once the blood has been oxygenated, the rewarming rate can proceed as fast as is convenient; however, further clinical study will be necessary for confirmation.

Administration of 5 per cent dextrose in water prewarmed to 100°F (38°C) should be started and continued slowly, since blood glucose is not well utilized in a hypothermic patient. Because of poor absorption and possible temperature dependence, drugs, especially morphine, must be administered cautiously. Since the output of the adrenal cortex has been observed to decrease with hypothermia (Hume, Egdahl and Nelson, 1956), this factor may contribute to rewarming shock. Thus intravenous steroids may be of value; however, this is not supported by a recent clinical study (Woolf, 1972). Because frequent rewarming complications are pulmonary edema and subsequent pneumonia, antibiotic coverage is warranted in hypothermic patients.

In hypothermic animals, low molecular weight dextran has been reported to decrease erythrocyte aggregation and blood viscosity and to decrease the incidence of cardiac arrhythmia (Fukusumi and Adolph, 1970); it is reported to improve the microcirculatory status in humans (Löfström, 1957). Vasopressor drugs, to control peripheral vasodilation, have been used in the past, but no definite benefit has been observed. Intravenous lidocaine may be useful for cardiac arrhythmias, and a defibrillator must be available should fibrillation supervene. Since electrical defibrillation is not usually successful with cardiac temperatures below 82.5°F (28°C) (Lloyd, 1971; Towne and coworkers, 1972), cardiac massage and artificial respiration must be maintained until the core temperature can be raised.

Hypothermia and Short Exposure to Cold. If, upon reaching the hospital, the patient is conscious and has a rectal temperature of 93°F (34°C) or higher, the exposure time probably was short. A patient of this type could be rapidly rewarmed, and this can be done by immersion in warm water at 104°F (40°C). However, rewarming by immersion may not always be desirable, as, for example, when major injuries coexist; effective cardiorespiratory resuscitation measures are made more difficult should this become necessary. Alternatively rapid rewarming can be achieved, though less effectively, with heating blankets and a heating mattress. The treatment is the same as that recommended for the patient being slowly rewarmed.

If frozen tissue coexists with hypothermia, it should be noted that the core temperature must be elevated to near normal levels before the local rewarming measures described earlier will be optimally effective. Despite the method of rewarming employed, the mortality rate after accidental hypothermia is high, ranging from 40 to 80 per cent in many series (Fernandez, O'Rouke and Ewy, 1970; Gregory, 1972); therefore, local cold injuries are of secondary priority. Regardless of the general physical appearance, the rectal temperature should be obtained in every cold-injured patient to detect possible subclinical hypothermia.

In recent years a small experience with new forms of rewarming procedures for hypothermic patients has been reported and deserves mention. Rewarming "internally" rather than by externally applied heat could theoretically eliminate the problem of peripheral vasodilation. Internal warming has been attempted in a variety of ways, including thoracotomy and direct warming of the mediastinum with heated physiologic saline solution (Linton and Ledingham, 1966) and peritoneal dialysis with warmed solutions (Lash, Burdette and Ozdil, 1967). Other methods attempted are extracorporeal circulation systems, incorporating a heat exchanger with either hemodialysis equipment (Davies, Millar and Miller, 1967) or cardiopulmonary bypass equipment (Towne and associates, 1972), and centripetal carotid infusion (Rogers and Hillman, 1970). Inhalation of heated gases administered with anesthesiology equipment has also been recently used (Henderson and Pettigrew, 1971) and would appear to hold the most promise. This technique, as described by Lloyd (1971), allows sufficient portability to permit initiation of rewarming prior to evacuation with continuation of treatment throughout the transfer to a hospital facility, while at the same time providing oxygenation for the patient. These above techniques of rewarming must be subjected to further clinical trials before their use can be advocated.

REFERENCES

Adolph, E. F.: Some differences in responses to low temperatures between warm-blooded and cold-blooded vertebrates. Am. J. Physiol., *166*:92, 1951.

Alexander, L.: Item No. 24, File No. 27-37 (Combined Intelligence Objectives Subcommittee, U.S. Army, July, 1945); Reported by Gagge, A. P., and Herrington, L. P.: Physiologic effects of heat and cold. Am. Rev. Physiol., 9:409, 1947.

Allison, F., Smith, M. R., and Wood, W. B.: Studies on the pathogenesis of acute inflammation: Inflammatory reaction to thermal injury as observed in the rabbit ear chamber. J. Exp. Med., *102*:655, 1955.

Bellman, S., and Adams-Ray, J.: Vascular reactions after experimental cold injury; a microangiographic study on rabbit ears. Angiology, 7:339, 1956.

Bellman, S., and Strombeck, J. O.: Transformation of the vascular system in cold-injured tissue of rabbit's ear. Angiology, *11*:108, 1960.

Bergentz, S. E., Gelin, L. E., and Rudenstam, C. M.: Intravascular aggregation of blood cells following intravenous infusion of fat emulsion. Acta Chir. Scand., *120*:115, 1960.

Bergentz, S. E., Eiken, O., and Nilsson, I. M.: The effect of dextran of various molecular weights on the coagulation in dogs. Thromb. Diath. Haemorrh. 6:15, 1961.

Bergman, H. J.: Platelet agglutinability as a factor in hemostasis. Second European Conference on Microcirculation, Pavia, 1962. Bibl. Anat., 4:736, 1964.

Bigelow, W. G., Lindsay, W. K., and Greenwood, W. F.: Hypothermia. Ann. Surg., *132*:849, 1950.

Blair, J. R.: Sequelae to cold injury in one hundred patients. *In* Vierech, E. (Ed.): Proceedings Symposia on Arctic Biology and Medicine. IV. Frostbite. Fort Wainwright, Alaska, Arctic Aeromedical Laboratory, 1964, pp. 321–355.

Block, M.: Cerebral effects of rewarming following prolonged hypothermia. Brain, 90:769, 1967.

Campbell, R.: General outcooling and local frostbite. *In* Viereck, E. (Ed.): Proceedings Symposia on Arctic Biology and Medicine. IV. Frostbite. Fort Wainwright, Alaska, Arctic Aeromedical Laboratory, 1964, p. 251.

Davies, D. M., Millar, E. J., and Miller, I. A.: Accidental hypothermia treated by extracorporal blood-warming. Lancet, *1*:1036, 1967.

Davis, L., Scarff, J. E., Rogers, N., and Dickinson, M.: High altitude frostbite; Preliminary report. Surg. Gynecol. Obstet., 77:561, 1943.

Deykin, D.: Emerging concepts of platelet function. New Engl. J. Med., *290*:144, 1974.

Duguid, H., Simpson, R. G., and Stowers, J. M.: Accidental hypothermia. Lancet, 2:1213, 1961.

Eiseman, B., and Spencer, F. C.: Effect of hypothermia on the flow characteristics of blood. Surgery, 52:532, 1962.

Fernandez, J. P., O'Rourke, R. A., and Ewy, G. A.: Rapid active external rewarming in accidental hypothermia. J.A.M.A., *212*:153, 1970.

Freeman, J., and Pugh, L.: Hypothermia in mountain accidents. Int. Anesthesiol. Clin., 7:997, 1969.

Friedman, N. B., Lange, K., and Weiner, D.: The pathology of experimental frostbite. Am. J. Med. Sci., *213*:61, 1947.

Fruehan, A.: Accidental hypothermia. Arch. Intern. Med., *106*:218, 1960.

Fuhrman, F. A., and Crismon, J. M.: Studies on gangrene following cold injury. VII. Treatment of cold injury by immediate rapid rewarming. J. Clin. Invest., 26:476, 1947.

Fukusumi, H., and Adolph, R. J.: Effect of dextran exchange upon the immersion hypothermic heart. J. Thorac. Cardiovasc. Surg., 59:251, 1970.

Gelin, L. E.: Anemia of injury. Acta Chir. Scand. (Suppl.), *210*:83, 1956.

Gregory, R. T.: Treatment after exposure to cold. Lancet, *1*:377, 1972.

Hakstian, R. W.: Cold-induced digital epiphyseal necrosis in childhood (systemic focal ischemia necrosis). Can. J. Surg., *15*:168, 1972.

Henderson, M. A., and Pettigrew, R. T.: Induction of controlled hyperthermia in treatment of cancer. Lancet, *1*:1275, 1971.

Hillman, H.: Treatment after exposure to cold. Lancet, *2*:1257, 1971.

Hillman, H.: Treatment after exposure to cold. Lancet, *1*:140, 1972.

Hume, D. M., Egdahl, R. H., and Nelson, D. H.: The effect of hypothermia on pituitary ACTH release and on adrenal cortical and medullary secretion in the dog. *In* Dripps, R. D. (Ed.): Physiology of Induced Hypothermia. Washington, National Academy of Sciences—National Research Council, 1956, p. 170.

Kattlove, H. E., and Alexander, B.: The effect of cold on platelets. I. Cold-induced platelet aggregation. Blood, *38*:39, 1971.

Killian, H.: Das Wesen der Kälteschäden. Schweiz. Med. Wochenschr., *79*:1262, 1949.

Kinmouth, J. B., Rob, C. G., and Simeone, F. B.: The cryopathies. *In* Vascular Surgery. London, E. Arnold, 1962, pp. 164–182.

Knize, D. M., Weatherley-White, R. C. A., and Paton, B. C.: Use of antisludging agents in experimental cold injuries. Surg. Gynecol. Obstet., *129*:1019, 1969a.

Knize, D. M., Weatherley-White, R. C. A., Paton, B. C., and Owens, J. C.: Prognostic factors in the management of frostbite. J. Trauma, *9*:749, 1969b.

Kreyberg, L., and Hanssen, O. F.: Necrosis of whole mouse skin *in situ* and survival of transplanted epithelium after freezing to −78°C and −190°C. Scand. J. Clin. Lab. Invest., *2*:168, 1950.

Kulka, J. P.: Histopathologic studies in frostbitten rabbits. *In* Ferrer, M. I. (Ed.): Cold Injury. New York, Josiah Macy, Jr., Foundation, 1956, p. 97.

Kulka, J. P.: Microcirculatory impairment as a factor in inflammatory tissue damage. Ann. N.Y. Acad. Sci., *116*:1018, 1964.

Lash, R. F., Burdette, J. A., and Ozdil, T.: Accidental hypothermia and barbiturate intoxication. A report of rapid "core" rewarming by peritoneal dialysis. J.A.M.A., *201*:269, 1967.

Linton, A. L., and Ledingham, I. M.: Severe hypothermia with barbiturate intoxication. Lancet, *1*:24, 1966.

Lloyd, E. L.: Treatment after exposure to cold. Lancet, *2*:1376, 1971.

Löfström, B.: Changes in blood volume in induced hypothermia. Acta Anes. Scand., *1*:1, 1957.

Lovelock, J. E.: The denaturation of lipid-protein complexes as a cause of damage by freezing. Proc. R. Soc. (Biol.), *147*:427, 1957.

Lutz, B. R.: Intravascular agglutination of the formed elements of the blood. Physiol. Rev., *31*:107, 1951.

Maggio, E.: Microhemocirculation. Springfield, Ill., Charles C Thomas, Publisher, 1965, pp. 95–118.

Majno, G., Schoefl, G. C., and Palade, G. E.: Effect of histamine and serotonin on vascular permeability. Fed. Proc., *20*:119, 1961.

Markert, C. L.: Lactate dehydrogenase isozymes: Dissociation and recombination of subunits. Science, *140*:1329, 1963.

Mazur, P.: Studies on rapidly frozen suspension of yeast cells by differential thermal analysis and conductometry. Biophys. J., *3*:323, 1963.

Mazur, P.: Causes of injury in frozen and thawed cells. Fed. Proc., *24*(Suppl. 14–15):5, 1965.

Merrill, E. W., Gilliland, E. R., and Lee, T. S.: Blood rheology; effect of fibrinogen deduced by addition. Circ. Res., *18*:437, 1966.

Merryman, H. T.: Mechanisms of freezing in living cells and tissues. Science, *124*:515, 1956.

Merryman, H. T.: The exceeding of a minimum tolerable cell volume in hypertonic suspension as a cause of freezing injury. *In* Walstenholme, G., and O'Connor, M. (Eds.): The Frozen Cell. London, J. and A. Churchill, 1970, p. 51.

Mills, W. J., and Whaley, R.: Frostbite: A method of management. *In* Viereck, E. G. (Ed.): Proceedings Symposia on Arctic Biology and Medicine. IV. Frostbite. Fort Wainwright, Alaska, Arctic Aeromedical Laboratory, 1964, p. 127.

Mills, W. J., Whaley, R., and Fish, W.: Frostbite: Experience with rapid rewarming and ultrasonic therapy. Alaska Med., *3*:28, 1961.

Molnar, G. W.: An evaluation of wind chill. *In* Horvath, S. M. (Ed.): Cold Injury. New York, Josiah Macy, Jr., Foundation, 1958, p. 175.

Moran, T.: Critical temperature of freezing living muscle. Proc. R. Soc., B, *105*:177, 1929.

Mundth, E. D.: Studies of the pathogenesis of cold injury. Microcirculatory changes in tissue injured by freezing. *In* Viereck, E. G. (Ed.): Proceedings Symposia on Arctic Biology and Medicine. IV. Frostbite. Fort Wainwright, Alaska, Arctic Aeromedical Laboratory, 1964, pp. 51–72.

Mundth, L. D., Long, D. M., and Brown, R. B.: Treatment of experimental frostbite with low molecular weight dextran. J. Trauma, *4*:246, 1964.

Orr, K. O., and Fainer, D. C.: Cold injuries in Korea during the winter of 1950–1951. Medicine, *31*:177, 1952.

Osborn, J. J.: Experimental hypothermia: Respiratory and blood pH changes in relation to cardiac function. Am. J. Physiol., *175*:389, 1953.

Pirozynski, W. J., and Webster, D. R.: Effect of hyaluronidase in edema following experimental cold injury. Proc. Soc. Exp. Biol. Med., *80*:306, 1952.

Quintanella, R., Krusen, F., and Essex, H.: Studies on frost-bite with special reference to treatment and the effect on minute blood vessels. Am. J. Physiol., *149*:149, 1947.

Radomski, M. W.: Response of lipoprotein lipase in various tissues to cold exposure. Am. J. Physiol., *220*:1852, 1971.

Robb, H. J.: Microvascular response to trauma. J. Trauma, *3*:407, 1963.

Rogers, P., and Hillman, H.: Increased recovery of anesthetized hypothermic rats induced by intracarotid infusion. Nature (Lond.), *228*:1314, 1970.

Sandison, J. C.: Observation on the circulating blood cells, adventitial (Rouget) and muscle cells, endothelium and macrophages in the transparent chamber of the rabbit ear. Anat. Rec., *50*:355, 1931.

Schatzki, R.: Roentgenologic changes in bones following cold injury in man. *In* Ferrer, M. I. (Ed.): Cold Injury. New York, Josiah Macy, Jr., Foundation, 1956, p. 37.

Shikama, K., and Yamuzahi, I.: Denaturization of catalase by freezing and thawing. Nature (Lond.), *190*:83, 1961.

Shumaker, H. B., Jr., Radigan, L. R., Ziperman, H. H., and Hughes, R. R.: Effect of Rutin and Benadryl with some notes on plaster casts and the role of edema. Angiology, *2*:100, 1951.

Skjorten, F.: Studies in the ultrastructure of pseudopod formation in human blood platelets. I. Effect of temperature, period of incubation, anticoagulant and mechanical force. Scand. J. Haematol., *5*:401, 1968.

Smith, A. U.: Biological effects of freezing and supercooling. *In* Effects of Subzero Temperature on Animal Cells and Tissues. Baltimore, Williams & Wilkins Company, 1961, p. 411.

Stowell, R. E., Young, D. E., Arnold, E. A., and Trump, B. F.: Structural chemical, physical and functional alterations in mammalian nucleus following different conditions of freezing, storage and thawing. Fed. Proc., *24*(Suppl. 15):5, 1965.

Swank, R. L.: Changes in blood produced by a fat meal and by intravenous heparin. J. Physiol., *164*:798, 1951.

Talbott, J. H., Consolazid, W. V., and Pecora, L. J.: Hypothermia. Arch. Intern. Med., *68*:1120, 1941.

Tishler, J. M.: The soft tissue and bone changes in frostbite injuries. Radiology, *102*:511, 1972.

Towne, W. D., Geiss, W. P., Yanes, H. O., and Rahimtoola, S. H.: Intractable ventricular fibrillation associated with profound accidental hypothermia — Successful treatment with partial cardiopulmonary by-pass. New Engl. J. Med., *287*:1135, 1972.

Trump, B. F., Young, D. E., Arnold, E. A., and Stowell, R. E.: Effects of freezing and thawing on the structure, chemical constitution and function of cytoplasmic structure. Fed. Proc., *24*(Suppl. 15)S-144, 1965.

Virtue, R. W.: Hypothermic Anesthesia. Springfield, Ill., Charles C Thomas, Publisher, 1955.

Weatherly-White, R. C. A., Sjostrom, B., and Paton, B. C.: Experimental studies in cold injury. J. Surg. Res., *4*: 17, 1964.

Weatherley-White, R. C. A., Knize, D. M., Geisterfer, D. J., and Paton, B. C.: Experimental studies in cold injury. Surgery, *66*:208, 1969.

Whayne, T. F., and DeBakey, M. F.: Cold Injury, Ground Type. Washington, U.S. Government Printing Office, 1958.

Woolf, P. D.: Accidental hypothermia: Endocrine function during recovery. J. Clin. Endocr., *34*:460, 1972.

Zingg, W.: The management of accidental hypothermia. Can. Med. Assoc. J., *96*:214, 1967.

Zweifach, B. W.: Functional Behavior of the Microcirculation. Springfield, Ill., Charles C Thomas, Publisher, 1961, p. 105.

CHAPTER 20

RADIATION EFFECTS

Biological and Surgical Considerations

STEPHAN ARIYAN, M.D.,
AND THOMAS J. KRIZEK, M.D.

On a cold and wintry evening in Bavaria in January, 1896, Rudolph Albert von Kölliker, an 80 year old biologist, stood before a strange machine, placed his hand on the glass part of the machine, and waited as Wilhelm Konrad Roentgen (1845–1923) pressed the electric switch. A red light appeared, and a photographic plate was exposed. When a few minutes later the picture was developed, it showed clearly the bones of von Kölliker's hand against the soft tissue background. When this was reported the next day in the press, the world learned of a "new kind of ray." Because its characteristics were unknown, it was labeled "X"—X-ray.*

Roentgen's discovery (1895) actually occurred several months earlier when he observed a greenish glow near a Crookes tube which had the ability to penetrate solid matter and expose photographic plates. The discovery ushered in the era of modern medicine, pro-

vided a diagnostic tool without which some specialties could not exist, and offered a therapeutic modality which has cured disease and alleviated the suffering of untold thousands. However, like many other potent agents, its use may be attended by accidental injury or serious side effects. The first cases of acute radiation dermatitis were reported within a year (Daniel, 1896). Soon thereafter, the effect of chronic exposure to small doses of radiation was noted as skin cancer on the hand of a technician, who had been demonstrating this new "X-ray" for four years (Frieben, 1902).

The discovery of additional injuries identified over the years has led to a high degree of protection for and awareness on the part of those likely to be chronically exposed. There remain several circumstances in which the effects of radiation require or influence the care provided by reconstructive surgeons: (a) patients accidentally exposed to high doses of radiation, from either industrial accidents or war; (b) patients who require surgery after either planned preoperative therapeutic radiation or radiation therapy failure; (c) patients who develop radiation injury either shortly after or many years after therapeutic radiation.

---

*"X," the twenty-fourth letter of the English alphabet, has origins unknown prior to its appearance in the Greek alphabet. In mathematics, the symbol X has long been used to represent the unknown quantity.

ETIOLOGY

In contrast to other forms of radiation such as visible light or infrared, the effects of radiation therapy are due to "ionizing radiation." This means simply that photons are delivered which have sufficiently high energy to ionize and break chemical bonds. Photons are small packages of energy, of which there are several types.

Alpha Particles. These particles are relatively large, are positively charged, and are, in fact, helium nuclei. Because of their relatively large mass, they are stopped by 2 to 9 cm of air. None can pass through a thin sheet of paper. Radium and radioactive isotopes, when injected or taken orally, will emit alpha particles into surrounding tissues.

Beta Particles. These are negatively charged particles with very small masses traveling at very high speeds. They are actually electrons. With their high speeds, they may penetrate up to 1 cm of tissue but are easily stopped by thin sheets of metal. They are therapeutically useful in thin and superficial layers of tissue and are used, for example, in the electron beam therapy of mycosis fungoides.

Gamma Rays. These are uncharged photons of energy traveling at the speed of light. They have the ability to penetrate to deep layers of tissue and have a therapeutic value. They are a product of the natural decay of radioactive material, e.g., radium and cobalt-60.

Roentgen or X-rays. These are identical in basic properties with gamma rays but are produced artificially by the bombardment of electrons onto a tungsten target, from which the X-rays are emitted. For practical purposes, gamma and X-rays are the same.

Orthovoltage. Orthovoltage refers to the range of radiation particles whose energy is less than a million volts, generated by machines delivering energy in the range of 80,000 to 400,000 volts, or 80 to 400 kilo electron volts (kev).

Supervoltage. Supervoltage describes the range of particles or radiation whose energy exceeds a million volts. These are generated by particle accelerators such as the betatron, cyclotron, or linear accelerator. The usual therapeutic range is between 4 and 8 million electron volts (Mev). The recently introduced Sagittaire units will deliver energy in excess of 22 million electron volts (Mev).

Rad. The rad is the most common unit of measurement in therapeutic radiation. It does not represent the energy that leaves the machine but rather the energy absorbed per unit mass of irradiated tissue from the ionizing particles. This is calculated from the known energy source, the distance to the tissue, and the types of tissue irradiated. One rad represents 100 ergs absorbed per gram of tissue irradiated. This concept of volume of tissue is most important. It is, for example, meaningless to say that a patient who has received 6000 rads to his tongue, 4000 rads to his neck, and 4000 rads to his chest has received 14,000 rads. It is like saying that a five-room house has a temperature of 350° F because the temperature of each room is 70° F. The volume of tissue must be identified.

BIOLOGICAL EFFECTS OF RADIATION

The total effect of radiation on tissues is not thoroughly understood. Ionizing radiation damages biological material in a unique way, unlike mechanical, thermal, or chemical injury, and it is probably a confusing misnomer to label it a "burn." The effects at the molecular level are both random and an "all or none" phenomenon. The resultant damage to a cell is determined by the relative importance of the destroyed molecule to the function of the cell. In the dose range encountered clinically (1000 to 10,000 rads), the biologically significant damage is that which occurs to DNA. Most of this damage can be repaired, and enzymatic processes may continue. However, genetic information is lost, and the cell loses its ability to divide indefinitely and produce a clone.

The clinical significance of this is clear. At doses 100 to 1000 times the usual therapeutic dose, rapid dissolution of cells occurs, and there are early gross and microscopic alterations in tissue. In the therapeutic range, there are no such clinical or microscopic changes until that time at which the injured cells attempt to divide, often many weeks later. In rapidly dividing cell populations, such as lymphocytes or intestinal mucosal cells, the effects may be manifest within hours or days. In populations of cells such as neurons or striated muscle which do not normally reproduce, even though the radiation may have destroyed the same genetic information in the DNA, the effect is never clinically or microscopically observed since the cell usually does not replicate. These tissues are therefore said to be "radioresistant."

The ability of tissue to repair itself after radiation injury is related entirely to the population of surviving cells. The biology of tumors is such that the tumor cells are turning over more slowly and are less numerous than the surrounding normal tissue. Since they are more numerous and have a rapid turnover rate, the surrounding normal cells are able to repopulate the area and allow healing to occur, even though some of their population has been destroyed in the same random fashion as tumor cells. If this were not the case, all therapeutic radiation of tumors would result in a residual open wound as the tumor disappeared.

DIAGNOSIS

A complete description of the problem or injury related to radiation requires documentation of a number of factors. The evaluation should include (a) a description of the area or region which has been exposed to radiation; (b) an assessment of the total dose which has been absorbed by the tissue; (c) the duration of the exposure to the radiation (hours, days, weeks); and (d) a description of the source of the radiation.

For example, when a patient who has received therapeutic radiation to a tongue lesion is being evaluated, an appropriate description would state that the patient received "6000 rads to his oral cavity and upper neck, in 30 treatments, over a 40-day period using a 6 Mev linear accelerator, ending 3 months ago."

LOCAL EFFECTS OF RADIATION INJURY

The local effects of radiation injury may be grouped for purposes of discussion into three major categories: acute, subacute, and chronic radiation injury.

Acute Radiation Injury. Acute radiation injury is usually the result of accidental injury, such as in industry, and will most often involve orthovoltage radiation. Exposure to a high dose of radiation in a short period of time (for example, 5000 to 10,000 rads in one day) produces injury of the skin and local tissues which resembles thermal burns in appearance but differs from burns by evolving more slowly and deeply. These changes were well described in a treatise by Warren (1943). The basal cells, which must divide regularly to maintain the epidermis, are damaged and show mitotic derangement immediately. In response to this injury, a transitory erythema may develop within minutes and may recur in cyclic waves. The recurrent nature of this erythema is not well understood.

The erythema is soon accompanied by edema, itching, and pain. These are followed by "dry desquamation" (scaling and flaking), "wet desquamation" (blistering and weeping), and sloughing and ulceration of the skin. There may be ischemic necrosis of the underlying tissue, as well as progressive, diffuse, obliterative endarteritis (Knowlton and associates, 1949; Upton, 1968). The chronic vasculitis causes pain of an unrelenting nature. The most serious sequelae to the vasculitis are progressive tissue ischemia, secondary infection, and necrosis (see Figs. 20–1 and 20–2).

Subacute Radiation Injury. This may result from the administration of repeated doses of lower intensity radiation over a longer period of time. There is also an erythema of the skin with associated edema. Mucous membranes may become inflamed. There is usually no ulceration or necrosis, and the edema and erythema subside over a period of several weeks. Following an interval of several months, the skin and subcutaneous tissue become thickened and harden into a "woody induration"; the skin subsequently develops a darker pigmentation. These changes are usually seen in the therapeutic ranges of radiation therapy, particularly when it has been delivered by orthovoltage machines.

Chronic Radiation Injury. Chronic radiation damage results from repeated low dose exposures to radiation, often over a long period of time. It has historically occurred as an occupational hazard in X-ray technicians and dentists. It can also be observed many years later in those who received therapeutic radiation, often, tragically, for benign disease. The chronic changes may progress to the most serious of sequelae, namely malignant transformation of skin, soft tissue, or bone.

The histologic changes which occur through

these phases are the same as for acute and subacute radiation injury but vary in time of evolution and intensity with the type of injury (Allen, 1954). Changes in the epidermis include early swelling of the prickle cell layer, edema of the basal cell layer and increased melanin production. Large nuclei first appear, followed by hyperkeratosis, acanthosis, and finally atrophy of the epidermis. The effects on the dermis are even more profound. In the acute phase there is edema and vesiculation of the upper dermis, which may lead to separation of the epidermis or subsequent dense scarring. There is progressive atrophy of hair follicles, sebaceous glands, and eccrine glands. Loss of elastic fibers and severe fibrosis may also be observed.

The most profound changes, and those of greatest concern to the surgeon, are the alterations in vascularity. An initial vasodilatation is followed by fibrinoid necrosis of vessel walls and thromboses. The end result is an obliterative endarteritis with chronic ischemia. The vascular changes pose the greatest challenge to the reconstructive surgeon.

"The effects of surgery are permanent...the effects of radiation are permanent, continuous, and progressive."

— Anonymous

SYSTEMIC EFFECTS OF RADIATION INJURY

In contrast to radiation administered to local areas of the body, intense whole-body radiation, as in those who were exposed to the atomic bombs, results in "radiation sickness." The latter may be separated into three phases — prodromal, latent, and main.

Prodromal Phase. This phase is characterized by gastrointestinal symptoms of anorexia, nausea, vomiting, and diarrhea. The dose necessary to cause the symptoms varies among individuals but is in the range of 50 rads total body dosage.

Latent Period. This is the period of time which is necessary for the depletion of cells irreparably damaged by the radiation. It is only after this interval that their sustained disturbances are manifest. The rapidity with which the cells are depleted depends on the dose and the tissues involved and may last hours to weeks.

Main Phase. This phase of the syndrome begins as the effects of the depletion of the cells during the latent phase become clinically manifest. The degree depends on the number of immature cells remaining to preserve or restore function. However, severe radiation damage to the brain or cardiovascular systems (20,000 rads) may result in death within minutes to hours. In the absence of such damage, death in severe injuries usually results from irreparable bone marrow or intestinal injury. It is estimated that 2000 rads to the whole body results in fatal enteritis within two weeks (Upton, 1968). Damage to the other tissues is usually of secondary importance in such severe radiation injuries.

MALIGNANT TRANSFORMATION

Ionizing radiation not only cures cancer but also may cause it. The conditions that set the stage for malignant transformation may be chronic inflammation, chronic exposure to radiation, or a combination of these. Laboratory studies in animals have suggested a co-carcinogenic effect of inflammation and radiation. Radiation administered to wounds chronically infected with bacteria (Lacassagne and Vinzent, 1929a, b) or chronically inflamed by sterile foreign bodies (Lacassagne, 1933; Burrows and Clarkson, 1943) has led to the development of sarcomas, while none developed in control animals exposed to radiation alone.

Chronic or repeated exposure to radiation has also been shown to have a carcinogenic effect on tissues. This phenomenon was demonstrated by Hoffman (1925) and Martland (1925, 1931) in the radium watch dial painters who were exposed to repeated bombardment by alpha particles. The dial painters swallowed the radium in the fluorescent paint when they pointed the brush tips on their tongues. The radium was absorbed and deposited in bones and emitted radioactive alpha particles continually. High levels of radiation located in the maxilla apparently disposed to malignancy in the mucous membranes of the sinuses (Warren, 1970). Warren also felt that this type of carcinogenesis, resulting from the chronic inhalation of radioactive gas in the air, was the cause of the bronchogenic carcinomas seen in the uranium miners of Colorado and the pitchblende miners of Europe (Ludewig and Lorenser, 1924). In addition, it has been noted that individuals receiving repeated small doses of radiation over long periods, such as physicians, dentists, radiologists, and technicians, have a higher incidence of skin cancer (Teloh, Mason and Wheelock, 1950; Huerper, 1954) and leukemia (Ulrich, 1946; Warren, 1956; March, 1961).

Acute or short-term exposure may also be associated with malignant transformation of the tissue within the irradiated field. Through the joint efforts of the Atomic Bomb Casualty Commission of the United States and the Japanese National Institute of Health, extensive studies, conducted over 25 years, of the Japanese survivors of the atomic bombs have led to the conclusion that there is a greater incidence of leukemia and thyroid carcinoma among the exposed people (Brill, Tomonaga and Heyssel, 1962; Socolow and coworkers, 1963; Zeldis, Jablon and Ishida, 1964; Miller, 1969). Furthermore, Simpson and Hempelmann (1957) showed an association between thyroid carcinoma and the radiation treatment of thymic enlargement. Well-controlled reviews (Pifer and coworkers, 1963; Toyooka and coworkers, 1963) of 2800 children treated with X-rays for thymic enlargement between 1926 and 1957 in an upstate New York county revealed a significantly higher frequency of thyroid carcinoma and leukemia than in untreated siblings or in the general population of children in the same area.

The potential for malignant transformation of soft tissue and bone in an area of radiation injury is of particular concern. Although the skin and soft tissue may be surgically replaced, it might be hazardous if the danger of subsequent development of osteogenic sarcoma in the underlying irradiated bone were high. A review of the 129 cases of osteogenic sarcoma following radiation reported in the literature indicates that the chances of malignant transformation must be very small (Krizek and Ariyan, 1973). Among these cases, 20 followed radium ingestion (radium dial painters), 35 followed radiation for chronic inflammation (co-carcinogen effect?), and 74 followed treatment of benign or malignant neoplasm. However, as Kilgore and Abbott (1938) have emphasized, malignant transformation must not be considered unless histologic evidence of nonmalignancy has been obtained prior to radiation. In fact, Cahan and associates (1948) have listed several criteria which should be operative before one considers radiation to be responsible for malignant transformation. These criteria are:

1. There should be histologic evidence that there was no malignancy present prior to the radiation.

2. The malignancy must occur within the field exposed to radiation.

3. There should be a reasonable latent period.

4. The malignant change should be confirmed histologically.

It is clear from this list that all but 20 of the reported cases of osteogenic sarcoma do *not* meet the criteria.

Osteogenic sarcoma is among the least common forms of cancer, with an incidence in the normal population of 1 per 100,000 (Hatfield and Schulz, 1970; Warren, 1970). In fact, Warren points out that this rate has been decreasing over the past 20 years, at a time when radiation fallout has been increasing. Burch (1960) and Newcombe (1957) have attempted to extrapolate the incidence of carcinogenesis but have been unsuccessful because the data were too scanty. Compared to the millions of people exposed to or treated by radiation who have survived a long latent period, the incidence must be small, if it is indeed any higher than the incidence of such sarcomas in the population at large.

OSTEORADIONECROSIS

Since first described a half century ago by Ewing (1926), osteoradionecrosis ("radiation osteitis") has been a dilemma to both radiotherapist and surgeon. He felt that the changes seen in bone, particularly in the mandible and pelvis, were related to vascular damage, rendering the bones more susceptible to infection and trauma. Several reviews indicate that this problem has been in no way resolved by newer techniques and modalities for delivering radiation (Bragg, 1970; Kim, 1974), and an incidence of mandibular osteoradionecrosis as high as 10 to 30 per cent has been reported for head and neck cancer patients treated by radiation (Rankow and Weissman, 1971). Although the influence of infection and trauma are probably operative, the changes in vascularity appear to be of paramount importance. It is of interest that disuse atrophy may also play a role (see Fig. 20–3), and adequate resurfacing, particularly with blood-bearing flap tissue, may reverse the apparently established "osteoradionecrosis" (see Figs. 20–4 and 20–5).

In addition to the dose of radiation, other factors influencing the development of mandibular radionecrosis include the size of the tumor treated, the proximity of the tumor to bone, the state of oral hygiene, and the number of dental extractions. Exposure of the bone to the oral cavity during or after radiation therapy is a common prelude to radionecrosis. When dental extractions are accomplished and healing is proceeding prior to radiation, and when oral hygiene is meticulously maintained during radiation, the chances of radionecrosis are dramatically reduced. The most prominent surgical contribution to the prevention of osteoradionecrosis is soft tissue coverage over the affected bone.

GENERAL PRINCIPLES OF TREATMENT

There are several distinct circumstances in which the surgeon will be called upon to treat the effects produced by radiation. The approach will vary, depending on the nature of the problem, the site of involvement, and the phase of the injury (i.e., acute, subacute, chronic). The most common categories of problems are outlined below, and several illustrative cases are presented.
1. Acute radiation injury
2. Planned surgery after therapeutic radiation
3. Radiation ulcers
4. Malignant transformation

Acute Radiation Injury

Acute radiation injury is most often due to an industrial accident and usually involves the extremities, particularly the hands. The diagnosis is critical. To establish a diagnosis, the amount of radiation to the total body and to the involved local tissues should be known. The assistance of a radiation therapist and radiation physicist is mandatory. The circumstances of the injury are reconstructed, the time of exposure estimated, and dosimetry studies carried out (often with water phantoms). Data will indicate the amount of radiation absorbed per volume of tissue. For example, in the cases subsequently illustrated, such studies provided information concerning surface dose and exposure of underlying soft tissue and bone. The management of total body radiation is nonsurgical and beyond the scope of this discussion.

The initial approach is conservative. The

local effects of radiation are progressive, and the extent of injury may not be readily apparent during the early phase. The outstanding clinical finding is pain, to such a degree that hospitalization is mandatory. Large doses of narcotics and sedatives are required, and narcotic addiction is a not uncommon sequela of the injury. Local skin care with bland ointments and steroid creams may provide some relief.

Since these injuries often involve the hands, the principles of managing the acutely injured hand should not be ignored simply because it is a radiation injury. Splinting will often be necessary to maintain position: the metacarpophalangeal joints in full flexion and interphalangeal joints in extension, with the wrist above the neutral position. Splinting maintains position, but it is motion that preserves function; hydrotherapy and range of motion exercises are mandatory, even in the face of severe pain.

The conservative approach may be all that is required, and Brown, McDowell, and Fryer (1949a, b) and Brown and Fryer (1956, 1957, 1965) have reported large series of patients so managed. However, in more severe injuries, skin breakdown begins in the first few weeks. Open wounds, secondary infection, and ischemia potentially set in motion a cycle of ulcer, infection, necrosis, and additional ulcers and necrosis, leading finally to gangrene. Lanzl, Rozenfeld, and Tarlov (1967) have predicted the inevitability of this cycle and progression and have advised early amputation. The infection appears to be the key factor in triggering the cycle: an ischemic wound, infected often with *Pseudomonas aeruginosa*, not unlike that seen in thermal burns. The ischemic wound, isolated from the bloodstream (and from systemically administered antibiotics), should be treated like a burn with appropriate topical antibacterials.

No surgery is indicated until the wound passes into the subacute phase, characterized by the disappearance of much of the erythema and edema. At such time, wide excision of the involved tissue should be accomplished. Even the margins and the bed will admittedly also have been exposed to radiation. Since there is some evidence that this tissue, although viable and still vascular, has a diminished resistance to infection, systemic antibiotics prior to, during, and for 48 hours after surgery are indicated.

The *sine qua non* to successful management is adequate soft tissue coverage. Except in the most exceptional circumstances, in which tendons, bone, or joints are actually exposed, the use of split-thickness skin grafts is the treatment of choice. Since bleeding from these wounds may be troublesome and difficult to control, a delayed grafting technique (see Chapter 6) is employed, unless one is very confident of hemostasis. The open wound is covered with a biological dressing (allograft, amnion, or xenograft), and the patient is returned to the operating room in 24 to 48 hours for the definitive application of skin grafts. The grafts should be of medium thickness and without "pie-crusting"; mesh grafts have no place in the treatment of radiation lesions. Postoperative care is similar to that of a thermal burn, and in the case of the hand, motion should be started by the fifth postoperative day. The most remarkable feature of the treatment is the immediate, dramatic relief of pain which the patient experiences.

The patient deserves a conscientious followup. Although the incidence of osteogenic sarcoma is small, routine (annual) radiologic examination of the part is indicated. The early radiographic changes sometimes seen in the bones may be due to disuse atrophy, not to osteoradionecrosis, and may totally revert to normal after adequate resurfacing.

Case 1: Acute Radiation Injury of the Hand (19,500 rads). A 43 year old male was exposed to 19,500 rads (dominant right hand) for

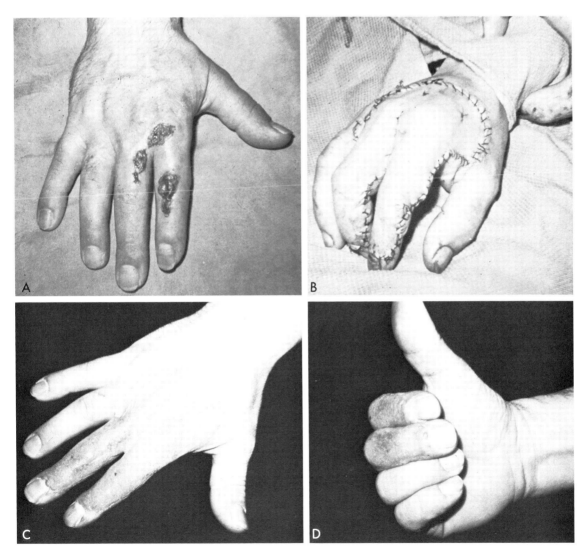

FIGURE 20–1. *A,* Massive radiation injury with skin necrosis three months after exposure to 19,500 rads. *B,* Wide area of excision and split-thickness skin graft coverage. *C, D,* Fifteen months after surgery, with full range of painless motion.

over several hours from an industrial 110-kev fluoroscope. He initially complained of "dermatitis," with itching and erythema over the dorsum of his index and middle fingers, symptoms which occurred within a few hours. He had further signs of radiation injury, with pain and breakdown of the skin over the subsequent ten days.

Prior to his surgical consultation, he had been treated by immobilization of the hand. The hand was treated with topical antibiotics, which resulted in healing of the weeping wounds, only to be followed by local skin breakdown (Fig. 20–1). When consulted three months after his injury, he had essentially no range of motion in the index finger and little motion in the middle finger. A biopsy was taken (Fig. 20–2), and this showed ulceration and the fibrinoid necrosis with vascular dilatation and arteriolar thickening that is usually seen in radionecrosis.

He was initially treated with analgesics and whirlpool therapy, accompanied by active and passive range of motion exercises. The hand

was placed in a dynamic splint with improvement of the range of motion. Two weeks after this therapy commenced, excision of the skin over the dorsum of the index and middle fingers and about half of the dorsum of the hand was accomplished. Active bleeding was observed in the wound bed, which was covered with a medium sized split-thickness skin graft (see Fig. 20–1, *B*).

Motion was again instituted with physical therapy after surgery, and the patient returned to work two months following surgery. At the end of one year, he had full range of motion (see Fig. 20–1, *C* and *D*).

The radiographic findings of his hand prior to surgery (Fig. 20–3) revealed demineralization and cystic degeneration, particularly adjacent to the interphalangeal joints. The findings were interpreted as being typical of osteoradionecrosis. Four months later, after motion had been restored and the wounds were healed, the radiographs were interpreted as being normal.

The patient is now at work four years after

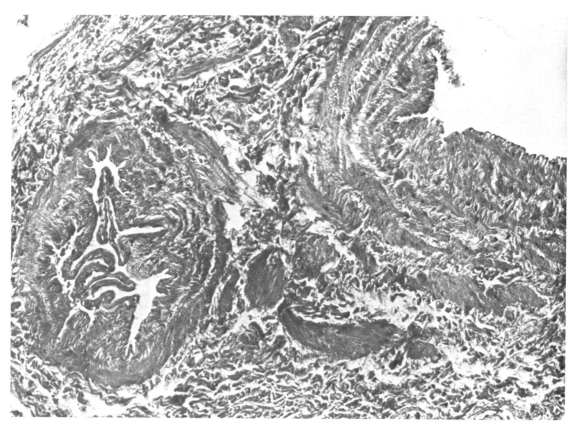

FIGURE 20–2.   Histologic appearance of radiation injury. Note fibrinoid necrosis, vascular dilatation, and arteriolar thickening.

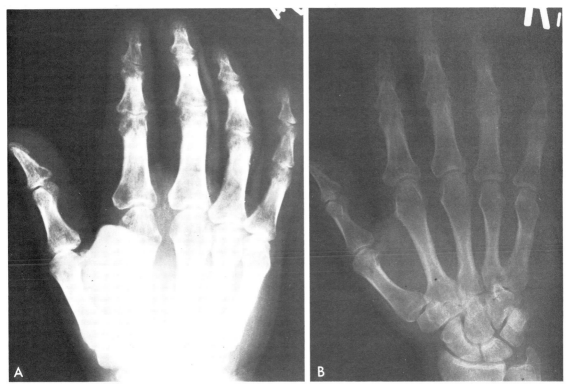

FIGURE 20–3. Radiographs of the hand seen in Figure 20–1. *A*, Preoperative film read as osteoradionecrosis. *B*, Four months following resurfacing, the bones appear normal.

injury and has a functional hand. Occasional arthritic-type pain is relieved with salicylates, and the radiographs remain normal.

Case 2: Acute Radiation Injury of the Hand (250,000 rads). A second patient, involved with the same faulty machine as in Case 1, was a 45 year old female who was exposed to 250,000 rads to both hands over a period of less than three hours. Additional calculations showed that a dose of 25,000 rads had been absorbed by the bone. She was initially treated in the same manner as the other patient prior to her transfer for surgical care, three months after the injuries. She had constant and excruciating pain and dry erythematous dermatitis over the dorsum of both index fingers and the tip of the left thumb (Fig. 20–4, *A*).

She was treated with active and passive range of motion exercises in whirlpool. The involved skin was excised down to the extensor mechanism over the dorsum of the right index and middle fingers; part of the dorsum of the hand was also resected (Fig. 20–4, *B, C*). Since the tendons were exposed and the blood supply of the bed did not appear satisfactory, the wound was covered with an undelayed deltopectoral flap (Fig. 20–4, *D*). Following excision of the ischemic tissue and covering of the wound, there was immediate and complete relief of pain.

Six weeks later, with return of functional range of motion to the right hand, the left hand was surgically treated. Since the ulceration of the left index finger involved not only the cutaneous surface but also the extensor tendon mechanism and the joint as well, a ray amputation was performed. In addition, the skin was removed over the thumb, first web space, and dorsum of the hand (Fig. 20–4, *E*). The wound was covered with a deltopectoral flap from the contralateral side.

After division, the flaps of both hands were revised and subsequently defatted. There was gradual increase in the ranges of motion in both hands (Fig. 20–4, *F* to *I*). The patient has been followed for four years with no evidence of pain. Recent X-rays showed no evidence of inflammatory or necrotic changes of the bone. An arteriogram that had been performed just prior to surgery had demonstrated marked diminution of flow to the digital arteries, and

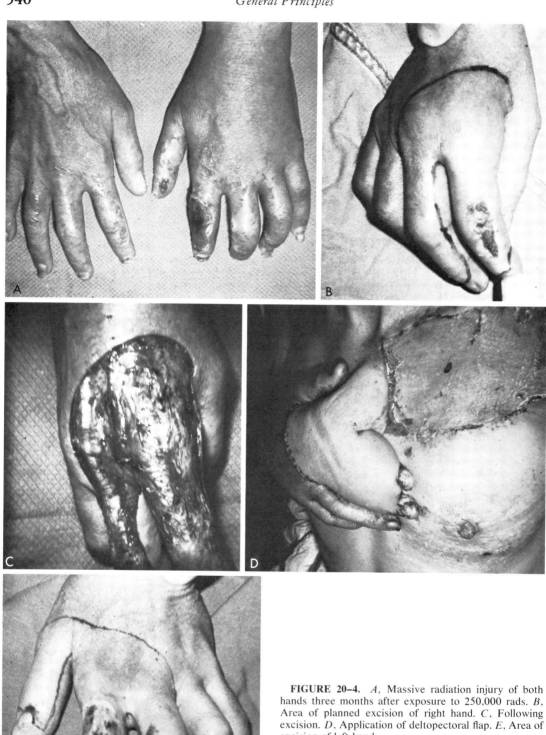

FIGURE 20–4. *A*, Massive radiation injury of both hands three months after exposure to 250,000 rads. *B*, Area of planned excision of right hand. *C*, Following excision. *D*, Application of deltopectoral flap. *E*, Area of excision of left hand.

Illustration continued on opposite page

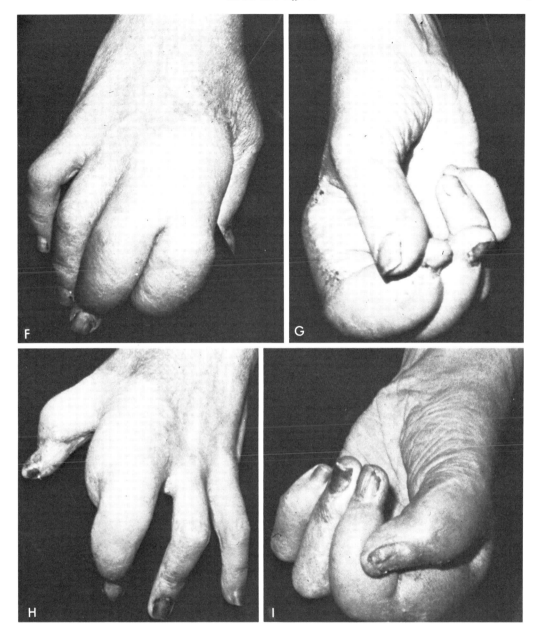

FIGURE 20–4 *(Continued).* *F, G,* Resurfaced right hand with adequate function 15 months following surgery. *H, I,* Resurfaced left hand.

precapillary arteriovenous shunts (Fig. 20–5). One year later, however, a repeat arteriogram showed revascularization and satisfactory blood flow throughout the hand.

Planned Surgery after Radiation Therapy

Therapeutic radiation followed by definitive surgery is a common approach to the manage-

ment of head and neck cancer in many centers. The rationale, even if not yet documented by valid statistical data to show improved survival, is predicated on solid reasoning. Surgical failures in head and neck cancer are related to the inability to provide adequate margins of resection. Radiation therapy fails because of an inability to control the large volume of tumor located centrally.

An understanding of radiation biology and

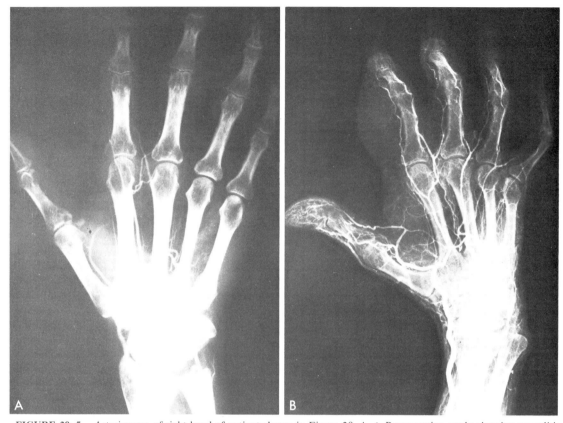

FIGURE 20–5. Arteriogram of right hand of patient shown in Figure 20–4. *A,* Preoperative study showing vasculitis and poor circulatory flow. *B,* At one year, vascularization is normal.

radiation effects provides the basis for the surgical approach in these circumstances. Several principles are involved:

1. Radiation therapy reduces bulk and renders it technically feasible to remove "inoperable" cancers; it does *not* make them more curable.

2. The volume of tissue which must be removed for cure is exactly the same after radiation therapy as it was before treatment.

3. The rate of disappearance, or lack of shrinkage in tumor size, has nothing to do with its "response" to radiation.

4. The surgical approach to head and neck cancer must be altered when operating in radiated fields.

If we conceive of a room (a tumor) full of balloons (tumor cells) and place ourselves in one corner with a bushel basket full of darts (rads), we have an appropriate analogy. As we stand blindfolded throwing darts (rads), we will begin breaking balloons. In the beginning we will break many balloons (tumor cells), and after 1000 darts (rads), we will have broken 90

per cent of them. After another 1000 darts (rads), we will have destroyed another 90 per cent of whatever is left. Success is based solely on random chance. If the room (tumor size) is small, the balloons (cells) few, and the darts (rads) many, we always succeed. Conversely, if the room is large, we are only partially successful. The same is true of tumors. By random chance, each 1000 rads kills about 90 per cent of cells, and 4000 rads will bring us to 99.9 per cent. However, just like the room, the *volume* in which the cells are contained does not change, and the cells may well be anywhere in that volume. For that reason, if the tumor was too large to operate on for cure before treatment, it probably still is. So, too, the appearance of the tumor means little. If it is rapidly dividing, it may disappear quickly, and if 90 per cent of the tumor cells are killed following each 1000 rads, it may disappear completely. We should note that the more anaplastic a tumor is, the more rapidly it divides (disappears). However, we know that no squamous cell cancer is ever cured with much less than

6000 rads. If it is dividing slowly, it may remain unchanged throughout the entire course of treatment, even though it is cured.

If one makes the decision to employ radiation therapy, it should be recognized that curability by surgery and the operation required for this should be determined *before* radiation therapy. Evaluation during therapy is deceptive because the rate of tumor disappearance is deceptive. Finally, the surgical approach must be altered because of changes in the tissues.

As the evolution of the radiation effect is developing as outlined above, the acute, edematous phase is the least favorable time for surgery. At this time, bleeding is extensive, and the tissues are prone to infection. Like any acutely inflamed tissue, meaningful fibroplasia does not occur until the inflammation subsides. In addition, the chronic phase of radiation injury is one of ischemia and dense fibroplasia, another period unfavorable for surgery. Timing is therefore critical, and the surgery should be performed after the acute inflammation subsides but before the time of dense fibroplasia and ischemia (and also before the tumor begins to recover and grow again). An adequate rule of thumb is to wait a week for each week the therapy was given. It would also seem that 4000 rads administered preoperatively can accomplish most of what 6000 rads can and with considerably less damage to tissue. The authors prefer to deliver 4000 rads over four weeks (five daily treatments of 200 rads each per week), followed by a delay of four weeks prior to surgery.

The principles of surgery which are altered by radiation therapy include the following:

1. The use of primary closure in the mouth or in the hypopharynx should be restricted to those situations in which there is no tension on the suture line.

2. Flap tissue (local, forehead, deltopectoral, etc.) should be used whenever the defect does not allow closure without tension, or when there is exposed bone.

3. Skin grafts should be employed only in areas which are not mobile (maxillary defects, cheek, etc.).

4. Neck dissection should be made through incisions which do not require a closure along the carotid artery.

5. Radiated tissue has diminished resistance to infection, and systemic antibiotics are routinely indicated.

6. Immediate bone grafts in irradiated beds are rarely successful.

It should be again noted that preoperative radiation does not yet have valid statistical confirmation as a therapeutic plan superior to other approaches.

Radiation Ulcers

Radiation ulcers are usually associated with prior therapeutic radiation rather than with accidental injury. Their distribution, therefore, is related to the areas where tumors are most commonly treated with therapeutic radiation, e.g., the oral cavity, neck, chest wall, anterior axillary fold, sacral region, and inguinal region.

The pathophysiology is not dissimilar to acute radiation injury and involves local ulceration, secondary infection, and finally necrosis. The symptoms and signs are similar to those of other ulcers but are characterized by the inordinate amount of pain that accompanies ischemia. The margins of such ulcers, although viable, are usually severely compromised and often cannot be employed as part of the reconstruction.

The principles of therapy are as above: local wound care, control of infection with topical antibacterial agents, resection of the ulcer bed and margins of the wound (usually resection of much of the original field of radiation is indicated), and finally adequate soft tissue coverage. In the oral cavity, particularly in the presence of osteoradionecrosis of the mandible, resection of the ulcer and necrotic bone allows sufficient collapse of adjacent tissue so that primary closure can be effected. On occasion, the underlying tissue bed is suitable, and a split-thickness skin graft will suffice (see Fig. 20–6). However, the principal indications for flap coverage as outlined by Robinson (1975) are appropriate:

(a) For coverage of exposed, or potentially exposed, vital structures—large vessels, nerves, tendons, bones, cartilage, peritoneum, pleura, or dura.
(b) To provide a moving or gliding surface for tendons or joints.
(c) As a cover through which future reconstructive procedures can be accomplished.
(d) For filling out contours, or for filling in cavities.
(e) To allow more motion in kinetic areas.

Case 3: Radiation Ulcer — Sacral Region (Split-Thickness Skin Graft). An example of this type of injury is seen in a 50 year old female with an adenocarcinoma of the uterus which was treated by hysterectomy. Following surgery, she had radium implant and external

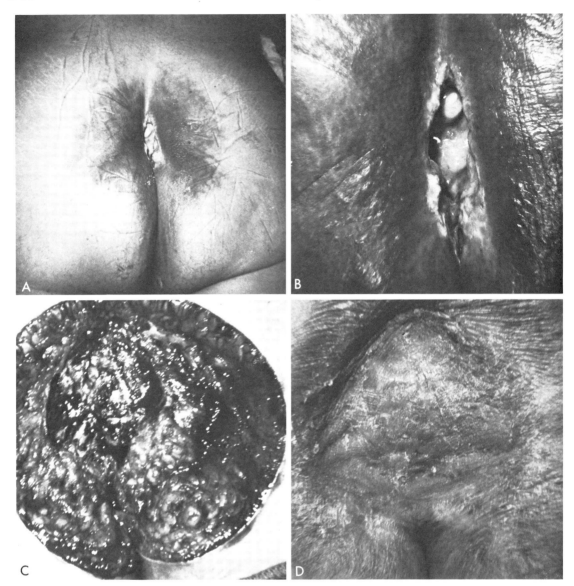

FIGURE 20-6. *A*, Hyperpigmentation and central ulcer in an area of skin exposed to radiation injury. *B*, Close-up view of ulcer. *C*, All ischemic tissue was excised to healthy skin margins. *D*, Appearance of skin graft at one year.

beam radiation of 4000 rads via double-opposing ports measuring 15 × 12 cm. An erythematous reaction in the gluteal crease subsequently resulted in early breakdown of the skin over the area. The area was hyperpigmented 18 months later, with a central ulcer that would not heal (Fig. 20–6, *A*, *B*).

The entire area was excised beyond the margins of pigmentation and beyond the area of vasculitis and ischemia. The excision was extended down to the sacral fascia, and there appeared to be healthy skin at the margins of

resection (Fig. 20–6, *C*). The wound was packed with saline-soaked gauze until adequate granulation tissue filled the bed, and a split-thickness skin graft was applied to the wound (Fig. 20–6, *D*). The patient is pain-free and the area remains healed two years later.

Case 4: Radiation Ulcer — Sacral Region (Rotation Flap). A 55 year old male had received preoperative radiation for an adenocarcinoma of the rectum. Several weeks after an abdominoperineal resection, the perineal wound broke down and failed to heal (Fig. 20–7, *A*). The ulcer measured 2 × 3 cm across and was 5 to 6 cm deep. There was an additional problem in that there had already been disruption of the suture line and the wound was deep (Fig. 20–7, *B*). Following excision of the lesion, the cavity was filled by the rotation of gluteus maximus muscle flaps (Fig. 20–7, *C*); cutaneous coverage was achieved by the rotation of a large buttock flap (Fig. 20–7, *D*). Since the tissues of the flap were outside the portals of radiation, they had a healthy blood supply and healed readily (Fig. 20–7, *E*). The patient remained pain-free without wound problems until his demise 18 months later from metastatic disease.

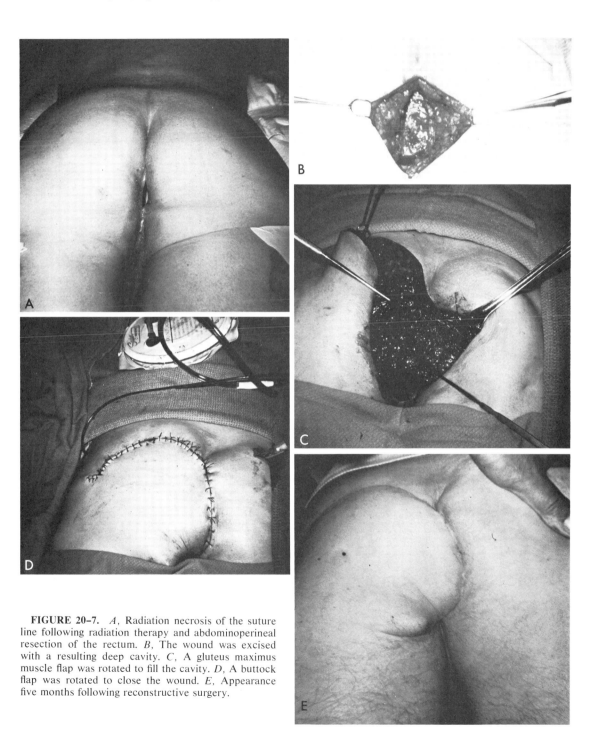

FIGURE 20–7. *A*, Radiation necrosis of the suture line following radiation therapy and abdominoperineal resection of the rectum. *B*, The wound was excised with a resulting deep cavity. *C*, A gluteus maximus muscle flap was rotated to fill the cavity. *D*, A buttock flap was rotated to close the wound. *E*, Appearance five months following reconstructive surgery.

Malignant Transformation

It is well documented that low dose chronic exposure or even therapeutic radiation may result in malignant degeneration of the skin after an interval of many years. The involved sites are related to the reason for exposure, either occupational (hands) or for the treatment of acne or hirsutism (face, upper neck). Carcinoma of the thyroid has also followed radiation to the thymus.

The pathophysiology appears to be the same as for other similar injury-induced malignancies, such as burn scar carcinoma (Marjolin's ulcer). The chronic radiation changes render the tissue ischemic and susceptible to injury with easy breakdown; any subsequent reparative process is difficult or lacking. As the tissue progresses through the stages of atrophy, pseu-doepitheliomatous hyperplasia, and finally carcinoma, the accessibility of the lesion allows for early diagnosis and early treatment. Since many of the lesions are superficial, topical chemotherapy may be effective. Ulcerated lesions, however, require excision and closure. Though infrequent, a postirradiated site with multiple cancers and a wide area of breakdown is among the most challenging reconstructive problems, often requiring resurfacing of large areas of the face. Split-thickness skin graft coverage is usually effective, if not an esthetic triumph.

Deeply invasive malignancy should be treated in a manner similar to other squamous cell carcinomas. Since the resected area is comparable to that seen with radiation ulcers, a similar approach and decision regarding flap coverage are appropriate.

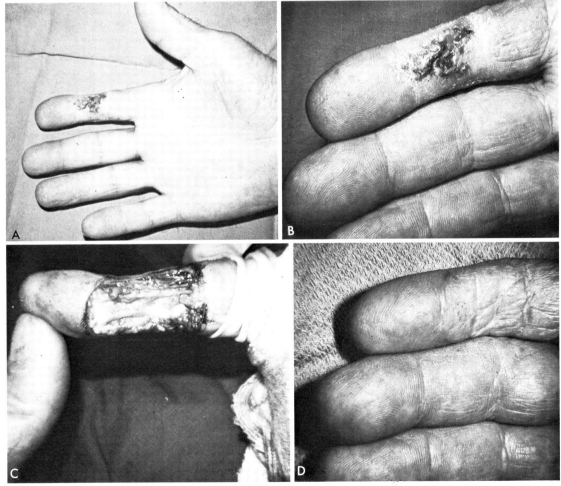

FIGURE 20–8. *A,* Ulceration over the middle phalanx of the index finger in an oral surgeon exposed to radiation over a prolonged period of time. *B,* Extensive chronic skin changes. *C,* The entire volar aspect of the middle phalanx was excised. *D,* One year following coverage with a cross-finger flap.

Case 5: Radiation-Induced Squamous Cell Carcinoma of the Finger.

An oral surgeon with a chronic radiation exposure of the index finger of his dominant right hand had a ten year history of intermittent scaling and breakdown on the volar aspect of the finger. A nonhealing ulcer developed (Fig. 20–8, *A*). Examination showed a considerable amount of radiation changes over the volar aspect of the middle phalanx (Fig. 20–8, *B*). A biopsy revealed squamous cell carcinoma.

This lesion was treated by wide excision of the skin of the volar aspect of the finger and the skin over the middle phalanx (Fig. 20–8, *C*). The defect was covered with a cross-finger flap (Fig. 20–8, *D*). The wound healed without difficulty, and the patient has not had any further skin breakdown over a follow-up period of five years.

CONCLUSION

In this era of modern radiotherapy, the problems associated with the indiscriminate treatment of benign disease have diminished. The skin-sparing effects of supervoltage therapy make the problems associated with orthovoltage treatment less frequent. A heightened awareness has protected the workers in this field from the disasters that befell their predecessors. However, this potent agent, usually employed for otherwise incurable disease, may result in complications. The reconstructive surgeon can often lend a hand.

An understanding of radiobiology and the pathophysiology of the injury, followed by the appropriate disposition of surgical principles, can help to alleviate the suffering of many unfortunate patients.

REFERENCES

Allen, A. C.: The Skin. St. Louis, Mo., C. V. Mosby Company, 1954.

Bragg, D. G., Homayoon, S., Chu, F. C. H., and Higinbotham, N. L.: The clinical and radiographic aspects of radiation osteitis. Radiology, *97*:103, 1970.

Brill, A. B., Tomonaga, M., and Heyssel, R. M.: Leukemia in man following exposure to ionizing radiation. A summary of the findings in Hiroshima and Nagasaki, and a comparison with human experience. Ann. Intern. Med., *56*:590, 1962.

Brown, J. B., and Fryer, M. P.: Report of surgical repair in the first group of atomic radiation injuries. Surg. Gynecol. Obstet., *103*:1, 1956.

Brown, J. B., and Fryer, M. P.: Reconstruction of electrical injuries, including cranial losses. With preliminary report of cathode-ray burns. Ann. Surg., *146*:342, 1957.

Brown, J. B., and Fryer, M. P.: High energy electron injury from accelerator machine. Radiation burns of chest wall and neck. 17-year follow up of atomic burns. Ann. Surg., *162*:426, 1965.

Brown, J. B., McDowell, F., and Fryer, M. P.: Radiation burns, including vocational and atomic exposures. Treatment and surgical prevention of chronic lesions. Ann. Surg., *130*:593, 1949a.

Brown, J. B., McDowell, F., and Fryer, M. P.: Surgical treatment of radiation burns. Surg. Gynecol. Obstet., *88*:609, 1949b.

Burch, P. R. J.: Radiation carcinogenesis: A new hypothesis. Nature, *185*:135, 1960.

Burrows, H., and Clarkson, J. R.: The role of inflammation in the induction of cancer by x-rays. Br. J. Radiol., *16*:381, 1943.

Cahan, W. G., Woodard, H. Q., Higinbotham, N. L., Stewart, F. W., and Coley, B. L.: Sarcoma arising in irradiated bone. Cancer, *1*:3, 1948.

Daniel, J.: The x-rays. New Science, *3*:562, 1896.

Ewing, J.: Radiation osteitis. Acta Radiol., *6*:399, 1926.

Frieben, E. A.: Cancroid des rechten Handrückens nach langdauernder Einwirkung von Rontgenstrahlen. Fortschr. Roentgenstr., *6*:106, 1902.

Hatfield, P. M., and Schulz, M. D.: Postirradiation sarcoma. Including five cases after x-ray therapy of breast carcinoma. Radiology, *96*:593, 1970.

Hoffman, F. L.: Radium (mesothorium) necrosis. J.A.M.A., *85*:961, 1925.

Hueper, W. C.: Recent developments in environmental cancer. Arch. Pathol., *58*:475, 1954.

Kilgore, A. R., and Abbott, L. C.: Sarcoma following benign bone lesions. West. J. Surg., *46*:348, 1938.

Kim, J. H., Chu, F. C. H., Pope, R. A., Woodard, H. Q., Bragg, D. B., and Homayoon, S.: Time dose factors in radiation induced osteitis. Am. J. Roentgenol. Radium Ther. Nucl. Med., *120*:684, 1974.

Knowlton, N. P., Leifer, E., Hogness, J. R., Hempelmann, L. H., Blaney, L. F., Gill, D. C., Oakes, W. R., and Shafer, C. L.: Beta-ray burns of human skin. J.A.M.A., *141*:239, 1949.

Krizek, T. J., and Ariyan, S.: Severe acute radiation injuries of the hands. Plast. Reconstr. Surg., *51*:14, 1973.

Lacassagne, A.: Conditions dans lesquelles out été obtenus, chez le Lapin, des cancers par action des rayons X sur des foyers inflammatoires. C. R. Soc. Biol., *112*:562, 1933.

Lacassagne, A., and Vinzent, R.: Action des rayons X sur un foyer infectieux local, provoqué chez le Lapin par l'injection de Streptobacillus caviae. C. R. Soc. Biol., *100*:247, 1929a.

Lacassagne, A., and Vinzent, R.: Sarcomes provoqués chez des Lapins par l'irradiation d'abscès à Streptobacillus caviae. C. R. Soc. Biol., *100*:249, 1929b.

Lanzl, L. H., Rozenfeld, M. L., and Tarlov, A. R.: Injury due to accidental high-dose exposure to 10 MeV electrons. Health Phys., *13*:241, 1967.

Ludewig, P., and Lorenser, E.: Untersuchungen der Grubenluft in den Schneeberger Gruben auf den Gehalt an Radium emanation. Strahlentherapie, *17*:428, 1924.

March, H. C.: Leukemia in radiologists, ten years later: With review of pertinent evidence of radiation leukemia. Am. J. Med. Sci., *242*:137, 1961.

Martland, H. S.: The occurrence of malignancy in radioactive persons. A general review of data gathered in the study of the radium dial painters with special reference to the occurrence of osteogenic sarcoma and the interrelationship of certain blood diseases. Am. J. Cancer, *15*:2435, 1931.

Martland, H. S., Conlon, P., and Knef, J. P.: Some unrecognized dangers in the use and handling of radio-active substances: With special reference to the storage of insoluble products of radium and mesothorium in the reticulo-endothelial system. J.A.M.A., *85*:1769, 1925.

Miller, R. W.: Delayed radiation effects in atom-bomb survivors. Major observations by the Atomic Bomb Casualty Commission are evaluated. Science, *166*:569, 1969.

Newcombe, H. B.: Magnitude of biological hazard from strontium-90. Science, *126*:549, 1957.

Pifer, J. W., Toyooka, E. T., Murray, R. W., Ames, W. R., and Hempelmann, L. H.: Neoplasms in children treated with x-rays for thymic enlargement. I. Neoplasms and mortality. J. Natl. Cancer Inst., *31*:1333, 1963.

Rankow, R. M., and Weissman, B.: Osteoradionecrosis of the mandible. Ann. Otol. Rhinol. Laryngol., *80*:603, 1971.

Robinson, D. W.: Surgical problems in the excision and repair of radiated tissue. Plast. Reconstr. Surg., *55*:41, 1975.

Simpson, C. L., and Hempelmann, L. H.: The association of tumors and roentgen ray treatment of the thorax in infancy. Cancer, *10*:42, 1957.

Socolow, E. L., Hashizume, A., Nerishi, S., and Niitani, R.: Thyroid carcinoma in man after exposure to ionizing radiation. A summary of the findings in Hiroshima and Nagasaki. New Engl. J. Med., *268*:406, 1963.

Teloh, H. A., Mason, M. L., and Wheelock, M. C.: A histopathologic study of radiation injuries of the skin. Surg. Gynecol. Obstet., *90*:335, 1950.

Toyooka, E. T., Pifer, J. W., Crump, S. L., Dutton, A. M., and Hempelmann, L. H.: Neoplasms in children treated with x-rays for thymic enlargement. II. Tumor incidence as a function of radiation factors. J. Natl. Cancer Inst., *31*:1357, 1963.

Ulrich, H.: Incidence of leukemia in radiologists. New Engl. J. Med., *234*:45, 1946.

Upton, A. C.: Effects of radiation on man. Annu. Rev. Nucl. Sci., *18*:495, 1968.

Warren, S.: Effects of radiation on normal tissues. XIII. Effects on the skin. Arch. Pathol., *35*:340, 1943.

Warren, S.: Longevity and causes of death from irradiation in physicians. J.A.M.A., *162*:464, 1956.

Warren, S.: Radiation carcinogenesis. Bull. N. Y. Acad. Med., *46*:131, 1970.

Zeldis, L. J., Jablon, S., and Ishida, M.: Current status of ABCC-NIH studies of carcinogenesis in Hiroshima and Nagasaki. Ann. N. Y. Acad. Sci., *114*:25, 1964.

CHAPTER 21

PSYCHIATRIC ASPECTS OF PLASTIC SURGERY

Eugene Meyer, M.D.,
and Norman J. Knorr, M.D.

Plastic surgery and the special aspect of corrective (cosmetic) surgery raise psychologic, social, and ethical considerations to an extent not encountered in other surgical fields. There can be general agreement that the psychology of the patient and the patient-physician relationship are of primary importance in plastic surgery, whether or not collaboration of the psychiatrist in the work of the plastic surgeon is a necessary consequence of these facts. As does every physician, the plastic surgeon necessarily enters the field of psychologic motivation, the personal meanings of illness and deformity, and the life situations of the patients seeking his help. In the field of elective corrective surgery, these factors are primary in the patient's seeking surgical help and the surgeon's undertaking the operations. Kolle's comment on corrective nasal surgery in 1911 describes a situation that still exists: "For some unaccountable reason the latter art has not yet met with the general favor the profession should grant it . . . yet the results have added much to the comfort and happiness of the patient."

The psychologic and emotional satisfaction of the patient have been among the stated goals of plastic surgeons for centuries. Tagliacozzi stated in 1597, "We restore, repair and make whole those parts of the face which nature has given, but which fortune has taken away, not so much that they may delight the eye but that

they may buoy up the spirits and help the mind of the afflicted" (Edgerton, 1961). Much later Roe, who first described his technique of rhinoplasty in 1887, commented, "We are able to relieve patients of a condition which would remain a lifelong mark of disfigurement, constantly observed, forming a never-ceasing source of embarrassment and mental distress to themselves, amounting in many cases, to a positive torture, as well as often causing them to be objects of greater or less aversion to others."

Improvement in a patient's mental illness as a result of surgery was first suggested in a statement by John Staige Davis. Plastic surgery, he said, "deals with the repair of defects and malformations either congenital or acquired; with the restoration of function and comfort; and, incidentally, with improvement of appearance and consequent relief of certain psychoses due to consciousness of deformity" (Edgerton, 1961). While the term "psychoses" is obviously used by Davis in a loose sense, he clearly suggests a favorable influence on mental illness by means of plastic surgery. In this and other similar comments lies an essential difference in the goals of plastic surgery as distinguished from the commonly accepted indications for other surgical procedures.

Doubts about the substantial rather than the temporary or superficial value to the patient of cosmetic surgery can only be answered by systematic long-term follow-up of patients undergoing such surgery. Such data are just beginning to be available, and a preliminary report is given in Chapter 22.

THE CONCEPT OF DEFORMITY

Comprehensive understanding of deformity must include several categories of data. These are: (1) social and cultural attitudes; (2) intra-familial attitudes and reactions; (3) individual and intrapsychic attitudes. In every case of deformity, all three levels of consideration are relevant. Deformity affects individual and group behavior, and individual and group behavior reacts on the subjective sense of deformity of the individual.

Social and Cultural Attitudes

Every physician is both a product of and a changer of the culture in which he lives. Cultural attitudes toward deformity and disability are important considerations in the care and treatment of patients by the plastic surgeon. In some cultures the physical form of children is shaped by binding the feet or molding the head of the child so as to produce a desired physical result (Porter, 1887). Mason (1887) has reviewed the deforming of the heads of children among American Indians. The "Flat-Head" Indians derived their name from this practice. Mason cited a Russian author of the nineteenth century, Pokrooski, who reviewed the practices of "tattoo, depilation, piercing the nose, the ears, the lips or the cheeks; filing and removing the teeth, castration, circumcision and similar mutilations; corset, Chinese feet, high-heeled boots, etc."

It is of particular interest that ceremonial and religious rites marking the transition from adolescent to adult status often have included various mutilations, using scarring, piercing of arms, amputation of fingers, depilation, or tattooing (Gould and Pyle, 1897). What would appear to be grossly mutilating procedures to a person of one culture are desirable marks of status—something to be proud of—for those of another culture.

In sharp contrast, in many more primitive societies the child who is grossly deformed at birth is either left to die or otherwise disposed of. Among nomadic Arab groups in North Africa, deformity arouses intense feelings of horror and revulsion which result in social isolation of the individual (Meyer, 1943).

In some cultures the deformed child and the grossly irrational individual are subjected to equal treatment—the individual somehow simply "disappears" (Crane, 1960). It would appear that a culture that is extremely marginal in economic status, one in which obtaining and distributing food is a primary occupation of all concerned, cannot afford the additional burden of a permanently crippled or deformed individual, whether the deformity be in physical or mental function.

It is well to bear in mind these facts when considering the psychologic and social aspects of the deformed or crippled individual in more sophisticated, developed, or so-called civilized societies. Many individuals in these countries manifest adverse reactions to deformity though these are often overlooked and rarely acknowledged. Macgregor and coworkers (1955) point out, "It is not unusual to see horror or disgust reflected in the expression of one who looks upon a grossly disfigured person and to hear seconds later such a remark as 'Oh that poor man.'" The cruelty of young children to a crippled schoolmate is another case in point. The more polite version of social alienation in the attitudes and reactions of people in civilized countries is no less painful and real to the person who is the target of such responses.

A meeting point of individual and cultural attitudes lies in the association of deformity with evil, degenerate, or antisocial behavior. The classic example from literature is dramatically demonstrated in Robert Louis Stevenson's "Dr. Jekyll and Mr. Hyde." The same theme is described by Shakespeare in Richard III:

> "I, that am curtail'd of this fair proportion,
> Cheated of feature by dissembling nature,
> Deform'd, unfinish'd, sent before my time
> Into this breathing world, scarce half made up,
> And that so lamely and unfashionable
> That dogs bark at me as I halt by them;
>
> And therefore, since I cannot prove a lover,
> To entertain these fair well-spoken days,
> I am determined to prove a villain,
> And hate the idle pleasures of these days."

Kolb (1954) pointed out the frequent literary characterization of the limb amputee as a terrifying and threatening individual, citing Melville's Ahab, Stevenson's Long John Silver, Barrie's Captain Hook, and Poe's General A.B.C. Smith. Rickman (1940) suggested that deformity and ugliness induce reactions of horror, dislike, and avoidance because they remind mankind of its capacity for hate and destructiveness.

The question of whether criminal behavior may result from social isolation and rejection by others in the experience of the grossly deformed individual is not only a literary topic. Pick's (1948) pioneering work in correction of deformity in penitentiary inmates suggests that such surgery is helpful in the rehabilitation of the criminal, whatever the contribution of deformity to crime. More recently Masters (1962) has reviewed photographs of persons convicted of various criminal acts. He reported a significantly higher incidence of various types of facial deformity in five major categories of crime.

Cultural influences on the individual's sense of deformity are also of consequence in patients who seek cosmetic plastic surgery. Several studies have reported a high incidence of foreign-born parents in patients seeking rhinoplasty (Meyer and associates, 1960; Jacobson, Edgerton, Meyer and Canter, 1960; Hill and Silver, 1950). The Jewish patient who seeks corrective nasal surgery raises the question of racial identification as motivation for seeking surgery. The superficially plausible idea that such patients wish to obscure their religious-racial affiliation is not borne out by detailed knowledge of these patients. In the great majority of cases they do not wish to dissociate themselves from either their religious affiliations or their current social milieu. They wish rather not to be stereotyped as "alien" or in other derogatory fashion and want to be associated with the accepted standards of "beauty." The fact that a substantial number of patients in Israel seek corrective nasal plastic surgery supports these observations (Neumann, 1960; Macgregor, 1967).

Cultural prejudices in respect to old age are relevant to motivations of other patients seeking cosmetic procedures. Patients seeking rhytidoplasty frequently have professional reasons for avoiding being characterized as "old." The prejudice against employment of the elderly person and the practical importance of appearance in a variety of jobs are frequently an important part of the quest for "face-lift" operations.

Intrafamilial Aspects of Deformity

Intrafamilial ramifications of deformity deserve separate consideration. Macgregor and Schaffner (1950) have pointed out how parental attitudes toward deformity in a child mold the child's own reactions. Children are frequently told that congenital defects are the result of "falls" or other accidental trauma. Such deceptions derive from reactions of guilt and shame on the part of parents and complicate life enormously for the child, who learns he must go along with such pretenses. "The deformed child is rejected on grounds that his deformities are due to 'sins of the fathers,' 'punishment for wrongdoing,' 'incestuous parentage,' etc." (Kolb, 1959).

Fostering realistic attitudes on the part of parents toward deformity and its residuals in the growing child and in the adolescent, though taken for granted, is a neglected area of systematic study. As Kolb (1959) stated, "The influence of family attitudes on the development of disturbed body images has been neglected in study and practice. In point of fact, however, the capacity for a satisfactory social adaptation among those with bodily defects depends more upon the family and cultural attitudes toward body structures than upon the presence of the defect." Kolb's review of this topic is well worth special attention by the interested surgeon. The Hampsons and Money (1955) have investigated children with endocrine dyscrasias and anatomic abnormalities of genital development. Their reports emphasize the great extent to which even gender role behavior is learned rather than determined by endocrine or instinctual influences.

Intrafamilial responses to deformity also have significance when patients seek anatomic corrections primarily because of a wish to please someone in their immediate family, generally the spouse, or because of rivalrous or envious feelings toward a sibling. Neither of these motivations is, in itself, a valid indication for surgery, and they are apt to be concealed by the patient. When motivation for operation is primarily the instigation of others, there is legitimate basis for refusing operation, or at the very least, for substantial deferral (Macgregor and Schaffner, 1950; Jacobson and associates, 1960).

Individual and Intrapsychic Attitudes Toward Deformity

Understanding what pushes a patient to seek the help of a plastic surgeon at a particular time in his life requires comprehension of complex and often unconscious or hardly conscious emotions and ideas in the patient.

A chronology of reactions to congenital deformity according to age has been described (Knorr and associates, 1968). Children with congenital deformities of the face do not recognize that they are deformed until about 4 years of age. Recognizing deformities of the trunk or extremities, particularly of the hands, probably occurs earlier. Identifying themselves as deformed is probably the result of physical maturing and managing to look into the mirror as well as becoming more observant and sensitive to the physical features of other persons. Outside stimulation and the environmental reaction to deformity impinges upon the child when he seeks playmates beyond the home and begins nursery school or kindergarten. Young children are frequently cruel in their attitudes to a deformed child, and the first signs of reaction to rejection — withdrawal and depression — occur in a deformed child at the age of 4 to 6 years. When the child is 6 or 7 years of age, the facial deformity has less personal significance, and there tends to be more of a focus on the deformity of the extremities. This continues until age 10 or 11, for the child is more interested in playing and developing manual skills than he is in personally interacting with others through his physical appearance. With puberty, the child becomes progressively more interested in his physical appearance, and the face again assumes paramount importance. The parents of a deformed child are frequently surprised when a child who had seemingly adjusted well to his facial deformity asks for help in obtaining further medical assistance to improve his appearance. The guilt reactions which these parents experienced years earlier for giving birth to a deformed child are restimulated as the family again focuses on the child's deformity.

There are differences in the emotional reactions of congenitally deformed children and those of the child who sustains traumatic deformity (Knorr and Meyer, 1970). When traumatic injury is sustained at a very early age, the resulting deformity is incorporated into the body image, and the child will behave as if he were congenitally deformed. When trauma occurs later, after age 3 or 4, the child will be more reactive to the deformity and will experience more anxiety and depression in adjusting to his deformity. One area of major difference between the congenitally deformed child and the traumatically deformed child is expectation of surgery. The congenitally deformed child is appreciative of surgery but suggests that he will always be different from normal children regardless of what the surgeon can achieve, while the traumatically deformed child may have fantasies of the surgeon's restoring his deformed anatomy to a completely normal state. This latter fantasy will frequently lead to difficulties between the patient and the surgeon. The surgeon must carefully prepare the deformed child for what can be realistically expected from surgery.

In the spectrum of deformity, there is a gradation between two apparent extremes. There are those "objective" deformities concerning which any jury would probably agree that "something should be done." Then there are those "subjective" deformities about which there would be no such agreement or even failure to perceive the person as deformed. Gross deformities, congenital or traumatic, are apt to be taken at face value — i.e., as sufficient and obvious motivation for seeking plastic surgery. It is well to remember that unconscious meanings attach to obvious deformity as a result of the pre-injury personal history of the individual or the symbolic meanings of the part of the body involved.

The terms "objective" and "subjective" deformity are misleading in that the patient whose deformity is purely subjective may experience as much or more distress than the patient with obvious deformity. In the case of the patient with a highly personal sense of deformity, there is, however, a much greater likelihood of unconscious factors playing a substantial role in his quest for surgery. In patients seeking corrective plastic surgery, one might better speak of surgical correction of the perceived body or the body image. The quest for corrective surgery is commonly associated by the patient with impairment of psychosocial functioning. Patients frequently state explicitly that they hope for greater ease in their work, social, or family situations. The surgeon inevitably must assess the realism of the patient's hopes and expectations. Not only must he consider whether or not the changes requested are technically feasible, but also whether increased happiness and effectiveness of the patient can be expected to follow. This places the surgeon squarely in the field of motivation and personality function — the field of psychiatry itself.

THE SURGEON-PATIENT RELATIONSHIP

When a patient places his life and future appearance in the hands of another — the surgeon — he expresses a high degree of trust in the technical competence of the surgeon and, more important, in the enduring concern of the surgeon for his health and welfare.

The plastic surgeon is undoubtedly the best witness, through his personal experience, of the importance of the physician-patient relationship. The psychiatrist with experience in the field of plastic surgery may, however, delineate certain aspects of this relationship as seen by a third party observer whose particular job is the understanding of personality function. In so doing, he must acknowledge the spirit of scientific objectivity that prompts a surgeon to invite close collaboration and inspection of his work with patients.

The patient who consults the plastic surgeon, whether his deformity be major or minor, knows only his subjective distress, his physical and social disability, and his hopes for greater happiness and ease of functioning as a result of surgery. Patients who have undergone surgery sometimes date the onset of their improvement from the first meeting with the surgeon. They relate this fact to the surgeon's acceptance of their sense of deformity and his assumption that the wish for a change in appearance is reasonable and perhaps feasible. Patients feel understood by the surgeon's initial acceptance, and their hope for change is made legitimate by all the assumptions built into the surgeon's methods of obtaining a history and examining the patient. Feelings of relief and renewed hope experienced by patients in their initial contact with the surgeon highlight the powerful therapeutic role of the patient's expectations and the personal contact with the surgeon.

The basic requirements of a working relationship between patient and surgeon can be summarized as (1) trust and (2) communication (Meyer and Mendelson, 1961). Although this is true of all physician-patient relationships, the sometimes long and arduous course of reconstructive and corrective surgery requires special attention to those dimensions. Trusting a surgeon with their external appearance is of greater significance for many people than trusting him to deal with inner or hidden bodily functions.

The surgeon must always know the special aspects of the patient's personality and his social and cultural background, as well as the details of his current life situation. A satisfactory correspondence must exist between the surgeon's and the patient's expectations in respect to any surgical procedure which might be undertaken. The patient not only must be told the actual facts of what the surgeon can do, but also he must really hear what is said.

This applies with particular force to the operative procedure itself and to the details of the immediate postoperative period. Patients may and frequently do have highly distorted or fantasy-endowed conceptions of the surgical procedure in spite of what they have been told.

One common distortion of the surgical procedure exaggerates the painful and traumatic aspects. The commonest underlying fantasy is that of death and rebirth or re-creation. The patient is, in fact, undergoing a true crisis of identity, and some measure of hope for a new start or a new beginning is almost inherent. General anesthesia may contribute to such fantasies.

At the other extreme, the operation may be conceived of as a magically painless, almost nontraumatic procedure. The patient, therefore, reacts with shock, surprise, anxiety, and even a sense of betrayal to the normal exigencies of the postoperative period. In the main, these are patients with little or no previous experience of surgery. Occasionally a patient who reacts thus has been deceived by his parents, in childhood, into going to the hospital for "an examination," which turned out to be a tonsillectomy. Such painful experience, linking betrayal and painful surgery, has been completely repressed. It is "remembered" in the form of a later postoperative reaction of undue anxiety, indignation, and irrational reproaches to the plastic surgeon.

The less conscious and unconscious symbolic meanings of an operation are inevitably present and not abnormal in themselves. Trouble ensues only when these unconscious fantasies skew the patient's expectations of surgery to a major extent, and there is a wide gap between fantasy and fact. The best cure for such situations is prevention. This requires that the surgeon not only inform the patient of the facts but also ascertain carefully that the patient has fully digested what he or she has been told. Of particular importance is the patient's past experience of other surgical procedures and convalescence and the degree of realism and mature appreciation of others shown by the patient in other aspects of his living.

Demanding, excessively anxious or distrustful patients often elicit quite human, reciprocal responses of annoyance and irritation in physicians and nurses. If possible, it is best to read the signs of these reactions as a fair sample of the patient's troubled situation. Even an emotionally disorganized patient is capable of observing the fact that his behavior antagonizes those in whose hands rest his health and future. Frequently the feedback to the patient of these reactions of physicians and nurses tends to aggravate his basic anxiety and its behavioral consequences (Meyer and Mendelson, 1961). To break up such vicious circles, the surgeon must sit down with his patient and attempt to unravel the sources of his fears, rational and irrational. Such an attempt restores a sense of better perspective for the surgeon as well as the patient, thus avoiding hasty decisions or expressions which may later be viewed with chagrin.

One other and quite different aspect of the surgeon's experience may lead to errors in judgment. An experienced surgeon has suggested the term "Pygmalion complex" to indicate that experience with feelings of deep and genuine gratitude from patients may tempt the surgeon into states of overconfidence. Undue shortcuts in his usual approach to patients may result in decisions made without due consideration. The difference between the *desire* to cure and the *need* to cure is one with which all physicians should be acquainted. Cultivation of honest self-scrutiny in this matter is the duty of all members of the medical profession.

The Disgruntled Patient

The disgruntled or litigious patient deserves some special comment. The motivations of such patients are complicated by legal advisors, the quest for monetary gain, and other factors. The soil on which lawsuits are grown is the physician-patient relationship. The angry, disgruntled, and accusatory patient complains as much or more of the *interpersonal* aspects of his treatment as of its technical aspects. Thus a young woman dying of leukemia angrily criticized her physician for withholding the news of her serious condition and added "He has absolutely no tact!" On query, she added "Tact is knowing who you're talking to."

The plastic surgeon who quickly or hurriedly agrees to operate runs the risk, at the very least, of being untactful — of not knowing on whom he is operating. Borderline or frankly paranoid people may and often do keep this aspect of their psychopathology well hidden until provoked by some threat that adds to their insecurity or sense of helplessness. An average expectable postoperative complication can be negotiated if the patient has an established framework of trust in his physician. If the patient is characteristically suspicious and

distrustful, anything but the smoothest operative and postoperative course may aggravate his latent paranoid psychopathology.

It should be emphasized that temporarily held paranoid attitudes are an extremely common phenomenon in frightened and disorganized patients on medical and surgical wards (Meyer, 1962). Fears of being poisoned, experimented on, and otherwise harmed are characteristic of many brain-damaged and anxious patients (Weinstein and Kahn, 1953). While the person with paranoid attitudes distorts the meaning of ordinary events, his "craziness" lies more in what he *fails* to see or register rather than in the total inaccuracy of what he is anxious or angry about. An untended physician-patient relationship leaves a vacuum of uncertainty that is filled by the suspicious and distrustful person with his own worst expectations.

An enduring grudge reaction that settles on the physician or surgeon can almost never breed in an atmosphere in which genuine, unhurried attempts to appreciate the patient as an individual person have been made, when the operative and postoperative situations have been fully explained, and when the patient, though disappointed, knows he has been treated with respect and concern.

THE POSTOPERATIVE PERIOD

Postoperative reactions of acute emotional disturbance are not uncommon in patients undergoing surgical procedures of various sorts. Transient emotional upsets in the immediate postoperative period are rather common in patients undergoing corrective surgery. Fifty-five per cent of 68 consecutive patients undergoing various corrective procedures were reported as showing some degree of acute transient emotional disturbance postoperatively (Edgerton, Jacobson and Meyer, 1960). The majority of these reactions occur around the third postoperative day and are almost predictable, should the surgeon be called away from the city at this time. Anxiety and depressive reactions are the commonest form these upsets take. Rather abrupt and, to the patient, unexplained episodes of crying spells, feelings of worthlessness, poor appetite, and poor sleep are rather characteristic of patients undergoing augmentation mammaplasty (Edgerton, Meyer and Jacobson, 1961). In patients undergoing corrective nasal plastic surgery, postoperative reactions are apt to take the form of apprehension, jitteriness, undue fearfulness, and marked sensitivity to pain incurred in the course of surgical dressing.

Rarely a patient may experience anxiety to the point of depersonalization, complaining of things "not feeling real," of feeling "wooden," "not here," and so on. Along with grossly disturbed behavior, feelings of acute depersonalization should be viewed as a psychiatric emergency. Although such feelings may subside spontaneously, the patient who experiences acute depersonalization may make sudden and unpredicted suicidal or assaultive attempts.

Postoperative emotional upsets are, however, generally susceptible to reassurance, judicious use of sedation, the help of special nurses for brief periods and, above all, discussion with the attending surgeon. A psychiatrist who has seen the patient during the preoperative period can be particularly helpful at such times. Patients frequently are able to vent their irrational fears more easily to the psychiatrist than to the surgeon whom they expect to condemn and disapprove childish thoughts and feelings.

Understanding these temporary psychologic upsets is of practical importance in their management, but also of theoretical interest. Patients undergoing plastic surgery, especially those with longstanding deformity, either congenital or acquired, are risking a change in identity. Change in physical appearance means change in the body image — the basic anchor or underpinning of the sense of identity. During the immediate postoperative period the patient is necessarily in a period of intense uncertainty. He has let go of one version of his physical appearance and must be uncertain of his future appearance and the reactions of people he has known.

Symbolic and intrapsychic meanings of corrective procedures can also result in an occasional reaction of immense satisfaction and pleasure on the part of a patient in this period of ambiguity. Thus one adolescent patient undergoing corrective nasal surgery commented in the immediate postoperative period as follows:

"It comes out inside of you. I don't know how you're going to tell it to anyone else. It's as if you were living your whole life behind a veil, and suddenly the veil is pushed aside and you can see people for the first time as they really are — as you always suspected they were; but you never came close enough to find out. I know I never did" (Meyer and associates, 1960).

Identity crises are part of normal growth and development, as Erikson has suggested (1956). Turbulence and emotional lability are characteristic of these normal crises, whether in adolescence, in middle age, or at the age of retirement. These normal crises, however, are stretched out over long periods of time, whereas a surgically induced crisis involving the physical body and the body image is compressed into a very brief period. The fact that the technical aspects of a surgical procedure may be minor in the eyes of the surgeon should not obscure the fact that, in psychologic terms, minor surgery can be a major event. It is indeed this very fact that may well be an important element in favorable changes in personality during the later postoperative period.

PLASTIC SURGERY AND THE NEUROTIC OR PSYCHOTIC PATIENT

When a surgical procedure is indicated as a result of a threat to the patient's life, a disturbed mental state in the patient is not considered a contraindication to surgery. Longstanding neurosis or psychosis may dictate special necessities in terms of the patient's pre- and postoperative care but will not influence the recommendation for surgery.

The situation is quite different when a neurotic or technically psychotic person seeks surgical correction of a minor deformity. Here the question is whether the patient's total situation will be benefited by surgery or whether the wish for operation is itself a symptom, the correction of which will do no good or may even aggravate the patient's mental illness.

Some psychiatrists have taken the extreme view that all corrective surgery is simply an indulgence of neurosis or of infantile and narcissistic wishes for an empty "movie star" version of beauty. Meerloo (1956), for example, portrayed a grim sequence of psychologic disorders in several women following plastic surgery. More systematic studies by psychiatrists of plastic surgical results report a high incidence of psychiatric disorder but have also reported high levels of satisfactory results (MacKenzie, 1944; Barsky, 1956; Edgerton, Jacobson and Meyer, 1960).

The statement is generally made that when neurosis or psychosis is "reactive" to the deformity, the surgeon may safely undertake surgical procedures if the changes requested are technically feasible (Barker and Smith, 1939; Barsky, 1956; Titchener and Levine, 1960). Another frequent observation is that the more explicit the deformity, the more pleased the patient is apt to be with the result. Concern about minor deformities is often taken to be prima facie evidence of neurotic disposition. A number of studies have stressed the need for close collaboration between the plastic surgeon and psychiatrist in the selection of patients, in the evaluation of postoperative emotional upsets, and in the presentation of the alternative of psychotherapy to patients who should not be operated upon or who seek further operations for minor defects (Barker and Smith, 1939; Barsky, 1956; Jacobson, Meyer and Edgerton, 1961).

While opinions from a variety of sources, thus briefly summarized, are in considerable agreement on broad outlines, the problem of applying to an individual patient generalities that hold for a group of patients is far from easy. Jacobson, Meyer and Edgerton (1961) suggested that the psychiatrist may be of value to the plastic surgeon in four basic ways: (1) identification of severe personality problems; (2) clarification of the patient's expectations and motivations for seeking plastic surgery; (3) definitive psychotherapeutic intervention as an alternative to surgery; and (4) facilitation of healthy psychologic development initiated or catalyzed by the surgical procedure. While the technical definition of a patient as neurotic or psychotic is not necessarily a contraindication to an elective surgical procedure, the undertaking of surgery in such patients should be highly selective and calls for informed and available psychiatric assistance in all cases.

Patients who represent the extremes of psychologic health and illness are not difficult to delineate and recognize. The grossly and manifestly psychotic patients whose complaints of deformity are clearly bizarre, and whose behavior corresponds, are not hard to spot. Thus, a psychotically depressed and paranoid 43 year old schoolteacher presented herself to a plastic surgeon with complaints of prominent veins on the dorsum of one thumb which she wished removed because "they make me look so masculine." Similarly, certain schizophrenic patients may present themselves with requests for plastic surgery and quickly reveal grandiose, unrealistic, or delusional ideas concerning the origin of the deformity and their expectations from the surgery. An unhurried

discussion with such patients is often sufficient to suggest to the surgeon that the complaint of deformity is simply one focus in a pattern of schizophrenic disorder.

At the other extreme are the stable individuals who present themselves for correction of obvious deformities or displeasing impairments of facial symmetry and form. A measure of anxiety and guilt about seeking surgical change in appearance is normal, but once this is surmounted, these patients give a coherent account of their distress, the circumstances under which they feel handicapped or self-conscious, and the development of the sense of deformity. They generally put maximum emphasis on the hope that the operation will help them feel better about themselves, and, if this can occur, they expect to be able to have greater ease and better function in some of their dealings with others. This primary expectation of change in *self*-perception is characteristic whether or not the patient has actually experienced teasing, ridicule, avoidance, or worse at the hands of other people. This contrasts sharply with the vaguely expressed, magical expectations of the severely schizoid or schizophrenic person that surgery will promote change in the attitudes or responses of other people, following which the patient will be able to feel better liked and more secure.

Thus, in respect to patients representing the extremes of the mental health spectrum, it is certainly true, as Blair and Brown (1931) have stated, that "the experienced man is not apt to make a grave mistake."

Borderline patients or patients who do not follow general rules evolved by common sense and experience are those who need better definition. Thus Hollender (1956) described a 38 year old man whose complaints of deformity were objective enough, but in whom the chief motivation for operation was displaced and symbolized guilt over sexual transgressions. The surgical result was not and could not be satisfactory to such a patient. Palmer and Blanton (1952) described cases of traumatic nasal deformity in a 16 year old girl and a 17 year old boy in whom the coexisting neurosis was so longstanding and severe as to require definitive psychotherapy as well as surgical intervention. As a result of definitive studies of patients suffering from facial deformity, Macgregor and her coworkers (1955) warned against operating on the psychotic patient. However, they also cite the case of a schizophrenic woman who apparently benefited in striking fashion from nasal surgery. Stern, Fournier and LaRivière (1957) described a severe postoperative psychotic depression in a 26 year old woman following corrective surgery of the nose. Stern, Doyon and Racine (1959) also stated that preoccupation with the shape of the breast "has always to be taken as a serious sign" and cite cases in which such preoccupations were associated with severe depressive reactions.

These reports of relatively small numbers of patients are difficult to evaluate because of bias in selection of the sample. Psychiatrists are apt to see the most disturbed group of patients who contemplate or have undergone plastic surgery. Surgeons, on the other hand, often do not have the facility or inclination to encourage patients to reveal some of the more disturbed aspects of their personalities. Patients who seek operations are also quite likely to obscure the less fortunate aspects of their functioning because they correctly enough expect that these would prejudice the surgeon in respect to operation.

One study of 98 consecutive patients presenting themselves for various corrective procedures reports that 70 per cent were assigned a psychiatric diagnosis. Sixteen per cent of this sample were psychotic, 20 per cent were neurotic and 35 per cent were assigned a diagnosis of personality trait disorder (Edgerton, Jacobson and Meyer, 1960). A later report by Jacobson, Meyer and Edgerton (1961) described 120 patients with minimal deformity and 37 patients with moderate to severe deformity who were referred for psychiatric evaluation. Of 120 patients with minimal deformity, 40 were felt to be in need of psychotherapy, and 32 patients underwent psychotherapy. Thirty-seven patients with moderate to severe deformity were also referred to the psychiatrist during the same two year period (1957–1959) because they represented "typical" or "difficult" problems in reconstructive surgery. Ten of these 37 patients had brief psychotherapy, and four more either refused or were unable to undertake it. It should be emphasized that these figures are derived from a research project in connection with which a psychiatrist is readily available. Nevertheless, it is impressive that one-third of 157 patients requiring the services of the plastic surgeon were in need of definitive psychiatric help. When psychiatric help was readily available, 42 of the 54 patients to whom psychotherapy was recommended accepted this recommendation.

DEFINITION AND MANAGEMENT OF THE PROBLEM PATIENT IN PLASTIC SURGERY

The results of technically successful plastic surgery are highly satisfactory to the patient in a substantial majority of instances. While long-term follow-up studies are necessary to establish just *how* the subjective satisfaction of the patient can be translated into more effective living, there is no doubt that subjective happiness and a sense of greater freedom to participate in various areas of living is reported by many patients.

Because the advisability of undertaking plastic surgery depends so much on the individual case, it is well to delineate, as far as may be, the kinds of cases and situations in which surgery may be contraindicated or undertaken only with special precautions.

The Type of Operation Requested

The most controversial category of patients seeking the services of the plastic surgeon is the patients seeking corrective surgery. A special study of 33 male patients requesting various facial operations, chiefly rhinoplasty, reported 13 of these patients were diagnosed as psychotic and four patients as severely neurotic (Jacobson and associates, 1960). Selected patients in this series underwent surgery, but evaluation of postoperative results showed minimal to modest improvement in the patient's effectiveness in living.

As a result of this study, the suggestion is made that psychiatric consultation is advisable for the *male patient seeking corrective surgery*. This recommendation is based on the high incidence of major psychiatric disorder which may pass unrecognized, and the general utility of the psychiatrist to the patient, if surgery is undertaken. In the male patients seeking corrective surgery, one finds the highest incidence of schizoid or schizophrenic persons whose hopes and expectations of the operation are apt to be excessive or even magical.

Many of these patients in childhood have had major and longstanding difficulties in their relationships with both parents. A lack of opportunity to achieve useful identifications with parents results in much generalized social anxiety and emotional withdrawal during the early years of development and adolescence. Heterosexual adjustment is apt to be defective and conflicted. The schizoid patient, in short, may suffer from lack of maturing interpersonal experience as much as or more than he has suffered from intensely conflicted experience.

In this setting, therefore, it is understandable that technically successful surgery is not apt to bring obvious change in the patient's capacity for effective living. Reactions of disappointment may bring repeated requests for further surgical correction of minor imperfections in the quest for "the perfect result." Careful preoperative evaluation of the male patient who seeks cosmetic surgery may alert the surgeon to the possibility that he is working in an unfavorable interpersonal field.

In recent years male patients have been seeking cosmetic surgery to remedy signs of aging. Competition for employment, particularly among executives of corporations and companies, places emphasis upon youth. The findings of Jacobson and his associates (1960) may require revision in the light of this new phenomenon.

Augmentation mammaplasty is an elective surgical procedure that evokes strong emotional bias. Patients with severe congenital deformities of a single breast or of the chest wall or deformity secondary to severe cystic disease provoke less controversy than do patients with a history of small breasts since adolescence who complain of ptosis and a sense of deformity after childbearing. The latter group constitute a substantial majority of the patients requesting augmentation mammaplasty.

Psychiatric evaluation of 68 patients seeking augmentation mammaplasty revealed a high incidence of latent depression and hysterical traits. Nevertheless, follow-up studies of one to eight years' duration have revealed that the majority of women report lasting satisfaction following augmentation mammaplasty. The most comprehensive report of such surgery concludes, however, with the following comment: "We feel strongly that, in spite of very encouraging results in many patients, the unresolved question of polymer carcinogenesis and the turbulent emotional potential of these patients both serve to warn the surgeon not to embark on a 'full speed ahead' program of augmentation mammaplasty. A few more years of experience will help to clarify the safety and long-term effects of this interesting type of plastic surgery" (Edgerton and coworkers, 1961). The reader is referred to Chapter 89 for current attitudes on augmentation mammaplasty.

A more recent study by Baker and associates (1974), consisting of in-depth psychiatric interviewing in one group and completion of a postoperative questionnaire in another group of patients who had undergone augmentation mammaplasty, showed that the average female was a married, educated, middle-class mother in her early thirties. Strong feelings of self-consciousness and sexual inadequacy had been present since adolescence. Disturbances in marital relationships were common. Many reported their small breast size had a negative influence on sexual breast play.

Another psychologic uncertainty for the surgeon and potential hazard for the patient is related to the degree of depression that may be present in the patient who requests plastic surgery for various *facial blemishes, scars, or acne.* Depression and social withdrawal may result from deformity and ugliness, as is so beautifully illustrated in Paul Gallico's story "The Snow Goose" (1953). Involutional depressive reactions in middle-aged patients may focus on evidence of aging or ugliness of facial features. The sense of deformity in these cases is a manifestation of an otherwise well hidden and serious depressive state. Complaints referable to particular foci, such as excess skin and sagging fat pockets of the eyelids, are particularly liable to be associated with significant degrees of depression. Routine, informed, and systematic questioning in respect to the past experiences of depressive reactions will be most helpful in such cases.

Recovery from depressive states can apparently be facilitated by plastic surgery. The severity and duration of the depressive reaction requires careful psychiatric evaluation. Surgeons should be reminded that somatic delusions may occur in severe depressive states as well as in schizophrenic reactions. Specific psychiatric treatment may be indicated as a preliminary to surgery, as an adjunct to surgery, and as the alternative to surgery.

A small number of young female patients with complaints of pain and disability referable to the temporomandibular joint are apt to be particularly troublesome from the psychologic standpoint. Whether the psychologic disability is primary or secondary to physical problems is frequently difficult to ascertain. Drug addiction, bitter resentment, and paranoid trends in these patients can handicap treatment and complicate the evaluation of surgical results.

Evidence from the Patient's History

A comprehensive, systematic history is of central importance to the genuine understanding of the patient's request or need for plastic surgery. This labors an obvious point, but the specific, often evident, nature of a physical defect or deformity frequently leads to sketchy surveys of the patient's general medical health record. Specific inquiry into nervous disorder and symptoms of anxiety and depression initially takes some extra time but saves time in the long run (Whitehorn, 1944). The history of such symptoms or illness usually is not volunteered by the patient and must be specifically investigated.

Histories of multiple surgical experiences interspersed with disabling medical illness may warn the surgeon that he is dealing with a surgically addicted patient whose capacity for healthy living is minimal. Some patients may in fact stabilize themselves against an overt psychotic decompensation by active solicitation of surgical procedures or hysterically talented simulations of medical and surgical illness.

A 50 year old patient was seen five years after a chemical burn produced an ulcer involving the inner aspect of the left foot and ankle. Dermatologic treatment had failed to result in improvement and the patient was eventually referred to the Department of Plastic Surgery. From 1953 through 1958 the patient was admitted 12 times to surgical wards for a variety of procedures. These were initiated by a left lumbar sympathectomy with excision of the ulcer and split-thickness skin grafting. The graft failed to take and became secondarily infected. In 1955 the ulcer was again excised and a cross-leg flap was effected from the right side to the left ankle because of recurrent folliculitis. Two subsequent admissions for severe dermatitis were followed by a further excision of the hair-bearing surface of the flap and application of a split-thickness graft (1957). Because it was felt that the patient might be irritating the site of the graft, a cast was applied and during this admission the patient showed better healing than previously. While still in the hospital, however, the patient's crutches slipped, he fell and suffered an intertrochanteric fracture of the left femur. This required removal of the cast from his ankle and again the dermatitis recurred with breakdown of the graft.

In desperation, the surgeons contemplated the possibility of a below-knee amputation of the patient's left leg. At this point the patient was referred for psychiatric consultation for the second time. The consulting psychiatrist advised strongly against operation, feeling that this patient was actively seeking an amputation. Accordingly, the surgeons of the Department of Plastic Surgery refused this operation, but at a later date amputation was undertaken on the general surgical service. The patient recovered fairly well from the procedure but had a good deal of stump pain. Nine months after amputation, the patient fell down the cellar steps of his house and fractured his jaw.

This patient was seen by psychiatrists on two occasions. Separate evaluations concluded that the patient was an immature, histrionic, and passive person who used his disabilities as a complaint against the world. He portrayed himself as a brave sufferer who was completely cooperative with all physicians and surgeons. While overtly commending his physicians, it was also perfectly clear that his praise of doctors was mixed with a great deal of covert blame. Although he had collected substantial funds because of his initial industrial accident, he had lived a marginal financial existence since that time, to the great detriment of his wife and children.

The practical management of such patients is extremely difficult. They evade and refute all suggestions of psychotherapy. In a quieter way, they resemble the more dramatic cases described under the title "Munchausen's syndrome" (Chapman, 1957).

A review of patients who request repeated cosmetic surgical procedures revealed a syndrome involving borderline or ambulatory psychotic patients who are "insatiable" in seeking physical changes in their anatomy, usually the facial region (Knorr and coworkers, 1967). These patients are usually male, aged 17 to 39, and unmarried. Additional characteristics include low self-esteem, emphasized by statements indicating a chronic history of lack of confidence, feelings of worthlessness, feelings of social inadequacy, and a propensity for frequent episodes of depression; hyposexuality, demonstrated by a history of minimal heterosexual and masturbation experience; grandiose ambitions for future accomplishments for which the patient has little qualification and background; failure to develop meaningful and long-term personal relationships; an extreme obsession with appearance and the need for surgery to the point of preventing the patient from engaging in any constructive endeavors; an attitude of passivity and obsequiousness toward the surgeon which may turn to overt aggression and legal threats if the surgeon elects not to operate or if the patient feels the surgical result is unsatisfactory; high anxiety in the patient that the surgeon does not understand the patient's request, a situation leading to frequent letters and telephone calls to the surgeon; the patient compulsively showing photographs and drawings to the surgeon concerning the physical alterations he hopes to obtain; a vagueness involving the patient's motivation for surgery, but with strong expressions of emotional and social urgency; and finally, dissatisfaction with surgery after an initial period of postoperative enthusiasm and a request for further surgery. A survey of the American Society of Plastic and Reconstructive Surgeons concerning the treatment of these patients revealed that some 38 per cent of the 325 members who responded to the questionnaire indicated that some treatment success is possible with a few patients when psychiatric evaluation and therapy accompanied surgical treatment. The remaining respondents felt that surgical treatment did not benefit these patients.

With the best treatment, the chances of rehabilitation are very poor. It may be that a small fraction of such patients are the lot of any conscientious plastic surgeon. Only careful combined surgical and psychiatric evaluation can determine the point at which further surgical efforts are no longer the answer to the patient's symptoms and complaints.

Such patients are fortunately infrequent, but their early recognition can spare the patient unnecessary surgery and may spare the surgeon unnecessary worry and frustration.

Evidence from the Surgeon's Assessment of the Patient's Psychologic and Emotional State

The plastic surgeon must and inevitably does develop his own rapid methods of evaluating the emotional stability and degree of mental disorder in his patients. There is little difficulty in the recognition of the obviously and grossly psychotic person whose complaints are bizarre, who expects the impossible, and whose manner communicates extreme lability of emotions. In psychiatric slang, the terms "pseudo-neurotic schizophrenia" and "smiling depression" convey the fact that major mental illness does not always express itself in obvious fashion.

It is well to state that the most expert psychiatrist may have a difficult time in assessing the nature and extent of mental illness in his patients. Estimates of the prevalence of significant emotional symptoms in various patient populations vary from a minimum of 25 per cent to an incredible 80 per cent (Hamman, 1939; Kaufman and Bernstein, 1957). Systematic inquiry will assist the surgeon in the better definition of situations of uncertainty in which it would be at best risky to operate and in which he may then counsel substantial deferral of surgery or psychiatric consultation or both. The surgeon should routinely seek to evaluate the following psychiatric syndromes and ways of living which are apt to be presented as complaints of physical deformity.

1. The Hidden Psychotic Patient. Complaints of somatic deformity are frequent in the incipient stages of certain schizophrenic reactions. Delusions of body odor may be translated into complaints in respect to the patient's nose. Systematic inquiry into the recent years of the patient's life will reveal progressive social isolation and fears of general inadequacy. Vagueness and multiplicity of the patient's complaints and preoccupation with minor though real dyssymmetries are characteristic.

A 30 year old electronics engineer requested rhytidoplasty because a drastic program of weight reduction left his face looking "old and tired." The physical basis of his complaints was objective enough, but the vagueness of his expectations and the social ill ease of his manner led to psychiatric referral. In discussion with the psychiatrist, the patient expanded on his sense of deformity, saying that he also wished the plastic surgeon to transplant hair on his receding hairline. He had started his program of restoring his youthful appearance by requesting a procedure he knew was more acceptable to surgeons. Once operated upon, the patient expected he could persuade the surgeon of the value of the more "experimental procedure."

2. The Patient With Major Emotional Disturbance Associated With Residual Congenital Deformity. The critical influence of life situations on the subjective sense of deformity is well illustrated in patients who tolerate clearcut anatomic abnormalities until some important defeat or rebuff occurs in their living. At this point, depressive feelings are apt to involve renewed self-consciousness of deformity and lead to requests for surgery.

A 26 year old single office worker presented with the complaint of deformity of her lip and nose. She appeared to be a rather shy and attractive young woman who was born with a double cleft lip, but no cleft of the palate. She was first operated on for this deformity at the relatively late age of 11 years and further surgery was undertaken at the ages of 13 and 14 years. Following these procedures, the patient had made a reasonably happy social and work adjustment. She became engaged to be married, but the young man broke the engagement. The patient then fell into a state of severe depression and for the first time in 12 years became extremely self-conscious. Because of the obvious residual deformity, correction of the patient's nose was first undertaken. Six months later, revision of the scars of her lower lip and realignment of the nasal septum were effected.

While it was intended that the patient see a psychiatrist prior to surgery, this did not take place. The psychiatrist was asked to see the patient as a matter of interest after her second operative procedure. In retrospect, it became quite clear that the patient had experienced a severe depressive reaction. This had been present at the time of her first operation and had gradually improved over the months between her two operations. Among the patient's symptoms had been a weight loss of 20 pounds, crying spells, poor sleep, suicidal thoughts, and an inability to concentrate. Because of these symptoms, she had resigned her job. At the time of the psychiatric interview, the patient was almost completely recovered from her depressive reaction and looked forward with interest to life and activity in another city.

It is a fair assumption that this patient would not have sought plastic surgery had she not become depressed over her broken engagement. Similar examples have been seen of young women who come for corrective surgery of the nose or breast and are found to be depressed or insecure over a recent crisis in living. If operation is deferred, in some cases, improvements in the patient's life situation may take place, with a decision to forego an operation. In situations of uncertainty, deferral of operation and review of the situation with a psychiatrist will increase the chances of the best decision respecting surgery.

3. The "Somatizing" Patient. A sense of embarrassment or self-consciousness about physical appearance is normal in adolescence. The physical changes at the time include rapid growth and changes in facial configuration, with growth of the nose as well as development of secondary sexual characteristics. The adolescent must lose the sense of himself as a child and develop a new physical image of himself as an adult. In normal development, there is de-forming of the physical image as child and re-forming of a new image as adult. These changes in body image are inevitably interwoven with the simultaneous changes in psychosocial status—the move toward heterosexual interests and the conflicted advance and retreat toward adult freedoms and responsibilities.

In addition to this normal unification of physical and social representations of self, some children are literally taught to retreat to physical expressions or symptoms in response to psychosocial conflicts. This can be done in various ways, most often by parents who are themselves physically anxious and overconcerned. Such patients are by no means malingerers. The retreat to physical symptoms is more apt to involve abdominal pain, concerns about the heart, or frankly hysterical symptoms. Occasionally such patients focus on a part of the face as deformed and request plastic surgery. In these instances, the complaint of deformity is almost entirely a symbolic communication of interpersonal distress, and operation in such cases must inevitably result in dissatisfaction.

A 30 year old married woman sought plastic surgery two months after her father's death. She requested that the "bump" on the side of her nose be removed. There was an obvious though not severe structural abnormality which the patient attributed to an injury in childhood. The surgeon undertook the operation and achieved an excellent result, not only by his own standards, but in the opinion of family and friends.

As soon as she saw the operative result, the patient became tearful, depressed, and angry, saying that the surgeon had "taken away" her nose and that she wanted

only the bump removed. She pressed for immediate reoperation to give her back the nose she had lost. Rightly enough, the surgeon counseled delay, but the patient continued to be depressed and unhappy and agreed to wait only with great reluctance. A consulting psychiatrist reinforced the wisdom of the plastic surgeon's advice. Fortunately, her family and friends did likewise (McClary, 1962).

In this instance, the patient's complaint of deformity was an expression of a conflicted and unresolved grief reaction to her father's death. The liberation of her conflicted grief followed the operation but fastened onto the surgical result and the surgeon rather than the loss of the patient's father.

4. Severe Deformity and Severe Personality Disturbance. A gross deformity impairing physical function can occur in a person who is obviously severely disturbed, if not psychotic. In such circumstances an operative procedure always involves some risk of failure or of postoperative complication. The prospect of tipping a marginally adjusted person into overt and severe psychosis must always induce uncertainty and anxiety. Such cases call for close psychiatric collaboration in order to prepare the patient for operation and to facilitate management of the postoperative period.

A 30 year old single woman of foreign-born parentage first developed a lymphedematous swelling of the right leg at the age of 13. This increased over the years, and when she first applied for treatment she was unable to wear a shoe on the right foot. The skin on her right ankle was beginning to abrade, and there was some question as to whether the patient would be able to hold her job.

A variety of treatments had been tried for the patient's lymphedema praecox. None of these had proved effective. The patient was extremely self-conscious about her deformity, which hindered all normal social activities. Otherwise very attractive, the patient had been engaged twice and the relationship broken off in both cases. The patient's deformity was a source of much contention within the family, and the patient expressed concern that if the contemplated surgery did not go well, she would be blamed by her parents for making matters worse.

It was quite clear that the patient was also an extremely labile and potentially quite disturbed person. A surgical colleague to whom she had initially applied for treatment strongly advised against undertaking major surgery. The psychiatric impression was that the patient was indeed a highly disturbed individual, although she was able to function satisfactorily in her job, except for the threat posed by her physical disability. It was evident that there was a real possibility of further severe emotional upset and overt psychosis in the course of the surgical procedures. The patient's ability to hold a job seemed to be the central stabilizing element in her psychologic adjustment. It was therefore thought that the risk of a postoperative psychosis was justified if certain previous conditions could be met.

For such a patient to undergo surgery without full consent and backing from her parents seemed extremely unwise. Her parents were asked to come to the hospital and talk with both the plastic surgeon and the psychiatrist prior to surgery. Thereafter a radical resection of the lymphedematous tissue of the right lower extremity was undertaken in two stages. The lymphedematous tissue of her right lower leg and foot was substantially reduced in the first operation, and 48 hours later a split-thickness skin graft of the right lower extremity was effected.

Postoperatively, the patient became intensely disturbed. She was noisy, tearful, angry, accusatory of the nurses and physicians. In spite of careful preoperative explanations, the patient had the delusion during this period that all the tissue of her right lower leg had been removed and that only the bone remained. Her acute psychosis lasted for only a few days and her later convalescence was slow but uneventful.

The patient required two more minor procedures at later dates, in the course of which there was no emotional disturbance. The psychiatrist continued to see the patient whenever she returned to the hospital either for follow-up visits or for these procedures. Six years after the first operation the patient is satisfied with the operative result and her mental state is improved.

The story of this patient underlines the fact that even the most severely disturbed patients may undergo major surgery without serious or lasting aggravation of their mental state. It should be added that free and detailed discussion between the surgeon and psychiatrist is essential before an operation can be agreed upon. The greatest hazard to severe psychologic decompensation in the postoperative period lies in situations in which no one knows how mentally disturbed the patient really is in the preoperative period. The disturbed patient then has two tasks in the course of surgery. The first is to undergo the normally severe uncertainties and anxieties that anyone must feel. The second task is to continue to hide his severe mental disorder under conditions of great stress. When the patient knows that the significant people in the environment realize the extent of his emotional or mental illness, the chances for a major disturbance in the postoperative period are greatly reduced.

THE PSYCHOSOCIAL SEQUELAE TO PLASTIC SURGERY

Linn and Goldman (1949), reporting on 58 patients seeking corrective nasal surgery, first clearly stated that such patients are actively seeking to rid themselves of neurotic self-preoccupations. In their observations, the patient after the operation is free to think of other things and "The energy thus liberated becomes available to the individual for more effective adjustment in life."

Linn's conception finds confirmation in statements such as the following one written by a 34 year old married woman more than five years after augmentation mammaplasty.

"I'm sure it helped me from the confines of my own little world. I think in new terms of myself as a person – not as an odd or 'different' creature. I feel like a woman who can take her place in life without apologizing or making excuses to myself or anyone else. . . ."

The patient cited was one of 32 patients interviewed or followed up by questionnaire five to ten years after augmentation mammaplasty. These patients, as a group, reported a high level of satisfaction with the operative results (Edgerton, Meyer and Jacobson, 1961).

The need for long-term follow-up is particularly true of patients operated on for various cosmetic reasons or for minor deformity (see Chapter 22). Subjective responses of pleasure or increased self-esteem reported by many patients in the first postoperative year are real enough. But some reports of individual patients or of small, unselected groups of patients have suggested that aggravation of mental disorder may follow plastic surgery. Meerloo (1956) reported a "schizophrenia-like syndrome" characterized by depersonalization and emotional withdrawal in several women following plastic surgery. He speaks of an "epidemic of plastic surgery – going on among teenagers – often forced to such operations by their parents or the example of a beautified friend."

Only long-term follow-up of significantly large groups of patients can answer the criticisms stated and implied by Meerloo. Neglect of such follow-up paradoxically *minimizes* the significance of plastic surgery in the life of the patient – the potentially lasting good results as well as the occasional bad result.

It appears that surgical alteration of the body part felt as ugly or deformed does indeed free-up energy for constructive use in many patients. In psychiatric terms, this process corresponds to what is described by the awkward term "derepression," the evidences for which are seen in the acute, emotionally turbulent postoperative reactions. The process that frees-up energy and feelings may, however, be more than the patient can handle, and adjuvant psychotherapy will then be required to help the patient best utilize his new situation.

With the best screening, occasional patients will be exposed to disappointment and aggravation of their preexisting neurotic symptoms. The patient who is attempting to stave off a major psychologic decompensation may succeed temporarily or not at all in this goal. If psychologic decompensation occurs after surgery, post hoc propter hoc reasoning will assume the psychosis to be caused by surgery — which may or may not be the case.

A less dramatic but more important reason exists for long-term follow-up studies. Willingly or not, the plastic surgeon enters the emotional life and development of the patient in a significant way. The patient seeking elective cosmetic surgery seeks actually for greater emotional and intellectual freedom. What he does with the increased freedom or the surgical push into greater participation in living therefore does become the business of the surgeon.

The patient undergoing plastic surgery presents a unique opportunity for deeper understanding of human psychology. Further psychiatric collaboration with interested plastic surgeons should bring greater assurance to the work of the plastic surgeon and a sharper appreciation of patients who will benefit from his skills.

CONCLUSIONS

1. The concept of deformity must be considered in the light of cultural, intrafamilial, and individual psychologic determinants.

2. Individual psychologic factors and the surgeon's clinical judgment of the individual case are of primary importance in decisions concerning operation.

3. Cultural and intrafamilial attitudes will facilitate or inhibit the patient's sense of deformity and the individual motivations for plastic surgery.

4. The importance of psychologic issues in the patient seeking plastic surgical procedures requires a more conscious and careful appreciation by the surgeon of his personal significance to the patient.

5. The sensitivity of patients undergoing plastic surgery to the state of the surgeon-patient relationship is stressed, particularly in respect to the immediate postoperative period.

6. The less obvious the deformity of the patient, the greater the chance of highly personal, symbolic, or unconscious meanings attaching to the sense of deformity and to the surgical procedure. Such situations call for the most explicit definition to the patient of what the surgeon can do, and of the anticipated operative and postoperative situations.

7. Informed and detailed questioning in respect to depressive symptoms and states of psychosocial and familial disorganization provides the best indices of a need for caution in respect to elective surgery.

8. The problem patient has been delineated in terms of (a) the type of operation requested, (b) the age and sex of the patient, (c) the patient's previous medical and surgical history, (d) the manner in which the patient conducts himself in an interview, and (e) the surgeon's assessment of the patient's psychologic state.

9. The objective value of the surgeon's uncertainty as a basis for psychiatric referral is emphasized. Many severe neurotic and some psychotic patients do not intrude their psychopathology on the plastic surgeon. These patients should ideally be referred for psychiatric evaluation and consideration of psychotherapy whether or not they are operated upon.

10. Severely disturbed or even psychotic patients can undergo indicated surgical procedures if they have the support of a psychiatrist prior to, during, and after the surgical procedure. If the patient knows his capacity for disturbed behavior is appreciated by his physicians, the chances of its occurrence are substantially reduced.

11. Surgical-psychiatric collaboration in the study of patients during the pre- and postoperative period is feasible when the surgeon believes that it is useful or necessary and the psychiatrist has the interest and takes the time to develop appreciation of the surgeon's work.

12. Because of the serious psychologic implications for the life of the patient, long-term (five-year) follow-up studies are needed.

REFERENCES

Baker, J. L., Kolin, I. S., and Bartlett, E. S.: Psychosexual dynamics of patients undergoing mammary augmentation. Plast. Reconstr. Surg., *53*:652, 1974.

Barker, W. Y., and Smith, L. H.: Facial disfigurement and personality. J.A.M.A., *112*:301, 1939.

Barsky, A. J.: Psychosomatic Medicine and Plastic Surgery. Chapter 9, *In* Cantor, A. J., and Foxe, A. N. (Eds.): Psychiatric Aspects of Surgery. New York, Grune & Stratton, 1956.

Blair, V. P., and Brown, J. B.: Nasal abnormalities, fancied and real. Surg. Gynecol. Obstet., *53*:797, 1931.

Chapman, J. S.: Peregrinating problem patients — Munchausen's syndrome. J.A.M.A., *165*:927, 1957.

Crane, P.: Personal communication, 1960.

Davis, J. S.: Quoted by Edgerton, M. T., 1961.

Edgerton, M. T.: Plastic Surgery: Past and Present (read at Johns Hopkins Medical History Club, April 7, 1961).

Edgerton, M. T., and McClary, A. R.: Augmentation mammaplasty, psychiatric implications and surgical indications (with special reference to use of the polyvinyl alcohol sponge (Ivalon)). Plast. Reconstr. Surg., *21*:279, 1958.

Edgerton, M. T., Jacobson, W. E., and Meyer, E.: Surgical-psychiatric study of patients seeking plastic (cosmetic) surgery: Ninety-eight consecutive patients with minimal deformity. Br. J. Plast. Surg., *13*:136, 1960.

Edgerton, M. T., Meyer, E., and Jacobson, W. E.: Augmentation mammaplasty. II. Further surgical and psychiatric evaluation. Plast. Reconstr. Surg., *27*:279, 1961.

Erikson, E. H.: The problem of ego identity. J. Am. Psychoanal. A., *4*:56, 1956.

Gallico, P.: The Snow Goose. New York, Alfred A. Knopf, 1953.

Gould, G. M., and Pyle, W. L.: Anomalies and Curiosities of Medicine. Philadelphia, W. B. Saunders Company, 1897.

Hamman, L.: The relationship of psychiatry to internal medicine. Ment. Hyg., *23*:177, 1939.

Hampson, J. L., Hampson, J. G., and Money, J.: The syndrome of gonadal agenesis (ovarian agenesis) and male chromosomal pattern in girls and women: Psychologic studies. Bull. Johns Hopkins Hosp., *97*:207, 1955.

Hill, G., and Silver, A. G.: Psychodynamic and esthetic motivations for plastic surgery. Psychosom. Med., *12*:345, 1950.

Hollender, M. H.: Observations on nasal symptoms: Relationship of the anatomical structure of the nose to psychological symptoms. Psychiat. Quart., *30*:375, 1956.

Jacobson, W. E., Edgerton, M. T., Meyer, E., Canter, A., and Slaughter, R.: Psychiatric evaluation of male patients seeking cosmetic surgery. Plast. Reconstr. Surg., *26*:356, 1960.

Jacobson, W. E., Meyer, E., and Edgerton, M. T.: Psychiatric contributions to the clinical management of plastic-surgery patients. Postgrad. Med., *29*:513, 1961.

Kaufman, M. R., and Bernstein, S.: A psychiatric evaluation of the problem patient. J.A.M.A., *163*:108, 1957.

Knorr, N. J., and Meyer, E.: The burned child: Psychological considerations. *In* Debuskey, E. (Ed.): The Care of the Chronically Ill Child. Springfield, Ill., Charles C Thomas, Publisher, 1970.

Knorr, N. J., Edgerton, M. T., and Hoopes, J. E.: The insatiable cosmetic surgery patient. Plast. Reconstr. Surg., *40*:285, 1967.

Knorr, N. J., Hoopes, J. E., and Edgerton, M. T.: Psychiatric-surgical approach to adolescent disturbance in self-image. Plast. Reconstr. Surg., *41*:248, 1968.

Kolb, L. C.: The Painful Phantom, Psychology, Physiology and Treatment. Springfield, Ill., Charles C Thomas, Publisher, 1954.

Kolb, L. C.: Disturbances of body-image. *In* American Handbook of Psychiatry. New York, Basic Books, Inc., 1959, Chapter 38, p. 749.

Kolle, F. S.: Cosmetic and Plastic Surgery. New York, D. Appleton & Co., 1911, Chapter XV, p. 339.

Linn, L., and Goldman, I. B.: Psychiatric observations concerning rhinoplasty. Psychosom. Med., *11*:307, 1949.

McClary, A. R.: Personal communication, 1962.

Macgregor, F. C.: Social and cultural components of persons seeking plastic surgery of the nose. J. Health Social Behavior, *8*:125, 1967.

Macgregor, F. C.: Social and psychological considerations. *In* Rees, T. D., and Wood-Smith, B. (Eds.): Cosmetic Facial Surgery. Philadelphia, W. B. Saunders Company, 1973, pp. 27–73.

Macgregor, F. C., and Schaffner, B.: Screening patients for nasal plastic operations: sociologic and psychiatric considerations. Psychosom. Med., *12*:277, 1950.

Macgregor, F. C., Abel, T. M., Bryt, A., Lauer, E., and Weissmann, S.: Facial Deformities and Plastic Surgery: A Psychosocial Study. Springfield, Ill., Charles C Thomas, Publisher, 1955, p. 63.

MacKenzie, C. M.: Facial deformity and change in personality following corrective surgery. Northwest. Med., *43*:230, 1944.

Mason, O. T.: Cradles of the American aborigines. Smithsonian Report, Smithsonian National Museum, p. 161, 1887 (Part II).

Masters, F.: The Quasimodo Complex. Paper read at Am. Assoc. of Plastic Surgeons, San Diego, Calif., May 9, 1962.

Meerloo, J. A. M.: The fate of one's face. Psychiat. Quart., *30*:31, 1956.

Meyer, E.: Personal observation, 1943.

Meyer, E.: Disturbed Behavior on Medical and Surgical Wards: A Training and Research Opportunity. *In* Masserman, J. (Ed.): Science and Psychoanalysis. Vol. V. New York, Grune & Stratton, 1962, p. 181.

Meyer, E., and Edgerton, M. T.: Psychology of patients seeking plastic surgery. Bull. Johns Hopkins Hosp., *100*:234, 1957.

Meyer, E., and Mendelson, M.: Psychiatric consultations with patients on medical and surgical wards: Patterns and processes. Psychiatry, *24*:197, 1961.

Meyer, E., Jacobson, W. E., Edgerton, M. T., and Canter, A.: Motivational patterns in patients seeking elective plastic surgery, I. Women who seek rhinoplasty. Psychosom. Med., *22*:193, 1960.

Neumann, Z.: Personal communication, 1960.

Palmer, A., and Blanton, S.: Mental factors in relation to reconstructive surgery of nose and ears. A.M.A. Arch. Otolaryngol., *56*:148, 1952.

Pick, J. F.: Ten years of plastic surgery in a penal institution, preliminary report. J. Internatl. Coll. Surg., *11*:315, 1948.

Porter, J. H.: Notes on the artificial deformation of children among savages and civilized peoples. Smithsonian Report, Smithsonian National Museum, p. 213, 1887 (Part II).

Rickman, J.: On the nature of ugliness and the creative impulse. Internatl. J. Psycho-analysis, *21*:294, 1940.

Roe, J. O.: The deformity termed "pug nose" and its correction by a simple operation. Med. Rec., *31*:621, 1887.

Shakespeare, W.: The Tragedy of King Richard III. The Works of Shakespeare, Edited by I. Gollancz. London, J. M. Dent & Co., 1900, Act I, Scene I.

Stern, K., Fournier, G., and LaRivière, A.: Psychiatric aspects of cosmetic surgery of the nose. Can. Med. Assoc. J., *76*:469, 1957.

Stern, K., Doyon, D., and Racine, R.: Preoccupation with the shape of the breasts as a psychiatric symptom in women. Can. Psychiat. Assoc. J., *4*:243, 1959.

Stevenson, R. L.: Dr. Jekyll and Mr. Hyde. The Folio Society, London, 1948.

Titchener, J. L., and Levine, M.: Surgery as a Human Experience. New York, Oxford University Press, 1960.

Weinstein, E. A., and Kahn, R. L.: Personality factors in denial of illness. Arch. Neurol. Psychiat., *69*:355, 1953.

Whitehorn, J. C.: Guide to interviewing and clinical personality study. Arch. Neurol. Psychiat., *52*:197, 1944.

CHAPTER 22

A SOCIAL SCIENCE APPROACH TO THE STUDY OF FACIAL DEFORMITIES AND PLASTIC SURGERY

FRANCES COOKE MACGREGOR, M.A.

This chapter consists of three parts, each of which is derived from a long-term study of the social, psychologic, and cultural implications of facial deformities. The first part deals with traumatic injuries of the face. The second considers cosmetic defects and the types of problems surgeons may encounter in dealing with persons seeking corrective surgery. The third part is a preliminary report of a 20-year follow-up study of patients who had undergone reconstructive plastic surgery.

SOCIAL AND PSYCHOLOGIC PROBLEMS ASSOCIATED WITH TRAUMATIC INJURIES TO THE FACE

Of the many disabilities or handicaps which can afflict man, facial disfigurement is one of tragic proportions. It is a misfortune compounded by a special irony in that it is rarely physically disabling. It does not inherently restrict one's ability to perform the normal activities of daily living, as in the case of one who is blind or crippled by arthritis or heart disease. Yet it is a handicap with such social and psychologic ramifications that one readily understands the anguish of the grossly disfigured patient who cried: "What is my crime? I have two legs, two hands, two eyes. I can talk, I can think, and I can work. It is only because of the way my face looks that I am prevented from getting a decent job or living a normal life. I can't even eat in a restaurant or travel in a bus. People stare at me. I spend most of my time in my room. I would be better off dead."

The magnitude of despair reflected in these words is not the overreaction of a neurotic patient to his disfigured face but a realistic response to a social fact. Actually the position of the disfigured person in our society is similar to that of other minority group members. Like others who deviate from the majority, his position is socially marginal (Macgregor and co-workers, 1953).

This adversity stems from the almost obsessive concern with physical attributes in our

565

highly competitive society. An attractive face is seen as a highly important ingredient for attracting a mate, obtaining a job, and being successful. Indeed, as the role of visual impression grows in importance, external appearance becomes a major concern of the public image makers; the politician's fate may be influenced by the cut of his hair or the skill of his make-up man. As the tolerance for faces that are marred or ugly to look at is so low, the person with a conspicuous defect may be more handicapped socially and economically than one who has lost an arm or a leg.

But the matter of esthetic standards and preferences is not all that operates to the disadvantage of the facially disfigured. More subtle perhaps but of profound importance is the unique sociologic function of the face in the interaction and relationships of man.

The Face: Social Significance. The face is that part of the human body upon which we tend to depend most for clues about each other. Not only does it represent one's personal identity and the region of one's selfhood, but also from its contour, features, and expressions judgments are made about personality and character. In the briefest encounter the face becomes a vehicle for personal impressions, a basis for antipathy or sympathy, and a precipitant of a train of thought to further knowledge of the other. Intimately connected with communication, the face is the area upon which we focus attention — receiving and interpreting signals from the eyes, mouth, and other expressive features — forming notions about the person himself, his feelings, attitudes, and attributes. In short, the face is a symbol by which one tries to bridge the gap between one's mind and that of the other person. "The union and interaction of individuals is based upon mutual glances. This is perhaps the most direct and purest reciprocity which exists anywhere. . . . So tenacious and subtle is this union that it can only be maintained by the shortest and straightest line between the eyes, and the smallest deviation from it, the slightest glance aside, completely destroys the character of this union. . . . The interaction of eye to eye dies in the moment in which the directness of function is lost. But the totality of social relations of human beings, their self-assertion, and self-abnegation, their intimacies and estrangements, would be changed in unpredictable ways if there occurred no glance of eye to eye" (Simmel, 1908).

Patients' Reactions and Adjustments to Facial Disfigurement

So closely is the face tied to the core of the self that any visible damage to it, minimal or severe, is normally accompanied by a pervading sense of shame and loss. The victim wants to hide his defect and to avoid being looked at, a reaction that reflects the symbolic values society attaches to the face and that are implicit in such terms as "shamefaced," "face the world," "lose face," "face value," and "your face is your fortune." The pity, curiosity, and revulsion that others manifest at the sight of the facially disfigured person — reactions that not only are demoralizing but also can have a seriously disorganizing effect on him and his life situation — are grievously traumatic to his ego.

The initial reaction of a person to any damage to his face is commonly one of acute distress, which may be followed by periods of mourning and prolonged depression. Aware as he is of the devaluative attitude of society toward persons whose faces are marred or unsightly, the patient tends to carry over and ascribe these same values to himself. Depending on his personal reactions to those with facial deviations prior to his own disfigurement, he anticipates rejection and being stared at or pitied.

To the extent that the victim of facial trauma sees shock or sorrow in the eyes of those around him, his self-devaluation and sense of loss will deepen. Even before he sees himself in a mirror he may receive clues as to the degree of damage. "From the way my face felt, and the daily attention I received from specialists brought in for consultation," said one seriously injured woman, "I knew my face was ruined. And there were the things I overheard — the nurses saying 'poor girl,' and the tone of extreme pity in the voices of my family and friends. There was no doubt in my mind as to what had happened. I felt dead inside." And a young war victim whose jaw had been shot away said, "I can still remember the look my lieutenant gave me when I was carried past him. That look froze me and filled me with panic."

So psychologically traumatizing is the sight of one's face which is no longer what it was that it is not unusual for the victim of severe injury to entertain thoughts of suicide or drastic alterations of life plans. "When I first saw myself in the mirror, I decided I could do one of three things," said a young woman whose face had been grossly disfigured in an automobile accident. "I could kill myself; I could enter a cloister, where I would be hidden from the world and could work; or I could go back into the world I knew and begin another life as an ugly woman."

In the case of individuals who have a history of emotional instability, disfigurement may precipitate a crippling neurosis. A 24 year old medical student who had a history of colitis and chronic anxiety became an invalid following the reconstruction of her nose, which had been disfigured by an explosion while she was living abroad. When she came to the United States, she remained a recluse for two years. She was obsessed by the distorted appearance of her nose and the scars on her arm and forehead resulting from skin flaps. She feared people would think she was a "victim of lues." In addition, she complained of numbness of her legs, migraine headaches, upset stomach, fatigue, and nightmares, all of which she recognized as psychosomatic manifestations. To facilitate breathing and prevent further contracture of scar tissue, tubes were inserted into her nostrils. But to her this was a minor problem. "I wouldn't care if I couldn't breathe well my whole life. It's the way I look that matters. It's on my mind all the time. I suffer tremendous fatigue and have such anxiety facing people. I'm afraid of new people and I won't go anywhere." Several months of psychotherapy were necessary before her request for corrective surgery could be considered.

There are individuals who despite their conspicuous disfigurement show extraordinary fortitude in their initial determination to go on as before. Irrespective of the psychologic mechanisms which may be operating, such as denial, fantasy, or feelings of omnipotence, the unrelenting assault upon the ego is such that, once these patients have left the protective walls of the hospital, their resistance is difficult to maintain. The war victim referred to previously, for example, was pleased with what the surgeons had accomplished, considering the extent of the original injury. Though further surgery would be required to improve both the appearance and functional impairment of his mouth, he left the hospital in high anticipation of returning to his family and resuming his normal life. "I was not self-conscious at all," he said, "except when eating, and I knew that would be fixed up soon." But first there were his sister's tears when she saw him, and the pronounced dismay of his parents to which he responded by trying to make light of his de-

formity. His confidence quickly disappeared, however, under the impact of people's reactions on the street. "I had not counted on the curiosity of men when I thought of coming back to normal life." Though he tried to ignore their remarks, glances, and pity, a series of unpleasant incidents finally forced him to stay home until such time as he could be "completely repaired."

While withdrawal and self-imposed isolation are more typical responses of persons with conspicuous facial deformities, the reaction and adjustment, in rare instances, may be the converse of those just described. J.M. had had a history of personality disorganization and social maladjustment for most of his 22 years. Treatment for neurosis in the Army, gambling, drinking, desertion and nonsupport of his wife, and suspected homosexuality had characterized the years preceding his accident. An angry acquaintance threw acid in his face, causing irreversible scarring and loss of one eye and part of an ear. Surprisingly, J.M. showed no evidence of depression, a reaction that had been anticipated. Between hospital admissions, he set about reorganizing himself and his life to the extent of returning to his wife and becoming more responsible and conforming. He explained his behavioral changes thus: His whole family had been "jinxed" in one way or another before and since leaving Ireland. Bad luck pursued them, but this accident, he said, had "ended the family jinx and from now on things will be better." He was able to give his adversity a positive and unique twist.

Some Problems of Rehabilitation

Theoretically, rehabilitation of the disfigured person begins when he enters the hospital. Plans include surgery, and, if indicated, prosthetic aids, teaching, and vocational training. The goal of all is to return the patient to his family, job, and society. But the path to rehabilitation is often complicated. Healing processes for any given surgical procedure differ among individuals, and in correcting a primary defect the surgeon may be obliged to create a secondary one. Predictions of esthetic results are difficult to make, for there are limitations to what even the most skillful surgeon can achieve.

Many factors that contribute to success or failure in rehabilitating the facially disfigured are not necessarily related to the degree of surgical repair or restoration but rather to the patient's emotional and psychologic needs and how he perceives his situation. The surgeon's definitions and interpretations of "success" and "failure," therefore, may differ from those of the patient. Although function may be restored, "success" from his frame of reference is not achieved if the cosmetic results do not restore his self-image and provide him with the anonymity he craves. To the degree that he evokes negative reactions he remains stigmatized.

Long-term or multistaged procedures can be especially demoralizing for the plastic surgery patient. Both hospitalization and surgical procedures, whether simple or complicated, normally produce anxiety. In addition to apprehension about physical pain and days of immobilization and discomfort, there are the uncertainty and concern about the esthetic outcome, on which the patient feels his future way of life may depend. Improvement may not be immediately noticeable. Indeed, he may look even worse during staged surgical procedures when, for example, tubed skin flaps are employed or an eye is removed.

After each phase of the overall plan of reconstructive surgery, time is required for healing before an evaluation of progress can be made and additional steps planned. During these intermediate waiting periods, the patient alternates between hope and despair. Some patients, imprisoned behind the shocking facade of a temporary but necessary appliance or forehead flap, remain in seclusion. Others, for whom there is the added indignity and humiliation of drooling or speech impairment, find the normal pursuits of society intolerable. Rage, frustration, and discouragement beset them, feelings frequently reinforced by their families, who like the patients have had no conception of the problems, complications, and time involved in facial restoration. When only a limited amount can be accomplished at each successive stage with no dramatic improvement apparent, patients become despondent. As one patient remarked: "You keep thinking 'just one more operation,' and then afterwards you get discouraged because you don't look so different. I don't think I can take any more." "The whole process of facial reconstruction is slow and tedious," commented another patient who had undergone several reconstructive procedures for her mutilated nose. "It exhausts the patient physically and emotionally and it

requires courage and will power to endure. It is truly a common struggle of the surgeon, the patient, and the nurses."

For the person who must accept a prosthetic device designed to conceal or replace a lost part of the face, adjustment is difficult and emotionally taxing. Besides the deep psychologic implications of a prosthesis on the maintenance of body integrity and the self-image, there is the fear of being unmasked should the appliance become dislodged.

Throughout the often prolonged and complicated road in the struggle toward total rehabilitation, a high degree of motivation is essential. To help the patient maintain his motivation, the support and understanding of the surgeon, staff, relatives, and friends are of inestimable value.

Interpersonal Relations: Communication

The very nature of surgery as a specialty requires of the surgeon that the technical and medical-surgical aspects in each case be given priority in his considerations. What is the immediate problem to be tackled? What surgical procedure is indicated to repair, reconstruct, or alter that part of the body which is distressing the patient?

The training of interns and residents in surgery, in contrast to that in other medical specialties, is perforce concerned with gaining experience and developing technical skills in the operating room. Because interpersonal relationships with surgical patients tend to be viewed as having little relevance, the social, psychologic, and cultural aspects of surgical care as determining factors in the patient's perception of his situation—his fears, needs, expectations, and emotional state—receive little attention in surgical training programs.

It has been observed that surgery as a career specialty is chosen by persons predisposed toward action and challenged by the intricate technical aspects of procedures to solve problems, in preference to specialties requiring close social interchange and communication with patients. Whether it is the result of the educational program or the orientation values of the surgeon trainee—there is evidence that both seem to play a part—the fact remains that in general the young surgeon perceives the doctor-patient relationship as peripheral to the role and function of a surgeon (Kutner, 1958).

In reality, however, success in management, treatment, and rehabilitation of the disfigured patient is determined in no small measure by the kind of relationship established between him and his doctor. Mutual trust and respect and clear lines of communication are essential ingredients both for preparing the patient psychologically for surgery and for maintaining a sound relationship with him until he is discharged. This ideal objective is not always achieved. Some patients are hard to handle. There are those who vacillate—who are late for their appointments or do not keep them. Others fail to comply with the prescribed medical regimen. Some are demanding and complain constantly, or become recalcitrant or even hostile. Others may discharge themselves from the hospital or fail to go through with the planned additional procedures. Tensions and conflicts may arise between patients and staff members, or between patient and surgeon, and communication breaks down altogether.

When such situations occur, the surgeon understandably is frustrated. He may become irritated, discouraged, even disgusted. The patient will in all likelihood be labeled as "uncooperative," "stubborn," or a "personality problem." When his behavior is viewed as difficult, deviant, or seemingly inappropriate, the tendency is to interpret it from a psychologic perspective, as an idiosyncratic feature of his personality. He may be referred to a social worker or psychiatrist, whose psychologic orientations (frequently Freudian) lead him to focus on the personality and to interpret behavior in terms of repression, hostility, guilt, neurosis, psychosis, and so forth. While it is true that deviant behavior may be symptomatic of an underlying emotional disturbance, it is equally true—and more often than is generally recognized—that the explanations are to be found on cultural and sociologic levels.

Particularly in large urban centers where the character of the patient population is heterogeneous, surgical services are likely to be dispensed across boundaries of ethnicity and social class. As a consequence, patients represent a wide range of sociocultural differences that play an important role in reactions to illness and hospitalization and in the patients' attitudes and responses toward management, treatment, and rehabilitation. If these differences are neither understood nor considered, the management and therapeutic outcome may be adversely affected (Macgregor, 1960). The following are two examples.

Mr. G. was born and reared in Spain but for the past nine years had been a university instructor in the United States. Several months before consulting a plastic surgeon, he had incurred numerous facial scars in a motorboat accident. These extended over the right side of his nose, leaving an indentation in his right cheek and the right frontal-temporal region. There was also some scarring of his eyelids.

The first operation involved excising and suturing the scar over the right temporal region. The surgeon's next concern was repairing the markedly damaged nose. However, Mr. G. declined the operation on the grounds that the correction of his nose could be postponed. "What bothers me the most," he said, "is the sagging of my eyelid. It seems as though my eyes have lost their sparkle and life. The importance of the eyes lies in their brilliance and what they convey to another, and mine look tired and blah."

In view of the esthetic contrast between the slight eye defect and the conspicuous nasal scars, the patient's attitude was, in the surgeon's frame of reference, unrealistic and bizarre. On the basis of a personality evaluation by a psychiatrist, Mr. G. was diagnosed as having an obsessive character disorder with narcissistic tendencies. Considered in the context of his social and cultural milieu, however, his reaction was not so strange. In Spain, the eyes have special social significance. Described by Cervantes as "silent tongues," they play a predominant role for the Spaniard in communication, particularly in flirtations between the sexes. Much signaling is done with them. They are "the windows of the soul"—so much so that the Spaniard is said to be far more affected by the quality of the gaze than he is by the color of the eyes (Ellis, undated). This high value which Spanish-speaking people place upon the eyes as opposed to other facial features was the determining factor in Mr. G's reaction and accounted for the difference in priority accorded the surgical procedures by patient and surgeon.

Failure to understand behavior that is culturally determined not only may result in making erroneous judgments but also may lead to a diagnostic error. An 18 year old Puerto Rican was refused surgery by the clinic surgeons and referred to a psychiatrist because they considered him psychologically disturbed. Their rationale was based on his apparent overreaction to a small x-shaped scar just above the eye, the result of having been accidentally hit by a chair during a brawl at a public dance. What they did not appreciate was the symbolic significance the scar had for this patient.

Among lower class Puerto Ricans in New York City, pimping, prostitution, and drug peddling were and are commonplace. Fights are frequent, and a customary form of revenge is to slash the adversary's face with a knife or a broken bottle. The object is to leave a permanent scar, which marks him as a "double-crosser." An intense stigma is attached to such scars, and persons who have them are viewed with contempt.

Coming as he had from an upper class family in Puerto Rico, this patient was particularly chagrined. He had already felt the impact of social disapproval from other Puerto Ricans and believed he had disgraced his family name. He dared not return to Puerto Rico with the scar. With the greatest urgency, therefore, he pleaded with the doctors to "remove" it. Their eventual realization that his insistence on plastic surgery did not stem from an emotional disturbance but was a legitimate request made it possible to rectify the original diagnostic error (Macgregor, 1960).

Of equal importance to the knowledge of a patient's cultural background is an awareness of the role played by social class factors in behavior and interpersonal relations. By and large, members of the health professions stem from middle class backgrounds, and their expectations of how patients "should" behave reflect their own standards and values. Hence they sometimes become irritated or impatient when dealing with lower class patients whose attitudes do not conform to what is deemed proper or acceptable. In teaching hospitals where clinic patients tend to represent minority groups and lower socioeconomic levels, the status gap between surgeon and patient is apt to be wide. Consequently, misunderstandings and problems of communication are frequent.

Physicians are regarded with awe, and in their presence many lower class patients are embarrassed by the marked differences in formal education and socioeconomic status. In their insecurity and apprehension, they become confused and inarticulate. Their failure to comply with expected middle class modes of conduct and ritualized forms of courtesy sometimes leads medical personnel to misinterpretations and negative judgments. These may be compounded by the commonly held stereotypes of lower class patients as being unintelligent and shiftless because they are poor or do not speak English.

In their studies of doctor-patient relationships, social scientists have observed that the doctor's perception of patients' socioeconomic status—and the level of knowledge and other characteristics he associates with it—influences to a considerable degree the amount of time he spends with them and the amount of information he communicates about treatment, possible complications, and prognosis. Because education is often equated with intelligence and the capacity to adjust, patients perceived as having middle or upper class status are more likely than the less educated to be credited with ability to comprehend medical explanations.

Physicians not infrequently underestimate patients' knowledge and capacity to understand. For example, a study aimed at measuring physicians' judgments about patients in an outpatient clinic showed that of the 89 doctors who participated, 81 per cent tended to underestimate the level of knowledge of the clinic patient population. Those who seriously misjudged patients' knowledge tended to spend less time discussing the patient's problems with him than did those whose evaluations were more accurate (Pratt and associates, 1958).

The effect upon the patient who receives only cursory information because he is perceived as ill-informed or unable to understand is that he reacts "either by asking uninspired questions or refraining from questioning the doctor at all, thus reinforcing the doctor's view that the patient is ill-equipped to comprehend his problem, and further reinforcing the doctor's tendency to skirt discussion of the problem. Lacking guidance by the doctor, the patient performs at a low level; hence, the doctor rates his capacities as even lower than they are" (Pratt and associates, 1958).

Though the findings of the above study were not conclusive, they substantiate my observations of the interaction between plastic surgeons and patients; namely, that the patient who is given a thorough explanation throughout the stages of his treatment not only tends to participate more actively and effectively with the surgeon but also is more likely to accept the plans and goals for rehabilitation.

Patient Management and Precautionary Measures

Sources of patients' apprehension, dissatisfaction or hostility, or their lack of cooperation in the treatment and rehabilitation program, can often be controlled if medical and nursing personnel are sensitized to the psychologic effects of treatment and management. More often than one might suspect, those aspects of their surgical experiences that patients find most disturbing and tend to remember longest are not the surgical procedures per se but the particular commissions or omissions in their management. Following are some examples with suggested precautionary measures.

Discussing Procedures in Front of Patients. During hospital rounds and clinic evaluation of patients, physicians routinely discuss in the patients' presence the disfigurements and possible surgical procedures. Important as this practice is for teaching purposes, it is for many persons a frightening experience, if not psychologically traumatic. For most people, especially those of certain cultural and ethnic backgrounds, a hospital is a place to be avoided if possible. Even when a patient comes to the hospital clinic to request an operation, he regards the idea of surgery with all it implies — the anesthetic, "being cut," "pain" — with varying degrees of dread.

While the patient under consideration may be sitting quietly in the examining chair, his face expressionless and seemingly unperturbed, it is often forgotten that he is highly sensitive to every word or sign that has — or that he thinks has — reference to him. Technical language, though certainly preferable to an alarming lay vocabulary, can (by the very fact that it is technical and incomprehensible for most) cause some patients to conclude that their cases have potentially dangerous aspects which the doctors don't want them to know about. Discussion of surgical procedure, interspersed with such anxiety-producing words as "incision," "scalpel," "detach" and "split" (not to mention the effect of voice tones, facial expressions, and gestures), may leave a lasting impression.

Signs of indecision and discussions in front of patients about alternate methods of treatment, or conflicting opinions among staff members, should be avoided. Not only is anxiety heightened, but also the patient's confidence in the surgeon and his associates may be undermined. In general, patients are not accustomed to and often misinterpret the technical dialogue, questions, and exchanges among surgeons and trainees about diagnoses and procedures that are routine features of teaching hospitals. In hearing only part of what is said and not understanding all, panic may be generated by the slightest comment or gesture which the patient construes as having dire implications for him.

Withholding Facts for Which the Patient Should Be Prepared. Under any circumstances, the sight of one's surgically mutilated face is a shock, which can be compounded by the outcome and residual effects about which the patient has not been forewarned. For example, when radical surgery is required to remove a malignancy, he should be as thoroughly prepared as possible for the expected extent of disfigurement and degree of improvement that can be anticipated. In one instance a patient was only told that because of a malignant growth he would have to have his eye removed. Though he was devastated by the thought of losing his eye, his fear of cancer was even greater and he readily agreed to an operation. He said he assumed that his eye would be replaced by an artificial one. He underwent an exenteration of the orbit and resection of the maxilla necessary to eradicate the cancer. On his third postoperative day he went to the bathroom. "When I saw myself in the mirror, I screamed," he said. "I realized I was looking into my own skull. I thought, 'Heavenly Father, what have I done?' Then when I asked the surgeon about a prosthetic eye, he said: 'You can't have one — you have no socket.' Just like that! I said: 'My God, how am I going to live? How am I going to work again?'" An additional and unexpected blow was the discovery that he would be deprived of his upper denture for an extended period of time because of the time delay in the preparation of the palatal defect and the construction of an obturator by the prosthodontist. This complication prevented returning to his job, even though the orbital cavity was covered by a patch. Totally unprepared for these surgical sequelae, he went into severe depression.

Minimizing Patients' Disfigurements. Another preventable psychologic hazard is the deliberate minimizing of a patient's disfigurement by medical personnel in an effort to spare him further pain. While this measure may be temporarily palliative, it only serves to increase the traumatizing effect when he sees himself in the mirror for the first time. For instance, a 45 year old truck driver was severely burned on the face, hands, and body in a highway crash. In addition to loss of hair and eyelashes, part of his right ear was missing.

He was taken to a small hospital. Though he

knew he was hurt, he didn't realize how badly. "I kept thinking to myself," he said, "'it won't be too long and I'll be out of here.'" The demeanor of the hospital personnel contributed to his optimism. "Everybody stopped in to see me—the nurses from other floors, when they went off duty, doctors on their way to see other patients. They all seemed to say: 'Don't worry—everything will be fixed in no time at all.' The doctors said: 'Don't worry, we'll get you fixed up again.'"

The patient had planned to be married soon, and even while in the hospital he continued with the arrangements. One day, when a nurse had him in a wheelchair, he insisted that he could go to the bathroom alone—the first time he had been on his feet long enough to do so. Worried because he didn't come out, the nurse went in after him. She found him frozen in front of the mirror. He was seeing himself for the first time since the accident. He said: "I'm a Frankenstein—that's what I am. I'm a monster." He called his marriage off and never spoke of it again. Later, recalling the shock of seeing himself, he said: "I had no idea I was that bad off. The bottom dropped out of my stomach. I felt like—you know—bang!" (and, putting his hand to his temple, he pulled an imaginary trigger). "I knew everything I was used to at the time was gone. My good times are over. I know that" (Schoepf, 1968).

Failure to Ascertain Patients' Expectations. Another roadblock often encountered by medical personnel stems from the patients' exaggerated expectations of what plastic surgery can do for them. The miracles attributed to cosmetic surgery by popular magazines, press releases, and films, not to mention the "amazing transformations in personality" that are also said to take place, have unfortunately given the general public an impression of achievements that are not always commensurate with the facts. In our research, we found that even some medically sophisticated laymen have unrealistic beliefs and expectations about the wonders plastic surgery can accomplish (Macgregor and associates, 1953). In relatively reputable periodicals one finds such titles as "How to Get a New Face" and "New Faces, New Lives." From such articles people gain the notions that scars can be completely eradicated, broken faces fixed like new, or hemangiomas erased with ease. The potential complications and problems in surgical reconstruction, the possibility of developing keloids,

or the color and texture differentiations that can result from skin grafting are not discussed.

It is important, therefore, to ascertain first the patient's concept of a successful cosmetic outcome. His expectations may be quite different from what the surgeon assumes and may even exceed what the surgeon knows is possible. What can and cannot be accomplished should be made crystal clear to the patient. If risks are involved or technical problems make the outcome uncertain, he should be told in advance, to give him the privilege of being forewarned of possible results and of participating in the final decisions.

There will be instances, however, when full presentation of facts and acknowledgment by surgeons of doubtful results will not be *heard* by the patient, so convinced is he of success. In his wishful thinking, he endows the surgeon with omnipotent powers. One determined patient, for example, resisted all efforts by the residents and the chief surgeon to underscore the questionable outcome of a second operation which she was certain would eradicate her residual scars. Fixing her attention on the rows of surgical books in the room where she was being interviewed she said: "But I'm just sure the doctors will succeed. Look at all those books, and think how much they *know*."

Talking and Listening to Patients. More often than is generally recognized, patients' dissatisfaction and the litigations that sometimes develop are traceable to the surgeon's attitude, which is manifested by a lack of concern for and interest in the patient as a person. Whether the disfigurement is mild or severe, the patient, in seeking surgical help, is also asking for acceptance and empathy in understanding of his problem and fears.

A brusque or hurried manner on the surgeon's part generates frustration and despair, and should the operative and postoperative course be less than smooth, resentment may follow. On the other hand, as Meyer (1964) pointed out, "An enduring grudge reaction that settles on the physician or surgeon can almost never breed in an atmosphere where genuine, unhurried attempts to appreciate the patient as an individual person have been made, when the operative and postoperative situations have been fully explained, and when the patient, though disappointed, knows he has been treated with respect and concern."

It is of particular importance during the long and often arduous course of multiple surgical procedures to allow the patient to express him-self freely. By so doing, the surgeon gives him a sense of support and acceptance through which he can gain some strength to withstand his handicap. Refusal to discuss his feelings of discouragement or hopelessness, on the other hand, may actually intensify these feelings rather than lessen them.

Hope for the Patient

Despite the remarkable achievements of modern plastic surgery, seriously disfigured faces can rarely be restored to their pre-injury appearance. Even with surgical or prosthetic modifications, the results may be far from ideal to either doctor or patient. When nothing more can be gained by continuing surgical procedures, the physical phase of rehabilitation may be considered completed. The possibility that at some unforeseeable future date new techniques or discoveries may offer new hope is beside the point. The fact remains that, as far as can be determined in the light of current knowledge, the patient has a lasting residual disfigurement.

Psychologic rehabilitation then becomes the major goal. Hopefully from the beginning the patient has been prepared for what the surgeon knows will be a result that falls short of what everyone would wish. Such preparation can help to cushion the shock of the inevitability of permanent damage. Nevertheless, as long as a patient is required to return for further evaluation and surgical consideration, his hopes will continue to be bolstered.

An essential phase in the rehabilitation of any handicapped person is that of coming to terms with and accepting his disability. Withholding or avoiding the facts in an effort to spare him further suffering is for the most part motivated by humanitarian concern, but in the long run it may not be in his best interest. While hope and optimism are important psychologic crutches in the face of adversity, concealing information that he will eventually discover for himself is to delay or interfere with the process of rehabilitation.

Reluctance to present the patient with the facts is sometimes unconsciously motivated by the surgeon's need to avoid a painful experience. He rationalizes his sidestepping on the grounds that it is best for the patient. "We must not eliminate the element of hope," said one surgeon in explanation of his evasive re-sponses to a patient's questions about future possibilities. "It is better to leave the patient with some doubt about further improvement. Let him discover [the futility of additional surgery] slowly."

"Leaving the door open," for whatever reason, is sufficient justification for many patients to postpone the immediate task of coping constructively with reality. One teenager, for example, delayed his college entrance for two successive years because he insisted upon waiting for the completion of experimentation which his surgeon had said *might* lead to the development of a technique that could eventuate in the patient's improvement.

There are no unequivocal rules about what and how much to tell patients. Decisions must be made on an individual basis. In special circumstances the removal of all hope could be psychologically disastrous. In general, however, as studies of psychologic adjustment to physical handicaps have shown, the mature individual is both capable and desirous of knowing the facts. The sooner he comes to terms with and accepts his situation, the more likely he is to begin the work of adjustment (Wright, 1960; Davis, 1963).

SELECTION OF COSMETIC SURGERY PATIENTS: SOCIAL AND PSYCHOLOGIC CONSIDERATIONS

The legitimization of cosmetic surgery by our society and by the medical profession in particular is relatively recent. Originally sought and performed furtively, plastic surgery for cosmetic purposes is as acceptable today as orthodontics, hair coloring, or any other form of personal enhancement. No longer is it regarded as a luxury reserved for "vain" wealthy women or aging actors but rather as a social or economic necessity (Macgregor, 1971).

The changing attitudes toward cosmetic surgery and the increasing demands for it have resulted from several factors. Dominant among these are the high premium on physical attributes and the cultural pressure to conform. As the role of visual impression grows in importance, appearance becomes of major concern. "Exposure" is now a formula for getting ahead, and the face is one's passport.

Another factor is the current devaluation of the middle and older age groups in what has become a youth culture. With respect to employment, this trend, coupled with the traditional view that as a man ages he becomes incompetent, has created problems of such proportions that aging signs such as wrinkles, baggy eyes, jowls, or a double chin are impediments that prevent many persons from obtaining or holding jobs, regardless of their capability.

Further impetus to the demand for cosmetic surgery has been given by research findings on the social and psychologic consequences of facial disfigurement, namely, that existing stereotypes—mostly negative or stigmatic—about the personality or character of a person with a receding chin, hook nose, malformed ears, or facial scars can adversely affect his mental health and life chances.

While in many ways beneficial to the patient and surgeon alike, the legitimization of cosmetic surgery has nonetheless been associated with hazards and complications. The public today is sophisticated about medical care and is critical in evaluating the end result. When dissatisfied, patients are outspoken about their rights and do not hesitate to seek legal aid. The plastic surgeon therefore is more vulnerable than ever. His difficulties are not necessarily related to surgical skill but lie in the area of human relations and communication. He must deal with a heterogeneous patient population, representing a wide range of sociocultural differences. The matter of correct evaluation and selection of candidates is beset with pitfalls for both him and his patients.

Unfortunately, there exists no "personality profile" or statistical chart by which one could learn in seconds whether a patient will be a psychologic risk: for instance, his real motivation for surgery, whether he will cooperate or pose a management problem, his subjective expectations, whether he will be punitive or litigious if the surgery is not totally successful. At best, a personality profile is a concept that rests on normative assumptions, and while statistical frequency may be interpreted as statistically "normal," it does not follow that the patient is "normal" in a mental health sense. Even if one had a chart covering all types of personalities with mathematical weighting of characteristics which, when submitted to statistical analysis, would indicate or contraindicate surgery, other variables (social class and ethnicity, for example) would still make such an instrument one of dubious value.

What Can Go Wrong and Why?

Since lack of relevant information not only is one of the major causes of errors in evaluation but also is the source of misunderstandings in the management of soundly selected patients, the importance of knowing the individual cannot be overemphasized. To know him well enough to decide judiciously whether or not to operate often takes more interviewing time than many surgeons feel is either possible or essential.

For example, it is generally assumed that when a cosmetic defect about which a patient complains is evident and operable, it is both unnecessary and unprofitable to investigate or discuss with him his problems, motives, and expectations. This assumption is erroneous. In contrast to the conspicuously disfigured patient, whose needs are obvious, the one who presents a "minor" defect requires particular attention. The former's complaints are situationally real, while with the latter one cannot be sure.

Special Problems of Cosmetic Surgery Patients

As evidenced by research findings (Macgregor, 1971), patients with slight defects tend to assess them as more conspicuous than they are and are also apt to be the most demanding. Additionally, the smaller the defect that troubles the patient, the more likely he is to focus on minute details and to magnify any residual imperfections during the postoperative period.

Cursory consultations with such patients seldom expose their underlying motives. Reasons such as wanting to look better and wanting to get or hold a job or a spouse are so highly sanctioned today as to obviate questioning. In many instances the stated reasons may be the true ones. But in as many others, the stated reasons can be oversimplifications or but a lesser element in motivation for the request. For example, one investigation of rhinoplasty patients showed that, while not verbalized to the surgeons, a dominant factor in the requests of approximately half of the 89 persons interviewed was the desire to reduce or eradicate ethnic visibility (Macgregor, 1967).

It is not uncommon that the presenting complaints of patients with mild or moderate deformities are symptomatic of emotional disturbance unrelated to the deformity (Macgregor and Schaffner, 1950). In a psychiatric analysis of women seeking rhinoplasty, Meyer and his associates (1960) concluded that preconscious and unconscious factors play an important part in patient motivation, and interpretations of these center around the following: conflicts in sexual identification; ambivalence in patients' identifications with parents; the symbolic (sexual) meaning of the nose and the wish for surgery; concepts of body image; and the incidence of psychopathology among patients.

Some unstable individuals select one body part which they claim to be ugly or deformed as an unconscious method of avoiding their own personality shortcomings. They are convinced that this single flaw causes all their problems and that plastic surgery will magically transform their lives. In a study of 50 rhinoplasty patients, Linn and Goldman (1949) found a high incidence of neurosis, while Jacobson and associates (1960) found that the male patient seeking surgery for mild congenital deformity is apt to have serious emotional illness. According to Knorr, Hoopes and Edgeton (1968), many adolescent and adult females who request breast augmentation exhibit hysterical character traits and are prone to depression.

In addition to the person who presents a single complaint, it is not unusual to meet in one's practice a patient obsessed with real or imagined defects who shifts attention from one body part to another. The patient moves from one surgeon to another seeking relief; the end result is often disastrous. The following case is illustrative and also underscores the importance of careful interviewing prior to acceptance of any patient.

Miss G., age 30, was convinced that her slightly large nose was the source of all her problems. The surgeon accepted her request for rhinoplasty without attempting to review her history or to learn what she expected of surgery. Though he considered his results good, she disagreed and demanded a second operation and then a third. When he refused her a fourth procedure, she sought other surgeons. Two consultants told her that further surgery was not advisable. Another, recognizing her disturbed state, suggested psychotherapy, but Miss G. argued that her first doctor had not thought she was "crazy," since he had agreed with her and operated three times. When she was at still another surgeon's office, she be-

lieved her nose was actually disfigured and was highly agitated. To the social scientist who interviewed Miss G. it was apparent that she needed immediate psychiatric care. She resisted this idea, but a few days later was committed to an institution because she had become violent and threatened suicide.

Had Miss G.'s first surgeon taken time to talk with her, he would have found strong evidence that her complaints were symptomatic of emotional illness and that psychiatry, not surgery, was indicated. In adolescence she had been obsessed with what she considered her "ugly" complexion (acne). Spending hours in front of the mirror, she aggravated the condition with heavy make-up. Because of this preoccupation and her refusal to go out socially she was a problem to her family. When the acne finally subsided, she became absorbed with the size of her breasts. Though they were not abnormally large, she underwent reduction mammoplasty. She next focused upon her nose, blaming it for her unhappiness and difficulties with others. By accepting her for rhinoplasty, the surgeon unwittingly validated her complaint, with results that eventuated in a complete nervous breakdown.

Criteria For Rejecting Candidates

Most plastic surgeons have rules of thumb for deciding that a person is a risky candidate psychologically. Although they are generally an aid in patient evaluation, strict adherence to these criteria can preclude objective judgment and thereby deprive some people of the attention they deserve.

History of Psychiatric Treatment. Because symptom removal has long been regarded by psychiatry with suspicion, a common caveat is a history of psychiatric treatment. As already indicated there is good reason to examine each potential patient's emotional status. However, not all forms of neurosis result from basic personality disturbances. Some may be realistic responses to external situations. Yet for most surgeons, the fact that a person has a record of emotional instability makes him immediately suspect, even when his complaint is valid. There is doubt whether surgery will satisfy him, whether he will become a management problem, or whether surgery will precipitate a psychologic breakdown. His chances of being accepted are even less if he has the reputation of being hostile or a "personality problem."

J.B., aged 22, was such a person. When first seen by plastic surgeons in a Veterans Administration Hospital, where he had been admitted for a complaint diagnosed as "psychosomatic," he was arrogant and defensive and had untenable relationships with both personnel and patients. The surgeons described him as a "pain in the neck."

To a psychiatrist, J.B. had disclosed his feelings about his face and how it interfered with his relationships. He had what has been called the "FLK syndrome" (funny looking kid). His large ears stood out from the sides of his rather small head. His upper jaw protruded, making the teeth so prominent that he could not bring his lips together. In contrast, the lower jaw was retruded.

Otoplasty was approved, but additional surgery and orthodontic treatment were discouraged lest these trigger a psychotic episode. In any event the surgeons regarded J.B. as "too difficult" and predicted he would be "a lot of trouble." The psychiatrist didn't consider J.B.'s appearance significant in the etiology of his personality disorder and was skeptical about the psychologic effectiveness of surgery. One resident surgeon, however, was inclined to operate. Because of conflicting opinions, the patient was referred to the social scientist member of the rehabilitation team.

A review of J.B.'s life history showed that his emotional problems had stemmed in large measure from ridicule and social rejection. At school his peculiar face on his small, thin body provoked the nicknames of "long-legged spider," "elephant ears," and "buck teeth" — epithets that he ruefully admitted were "appropriate, but this makes an impression. I always looked odd, and, therefore, I was considered odd."

When he became interested in girls, his frustration continued. "I used to go up to a girl at a dance, but I was always rejected. When I was young, everyone else went out with girls — I didn't."

Convinced that he would have to go through life looking "odd," his efforts to cope with a hostile environment took several forms. He developed "a very short, sharp tongue;" he rationalized leaving school on the grounds that he was "creative" and so musically gifted that he didn't need formal training. Since he was "talented," his looks were not "the most important." To cover his real feelings of in-

feriority and insecurity, he became arrogant and "put on an air of superiority and supersecurity." His isolation from others, he convinced himself, was self-imposed, since he had "superior intelligence and most other people were boring and unintelligent." Though his evaluation of his appearance was realistic, the defenses and stratagems he used to cope with his situation led only to further social rejection, withdrawal, and severe maladjustment.

J.B.'s growing intolerance of others multiplied his problems when he was drafted into the army. Hating it, he manifested symptoms such as shortness of breath and inability to perform routine physical activities. After hospitalization for bronchitis and pneumonia, he refused to return to duty. Placed in a mental hospital, he was eventually given a psychiatric discharge.

His behavior at the VA hospital where he had undergone otoplasty tended to substantiate the surgeons' impressions of J.B.'s instability. His neurosis, however, was situational, and his days were fraught with unmitigated humiliation. Surgery could not be expected to heal his psychic wounds, but correction of his appearance would remove a stigmatic barrier to his relations with others and help him to gain some self-esteem. For these reasons the social scientist endorsed surgery.

Postoperatively there was a striking change in J.B.'s face. His dress was also striking: "mod" clothes, square gold-rimmed glasses, and ornate rings. He was delighted with the surgical results. He had begun to date and for the first time spoke hopefully of marriage. While his improved appearance gave him an almost immediate sense of well-being and more confidence when meeting people, he had sufficient insight to realize that he lacked the skills of normal social interaction.

"It will take a lot more time being with people to change from the way I was before. Because I kept to myself, I have to learn how to act around people. It's not that I'm not fairly well mannered and so on, but I can't carry on a conversation. There seem to be certain intricacies in human relationships that you have to learn before you can actually get along."

J.B. obtained a job as assistant nurse in a department of physical medicine. He found the patients interesting and enjoyed his work. Within a few months his former hostility and arrogance had almost vanished.

Possibility of Litigation. Another criterion for rejecting candidates is the possibility of punitive action by those who may find fault with the postoperative results, even though these may be satisfactory from the surgeon's point of view. In a specialty that has one of the highest records for malpractice suits, surgeons are perforce wary of accepting any patient who they suspect may retaliate if his expectations are not fulfilled. Patients who have had cosmetic surgery elsewhere, but who wish additional operations, tend to be viewed with caution. Blame, derogatory remarks about the original doctor, and vindictive attitudes are seen as red flags, while any hint of legal action is so threatening that most surgeons close the door on further consideration of the patient's needs. This fear, realistic and justifiable as it may be in some cases, is so generalized that some patients who merit help are denied it. Caught in the rigid system of medical values and the stigma attached to those who seek any form of retribution, such persons are left to work out their problems alone. Even experienced specialists may make injudicious decisions when biases have priority and positions are taken without an effort to ascertain the facts.

A case in point is that of S.F. In infancy a skin infection on her nose had left conspicuous pitting, about which she became exceedingly self-conscious. At age 24, she consulted a plastic surgeon who performed dermabrasion and rhinoplasty, which unfortunately resulted in further scarring and also notched alae. Four years later she requested evaluation at a plastic surgery clinic and was accepted for another dermabrasion. Dubious about this procedure because of its previous failure to eradicate the pitting, she asked instead for a skin overgraft. Although advised of the risk involved (possible scarring and a differentiation in skin color), she chose to take the chance, preferring this possible outcome to the pitting. Moreover, she volunteered to sign any document exonerating the surgeons should the operation fail.

While awaiting arrangement of her surgical appointment, S.F. mentioned to another patient that she had sued her first surgeon. The recipient of this information, an "old patient," told the head nurse. The surgeon's immediate reaction was to cancel the operation.

The story about the lawsuit was correct, but S.F. had not instigated it. While she had been disappointed with the surgical results, so had the surgeon. Two days before operating he had

broken his leg. According to S.F. he was in great pain and therefore had not done "as good a job as he might have. I felt sorry for him and I didn't blame him for what happened. He even offered to perform another operation." At the time S.F. was a secretary in a law firm. It was her employer who instituted procedures on her behalf, on the grounds that the surgery had been "botched up." She described the trial as "a terrible ordeal. I would never want to go through anything like it again." She still felt sorry for the surgeon and held no grudge. Her employer, however, had persisted and won the suit.

When the details of this case were reported to the surgeon who had refused to operate, S.F. was brought to the clinic conference for re-evaluation. While several members of the group favored surgery, others more skeptical and worried about legal action vetoed the idea. The patient, whose hopes had been raised, left the clinic in tears.

Surgeons' Motivations

Though the plastic surgeon may sometimes be overly cautious in selection, he may also err on the side of suggesting surgery. For instance, his high sensitivity to the slightest deviation or asymmetry and his zeal to make "beautiful people" may tempt him to propose esthetic improvements. Referred to as the "pygmalion complex," this enthusiasm to make alterations is a potential pitfall and can obscure the difference between "desire to cure and the need to cure" (Meyer, 1964). Surgeons' suggestions may also be motivated by professional self-interest, such as eagerness to obtain operating experience or to recruit patients.

While in some instances correction can be safely initiated and should be, the surgeon needs to be conscious of his motivations. To suggest that an individual's appearance can be improved is to point up a deficiency, a responsibility that must be carefully weighed. Should the person be nonreceptive, he will only be disconcerted. On the other hand, he may be more than ready to comply; but if he is dissatisfied with the outcome, the doctor may have to bear the full onus.

Such a consequence was aborted in the case of R.L., aged 39, who said she had come to the clinic because the previous week, while she was being treated in the otolaryngology clinic for a sinus infection, a plastic surgery resident observed that a rhinoplasty would improve her appearance. She asserted she had never thought of having an operation, but "since the doctor thought it would be a good idea" she was "willing" to have it.

Interviewing disclosed that R.L. actually had long desired to have her nose altered but had refrained for fear the results would fall short of her standards of perfection. In the event of an imperfect result, she would have only herself to blame, a situation that she seemed psychologically unable to handle. Discussion of her work experience and social relationships revealed a vindictive need to hold others responsible whenever she failed. Fortuitously, in this instance, the resident's casual suggestion of a rhinoplasty had provided a solution to her dilemma. Should the operation fail to fulfill her hopes, he could be a convenient scapegoat. Considering the psychologic hazard involved, it was decided not to operate.

Conflicting Concepts of "Success"

Another source of problems in cosmetic surgery is the dichotomy between the surgeon's concept of a satisfactory result and the patient's expectations. Since the surgeon's training is necessarily concerned with reconstruction or correction that approximates in form and contour the anatomic "ideal" — nose, chin, ear, or breast — he assumes that the patient has the same objective. That there are cultural variations in concepts of the "ideal" may be forgotten. Confident in his judgment of what can and should be done, the surgeon is dismayed and puzzled when a patient views technically successful results as disappointing.

Arbitrary ascription of physicians' standards in the controversial area of cosmetic surgery, where patients' responses are so often the criteria for "success," is to invite complications, as shown in the following case. Tired of being called "ski snoot" and being teased about her "Bob Hope" nose, 29 year old N.H. requested correction of its retroussé tip. The surgeon achieved what he considered an excellent result, but N.H. first wept hysterically, then became depressed. Though the modified tip pleased her, she had not expected the elimination of a slight dorsal concavity. To her this was a calamity because she was Irish and extremely proud of her heritage. Equating "Irishness" with a turned-up nose, she had tacitly valued the dorsal curvature.

The surgeon's perception and creation of the "best" esthetic effect — in this instance, a straight dorsum — destroyed what the patient prized — her Irish identity.

Preoperative consensus could forestall such deleterious outcomes. Of central importance to satisfactory results as well as doctor-patient relationships is a clear understanding of the patient's perception of his defect, what it *means to him,* and what he expects surgery to achieve esthetically. The surgeon should insist on as much specificity as possible from patients about what they want or do not want done and why and, in turn, explain as definitively as he can what alterations he has in mind.

Reliance on Other Professionals

Because of the exigencies of treatment, it is important for plastic surgeons to have other professionals available for consultation in making judgments in the patient's best interests. Most medical centers have psychiatrists, clinical psychologists, and psychiatric social workers available for referral and consultation, and it has become customary to turn to these specialists when questions arise regarding psychologic diagnosis and management. They are also the ones most often included as participants in rehabilitation and research programs. Their use of such methods as interviews, psychologic tests, and projective techniques often provides useful adjunctive information and insights in the team approach to comprehensive care.

In depending on these disciplines for psychosocial evaluations and solutions to behavioral problems, the plastic surgeon should also be cognizant of certain limitations. The traditional training of psychiatrists, psychologists, and social workers is rooted in Freudian theory and individual psychology, and as such has focused on personality development, the unconscious, and the intrapsychic processes of persons who manifest some form of psychopathology or behavior considered abnormal. This orientation, aimed at understanding the individual, is concerned primarily with such idiosyncratic features as his emotional life, personality structure, primary sexual identification, and the like. Interpretations of behavior considered deviant (which implies the existence of norms) tend to be couched in negative terms: repression, guilt, hostility, fixation, neurosis, and so on. Such interpretations fail to consider the person in the context of his social, cultural, and religious background, the influence of the social world in which he lives, and the impact of these factors on his attitudes and behavior.

Today the narrowness and shortcomings of the individual psychologic approach to behavior are recognized, and there is increasing attention to broader perspectives that include those of sociology and anthropology. According to the noted psychiatrist Jurgen Ruesch (1966), the emphasis must "shift away from man as an isolated entity and towards consideration of man in his environment." His social needs and his interdependence with his environment, including interaction with his surroundings, must be considered. In a similar vein Murphy (1968) states, "The conception of personality as a self-contained . . . whole . . . goes badly with the world of reality."

For the person with cosmetic defects, his "world of reality" has unique import and must be taken into account. A facial flaw in particular can have profound consequences for his personal adjustment and social interaction. Frequently, his problems are sociogenic rather than psychogenic. Referral to the psychiatrically oriented, therefore, for diagnosis and solution of a patient's problems is not always the answer. Two patients illustrate this point.

C.A., a young mother of three, had incurred a slight facial scar in a car accident. In view of her low socioeconomic level and her established role as a housewife, her intense anxiety about her appearance seemed to the surgeons disproportionate and symptomatic of emotional disturbance. It was suggested that she required the services of a psychiatrist more than she did a plastic surgeon. C.A. happened to be Puerto Rican, and interviewing by a social science researcher revealed that indeed she had reason to be disturbed. In her sociocultural milieu, a scar on a woman's face is a sign that one has been branded for unfaithfulness. She was distressed more for her husband, whom she loved, than she was about herself, since his acquaintances were assuming he had slashed her cheek because she had committed adultery. The stigma which Puerto Ricans attach to such scars was the sole reason both for her visit to the clinic and for what the surgeons had perceived as an "overreaction." Fortunately in this instance a serious diagnostic mistake was averted.

Sarah was a 14 year old girl whose lack of psychologic readiness for surgery was the subject of a clinic conference. The surgeon suggested that the excessive anxiety of the mother was a factor in the child's resistance to a minor operation. The psychiatrist who had been called in to see Sarah declared that in his opinion the mother was not so much anxious as blatantly hostile toward her daughter. What kind of mother was it, he asked, who would slap her child's face on learning that the child's menses had begun? This fact he had learned from Sarah herself while questioning her about the menarche. For him this was substantial and sufficient evidence of the mother's hostility, even cruelty. What he failed to take into consideration, or to explore, was the possibility that there might be some other explanation for the mother's behavior.

Both Sarah and her mother were Orthodox Jews from Eastern Europe, among whom it is the custom for the mother to slap her daughter's face at the time of the menarche "to bring roses to the cheeks," or to bring good luck. By assessing behavior in terms of his own cultural standards of what is normal or abnormal, the psychiatrist was led to a false interpretation. The mother's behavior in this situation was not aberrant. Because it was a custom of their culture, it had no deeper psychologic implication for the child than the ritualistic and facetious spanking an American child is given on his birthday (Macgregor, 1960).

In using the services of other professionals, plastic surgeons should have a knowledge of and weigh their special orientations and biases. Indiscriminate and unquestioning reliance on any single discipline for interpretations of behavior can make for judgmental errors. On the other hand, appreciation of the training, value orientation, role, and function of each specialist enables the surgeon to make optimal use of all whom he may have occasion to consult.

TWENTY YEARS AFTER PLASTIC SURGERY: A PRELIMINARY REPORT

The following is a preliminary report of a longitudinal study of 16 plastic surgery patients of the Institute of Reconstructive Plastic Surgery, New York University Medical Center, who were participants in two separate research projects on the social and psychologic implications of facial disfigurement and plastic surgery. The first of these was an exploratory study of 41 plastic surgery patients in 1946–47 (Macgregor, 1947) and part of the year 1948–49. The other was a study of 74 patients in 1949–52 by an interdisciplinary team consisting of a plastic surgeon, a sociologist, a psychiatrist, two clinical psychologists, and a home investigator with anthropologic training (Macgregor and associates, 1953).

The latter project had been organized to continue on a more intensive and comprehensive scale the research begun in the original study. Its overall purpose was to investigate the sociologic, psychologic, and cultural aspects of facial disfigurement; the relationship of disfigurement to personality structure and development; the significance of it in interpersonal relations and social adjustment; and the effects of plastic surgery on this adjustment.* Both studies included patients with congenital deformities and disfigurements resulting from trauma or disease that ranged in appearance from barely noticeable to very conspicuous.

In both reports of our findings and recommendations the need to assess the long-range effects of plastic surgical intervention or facial disfigurement was stressed. Our postoperative follow-up studies had ranged roughly from 3 months to $2^{1}/_{2}$ years, a period considered to be insufficient for making unqualified statements about long-range outcomes and modes of adjustment, particularly in cases in which complete restoration was not possible. For example, in terms of patients' satisfaction with their appearance postoperatively, it was noted that they often express satisfaction with a noticeable but relative improvement in their appearance, and indeed they may experience a rise in self-esteem. However, with the passage of time, changing life situations, and the continuing reality of a visible and uncorrectible defect, related problems persist or new ones emerge. To be sure, in many cases a goal is attained; the patient is able to appear in public with less fear of being conspicuous; he even marries and has children. In short, he is able to live a more "useful" and "better" life—a major objective of rehabilitation programs. But the question remains: How and at what cost to the patient in terms of the *quality* of his life?

The 20-Year Study

The plans for the follow-up study required face-to-face interviews of our former patients. At no time would they receive questionnaires—the method of choice in many follow-up studies—with such fill-in items as education, employment, income, marital status, degree of satisfaction with appearance, life situation, and so on. Important and necessary as such information is, it would not disclose much about personality dynamics, interpersonal relations, and processes of social adjustment. Moreover, to learn more about what patients think and feel, long experience had proved the unquestionably greater value of intensive and nondirective interviewing, as opposed to questionnaires filled in by respondents at a distance. The structured interview during which questions are read to respondents and their answers checked off in a box or on a five-point scale is similarly deficient.

A very special advantage of the informal interview is that it allows one to explore particular areas and pursue clues which patients often inadvertently or unconsciously provide. As is well known, a great deal of communication in face-to-face relationships takes place not by the spoken word but on kinesthetic and paralinguistic levels. The trained observer can note and record such expressive behavior as facial and postural changes, and other nonverbal responses and signs which often reveal more than what is being said. For example, a patient may respond to a question in one way but disclaim or modify it by a gesture, an expression, or a shift in his body (Birdwhistell, 1970). Initially in the interview he may withhold information or deny certain feelings and experiences; he may exaggerate or play down the extent to which his disfigurement affects him, while the position and tonus of his entire body belie his verbal statement. It is only when he feels more confident and at ease—and this may be toward the end of the interview or even several interviews later—that he is ready to voice his thoughts and feelings.

In social scientific research on problems of the physically disabled, the prevailing attitude is that the data and understanding derived from a few cases are not representative. Sociologists in particular tend to lean heavily on large-scale surveys that can be quantified and which may produce "statistically significant," if disparate, pieces of information about human behavior. Yet to understand some facets of human experience and the human being himself that cannot be handled or told statistically, other methods such as observation, description, and interpretation—those traditionally used by the anthropologist—are useful. By giving attention

---

*For a detailed report see Macgregor, F. C., Abel, T., Bryt, A., Lauer, E., and Weissman, S.: Facial Deformities and Plastic Surgery: A Psychosocial Study. Springfield, Ill., Charles C Thomas, Publisher, 1953.

to the life histories of a few, one can retain what is personal and intimate—the human struggle and what it means to be visibly impaired—while 100 or 200 case studies are apt to be compressed into aseptic reports consisting of categories, charts, and numbers from which the magnitude and complexities of such afflictions cannot possibly be appreciated.

It was not my purpose to do a quantitative study or to be primarily concerned with what is or is not statistically significant; I hoped to "zero in" on a few cases in depth—persons whose problems, anxieties, modes of adjustment, and the like are not dissimilar to those of other disfigured persons, but whose experiences merely vary in kind or amount. In a qualitative study, nevertheless, it is useful to have quantitative checks. Fortunately, these were provided by my data from previous interviews with more than 300 patients and their relatives, as well as supplementary data obtained from the hundreds of other patients whom I had observed or interviewed informally.

The response of the former patients whom we succeeded in locating was surprisingly enthusiastic. Granted, they had cooperated in the original research, but this was no guarantee that they would do so again. Before, their situations were quite different. At that time they were patients seeking or undergoing plastic surgery. They were troubled about immediate and specific problems, and they found it helpful or at least bearable to talk to professionals who were directly concerned about their welfare. But this was 20 odd years ago, and it would be understandable if they were less than anxious to relive or dredge up painful memories or to discuss the years given to adjustment and coming to terms, if indeed they had. But our misgivings were unfounded. All those within reasonable traveling distance responded to our request.

In the original studies we had accumulated voluminous records on these 16 patients. The estimated number of interview and observation hours ranged from 15 to 68, with an average of 27 hours per person. On all but three, there were psychiatric and psychologic reports in addition to the sociologic reports. And there were the reports of the anthropologist-home investigator, which contained first-hand observations of patients and their families in their homes, schools, and day-to-day surroundings—the kind of valuable information unobtainable in an office or hospital setting (Macgregor and associates, 1953).

TABLE 22–1. *Distribution of Patients According to Age, Sex, Marital Status, and Severity of Disfigurement*

		ORIGINAL STUDIES (1946–47, 1949–52)		FOLLOW-UP STUDY (1971–73)	
Age (Years)	1½–12	5		20–29	3
	13–20	4		30–39	4
	21–30	6		40–49	6
	31–40	1		50–59	3
		16			16
Sex	Male	8			
	Female	8			
		16			
Marital Status	Single	14		Single	3
	Married	2		Married	13
		16			16
Severity of Disfigurement	Slight			Slight	2
	Moderate			Moderate	7
	Marked	9		Marked	5
	Gross	7		Gross	2
		16			16

Characteristics of the Group

At the point of entry into the original studies, the age range of patients was from 18 months to 33 years (Table 22–1). Five patients were under 12, five under 20, five under 30, and one under 40. There were eight males and eight females, two of whom were married. As to the severity of their disfigurements, nine patients were classified as "marked" and seven as "gross."

As shown by Table 22–2, the group was highly diversified in other respects. While there was a proportionately high percentage of Jews,* most of whom were of eastern European background, a variety of nationalities and religions were represented. There were also differentials in family income levels, which ranged from high to low in almost equal distribution.

At the time of the follow-up study (1971–74), the age range within the group was from 22 to 58 (Table 22–1). Three were in their twenties,

---

*Of the original 44 patients, there were 18 Catholics, 13 Protestants, 12 Jews, and one patient with no affiliation. Why, 20 years later, we were able to locate proportionately more Jewish patients than Catholic or Protestant I am unable to explain.

TABLE 22–2. *Social Characteristics of Patients (at time of original study)*

ETHNOCULTURAL BACKGROUND	
Jewish	9
Italian	2
Scandinavian	2
Polish	1
Latin American	1
English	1
	16

IMMIGRANT STATUS	
Foreign born	7
Immigrant parents	4
Immigrant grandparents	5
	16

RELIGION	
Jewish	8
Catholic	5
Protestant	2
No affiliation	1
	16

SOCIO-ECONOMIC STATUS ESTIMATED FAMILY INCOME	
High	5
Middle	6
Low	5
	16

One patient of Jewish background became a Catholic.

four in their thirties, and nine were over forty. Thirteen were married, twelve of whom had children. Four, all women, whose faces were still noticeably marred, had been divorced but were now remarried.

The classification of severity of the deformity was made when they first entered the study. Since the surgical and cosmetic problems they presented were complex (many had multiple deformities), all of them would require a series of plastic surgery operations. Some had had a number of operations prior to the study. Others began the first of several corrective procedures and were completed within the time frame of the study. But more than half of the patients would undergo additional surgery in the ensuing years.

As one would expect, there were noticeable transformations or alterations in the cosmetic effect, and with reentry into the follow-up study most of the patients were reclassified. Thus we find that of the 16, nine could be moved into the slight or moderate category (Table 22–1). Of the seven patients originally classified as grossly deformed, five were now evaluated as marked. The degree of disfigure-

ment of one unfortunate patient, however, originally classified as marked, was now evaluated as gross. Her mother, too impatient to follow the surgeon's advice, had sought and received surgery for her daughter in another country with disastrous results.

Preliminary Findings

The one obvious characteristic which this heterogeneous group of individuals had in common—and for more than two decades—was a facial disfigurement. Yet despite this serious social handicap, they had, according to numerical count, done remarkably well (Table 22–3).

Practically all were now self-supporting (or supported by a spouse) and married. Educationally their record was good: all but four had completed high school, and seven had college or graduate degrees. While these achievements were heartening from a rehabilitation standpoint, it was but the tip of the iceberg; only from the patients' detailed reports did one gain some real insight into the quality of the lives of those with facial stigmata.

As we near the completion of the follow-up interviews and the analysis of data, there are beginning to emerge some trends and behavioral patterns related to disfigurement and prolonged social and psychologic stress, coping systems, social adjustment, types of life compromises (occupations, marriage partners,

TABLE 22–3. *Occupational Status and Education at Time of Follow-up*

OCCUPATIONAL STATUS	
Professional, proprietor, managerial	3
Clerical and sales	1
Skilled	4
Unskilled	2
Housewives	3
Unemployed	1
Graduate students	2
	16

EDUCATION		
Graduate degree	5	(2)*
College graduate only	2	
Post high school	1	
High school graduate only	4	
Some high school	4	
	16	

*Parentheses indicate those still in school.

and life goals), and factors that impede or enhance a facially handicapped person's chances of realizing his potential. Because it is both premature and outside the scope of this chapter to deal with all these emerging patterns, I will touch briefly on a few of the immediate findings. Of the measurable items, one of the striking findings concerns marital patterns. Of the 13 patients who were married, the disfigurement, in all but one instance, played a decisive role in the selection of the partners. Because opportunities for dating and marriage were either nonexistent, limited, or perceived as limited, all but one of these 13 had married someone from a lower social class or educational level, someone from another religion, or (in four instances) a person who was also handicapped. They seemed to feel, as they indicated, that they must be content with any willing partner. Women patients tended to accept a marriage proposal to "prove" to themselves that they were attractive as women, while the men, unable to win a woman of their choice, settled for "second best."

Another salient feature was the strong orientation of so many members of the group toward helping other disadvantaged persons. These included alcoholics and drug addicts, the mentally ill, crippled and retarded children, ghetto youths, the aged, war veterans, and the facially disfigured. Of the ten patients who were so engaged (part or full time), it was noted that there seemed to be a relationship between the severity of the disfigurement or its psychologic consequences and the selection of activity. For example, the most severely disfigured person wanted to work with retarded children, who presumably would not find her appearance repelling. Three of the most "normal" looking patients (all had residual ear malformations which wigs, modern hair styles, or prosthetics helped to conceal) were counselors or community workers. Hospital and nursing home settings appeared to provide a more secure environment for five patients with marked disfigurements, while the two patients who worked in psychiatric institutions were those who had previously undergone psychotherapy for severe emotional disorders associated with their appearance.

Although much of the data is yet to be analyzed, it is more than apparent that the quality of the lives of these particular individuals has been greatly affected by their disfigured faces, causing them to make extraordinary life compromises. Although their modes of adaptation and their coping systems have varied, the fact that they all have, to a greater or lesser degree, been able to maintain their psychologic equilibrium and their integrity is a statement of their astonishing reserves.

REFERENCES

Birdwhistell, R. L.: Kinesics and Context: Essays on Body Motion Communication. Philadelphia, University of Pennsylvania Press, 1970.

Davis, F.: Passage Through Crisis: Polio Victims and Their Families. Indianapolis, Bobbs-Merrill Company, Inc., 1963.

Ellis, H.: The Soul of Spain. Boston, Houghton Mifflin Company, printed in Great Britain (undated).

Jacobson, W. E., Edgerton, M. T., Meyer, E., Canter, A., and Slaughter, R.: Psychiatric evaluation of male patients seeking cosmetic surgery. Plast. Reconstr. Surg., 26:356, 1960.

Knorr, N. J., Hoopes, J. E., and Edgerton, M. T.: Psychiatric-surgical approach to adolescent disturbance in self-image. Plast. Reconstr. Surg., 41:248, 1968.

Kutner, B.: Surgeons and their patients. In Jaco, E. G. (Ed.): Patients, Physicians and Illness. Glencoe, Ill., The Free Press, 1958, pp. 384–397.

Linn, L., and Goldman, L. B.: Psychiatric observations concerning rhinoplasty. Psychosom. Med., 11:307, 1949.

Macgregor, F. C.: The Sociological Aspects of Facial Deformities. Unpublished Master's thesis, University of Missouri, 1947.

Macgregor, F. C.: Some Psycho-social problems associated with facial deformities. Amer. Sociol. Rev., 16:629, 1951.

Macgregor, F. C.: Social Science in Nursing: Applications for the Improvement of Patient Care. New York, Russell Sage Foundation, 1960, pp. 19, 20; 23, 24.

Macgregor, F. C.: Social and cultural components in the motivations of persons seeking plastic surgery of the nose. J. Health Soc. Behav., 8:125, 1967.

Macgregor, F. C.: Symposium on cosmetic surgery. Surg. Clin. North Am., 51:289, 1971.

Macgregor, F. C.: Transformation and Identity: The Face and Plastic Surgery. New York, Quadrangle Press, The New York Times Book Company, 1974.

Macgregor, F. C., and Schaffner, B.: Screening patients for nasal plastic operations: Some sociologic and psychiatric considerations. Psychosom. Med., 12:277, 1950.

Macgregor, F. C., Abel, T. M., Bryt, A., Lauer, E., and Weissmann, S.: Facial Deformities and Plastic Surgery: A Psychosocial Study. Springfield, Ill., Charles C Thomas, Publisher, 1953.

Meyer, E.: Psychiatric aspects of plastic surgery. In Converse, J. M. (Ed.): Reconstructive Plastic Surgery. 1st Ed. Philadelphia, W. B. Saunders Company, 1964, p. 371.

Meyer, E., Jacobson, E. E., Edgerton, M. T., and Canter, A.: Motivational patterns in patients seeking elective plastic surgery. I. Women who seek rhinoplasty. Psychosom. Med., 22:193, 1960.

Murphy, G.: Cited in Norbeck, E., Price-Williams, D., and McCord, W. M. (Eds.): The Study of Personality: An Interdisciplinary Appraisal. New York, Holt, Rhinehart and Winston, 1968.

Pratt, L., Seligman, A., and Reader, G.: Physicians' views on the level of medical information among patients. *In* Jaco, E. G. (Ed.): Patients, Physicians and Illness. Glencoe, Ill., The Free Press, 1958.

Ruesch, J.: The future of psychologically oriented psychiatry. *In* Masserman, J. H. (Ed.): Sexuality of Women. New York, Grune & Stratton, 1966, pp. 144–163.

Schoepf, B.: Personal communication, 1968.

Simmel, G.: Soziologie. Leipzig, Dunchir und Humblst. 1908, pp. 646–651; cited in Park, R. E., and Burgess, E. W.: Introduction to the Science of Sociology. Chicago, University of Chicago Press, 1924, p. 358.

Wright, B. A.: Physical Disability: A Psychological Approach. New York, Harper and Bros., 1960.

CHAPTER 23

THE ROLE OF THE ANESTHESIOLOGIST IN PLASTIC SURGERY

Seamus Lynch, M.D.

The administration and management of anesthesia for plastic surgery present many problems seldom encountered in the general practice of anesthesia. The popular anesthetic agents have many limitations in their application in plastic surgery. Several techniques acceptable in general surgery are of little value in plastic surgery. For example, much of the endotracheal equipment used in general surgery is bulky and must be modified to meet the need for unobtrusive anesthetic methods in plastic surgical procedures of the head and neck region. Bleeding, even in small amounts, can be of grave concern to the plastic surgeon, since it may be critical to the success or failure of the operation. The anesthesiologist, therefore, should make special efforts to avoid any factors that may contribute to increased bleeding during general anesthesia.

PREOPERATIVE EVALUATION

Before operation, it is essential that the patient undergoing plastic surgery is visited and examined by the anesthesiologist. The usual purpose of this visit is to gain the confidence of the patient and to relieve his fears and anxie-

ties, but it is also at this time that the anesthesiologist learns the exact nature of the operation. He can then plan the proper placement of the intravenous infusion, the position of the endotracheal tube (nasal or oral), and the location of the anesthesia machine. This advance planning will eliminate confusion in the operating room and give the surgeon maximum freedom within the surgical field. A thorough examination of the patient's airway is also made; this is particularly important in patients with deformities or tumors of the head and neck and may even include examination by laryngeal mirror of the hypopharynx and glottis, if conditions warrant. Such an examination will guide the anesthesiologist in his choice of the technique and method of induction. Many potential errors in the induction of anesthesia can be avoided by such preoperative evaluation and planning.

Many plastic surgery patients are children who must undergo several operations. In these patients, the preoperative visit is probably more important than the premedication, regardless of the drug and dosage administered. Remarkable cooperation can be achieved with children by the anesthesiologist who takes the time in his preoperative visit to gain their confidence and friendship.

585

PREMEDICATION

The patient who has been properly premedicated arrives in the operating room in a drowsy, amnesic, and cooperative state, free of any circulatory or respiratory depression. This optimum condition usually can be achieved by a combination of drugs; because of their pharmacologic activity, each drug plays an important role in the final effect.

Barbiturates. A short-acting barbiturate, such as secobarbital (Seconal) or pentobarbital (Nembutal), 50 to 100 mg, is an ideal hypnotic agent. It is given orally 90 minutes prior to induction of anesthesia.

Narcotics. Morphine sulfate, 8 to 10 mg, and meperidine (Demerol), 50 to 100 mg, are the commonly used narcotics. They enhance the sedative effect of barbiturates and, because of their analgesic action, reduce the amount of anesthetic agent necessary during the course of the surgical procedure.

Belladonna Alkaloids. Atropine sulfate and scopolamine hydrobromide, 0.4 to 0.6 mg, are important factors in a proper preoperative medication regimen. Their primary value is in drying secretions in the airway. They also diminish the reflex activity of the pharynx, larynx, and heart. Because it is a superior drying agent and has an important specific amnesic effect on the patient, scopolamine is preferred. Atropine sulfate, however, effects greater control on the reflex activity of the myocardium. The narcotic and belladonna drugs are miscible and are administered by subcutaneous or intramuscular injection one hour prior to surgery.

Tranquilizers. The addition of a phenothiazine derivative, such as prochlorperazine (Compazine), 10 to 20 mg, or perphenazine (Trilafon), 5 to 10 mg, enhances the hypnotic effects of the barbiturate and narcotic without producing significant hypotension. As shown by Bellville and coworkers (1960), their particular value is in their potent antiemetic properties, since a reduction in the incidence of postoperative nausea and vomiting is best for both patient and surgeon. The patient has a smooth, pleasant emergence from the anesthetic, and the surgeon need not contend with vomitus-soaked dressings.

The premedication of a child can be accomplished satisfactorily with reduced doses of the above-mentioned drugs. If a child cannot swallow a capsule, the barbiturate can be effectively administered as a rectal suppository, in a dose of 60 to 120 mg.

Valium is a benzodiazepine derivative. It is an effective tranquilizer in a 10- to 20-mg dose injected intramuscularly. It is also a useful adjunct for the relief of skeletal muscle spasm. The patient under Valium is relaxed and calm and has a significant degree of amnesia. Its main drawback is that there is a small incidence of phlebitis when it is administered intravenously.

Innovar is a combination, in a 50:1 ratio, of a tranquilizer and a short-acting narcotic analgesic. Droperidol (Inapsine) is the tranquilizer and neuroleptic agent and fentanyl (Sublimaze) the narcotic. Each cubic centimeter contains fentanyl (Sublimaze), 0.05 mg, and droperidol (Inapsine), 2.5 mg. Innovar can be used intramuscularly as premedication or intravenously during surgery to produce the state of neuroleptanalgesia (Fox and Fox, 1966). The neuroleptic state is characterized by mental withdrawal; hypomotility, a disinclination to move; homeostatic stabilization by blockade of the adrenergic receptors; and potent antiemesis.

Pentazocine (Talwin) is a potent analgesic. Talwin, 30 mg, is usually equivalent in effect to morphine, 10 mg, or meperidine, 75 to 100 mg. Analgesia occurs within 15 to 20 minutes after intramuscular injection and should last three hours. The usual narcotic antagonists such as nalorphine or naloxone (Narcan) are not effective in reversing the respiratory depression caused by Talwin. Although it is not controlled as a narcotic, dependency on it can occur.

Propranolol (Inderal) is a β-adrenergic blocking agent which is used in the treatment of supraventricular cardiac arrhythmias, such as atrial fibrillation, flutter, and paroxysmal tachycardia. Its main interest to the anesthesiologist is its use in the aftercare of the patient who has had a myocardial infarct and in the treatment of those patients with angina pectoris, as propranolol blocks the ability of catecholamines to increase myocardial work and oxygen consumption. With propranolol there is a depression of A-V conduction and direct myocardial depression; caution is warranted when one is anesthetizing patients who are being treated with this drug. Propranolol is dispensed as tablets, 10 to 40 mg. The daily maintenance dose is 20 to 80 mg. It is available also in ampule form for intravenous use, 1 mg per ml. The intravenous dose is 0.5 ml to a maximum of 4 ml.

ANESTHETIC AGENTS

Thiopental sodium (Pentothal sodium) is a versatile agent for use in plastic surgery, with few contraindications to its use. Contrary to popular belief, it is not a true anesthetic. As it belongs to the barbiturate family of drugs, thiopental sodium has no analgesic effect within its clinical range. When combined with a low potency, nonflammable agent such as nitrous oxide, it can produce excellent anesthesia for a wide range of plastic surgical procedures. Such a combination allows the free use of electro-coagulation. Neither Pentothal nor nitrous oxide sensitizes the heart to the arrhythmic effects of epinephrine; indeed, Pentothal affords protection against such effects. It is apparent that this combination of agents allows the surgeon wide latitude in his surgical technique and provides the patient with a safe and smooth anesthesia.

Cyclopropane is of little value in plastic surgery. It is highly flammable, and the use of epinephrine is contraindicated during its administration, because of the frequent occurrence of severe ventricular arrhythmias. McLoughlin (1954) demonstrated that cyclopropane increases the amount of bleeding in the wound. Its use should be reversed for patients in shock from hemorrhage. In hypovolemic shock cyclopropane is the agent of choice.

Halothane (Fluothane) is a valuable agent, particularly in children. It is nonflammable, allowing the free use of electrocoagulation. It obtunds the pharyngeal, laryngeal, and tracheal reflexes in light planes of anesthesia so that coughing and straining are rarely encountered. Currently there is a difference of opinion as to whether epinephrine can be used safely during the administration of halothane (Katz and coworkers, 1962). The author employs halothane freely for the maintenance of anesthesia, without restricting the concomitant use of epinephrine. However, the concentration should not exceed 1:100,000. Significant cardiac irregularities have not occurred in our experience. It is of particular value in cleft lip and palate operations, as the arousal time is very short and emergence delirium quite rare.

Succinylcholine chloride is a short-acting muscle relaxant whose primary value is its ability to relax the patient's jaw, pharynx, and larynx to facilitate atraumatic intubation of the trachea. Since its action is not selective for those muscles, the patient is totally paralyzed for the duration of its effect. Prior to intubation and immediately following, therefore, the anesthesiologist must maintain respiration for the patient until spontaneous respirations return, usually after a period of five to ten minutes.

Since prolonged muscle relaxation is rarely required during plastic surgery, d-*tubocurarine* is not frequently used. In the patient who is prone to cough or in the hypermetabolic patient who requires heavy doses of anesthetic agents to provide acceptable operating conditions, curare can provide a much smoother anesthetic course by paralyzing voluntary muscle activity. Assisted breathing is always necessary when curare is administered.

Methohexital sodium (Brevital) is a very short-acting barbiturate. It differs chemically from the established barbiturate anesthetics in that it contains no sulfur. It is used in a 1 per cent solution. The usual induction dose is 5 to 12 ml (50 to 120 mg), which produces anesthesia for five to seven minutes.

Methoxyflurane (Penthrane) is a halogenated ether which is nonflammable and nonexplosive. It is a valuable agent, but its odor is usually considered unpleasant by the operating room personnel. Induction is much slower than with halothane. Due to the occasional occurrence of high-output kidney failure (Crandell and coworkers, 1966), it should not be used for operations on the elderly or on patients in whom prolonged surgery is anticipated.

Ketamine hydrochloride is an intravenous or intramuscular anesthetic which produces a profound dissociated sleep. Muscle tone of the tongue and pharyngeal muscles remains as in the awake state, and the respiration is not depressed, so that the endotracheal tube and controlled respiration are rarely needed. It would seem to be the ideal anesthetic for plastic surgery. Unfortunately, blood pressure and pulse rates are elevated with ketamine, and there is increased bleeding in the surgical wound. Its main drawback is the high incidence of delirium, nightmares, delusions, and schizoid reactions during the awakening period associated with its use. It seems to distort the perception of time. Such an unpleasant experience may last only a few seconds, but to the patient it seems to go on for hours. This "nightmare" anesthetic has no place in plastic surgery.

Enflurane (Ethrane) is also a halogenated ether. It is nonflammable and nonexplosive. Although induction is slower with this drug than with halothane, it provides excellent working conditions for the plastic surgeon. Controlled hypotension is readily achieved when required to produce a relatively bloodless surgical field. However, if the depth of anesthesia is excessive, motor activity may be encountered, consisting of twitching or "jerking" of various muscle groups. This complication is self-limiting and can easily be terminated by lowering the anesthetic concentration. Compatibility of enflurane with epinephrine seems to be equivalent to that seen with halothane.

NEUROLEPTANALGESIA

Neuroleptanalgesia is a condition of induced narcosis which produces profound analgesia and psychomotor sedation, while allegedly leaving the cortical cardiovascular functions intact. The principal application of neuroleptanalgesia in plastic surgery is as a supplement to local anesthesia. Although the combination of any narcotic and any tranquilizer may produce the condition of neuroleptanalgesia, the drug Innovar has become almost synonymous with this state of induced psychic indifference. It is of interest that when Innovar is properly administered the patient can cooperate and respond to questions, yet when he is not stimulated by conversation, the neuroleptic state of calm detachment returns. Operations such as blepharoplasty, facial plasty, and revision of scars lend themselves to this technique, as regional anesthesia is so readily established by the surgeon.

The patient is premedicated in the usual manner. On arrival in the operating room, an intravenous infusion is started and Innovar is injected in increments of 0.5 to 1 ml through the infusion tubing until the patient is in the neuroleptic state. At this time, should there be any signs of respiratory obstruction, a soft nasal airway is inserted and the head is adjusted for optimum breathing. At this time, the surgeon administers the local anesthetic and operates. If the patient shows signs of awareness or movement, additional 0.5-ml increments of Innovar are given. For example, during a blepharoplasty, the tugging during the extirpation of the herniated fat usually elicits a pain response. At this phase of the operation, the anesthesiologist should anticipate this pain response and administer an additional 0.5 ml of Innovar. It must be stressed that Innovar is composed of a potent narcotic and a tranquilizer and should be used only when the patient's vital signs are constantly monitored by an anesthesiologist who is prepared, at a moment's notice, to institute endotracheal intubation, controlled respiration and cardiopulmonary resuscitation.

Innovar also can be used for the establishment of the total anesthetic state should endotracheal intubation be required for the safety of the patient. Here, induction is by thiopental and succinylcholine, as described elsewhere. Anesthesia is maintained with nitrous oxide by inhalation and with intermittent injections of Innovar in increments of 0.5 to 1 ml. This technique is of special value in the patient for whom halothane may be contraindicated, for example, a patient with a history of liver disease (Bunker and coworkers, 1969).

If there is any need to move the patient's head, the surgeon ought to alert the anesthesiologist, so that a deeper plane of anesthesia can be established before the repositioning is done. Otherwise bucking will surely occur, resulting in increased bleeding in the wound. With halothane, on the other hand, the surgeon is virtually guaranteed that the patient will not cough or buck. Such a guarantee cannot be made for Innovar.

A satisfactory alternative is the supplementation of local analgesia with a combination of diazepam (Valium) and meperidine (Demerol). Diazepam, 10 mg, is injected intravenously as soon as the intravenous infusion is established. Meperidine is then given to the patient in a solution containing 10 mg per ml. The solution is injected intermittently in 1-ml increments until the appropriate neuroleptic state is achieved.

AIRWAY MANAGEMENT

By its very nature, an operation in the head or neck region demands the use of an endotracheal tube to provide a free and unobstructed airway, even in the presence of blood in the pharynx, and to enable the anesthesiologist to be at a considerable distance from the surgical site. If resuscitation is necessary during the course of the surgery, it can be instituted immediately, thereby avoiding dangerous delays. In expert hands, complications from the use of an endotracheal tube are rare and of minor significance.

Oral Intubation. This is a simple technical procedure which is performed quickly and atraumatically while the patient is totally relaxed by succinylcholine. It is important to use an adequate dose of this drug (60 to 100 mg). Smaller amounts do not produce complete relaxation, and pressure from the laryngoscope blade can damage the incisors or produce tears of the soft tissues in the hypopharynx. As its duration of action is directly related to its dose level, recovery from a small dose of succinylcholine is rapid. Such a quick return of muscle activity following intubation does not allow sufficient time for the topical anesthetic agent to attain its peak effect, and there is a resulting straining and coughing with the endotracheal tube in place. This relaxant, in amounts of 20 to 60 mg, can be safely used for the intubation of a child. Oral intubation is used on all patients undergoing surgery of the head, with the exception of intraoral and perioral operations or those procedures associated with intermaxillary wiring.

Nasal Intubation. The nasal technique is preferable for all intraoral operations, since it leaves the surgical field completely free for the surgeon. It is a more difficult intubation, however, and there is always the possibility of inducing troublesome epistaxis. To avoid this complication, it is advisable to shrink the nasal mucosa and turbinates with cocaine hydrochloride (4 per cent) prior to the insertion of a nasal tube. The use of this method should be avoided in children, because of the varying amounts of adenoid tissue in the nasopharynx.

Blind-Awake Nasal Technique. The blind technique is generally reserved for the patient presenting a difficult airway problem, such as large lesions of the oral cavity, reconstruction following extensive cancer surgery on the jaw and neck, trismus, jaw malformations, or the wired jaw; each of these conditions requires establishment of the airway through intubation before general anesthesia is induced. Following the application of a topical anesthetic to the airway, the tube is inserted through the nose and nasopharynx into the oropharynx. From this point on, the tube is advanced into the trachea by utilizing, as the only guide, the intensity and pitch of the breadth sounds emanating from the lumen of the tube. As soon as the tube is in place, anesthesia can be safely induced. If the operator is unhurried and gentle, there is minimal discomfort to the patient.

The immediate postoperative period is fraught with danger whenever the mandible is immobilized by intermaxillary fixation. While the patient is emerging from anesthesia, blood, mucus, and vomitus are difficult to remove from the pharynx, for suction can be accomplished only through the nose by means of a nasal catheter. In order to prevent aspiration into the lungs, it is essential that the endotracheal tube remain in the trachea until the patient has completely recovered from the anesthetic. When the endotracheal tube is removed, a soft nasopharyngeal airway is inserted to facilitate further suction until the patient is completely able to eliminate his own airway secretions. Extreme care must be taken to insure the patency of this airway.

Attention to Detail

Reduction in Bulk of Equipment. One of the problems most annoying to the plastic surgeon in attempting to operate on a face is the presence of large, bulky equipment encroaching on the operative field. To keep bulk at a minimum, it is preferable to use a soft rubber Magill endotracheal tube with a curved metal adapter at its proximal end. The tube is cut to exact length so that, following insertion, only the metal piece, resting on the lower lip or the

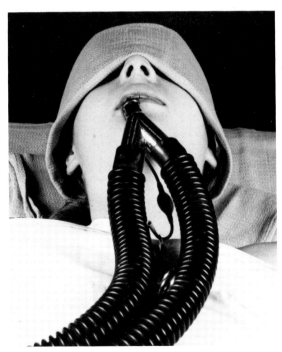

FIGURE 23–1. Oral intubation for operations on the upper face and head.

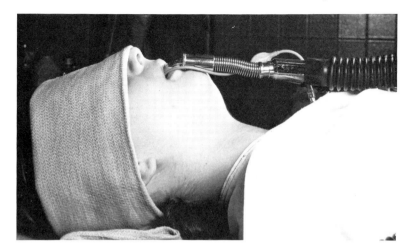

FIGURE 23-2. Oral intubation showing the cylindrical extension piece.

dorsum of the nose, is visible. The metal piece, in turn, is connected to a small, cylindrical, malleable connecting piece and then to the hoses leading from the machine. The hoses are extra long, allowing the anesthesiologist to sit at the foot of the table in the case of oral intubation, or far behind the head in the case of nasal intubation. A minimal number of short adhesive strips are used to secure the tube. If distortion of the face is a problem to the surgeon, adhesive is not used, since distortion is virtually eliminated when the tube lies freely. It is also unwise to affix the tube in operations in which it is necessary for the surgeon to move the tube from side to side, as in the case of full-face dermabrasion (Figs. 23-1 to 23-3).

Carbon Dioxide Retention. Depressed respiration produces an elevated blood carbon dioxide level. By its direct vasodilating effect, this in turn increases the amount of oozing in the surgical field. It is therefore important that the patient's ventilation be augmented at all times by the technique of assisted or controlled respiration. Carbon dioxide tension also plays a role in the reduction of cerebral edema during craniofacial surgical procedures.

Airway Obstruction. The fact that the patient has been sucessfully intubated does not guarantee that the airway will remain patent for the duration of the anesthesia. Under certain conditions the tube may become kinked by hyperextension or hyperflexion of the neck. The lumen may be partially or completely occluded by a blood clot or inspissated mucus from within, or by the pressure of retractors or pharyngeal packs from without. When total obstruction occurs, it is readily diagnosed and remedied because breathing ceases.

Unfortunately, when the obstruction is not complete and a partial airway remains, only the alert anesthesiologist will be aware of the situation and be able to take the necessary steps to relieve the obstruction. When it remains uncorrected, the patient must exert considerable effort to overcome the increased re-

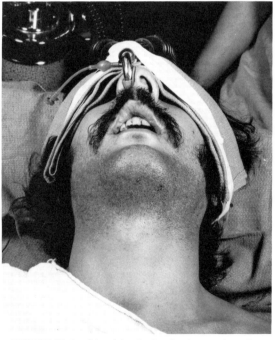

FIGURE 23-3. Nasal intubation for intraoral, perioral, and neck operations.

sistance to breathing. This results in an annoying oozing of blood in the surgical field. The increased bleeding is due to the elevation of the venous and arterial pressures and the increase in the level of carbon dioxide in the blood. Any sudden change in the amount of bleeding in the wound warrants immediate inspection of the airway.

Coughing. Coughing and straining with the endotracheal tube in place produce an elevation in blood pressure and a rise in peripheral venous pressure, resulting undoubtedly in increased bleeding. It can even cause a recurrence of bleeding in areas already under hemostatic control. It is essential that the anesthesiologist institute adequate topical anesthesia of the larynx and trachea and that he maintain a proper depth of anesthesia. On the other hand, the surgeon should be aware of the fact that an otherwise smooth anesthesia can be marred by abrupt repositioning of the head and neck. These actions tend to move the tube and invariably lead to coughing and straining. The surgeon should forewarn the anesthesiologist of his intentions, so that the anesthesiologist may either deepen the level of anesthesia or administer small amounts of a short-acting muscle relaxant. The move can then be made without fear of causing unnecessary complications.

Premature Recovery. In abdominal or chest surgery, it may be desirable to have the patient wide awake at the end of the operation. In plastic surgery this is to be avoided. Application of the dressing is of great importance to the success of the operation. It is almost impossible to apply a dressing properly when the patient is coughing, vomiting, or resisting vigorously. Straining may also cause bleeding under a skin graft. To maintain quiescence until the end of the operation, either an adequate depth of anesthesia must be maintained until the completion of the dressing, or a small amount of succinylcholine must be administered.

Recovery Period. In the recovery room the patient is watched closely by the anesthesia and recovery room staffs for signs of airway impairment, particularly when the operation is in the region of the oral cavity or if the dressings encroach, by pressure, on the neck. If there are signs of a delirious emergence from anesthesia, it may be controlled by the intravenous injection of a mixture containing meperidine,

10 mg, and perphenazine, 1 mg, in each cubic centimeter. One cubic centimeter is given at five-minute intervals until the desired effect is attained. This allows a quiet, relaxed awakening which is greatly appreciated by the surgeon, the patient, and the nursing staff.

Laryngeal Edema. This infrequent but serious complication of tracheal intubation usually occurs in children. Because of the small diameter of the child's larynx, a minute amount of mucosal edema greatly reduces the cross-sectional area, producing varying degrees of respiratory obstruction. This condition is readily diagnosed by the croupy cough, restlessness, and respiratory stridor with retraction of the chest wall on inspiration. The diagnosis should be made before cyanosis is evident. Treatment consists of placing the child in a croupette with a high oxygen and moisture content. To reduce restlessness, sedation is induced with a barbiturate administered either by injection or by rectal suppository. Prednisolone, 12.5 to 25 mg, or dexamethasone (Decadron), 2 to 4 mg, by intramuscular injection, is effective in reducing the edema and may be repeated in three hours. However, if symptoms persist and there is a rise in pulse rate, tracheotomy should be performed without further delay.

The careful anesthesiologist can virtually eliminate the occurrence of laryngeal edema by using a sterile endotracheal tube of the proper diameter. If the tube does not pass freely through the larynx, it should be discarded and one of smaller diameter introduced. Coughing while the tube is in place can be prevented by maintaining the proper depth of anesthesia. The surgeon should avoid frequent changes in the position of the child's head, as this can produce considerable irritation to the laryngeal cords. If these precautions are observed, laryngeal edema should be a rare occurrence.

THE BLEEDING PROBLEM

Modern anesthesia favors light planes of anesthesia and stresses the dangers of inhalational and intravenous anesthetic agents. However, deep anesthesia has the value of reduced peripheral circulation and thus a relatively bloodless field. Unfortunately, the higher morbidity rate associated with deep anesthesia far outweighs this advantage. With the lighter levels used today, the peripheral blood flow is greatly increased; this is probably one of the major reasons why local anesthesia is favored by the plastic surgeon. There is no doubt that there is less bleeding in the conscious patient under local anesthesia than in a similar patient undergoing general anesthesia. This point is clearly demonstrated by the data in Table 23–1.

INDUCED HYPOTENSION

Because of the facts discussed above and the increasing demand by patients for general anesthesia, efforts have been made to produce a dry, bloodless field in the anesthetized patient. The most dramatic approach is the application of induced hypotension to general anesthesia in plastic surgery. This technique has been fostered by Enderby (1958) in England.

Hypotension is induced by drugs that cause generalized peripheral vasodilation. Combined with posture, such as the head-up position for operations in the head and neck, hypotension allows pooling of the blood in the dependent areas away from the surgical site. The venous return to the heart is reduced and the cardiac output falls, vastly reducing the amount of bleeding in the surgical wound. Vasodilation is produced by drugs that block the autonomic ganglia. Those commonly used are hexamethonium (C6), pentolinium tartrate (Ansolysen), trimethaphan camphorsulfonate (Arfonad), homatropinium (Trophenium) and sodium nitroprusside.

An important part of the technique advocated by Enderby is controlled respiration.

TABLE 23–1. *Blood Flow (ml) in the Awake State, Under Light Anesthesia, and Under Deep Cyclopropane Anesthesia*

	CONSCIOUS	LIGHT ANESTHESIA	DEEP ANESTHESIA
Skin flow	250	1000	500
Muscle flow	500	1500	750
Kidney	1400	900	250
Liver	1400	900	400
Brain	750	750	500
Coronary	400	400	400
Cardiac output	4700	5450	2750

Tabular material reproduced by kind permission from A Practice of Anaesthesia (1960) by W. D. Wylie and H. C. Churchill-Davidson. London: Lloyd-Luke (Medical Books).

Positive pressure applied to the airway through intermittent manual pressure on the rebreathing bag, by raising the intrapleural pressure, can further reduce the venous return to the heart. This technique has a marked hypotensive effect when used in combination with the ganglion-blocking agents.

Halothane and Hypotension. Halothane produces hypotension by causing generalized peripheral vasodilation and by reducing the cardiac output. The action of halothane is probably due to a diminished sympathoadrenal response as the norepinephrine effect on the myocardium is reduced (Severinghaus and Cullen, 1958; Enderby, 1960; Black and McArdle, 1962). The author has employed this property of halothane in a series of 750 patients undergoing plastic surgery in whom induced hypotension was deemed desirable.

The patient is premedicated in the usual manner and induced with thiopental. Following intubation, the patient is placed in a 20- to 30-degree head-up tilt, and administration of halothane in oxygen in a semiclosed system is begun. A sufficiently high concentration is administered to reduce the blood pressure to the desired level. The concentration may vary from 1 to 3 per cent, depending upon the individual response of the patient. At this time, the surgeon infiltrates the surgical field with a mixture containing procaine, 0.5 per cent, and epinephrine, 1:200,000. The purpose of this infiltration is twofold. (1) In light planes of general anesthesia, surgical stimuli tend to elevate the blood pressure. Procaine, by blocking these stimuli, allows a significantly lower concentration of halothane to be used in attaining the desired level of hypotension. (2) Epinephrine, by its vasoconstrictor effect, eliminates the need for profound hypotension, that is, below 60 mm Hg. It must be stressed that higher concentrations of epinephrine are unnecessary and dangerous. There were no serious arrhythmias in our series with the above regimen. However, in four patients in whom 1:35,000 epinephrine was used inadvertently, hypertension, tachycardia, multiple ventricular extrasystoles, and ventricular tachycardia were noted.

Following surgical incision, an evaluation of the bleeding in the wound is made, and the blood pressure is lowered by increasing the inhaled concentration of halothane to achieve the minimal reduction compatible with the control of bleeding. Systolic levels of 60 to 70 mm Hg are easily maintained and give a satisfactory bloodless field in the majority of cases. It has been noted, however, that, in the corrective nasal plastic operation and in scalp and forehead flap operations, a more profound hypotension is necessary to control bleeding. In such cases, the systolic blood pressure is reduced below 50 mm Hg.

In 15 per cent of our cases, halothane used alone did not lower the blood pressure sufficiently. Rather than incorporate the use of controlled respiration, a small amount of Arfonad (50 to 150 mg) is administered by infusion. This rapidly produces the required blood pressure level. As halothane potentiates the action of the ganglion-blocking agents, very small amounts of Arfonad are required in its presence (Enderby, 1960).

When the operation is completed, the level of anesthesia and hypotension is maintained until after the dressings are applied. The patient is transported to the recovery room and retained there in the same degree of head-up tilt as in the operating room. Oxygen is administered by oral or nasal catheter until the patient has reacted fully. The blood level of halothane is rapidly reduced as soon as administration of this agent is stopped, and the blood pressure gradually returns to normal within one hour. It has not been found necessary to restore the blood pressure by the use of vasopressors.

This technique has been administered to patients varying in age from 16 to 83 years. There has been no complication associated with hypotension, and there were no deaths.

Dangers of Induced Hypotension. Cerebral thrombosis, hemophilia, thrombosis of the central retinal artery, coronary thrombosis, oliguria, anuria, and postoperative hemorrhage have been reported as complications of induced hypotension.

Hampton and Little (1957) reported 42 deaths in 21,000 patients undergoing hypotensive anesthesia in Great Britain, an incidence of 1 in 500. Enderby (1961), on the other hand, noted nine deaths in 9000 cases, or 1 in 1000 mortality; however, these occurred early in the series, and there were no deaths in the last 3000 cases. As a comparison, the mortality rate from anesthesia without induced hypotension in the United States is approximately 1 in 2000. The increased morbidity and mortality would seem to be sufficient reason to reserve this technique for those cases in which the risk of death from massive hemorrhage exceeds that from induced hypotension.

On the other hand, the surgeon should realize that the skilled anesthesiologist who has experience with this technique can safely apply induced hypotension without a significant increase in danger to the patient (Enderby, 1961; Linacre, 1961). It is, however, such an exacting and demanding technique, with so little margin for error, that it cannot be recommended for general use.

CLEFT PALATE AND LIP OPERATIONS

A noted pediatric anesthesiologist (Smith, 1959) has set down exacting conditions for the anesthetic management of children undergoing cleft palate and lip operations. He stated, "The apparatus must not involve increased resistance or dead space, and it must not interfere with the surgeon or contaminate the field, but should provide means of assisting or controlling the child's respiration."

This is, indeed, a difficult order to fill. Cleft palate and lip operations demand that the surgeon should be prepared to share the surgical field with the anesthesiologist if the patient's safety is to remain of prime concern. Unfortunately, extensions to the endotracheal tube cannot be used, since these additions merely increase the dead space and resistance to breathing. Such a physiologic insult is poorly tolerated by infants and young children. A satisfactory compromise is achieved by using the equipment shown in Figure 23–4, which allows the anesthesiologist complete control without intruding upon the surgical field.

Cleft lip and palate operations can be done readily in the presence of an oral endotracheal tube which is placed either in the groove of a Dott or Dingman gag or within the lingual groove and brought out at the side of the mouth, where it is joined to a nonrebreathing valve, and thence to the source of the anesthetic agents. Cardiorespiratory action is monitored by a stethoscope fastened to the precordium or by an electronic pulse monitor. Halothane has proved to be a valuable agent for this procedure, as the gag reflex is obtunded in light planes of anesthesia. Induction is quite short and recovery is extremely rapid. At the completion of surgery, great care is taken to remove all blood and secretions from the oropharynx, as a minute clot of blood remaining in the hypopharynx may be aspirated with fatal results.

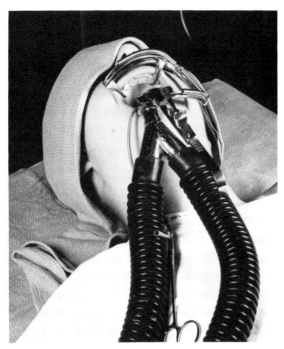

FIGURE 23–4. Demonstration of the Kilner-Dott gag in place for palate surgery. Although the child is intubated via the oral route, the tube and associated equipment are unobtrusive.

In cleft palate and pharyngeal flap operations, particularly in adolescent and adult patients, blood loss may be large. The anesthesiologist should be prepared to transfuse blood during these operations.

REGIONAL ANESTHESIA

When local anesthesia is chosen, it is usually administered by the surgeon who simply infiltrates the surgical area with one of the more popular anesthetic agents. However, as in the case of an operation on the hand or forearm or on the abdomen or lower extremities (particularly where large areas are involved), it may be advisable to have the anesthesiologist administer the regional anesthetic to the patient by the brachial plexus, the spinal, or the epidural route.

Brachial Plexus Block. This valuable method of anesthesia has never been widely accepted by surgeons because of the relatively high incidence of failures, delayed onset of action, and pneumothorax. Since the introduction

of the axillary approach by Burnham (1959), pneumothorax as a complication has been eliminated (Brand and Papper, 1961). The incidence of failures depends entirely upon the experience of the anesthesiologist with this technique; with the use of agents such as lidocaine (Xylocaine) and mepivacaine (Carbocaine), the onset is rapid and the anesthetic effect profound and prolonged. This method of anesthesia, when combined with a tourniquet, presents the ideal operating conditions for surgery of the forearm or hand. The details of the technique of axillary block were outlined by Abadir (1970). When sedative doses of thiopental sodium are added, it may be used successfully, even on the apprehensive patient. It is undoubtedly the method of choice for operations in the forearm or hand when the patient has recently ingested food.

Spinal and Epidural Blocks. For operations on the abdomen or lower extremities, spinal and epidural blocks are frequently used and, like the brachial plexus block, are the methods of choice for emergency surgery when the patient has a full stomach. The spinal technique has the advantage of rapid onset of profound anesthesia, but, unfortunately, there is a 5 to 10 per cent incidence of postoperative headache. This is probably due to leakage of the cerebrospinal fluid through the opening made by the needle. The use of a small needle (26-gauge) reduces the incidence of headache to about 1 per cent, but considererable skill is needed to introduce the needle subdurally.

Epidural block is accomplished by introducing local anesthetic agents into the epidural space. As the dura is not punctured and there is no leakage of fluid, postoperative headache cannot occur. The epidural block is technically more difficult to perform than the spinal block, and the ensuing anesthesia, though adequate, is not as profound. The apprehensive patient may safely be sedated with thiopental sodium or Valium during the course of these blocks. This knowledge allows the patient to accept regional anesthetic procedures more readily, as the desire for sleep while in the operating room is common.

Complications of Local Analgesia. The toxicity of local anesthetic agents is so well documented in the literature that review would be redundant here. When a patient under local analgesia exhibits signs of toxicity, such as tremors, jactitations, and convulsions, or in the event of a sudden loss of communication, a change in blood color, or lack of bleeding, the surgeon should assume that there is something seriously wrong with the patient. The patient should be undraped, and his pulse, blood pressure, and respiration should be checked. Should any of the vital signs be significantly diminished or absent, the surgeon must institute the following actions:

1. Establish an airway by lifting the chin or pulling the tongue forward. Should this not improve the situation, insert an oral or a nasopharyngeal airway, apply oxygen, and institute controlled intermittent positive pressure breathing.

2. If the blood pressure is severely reduced (below 80 mm Hg systolic), a vasopressor should be injected intravenously. Ephedrine, 25 to 50 mg, is excellent under these circumstances.

3. If neither pulse nor blood pressure is measurable, closed chest cardiac massage must be instituted along with controlled positive pressure breathing. After an anesthesiologist and resuscitation equipment have arrived, the surgeon should then consider pharmacologic therapy, such as epinephrine, bicarbonates, and osmotic therapy, together with hypothermia, electrocardiography, and, if necessary, cardiac defibrillation.

Complications directly related to local anesthetic agents are quite rare, when used in their recommended volumes and concentrations. The most frequently observed problems during local analgesia are iatrogenically induced and relate to the abuse of the various drugs commonly used as premedicants, and the intravenous supplementation of such medications during the operative procedure.

Premedication for patients having surgery with local analgesia should be such that a calm, cooperative and relaxed state is achieved, yet the ability to communicate is retained. However, all too frequently various degrees of stupor and, indeed, outright coma are induced by massive doses of barbiturates, tranquilizers, narcotics and neuroleptics. Such overmedication of patients produces bradypnea and hypopnea leading to hypoxia, hypercarbia and hypotension. It is clinically manifest as the pale, clammy patient who bleeds little, is frequently restless, and has lost the ability to communicate intelligently. Should these symptoms occur, the measures described above must be instituted rapidly.

It is important to realize that the effects of tranquilizers and barbiturates cannot be reversed pharmacologically. Narcan is an effective antagonist only against the narcotic drugs.

Finally, the surgeon who elects to operate under local analgesia is responsible for monitoring the vital signs. Such monitoring may be achieved by electronic means or by the presence of an anesthesiologist.

REFERENCES

Abadir, A.: Anesthesia for hand surgery. Orthop. Clin. North Am., *1*:205, 1970.

Bellville, J. W., Bross, D. D. J., and Howland, W. S.: Postoperative nausea and vomiting. Clin. Pharmacol. Ther., *1*:590, 1960.

Black, G. W., and McArdle, W.: Effects of halothane on the peripheral circulation in man. Br. J. Anaesth., *34*:2, 1962.

Brand, L., and Papper, E. M.: A comparison of supraclavicular and axillary techniques for brachial plexus blocks. Anesthesiology, *22*:226, 1961.

Bunker, J. P., Forrest, W. H., Jr., Mosteller, F., and Vandam, L. D. (Eds.): The National Halothane Study—A Study of the Possible Association between Halothane Anesthesia and Postoperative Hepatic Necrosis. National Institutes of Health, National Institute of General Medical Sciences, Bethesda, 1969.

Burnham, P. J.: Simple regional nerve block for surgery of the hand and forearm. J.A.M.A., *169*:941, 1959.

Crandell, W. B., Pappas, S. G., and Macdonald, A.: Nephrotoxicity associated with methoxyflurane anesthesia. Anesthesiology, *27*:591, 1966.

Enderby, G. E. H.: The advantages of controlled hypotension in surgery. Br. Med. Bull., *14*:1, 1958.

Enderby, G. E. H.: Halothane and hypotension. Anaesthesia, *15*:25, 1960.

Enderby, G. E. H.: A report on the mortality and morbidity following 9,109 hypotensive anesthetics. Br. J. Anaesth., *33*:109, 1961.

Fox, J. W. C., and Fox, E.: Neuroleptanalgesia: A review. North Carolina Med. J., *27*:471, 1966.

Hampton, L. J., and Little, D. M.: Results of questionnaire concerning controlled hypotension in anaesthesia. Lancet, *2*:772, 1957.

Katz, R. M., Matteo, R. S., and Papper, E. M.: Injection of epinephrine during general anesthesia with halogenated hydrocarbons and by cyclopropane in man. Anesthesiology, *23*:597, 1962.

Linacre, J. L.: Induced hypotension in gynecological surgery. Br. J. Anaesth., *33*:45, 1961.

McLoughlin, G.: Bleeding from cut skin and subcutaneous tissue surfaces during cyclopropane anaesthesia. Br. J. Anaesthiol., *26*:84, 1954.

Severinghaus, J. W., and Cullen, S. C.: Depression of myocardium and body O_2 consumption with Fluothane in man. Anesthesiology, *19*:165, 1958.

Smith, R. M.: Anesthesia for Infants and Children. St. Louis, Mo., C. V. Mosby Company, 1959.

Wylie, D., and Churchill-Davidson, H. C.: A Practice of Anesthesia. Chicago, Year Book Medical Publishers, 1960.

INDEX

Note: Page numbers in *italics* refer to illustrations. Page numbers followed by the letter "t" refer to tables.

Abbé lip flap. See Flap, Abbé.
Abbé operation, in upper lip defects, 1549–1552
  in vermilion border defects, 1575, 1576, *1576*
Abdomen
  as donor site for dermis-fat graft, *260*
  as donor site for flaps, 212–215, 3747, *3747*, 3748, *3748*
  as donor site for full-thickness skin grafts, 164, 165
  as donor site for split-thickness skin grafts, 176, *176*
Abdominal adiposity, 3801–3811
"Abdominal apron," *3731*
Abdominal flap. See *Flap, abdominal.*
Abdominal incisions, 3729, 3730
Abdominal wall
  anterior, anatomy of, 3727–3729
    embryology of, 3741, *3742*, 3743, *3743*
  circulation of, 3729
  deficiencies and defects of, 3741–3747
  dermolipectomy of, 3800–3811
    age of patients undergoing, 3810t
    complications of, 3811t
    history of, 3800, 3801, *3802*
    indications for, 3809t
    Pitanguy surgical technique of, 3802–3809
    results of, *3808, 3809*, 3809t, 3810, *3810*, 3810t, 3811, *3811*, 3811t, *3812*
    surgical principles of, 3801, 3802
  gas gangrene of, 3739–3741
  hernias of, 3730, 3731, *3731*
  layers of, 3728
  lymphatic drainage of, 3729
  muscles of, 3728, 3729
  nerves of, 3729
  reconstructive surgery of, 3727–3762
    de-epithelized skin flaps in, 3736, *3737*
    fascial grafts in, 3735, 3736, *3736*
    musculofascial flaps in, 3732–3735
    of acquired defects, 3731–3741
    prosthetic support in, 3737–3739, *3739*
    skin grafts in, 3737
Abductor digiti minimi muscle, flap of in foot, 3558, *3558*
Abductor hallucis muscle, mobilization of for flap, *3556*, 3557
Abscess formation, following corrective surgery of jaws, 1468, 1469
Acanthotic ameloblastoma, of jaws, 2550, *2551*

Acenocoumarin, in microvascular surgery, 367
Acinic cell carcinoma, of parotid gland, 2528, 2529
Acland microvascular clamp, 344, 345, *345*
Acne scars, dermabrasion for, 446, 447
Acral absence, 3329–3331
Acrocephalosyndactyly. See *Apert's syndrome.*
Acrocephaly, in Crouzon's disease, 2468, *2468*
Acrochordon, 2791, *2791*
Acromiocervical flap, *1654*
Acromiopectoral flap, 1267, *1655*
Acrylic resin implants, 392
Acrylic resin splint, 1477, *1478, 1479*
  in correction of jaw deformities, 1301, *1301, 1302*
  in maxillofacial prosthetics, *2920*
Actinic keratosis. See *Keratosis, actinic.*
Adamantinoma, of jaws, 2547–2552
Adenocarcinoma, adenoid cystic, of parotid gland, 2528, *2528, 2529, 2532*
  total glossectomy for, *2612*
Adenoid cystic adenocarcinoma, of parotid gland, 2528, *2528, 2529, 2532*
Adenoid cystic carcinoma, of maxilla, *2726*
Adenoides cysticum, basal cell, *2820*
  epithelial, 2874, 2875
Adenoma, of scalp, *2764*
  sebaceous, 2875
Adhesions, around sutured nerves and tendons, fat transplants in, 255, 256
  in tendon, 284
  peritendinous, 99, *100*
Adhesive strips, for wound closure, 640, 641, *645*
Adipose cells, behavior of in fat grafts, 251, 252, *252–258*
Adipose tissue, reaction of to silicone, 397, 398, *398*
Adipose tissue grafts. See *Fat, transplantation of.*
Adiposity, abdominal, 3801–3811
Adnexa oculi, deformities of, 858–946
  general anatomical considerations in, 859, 860
  general operative considerations in, 867–869
Adrenal cortical hyperplasia, congenital, female hermaphroditism in, 3936, *3936*, 3944–3953
Adrenal steroids, and immunosuppression, 138
Adrenocorticotropic hormone (ACTH), in thermal burn, 485
Advancement flaps. See *Flaps, advancement.*
Aegineta, Paulus, 4, 5

Aeroplast, use of in splinting of nose, 1087, 1088, *1089*
Aging
 of dermis, 1874
 of epidermis, 1874
 of face. See *Face, aging.*
 of skin, 1873–1875
 of subcutaneous tissue, 1875, *1875*
 premature, diseases of, 1877
Airway establishment, in thermal burns, 477, 478
Airway management, in maxillary fractures, 700
 in plastic surgery, 588–591
Airway obstruction, following maxillary fractures, 707
Akiyama prosthesis, for mammary augmentation, 3697
Ala. See *Nasal ala.*
Alar groove, 1042, *1042*
Alkylating agents, and immunosuppression, 138
 and rare craniofacial clefts, 2122
Allele, 139
Allogeneic, 141
Allograft(s), 126
 bone, immune response to, 323, 324
  in restoration of continuity of mandible, 1474
 cartilage, 306–308, *310*
 definition of, 52, 156
 fascia, 263
 fat, 254, *258*
 skin, 188
  after thermal burn, 503, 505
  in cranial defects, *829*, 830
 tendon, 284–288
 vascularization of, 157, 159–163
Allograft rejection reactions, skin, 128, 129
Alpha methyl tyrosine, 3769, 3770
Alpha particles, 532
Alveolabial sulcus, formation of, *1945*, 1946
Alveolar fractures, 697, 700, *701*
 in children, 800, *802*, 805
Alveolar nerve, 1470
Alveolar process, 2315
 reconstruction of, *1510*, 1511, *1511*, *1512*, 1513, *1513*
Alveolar ridge, restoration of in mandibular reconstruction, 1503–1507
Alveolar structures, fractures of, 664, 665, 697, 700, *701*
Alveolus, lower, tumors of, nasolabial flaps in reconstruction of, *2683*
 squamous cell carcinoma of, *2656*
 tumors of, forehead flap in, 2668, 2669, *2669*
Ameloblastic fibroma, of jaws, 2552, *2552*, 2553
Ameloblastomas, of jaws, 2547–2552
 of mandible, 2634, *2636*
  recurrent, 2622, *2623*, 2624
β-Aminopropionitrile (BAPN), 93, 94, 284
Aminopterin, 2122
Amniocentesis, and genetic counseling, 121
Amputation
 and traumatic neuroma, 3149–3151
 digital, major, 3144, 3145
 high thigh, and leg filleting, for multiple pressure sores, 3795, *3795*
 Krukenberg, 3096, *3098*
 of auricle. See *Auricle, amputated.*
 of fingertip, 3144, *3145*
 of hand. See *Hand, amputation of.*
 of penis, *3915*
 of thumb, 3355. See also *Thumb, traumatic loss of.*
 of toes, *3536*
 palmar, *3147*, 3148, *3148*, 3149, *3149*

Anastomoses, lymphaticovenous, 384–388
 microvascular. See *Microvascular surgery.*
"Andy Gump" deformity, 2631, *2634*, 2643, 2692, 2694
Anemia, after thermal burn, 485
 Fanconi's, radial ray deficiency in, 3334
 with pressure sores, 3774
Anesthesia
 block, in corrective rhinoplasty, 1063
 for fractures of nasal bones and cartilages, 726, *727*
 in acute hand injuries, 3009–3012
 in cleft lip and cleft palate, repair, 593, 594, *594*, 2020, 2094
 in contractures of cervical region, 1644
 in esthetic blepharoplasty, 1881
 in facial injuries, 626, 627, *627*
 in head and neck surgery, 2589, 2590, 2590t
 in nasal corrective surgery, 1059–1063
 in oromandibular tumor surgery, 2589, 2590, 2950t
 in plastic surgery, 587, 588
 in replantation surgery, 3246
 in skin grafting after thermal burns, 494, 495
 infiltration, in corrective rhinoplasty, 1061, 1062, *1062*, 1063
 of infraorbital nerve, 791, 1001, *1001*, 1002
 regional, of auricle, *1673*
  of eyelids, 867
 topical, in corrective rhinoplasty, 1061, *1061*, 1062
Anesthesiologist, role of in plastic surgery, 585–595
Aneurysm, arteriovenous, of jaws, 2567, *2567*, 2568
 simulating neoplasm, in hand, 3483, *3484*
Angioma, cherry, 2792, *2792*
 of hand and forearm, 3482, *3483*
 sclerosing, 2790, *2790*, 2791
Angioma racemosum, 2866
Angiosarcoma, of jaws, 2569, *2569*, 2570
Angle's classification of malocclusion, 1292, *1292*, 1293
Ankylosis, complete bilateral fibro-osseous, 682, *683*
 temporomandibular joint. See *Temporomandibular joint ankylosis.*
Annular grooves, of hand, 3328, *3328*, 3329
Anophthalmos, 962–968
 ocular prostheses in, 2942, 2943, *2945*
 operative procedure for correction of, 2460, *2461*, 2462
Anorectal malformations, 3825–3969
Anorectal prolapse, with exstrophy of bladder, 3871, *3873*
Anotia, 1676, 1677, *1677*
Anthelical fold, restoration of, in treatment of prominent ear, 1711, *1711*, 1712
Anthropometric landmarks, 1289, *1290*
Anthropometric points of face, 27, 28, *28*
Antia method of bilateral cleft lip repair, 2086, *2086*
Antibodies, and allograft rejection, 134, 135, *135*
Anticoagulants, in replantation surgery, 3256, 3257
Anticoagulation, in microvascular surgery, 365–370
Anticonvulsants, and rare craniofacial clefts, 2122
Anticubital flexor crease, as donor site for full-thickness skin grafts, 165
Antigens, and genes, 140–147
 lymphocyte-defined (LD), 130, 131, 142–147
 transplantation, 129
Antilymphocyte globulin (ALG), 137, 138
Antilymphocyte serum (ALS), 137, 138
Antimetabolites, and immunosuppression, 138
 and rare craniofacial clefts, 2122
Antisludging agents, in treatment of cold injury, 524–526
Antrum, gastric, free revascularized transplantation of, in pharyngoesophageal reconstruction, 2711, *2711*

Apertognathism. See *Open bite.*
Apert's syndrome, *31, 33,* 832, 2321–2327, 2407, 2465, 2466
  anatomical pathology in, 2468–2472
  calvarium in, 2468, 2469, *2469*
  coronal synostosis in, 2495
  cranial fossa and orbits in, 2469–2471
  etiopathogenesis of, 2321, 2322
  extremity and skeletal deformities in, 2322–2326, *2326,* 2327, 2472, *2472*
  facial deformities in, 2324, 2472
  history of, 2321
  Le Fort III osteotomy in, 2477, 2480
  maxilla in, 2471, 2472
  neurosurgery in, 2324, 2325
  ocular deformities in, 2322, *2323,* 2471
  orbital hypertelorism in, 2437, *2439, 2443*
  physical characteristics of, 2322–2324
  preoperative cephalometric planning in, 2482, *2484*
  ptosis of upper eyelid in, 2472, 2485
  reconstructive surgery in, 2325–2327
  skull deformities in, 2322, *2326*
  syndactyly in, 3311, 3313–3319
  treatment of, 2324–2327
Apical ectodermal ridge (AER), and hand and limb deformities, 3308, 3309, *3309,* 3310
Aplasia cutis congenita, 827, 828
Apocrine sweat glands, *153,* 155
Arch and band appliances, in maxillofacial prosthetics, 2920, *2920,* 2921
Arch bar fixation, 649–651, *651–653*
  in jaw deformities, 1300, *1301*
  in mandibular fractures, 669, *669,* 670
  in maxillary fractures, 700–702
Arch bars, prefabricated, in mandibular fractures, 665, 667, *667*
Arch wires, banded dental, in mandibular fractures, 667, *668,* 669
  cable, in fixation of facial bone fractures in children, 800, *801*
    in mandibular fractures, 667, *668*
Areola, simulation of by tattooing, *3722,* 3723
Areola-nipple complex, reconstruction of after radical mastectomy, *3716–3719,* 3720–3723
Arhinencephaly, 2128
  orbital hypotelorism in, 2462, *2462,* 2463, *2463, 2464*
  with median cleft lip, *1180,* 1181
Aries-Pitanguy technique of breast reduction, 3667, *3668, 3669*
Arm. See also *Extremity, upper.*
  thoracobrachial flap in repair of, 215, *215*
Arm flap technique, of nose repair, 5, 6
Arrector pili muscle, 154, 155
  in dermis graft, *249*
Arsenical keratoses, 2858, 3456
Arterial flaps, 194, *194,* 217
Arterial occlusion, in microvascular replants, 371
Arterial repair, microvascular, 358, *358–362*
Arteriovenous aneurysm, of jaws, 2567, *2567, 2568*
Arteriovenous fistula, of hand, *3483*
Artery(arteries)
  auricular, 1521
  direct cutaneous, 193, *193*
  epigastric, 3041, *3042*
  facial, transverse, 1779
  lingual, distribution of, 2701, *2701*
  microvascular repair patency rates for, 353, 353t, 354
  musculocutaneous, 193, *193*

Artery(arteries) *(Continued)*
  occipital, 1779
  of abdominal wall, 3729
  radial, 2976
  stylomastoid, 1779
  superficial temporal, 1779
    and forehead flap, 217, *217*
  ulnar, 2976
Artery island flap, 959, *961, 962*
Arthritis, of hand, 3507–3518
  correction of early ulnar drift in, 3514, 3515, *3515*
  degenerative, 3507–3511
  digital joints in, 3515–3517
  gouty, 3511, *3511*
  intrinsic muscle release in, 3514, *3514*
  muscles in, 3513–3515
  rheumatoid, 3511–3518
  surgical treatment of, 3512–3518
  synovectomy for, 3512, 3513
  tendons and tendon sheaths in, 3512, 3513
  thumb in, 3517, 3518
Arthrodesis, small joint, in arthritic hand, 3510, 3511, *3511*
Arthroplasty, in arthritic hand, 3508, 3516
Arthrosis, temporomandibular, 1529, *1529*
Articular disc, 1521, 1522, *1522*
Asche forceps, for reduction of nasal fractures, 727, *727,* 728, *785*
Asche metal, in splinting of nose, 1087, *1087, 1088*
Ascites, chylous, 3586, *3587*
Ascorbic acid depletion, and wound healing, 92, 93
Ashley operation, in repair of lower lip defect, 1567, 1568, *1568*
Ashley prosthesis, for mammary augmentation, 3697, 3698
L-Asparaginase, and immunosuppression, 138
Asphyxia neonatorum, 1165
Aspirin, and craniofacial clefts, 2123
  in microvascular surgery, 367
Atheroma, 2784–2786
Atriodigital dysplasia, 3334
Atropine absorption test, of flap circulation, 195
Auditory canal, external, stenosis of, 1735, *1735,* 1736
Auditory meatus, external, 2309
Aufricht retractor, 1070, *1070*
Auricle. See also *Ear.*
  amputated, replantation of, 1725–1732
    as composite graft, 1728, 1731, 1732, *1734*
    dermabrasion and, 1727, 1728, *1731*
    microsurgery and, 1732
    upon removal of medial auricular skin and fenestration of cartilage, 1728, *1732*
    with auricular cartilage, 1727, *1729, 1730*
    with auricular tissue as composite graft, 1727, *1728*
    with auricular tissue attached by narrow pedicle, *1726,* 1727, *1727*
  anatomy of, 1672, *1672, 1673*
  avulsion of, *1747*
  deformities of, 1671–1773
    acquired, 1724–1768
      amputation, 1725–1732
      full-thickness, 1744–1768
        following trauma, 1744–1750
        partial, 1750–1761
      with loss of auricular tissue, 1736–1743
      without loss of auricular tissue, 1732–1736
    burn, 1636

Auricle *(Continued)*
 deformities of, congenital, 1671–1724
  classification of, 1675, 1676, 1676t
  diagnosis of, 1675, 1676, *1676*, 1676t
  etiology of, 1674, 1675
  hearing improvement after middle ear surgery in, 1722, 1722t, 1723
  indications, contraindications, and timing of middle ear surgery in, 1719–1724
 in mandibulofacial dysostosis, treatment of, 2419, 2422
 embryology of, 1672–1674, 2307, *2308*, 2309
 full-thickness defects of, auricular cartilage in reconstruction of, 1753–1755
  costal cartilage in reconstruction of, 1755–1758
 hypoplasia of, complete. See *Microtia.*
  of middle third, 1705, *1706*
  of superior third, 1705–1710
 injuries of, 637, *642*
 prominence of, 1710–1718
 reconstruction of, history of, 1671, 1672
 reduction of, *1718*, 1719
 regional anesthesia of, *1673*
 sensory nerve supply of, *1673*
 Tanzer's method of reconstructing, *1684*
 tumors of, benign, 1766, 1767
  malignant, 1768, *1768*
Auricular artery, 1521
Auricular cartilage. See *Cartilage, auricular.*
Auricular fistulas and cysts, 2877
Auricular graft. See *Graft, auricular.*
Auricular loss, major, following trauma, 1744–1750
 partial, 1750–1761
  auricular cartilage in reconstruction of, 1753–1755
  composite grafts in, 1750, *1751*, 1752, *1752*
  costal cartilage in reconstruction of, 1755–1758
Auricular muscle, 1782
Auricular nerve, posterior, 1777
Auricular prosthesis, in auricular reconstruction following trauma, 1750
Auricular skin, loss of, 1736, *1736*, *1737*
Auricular tissue, as composite graft, replantation of, 1727, *1728*
 attached by narrow pedicle, replantation of, *1726*, 1727, *1727*
Auriculotemporal syndrome, following parotid tumor surgery, 2538
Autogenous transplants, in treatment of orbital fractures, 995–997
Autograft(s), 126
 cartilage, 304–306
 definition of, 52, 156
 fascia, 263
 fat, 252, 253
 in breast reconstruction, 3716
 skeletal muscle, 297, 298
 skin, split-thickness, in cranial defects, 830, *830*
 tendon, 278–284
 vascularization of, 157, 159–163
Avulsion injuries
 of auricle, *1747*
 of eyelid, 872–874
 of face, 635, 636, *639*, 640
 of fingers, 3144, *3146*
 of penis, 3905–3908
 of scalp, 832–837, *838–840*
 ring, 3019, *3020*, 3021, *3021*
 timing of skin replacement in, 225
Axial pattern flap. See. *Flap, axial pattern.*

Axilla, burns of, 3391–3393, *3394–3397*
Axillary contractures, correction of, 3393, *3393–3397*
Axonotmesis, 1784, 2986
Azathioprine, and immunosuppression, 138

B cells, 133, 134
Badenoch urethroplasty, *3889*
Band and arch appliance, in fixation of facial bone fractures in children, 800, *802*
Banded dental arch, in mandibular fractures, 667, *668*, 669
Banding techniques, in identification of chromosomes, *110*, 111, *111*, 112, *112*, *113*, *114*
Bands, constricting, congenital, 419, 420, *421*
 of lower extremity, 3527, *3528*
Barbiturates, 586
Barr bodies, 108, *108*, 109, 3932, *3933*
Barraquer-Simons disease, silicone fluid injections in, 2348
Barsky technique of bilateral cleft lip repair, 2084, 2085, *2085*, 2086
Barter principle, 45
Basal bone, mandibular and maxillary, growth of, 1993, *1993*, 1994, *1994*
Basal cell epithelioma, 2806–2810, 2819–2828
 early, 2819, 2820
 histology of, 2822–2828
 morphea-like or fibrosing, 2821, 2824, 2831
 multicentric, 2820, *2821*
 nevoid, 2822
 noduloulcerative, 2821, 2824, 2831
 of cheek, *2823*, *2827*
 of craniofacial skeleton, 2757, 2758, *2758*, *2759*
 of ear, *2773*
 of eyelids, 879, 880
 of face, *2821*
 of hand and forearm, 3460
 of nasolabial fold, *2758*
 of nose, 1192, 1193, *1262*, 1263, *2824*, *2825*, *2892*
  repair of by median island forehead flap, *1234*
 of upper lip, *2826*, *2827*
 pigmented, 2820, 2821, 2824
 reconstruction of nasal defect after radiation for treatment of, 1254, *1254*, 1255
 recurrent, chemosurgery for, 2833, *2884*
 repair of lateral nasal wall defect due to, *1251*
 roentgen ray therapy of, 2809, 2810
 superficial, 2821
 treatment of, *2823*, 2824, *2824*, *2825–2827*, 2828
 types of lesions of, 2819–2822
Basal cell papilloma, 2781–2783
Basosquamous carcinoma, chemosurgery for, *2885*
 of skin, 2828
Bauer, Trusler, and Tondra method of bilateral cleft lip repair, 2073, *2073*, 2074, *2074*, 2075, *2075*
BCG vaccine, in treatment of malignant melanoma, 2852
 in treatment of skin cancer, 2839
Beard's modification of Fasanella-Servat operation, 925, *925*
Beau's lines, 2978
Bedsore. See *Pressure sore.*
Belladonna alkaloids, 586
Bell's phenomenon, in Möbius syndrome, 2328, *2329*
Bennett's fracture, 3048, *3048*, 3049, *3049*
Bernard operation, in repair of lower lip defect, 1568, 1569, *1569*

Berry syndrome. See *Mandibulofacial dysostosis.*
Beta particles, 532
Biceps femoris muscle flap, in pressure sore, *3788*
Biceps femoris myocutaneous flap, 3561, *3561*, 3562
Biesenberger-McIndoe operation for breast reduction, 3670, *3671*, 3672, *3672*, *3673*
Bi-lobed flap, 206, *208*, 1583, *1586*
Bimaxillary protrusion, 1295, 1428, *1428*
  surgical-orthodontic treatment of, 1436–1439
Binder's syndrome, 2465, *2466*, *2467*
Bipedicle flap. See *Flap, bipedicle.*
Bipolar coagulation, 345, 346
Bite-blocks
  in jaw deformities, 1301, *1302*
  in mandibular fractures, 672, 673, 680, *680*
  in maxillofacial prosthetics, 2920, *2920*, 2921
  maxillary, 1475, *1476*
Bladder, exstrophy of, 3830, 3862, 3871–3879
  bilateral iliac osteotomy in, 3874, *3874*
  etiology and incidence of, 3873
  treatment of, 3873–3879
Blair, Vilray Papin, 13, 14, 15, *15*
Blair knife, 173, 174
Blair suction box, 14
Blair-Brown-McDowell repair of cleft lip, 2017, 2019 *2026*, 2027, 2032, 2035, *2036*, 2037
Blepharochalasis, 1878, *1879*
Blepharodermachalasis, construction of supratarsal fold in, 954, 955
Blepharophimosis, 944–946
Blepharoplasty, corrective, combined with face lifting, 1912
  esthetic, 1877–1898
    anesthesia in, 1881
    complications of, 1893–1898
    photographs in, 1881
    planning of operation in, 1881
    preoperative examination in, 1880, 1881
    technique of, 1881–1893
      in lower eyelids, *1886*, *1887*, 1888, 1889, *1889*
      in upper eyelids, *1882*, *1883*, *1884*, 1885, 1889, *1890*
      muscle flap, 1889, 1890, *1891*, 1892
      skin marking in, 1881–1885
      variations in, 1892, *1892*, 1893
Blepharoptosis, acquired, surgical treatment of, 920–940
  following orbital fractures, 791
  frontalis suspension for, 931, 936–940
Blindness, following esthetic blepharoplasty, 1897, 1898
  following maxillary fractures, 707, 708
  following orbital and naso-orbital fractures, 790, 791
Blood, coagulability of, 350, 351
Blood flow, disturbances of, and thrombosis, 354, *355*
Blood supply, of tendon, 267, 268, *268*, 269, *269*
Blowout fracture, of orbital floor. See *Orbit, floor of blowout fractures of.*
Body, length of in relation to head, 34, *38*
Body image, 27
Bolus tie-over grafting, in intraoral tumor surgery, 2655–2657, *2658*
Bone(s)
  avascular necrosis and osteitis of, in mandibular fractures, 693
  basal, mandibular and maxillary, growth of, 1993, *1993*, 1994, *1994*
  biological principles in healing of, 101, 102
  cancellous, autogenous, 101
    autograft of, 324, 326
    coarse, 314, *314*
  chondral, 313

Bone(s) *(Continued)*
  compact cortical, 313, 314, *314*
    autograft of, 324, *325*
  cranial, 823, 824, *824*, 2313
  ethmoid, 2431, *2432*, 2433
  facial. See *Facial bones.* 796–814
  frontal, contour restoration of, 851, 854
    fixation of bone graft into, 1147
    fracture of, *1025*
    nasal spine of, 1042, *1044*
    repair of full-thickness defects of, 845–855
    surgery of, in Crouzon's disease, 2485
    tumors of, craniofacial surgical techniques in, 2490
  inorganic implants over, 405, *406*, *407*, *408*
  mesenchymal, 313
  nasal. See *Nasal bones and cartilages.*
  of hand, 2957–2961
    tumors of, 3496–3500
  remodeling of, 315
  sphenoid, 2431, *2432*
  temporal, 1521
    cancers of, 2770–2772
  transplantation of, 313–339. See also *Graft, bone.*
    allografts and xenografts, immune response to, 323, 324
      in restoration of continuity of mandible, 1474
    clinical aspects of, 324–338
    history of, 317–323
Bone cavities, in lower extremity, 3523
Bone chips, cancellous, in restoration of continuity of mandible, 1473, 1474
Bone cyst, simple (traumatic), of jaws, 2563, *2564*
Bone deformities, in Romberg's disease, 2338, 2339
Bone deposition and resorption, 315
"Bone flap operation," in cleft palate repair, 2092
Bone graft struts, tibial, in reconstruction of sternal defects, 3629, *3629*
Bone grafts. See *Grafts, bone.*
Bone induction principle, 101
Bone necrosis, following corrective surgery of jaws, 1469
Bone plate fixation, in mandibular fractures, 676, 677, *677*, *678*
Bony orbits, 2433–2435
Boo-Chai classification of craniofacial clefts, 2126, *2126*
Boutonnière deformity, 2998, 3173–3715
Bowen's disease, 2810, 2811, *2811*, 2853, 2856
  nails in, 2980
  of hands and forearm, 3459
Brachial flap, 1199, 1266, 1267, *1267*
Brachial plexus or axillary block, 594
  in acute hand injuries, 3010
Brachydactyly, 3331–3333
Brain weight and shape, increase in, 2493, *2493*, 2493t
Branchial arches, early development of, 2902, *2903*
Branchial cysts and fistulas, 2876, 2877, 2908–2914
  clinical features of, 2908, 2909, *2909*
  differential diagnosis of, 2911, 2912, *2912*
  etiology of, 2909, 2910, *2910*
  pathology of, 2910, 2911, *2911*
  treatment of, 2912–2914
Branchial membranes, mesodermal reinforcement of, 1942–1944
Branchiogenic carcinoma, 2914–2916
Brand plantaris tendon stripper, 275, *276*
Breast(s)
  blood supply to, 3663, 3664
  carcinoma of, 3653, 3654
  developmental anomalies in, 3706, *3706*, 3707
  lymphatic drainage of, 3664
  nerve supply to, 3664

Breast(s) (*Continued*)
pigeon. See *Pectus carinatum.*
plastic surgery of, 3661–3726
history of, 3661–3663
ptosis of, *3812*
reconstruction of after radical mastectomy, 3611–3623,
3710–3723
areola-nipple complex in, *3716–3719,* 3720–3723
autografts in, 3716
contralateral remaining breast in, 3723
distant skin flaps in, 3715, *3715,* 3716
indications for, 3711, 3711t
inorganic implants in, 3716, 3720
labia minora grafts in, *3717,* 3721, 3723
local skin flaps in, *3712, 3713, 3713, 3714*
replacement of absent glandular, adipose tissue and
muscle in, 3716–3720
replacement of missing skin in, 3713–3716
timing of, 3711, 3712
types of procedures in, 3712–3723
surgical anatomy of, 3663, 3664
Breast augmentation mammaplasty. See *Mammaplasty,*
augmentation.
Breast deformities, classification of, 3664, 3664t, 3665
Breast flap, in chest wall reconstruction, 3615–3617,
3618
Breast reduction mammaplasty and mastopexy,
3665–3689, *3809*
complications of, 3688, 3689
in Klinefelter's syndrome, *3963*
indications for operation in, 3665
preoperative planning and selection of operation in,
3665, 3666
technique of, 3666–3684, *3685–3687*
Brent's technique for eyebrow reconstruction, 957, *958*
Brephoplasty, 52
Brevital, 587
Bridge flap, 895–898, *1557*
Brooke's tumor, 2874, 2875
Brown air-driven dermatome, 495, *495*
Brown electric dermatome, 167, *167*
Browne technique of repair of hypospadias, 3848, 3850,
3850
Browne's procedure for reconstruction of urethra, 3841,
3841, 3842, *3842*
Bruxism, and temporomandibular joint pain, 1524
Buccal branches, of facial nerve, 1778
Buccal mucosa, carcinoma of, *2674, 2677*
squamous cell, *2608, 2658, 2659*
tumors of, 2607, *2608, 2609*
forehead flap in, 2671–2673
Buccal sulcus, restoration of in mandibular reconstruction,
1503–1507
Buccinator muscle, 1781
Buccopharyngeal membrane, 2303
Bucknall's procedure for reconstruction of urethra, 3839,
3840
Bunnell, Sterling, 18, 20
Burn(s)
axillary contracture following, four-flap Z-plasty in,
60, *61*
contraction vs. contracture in, 3370
electrical, 469, *469,* 512, 513, 1596
of perioral region, 1639, 1640
facial. See *Facial burns.*
lye, 1603
of axilla, 3391–3393, *3394–3397*
of elbow, 3391–3399
of hand. See *Hand, burns of.*

Burn(s) (*Continued*)
of upper extremity, 3368–3402. See also *Hand, burns*
of.
thermal, age of patient in, 469, 470
allografts following, 503, 505
anemia in, 485
antibiotic therapy in, 483
associated injury or concurrent disease in, 471, 472,
472t
auricular reconstruction after, 1746
central venous pressure in, 481
classification and diagnosis of, 465–472
complications of, 506–510
convalescence and rehabilitation after, 510–512
degree classification of, 466–469
depth of, 466–469
emergency sedation in, 478
endocrine changes in, 475, 476
establishment of airway in, 477, 478
etiology of, 465
exposure therapy in, 493
extent of body surface involved in, 466, *466,* 467
fluid replacement therapy in, 478–482
grafting procedures in, 493–505
historical aspects of, 464, 465
immediate hospital care followng, 476–487
infection of, 508, 509
insertion of indwelling catheter in, 481, 481t
local wound management in, 486, 487, *487, 488*
loss of circulating red cells in, 474, 475
metabolic changes in, 475
morbidity of, 472, *472,* 473
mortality from, 470t, 471t
musculoskeletal changes in, 475, 476t
nutritional requirements in, 483, 484
occlusive dressings in, 492, 493
of hand. See *Hand, burns of.*
pathophysiology of, 473–476
positioning and exercise of patient with, 484
postgrafting phase in treatment of, 505, 506
pregrafting phase of wound management in, 491–493
psychologic aspects of, 485, 486
renal failure in, 481, 482
respiratory tract in, 507, 508
scar contracture of cervical region in, 1644, *1645,*
1646, 1649
shock phase of, 506, 507
silver nitrate in treatment of, 488, 488t, 489, *489,*
489t, 490
silver sulfadiazine in treatment of, 491, 491t, 492t
Sulfamylon in treatment of, 490, 490t, 491
surface water loss in, 474, 474t
tetanus prophylaxis in, 482, 483
thinned helical border secondary to, *1737*
topical agents for, 487–493
use of ACTH and cortisone in, 485
xenografts following, 505
wound healing following, 1596–1601
Burn eschar, electric dermatome in removal of, 173
Burn scar contracture, of lower lip, *1560,* 1561, *1561*
of upper lip, 1545, *1545*
Burn scars
circumferential, decompression of, 486, 487, *487, 488*
dermabrasion for, 447, *451, 452*
hypertrophic, treatment of, 1640, 1641
treatment of, 1614, 1617, *1617*
Burn septicemia, 508, 509
Burn shock, fluid replacement therapy for, 478–482
Burn toxin, 476

Burn wound, excision of, 493, *494*
Burow's triangle, 205, *206*, 208, *208*
Buschke-Lowenstein tumor, 2778
Buttocks, dermolipectomy of, 3811–3820
  drooping, correction of, 3818, *3818*
Button-hole incision, for cancellous chips, 330

C-banding, *110*, 111
C-osteotomy, for elongation of mandible, 1367, 1368, *1369*, 1370
Cable arch wire, in fixation of facial bone fractures in children, 800, *801*
  in mandibular fractures, 667, *668*
Cable graft, of nerves, 3231
Calcaneal ulcer, *3559*
Calcification, 101, 102
  role of ground substance in, 316, 317
Calculi, of salivary glands, 2542, *2543*
Caldwell position, 611, *612*
Callus, plantar, 3529
Calvarium, deformities of, 822–857
  in Crouzon's disease and Apert's syndrome, 2468, *2468*, 2469, *2469*
Camille Bernard operation, in repair of lower lip defect, 1569, *1569*
Camper's fascia, 3728
Camptodactyly, 3326, *3327*
Canaliculodacryocystorhinostomy, 986, 987
Canaliculus, 313
  repair of, 813
  transection of, 983, *983*
Cancellous bone, autogenous, 101
  coarse, 314, *314*
Cancellous bone autograft, 324, 326
Cancellous bone chips, button-hole incision for, 330
Cancer
  epidermoid, of maxillary sinus, 2767, *2769*
  fungating, of cheek and nose, deltopectoral flap in, *2746*, 2747
  in scars, 415, 2819
  mammaplasty and, 3708–3710
  of cheek, double flap in, *2627*
  of chin, *2632, 2633, 2634*
  of cranium, 2763
  of ethmoid sinus, 2767, *2768*
  of floor of mouth, 2609–2613, 2620, *2620*
  of head and neck, surgical treatment of, 2509–2520
  of hypopharynx, 2698
  of laryngopharynx, 2698
  of mastoid, 2770
  of middle ear, 2770
  of nasopharynx, 2697, 2698
  of oropharynx, 2698
  of paranasal sinuses, 2767–2770
  of pharynx, 2697, 2698
  of scalp, 2763–2767
  of temporal bone, 2770–2772
  of tongue, 2609–2613, *2628, 2629, 2634*
  of tonsil and floor of mouth, 2609–2613
  radiation and, 534, 535, 546, *546*, 547
  skin. See *Skin cancer* and *Skin, tumors of.*
Cancer center, 2512
Cancer team, interdisciplinary, 2512, 2513, 2516, 2517
Caninus muscle, 1781
Canthal buttons, acrylic, 1022, *1022*
Canthal defects, excision of, with healing by second intention, 903, *904*
Canthal tendons, medial and lateral, *859, 863, 864*

Canthopexy, 1012–1020
Canthoplasty, lateral, in Crouzon's disease, 2485
  medial, 1012, 2485
    in orbital hypertelorism, 2453, *2454*
Canthus, lateral, antimongoloid slant of, correction of, 1921, 1922
  deformities of, 1001
  medial, deformities of, 1001
    forward displacement of by burn contractures, 1630, *1630*
    left, *1006*
    superficial structures of, *1005*
Canthus inversus, after naso-orbital fracture, medial canthoplasty for, 1018, *1019*, 1020
Capillary bed, diffusion of fluids in, 3568, *3568*
Capillary hemangiomas. See *Hemangiomas, capillary.*
Capillary refill time, in microvascular surgery, 370
Capitate, *2968*, 2969
Caput medusae, 3729
Carbon, elemental, as implant, 410
Carcinoma
  acinic cell, of parotid gland, 2528, 2529
  adenoid cystic, of maxilla, *2726*
  anaplastic, of orbitomaxillary region, *2727*
  basal cell. See *Basal cell epithelioma.*
  basosquamous, 2828, *2885*
  branchiogenic, 2914–2916
  chronic radiodermatitis and, 2856
  epidermoid, 2812–2814
    in burn, scar, 81, *82*
  intraoral, mandible in. See *Mandible, in intraoral carcinoma.*
  mucoepidermoid, of maxillary sinus, *2585*
    of parotid gland, 2528, *2529*
  of angle of mouth, *2674*
  of breast and chest wall, 3653, 3654
  of buccal mucosa, *2608, 2658, 2659, 2674, 2677*
  of skin. See *Skin, tumors of, Carcinoma and Skin cancer.*
  sebaceous gland, 2875, 3464
  squamous cell. See *Squamous cell carcinoma.*
  verrucous, 2778, 2779
Carotid artery rupture, following oropharyngoesophageal reconstructive surgery, 2754
Carotid body tumor, 2638, 2639
Cardiopulmonary function, in pectus excavatum, 3635, 3636
Carpal navicular, 2969
Carpal tunnel, calculation of motor conduction velocity through, 2983t
  flexor tendon injuries in, 3070, *3071*
  nerve and tendon injuries in, 3210, *3211*, 3212, *3212*
Carpal tunnel syndrome, 3428–3437
  anatomy and pathology of, 3429, *3429*, 3430, *3430*
  diagnosis of, 3432, 3433, *3433*
  differential diagnosis of, 3433
  history of, 3428, 3429
  pathogenesis of, 3430–3432
  results and complications of, 3435, 3437
  treatment of, 3433–3435
Carpals, dislocation of, 3044–3047
Carpenter syndrome, 2468
Carpometacarpal joint, first, arthritic changes in, 3507, 3508
Carpue, Joseph, 7, 8
Carpus, 2967, 2969
Cartilage
  auricular, in reconstruction of auricle, 1753–1755
    in reconstruction of philtrum, *2171*
    loss of, 1743, *1743*
    replantation of, 1727, *1729, 1730*

Cartilage *(Continued)*
  autogenous, reconstruction with in microtia, 1683–1696
  deformation of, 302–304
    in Romberg's disease, 2338, *2338, 2339*
  ear, transplantation of, 306–308
  human, polymorphism of, 301, 302, *302*
  Meckel's, 815, *816,* 817, *818,* 2369, 2370
  of hand and forearm, tumors of, 3496–3500
  preserved, in repair of microtia, 1701, 1702
  Reichert's, 2369, 2370
  rib, 303–305, *305, 306*
  transplantation of, 301–312. See also *Graft, cartilage.*
    allografts, 306–308
      in repair of microtia, 1701
    autografts, 304–306
    in nose, 1148–1150
    in Romberg's disease, 2342, 2343, *2343*
    storage in, 308
    xenograft, 307
      in correction of mandibulofacial dysostosis, 2414, *2415*
Cartilage implants, dead, behavior of, 308, 309
Cast cap splint, *657, 669*
Castroviejo dermatome, 173, *173,* 917, *918*
Catgut implants, 392
Cauliflower ear, 1732, 1735
Cavernous hemangioma, 2793, *2793, 2866, 2866–2868*
Cebocephaly, 1179, *1180,* 1181
  orbital hypotelorism in, 2462, *2463*
Cecil-Culp technique of repair of hypospadias, 3850, *3851*
Cell survival theory, of fat grafts, 251
Celsus, 4, *4,* 261
Cement, 313
Cementoma, of jaws, 2555, *2555, 2556*
Cephalometry, 1293, 1294, *1294, 1295,* 1296t, 1298, *1300*
  in mandibular micrognathia, *1345, 1346,* 1347
  in mandibular prognathism, *1311, 1312*
  in maxillary deformities, 1425, *1425*
  in orbital hypertelorism, 2457, 2458, *2458, 2459*
Ceramics, porous, as implants, 410
Cerebral anomalies, in craniofacial microsomia, 2375, 2376
Cerebrospinal fluid rhinorrhea or otorrhea, following maxillary fractures, 700
  following orbital fractures, 791, 792
Cervical branches, of facial nerve, 1778
Cervical cleft and web, midline, congenital, 1661, 1664, *1664*
Cervical flap. See *Flap, cervical.*
Cervical region, deformities of, 1643–1670
  complete contractures, 1644–1658
    anesthesia in, 1644
    excision of scar in, 1644, *1646, 1647,* 1648, *1648, 1649*
    microvascular surgery in, 1654, *1658*
    postoperative care in, 1650
    preparation of mold of neck in, 1650
    skin flaps in, 1652–1654, *1654–1657*
    skin grafting in, 1648, 1650, 1654, 1658
    splint in, 1650–1652
  congenital midline cleft and web, 1661, 1664, *1664*
  congenital muscular torticollis, 1664–1668
  congenital webbing of neck, 1659–1661
  limited contractures, 1658, *1659*
  scar contractures, 1643, 1644, *1645*
Cervical sinus, 2306, 2903, *2903*
Cervical-aural fistulas, 2913, 2914, *2914*
Cervicofacial nerve, 1777

Cheek(s)
  basal cell epithelioma of, *2823, 2827*
  cancer of, double flap in, *2627*
  deformities of, 1579–1593
    burn, 1636, *1637*
    full-thickness, 1587–1593
    superficial, 1579–1587
  deltopectoral flap in resurfacing of, *2746, 2747*
  embryonic development of, 2313
  melanoma of, *2630*
  tumors of, combined forehead and deltopectoral flaps in, *2672, 2674*
Cheek flap. See *Flap, cheek.*
Chemabrasion. See *Chemical planing.*
Chemical planing, 454–462. See also *Chemosurgery.*
  agents and toxicology in, 454–456
  contraindications to, 461, 462
  indications for, 460, *460,* 461, *461*
  mode of action in, 456
  results of, 459, 460
  technique of, 456–459
Chemocheck, 2888
Chemosurgery. See also *Chemical planing.*
  for recurrent basal cell epithelioma, 2883, *2884*
  for skin cancer, 2830, 2880–2894
    chemocheck in, 2888
    cure rate in, 2887, 2888, 2888t
    fresh tissue technique of, 2886, *2887*
    historical background of, 2881
    in periorbital region, 2884, 2886
    indications for, 2881–2886
    on ear, 2884
    on face, repair of defects after, 2889–2894
    on nose, 2883, 2884, *2884, 2885, 2892*
    technique of, 2881, *2882, 2883*
  in eyelid defects, 903
  Mohs, for skin cancer, 2830
    for tumors of nose, 1193, 1194
    scalping flap for nasal reconstruction following, 1251, *1252*
Chemosurgery unit, 2889, *2889*
Chemotactic factor, 134, *135*
Chemotherapy, of malignant melanoma, 2853
  of parotid gland, 2536
  of skin cancer, 2838, 2839, *2839*
Cherubism, 2559–2561
Chest, funnel. See *Pectus excavatum.*
Chest wall, tumors of, 3652–3657
Chest wall dehiscence, 3633
Chest wall reconstruction, 3609–3660
  after tumor excision, 3652–3657
  closure of pleural space in, 3617, 3621, *3622,* 3623, *3623–3625*
  distant flaps in, 3614–3617
  extent of radiation damage and, 3611, *3612*
  in pectus carinatum, 3646–3652
  in pectus excavatum, 3633–3645
  local flaps in, 3611, *3613,* 3614, *3614*
  of sternal defects, 3628–3631
  preoperative planning in, 3611
  prosthetic implants in, 3627, 3628
  rib as stabilizing factor in, 3623, *3626, 3627, 3627*
Chilblains, 517
Chimerism, 136, 137
Chin
  cancer of, *2632, 2633, 2634*
  deformities of, 1382–1404
    anatomical considerations in, 1383, 1384
    burn, 1636–1638
    macrogenia, 1404

Chin *(Continued)*
  deformities of, microgenia, 1384–1404
  embryonic development of, 2311
Chin augmentation, *1057, 1058, 1059*
  combined with face lifting, 1916, 1917, *1918*, 1919, *1919*
  in microgenia, 1384, 1385
Chlorpromazine, in microvascular surgery, 352
Choanal atresia, 2239
  congenital, 1163–1169
    bony, bilateral, 1184
    clinical manifestations of, 1164, 1165, 1165t
    diagnosis of, 1165, 1166
    embryology and anatomy of, 1164
    history of, 1163, 1164
    incidence of, 1164
    treatment of, 1166–1169
Chondral bone, 313
Chondritis, post-thermal, 1604, 1605
Chondrocranium, 2313
Chondrocutaneous graft, 883–891
Chondrocyte, 301, 302, *302*
  antigenicity of, 306, 307
Chondroectodermal dysplasia, polydactyly in, 3320
Chondroma, of hand and forearm, 3497, *3498,* 3499
  of jaws, 2566
  of rib cage, 3652
Chondrosarcoma, of maxilla, 2575, *2575*
Chorda tympani, 1777, 1786
Chordee, correction of in hypospadias, 3836, *3836, 3837*
  without hypospadias, 3847, *3847,* 3848
Choroidal fissure, 2304
Chromatin, sex, 108, 109, 3932–3934
  structure and function of as it relates to DNA, 116, 117
Chromosomal abnormalities, and congenital malformations, 108–115
Chromosome karyotype, 3934, *3935, 3936*
Chromosomes, 139, 140
  in sex identification, 3930, 3931
  sex, 3932, 3933, *3934*
Chronaxie, 1787
Chylous ascites, 3586, *3587*
Chylous fistula, following oropharyngoesophageal reconstructive surgery, 2752
Cialit, in preservation of tendon, 287
Cicatricial ectropion, 909–911
Cicatricial entropion, 914
Cicatrix. See *Scar.*
Circulation, plasmatic, 157, 158
Circulatory disabilities, in lower extremity, 3523–3526
Cisterna chyli, obstruction of, 3586, *3587,* 3588, *3588, 3589*
Clamps, microvascular, 344, *344,* 345, *345*
Class III malocclusion, 1418, *1418, 1459, 1460*
Claw hand, 2975, 3206, 3207, *3207,* 3279
  splinting in, 2998
Clear cell hidradenoma, of eyelids, 879
Cleavage lines, 76, 77
Cleft(s)
  craniofacial, midline, 2119, 2120, *2120*
    rare. See *Craniofacial clefts, rare.*
  facial, 2117, 2119, *2119,* 2128, 2128t, 2129, 2312
  hyomandibular, 2311
  interdigital, cicatricial webbing of, in burns of hand, 3377
  median, false, 2132, *2133*
  naso-orbital, *2460*
  of mandibular process, 2120, 2121
  of maxillary process, 2121

Cleft lip. See also *Cleft lip and palate* and *Cleft lip and nose.*
  bilateral, muscles of, 1970–1975
    with bilateral cleft of primary palate, 2048–2089
      closure of clefts one side at a time in, 2057, *2057,* 2059
      complications of repair of, 2086–2088
      diagnosis of, 2049
      incidence of, 2048
      techniques of lip repair in, *2058,* 2059–2086
        adaptation of Tennison unilateral cleft lip incision, *2069,* 2070–2073
        Barsky technique, 2084, 2085, *2085,* 2086
        Bauer, Trusler, and Tondra method, 2073, *2073,* 2074, *2074,* 2075, *2075*
        Manchester method, 2078, *2079,* 2080
        Millard methods, 2075–2078
        primary Abbé flap, 2086, *2086*
        Skoog method, 2078, *2080,* 2081, *2081*
        Spina's method, 2083, *2083, 2084*
        straight line closure, *2058,* 2059–2067, *2068, 2069*
        Wynn method, 2081, 2082, *2082,* 2083
      treatment of, 2049–2059
        control of protruding premaxilla in, 2050–2059
        principles and objectives of, 2049, 2050
        timing of repair in, 2050
        use of prolabium in, 2050
    orbicularis oris muscle in, 2166, *2167*
    maxillary growth in, 2002
    median, 2134, *2134*
      with arhinencephaly, *1180,* 1181
    secondary deformities of, 2165–2176
      deficient buccal sulcus, 2171, 2172, *2172*
      excessively long lip, 2166, *2168, 2169*
      excessively short lip, 2166
      flattening of lip, 2166
      incomplete muscle union, 2166, *2167*
      malalignment of upper lip, 2172–2174
      reconstruction of philtrum in, 2169–2171
      tight upper lip, 2167, 2169, *2170*
      upper lip scars, 2176
      whistle deformity, *2173,* 2174, *2174, 2175,* 2176, *2176*
  unilateral, 2016–2047
    criteria for satisfactory repair of, 2025
    history of, 2016–2019
    methods of repair of, 2025–2032
    muscles of, 1967, *1967,* 1968, *1968, 1969,* 1970
    technique of various repairs in, 2032–2045
    treatment of, 2019–2025
      aftercare in, 2023
      anesthesia in, 2020
      dressings in, 2021, 2023
      extended operations in, 2023–2025
      positioning and marking of patient in, 2020, 2021
      preoperative feeding in, 2019, 2020
      surgical technique in, 2021, *2022*
      timing of operation in, 2020
Cleft lip and nose, secondary deformities of, 2176–2193
  bilateral, 2185–2193
    corrective surgery of, 2188–2193
    pathologic anatomy of, 2185, 2188, *2188*
  unilateral, 2176–2185
    corrective surgery of, 2179–2185
    pathologic anatomy of, 2176–2179
    timing of corrective nasal surgery in, 2179
Cleft lip and palate, 1930–1940. See also *Cleft lip, bilateral, with bilateral cleft of primary palate,* and *Cleft palate.*

Cleft lip and palate *(Continued)*
  anatomy of facial skeleton in, 1950–1965
  bilateral, complete, prenatal facial growth in, 1991,
    1991, 1992, *1992*
    embryology of, 1950–1957
      cause of premaxillary protrusion in, 1956, 1957
      development of bilateral cleft deformity in,
        1953–1956
      lip and columella in, *1951,* 1952
      maxillary segments in, 1952, 1953, *1954, 1955*
      nasal septum, premaxillae, and vomer in, *1951,*
        1952, *1953*
      premaxillary malformation in, 1950, 1951, *1951,*
        1952
    lip reconstruction in, 1999, *1999,* 2000, *2000, 2001*
    maxillary growth in, 2004
  causes of abnormal facial growth in, 2006–2011
  classification of, 1935–1937
  dentition in, 2217, *2218,* 2219, *2219, 2220*
  effect of lip reconstruction on maxillary complex in,
    1998, *1998*
  effect of palate reconstruction on maxillary complex in,
    2000–2002
  embryology of, 1941–1949
    classification and nomenclature in, 1946
  epidemiology of, 1937–1939
  facial growth in, 1989–2015
    effect of bone grafting on, 2011
    effect of orthodontics on, 2011
    effect of preoperative orthopedics on, 2011
    following surgical repair, 1996–2011
    in unrepaired cleft lip and palate, 1995, 1996, *1996*
    potential for, 1989, 1990
    prenatal, 1990–1992
    preservation of, 2094
  general growth in patients with, 1992, 1993
  genetic factors and, 1939
  history of, 1930–1935
  incidence of, 1937, 1938
  jaw and tooth relations in, 2006
  mandible in, 2215, *2216,* 2217
  maxilla in, 2214, *2214,* 2215, *2215*
  musculature of, 1966–1988
  operations for, anesthesia in, 593, 594, *594*
  orthodontics in, 2213–2234
    history of, 2213, 2214
    stages of treatment in, 2221–2231
      newborn period, 2221–2224
      period of adult dentition, 2230, *2230,* 2231, *2231*
      period of deciduous dentition, 2224–2229
      period of mixed dentition, 2229, *2229,* 2230, *2230*
  parental age and, 1938, 1939
  racial influences on, 1938
  sex ratio in, 1938
  speech problems in, 2246–2267
    compensatory mechanisms in, 2262, 2263
    diagnostic procedures in, 2263, 2264
    etiologic considerations in, 2260–2263
    historical aspects of, 2259
    nature of, 2257–2259
    surgeon's responsibility in, 2246, 2247
    therapy of, 2264, 2265
  unilateral, complete, maxillary growth in, 2003, *2003,*
    2004
    prenatal facial growth in, 1990, *1990,* 1991, *1991*
    embryology of, 1957–1963
      development of unilateral cleft skeletal deformity
        in, 1959, 1960, 1961, *1961*
      lip and columella in, 1959
      onset and rate of development of, 1961, 1962

Cleft lip and palate *(Continued)*
  unilateral, embryology of, premaxillary segment and
    nasal septum in, 1957, 1958, *1958,* 1959, *1959*
    Simonart's bar in, *1961,* 1962, *1962,* 1963
    vomer and palatal process in, 1959, *1960*
    lip reconstruction in, 1998, 1999, *1999*
  unrepaired, facial growth in, 1995, 1996, *1996*
Cleft palate, 2090–2115. See also *Cleft lip and palate*
  and *Cleft lip, bilateral, with bilateral cleft of*
  primary palate.
  bone grafting in, 2205–2212
    development of, 2206
    disenchantment with, 2206, 2207
    experimental studies of, 2207, 2208
    newer approaches in, 2209, 2210
    results of longitudinal studies of, 2207
    technique of, 2208, *2209*
    with osteotomy to correct maxillary hypoplasia,
      2208, 2209
  bony changes in, 1987, 1988
  counseling parents of patient with, 2090, 2091
  definition of, 2091
  early orthopedic treatment of, 2205
  embryology of, 1963, *1963,* 1964
  goals of surgery in, 2093, 2094
  history of, 2091–2093
  maxillary advancement in, 1447, *1447,* 1448, *1448*
  maxillary growth in, 2002, *2002,* 2003, *2003*
  muscle arrangement in, 1984, 1987, 1988
  secondary deformities of, 2194–2201
    maxillary, 2194–2198
    oronasal fistulas, 2198–2201
  submucous, 2104–2114
    anatomical findings in, 2111
    developmental shortening of palate in, 2113, *2113*
    diagnosis of, 2104, *2104, 2105,* 2106
    differential diagnosis of, 2106
    histologic findings in, 2111, *2111, 2112,* 2113
    history of diagnosis and therapy in, 2108, 2109
    incidence of in United States, 2106–2108
    palate length and mobility in, 2107, 2107t, 2108,
      2108t
    speech evaluation in, 2107, 2107t
    statistics on, from Prague Plastic Surgery Clinic.
      2109
    treatment of at Prague Plastic Surgery Clinic, 2109–
      2111
  surgery for, 2094–2103
    anesthesia in, 2094
    complications of, 2102, 2103
    formation of levator sling in, 2094, 2095, *2095*
    palatoplasty and primary pharyngeal flap in,
      2096–2102
    V-Y retroposition ("push-back") procedure in, 2095,
      2096, *2096, 2097*
Cleft palate prosthetics, 2283–2293
  evaluation of patient prior to, 2290
  indications for, 2284
  palatal lift appliance in, 2291–2293
  preparation of obturator in, 2284–2287
  types of obturators in, 2287–2290
    influence of patient's age on, 2291, *2291, 2292*
Cleft palate speech, history of surgery for, 2271–2276
Cleidocranial dysostosis, 2408
Clinodactyly, *3332*
Clip bar, in retention of maxillary prosthesis, 2934,
  2934
Clitoris, *3828, 3829,* 3831, *3833*
Cloaca, 3828, *3828*
  embryology of, 3829–3831

Cloacal membrane, 3828, *3828, 3831, 3832*
Clostridial myonecrosis, of abdominal wall, 3739–3741
Clotting system, and graft rejection, 135, *135*
Clubhand, radial, *3333*
Coagulation, bipolar, 345, 346
  during surgery, 350, 351
Cochlear duct, 2306
Cockleshell ear, 1705, *1707*
Coelst, M., 17, *20*
Coffin-Siris syndrome, 2980
Coisogenic, 141
Cold injury, 516–530
  body heat conservation and, 520, 521
  classification of, 516–520
  degree of, 516, 516t, 517, *517, 518*
  direct cellular injury in, 521, 522
  mental state and, 521
  microvascular insult in, 522–524
  mobility and, 521
  pathogenesis of, 521–524
  predisposing factors of, 520, 521
  race and climate and, 521
  treatment of, 524–528
  thawing in, 524, 525, 525t
Collagen
  changes in physical properties of, 93, 94
  deposition of, 94, 95
  in tendon, 266, 267, 269, 270
  structure and synthesis of, 86–89, 94, 95
Collagen fibers, 69, *70, 71, 72, 96, 97*
Collagen metabolism, factors affecting, 92, 93
Collagenase, tissue, 91
Collagenolytic enzyme, 91
Collagenous tissue, remodeling of, 89–92
Colles' fracture, Dupuytren's contracture after, 3407, *3407*
Collis procedure for repairing cleft lip, 2017, *2017*, 2028
Colon, flap of in oropharyngoesophageal reconstructive surgery, 2708, *2709, 2710*
Columella, 1042, *1042*, 1051, *1051*, 1052
  defects of, 1268–1271
    reconstruction of, 1269–1271
    retrusion of, 1095–1098, 1268, 1269, *1269*
  hanging, correction of, 1095, *1095*
  in unilateral cleft lip and palate, 1959
  lengthening of, in bilateral cleft lip repair, *2063, 2064,* 2066, 2067, *2068, 2069*
  retruded and retracted, correction of, 1095–1098, 1268, 1269, *1269*
  wide, narrowing of, 1093, *1094*
Columella-ala triangle, correction of, 1093, 1094, *1094, 1097*
Columnae adiposae, 155
Complement, 134, 135, *135*
Composite flaps, 223, 1503
Composite grafts. See *Grafts, composite.*
Concha, alteration of, in treatment of prominent ear, 1710, 1711, *1711*
Condylar hyperplasia, and unilateral mandibular macrognathia, 1378–1382
Condylar hypoplasia, 1375–1378
Condyle. See *Mandible, condylar process of.*
Condyloma, malignant, 2778, 2779
Coniotomy, 602, *602*
Conjunctiva, 865, *865*
  embryonic development of, 2312
Conjunctival flap, in connection of symblepharon, 916, *917*
Conjunctival graft, in correction of symblepharon, 916–918

Conjunctival irritation, following esthetic blepharoplasty, 1893, 1894
Conjunctivodacryocystorhinostomy, 987–989
Conjunctivodacryorhinostomy, 1016
Conjunctivorhinostomy, 1016
Connective tissue tumors, of jaws, 2567–2569
Constricting band, congenital, 419, 420, *421*
  of lower extremity, W-plasty in, 60, *62*
Contact inhibition, 80
Contraction
  in burn injury, 1596–1599
  of grafted skin, 182, 183
  scar, physical basis of, 415–420
  vs. contracture, 83, 3370
  wound, 79, 83–86
Contraction phenomenon, inter-island, 444
Contracture(s)
  adduction, of thumb. See *Thumb, adduction contracture of.*
  axillary, correction of, 3393, *3393–3397*
  burn scar, of lip, 1545, *1545, 1560,* 1561, *1561*
  complete, of cervical region, 1644–1658
  Dupuytren's. See *Dupuytren's contracture.*
  limited, of cervical region, 1658, *1659*
  muscle, in hand, 3126, 3128, *3129, 3130*
  scar, 430, 431, *432,* 434, 460, 1643, 1644, *1645,* 2966, *2967*
  Volkmann's, 3130–3137
  vs. contraction, 83, 3370
Contrast media, and microcirculation, 352
Conway technique of breast reduction, 3684, *3687*
Cornea, care of during surgery, 867–869
Corneal abrasion, following esthetic blepharoplasty, 1893, 1894
Coronal flap, for exposure in malunited naso-orbital fractures, 1020
Coronal synostosis, 2493, 2495, *2495, 2496, 2497*
  bilateral, correction of, 2495, 2497, *2497, 2498*
  unilateral, correction of, 2497, 2498, *2499–2502*
Coronoid process of mandible, fractures of, 688
Corrugator supercilii muscle, 1782
Cortical bone, compact, 313, 314, *314*
  autograft of, 324, *325*
Cortical osteotomy, in jaw deformities, 1304, 1305, *1305, 1306*
Corticosteroids, and immunosuppression, 138
  and rare craniofacial clefts, 2123
Cortisone, and wound contraction, 86, 93
  in thermal burn, 485
Cosmetic surgery, 12
  for aging face, 1868–1929
  social and psychologic considerations in selection of patients for, 573–579
Costal cartilage grafts. See *Graft, cartilage, costal.*
Cotton implants, 392
Coumarin, in microvascular surgery, 367
Coup de sabre deformity, in Romberg's disease, 2339, *2339,* 2340
Crane principle, 223
Cranial bones, embryonic development of, 2313
  growth of, 823, 824, *824*
Cranial cavity, evaluation of volume of, 2498, 2499
Cranial fossa, anterior, 2435, *2436*
  fractures involving, 739
  osteotomy of in orbital hypertelorism, 2450, 2452, *2452*
  in Crouzon's disease and Apert's syndrome, 2469–2471
  middle, 2435, *2436*
Cranial nerve anomalies, in craniofacial microsomia, 2376, *2376,* 2377

Cranial sutures, premature synostosis of, 831, 832,
    2465–2472
Cranial synostosis, 2465
Cranial vault, congenital absence of, 828–831
    reshaping of, 2492–2502, *2503–2506*
        complications of, 2502
Craniectomy, strip, for coronal synostosis, 2495, *2497*
    for sagittal synostosis, 2493, *2495*
Craniofacial anomalies, 2296–2358
Craniofacial clefts, rare, 2116–2164
        American Association of Cleft Palate Rehabilitation
            classification of, 2125, *2125,* 2126, *2126*
        Boo-Chai classification of, 2126, *2126*
        classification of, 2125–2131
        clinical varieties of, 2131, 2154
        description of, 2131–2154
        drugs and chemicals and, 2122, 2123
        embryologic aspects of, 2117–2121
        etiology of, 2121–2123
        incidence of, 2116, 2117
        infection and, 2122
        Karfik classification of, 2126, 2127t, 2128
        maternal metabolic imbalance and, 2122
        morphopathogenesis of, 2123–2125
        radiation and, 2121, 2122
        Tessier classification of, 2129–2131
            combinations of clefts No. 6, 7, and 8, 2149,
                2149, 2150, *2150*
            No. 0, 2131–2137
            No. 1, 2137, 2138, *2138, 2139*
            No. 2, 2138, *2139,* 2140, *2140*
            No. 3, 2140, 2141, *2141, 2142*
            No. 4, 2142, 2143, *2143,* 2144, *2144*
            No. 5, 2144, 2145, *2145*
            No. 6, 2145, 2146, *2146*
            No. 7, 2146–2148
            No. 8, 2149, *2149*
            No. 9, 2150, *2150*
            No. 10, 2150, *2151*
            No. 11, 2150
            No. 12, 2150, 2151, *2151*
            No. 13, 2151
            No. 14, 2152–2154
        treatment of, 2154–2160
Craniofacial disjunction, *697,* 698
Craniofacial dysostosis. See *Crouzon's disease.*
Craniofacial dysrhaphia, median, *2153,* 2154
Craniofacial microsomia, 1676, *1677,* 2124, 2125, 2359–
    2400, 2403, *2406*
    bilateral, 2391–2398
        surgical reconstruction of mandible in, 2394–2398
        variations of syndrome of, 2391, *2392–2394*
    clinical spectrum of syndrome of, 2360–2366, *2367,
        2368*
    differential diagnosis of, 2359, 2360
    ear deformity in, 2361–2366, 2374, 2375, *2375,* 2391,
        2392, 2393
    early vs. late reconstruction in, 2386, *2387–2391*
    embryology of, 2368–2370
    etiopathogenesis of, 2370
    history of, 2360
    incidence of, 2360
    jaw deformity in, 2361–2366, 2371–2373
    muscles of mastication in, 2374
    nervous system deformities in, 2375–2377
    pathology of, 2370–2377
    restoration of soft tissue contour in, 2385, 2386
    sex distribution of, 2360
    skeletal deformities in, 2373, 2374, *2374*
    soft tissue deformities in, 2377

Craniofacial microsomia *(Continued)*
    treatment of, 2377–2386
    unilateral vs. bilateral, 2361
Craniofacial skeleton, anatomy of, 2431–2436
    tumors involving, 2757–2775
        basal cell epithelioma, 2757, 2758, *2758, 2759*
        complications of, 2762, *2762,* 2763
        pathology of, 2757–2759, *2760, 2761*
        squamous cell carcinoma, 2758, 2759, *2760, 2761*
        treatment of, 2760, 2761
Craniofacial structures, midline, clefts of, 2119, 2120,
    2120
Craniofacial surgery
    complications following, 2490–2492
    designing the surgical procedure in, 2429
    extraocular and levator muscle function following,
        2485, 2486
    in Crouzon's disease and Apert's syndrome, 2465–2486
    in fibrous dysplasia, 2490, *2491*
    in malunited fractures of midface, 2488
    in orbital hypertelorism, 2436–2462
    in orbital hypotelorism, 2462–2465
    in traumatic hypertelorism, 2488
    in tumors of fronto-ethmoid area, 2490
    intraoperative monitoring in, 2429, *2430*
    postoperative period in, 2429, 2431, *2431*
    preoperative planning of, 2428, *2428,* 2429
    principles of, 2427–2508
    techniques of, applications of, 2488, *2489,* 2490, *2490*
Craniofacial surgery team, organization of, 2427–2431
Craniofacial suspension, in maxillary fractures, *704*
Craniopagus, 825, *825, 826,* 827, *827*
Cranioplast implants, 772, 790
Craniotelencephalic dysplasia, 2493, *2494*
Cranium
    advanced cancers of, 2763
    defects of, congenital, 824–832
        bone grafting in, 841–855
        traumatic, 838–845
    growth of compared to face, *800*
    phylogeny of, 823
Crease lines, 71, 72, 77
"Creep," 71
Cri du chat syndrome, syndactyly in, 3313
Cribriform plate, 2433, *2433*
    depressed, in orbital hypertelorism, 2437, *2440*
"Crocodile tear" syndrome, 1840
Cronin prosthesis, for mammary augmentation, 3697,
    3698, 3699, 3702, 3706
Cronin technique of columella lengthening in bilateral
    cleft lip repair, 2066, 2067, *2068, 2069*
Cronin technique of freeing nasal mucosa in cleft palate
    repair, *2100,* 2102
Cross-arm flap, 215, *216,* 217
Crossbite, 1295, *1298*
    anterior, in cleft lip and palate, *2230*
Cross-face nerve transplantation, reconstruction of face
    through, in facial paralysis, 1848–1864
Cross-finger flap, *216,* 217
Cross-leg flap, 217
Cross-zygomaticus muscle graft, in oral paralysis, 1846,
    1847, *1847*
Crouzon's disease, 832, 2315–2320, 2407, 2465, 2466
    anatomical pathology in, 2468–2472
    advancement osteotomy of mandibular symphysis in,
        2485
    calvarium in, 2468, *2468, 2469*
    coronal synostosis in, 2495, *2497*
    corrective nasal surgery in, 2485
    cranial fossa and orbits in, 2469–2471

Crouzon's disease *(Continued)*
  etiopathogenesis of, 2316
  facial deformities in, 2317, 2472, *2472*
  frontal bone surgery in, 2485
  history of, 2315, 2316
  hyponasality in, 1451, *1451*, 1452
  maxilla in, 2471, *2471*, 2472
  medial and lateral canthoplasties in, 2485
  neurologic disorders in, 2317, 2318
  neurosurgery in, 2318
  ocular deformities in, 2317, *2317*, 2471, *2471*
  operative procedures for correction of, 2472–2486
    types of osteotomies used in, 2473–2481
  physical characteristics of, 2316–2318
  preoperative cephalometric planning in, 2482, *2483*
  preoperative orthodontic planning in, 2482, *2482*
  ptosis of upper eyelid in, *2479*, 2485
  reconstructive surgery in, 2318–2320
  skull deformities in, 2316, 2317
  timing of surgery in, 2486, *2487*
  treatment of, 2318–2320
"Crown of thorns" appliance, 677, *678*, 702, *706*, 1372, *1372*
Cryobiologic preservation of skin, 181, 182
Cryosurgery, of actinic keratosis, 2803, *2803*
Cryotherapy, in multifocal intraoral tumor, 2651
Cryptorchidism, 3834
Cryptotia, 1709, *1709*
Crystallometry, liquid, in evaluation of flap circulation, 195
Cup ear, 1705–1709
Curettage and electrodesiccation
  of basal cell epithelioma, 2806–2809, *2810*
  of nevi, *2798*, 2799, *2799*, *2800*
  of seborrheic keratosis, *2783*, *2783*
  of skin cancer, 2830
  of warts, 2779–2781, 2876
Curling's ulcer, 509
Cutaneous flaps, 194, *194*
Cutaneous horn, 2858
Cutaneous sensation, neurohistologic basis of, 226
Cutaneous tags, 2791, *2791*
Cutis laxa, 1877
Cutler-Beard technique, 895–898
α-Cyanoacrylate adhesive implants, 393
Cyclophosphamide, and immunosuppression, 138
Cyclopia, orbital hypotelorism in, 2463, *2463*
Cyclopropane, 587
Cyclops, 1179, *1179*
Cylindroma, 2789, *2789*
  of parotid gland, 2528, *2528*, 2529, *2532*
Cyst(s)
  auricular, 2877
  bone, simple (traumatic), of jaws, 2563, *2564*
  branchial. See *Branchial cysts and fistulas.*
  dentigerous, ameloblastoma arising in, 2550, *2550*, *2551*, 2552, *2552*
    of jaws, 2564, *2564*
  dermoid, *2877*, 2878, *2878*
    of eyelids, 877
    of nose, 1170, *1170*, *1174*, 1175, *1175*, 1176, 1177
  epidermal and pilar, 2784–2786
    following dermal overgrafting, 184, *185*, 186
    in dermis grafts, 247, *247*, 248, *248*
  epithelial, of hand and forearm, 3450–3452
    of jaws, 2563–2565
  globulomaxillary, 2564, 2565, *2565*
  inclusion, of eyelids, 878, 879
  mucous, 2791, *2791*, 2792
    formation of, 1542

Cyst(s) *(Continued)*
  mucous, of hand and forearm, 3470, *3470*, 3471, *3471*
  myxoid, 2792
    of hand and forearm, 3470, *3470*, 3471, *3471*
  nasoalveolar, 2565
  nasopalatine duct, 2564, *2565*
  odontogenic, of jaws, 2563, 2564, *2564*
  of neck, congenital. See *Neck, congenital cysts and tumors of.*
  primordial, of jaws, 2563
  radicular, of jaws, 2565, *2565*
  salivary, following face lift operation, 1926
  sebaceous, 2784–2786, 2877, 2878
    of auricle, 1766
  silicone, 396, *396*
  skin, 2876–2878
  synovial, of hand and forearm, 3470
  thyroglossal duct, 2877, *2877*, 2905–2908
Cystadenoma lymphomatosum, papillary, of parotid gland, 2527, *2527*
Cystic hygroma, 2873, 2874
Cytoxan, in treatment of skin cancer, 2839

Dacron, 402, 405, *408*
Dacron implants, 392, 393, 401, 402
Dacryocystectomy, 984–986
Dacryocystitis, 983, 984, *984*
Dacryocystorhinostomy, 984–986, 1012–1020
Dautrey modification of sagittal-split osteotomy of ramus, *1329*, 1330–1334
Davis, J. Staige, 13, *15*
Davol disposable head dermatome, 173, *174*
De Quervain's disease, 3443, 3444, *3444–3446*
Decubitus ulcer. See *Pressure sore.*
Defect, apparent versus true, 24, *24*, 25
  principle of shifting of, 45, 46
Deformity (deformities)
  concept of, 550–552
  congenital, 104–125
    chromosomal abnormalities and, 108–115
    etiology of, 107–118
    genetic counseling for, 118–122
    history of, 104, 105
    incidence of, 106, 107
  developmental, of facial skeleton, 814–819
  evaluation of, 23–38
  facial, social science approach to, 565–584
  interpretation of, 26, 27
"Degloving" technique, *677*
  in mandibular malformations, *1307*, 1308, *1308*
  in mandibular micrognathia, *1349*, 1350
  midface, 1426, *1426*, 1427
  maxillectomy via, 2582, *2583*, 2584, *2584*, 2585, *2585*, *2586*
Deltopectoral flap. See *Flap, deltopectoral.*
Denasality, 2258
Denervation, of muscle graft, 294–299
Dental appliance, used with pressure dressing, in intraoral tumor surgery, 2652–2655
Dental casts, in correction of mandibular prognathism, 1312, *1313*
  planning of osteotomies for jaw malformations using, 1297, 1298, *1299*
Dental compound, use of in splinting of nose, 1087, *1087*, *1088*, *1089*
Dental lamina, 2313
  ectodermal, formation of, *1945*, 1946
Dental occlusion, 647, *647*, 648

Dental prosthesis, and skin graft inlay, in correction of
    microgenia, *1402*, 1403, *1403*, 1404
Dental wiring, in jaw fractures, 648–652
Dentigerous cyst, ameloblastoma arising in, 2550, *2550*,
    2551, 2552, *2552*
  of jaws, 2564, *2564*
Dentition, 646, 647. See also *Teeth.*
  as guide in reduction and fixation of jaw fractures, 648
  esthetic, cleft palate repair and, 2094
  in cleft lip and palate, 2217, *2218*, 2219, *2219*, 2220
  influence of on speech, 2261, 2262
  secondary, position of in skull, *797*, *798*, 799, 800
Dentoalveolar complex, in jaw deformities, 1292, *1292*,
    1293
Dentoalveolar osteotomy, in jaw deformities, 1304, *1304*
Dentoalveolar process, 648, *648*
  growth of, 1994, 1995
Denture, artificial, auxiliary means for increasing
      masticatory efficiency of, 2935, *2936*, 2937, *2937–
      2939*
    intermaxillary fixation using, in jaw deformities, 1301,
      1302
    temporary, as maxillary prostheses, 2929, *2931*, 2932,
      2932, *2933*
"Denture-splint," in intraoral tumor surgery, 2652–2655
Deoxyribonucleic acid. See *DNA.*
Depressor septi nasi muscle, 1051, *1051*, 1052, 1781
Dermabrasion, 442–454, 628, *628*, *630*
  and replantation of amputated auricle, 1727, 1728,
    1731
  complications of, 453, 454
  contraindications to, 451, 453
  equipment in, 445
  healing of abraded areas in, 443–445
  history of, 442, 443
  in malignancy, 453
  in rhinophyma, 1191
  indications for, 446–453
  limitations of, 450, 451
  of tattoos, 2815, *2816*
  operative procedure in, 445, 446
  postoperative care in, 446
Dermachalasis, 1878, *1879*, 1880
Dermal flap technique, in treatment of lymphedema,
    3597, *3600*, 3601, *3601*
Dermal overgrafting, 183–188
  dermabrasion and, in burn scars, 447, *451*, *452*
  for venous stasis ulcers of lower extremity, 3524,
    3525, *3525*, *3532*
  in burn scars, 1617, *1617*
  of calcaneal defect, *3532*
Dermatitis, radiation, and chest wall reconstruction, 3611,
    3612
Dermatofibroma, 2790, 2866, 2867
  of hand and forearm, 3472
Dermatofibrosarcoma, 2840
Dermatome(s)
  Brown air-driven, 495, *495*
  Brown electric, 167, *167*
  development of, 14
  for removal of split-thickness skin grafts, 167–173
Dermatopraxia, 88, 93
Dermatosis, irradiation, of hand and forearms, 3457,
    3457, *3458*, 3459
Dermatosis papulosa nigra, 2782
Dermis, 152, *153*, 154
  aging of, 1874
  and wound healing, 95
  transplantation of, 240–250
    histologic changes in grafts in, 246–249

Dermis *(Continued)*
  transplantation of, history of, 242–244
    in facial palsy, 1820
    in Romberg's disease, 2344, 2345
    operative procedure in, 244, 245, *245*, 246
Dermis-fat flap. See *Flap, dermis-fat.*
Dermis-fat graft. See *Graft, dermis-fat.*
Dermoepidermal junction, 154
Dermoid cysts, *2877*, 2878, *2878*
  of eyelids, 877
  of nose, 1170, *1170*, *1174*, 1175, *1175*, 1176, 1177
Dermolipectomy, 3800–3822
  of abdominal wall. See *Abdominal wall, dermolipectomy
    of.*
  of buttocks, 3811–3820
  of thighs, 3811–3820
  of upper extremity, *3819*, 3820–3822
Desmoid tumor, 2879
Desmosomes, 154
Dextran, in microvascular surgery, 369
  low molecular weight, 202
    in treatment of cold injury, 524, 526
Diabetes mellitus, and maxillary tumor surgery, 2587
Diazepam, 586
  and craniofacial clefts, 2123
Dieffenbach, 8
Dieffenbach operation, modified, in complete loss of
    lower lip, 1571, 1572, *1572*, 1573
Digastric muscle, 660, *661*
  anterior, 1782
Digital. See also *Finger.*
Digital amputations, major, 3143–3145
Digital extension, 3166–3180, *3181–3183*
Digital extensor-flexor system, 3166–3184
Digital flexion, 3183–3206
  factors in graft survival in, 3192–3206
  specific problems of tendon repair in, 3184–3192
Digital joint injuries, 3056, *3057*, *3058*
Digital joints, in arthritic hand, 3515–3517
  fusion of, 3510, 3511, *3511*
Digital necrosis, secondary to ischemia, *2967*
Digital nerve blocks, in acute hand injuries, *3011*, 3012
Digital nerves, results of grafting in, 3237
Digital posture, anomalies of, 3325, *3325*, 3326, *3326*,
    3327
Digital replantation, 3252–3256
  arterial anastomosis in, 3253, 3255, *3255*
  bone shortening in, 3253
  extensor tendon in, 3253
  flexor tendons and skin in, 3256
  indications for, 3252
  nerve repair in, 3256
  operative techniques in, 3252–3256
  results of, 3257–3259
  sequence of multiple digits in, 3262, *3262*, *3263*
  sequence of repair in, 3253, 3253t, *3254*
  vascular anastomoses in, 3253
  vein repair in, 3253
Digital shortening, disorders resulting in, 3331–3333
Digital tendovaginitis, stenosing, 3440–3443
Digits, supernumerary, surgical management of, 3319–
    3325
Dilator muscle, 1781
Dimethyl sulfoxide (DMSO), 198
Dimethyl triazeno imidazole carboxamide (DTIC), in
    treatment of malignant melanoma, 2853
β,β-Dimethylcysteine, 93, 94
Dimethylpolysiloxane. See *Silicone.*
Dingman approach, in reduction of fractures of zygoma,
    715, *716*

Dingman mouth gag, 2279
Diphenylhydantoin, 2122
Diploid number, 140
Diplopia, following blowout fracture of orbital floor, 757, 757t, 758, 992–995
  following esthetic blepharoplasty, 1893
Dipyridamole, in microvascular surgery, 365, 368, 369
"Dish-face" deformity, 1424, 1425, 2092
Disjunction, craniofacial, *697*, 698
Dislocations, in acute hand injuries, 3041–3060
Distant flaps. See *Flaps, distant.*
Distoclusion, 647, *647*, 1292, *1292*
Disulphine blue dye, in evaluation of flap circulation, 195
Diverticulum, Meckel's, 3728
DNA, and chromatin, 116, 117
  nature of, 115, 116, *116*
Dog-ear, removal of, 49, *53*
Doppler flowmeter, 199, 345
Dorsal flap, in chest wall reconstruction, *3613*
Dorsalis pedis flap. See *Flap, dorsalis pedis.*
Dorsum, of nose. See *Nasal dorsum.*
Drugs, immunosuppressive, 138
Drum dermatomes, 167–172
"Dry eye" syndrome, following esthetic blepharoplasty, 1896, 1897
Duct(s)
  cochlear, 2306
  Müllerian, 3828
  nasolacrimal, *980*, 981, 2307
  parotid, 630–632, *635*, *636*, 2543, 2544, *2544*
  salivary, 2542, 2543
  semicircular, 2306
  Stensen's. See *Stensen's duct.*
  submaxillary, 632
  thoracic, *3571*, *3577*, 3586–3590
  thyroglossal, 2877, *2877*, 2904–2908
  vitelline, 3278
  Wolffian, 3828, 3829
Dufourmentel, Léon, 16, 17
Duplay's method of reconstruction of hypospadias, 3838, *3838*
Duplay's method of reconstruction of urethra, 3837, *3837*
Dupuytren, 8
Dupuytren's contracture, 2995, 2998, 3403–3427, 3474, 3475
  associated diseases in, 3406, 3407
  complications of surgery for, 3415, 3424, 3425, *3425*
  dermal involvement in, 3416, 3417
  distribution of hyperplastic tissue in, 3415, 3416, *3416*
  dressing technique in, 3417, *3418*, 3419
  ectopic deposits in, 3411, 3412, *3412*
    surgery for, 3422, 3424
  etiology of, 3403–3406
  fasciectomy in, 3413, *3414*, 3419–3424
  genetic basis of, 3406
  injury and, 3407–3409
    age distribution in, 3408, *3408*
  intrinsic and extrinsic theories of pathogenesis of, 3410, *3411*
  local flap arrangement in, 3417, *3417*, *3418*
  management of skin in, 3415–3419
  manual labor and, 3408, 3409, *3409*
  myofibroblast in, 3405, 3406
  operative techniques in, 3419–3424
  palmar fasciotomy in, 3413, 3419, *3419*
  selection of operation in, 3413–3415
  skin incisions in, 3415
  skin replacement in, 3421, 3422, *3423*, *3424*
  structural changes in, 3409, 3410

Dura, congenital absence of, 828–831
  exposure of, following maxillary tumor surgery, 2588
Dural defects, fat grafts in repair of, 255
Dynamic lines of face, 1870, *1870*, 1871, *1871*, 1872, *1872*
Dyscephaly, 2407, *2407*
Dystonia canthorum, 942

Ear(s). See also *Auricle.*
  basal cell epithelioma of, *2773*
  burn involvement of, 1604, 1605
  cauliflower, 1732, 1735
  chemosurgery on, 2884
  cockleshell, 1705, *1707*
  concave "telephone" deformity of, *1717*, 1718
  constricted, 1705–1709
  cup or lop, 1705–1709
    in Möbius syndrome, 2327, *2328*
  development of reconstructive surgery of, 1724, 1725
  external, embryology of, 1673, 1674, *1674*, *1675*, 2307, *2308*, 2309
  form of, 34, *38*
  inner, embryology of, 1672
  lacerations of, *642*
  middle, cancers of, 2770
    embryology of, 1672, 1673, *1674*
    surgery of, in congenital auricular malformation, 1719–1724
  pocket, 1709, *1709*
  postchemosurgery reconstruction of, 2893
  prominent, 1710–1718
    complications in, *1717*, 1718
    pathology of, 1710, *1710*
    treatment of, 1710–1718
  shell, 1710, 1717, 1718
Ear cartilage, transplantation of, 306–308
Ear deformity, in craniofacial microsomia, 2361–2366, 2374, 2375, *2375*, 2391, *2392*, *2393*
Ear hillocks, 2313
Ear prostheses, 2948
Earlobe, reconstruction of, 1761–1766
Eave flap, 1703, *1704*, 1740, *1742*
Ecchondroma, of hand and forearm, 3499
Eccrine poroma, 2788, *2788*, 2789
Eccrine sweat glands, *153*, 155
Ectodermal cell masses, polarization of, in developing lip and palate, 1944–1946
Ectrodactyly, surgical management of, 3329–3331
Ectropion, 907–911, *912*, *913*
  following esthetic blepharoplasty, 1894
Edema. See also *Lymphedema.*
  acute, 3578, 3579
  chronic, 3579–3585
  laryngeal, after tracheal intubation, 591
  of hand, 3014, 3109–3111, *3112*, 3382, 3383
  pathophysiology of, 3578–3585
  regional, classification of, 3578
Edge-wise orthodontic and fixation appliance, in jaw fractures, 651, *656*
Edmonds operation for correction of chordee, 3836, *3836*
Effudex, in treatment of skin cancer, 2839
Ehlers-Danlos syndrome, 1876, *1876*
Elastic band, extraoral, for newborn with cleft lip and palate, 2223, *2223*
Elastic tissue, 154
Elastic traction, intraoral, 2053, *2053*, 2054
  with head cap, in bilateral cleft lip, 2052, *2052*, 2053

Elastin, 69, 70
  in tendon, 267
Elbow, burns of, 3391–3399
  repair of with abdominal flap, *214*
  ulcers of, 3792, *3793*
Electric dermatome, 172, 173
Electrical burns, 469, *469*, 512, 513, 1596
  of perioral region, 1639, 1640
Electrical current, and thrombosis, 352
Electrocutting current treatment, of rhinophyma, 2783,
  2784, *2784, 2785*
Electrodesiccation. See *Curettage and electrodesiccation.*
Electrodiagnosis, of hand, 2981–2989
Electrogustometry, 1787, 1788
Electromyography, 2981–2989
  in facial palsy, 1789–1791, *1792*
Ellis-van Creveld syndrome, polydactyly in, 3320
Enamel organs of teeth, 2315
Encephalocele, frontal, *2151, 2152, 2153,* 2154, *2154*
  of nose, 1169, *1170, 1172,* 1173–1175
Enchondroma, of hand and forearm, 3452, 3497, *3498,*
  3499
Endoneurium, 3216, *3216*
Enflurane, 587, 588
Enophthalmos, following orbital fractures, 757t, 758–761,
  790, 994–1000
Entropion, 913, 914, *915*
Enzymes, and immunosuppression, 138
Ephelides, 2797
Epiblepharon, 942–944, *944*
Epicanthal folds, following skin grafting of eyelids, *1628,*
  1629
  in naso-orbital fractures, correction of, 1011
Epicanthus, congenital and traumatic, 940–942
Epicranius, 822, *822,* 823
Epidermal appendage tumors, 2786–2788
Epidermal cysts. See *Cysts, epidermal.*
Epidermis, 152, 153, *153,* 154
  aging of, 1874
Epidermodysplasia verruciformis, 2779
  of hand and forearm, 3450
Epidermoid carcinoma, 81, *82,* 2812–2814
  of maxillary sinus, 2767, *2769*
Epidermoid cyst. See *Cyst, epidermal.*
Epidural block, 594
Epigastric artery, inferior, distant flaps based on in acute
  hand injuries, 3041, *3042*
Epigastric hernia, 3728
Epilepsy, Dupuytren's contracture in, 3406, 3407
Epineural suture, in nerves of hand, 3222
Epineurium, 3216, *3216*
Epiphora, 981
  following esthetic blepharoplasty, 1893
  in facial palsy, relief of, 1832–1834
Epispadias, 3832, 3862–3871
  etiology and incidence of, 3863
  female, 3868, *3870,* 3871
  repair of complete type of, 3868, *3869, 3870,* 3871
  repair of simple type of, *3865,* 3866–3868
  treatment of, 3863, 3866
  types of, 3863, *3864*
Epithelial cysts, of hand and forearm, 3450–3452
  of jaws, 2563–2565
Epithelial tumors, of hand and forearm, 3450–3464
Epithelioma
  basal cell. See *Basal cell epithelioma.*
  calcifying, benign, of Malherbe, 2787, 2788
    of hand and forearm, 3452, *3452*
  dermabrasion of, 450

Epithelioma *(Continued)*
  prickle cell, 2812–2814
  squamous cell. See *Squamous cell carcinoma.*
Epithelioma adenoides cysticum, 2874, 2875
Epithelium, function of, 79
Epithelization, 79–83
Epitrichium, 2312
Erythroplasia of Queyrat, 2811, 2812, *2812, 2853, 2854,*
  2855, 2856
Eschar, burn, removal of, 492
Escharotomy, of burned hand, 3383
Esophagus. See also *Oropharyngoesophageal reconstruc-*
  tive surgery.
  bypassing or replacement of by flaps, 2708, *2708, 2709*
  reconstruction of, deltopectoral flap in, 2739, *2740*
Esser, J. F. S., 17, *20*
Esthetic surgery, definition of, 4
  for aging face, 1868–1929
Estlander operation, in lower lip defect, 1565, 1567,
  1567, 1568
  in upper lip defect, 1553–1556
Etheron sponges, 407
Ethmocephaly, 1179
  orbital hypotelorism in, 2462, *2463*
Ethmoid bone, 2431, *2432,* 2433
Ethmoid plate, 1047, *1047*
Ethmoid sinus, 777, 778
  cancer of, 2767, *2768*
  horizontal widening of, in orbital hypertelorism,
    2437, *2440*
  tumors of, craniofacial surgical techniques in, 2490
Ethrane, 587, 588
Ethyl chloride, 442, 443
Eversion technique, of nasal tip exposure, 1106, *1106*
Ewing's sarcoma, of jaws, 2567, *2568,* 2569, *2569*
Excision(s)
  diamond, *434*
  multiple curve, of scars, *434,* 435, *435*
  partial, multiple, in scar revision, 434
    repeated, 64
  split-thickness, in scar revision, 434, 435
  step, *434*
  tangential, in burns of hand, 3387, *3387,* 3388
Excision and closure, in scar revision, 434
Exophthalmos, 970–980, 2502, *2505, 2506*
  in Crouzon's disease and Apert's syndrome, 2471, *2471*
Exostosis, osteocartilaginous, of hand and forearm, 3499
Extensor carpi radialis, 2961, 2969
Extensor digiti minimi tendon, 278
Extensor digitorum brevis muscle, 297, *297,* 298
Extensor digitorum brevis muscle graft, in eyelid paraly-
  sis, 1841, *1841–1842*
Extensor digitorum longus muscle, flap of in leg defect,
  3557, 3558
Extensor digitorum longus tendons to second, third, and
  fourth toes, 277, *277,* 278
Extensor indicis tendon, 278
Extensor pollicis longus, 2969
Extensor tendon deformities, in hand, 3325, 3326, *3326*
External oblique muscle, 3728
Extraocular muscle imbalance, 1000, 1001
  in maxillary fractures, 708
Extraocular muscle injury, 1009
Extraocular muscles, 752, *753*
Extratemporal facial nerve, *1775, 1776,* 1777, 1778, *1778*
Extremity, lower, 3519–3605. See also *Foot* and *Thigh.*
  anatomical arrangement of lymphatic channels in,
    3572–3577
  arterial disease in, 3525, 2526

Extremity (*Continued*)
  lower, as donor site of flaps, 217
    bone cavities in, 3523
    circulatory disabilities in, 3523–3526
    congenital anomalies of, 3527–3529
    lymphatic disease in, 3526
    lymphatics of, 3572–3574, *3574–3577*
    osteomyelitis of, 3526, 3527, *3527*
    reconstructive surgery of, 3521–3566
      muscle flaps in, 3549–3560
      myocutaneous flaps in, 3560–3563
      problems in, 3522–3530
      procedures used in resurfacing cutaneous defects in, 3530–3565
      skin flaps in, 3531–3549
        axial pattern, 3540–3542, *3543*
        distant, 3534–3540
        local, 3533, *3533*, 3534, *3534–3536*
        microvascular free, 3542–3549
      skin grafting in, 3531, *3531, 3532*
      wound closure by primary approximation in, 3530, 3531
    transfer of tube flap to, 212, *212*
    trauma to, 3522, 3523
    tumors of, 3526
    venous stasis ulcers in, 3523–3525, *3525, 3532,* 3552, 3553
  upper, 2951–3518. See also *Hand, Forearm,* and *Arm.*
    anatomical arrangement of lymphatic channels in, 3578, *3578*
    as donor site of flaps, 215, *216,* 217
    burned, 3368–3402. See also *Hand, burns of.*
    dermolipectomy of, *3819,* 3820–3822
    injury to resulting in acute ischemia of hand, 3085–3089
    lymphedema of, *3585, 3585,* 3586, *3586*
Extremity deformities, in Apert's syndrome, 2322–2324, 2472, *2472*
  in Crouzon's disease, 2472, *2472*
  in Romberg's disease, 2339
Eye deformities, in Möbius syndrome, 2328, *2330*
Eye sockets, unusually large, prostheses in, 2943–2946
Eyebrow(s)
  burn deformities of, 1618–1620, *1621*
  deformities of, 956–961
  distortion of, 956, *956*
  drooping, correction of, 1921, 1922
  island flap reconstruction of, 219, *219*
  position of, 31, *34*
  ptosis of, and hooding of upper eyelids, *1879,* 1880
Eyelash grafting, 894, 895, *895*
Eyelashes, embryonic development of, 2312
Eyelet method of intermaxillary fixation, 649, *649*
Eyelid(s)
  anatomy of, 860–867, 1878
  avulsion of, 872–784
  burn involvement of, 1603, 1604, 1620–1635
  Caucasian vs. Oriental, 950t
  deformities of, 858–946
    in mandibulofacial dysostosis, treatment of, 2416–2419, *2420–2422*
    requiring esthetic blepharoplasty, classification of, 1878, *1879,* 1880
  embryonic development of, 2312
  general operative considerations in, 867–869
  lacerations of, 869–874
  lower, reconstruction of, 884–886, 891–895
    vertical shortening of, 791, 1001
  Oriental, surgical correction of, 947–956

Eyelid(s) (*Continued*)
  paralyzed, fascial strips in, 1822, *1823, 1824*
    ipsilateral temporalis muscle reinnervation of graft in, 1841, *1841,* 1842
    Silastic rod reconstruction of, 1838, 1839, *1839, 1840*
    treatment of, 1841–1844
  position of, 32, *35*
  reconstruction of, 881–902
    indications for, 891
    of full-thickness defects, 883
    of lateral segment of lids, 898, 899, *900*
    of lower lid, 884–886, 891–895
    of medial segments of lids, 899, 901, *901, 902*
    of upper lid, 886–891, 895–898
    postchemosurgery, 2893, 2894
  regional anesthesia of, 867
  sensory innervation of, 865–867
  skin and subcutaneous fascia of, 861, *861*
  tumors of, 874–882
    benign, 874–879
    malignant, 879–881
  upper, as donor site for full-thickness skin grafts, 164
    construction of supratarsal fold in correction of, 954, *954*
    hooding of caused by ptosis of eyebrows, *1879,* 1880
    ptosis of, 918–920, 920t, 1009, *1011*
      in Crouzon's disease and Apert's syndrome, 2472, *2479,* 2485
    reconstruction of, 886–891, 895–898
    retraction of in Graves' disease, 978–980
Eyelid folds, asymmetric, construction of supratarsal fold in correction of, 955
Eyelid suture, occlusive, 868, *869*
Eyes, too high-set, 31, *34*

Face
  abrasions of, 628, *629, 632*
  aging, 1869–1877
    esthetic surgery for, 1868–1929
      historical background of, 1868, 1869
      preoperative considerations in, 1877
  anthropometric points of, 27, 28, *28*
  avulsed wounds of, 635, 636, *639, 640*
  basal cell epithelioma of, *2821*
  contusions of, 628, 629, *629, 639*
  embryology of, 2117, *2118,* 2296–2358
  esthetic units of, *1581, 1607*
  full-face view of, 37, *40*
  gunshot wounds of, 10
  hard and soft tissues of, in jaw deformities, 1289–1292
  injuries to. See *Facial Injuries.*
  lacerations of, 628–632, *633–636, 639*
  lateral and profile views of, 613, *615*
  matching left and right profile views of, 37, *41*
  multiple small glass cuts of, 643
  normal, growth of, 1993–1995
  paralysis of. See *Facial palsy.*
  postnatal growth of, 814, 815, *815, 816*
  proportions of, 29–35, *36*
    according to Leonardo's square, *2926*
  reconstruction of through cross-face nerve transplantation in facial paralysis, 1848–1864
  regional entities of, 26, *26*
  repair of postchemosurgery defects of, 2889–2894
  sarcoma of, deltopectoral flap in repair of, *2750*
  short, 1460–1466
  soft tissue wounds of. See *Soft tissue wounds, facial.*

Face *(Continued)*
  submental view of, 37, *40*
  three-quarter anterior view of, 37, *41*
  traumatic injuries to, social and psychologic problems
      associated with, 565–573
Face lift operation, 1898–1926
  additional operative procedures in cervical area in,
      1919–1921
  additional operative procedures in submental area in,
      1914–1919
  anatomy in, 1899–1901
  combined with corrective blepharoplasty, 1912
  in male patient, 1913, *1913*
  no dressing, 1912, 1913
  postoperative complications of, 1922–1926
  preoperative examination in, 1898, 1899
  secondary, 1912
  technique of, 1901–1922
      subplatysma approach in, 1911, 1912
      supraplatysma approach in, 1901–1914
  upper, 1909, *1909, 1910,* 1911
Face mask, elasticized, in burn injury, 1606, *1607*
Facial artery, transverse, 1779
Facial asymmetry, congenital, transplantation of dermis
      in correction of, *243*
  neonatal, 1786
Facial bones
  embryonic development of, 2313
  fractures of, and multisystem injuries, 733, 734
      clinical management of, 599–747
      in children. See *Facial injuries, in children, involving
          fractures of facial bones.*
      midfacial, 805–808
      panfacial, 732–741
      planning of treatment in, 608–624
      roentgenographic evaluation of, 610–624
Facial burns, 1595–1642
  contraction in, 1596–1599
  due to lye, 1603
  electrical, 1596
  exposure technique in, 1602, 1603, *1603*
  hypertrophic scars in, 1599–1601
  reconstruction of, 1609–1618
  respiratory tract involvement in, 1601, 1602
  skin grafting in, 1605, *1606*, 1611, 1612
  treatment of, 1601–1638
      during acute period, 1601–1605
      during chronic period, 1605–1618
      on auricle, 1636
      on cheeks, 1636, *1637*
      on chin and perioral area, 1636–1638
      on eyebrows, 1618–1620, *1621*
      on eyelids, 1620–1635
      on forehead, 1618
      on nose, 1636, *1636, 1637*
      on scalp, 1618
  wound healing following, 1596–1601
Facial clefts, 2312
  formation of, theories of, 2117, 2119, *2119*
  median, classification of, 2128, 2128t, 2129
Facial deformities, in Apert's syndrome, 2324
  in Crouzon's disease, 2317
Facial growth, in cleft lip and palate. See *Cleft lip and
      palate, facial growth in.*
Facial hyperplasia, 1382, *1383*
Facial injuries
  anesthesia in, 626, 627, *627*
  classification of, 608, *609*, 610
  cleaning of wound in, 623, 625

Facial injuries *(Continued)*
  clinical examination in, 608–610
  clinical management of, 599–747
  control of hemorrhage in, 607, *607*, 608
  delayed primary wound closure in, 625
  emergency treatment of, 601–608
  general considerations in definitive treatment of, 624–
      627
  in children, 794–821
      anatomical considerations in, 794, 795
      emergency treatment of, 796
      involving fractures of facial bones, 796–814
          complications of, 808
          compound, multiple, and comminuted, 808–814
          incidence of, 796, 798
          mandibular, 798–805
          maxillary, 805, 806
          nasal skeletal and naso-orbital, 806, 807
          zygoma and orbital floor, 807, 808
      involving soft tissue, 795, 796
      prenatal and occurring at birth, 795
  in infants, 795
  instrumentation for treatment of, 626
  photography in, 625, 626
  planning of treatment in, 608–624
  preoperative considerations in, 626
  prevention and control of shock in, 608
  roentgenographic evaluation of, 610–624
  soft tissue. See *Soft tissue wounds, facial.*
  tetanus prophylaxis in, 624, 625
  timing of treatment of, 600, 601
  treatment of soft tissue wounds in, 625
Facial microsomia, 1676, *1677*
Facial muscles, 1780–1782
Facial nerve
  abnormal function of, following parotid tumor surgery,
      2538
  anomaly of, 1721, *1721*
  cross-face transplantation of, 1848–1864
  exposure of in parotid tumor surgery, *2533,* 2534,
      2534, 2535
  extratemporal, *1775, 1776, 1777, 1778, 1778*
  intratemporal, 1775, 1777
  main branches of with peripheral area of distribution,
      1849
  neurectomy of, 1827
  repair of, 813, 814
  surgery of, 1794–1840
      extratemporal, 1795
      intratemporal, 1794, 1795
      nonsuture technique in, 1795, 1796, *1796*
      suture technique in, 1796–1798
  surgical exposure of, 1778, 1779
  types of branching of, 1779, *1780*
  vascular supply of, 1779, 1780
Facial nerve grafts, 1798–1805
  approach in, 1798
  choice of grafting procedure in, 1799, 1800
  cross-face nerve transplantation in, 1805
  nerve crossing in, 1800–1805
  nerve rerouting in, 1800
  preoperative considerations in, 1798, *1799*
Facial pain, post-traumatic, 741–745
Facial palsy, 1774–1867, *2839*
  anatomy of, 1775–1783
  autogenous muscle grafts in reconstruction of, 1841–
      1848
  bilateral, 1786
  choice of corrective procedure in, 1830, 1831

Facial palsy *(Continued)*
  clinical examination in, 1785, 1786
  complications of reconstructive procedures in, 1831, 1832
  congenital, bilateral. See *Möbius syndrome.*
  correction of palpebral deformities and relief of epiphora in, 1832–1834
  cross-face nerve transplantation in, *1859*
  dermis transplants in, 1820
  diagnosis of, 1785–1787
    in acute trauma, 1786, 1787
  electrodiagnostic tests in, 1787–1794
  etiology of, 1784, 1785
  excision of redundant skin in, 1828–1830
  external mechanical support for, 1839, 1840
  fascia transplantation in, 262, 1820–1823
  fascicular nerve grafting in, 1797, 1798, *1798*
  following face lift operation, 1925, 1926
  following parotid tumor surgery, 2537
  history of, 1775
  in craniofacial microsomia, 2376, *2376*
  inorganic implants in, 1819, 1820
  lid magnets in, 1838
  location of lesion in, 1786
  muscle transfers in, 1806–1819
  ocular signs in, 1786
  operations for, 2536
  palpebral spring for lid palsy in, 1834, *1834*, 1835, *1835*
  paradoxical lacrimation in, 1840
  pathology of, 1783, *1783*, 1784
  reconstruction in, 1805–1830
    of face through cross-face nerve transplantation, 1848–1864
    of lax oral sphincter, 1823–1826
  removal of antagonistic muscle pull in, 1826–1828
  Silastic rod reconstruction of paralyzed eyelid in, 1838, 1839, *1839*, *1840*
  special procedures in, 1832–1839
  supranuclear, 1786
  surgical simulation of wrinkles in, 1832
  unusual residuals of, 1840
  upper lid loading in lagophthalmos of, 1835–1838
Facial skeleton
  anatomy of in cleft lip and palate, 1950–1965
  developmental malformations of, 814–819
  growth of, 823, 824, *824*
  multiple and complex fractures of, 732–741. See also *Facial bones, fractures of.*
Facial wrinkles, surgical simulation of, 1832
Faciostenoses, 2315–2327
Fan flap, 1549, *1549*, 1565, *1566*
Fanconi's anemia, radial ray deficiency in, 3334
Fasanella-Servat operation, 923–929
Fascia
  of hand, examination of, 2966, 2967, *2967*
  preserved, 263–265
  Scarpa's, 3728
  transplantation of, 262–265
    in abdominal wall, 3735, 3736, *3736*
    in facial palsy, 1820–1823
    in Romberg's disease, 2344, 2345
  transversalis, 3729
Fascia lata, 332
  technique of removal of, 263, 264, *264*, 265, 1820–1823
  tensile strength of, 263
Fascia-fat graft, *254*, *255*
Fascicular nerve grafting, 3231, 3232
  in facial palsy, 1797, 1798, *1798*
  microsurgical, 1797

Fasciculi, choice of in cross-face nerve transplantation
    in facial palsy, 1861, 1862
  tendon, 267, *268*
Fasciectomy, in Dupuytren's contracture, 3413, *3414*, 3419–3424
Fasciitis, nodular, pseudosarcomatous, of hand and forearm, 3475
Fasciotomy, in Dupuytren's contracture, 3413, 3419, *3419*
Fat, transplantation of, 251–261
  allografts, 254, *258*
  autografts, 252, 253
    management of, 256–261
  cell behavior in, 251, 252, *252–258*
  contraindications to, 255, 256
  in augmentation mammaplasty, 254, *259*
  in mandibular hypoplasia, 2423, *2423*
  in Romberg's disease, 254, *258*, 2344, *2344*
  indications for, 254, 255, *258*, *259*
Fat-dermal grafts. See *Graft, dermis-fat.*
Faucial region, squamous cell carcinoma of, *2680*, *2681*
  tumors of, forehead flap in, 2669–2671
Feminizing testicularism, 3954–3956, *3957*
Fernandez technique, of Oriental eyelid correction, 955, *955*, 956
Ferris Smith technique, in upper lip defect, 1552, 1553, *1554*
Fiberoptic headlight, 1064, *1064*
Fiberoptic nasal endoscope, 2270
Fibroblasts, 88
  contractile, 283
  in tendon, 271
Fibroepithelioma, premalignant, 2822
Fibroma, 2879
  ameloblastic, of jaws, 2552, *2552*, 2553
  of thorax, 3654
  soft, 2791, *2791*
Fibroma durum, 2790, *2790*, 2791
Fibroma simplex, 2790, *2790*, 2791
Fibromatosis, juvenile, 3475
  of hand and forearm, 3474–3478
Fibrosarcoma, 2840
  in scar, 415
  neurogenic, of chest wall, 3652, *3652*
  of hand and forearm, 3489
  of mandible, 2637, 2638, *2638*
Fibrosis, subepidermal, 2866, 2867
Fibrous dysplasia, *1481*
  craniofacial surgical techniques in, 2490, *2491*
  of jaws, 2557–2561
Fibrous xanthoma, of hand and forearm, 3472, *3472*
Fibula grafts, microvascular, 382–384
Filarial lymphangitis, 3585
Finger(s). See also *Digital.*
  avulsion injuries of, 3144, *3146*
  crooked, 3326, *3327*
  extension-abduction and flexion-adduction of, *2968*, 2970, *2970*
  joints of. See *Digital joints.*
  shortened, disorders resulting in, 3331–3333
  squamous cell carcinoma of, chemosurgery for, *2885*, 2886
  trigger, 3512
Finger transfer, in reconstruction of thumb, 3355–3363, *3364*, *3365*
Fingernails. See *Nails, of hand.*
Fingertip amputations, 3144, *3145*
First and second branchial arch syndrome. See *Craniofacial microsomia.*
First and second branchial arches, structures derived from, 2369t

Fistula(s)
  arteriovenous, of hand, *3483*
  auricular, 2877
  branchial. See *Branchial cysts and fistulas.*
  cervical-aural, 2913, 2914, *2914*
  chylous, 2752
  following intraoral tumor surgery, 2687, 2688
  oronasal, in cleft palate, 2198–2201
  skin, 2876–2878
  thyroglossal duct, 2877, *2877*, 2905–2908
  tracheoesophageal, 2239
Fixation
  in mandibular reconstruction, methods of, 1474–1481
  in maxillofacial prosthetics, 2919–2921
  intermaxillary, 648–652, 701, *701*
  interosseous, in orbital hypertelorism, 2453, *2453*
Fixation appliances, buried, inert, in maxillofacial
      prosthetics, 2921
  in correction of jaw deformities, 1300, 1301, *1301, 1302*
  skeletal, external, biphase, *1476*, 1477, *1477–1480*
Flap(s)
  Abbé, 219, 1558, *1558*, 2167, 2169, *2170*
    in bilateral cleft lip repair, 2086, *2086*
    in cleft palate repair, 2195, *2195, 2196*
    in defects of vermilion border, 1575, 1576, *1576*
    in upper lip defects, 1549–1552
  abdominal, for nasal reconstruction, 1267, *1267,*
      1268, *1268*
    in elbow repair, *214*
    jump, in scalp defects, 837, *838, 839*
    tube, *210*, 3909–3913
      in reconstruction of penis, 3909, 3911, 3912,
        3912, 3913
  acromiocervical, in contractures of cervical region,
      1654
  acromiopectoral, in contractures of cervical region, *1655*
    for nasal reconstruction, 1267
  advancement, 4, *4*, 202–205
    bilateral, to close median defect of forehead, 1230,
      1230
    bipedicle, 205, *206*
    cheek, 1197, *1198*
    in reconstruction of helical rim, 1740, *1741*
    in upper lip defect, 1545, *1546*
    lateral, in eyelid reconstruction, 885, *885*
    mucosal, prolabial, 2172, *2172*
    of vermilion, muscle, and mucosa, in reconstruction
      of oral commissure, *1589*
    1–2, 204, *205, 1198*
      in burn scars, 1612, 1614, *1615, 1616*
      in repair of lower lip defect, 1563, *1563*
    orbicularis muscle, in reconstructed lower lip, 1577,
      1578, *1578*
    V-Y, 205, *206, 1564*, 1565, *1565*
      in pressure sores, 3781
      to prevent vermilion notching, 2174, *2176*
  arm, in nose repair, 5, 6
  arterial, 194, *194*, 217
  artery island, in eyebrow reconstruction, 959, *961, 962*
  axial pattern, 194, 217–223
    closure of abdominal wall defect with, *3732*
    definition of, 191
    in lower extremity, 3540–3542, *3543*
  bi-lobed, in repair of cheek defects, 1583, *1586*
    of Zimany, 206, *208*
  bipedicle, advancement, 205, *206*
    for elliptical defects, *3533*, 3534, *3534*
    in pressure sores, 3781, *3781*
    in repair of lower lip defect, *1562*, 1563
    mucosal, 1576, *1577*

Flap(s) *(Continued)*
  bipedicle, scalp, 1501, *1502*
    tongue, 2702, 2703, *2704*
    Tripier, in eyelid reconstruction, 885, *887,* 888
  brachial, Tagliacotian, 1199
    for nasal reconstruction, 1266, 1267, *1267*
  breast, in chest wall reconstruction, 3615–3617, *3618*
  bridge, Cutler-Beard, 895–898
    in lip defect, *1557*
  cervical, apron, for oropharyngeal lining, 2722, 2723,
      2723
    compound, for palatal reconstruction, 2723–2730
    in cheek defect, 1582, *1585*
    in columellar defect, 1269, 1270, *1270*
    in lower lip defect, 1562, *1562*
    in nasal reconstruction, 1267
    in oropharyngoesophageal reconstructive surgery,
      2717–2731
    in postchemosurgery defect of perioral region, *2893*
    visor-type, in mandibular tumor surgery, 2616, *2617*
  cervicofacial, in repair of cheek defect, *1592*, 1593
  cheek, advancement, 1197, *1198*
    in maxillary reconstruction, *1510*
    in upper lip defect, 1545, *1546*, 1552, *1553*
  closed carried, in chest wall reconstruction, 3617,
      3620, 3621
  composite, 223
    in mandibular reconstruction, 1503
  conjunctival, in correction of symblepharon, 916, *917*
  coronal, for exposure in malunited naso-orbital frac-
      tures, 1020
  cross-arm, 215, *216*, 217
  cross-finger, *3025, 3026, 3027, 3027–3029*
  cross-leg, 3534–3538, *3548*
  cutaneous, 194, *194*
  de-epithelized, buried, 254
    in reconstruction of abdominal wall, 3736, *3737*
  deltopectoral, 217, 218, *218*
    in burns of hand, 2747, *2747*
    in chest wall reconstruction, *3614*
    in intraoral tumor surgery, 2647, *2648*, 2649, *2649*
      design of flap in, 2674, *2675*, 2676
      division of flap and completion of insetting in,
        2681, 2682
      management of bridge segment in, 2679
      principle of, 2673, 2674, *2675*
      role of compared with forehead flap, 2684, 2685
      secondary defect in, 2681
      suture inside mouth in, 2679, *2681*
      transfer of to mouth, 2676–2679
    in laryngopharynx, 2735–2739
    in nasal reconstruction, 1267, 2746, 2747
    in oropharyngoesophageal reconstructive surgery,
      2731–2747, *2748–2750*
      external and two-layer reconstructions with, *2745,*
        2746, 2747, 2747–2750
    in oropharynx and mouth, 2739–2743, *2744, 2745*
    in soft tissue defects of mandible, 1500, *1500*
    in upper lip defect, *2748*
    microvascular, 377
  dermal, in treatment of lymphedema, 3597, *3600,* 3601,
      3601
  dermis-fat, 261
    free, in Romberg's disease, 2348
    in augmentation mammaplasty, 3690, 3691, *3692–*
      3694
    in pressure sores, *3788*
  distant, 212–217
    definition of, 191
    in acute hand injuries, 3035–3041

Flap(s) *(Continued)*
  distant, in breast after radical mastectomy, 3715, *3715,*
    3716
    in chest wall reconstruction, 3614–3617
    in cutaneous defects of nose, 1199
    in lower extremity, 3534–3540
    in postchemosurgery defects of face, 2891
    in skin cancer surgery, 2832
    in upper lip defects, 1546, *1547*
  dorsal, in chest wall reconstruction, *3613*
  dorsalis pedis, 219, 3540–3542, *3543*
    microvascular, 377, 378
  double, in head and neck surgery, 2624, *2624–2630*
    pendulum, in cleft lip repair, 2174, *2176*
    rotation, in pressure sores, 3781, *3781, 3790*
  eave, in auricular reconstruction, 1703, *1704,* 1740,
    1742
  Estlander, 1553–1556, 1565, 1567, *1567, 1568*
  fan, in lower lip defect, 1565, *1566*
    in upper lip defect, 1549, *1549*
  forehead, 217, *217*
    evolution of, 1210–1214
    Gillies up-and-down, *1213,* 1226
    in burned nose, *1637*
    in cheek defect, 1556, *1557, 1588, 1592,* 1593
    in columellar defect, 1270, *1270,* 1271, *1271, 1272*
    in cutaneous defects of nose, 1199
    in defects of buccal mucosa, 2671–2673
    in defects of faucial region, posterior third of tongue,
      and pharyngeal wall, 2669–2671
    in defects of side of tongue, lower alveolus, and floor
      of mouth, 2668, 2669, *2669*
    in defects of symphyseal region, 2673
    in ectropion of lower eyelid, 911, *912, 913*
    in head and neck surgery, 2626, 2631–2636
    in intraoral tumor surgery, 2647, *2647,* 2649,
      2657–2673
      basic technique of, 2662–2667
      principle of, 2657–2662
      prior delay and carotid ligation in, 2667
      role of compared with deltopectoral flap, 2684,
        2685
      tunnel in, *2663,* 2664, *2665, 2665,* 2667, 2668
      variations in technique of, 2667, 2668
      width of pedicle in, 2667
    in lip defect, 1556, *1557*
    in nasal reconstruction, 1226–1234
      complications of, 1264, 1266
      consecutive or combined use of scalping and median
        flaps in, 1245, 1246
    in oropharyngoesophageal reconstructive surgery,
      2716, 2716, 2717, *2717, 2718*
    in skin cancer surgery, *2832, 2833*
    island, clinical applications of, 1233, 1234, *1234,*
      1235
      in full-thickness dorsal nasal defects, *1252,* 1253,
        1253, 1254
      in nasal reconstruction, *1262*
      with subcutaneous tissue pedicle, for nasal
        reconstruction, 1231–1233
    median, 1199, *1213,* 1226, 1228–1231, *1241*
      clinical applications of, 1233, 1234, *1234, 1235*
      for relining nose, 1206, *1207, 1208*
      gull-shaped, 1256, *1257,* 1258, *1258,* 1259, *1259*
      in lateral nasal wall defects, 1250, *1250,* 1251,
        1251
      variations of, 1230, 1231
    oblique, *1213,* 1226, 1239, *1240,* 1241
    scalping, 1023, 1024, *1024, 1025,* 1199, *1213,* 1226,
      1234–1263

Flap(s) *(Continued)*
  forehead, sickle, 1226, *1227*
    adequate length in, 1239, *1239, 1240,* 1241
    avoiding tension in, 1241
    care of temporary scalp defect in, 1242, 1243
    establishing one-piece continuity in, 1241, 1242,
      1242
    in eyebrow reconstruction, 959, 961
    in foreshortened nose due to burns, *1280*
    in subtotal nasal reconstruction, 1244–1256
      following chemosurgical treatment, 1251, *1252*
      following extensive radiation, 1254, *1254,* 1255
      of full-thickness dorsal defects, *1252,* 1253,
        1253, 1254
      of large unilateral alar and lateral wall defects,
        1246–1250
      of lateral nasal wall defects, 1250, *1250,* 1251,
        1251
      "retouching" procedures in, 1255, *1255,* 1256,
        1256
    planning and design of, 1237, *1237*
    preliminary rhinoplastic reduction in, 1237, *1237*
    providing base for new nose in, 1241, *1241*
    repair of permanent forehead defect in, 1242
    return of pedicle in, 1243, *1243,* 1244
    technique of, 1237–1239
  supraorbital, horizontal, *1213,* 1223
  use of in different tumor sites, 2668–2673
  free, in pressure sores, 3781, 3782
    microvascular. See *Flap, microvascular free.*
  from opposite eyebrow, in eyebrow reconstruction,
    958, 959, *959*
  full-thickness, rectangular, in lip defect, 1558, *1558*
  groin, 218, *218*
    microvascular, *373, 374, 374, 376, 377*
  hinge, 200, 201, *201,* 1223, *1223, 1244*
  hypogastric, 218, *218*
  in acute hand injuries. See *Hand injuries, acute,*
    flaps in.
  in head and neck surgery, 2624–2636
  in mandibular tumor surgery, 2631, *2632, 2633,* 2634,
    2634
  in oromandibular tumors, 2624–2636
  Indian, *1213*
  island, 194, *194,* 195, 217, 219, *219,* 1199. See also
    Flap, forehead, island.
    arterial pedicle, in repair of cheek defect, 1582,
      1583, *1585*
    artery, in eybrow reconstruction, 959, *961, 962*
    in eyelid reconstruction, 882, *882*
    Millard, 2273, 2277
    neurovascular, 219, *219*
      in pressure sores, 3781, 3782
    with subcutaneous pedicle, 4, *4*
  island leg, for multiple pressure sores, 3796, *3796*
  jump, abdominal, in scalp defects, 837, *838, 839*
    in cheek defect, 1584, 1587, *1587*
    in chest wall reconstruction, 3617, *3620, 3621*
    in lower extremity, 3539, *3539,* 3540
  Langenbeck, *2200,* 2201, *2201*
  lip, Stein-Abbé, 223
  local, definition of, 191
    in acute hand injuries, 3027–3035
    in breast after radical mastectomy, *3712,* 3713, *3713,*
      3714
    in burn contractures, 1610, 1611
    in cheek defect, 1580–1582, *1583–1585*
    in chest wall reconstruction, 3611, *3613,* 3614, *3614*
    in cutaneous defects of nose, 1196, 1197, *1197, 1198*
    in Dupuytren's contracture, 3417, *3417*

Flap(s) *(Continued)*
  local, in knee, 3534, *3534*
    in lower extremity, 3533, *3533*, 3534, *3534–3536*
    in postchemosurgery defects of face, 2891
    in Romberg's disease, 2345–2348
    in scalp defects, 833, *835*
    in skin cancer surgery, 2831, *2832–2837*
    in upper lip defects, 1545, *1545*, 1546, *1546*, *1547*
  microvascular free, 54, 195, 222, 223, 372–379
    advantages of, 374, 375
    definition of, 191
    disadvantages of, 375
    donor site for, 376–378
    groin, *373*, 374, *374*, 376, *377*
      in contracture of cervical region, 1654, *1658*
    history of, 372, 373
    in lower extremity, 3542–3549
    in mandibular reconstruction, 1503
    indications for, 373, 374
    operative technique in, 378, 379
    postoperative management in, 379
    preoperative evaluation in, 375–378
  Millard island, 2273, 2277
  mucoperiosteal, 2199, *2199*, *2200*
  mucosal, bipedicle, 1576, *1577*
  mucosal apron, 1576, *1576*
  muscle, 299
    causes of necrosis in, 3560
    in anterior aspect of leg, *3557*, 3558
    in chest wall reconstruction, *3623–3625*
    in hip, 3549, 3550, *3550*, *3551*
    in knee, 3550, *3551*, *3552*
    in leg, 3550–3558
    in lower extremity, 3549–3560
      technique of, 3549
    in lower lateral third of leg, 3557, *3557*, 3558
    in lower part of lateral leg and ankle joint, 3558
    in pressure sore, *3788*, *3791*
    in sole of foot, 3558, *3558*, *3559*
    in trochanteric defect, 3549, 3550, *3550*, *3551*
  muscle-rib, in chest wall reconstruction, *3626*
  musculofascial, in reconstruction of abdominal wall,
      3732–3735
  myocutaneous, 219, *220*, *221*, 222
    gracilis, vaginal reconstruction by, 3926–3929
    in reconstruction of lower extremity, 3560–3563
  nasolabial, *1025*, 1026, 1197, *1197*
    in floor of mouth, 2683
    for relining nose, 1205, *1205*, 1206, *1206*, 1258, *1259*
    in columellar defect, *1270*, 1271
    in complete loss of lower lip, 1570, *1570*, *1571*
    in cutaneous defects of skin of nose, 1197, *1197*
    in full-thickness defects of lower portion of nose,
      1218–1220
    in intraoral tumor surgery, 2649, 2650, *2650*,
      2682–2684
    in lower lip defect, *1560*, 1561, 1569, *1569*
    in upper lip defect, 1545, *1545*, 1552, *1552*
  neck, horizontal, in oropharyngoesophageal
      reconstructive surgery, 2719–2723
    MacFee, 2679, *2680*, 2682
  omental, in chest wall reconstruction, 3614, 3615, *3615*
    transposition of in lymphedema, 3593
  osteoperiosteal, 2423, *2423*
  "over and out," in repair of cheek defect, *1589*, 1590,
    1590
  overlapping of, 223
  pectoral muscle, *3624*, *3625*
  pedicle, in burns of hand, 3375, *3375*, 3376, *3376*

Flap(s) *(Continued)*
    pedicle, in scalp defects, 833, *834*
    tube, in thumb reconstruction, 3365, *3366*, 3367
  pendulum, double, in cleft lip repair, 2174, *2176*
  periosteal, in chest wall reconstruction, *3627*
  pharyngeal, and maxillary advancement procedures,
      1452
    in cleft palate repair, 2274, *2275*, 2278, 2279
    primary, and palatoplasty, in cleft palate repair,
      2096–2102
  postauricular, in cheek defect, 1581, *1582*, 1584
    in helical reconstruction, 1739, *1739*
  preauricular, in cheek defect, 1581, *1582*
  quadrilateral, in upper lip defect, 1548, *1548*
  random pattern, 194, 202–217
    advancement. See *Flap, advancement.*
    direct, from a distance, 212–217
    rotation. See *Flap, rotation.*
    transposition. See *Flap, transposition.*
    tube. See *Flap, tube.*
  rectangular, in cheek defect, 1581, *1584*
    in cleft lip repair, 2018, 2019, 2027, *2027*, 2028, 2032,
      2033, 2037, 2038, *2038*, *2039*
  rotation, 206, 208, *208*
    delayed, in cheek defect, *1592*, 1593
    double, in pressure sores, 3781, *3781*, *3790*
    in acute hand injuries, 3034, 3035, *3036*
    in cheek defect, 1581, *1583*
    in chin soft tissue defect, 1500, *1501*
    in decubitus ulcer, scar in, 421, 422, *422*
    in eyelid reconstruction, 884–891
    in lower lip, 1500, *1501*, 1565, *1565*
    in median defect of forehead, 1230, *1231*
    in radiation ulcer, 544, 545, *545*
    in scalp defects, 828, *829*
    lateral, in lower lip defect, 1569, *1570*
  sandwich, of Moore and Chong, 2273, 2277
  scalp, 825, *826*, *830*, 834–838
    bifrontal (coronal), 845, *848*
      exposure of midface skeleton through, 1427
    bipedicle, in reconstruction of soft tissue defects of
      mandible, 1501, *1502*
    in burn deformity of eyebrows, 1619, 1620, *1620*,
      1621
    in eyebrow reconstruction, 959, *960–962*
    in treatment of baldness, 231, *231*
  septal, in repair of full-thickness defects of lower portion
      of nose, 1215, 1218, *1218*
  shoulder-back, in contractures of cervical region, *1656*
  sickle, in upper lip defect, *1547*
  skin, 152–239. See also general entries under *Flap.*
    age of patient and, 200
    classification of, 193–195
    definition of, 156
    delay of, 99, 196–198
    design of, 199, *199*
    direct, from a distance, 212–217
    division and insetting of, 201, 202
    failure in transfer of, 225, 226
    following resection of intraoral tumors, 2644–2650
    in burn contractures, 1612–1614
    in contractures of cervical region, 1652–1654,
      1654–1657
    in lower extremity, 3531–3549
    in oropharyngoesophageal reconstructive surgery,
      2715–2747, 2748–2750
    location of, 199, 200
    mechanical factors in, 200, *200*
    of marginal viability, salvaging of, 202

Flap(s) *(Continued)*
  skin, overgrafting of, 223
    overlapping of, 223
    principles of surgery involving, 199–202
    reinnervation of, 226–229
    sebaceous gland function in, 229
    suitability of, 223, 224
    sweat gland function in, 228
    tests of circulation of, 195, 196
    transfer of from a distance, 200, 201, *201*
    types of, 202–223
    vascular anatomy of, 191–193
    vascular augmentation or enhancement of survival of, 198
  sling, in auricular reconstruction, 1749, *1750*
  split-rib, in chest wall reconstruction, *3626*
  Stein-Kazanjian, in complete loss of lower lip, *1572,* 1573
  sternomastoid, in intraoral tumor surgery, 2645, *2646,* 2647
  subcutaneous, rotated, in reconstruction of philtrum, *2171*
  submandibular apron, in intraoral tumor surgery, 2645, *2646*
  supporting, in reconstruction of lower lip, 1559, *1560*
  "switch," of lower eyelid, in repair of upper lid defects, *889, 890, 890, 891, 892*
  tarsoconjunctival, 882, 891–902
    in mandibulofacial dysostosis, *2416,* 2419, *2420–2422*
    in severe burn ectropion, 1631, 1632, *1632–1635*
  temporal. See *Flap, forehead.*
  thenar, *216,* 217, 3027–3033
  thoracoabdominal tube, in chest wall reconstruction, 3617, *3619*
  thoracobrachial, 215, *215*
  thoracoepigastric (axilloabdominal), in contractures of cervical region, *1656*
  tongue, 1576, *1578*
    dorsal, anteriorly based, 2702, *2704*
      posteriorly based, 2701, 2702, *2702, 2703*
    in angle of mouth, *2674*
    in cleft palate repair, 2201
    in intraoral tumor surgery, 2645, *2645*
    in oropharyngoesophageal reconstructive surgery, 2700–2705
    tip-derived, 2703, 2705, *2705*
    transverse, bipedicle, 2702, 2703, *2704*
    ventral, 2705, *2706*
  total thigh, for multiple pressure sores, *3794*
  transabdominal, in contractures of cervical region, *1657*
  transposition, 205, 206, *207, 208*
    in acute hand injuries, 3034, 3035, *3036*
    in cheek defect, 1580, *1581, 1582, 1583*
    in chest wall reconstruction, *3613*
    in postchemosurgery defects of face, 2891, *2892, 2893*
    in upper lip defect, 1545, *1545, 1546, 1547*
  trapdoor, 1023, *1024, 1025, 1501*
    Z-plasty and W-plasty in repair of depressed scars of, 64
  triangular, in cleft lip repair, 2019, *2028,* 2038, 2039, *2040,* 2041, *2041,* 2043
  Tripier, bipedicle, in eyelid reconstruction, 885, *887,* 888
  tube, 14, 208–212
    abdominal, *210*
    elongation of tube in, 210, *210*
      in reconstruction of penis, 3909, 3911, 3912, *3912, 3913*
      in auricular reconstruction, 1739, *1739,* 1740, *1740, 1741*

Flap(s) *(Continued)*
  tube, in cheek defect, 1583, 1584, *1586, 1588*
    in lower extremity, 3538, *3538,* 3539, *3548*
    in pressure sores, 3780, 3781
    in Romberg's disease, 2345–2348
    in scalp defects, 837, *839*
    mucous membrane, 1576, *1576*
    pedicle, in thumb reconstruction, 3365, *3366,* 3367
    scapular, *211*
    thoracoabdominal, in chest wall reconstruction, 3617, *3619*
    transfer of, 210–212
    varieties of, 210, *210*
  tumbler, in pressure sores, 3781
  Zimany, 206, *208*
Flexor carpi radialis, 2961, 2969
Flexor digitorum longus muscle, mobilization of for flap, 3556
Flexor digitorum profundus, 2961, 2962
Flexor digitorum profundus tendon, division of distal to insertion of superficialis, 3073, 3075, *3076*
Flexor digitorum superficialis tendon, 278
Flexor hallucis longus muscle, mobilization of for flap, 3557
Flexor pollicis longus, 2962
Flexor pollicis longus tendon, injuries of, 3075, 3077, *3077*
Flexor tendon, composite allografts of, 287, 288
Flexor tendon grafts, 3193–3206
Flexor tendon injuries, elastic finger traction in, *2992,* 2994
Fluorescein dye tests, of flap circulation, 195
5-Fluorouracil (5FU), in treatment of skin cancer, 2803, 2804, *2804,* 2839
Fluothane, 587
Flying wing operation, 1138, *1139,* 1140
Fold of Douglas, 3729
Folic acid antagonists, and immunosuppression, 138
Follicular ameloblastoma, of jaws, 2550, *2551*
Follicular keratosis, inverted, of eyelids, 878
Fong's disease, 2980
Foot. See also *Extremity, lower.*
  dorsum of, anatomy of, *3541*
  immersion, 517
  muscle flap in defects of sole of, 3558, *3558, 3559*
Foot deformity, in Apert's syndrome, 2323, *2323*
Foot ulcers, 3792
Foramen cecum, 2904, *2905*
Forced duction test, 762, 763, *763*
Forceps, disimpaction, for maxillary fractures, 702, *705*
  for reduction of nasal fractures, 727, *727, 728*
Forearm. See also *Extremity, upper.*
  nerve injuries in, 3206–3212
  tendon injuries in, 3063, 3064, 3069, *3069,* 3070, 3206–3212
  tumors of. See *Hand and forearm, tumors of.*
Forehead, blood supply of, 1227, *1227*
  burn deformities of, 1618
  deformities of, 822–857
Forehead advancement, in correction of bilateral coronal synostosis, 2495, 2497, *2497, 2498*
Forehead flap. See *Flap, forehead.*
Forehead wrinkles, correction of, 1921
Forward traction test, 997, *998*
Fossa, glenoid, 1521
Four-flap technique of cleft palate repair, 2095, 2096, *2096, 2097*
Four-flap technique of Mustardé for correction of epicanthus, *940,* 941, *943*
Fovea radialis, 2969

Fracture(s)
  alveolar, 697, 700, *701*
    in children, 800, *802*, 805
  Bennett's, 3048, *3048*, 3049, *3049*
  blowout, of orbital floor. See *Orbit, floor of, blowout fractures of.*
  Colles', 3407, *3407*
  comminuted, 655, 676–679
    of nasal bones, 730, 731, *731, 732*
    of orbital floor, 775, 776
    of zygoma, 715–719
  complex, 655
  compound, 654, 655
    of limbs, timing of skin replacement in, 225
    of nasal bones, 731
  compound comminuted, of edentulous mandible, 691, 692
    of zygoma, 719, *720*
  condylar, in children, 802–805
  depressed, 655
  greenstick, 655, 796, 798
  Guérin's, 697, *697*
  impacted, 655
  Le Fort, 697, *697*, 698
  malunited, depressed, of zygoma, 1029–1031
    of nasal bones, 1130, 1131, *1131*
    orbital and naso-orbital, 989–1033
  nasal skeletal. See *Nasal bones and cartilages, fractures of.*
  naso-orbital. See *Naso-orbital fractures.*
  of condyle. See *Mandible, condylar process of, fractures of.*
  of facial bones. See *Facial bones, fractures of.*
  of hand. See *Hand, fractures and dislocations of.*
  of jaws. See *Jaws, fractures of.*
  of mandible. See *Mandible, fractures of.*
  of maxilla. See *Maxilla, fractures of.*
  of nasal bone graft, 1150
  of nasal bones and cartilages. See *Nasal bones and cartilages, fractures of.*
  of nasal septal framework, 725, *725*, 728–731
  of temporomandibular joint, 802–805
  of thumb, 3048, *3048, 3049*
  of tibia, 3527, *3527*
  of zygoma. See *Zygoma, fractures of.*
  orbital. See *Orbit, fractures of.*
  panfacial, 732–741
  simple, 654
  subcondylar, compound comminuted, 687
  supraorbital and glabellar, involving frontal sinus, 785, 788, 789
Fracture-dislocation, orbital, malunited, 1031, *1032*
Franceschetti-Zwahlen-Klein syndrome. See *Mandibulofacial dysostosis.*
Frankfort horizontal, 28, *28*, 1289, *1290*
Freckle(s), 2797
  melanotic, of eyelids, 878
Freeze-dried fascia, 263
Freezing, of skin, 181, 182
  of tendon, 285
Frenulum, 3832, *3833*
Freon, 443, 446
Frey syndrome, following parotid tumor surgery, 2538
Frohse, syndrome arcade of, 3446
Frontal bar, 2447, *2448*
Frontal bone. See *Bone, frontal.*
Frontal nerve, 866, *867*
Frontal sinus, 777, *778*
  fractures involving, 785, 788, 789
  in frontal bone defects, 848, 849, *851, 852, 853*

Frontalis muscle, 1782
  reanimation of, 1818
Frontalis suspension for blepharoptosis, 931, 936–940
Fronto-ethmoid area, tumors of, craniofacial surgery in, 2490
Frontonasal dysplasia, 2129
Frontonasal process, 2304
Frontonasal prominence, 2303
Fronto-occipital anteroposterior projection, 611, 612, *612*
Frostbite, 517, 519, *519*
Frown lines, glabellar, correction of, 1921
Fuchs position, 613, *615*
Funicular suture techniques, in nerves of hand, 3222
Fusion operation, in arthritic hand, 3508, 3510, 3511, *3511*

G-banding, 111, *111, 114*
Galactosemia, 119
Galea aponeurotica, 822, *822*
Galen, 261
Galvanic tongue stimulation, in facial palsy, 1787, 1788
Gamma rays, 532
Ganglion, of hand and forearm, 3469, 3470, *3470*
Gangrene, gas, of abdominal wall, 3739–3741
Gastric tube technique, reversed, 2707, *2708*
Gastrocnemius muscle, mobilization of for flap, 3553, 3554, *3554*
Gastrocnemius myocutaneous flap, 3563, *3563, 3564*
Gastrointestinal tract, transplantation of in oropharyngo-esophageal reconstructive surgery, 2707–2712
Gastroschisis, 3741–3747
  closure of abdominal wall in, 3746, 3747
  embryology of, 3741, 3743, *3743*
  preoperative management of, 3743, 3744
  surgical correction of, 3744–3746
Gene(s), 139
  and antigens, 140–147
  nature of, 115–117
Genetic counseling, 118–122
  amniocentesis and, 121
  medical ethics and law and, 121, 122
Genetics, basic, 139, 140, 140t
  histocompatibility, 129–131
  of transplantation, 139–147
Genioglossus muscle, 660, *661*
Geniohyoid muscle, 660, *661*
Genital folds, 3831, *3831*, 3832
Genital reconstruction, in transsexual, *3964*
Genital ridge, 3832
Genital swellings, 3831, *3831*, 3832
Genital tract anomalies, embryology of, 3831–3834
Genital tubercle, *3828, 3829*, 3831, *3831, 3832*
Genitalia, developmental anatomy of, 3936, 3937
  female, external, abnormalities of, 3922–3929
    historical aspects of, 3922, 3923
    operative technique in, 3923–3925
    pathogenesis of, 3923
    therapy of, 3923
    reconstruction of, 3925
  male, construction of in true hermaphroditism, 3944, *3946–3950*
    injuries to, 3902–3909
      complications in, 3908, 3909
      diagnosis of, 3904
      historical aspects of, 3903, 3904
      mechanism and etiology of, 3902, 3903, *3903*
      skin grafting in, 3905, *3905*, 3906
      treatment of, 3904–3908
    reconstruction of, 3902–3921

Genitourinary system, 3825–3969
embryology of, 3827–3834
Georgiade's external traction apparatus, 1372, *1372*
Georgiade's intraoral traction, 2053, *2053*, 2054
Germinal ridge, 3832
Giant cell reparative granuloma, of jaws, 2561, *2561, 2562, 2563*
Giant cell tumor, of bone, of hand and forearm, 3499, 3500
of tendon sheath of hand, 3472, *3472*, 3473, *3473, 3474*
Gigantomastia, operation for, 3676, 3684, *3685–3688*
Gillies, Harold Delf, 4, 10, 13, 14, 20, *20*
Gillies up-and-down flap, *1213*, 1226
Gilmer technique of intermaxillary fixation, 648, 649, *649*
Gingival incision, in mandibular malformations, 1307, *1307*, 1308
Glabellar fractures, 785, 788, *788*, 789
Glabellar frown lines, correction of, 1921
Glands
meibomian, 861
parathyroid, 2904, *2904*
parotid. See *Parotid gland.*
salivary. See *Salivary glands.*
sebaceous, *153*, 154, 155
submandibular, tumors of, 2538, 2539
sweat (eccrine and apocrine). See *Sweat glands.*
tarsal (meibomian), 861
thymus, 2904, *2904*, 2905
thyroid, 2904, *2904*
Glaucoma, closed angle, acute, following esthetic
blepharoplasty, 1897
Glenoid fossa, 1521
Glioma, nasal, 1169, 1170, *1170*, 1171, *1171*, 1173
orbital hypertelorism secondary to, *2459*
Globes, burn involvement of, 1603, 1604
Globulomaxillary cyst, 2564, 2565, *2565*
Glomus tumor, 2796, *2796*, 2869
of hand and forearm, 3485, *3485*, 3486, *3486, 3487*
Glossectomy, total, for cancer of tongue, tonsil, or floor
of mouth, 2612, *2612*
Glucose-6-phosphate dehydrogenase, 120
Gluteus maximus muscle flap, in pressure sore, *3791*
Glycosaminoglycans, 270
Gnathion, 28, 1289, *1290*
Gold implants, 392
Goldenhar's syndrome, 2121, 2360, 2408, *2408, 2409*
Gonadal sex, 3934–3936, *3937*
Gout, soft tissue deposits in hands in, 3478, *3479*
Gouty arthritis, of hand, 3511, *3511*
Gracilis myocutaneous flap, 3562, *3562*
vaginal reconstruction by, 3926–3929
Graft(s)
auricular, composite, 1269, *1270*, 1727, *1728*
elongation of foreshortened nose by, 1279, 1280, *1281*
for alar defects, 1220–1225
for pinched tip deformity, 1157
in repair of nasal defect, *640*
bone. See also *Bone, transplantation of.*
associated with elongation osteotomy, 1362, 1365, *1365*
cantilever, to provide nasal skeletal framework, 1259, *1260, 1261*
wired to nasal bones, 1143, 1144, *1144, 1145*
effect of on facial growth in cleft lip and palate, 2011
following mandibular resection, 2692–2694
iliac. See *Iliac bone graft.*
in bilateral cleft lip repair, 2067
in blowout fractures of orbital floor, 770, 772, *772*
in cleft palate patient, 2205–2210

Graft(s) *(Continued)*
bone, in conjunction with horizontal advancement
osteotomy of lower portion of mandible, 1394, *1394*, 1395
in conjunction with osteotomy and septal framework
resection, 1148, 1149
in cranial defects, conditions for success in, 841–845
in malunited fractures of zygoma, 1029–1031
in mandibular hypoplasia, 2423, *2423*
in mandibular reconstruction, 1473, 1474, 1480, *1480*, 1481, *1481*, 1482, 1485–1491, 2616–2618
associated with soft tissue loss, 1502
in mandibular tumors, 2616–2618
in maxillary reconstruction, *1510–1513*
in microgenia, 1385–1387
in naso-orbital fractures, 1012–1020
in naso-orbito-maxillary osteotomy, 1458, *1458, 1459, 1460*
in orbital fractures, 996, *996*, 997
in orbital hypertelorism, 2453, *2453*, 2454, 2455
in palatal and alveolar defects, 2201
in Romberg's disease, 2342, 2343, *2343*
in thumb reconstruction, 3365, *3366*, 3367
microvascular free, 379–384
in mandibular reconstruction, 1503
nasal, complications following, 1148–1150
fracture of, 1150
in children, 1145
multiple, 1145
with columellar strut, 1144, 1145
onlay, in treatment of maxillary micrognathia, 1441, *1441*, 1442, *1442*
primary, in mandibular reconstruction, 1483–1497
in naso-orbital fractures, 785, *786   787*
in panfacial fractures, 739–741, *742, 743*
secondary, after orthodontic treatment for cleft lip
and palate, 2231, *2231*
tibial, 326, 327, *327*
cartilage. See also *Cartilage, transplantation of.*
costal, for nasal contour restoration, 1147, 1148, *1148*
in auricular reconstruction, 1743, *1743*, 1755–1758
to provide nasal skeletal framework, 1259, *1262*, 1263
in conjunction with osteotomy and septal framework
resection, 1148, 1149
in microgenia, 1385–1387
nasal, complications following, 1148–1150
septal, 1129, *1129*, 1138
chondrocutaneous, composite, in eyelid reconstruction, 883–891
composite, 191
auricular, 1157, 1220–1225, 1269, *1270*, 1279, 1280, *1281*, 1727, *1728*
dermis-fat, 240–242, *243*
in alar defects, in children, 1225, *1226*
in eyelid reconstruction, 883–891, 902, 903, *903*
in full-thickness loss of nasal tissue, 1214
in partial auricular loss, 1750, *1751*, 1752, *1752*
of amputated auricle, 1728, 1731, 1732, *1734*
of skin and adipose tissue, for alar defects, 1225, *1225*
of skin and cartilage, for alar defects, 1220–1225
septal, as lining for median forehead flap in nasal
reconstruction, 1234, *1234, 1235*
in nasal reconstruction, *1246–1249*
skin-fat, to repair columellar defect, 1269, *1269*
wedge, in nasolabial reconstruction, 1224, *1224*, 1225
conjunctival, in correction of symblepharon, 916–918
dermis. See *Dermis, transplantation of.*

Graft(s) *(Continued)*
   dermis-fat, 240–242, *243*, 254, *254*, 255–257, *258*, 259,
      259, 260
      experimental, *252, 253*
      in augmentation mammaplasty, 3691, 3694, *3695,*
         3696
      in Romberg's disease, *2345–2348*
   eyelash, 894, 895, *895*
   fascia-fat, *254, 255*
   fascial. See *Fascia, transplantation of.*
   fat. See *Fat, transplantation of.*
   fibula, microvascular, 382–384
   flexor tendon, 3193–3206
      for eyebrow reconstruction, 957, *957,* 958, *958, 959*
      in acute hand injuries, 3023, *3024*
   "kebab," 2694
   labia minora, in reconstruction of breast after radical
      mastectomy, *3717,* 3721, 3723
   mesh, 174, 175, *175*
   microvascular free bone, 379–384
   mucosal, 176, 177, *177*
      in correction of symblepharon, 916–918, *918, 919*
      inlay technique of, 1503–1507
   muscle. See *Muscle grafts.*
   nerve. See *Nerve grafting.*
   olecranon process, 334
   osteoperiosteal, in defects of cranium, 838, 839
   pressure bolus, 2655–2657, *2658*
   quilted, in intraoral tumor surgery, 2657, *2659*
   rib, 334–338
      cantilever, in nasal reconstruction, 1264, *1265*
      in cranial defects, 839, 840
      in sternal defects, 3630, *3630*
      microvascular, 379–382
      split. See *Graft, split-rib.*
   scalp, in burn deformity of eyebrows, 1618, *1618,* 1619,
      1619
   sensitization to and recognition of, 132–134, *134*
   septal cartilage, 1129, *1129,* 1138
   skeletal muscle, 293–300
   skin, 54, 152–239
      after thermal burns, 493–505
         anesthesia in, 494, 495
         application of graft in, 496–498, *499*
         donor sites in, 495, *495,* 496
         skeletal traction in, 500–503, *504*
      birth of, 9
      causes of failure of "take" of 179, 180
      color changes in, 158, 159, 183
      combined composite scalp and full-thickness, in
         eyebrow reconstruction, 958
      comparative thickness of, 156, *156*
      contraction of, 95, *98,* 182, 183
      definition of, 156
      delayed, 179
      eyelid, contraction of, 1629
      following resection of intraoral tumors, 2644
      full-thickness, 157, 163–166
         donor sites for, 164, *164,* 165, *165*
         in baldness, 230, *230,* 231
         in postchemosurgery defects of face, 2890, 2891,
            2892
         in skin cancer surgery, 2831, 2832
         in strictures of male urethra, *3894*
         in oropharyngoesophageal reconstructive surgery,
            2715
         pressure dressings with, 165, 166, *166*
         removal of, 165, *165*
         use of, 164
      healing of donor sites in, 180, 181
      in abdominal wall, 3737

Graft(s) *(Continued)*
   skin, in acute hand injuries, 3023, *3024*
      in burn ectropion of eyelids, 1620, 1621, *1621,* 1622,
         1623
      in burns of hand, *3372,* 3374, 3375, 3387, *3387,*
         3388
      in cheek defects, 1579, 1580, *1581*
      in contractures of cervical region, 1648, 1650, 1654,
         1658
      in cutaneous defects of nose, 1197–1199
      in eyelid defect, 882, 883
      in facial burns, 1605, *1606,* 1611, 1612
      in lower extremity, 3531, *3531, 3532*
      in lower eyelid, 1623, *1627, 1628,* 1629
      in male genitalia, 3905, *3905,* 3906
      in mouth, 2651–2657
      in pressure sore, 3780
      in upper eyelids, 1622, 1623, *1624–1627*
      in upper lip defects, 1545, *1545*
      in urethra, 3842, *3843*
      mucosal. See *Graft, mucosal.*
      on dermal bed, 183–188
      pinch, 13, 14
      postoperative care of donor area in, 180
      proper thickness of, 95, 98, 99, *99*
      reinnervation of, 226–229
      sebaceous gland function in, 229
      split-thickness, 14, 156, 157, 166–188
         and wound contraction, 86
         application of, 177
         behavior of, 182, 183
         donor site for, 176, *176*
         formation of nipple by serial application of, *3722,*
            3723
         healing of donor sites in, 180, 181
         in chest wall reconstruction, *3622*
         in lower lip defect, *1561,* 1562
         in postchemosurgery defects of face, 2890
         in pressure sores, 3780
         in radiation ulcer, 543, 544, *544*
         in scalp avulsion, 832, *833, 834*
         in scrotal reconstruction, 3908
         in skin cancer surgery, 2832
         postoperative care of, 178
         pressure dressing for, 177
         removal of, 166–174
         revascularization of, 163
         storage of, 181, 182
         thick, 164, 165
         to cover defect of fat graft, 256, *260*
         without dressings (open), 178, 179
      suitability of, 223, 224
      survival of, phases of, 157–163
      sweat gland function in, 228
      Thiersch, 14
      types of, 163–191
      vascularization of, 157, 159–163
      within nose, 1200, 1201, *1201*
   split-rib, 315, 316, *316–320,* 334–338, 841, *841,* 842,
      849, 851, *854, 855*
      for mandibular reconstruction, 1485, 1490, *1490*
      in manibulofacial dysostosis, 2414, *2415, 2416*
      in Romberg's disease, *2343*
      versus iliac bone grafts, in mandibular reconstruction,
         1482
   tendon. See *Tendon, transplantation of.*
   trochanteric, 334
   vein, 356, *357*
   Wolfe, in Dupuytren's contracture, 3417, *3417, 3418,*
      3419, *3419,* 3422, *3423*
Graft rejection, small lymphocyte and, 132, 133

Granular cell ameloblastoma, of jaws, 2550, *2551*
Granular cell myoblastoma, 2796, 2797, *2797*
    of hand and forearm, 3473, 3474
    of tongue, 2622, *2622*
Granuloma, giant cell reparative, of jaws, 2561, *2561,*
        2562, 2563
    pyogenic, 2795, *2795*
        of eyelids, 878
        of finger, 3482, *3483*
Granuloma telangiectaticum, 2795, *2795*
Graphite, pyrolytic, 402
Graves' disease, orbital pathology in, 971–978
    upper lid retraction in, 978–980
Gravitational lines of face and neck, *1870, 1872, 1873,*
        1873
Greenstick fracture, 655, 796, 798
Groin flap, 218, *218*
    microvascular, *373, 374, 374,* 376, *377*
Ground substance, in tendon, 267, 270
    role of in calcification, 316, 317
Guérin's fracture, 697, *697*
Gunshot wounds, of face, 10
    of jaw, reconstruction of, 1472, *1472*
    of mandible, reconstruction of, 1498, *1498, 1499, 1500,*
        1502
Gynecomastia, 3707, 3708, *3708*
    in Klinefelter's syndrome, *3963*

Hagedorn's operation for cleft lip, 2018, *2018*
Hageman factor, 135
Hair, transfixing fibrous networks in skin, 70, *74*
Hair follicles, 154, 155
    in transplanted dermis, 247, 248, *248*
    tumors of, 2874, 2875
Hair loss, following face lift operation, 1924, 1925
Hair transplantation, for correction of baldness, 229–232
Half-Z technique, 58, *58*
Hall air drill, 445
Hall turbine dermatome, 173
Hallermann-Streiff syndrome, 2408
"Halo" appliance, 677, *678,* 702, *706,* 1372, *1372,*
        1537, *1537,* 2398
Halothane, 587
    and hypotension, 592, 593
Hamate hook, *2969,* 2970
Hamulus, in cleft palate, 1987, 1988
Hand, 2951–3518
    acute ischemia in, resulting from upper extremity
        injuries, 3085–3089
    amputations of, 3090–3096, *3097–3099,* 3143–3151,
        3154, 3155
        and traumatic neuroma, 3149–3151
        congenital, 3329–3331
        subtotal, 3146–3149
    arthritic. See *Arthritis, of hand.*
    burns of, 484, 485, 3368–3391
        adduction contracture of thumb in, 3376, *3376,*
            3377
        attenuation of extensor mechanism in, 3379, *3379*
        cicatricial webbing of interdigital clefts in, 3377
        complications of, 3380
        conservative therapy of with topical antibiotics,
            3372, 3373
        contraction and contracture in, 3370
        early care in, 3371, 3372
        flexion contractures in, 3371, *3372*
        interphalangeal joint deformities in, 3378, 3379
        joint stiffness in, 3370, 3371, *3371,* 3377, *3377,*
            3378, *3378*

Hand *(Continued)*
    burns of, of dorsal surface, acute, treatment of, 3390,
            3390, 3391, 3391
        debridement and early excision in, 3385, 3386,
            3386
        deep, 3388, 3389
        edema in, 3382, 3383
        escharotomy of, 3383
        evaluation of depth of burn in, 3389
        hypertrophic scars in, 3389
        immediate management of, 3381–3391
        immobilization, pressure dressing, and physio-
            therapy in, 3383, 3384, *3384*
        physiotherapy and hydrotherapy of, 3384, 3385
        positioning of hand in, 3385
        tangential excision and immediate grafting in,
            3387, *3387,* 3388
        topical treatment in, 3389
    pathology of, 3369–3371
    pedicle flaps in, 3375, *3375,* 3376, *3376*
    secondary contractures in, grafting in, *3372,* 3374,
        3375
    skin replacement in, 3373–3376
    splinting and physiotherapy in, 3379, 3380
    cicatricial contracture in, 2966, *2967*
    clasped, congenital, 3325, 3326, *3326, 3327*
    combined motor-sensory nerve conduction studies of,
        2984
    constraint of edema on mechanics of, 3109–3111,
        3112
    contracted web space in, four-flap Z-plasty in, 60, *61*
    digital necrosis secondary to ischemia in, *2967*
    direct electrical stimulation of muscle or nerve of, 2981
    disability evaluation of, 2976
    dorsum of, burns of. See *Hand, burns of, of dorsal*
        surface.
        deltopectoral flap in resurfacing of, 2747, *2747*
    dressings in, 2991–2995
    elastic finger traction in, *2992,* 2993
    examination of, 2964–2990
        electrodiagnostic, 2981–2989
            clinical application of, 2984–2989
            complications of, 2989
    extensor tendon deformities in, 3325, 3326, *3326*
    extrinsic extensor loss in, 3269–3275, *3276–3278*
    fixed unit of, 2958, *2958*
    fractures and dislocations of, 3041–3060
        anatomic reduction in, 3043, 3044, *3044*
        immobilization in protective position in, 3044, *3045*
        of carpals, 3044–3047
        of digital joints, 3056, *3057, 3058*
        of metacarpals, 3050–3053
        of phalanges, 3053–3056
        of scaphoid, 3047
        of thumb, 3048–3050
        open, 3056, *3058,* 3059, *3059*
        remobilization based on clinical evaluation in, 3044
        treatment of, 3041–3044
    function of, dynamics of, 2961, 2962
    indirect effects of injury on architectural dynamics of,
        3106, 3107, *3108*
    integument and fascia of, examination of, 2966, 2967,
        2967
    mangled, 3056, *3058,* 3059, *3059*
    motor nerve conduction studies of, 2982, 2983, *2983,*
        2983t
    muscles and tendons of, examination of, 2971–2974
    nails of. See *Nails, of hand.*
    needle electrode examination of, 2982, *2982*
    nerve and tendon entrapment syndromes of,
        3428–3448

Hand *(Continued)*
  nerve and tendon severance in, 3206, 3207, *3207*
  nerve grafting in, 3227–3240
  nerves of, examination of, 2974, 2975
    peripheral. See *Nerves, peripheral, of hand and forearm.*
  neuromuscular apparatus of, 2957–2961
  partially paralyzed, central nervous system adaptation in, 3303
    interphalangeal flexion in, 3275, 3278
    metacarpophalangeal flexion in, 3278–3280, *3281, 3282*
    restoration of power and stability in, 3266–3305
    restoration of power pinch in, 3301
    restoration of thumb opposition in, 3285–3301
    tendon transfer in, 3268, 3269, *3269*
    tenodesis in, 3303, 3304
  "position of function" of, 3385
    for arthrodesis of irreparable damaged joint, 3014
  primary and secondary nerve repair in, 3207–3209
  protective position of, in temporary immobilization, 3014, 3015
  reconstructive surgery of, 3103–3153
    amputations in, 3143–3151
    bones and joints of amputated parts used in, 3158, 3159, *3161*
    composite skin island transfer on neurovascular pedicle in, 3138–3142
    composite tissues of amputated parts used in, 3159, *3163, 3164,* 3165
    extrinsic flexor musculature in, 3130–3137
    fingernails of amputated parts used in, 3155, *3160*
    in wrist, 3112–3115
    intrinsic musculature in, 3124–3129
    nerves of amputated parts used in, 3155, 3156
    relationship of thumb to fixed unit of hand in, 3115–3124
    shifting local tissue for sensory deficit in, 3142
    skin of amputated parts used in, 3155, *3157, 3158, 3159*
    special structural considerations in, 3112–3137
    specific usable tissue in, 3155–3165
    tactile sense as consideration in, 3137–3142
    tendons of amputated parts used in, 3156, 3158
  repair of peripheral nerves in, 3215–3242
  replantation of amputated parts in, 3084, *3085, 3086*
  sensory nerve conduction studies of, 2983, 2984, *2984*
  skeleton of, 2957–2961
    examination of, 2967–2971
  splints in, 2991–2993, 2995–2999
  split (lobster), 3335–3337
  surgery of, 2953–2956
  surgical anatomy of, 2957–2963
  tactile sense in, 3137–3142
  tendons of. See *Tendons, of hand.*
  thermal burns of. See *Hand, burns of.*
  topographical aspect of, *2969, 2970*
  vessels of, examination of, 2976
Hand and forearm, tumors of, 3449–3506
  actinic keratosis, 3455, 3456, *3456*
  angiomas, 3482, *3483*
  arsenical keratosis, 3456
  basal cell epithelioma, 3460
  Bowen's disease, 3459
  calcified epithelioma of Malherbe, 3452, *3452*
  capillary hemangiomas, 3482, *3484*
  enchondroma, 3452, 3497, *3498,* 3499
  epithelial and tumor-like lesions, 3450–3464
    malignant, 3459–3464
    precancerous, 3455–3459

Hand and forearm *(Continued)*
  epithelial cysts, 3450–3452
  fibromatoses, 3474–3478
  fibrosarcoma, 3489
  ganglia, 3469, 3470, *3470*
  giant cell tumor of bone, 3499, 3500
  giant cell tumor of tendon sheath, 3472, *3472, 3473, 3473, 3474*
  glomus tumor, 3485, *3485,* 3486, *3486, 3487*
  granular cell myoblastoma, 3473, 3474
  hemangioendothelioma, 3488
  hemangiopericytomas, 3487, 3488
  histiocytoma, 3471, *3471,* 3472, *3472*
  irradiation dermatosis, 3457, *3457, 3458,* 3459
  Kaposi's idiopathic hemorrhagic sarcoma, 3488, *3488,* 3489
  keratoacanthoma, 3452, 3453, *3453, 3454*
  leiomyoma, 3481, *3481,* 3482
  lipoma, 3478, *3479,* 3480, *3480, 3481*
  liposarcoma, 3489, 3490
  lymphangioma, 3488
  malignant schwannoma, 3495, 3496, *3496*
  mesenchymoma, 3482
  metastatic, 3500
  myxoid (mucous) cysts, 3470, *3470,* 3471, *3471*
  myxoma, 3489
  neurilemoma, 3493, *3494*
  neurofibroma, 3494, *3494, 3495*
  of bone and cartilage, 3496–3500
  of nonepithelial soft tissues, 3468–3482
  of peripheral nerves, 3493–3496
  of vascular system, 3482–3489
  osteochondroma, 3499
  osteogenic sarcoma, 3499
  osteoid osteoma, 3499
  pigmented nevi and malignant melanoma, 3464–3468
  pseudosarcomatous nodular fasciitis, 3475
  rhabdomyosarcoma, 3490
  sarcomas of soft tissues, 3489–3491, *3492, 3493*
  seborrheic keratosis, 3453, 3455, *3455*
  squamous cell carcinoma, 3459, *3459,* 3460, *3460–3464*
  sweat and sebaceous gland, 3453, 3464
  synovial cysts, 3470
  synovial sarcoma, 3490, 3491, *3491–3493*
  warts, 3450, *3451*
  xanthoma, 3471
Hand deformities, congenital, 2976
  abnormal morphogenesis and, 3309, *3309,* 3310
  associated anomalies in, 3311, *3311,* 3312
  embryology of, 3307–3309
  genetics and, 3307
  incidence of, 3307
  surgical management of, 3306–3349
    annular grooves, 3328, *3328, 3329*
    in anomalies of digital posture, 3325, *3325,* 3326, *3326, 3327*
    in ectrodactyly, 3329–3331
    in longitudinal deficiency states, 3333–3348
    in polydactyly, 3319–3325
    in syndactyly, 3313–3319
    in transverse deficiency states, 3327–3331
    timing of, 3312, *3312,* 3313
  in Apert's syndrome, 2322–2325, *2326,* 2327, 2472, *2472*
  in Möbius syndrome, 2329, *2331*
Hand injuries, acute, amputations and prosthetic considerations in, 3090–3096, *3097–3099*
  anesthesia in, 3009–3012

Hand injuries (*Continued*)
  acute, antibiotics in, 3016, 3017
    dressings and early postoperative management in, 3015–3017
    due to radiation, 537–541, *542*
    edema in, 3014
    evaluation and diagnosis in, 3001–3009
    examination in, 2964, *2965, 2966*
    flaps in, 3023–3041
      cross-finger, 3025, *3026*, 3027, *3027–3029*
      distant, 3035–3041
      local, 3027–3035
      on permanent subcutaneous pedicles, 3033, 3034, *3034*
      thenar, 3027–3033
      transferred on specific neurovascular pedicles, 3034, *3035*
      transposition and rotation, 3034, 3035, *3036*
    foreign bodies in, 3018, 3019, *3020*
    fractures and dislocations in. See *Hand, fractures and dislocations of.*
    grafts in, 3023, *3024*
    immobilization in, 3014, 3015
    inflammation in, 3014
    injection, 3018, *3018, 3019*
    involving crushing of soft tissues, 3021, 3022
    involving fingernails, 3017, 3018
    lacerations, 3017
    management of, 3000–3102
    of nerves, 3009, 3078–3084
    of tendon, 3004–3009, 3060–3078
      blood supply and isolation in, 3062
      extensor, 3063–3068
      flexor, 3068–3078
      hematoma in, 3062
      motion and remobilization in, 3062, 3063
    of skin, *3003*, 3004, *3004*
    preoperative preparation and use of tourniquet in, 3012, 3013, *3013*
    protection of uninjured small joints in, 3013–3015
    ring avulsion, 3019, *3020*, 3021, *3021*
    skeletal, 3004, *3005*
      in children, 3059, 3060
    soft tissue injury in, 3017–3022
    soft tissue replacement in, 3023–3041
    thrombosis and embolization in, 3089, 3090, *3090, 3091*
    vascular, 3004, 3084–3090
  conservation of usable structures in, 3154–3165
Hand therapy, 3100–3102
Haploid number, 140
Hayton-Williams disimpaction forceps, 702, *705*
Head and neck, 597–2949. See also *Neck.*
  cancer of, surgical treatment of, 2509–2520
    history of, 2509–2511
    recent developments in, 2511–2514
    reconstructive techniques in, 2514–2519
  carotid body and vagal tumors of, 2638, 2639, *2639, 2640*
  embryonic development of, 2297–2315
  melanomas of, 2636, *2637*
  sarcomas of, 2636–2638
  tumors of, in children, 2622–2624
Head and neck surgery, anesthesia in, 2589, 2590, 2590t
  flaps in, 2624–2636
  tracheotomy in, 2590–2592
Head cap, in maxillary fractures, 701, *701*
Head frames, in mandibular fractures, 677, *678*
  in maxillary fractures, 702, *706*
Headlight, fiberoptic, 1064, *1064*

Hearing, preservation of in cleft palate repair, 2093, 2094
Hearing loss, and speech, 2262
Heberden's nodes, in arthritic hand, 3507
Heel ulcers, 3792
Heifetz clamps, 345, *345*
Helical rim, loss of, 1736–1740, *1741, 1742*
Helical tumor, wedge resection of, 1768, *1768*
Helix, deformity of, 1708, 1709
Hemangiectatic hypertrophy, 2793
Hemangioendothelial sarcoma, of chest wall, 3652, *3653*
Hemangioendothelioma, of hand and forearm, 3488
Hemangiomas, 2865–2868
  capillary, 2793, *2793*, 2794, 2795, *2865, 2865*, 2866
    of hand and forearm, 3482, *3484*
  cavernous, 2793, *2793*, 2866, *2866–2868*
  dermabrasion of, 449
  hyperkeratotic, 2795
  of eyelids, 874
  of jaws, 2567, *2567, 2568*
  of nose, 1170, *1176*, 1177, *1177*, 1178
  pathology of, 2794, 2795
  sclerosing, 2866, 2867
  senile, 2866
  syndromes associated with, 2867, 2868
  verrucous, 2795
  with thrombocytopenia, 2794, 2868
Hemangiopericytomas, 2869, *2869*
  of hand and forearm, 3487, 3488
Hemangiosarcoma, of hand and forearm, 3488
Hematoma
  and failure of skin graft, 180
  following corrective surgery of jaws, 1468, 1469
  following face lift operation, 1922–1924
  in acute hand injuries, 3062
  of nasal septum, 728, 730, *730*
  of orbit, following orbital fractures, 791
Hemicraniofacial microsomia. See *Craniofacial microsomia.*
Hemifacial atrophy, fat grafts in, 254, *258*
  progressive. See *Romberg's disease.*
Hemifacial hyperplasia, 1382
Hemifacial microsomia, 1676, *1677*
Hemimandible, reconstruction of, 1492, *1493, 1494*
Hemimaxilla, reconstruction of, *1511*
Hemolytic disease of newborn, 120
Hemoptysis, 3610
Hemorrhage, following corrective rhinoplasty, 1090
  following maxillary fractures, 700, 707
  primary, in mandibular fractures, 692
Henderson-O'Brien microvascular clamp, 344, *345*
Heparin, in microvascular surgery, 366, 367
Hermaphroditism, 3930–3969
  classification of, 3938–3941
  female, diagnosis of, 3946, 3951, *3951*
    differential diagnosis of, 3951, 3952
    treatment of, 3952, *3952*, 3953, *3953*
    with congenital adrenocortical hyperplasia, 3936, *3936*
  male, treatment of, 3953, 3954, *3954, 3955*
  true, construction of male genitalia in, 3944, *3946–3950*
    construction of vagina in, 3942–3944, *3945*
    diagnosis of, 3941, 3942
    surgical procedures in, 3942, *3942*
    treatment of, 3941–3944
Hernias, epigastric, 3728
  of abdominal wall, 3730, 3731, *3731*
Heterograft, definition of, 52, 156
Heterozygosity, 139
Hidradenitis suppurativa, 2879, 2880, *2880*

Hidradenoma, clear cell, of eyelids, 879
Hidradenoma papilliferum, 2789
Hinge flap, 200, 201, *201*, 1223, *1223*, *1244*
Hip, muscle flaps in, 3549, 3550, *3550, 3551*
Histamine dihydrochloride, 85
Histamine iontophoresis, 198
Histamine scratch test, of flap circulation, 195
Histiocytoma, 2790, *2790*, 2791, 2866, 2867
  of hand and forearm, 3471, *3471*, 3472, *3472*
Histocompatibility complex, major (MHC), 130, *131*,
    142, 145t
Histocompatibility genetics, 129–131
Histocompatibility systems, 141–147
Histocompatibility typing, 127, 128
HLA lymphocyte-defined (LD) system, 142, 143
HLA serologically defined (SD) system, 142, 142t
HLA serology, 128
HLA-D specificities, frequency of, 143, 144t
Hockey-stick incision, 1105, 1106
Hodgson-Toksu "tumble flap" repair of hypospadias,
    3852, *3853*
Holocrine glands, sebaceous, 155
Holoprosencephaly, *2120*, 2128, 2128t
  orbital hypotelorism in, *2463*
Holt-Oram syndrome, 3334
Homograft, definition of, 52, 156
Homozygosity, 139
Hood, George F., 14
Hormonal sex, 3937, 3938
Horn, cutaneous, 2858
Horn cell, anterior, metabolic changes in, 3217–3219
Horner's muscle, 862, *862*
Host cell replacement theory, of fat grafts, 251
"Hourglass" deformity, *2448*, 2449
Human form, proportions of, 29–35
Humby knife, *166*, 167, 173, 174
Hydrocortisone, in treatment of keloids, 430
cis-Hydroxyproline, 284
5-Hydroxytryptamine, 85
Hygroma, cystic, 2873, 2874
Hynes pharyngoplasty, *2272*
Hyoid arches, 2902, *2903*
Hyomandibular cleft, 2311
Hypernasality, 2258, 2268, 2269
Hyperpigmentation, 459
Hyperrhinolalia, 2258
Hypodermis, 155, 156
Hypogastric flap, 218, *218*
Hypoglossal-facial nerve anastomosis, 1800, *1801, 1802,
    1803, 1804*
Hypomastia, unilateral, 3706, *3706*, 3707
Hyponasality, 2258
Hypopharynx, cancer of, 2698
  reconstructive surgery of, 2697–2756
  tumors of, 2613, *2613, 2614, 2615*
Hypopigmentation, 459, 460
Hypospadias, 3831, 3845–3861
  complications in, 3859, 3860
  correction of chordee in, 3836, *3836, 3837*
  embryology of, 3846, 3847, *3847*
  historical aspects and evolution of techniques of
    treatment of, 3835–3844
  history of, 3846
  incidence of, 3846
  modern techniques for repair of, 3848–3852, *3853*
  pathologic anatomy of, 3845, *3845*
  postoperative care in, 3859
  reconstruction of urethra in, 3836–3843
  surgical treatment of, 3853–3859
  with and without chordee, 3847, *3847*, 3848

Hyporhinolalia, 2258
Hypotension, induced, 592, 593
Hypothenar muscles, 2961
Hypothermia, 519, 520, *520*
  hospital care for patient with, 526–528

IgG molecule, 134, *134*
IgM molecule, 134
Iliac bone autograft, 327–334
Iliac bone graft, *1025*
  following mandibular resection for cancer, 2618, 2622,
    2623, 2624
  for nasal contour restoration, 1141–1147, *1458*
  in cranial defects, 845, *848*, 849, *849, 850, 855*
  in microgenia, *1386*
  in Romberg's disease, *2343*
  versus split rib grafts, in mandibular reconstruction,
    1482
Iliac crest, ulcer of, 3792
Iliac lymphatics, obstruction of, 3588, *3589*, 3590, *3590*
Iliff's modification of Fasanella-Servat operation, 928,
    929
Immersion foot, 517
Immune response, to bone allografts and xenografts, 323,
    324
Immunity, mediators of, 134, 135, *135*
Immunoglobulins, 133, 134
Immunologic enhancement, 137
Immunologic tolerance, 136, 137
Immunologically privileged sites, 136
Immunosuppression, 137, 138
Immunotherapy, in treatment of malignant melanoma,
    2851–2853
Implantation, definition of, 53
Implants, cartilage, dead, behavior of, 308, 309, *310*
  inorganic, 392–412. See also *Prostheses.*
    acrylic resin, 392
    adhesives and glues, 393
    choice of prosthetic material in, 406–409
    definition of, 53
    effect of surgical technique in, 405, 406
    in augmentation mammaplasty, 3694–3698,
      3698–3702
    in auricular reconstruction following trauma, 1750
    in blowout fractures of orbital floor, 772, 773, *773*,
      789, 790
    in breast after radical mastectomy, 3716, 3720
    in cranial defects, 840, 841
    in facial palsy, 1819, 1820
    in mandibulofacial dysostosis, 2416, *2417, 2418*
    in microgenia, 1399–1403
    in microtia, 1696, 1699, 1701, *1701*
    in naso-orbital fractures, 772, 790
    in orbital fractures, 995–997
    in saddle-nose deformities, 1140, 1141, *1141*
    malignancy in, 409, 410
    metallic, 392, 393
    over bone, 405, *406, 407, 408*
    proplast, 402
    Silastic. See *Silastic implants.*
    silicone. See *Silicone implants.*
    synthetic, 393
Inbreeding, 141
Incision(s)
  abdominal, 3729, 3730
  button-hole, for cancellous chips, 330
  choice of site of, 43
  for radical neck dissection, 2593, *2593, 2594*

Incision(s) *(Continued)*
  gingival, in mandibular malformations, 1307, *1307*, 1308
  hockey-stick, 685, 1105, 1106
  Luckett, 1711, *1711*, 1712
  MacFee, in intraoral tumor surgery, 2649, *2649*, 2679, *2680*, 2685
  transfixion, in rhinoplasty, 1068–1070
    variations in, 1100, 1101, *1101*
  vestibular, labiobuccal, 1307, *1307*
Inclusion cyst, of eyelids, 878, 879
Inderal, 586, 587
Indian forehead flap, *1213*
Infection
  and failure of skin graft, 180
  and rare craniofacial clefts, 2122
  as contraindication to fat grafts, 255
  failure of flap transfer due to, 226
  following corrective rhinoplasty, 1090
  following corrective surgery of jaws, 1468, 1469
  following mandibular fractures, 693
  following maxillary fractures, 707
  in plastic surgery, 50, 51
  in replantation surgery, 3263
Infracture, in corrective rhinoplasty, 1081, 1083, *1084*
Infraorbital nerve. See *Nerve, infraorbital.*
Infrared thermography, in evaluation of flap circulation, 196
Inguinal crease, as donor site for full-thickness skin grafts, 165
Innovar, 586
Inorganic implants. See *Implants, inorganic.*
Inosculation, 157, 163
Integument. See *Skin.*
Interdental osteotomy, in correction of mandibular micrognathia, 1356, 1357
Interdigital clefts, cicatricial webbing of, in burns of hand, 3377
Interfascicular nerve grafting, 3231–3234, 3238, 3240
Inter-island contraction phenomenon, 444
Intermaxillary fixation techniques, 648–652
  in maxillary fractures, 701, *701*
Internal oblique muscle, 3728
Interorbital distance, classification of orbital hypertelorism on basis of, 2441, 2441t
  measurement of, 2437, *2439*
Interorbital space, 749, *749*, 777, *777*
  resection of median or two paramedian sections of bone from in orbital hypertelorism, 2450, *2451*
  widening of, 723, *725*
Interossei, in reconstructive surgery of hand, 3126
Interosseous fixation, in orbital hypertelorism, 2453, *2453*
Interphalangeal extension, 3014
Interphalangeal flexion, 3275, 3278
Interphalangeal joints, 2960
  arthritis of, 3508–3511
  deformities of, 2970, 2971, *2972*
    in burns of hand, 3378, 3379
  distal, extensor tendon injuries at, *3066*, 3067, *3067*, 3068
  proximal, extensor tendon injuries at, 3064–3067
    hyperextension of, *3173*, *3174*, 3175–3180, *3181–3813*
Intersex problems, 3930–3969
  treatment of, 3941–3965
Intersexuality, classification of, 3938–3941
Intraocular pressure, 1001
Intraoral appliances, in mandibular fractures, 689
Intraoral carcinoma, mandible in, 2688–2695

Intraoral tumors
  basic clinical management of, 2642
  bolus tie-over grafting following removal of, 2655–2657, *2658*
  direct suture closure of in single lesion, 2643, 2644
  pressure dressing using dental appliance following removal of, 2652–2655
  quilted grafting following removal of, 2657, *2659*
  reconstruction following excision of, 2642–2696
    deltopectoral flap in. See *Flap, deltopectoral, in intraoral tumor surgery.*
    dressings and suction in, 2685, 2686, *2686*
    fistula in, 2687, 2688
    flap necrosis in, 2687
    forehead flap in. See *Flap, forehead, in intraoral tumor surgery.*
    nasolabial flap in, 2649, 2650, *2650*, 2682–2684
    postoperative complications in, 2686–2688
    skin grafting in, 2651–2657
  reconstructive policy for in multifocal lesion, 2650, 2651
  reconstructive policy for in single lesion, 2643–2650
  skin flaps for repair of single lesion in, 2644–2650
  skin grafts for repair of single lesion in, 2644
Intratemporal facial nerve, 1775, 1777
Intubation, nasal, 589, *590*
  oral, 588, 589, *589*, *590*
Irradiation, of tendon, 285
Irradiation dermatosis, of hand and forearms, 3457, *3457*, *3458*, 3459
Ischial ulcers, 3784, *3785–3788*, 3789
Island flaps. See *Flap, island,* and *Flap, forehead, island.*
Isograft, definition of, 52, 156
Ivalon sponges, 407

Jalaguier's procedure for repairing cleft lip, 2017, *2017*, 2018, 2019
Jaws. See also *Maxilla* and *Mandible.*
  deformities of, 1288–1520
    acquired, 1288, 1289, 1470–1513
    complications following corrective surgery of, 1468–1470
    component concept of, 1289–1294
    congenital, 1288
    developmental, 1288–1470
      classification of, 1294, 1295, 1297t, *1298*
      diagnosis of, facial, 1295, 1298
      oral and dentoalveolar, 1298, *1299*
      orthodontics and surgery in, 1302–1305
      preoperative planning in, 1298–1300
    in craniofacial microsomia, 2361–2366, 2371–2373
    prosthodontics and surgery in, 1303
  epithelial cysts of, 2563–2565
  fractures of, 646–708
    importance of teeth in management of, 646–652
    malunited, 1470, 1471
    mandibular. See *Mandible, fractures of.*
    maxillary. See *Maxilla, fractures of.*
  giant cell reparative granuloma of, 2561, *2561*, *2562*, *2563*
  metastatic tumors to, *2571*, *2572*, *2572*
  multiple myeloma of, 2570, *2570*
  simple bone cyst of, 2563, *2564*
  tumors of, 2547–2573
    ameloblastic fibroma, 2552, *2552*, 2553
    ameloblastomas, 2547–2552
    angiosarcoma, 2569, *2569*, *2570*
    cementoma, 2555, *2555*, 2556

Jaws *(Continued)*
  tumors of, chondroma, 2566
    connective tissue, 2567–2569
    Ewing's sarcoma, 2567, *2568,* 2569, *2569*
    fibrous dysplasia, 2557–2561
    hemangioma, 2567, *2567, 2568*
    myxoma, 2554, *2554, 2555*
    odontomas, 2553, *2553, 2554*
    osseous, 2566, *2566, 2567*
    osteogenic sarcoma, 2566, *2566, 2567*
    osteoma, 2556, *2556, 2557*
Jaw skeleton, upper, reconstruction of, 1509–1513
Jaw surgery, corrective, in craniofacial microsomia,
  2377–2386
Jejunal segment, free revascularized transplantation of, in
  pharyngoesophageal reconstruction, 2708, 2709, *2710*
Joint(s)
  digital, fractures and dislocations of, 3056, *3057, 3058*
    in arthritic hand, 3515–3517
      fusion of, 3510, 3511, *3511*
  interphalangeal. See *Interphalangeal joints.*
  metacarpophalangeal. See *Metacarpophalangeal joint.*
  of hand, 2967–2971
  radiocarpal, 2961
  radioulnar, 2961
  Silastic implants in, 102
  stiff, biological processes in development of, 102
  temporomandibular. See *Temporomandibular joint.*
  transplantation of, 102
Jones tube, 1016
Joseph, 12
Joseph knife, *1102*
  modified, *1067,* 1068
Joseph periosteal elevator, *1102, 1103*
Joseph saw guide, 1103, *1103*
Joseph technique, of corrective rhinoplasty, 1065, 1066,
  1066
Joseph tip operation, 1106, 1107, *1107*
Jowls, correction of, 1921
Jump flap. See *Flap, jump.*

Kaposi's sarcoma, 2841
  of hand and forearm, 3488, *3488,* 3489
Karfik classification of craniofacial clefts, 2126, 2127t,
  2128
Karyotype, chromosome, 3934, *3935, 3936*
  human, *110, 111, 112, 113*
Kasabach-Merritt syndrome, 2794
Kaye method of correction of flattening of anthelix,
  1712, 1713
Kazanjian, 10
Kazanjian button, 651, *655*
Kazanjian extraoral traction appliance, *1371,* 1372
Kazanjian T-bar attachment, 679, *679*
"Kebab" graft, 2694
Keloid tendency, 422, *422*
Keloids, 89, *89,* 91, 92, 424–430
  characteristics of, 424
  etiology of, 427, 428
  incidence of, 427
  method of treatment of, 429, 430
  of thorax, 3654, *3654*
  pathology of, 424–427
  results of treatment of, 428, 429
  sternal, chemical planing of, 461
Keratinocytes, 154
Keratoacanthoma, 2814, 2815, *2815,* 2857, 2858
  of eyelids, 878
  of hand and forearm, 3453, *3453, 3454*

Keratoconjunctivitis sicca, following esthetic
  blepharoplasty, 1896, 1897
Keratosis (keratoses), 2856–2858
  actinic (senile), 2802–2804, 2857, *2857*
    of auricle, 1767
    of hand and forearm, 3455, 3456, *3456*
  arsenical, 2858
    of hand and forearm, 3456
  follicular, inverted, of eyelids, 878
  seborrheic, 2781–2783, 2857, *2858*
    of hand and forearm, 3453, 3455, *3455*
  solar, 2802
Keratosis plantaris, 3529, 3530
Keratotic lesions, dermabrasion of, 449, 450
Ketamine hydrochloride, 495, 587
Kidney, embryology of, 3828, 3829, *3829*
Kilner, T. Pomfret, 16, *20*
Kilner-Dott gag, 593, *594*
Kinin system, and graft rejection, 135, *135*
Kirschner wire fixation, in mandibular fractures, 676
Kleeblattschädel anomaly, 2466, 2493, *2494*
Klinefelter's syndrome, 109, 3707, 3931, 3934, 3938,
  3956, 3960, *3961–3963*
Klippel-Feil syndrome, radial ray deficiency in, 3334
Klippel-Trenaunay-Weber syndrome, 2793
Knee, local flap in, 3534, *3534*
  muscle flap in, 3550, *3551, 3552*
Knee ulcers, 3792, *3792*
Knife, button, curved, *1069*
  Joseph, *1067, 1068, 1102*
Koenig operation for cleft lip, 2018, *2018*
Krönlein-Berke operation for orbital decompression, 973,
  973, 974, 975
Krukenberg amputation, 3096, *3098*
Kuhnt-Szymanowski operation, 908, 2419

L-osteotomy, 1347, *1348*
Labia majora, 3832, *3833*
Labia majora skin, as donor site for full-thickness skin
  grafts, 165
Labia minora, 3832, *3833*
Labia minora grafts, in reconstruction of breast after
  radical mastectomy, *3717,* 3721, 3723
Labiobuccal sulcus, restoration of in mandibular
  reconstruction, 1503–1507
Labiobuccal vestibular incision, in mandibular
  malformations, 1307, *1307*
Labiogingival lamina, 2313
Lacrimal apparatus, repair of, 982–989
Lacrimal groove, 1043, *1043*
Lacrimal injuries, in naso-orbital fractures, *1006,* 1008,
  1009, *1010*
Lacrimal nerve, 866
Lacrimal sac, *980,* 981
Lacrimal system, defects of, 980–989
  anatomical considerations in, 980, *980,* 981
  excretory and developmental, 981, *981,* 982
Lacrimal system complications, following orbital
  fractures, 791
Lacrimal system lacerations, 632
Lacrimal system obstruction, in maxillary fractures, 708
Lacrimation, paradoxical, in facial palsy, 1840
Lacunae, 313
Lagophthalmos, 918
Lamina papyracea, comminuted, in naso-orbital
  fractures, 779, *780*
Langenbeck flaps, in cleft palate repair, *2200,* 2201, *2201*
Langer's lines, 39, 40, 71, 74, 76, *76,* 77, 417, *417,* 418
Lanugo, 154

Laryngeal edema, after tracheal intubation, 591
Laryngopharynx, cancer of, 2698
  deltopectoral flap in reconstruction of, 2735–2739
  reconstructive surgery of, 2697–2756
Laryngotracheal substitution, for retrocricoid pharynx, 2705–2707
Lateral anterior projection, 613, *615*
Laterognathism, 1294
  mandibular, 1373–1382, 1420, *1424*
Lathyrism, 93, 94
Latissimus dorsi muscle flap, in chest wall reconstruction, *3623*
Laurence-Moon-Biedl-Bardet syndrome, polydactyly in, 3320
"Lazy-T" method of treatment of ectropion, 908, 909, *909, 910, 911*
Le Fort classification of fractures, 697, *697*, 698
Le Fort I osteotomy, 1442–1445, *1454*, 1459
Le Fort 1½ osteotomy, 1445, 1446, *1446, 1449, 1450*, 2194, 2195, *2195*
Le Fort II osteotomy, 1454, *1454*, 1455
Le Fort III osteotomy, 1454, *1454*, 1466
  combined with Le Fort I osteotomy, 2488, *2488, 2489*, 2490, *2490*
    in Crouzon's disease, 2480
  in Apert's syndrome, 2477, 2480
  in cleft palate repair, 2195, 2197, *2197*
  through combined intracranial approach, in Crouzon's disease, 2476–2480
  through subcranial (extracranial) route, in Crouzon's disease, 2474–2476
Leadbetter urethroplasty, *3893*
Leg. See *Extremity, lower.*
Leiomyoma, of hand and forearm, 3481, *3481*, 3482
Leiomyosarcoma, 2840
Lemaitre, 12, *12, 13*
LeMesurier operation, 2166, *2168, 2169*
LeMesurier rectangular flap, in cleft lip repair, 2018, 2019, 2027, *2027*, 2028, 2032, 2033, 2037, 2038, *2038, 2039*
Lens vesicle, 2304
Lentigines, 2797
Lentigo maligna, 2805, *2805*, 2806, *2806*
Lentigo malignant melanoma, 2844, *2844*
Leser-Trélat sign, 2782
Leukocytes, polymorphonuclear, sex differences in, 3932, 3933, *3933*
Leukonychia, 2978
Leukoplakia, 2599, 2600, *2600*, 2804, *2804*, 2805
Levant frame, 1491, *1491*
Levator palpebrae superioris, *860, 861*, 864, *864*, 865, *865*
  action of, 948, 949, *949*, 950t
  repair of injuries to, 872
Levator resection, external, 930, 931, *932–935*
  for ptosis, 922–931
  of Jones, 929, 930, *930*
Levator sling, formation of in cleft palate repair, 2094, 2095, *2095*
Levator transplant procedure, in cleft palate repair, *2273*
Levator veli palatini muscle, *1977, 1978*, 1979–1981, *1982*, 1987, 1988
Lidocaine, 627
Limb, compound fracture of, timing of skin replacement in, 225
  lower. See *Extremity, lower.*
  upper. See also *Extremity, upper.*
    sensibility in, 2962, 2963
Limb deformities, classification of, 3310–3313

Limb replantation, 3243–3245, 3247–3252
  bone shortening in, 3247
  indications for, 3244, 3245, *3245, 3246*
  muscles and tendons in, 3247
  nerves in, 3250, *3250*, 3251, *3251*
  results of, 3257
  skin in, 3251, 3252
  vascular anastomoses in, 3247, 3250
Linea alba, 3728
Linea semicircularis, 3729
Lineae albicantes, 3728
Lineae semilunares, 3728
Lineae transversae, 3728
Lines of expression, 42, 43
Lines of maximal tension, 77
Lines of minimal tension, 42, *42*
  Z-plasty and, 56, 57, *57*, 58
Lines of minimum extensibility, 76
Lines of tension, 38–40
Lingual blood supply, 2701, *2701*
Linkage disequilibrium, 140
Lip(s)
  cleft. See *Cleft lip, cleft lip and nose,* and *Cleft lip and palate.*
  deformities of, 1540–1578
    congenital, 1540–1544
    techniques for repair of, 1544–1593
  double, congenital, 1543, *1543*, 1544
  in bilateral cleft lip and palate, *1951*, 1952
  in unilateral cleft lip and palate, 1959
  lacerations of, 636, 637, *641*
  lower, complete loss of, 1570–1573
    deformities of, 1559–1573
      associated with chin deformity and loss of section of mandible, 1573
      full-thickness, 1564–1570
        lateral, 1569, *1569, 1570*
        median, 1564–1569
      superficial, 1559–1564
    ectropion of, *1560*, 1561–1563
    entropion of, 1563, *1563*, 1564
    reconstructed, restoration of muscular function of, 1577, 1578, *1579*
    squamous cell cancer and leukoplakia of, *2600, 2603*
    squamous cell carcinoma of, *2834–2836, 2839*
    treatment of burn deformities of, 1638, *1638, 1639*
    tumors of, 2603–2607
  metastatic carcinoma to jaws from, *2573*
  muscles of, 1966–1975
  loosening of after treatment of lip sinuses, 1542, 1543
  proportions of, 33, *37*
  role of in speech, 2253
  upper, basal cell epithelioma of, *2826, 2827*
    complete loss of, 1556–1558
    deformities of, 1544–1558
      full-thickness, 1546–1558
        lateral, 1552–1556
        median, 1548–1552
      superficial, 1544–1546
    deltopectoral flap in defect of, *2748*
    ectropion of, 1544, *1545, 1546*
    embryonic development of, 2307
    lengthening of, 1558, *1559*
    reconstruction of columella using tissue from, 1269
    treatment of burn deformities of, 1636, 1637, *1637*, 1638
    tumors of, 2601, *2601, 2602*
Lip adhesion, in newborn with cleft lip and palate, 2223, *2224*

Lip adhesion operation, 2021, *2022*, 2032, 2033, *2033*
  in bilateral cleft lip repair, 2054, *2054*, 2055
Lip posture, competent and incompetent, 1291, *1291*,
  1292
Lip reconstruction, effect of on maxillary complex, 1998,
  1998
  in bilateral cleft lip and palate, 1999, *1999*, 2000,
    2000, *2001*
  in unilateral cleft lip and palate, 1998, 1999, *1999*
Lip sinuses, congenital, 1540–1543
Lip sulcus, 2314, 2315
Lip-furrow band, 2313
Lipoblastomatosis, 3480, *3481*
Lipodystrophy, silicone fluid injections in, 2348,
  2351–2353
  trochanteric, 3811–3820
Lipoidal histiocytoma, 2790, *2790*, 2791
Lipoma, 2878
  of hand and forearm, 3478, *3479*, 3480, *3480*, *3481*
  of thorax, 3656, *3656*, 3657
Liposarcoma, 2840
  of hand and forearm, 3489, 3490
Lister's tubercle, 2969
Lobectomy, in parotid tumor surgery, *2534*, 2535
Local flap. See *Flap, local.*
Lockwood's suspensory ligament, 864
Locus, 139
Lop ear, 1705–1709
Lower extremity. See *Extremity, lower.*
Luckett incision, 1711, *1711*, 1712
Lumbrical muscles, 2962
  in reconstructive surgery of hand, 3128, 3129, *3131*
    role of in finger extension, 3172
Lunate, dislocation of, 3045, *3046*
Lye burns, 1603
Lymph, flow of in disease states, *3570*
Lymph drainage, in tendon, 269
Lymph node dissection, in skin cancer surgery, 2832,
  2836
  regional, in malignant melanoma, 2849, 2850
Lymph nodes, popliteal, normal lymphangiogram of, *3575*
Lymphangiectasis, 2873
Lymphangiography, 3571, *3571*, 3572
Lymphangioma(s), 2796, 2873, *2873*, 2874, *2874*
  of eyelids, 874, *875*
  of hand and forearm, 3488
  of thorax, 3657, *3657*
Lymphangioma cavernosum, 2873
Lymphangioma cutis circumscriptum, 2873
Lymphangioma cysticum colli, 2873, 2874
Lymphangioma simplex, 2873
Lymphangioplasty, in lymphedema, 3593, *3594*
Lymphangiosarcoma, 2873
Lymphangitis, filarial, 3585
Lymphatic drainage, of abdominal wall, 3729
Lymphatic valve, 3567, *3568*
Lymphatics
  aplasia of, 3581, *3581*
  deep, of lower extremity, 3574, *3574–3577*
  foot, cannulation of, *3572*
  hypoplasia of, 3581, *3581*, 3582
  inguinal, iliac, and periaortic, *3576*
    obstruction of, 3588, *3589*, 3590, *3590*
  superficial, in lower extremity, *3553*, 3572, *3572*,
    3574, *3574*
  thigh, normal lymphangiogram of, *3574*
  varicose, 3582, *3582*
Lymphaticovenous anastomoses, 384–388
Lymphaticovenous shunts, in lymphedema, 3590, *3590*,
  3593, 3595

Lymphedema, 3567–3605. See also *Edema.*
  acquired, 3583
  anatomy of, 3571–3578
  congenital, 3579–3583
    increased intralymphatic pressures associated with,
      3570
  embryology of, 3567, *3568*
  experimental, 3590, *3591*, *3592*
  in neoplastic disease, 3583, *3584*, 3585, *3585*
  of upper extremity, 3585, *3585*, 3586, *3586*
  pathophysiology of, 3578–3585
  physiology of, 3567–3571
  treatment of, 3593–3602
    anastomosis of superficial to deep lymphatic system
      in, 3597–3601
    conservative, 3593
    excision of lymphedematous tissue in, 3595, *3596*,
      3597, *3597*
    lymphangioplasty in, 3593, *3594*
    lymphatic bridge procedures with pedicles in, 3593
    lymphaticovenous shunts in, 3593, 3595
    surgical, 3593–3602
    transposition of omental flap in, 3593
Lymphocyte, small, and graft rejection, 132, 133
Lymphocyte-defined (LD) antigen, 130, 131, 142–147
Lymphoid system, 131, 132, *132*
Lyophilization, of tendon, 285
Lysozyme, 1054

McBurney's point, 3728
MacFee incision, in intraoral tumor surgery, 2649, *2649*,
  2679, *2680*, 2685
MacFee neck flap, 2679, *2680*, 2682
McKenty elevator, *1133*
McKissock operation for breast reduction, 3676,
  3681–3683
Macrocheilia, 1544
Macrogenia, 1404
Macrogenitosomia precox, 3946
Macrognathia, mandibular, and condylar hyperplasia,
  1378–1382
Macromastia, *3809*
  mild to moderate, operation for, 3667, *3668*, *3669*
  moderate to severe, operation for, 3667–3676,
    3676–3683
  severe, operation for, 3676, 3684, *3685–3688*
Macrophage, 133
Macrotia, correction of, *1718*, 1719
Maffucci's syndrome, 2867, 2868
Magnesium sulfate, in microvascular surgery, 365
Major histocompatibility complex (MHC), 130, *131*, 142,
  145t
Malformations. See *Deformity.*
Malignancy, dermabrasion in, 453
  of inorganic implants, 409, 410
  radiation and, 534, 535, 546, *546*, 547
Malocclusion
  as cause of incompetent lip posture, *1291*
  Class III, *1459*, *1460*
  classification of, 647, *647*, 1292, *1292*, 1293
  in maxillary fractures, 700
Malunion, following corrective surgery of jaws, 1469
Mammaplasty, and cancer, 3708–3710
  augmentation, 3689–3704
    complications of, 3698, 3703, 3704
    fat grafts in, 254, *259*
    indications for, 3689, 3690
    methods of, 3690–3698

Mammaplasty (*Continued*)
  augmentation, methods of, dermis-fat grafts, 3691,
      3694, *3695, 3696*
    flaps of dermis-fat, 3690, 3691, *3692–3694*
    injection technique, 3690
    prosthetic implants, 3694–3698, *3698–3702*
  breast reduction. See *Breast reduction mammaplasty
      and mastopexy.*
Manchester method of bilateral cleft lip repair, 2078,
    2079, 2080
Mandible. See also *Jaws.*
  body of, bone grafting to reconstruct, 1485–1491
    combined step osteotomy and horizontal osteotomy
        of, 1357, 1358
    elongation by sagittal splitting of, 1358, *1359, 1360,*
        1361
    oblique lateral view of, *620,* 621
    osteotomies of in prognathism, 1317–1319
    techniques for lengthening of, 1353–1363
  condylar process of, 680, 681, *681,* 1521
    dislocation of, 687, 688
    evolution of operations on for prognathism, 1315,
        1316
    fractures of, 680–688
      classification of, 681, *681*
      diagnosis of, 681–683
      in children, 802–805
      roentgenography in, 683
      treatment of, 683–688
    hypermobility and dislocation of, 1526–1528
    osteotomies in for prognathism, 1319, *1320*
  coronoid process of, fractures of, 688
  duplication of, 2134, *2135*
  edentulous, fractures of, 688–692
  elongation osteotomies of body of, in mandibular
      micrognathia, 1347–1353
  embryology of, 2547
  evolution of operations on body of for prognathism,
      1313, 1315
  extraoral and intraoral approaches to body of, 1306–
      1308
  fibrosarcoma of, 2637, 2638, *2638*
  fractures of, 652–694
    Class I, treatment of, 665–670
    Class II, treatment of, 670–680
    Class III, treatment of, 688–692
    classification of, 653–656, *658*
    clinical examination of, 656–658
    complications of, 692–694
    compound comminuted anterior, treatment of, 669,
        669, 670, *670, 671*
    damage to teeth and alveolar structures in, 664, 665
    diagnosis of, 658–665
    direction and angulation of fracture line in, 662,
        663, *663*
    direction and intensity of traumatic force in, 664
    factors influencing displacement of fractured seg-
        ments in, 661–665
    in children, 798–805
    malunion of, 694, 1471
    nonunion of, 693, 694
    panoramic roentgenogram in, 624, *624*
    presence or absence of teeth in, 663, *663*
    respiratory complications of, 692, 693
    roentgenologic findings in, 659
    soft tissue at site of fracture and, 663, 664, *664*
    treatment of, 665–692
      with panfacial fractures, 739, *740, 741*
  growth of in patient with repaired cleft lip and
      palate, 2004–2006
  in cleft lip and palate, 2215, *2216,* 2217

Mandible (*Continued*)
  in intraoral carcinoma, 2688–2695
    conservative mandibular resection in, 2690–2692
    direct tumor spread to, 2688, 2689
    management of following mandibular resection,
        2692–2695
    osteotomy in, 2690
    pathologic aspects of, 2688, 2689
    surgical aspects of, 2689, 2690
    tumor spread to via inferior alveolar nerve, 2689
    tumor spread to via lymphatics, 2689
  in micrognathia, 1370
  median cleft of, 2134, *2134*
  muscles influencing movement of, 659, *659,* 660,
      661
  oblique lateral views of, *620, 621, 621, 622*
  occlusal inferosuperior views of, 619, *619, 620*
  osteogenic sarcoma of, 2637, *2637*
  osteomyelitis of, 693
  posteroinferior view of, 621, *622*
  postnatal growth of, 815–818
  ramus of. See *Mandibular ramus.*
  reconstruction of full-thickness defects of, 1472–1509
    alternative techniques of, 1502, 1503
    associated with loss of soft tissue, 1497–1502
    involving little soft tissue loss, 1481, *1481,* 1482
    methods of fixation in, 1474–1481
    primary bone grafting in, 1483–1497
    procedures to increase area of purchase for denture
        in edentulous mandible in, 1507–1509
    restoration of buccal sulcus and functional alveolar
        ridge in, 1503–1507
    restoration of continuity of mandible in, 1473, 1474
  resection of, in parotid tumor surgery, 2536
  skeletal osteotomy through, in jaw deformities, *1303*
  skeletal relationship of to maxilla, 1293, 1294, *1294,*
      1295, 1296t
  symphysis of, advancement osteotomy of, in Crouzon's
      disease, 2485
    oblique lateral view of, 621, *621*
  tumors of, 2547–2573, 2613, 2615–2621
    bone grafting in, 2616–2618
    flaps in, 2631, *2632, 2633, 2634, 2634*
    immediate reconstruction of, 2615, 2616, *2616, 2617*
    reconstruction following excision of, 2642–2696
    sulcus reconstruction in, 2618–2621
Mandibular arches, 2902
Mandibular asymmetry, *30*
Mandibular basal bone, growth of, 1993
Mandibular deviation, lateral, resulting from loss of bone,
    1382
Mandibular hypoplasia, 804, *804*
  in mandibulofacial dysostosis, treatment of, 2422–2424
Mandibular laterognathism, 1373–1382
  anterior open bite with, 1420, *1424*
Mandibular macrognathia, unilateral, and condylar
    hyperplasia, 1378–1382
Mandibular malformations, treatment of, 1306–1421
    surgical approach in, 1306–1308
Mandibular micrognathia, 1294, 1341–1373
  acquired, 1342
  bilateral, *1340, 1341,* 1342
  congenital, 1341, 1342
  developmental, 1342
  etiology of, 1341, 1342
  open bite with, 1421
  treatment of, 1344–1373
    contour restoration in, 1373, *1374*
    early surgical-orthodontic planning in, 1344
    elongation osteotomies of body of mandible in,
        1347–1353

Mandibular micrognathia (*Continued*)
  treatment of, operations on ramus to increase projection
    of mandible in, 1363–1373
    preoperative planning in, 1344–1347
    techniques for lengthening mandibular body in,
      1353–1363
    unilateral, 1342, *1343*
    variations of, and associated functional disturbances,
      1342–1344
Mandibular process, clefts of, 2120, 2121
Mandibular prognathism, 1309–1341
  children and adolescents with, 1338, *1339*
  classification of, 1309, 1310, *1311, 1312*
  etiology of, 1309
  surgical correction of, 1317–1340
    choice of procedure in, 1338–1340
    osteotomies of body of mandible in, 1317–1319
    osteotomies of condylar region in, 1319, *1320*
    osteotomies of ramus in, 1319–1334
  treatment of, 1310–1317
    evolution of techniques for, 1313–1317
    in edentulous patient, 1335–1338
    orthodontic versus surgical, 1310, 1312
    preoperative planning in, 1312, 1313, *1313, 1314*
  with microgenia, 1338
  with open bite, 1338, *1417,* 1418–1421
Mandibular prostheses, 2921–2928, *2929, 2930*
  in loss of lateral section of mandible, 2923–2928
  in loss of median section of major portion of body of
    edentulous or semiedentulous mandible, 2923,
    2925, 2926
Mandibular ramus
  evolution of operations on for prognathism, 1316,
    1316, 1317, *1317*
  extraoral and intraoral approaches to, 1308
  loose fragment of, intraoral fixation of, 1475, *1475*
  oblique lateral view of, 621, *621*
  operations on to increase projection of mandible,
    1363–1373
  osteotomies of for prognathism, 1319–1334
  reconstruction of, bilateral, 1495–1497
    bone grafting in, 1491, 1492, *1492, 1493*
Mandibular retrognathism, 1294, 1341–1373
Mandibulofacial dysostosis. See *Treacher Collins
  syndrome.*
Marcus Gunn test, 633, 635
Marginalis mandibularis, 1778
  reanimation of muscles supplied by, 1853, *1854,* 1855,
    1855
Marie-Sainton syndrome, 2408
Marlex mesh, 407
  in reconstruction of sternal defects, 3628, *3631*
Mass spectrometer, in evaluation of flap circulation, 196
Masseter muscle, *659,* 660, 1782, *1782*
  in craniofacial microsomia, 2374
Masseter muscle transposition, combined with fascial
  suspension, in facial palsy, 1807–1810
  electromyography in, 1791, *1791*
  in facial palsy, *1859*
Masseteric hypertrophy, benign, 1404–1406
Mastectomy
  radical, 3653, 3654
    defect after, 3711
    modified, 3710
    reconstruction of breast after. See *Breast, recon-
      struction of after radical mastectomy.*
  simple, 3710
  subcutaneous, with reconstruction, 3704–3706
  supraradical, 3710, 3711
Mastication, muscles of, 659, *659,* 660, 1782, *1782,*
  1783, 2374

Mastoid, cancer of, 2770
Mastopexy. See *Breast reduction mammaplasty and
  mastopexy.*
Maxilla. See also *Jaws.*
  adenoid cystic carcinoma of, *2726*
  anatomy of, 2435, 2436
  chondrosarcoma of, 2575, *2575*
  deformities of, 1421–1470
    classification of, 1422–1425
    dentoalveolar, 1422
      segmental osteotomies to correct, 1427, 1428
      surgical-orthodontic correction of, 1428–1439
    in cleft palate, 2194–2198
    preoperative planning and diagnosis in, 1425,
      1425
    skeletal, 1424, 1425
    surgical approach to, 1425–1427
  edentulous, fractures of, 703, 706, *706, 707*
  embryology of, 2547
  fractures of, 694–708
    airway management in, 700
    alveolar, 697, 700, *701*
    anatomical considerations in, 694–697
    and blindness, 707, 708
    cerebrospinal rhinorrhea or otorrhea in, 700
    classification of, 697, *697,* 698, *698*
    complications of, 707, 708
    control of hemorrhage in, 700
    etiology of, 698, 699
    examination and diagnosis of, 699, *699,* 700
    extraocular muscle imbalance in, 708
    in children, 805, 806
    lacrimal system obstruction in, 708
    malocclusion of teeth in, 700
    malunited or malpositioned, 702
    nonunion and malunion of, 708, 1471
    postoperative care of, 707
    pyramidal, *697,* 698, 702, *703, 704*
    roentgenographic findings in, 700
    transverse, 697, *697,* 700–702
    treatment of, 700–707
    vertical, 698, *698*
  growth of in patient with repaired cleft lip and palate,
    2002–2004
  in cleft lip and palate, 2214, *2214,* 2215, *2215*
  in Crouzon's disease and Apert's syndrome, 2471,
    2471, 2472
  reconstruction of, 1509–1513
  skeletal relationship of to mandible, 1293, 1294, *1294,
    1295,* 1296t
  squamous cell carcinoma of, 2574, *2575, 2586, 2653*
  tumors of, 2547–2573
    malignant, 2574–2588
      biopsy of, 2577
      classification of, 2574
      complications of surgery for, 2587, 2588
      etiology of, 2574
      examination and diagnosis of, 2576, 2577, *2577*
      incidence of, 2574
      local invasion of, 2575
      management of cervical metastases in, 2586
      metastases from, 2575, 2576
      pathology of, 2574–2576
      prognosis of, 2586, 2587
      roentgenologic examination of, 2576, *2577*
      treatment of, 2577–2586
        operative, 2578–2584
        radiation, 2585, 2586
Maxillary advancement, in cleft palate patients, 1447,
  1447, 1448, *1448*
  pharyngeal flaps and, 1452

Maxillary advancement *(Continued)*
 velopharyngeal incompetence following, 1451, *1451*, 1452, *1452, 1453*
Maxillary basal bone, growth of, 1993, *1993*, 1994, *1994*
Maxillary complex, effect of lip reconstruction on, 1998, *1998*
 effect of palate reconstruction on, 2000–2002
Maxillary displacement, in complete unilateral cleft lip and palate, 1990, *1990*, 1991, *1991*
Maxillary hypoplasia, 1295, 1424, *1447*
 bone grafting and osteotomy to correct, 2208, 2209
 cortical osteotomy in, *1305*
Maxillary micrognathia, 1295, 1424, 1439–1459
 choice of treatment methods in, 1440–1459
 onlay bone grafts in treatment of, 1441, *1441*, 1442, *1442*
 open bite with, 1411
 osteotomies in, 1442–1459
 prosthodontic treatment of, 1440, *1440*, 1441
Maxillary nerve, 866, 867
Maxillary osteotomies, teeth in, 1452, 1453
Maxillary process, clefts associated with, 2121
Maxillary prostheses, 2929–2937
 auxiliary means for increasing masticatory efficiency of artificial denture in, 2935, *2936*, 2937, *2937–2939*
 methods of retention of, 2932–2935
 temporary dentures as, 2929, *2931*, 2932, *2932*, *2933*
Maxillary protrusion, 1422
 associated with mandibular micrognathia, *1355*, *1356*, 1357, *1357, 1358, 1359*
 dentoalveolar, surgical-orthodontic correction of, 1428–1433
Maxillary retrognathism, 1295, 1424
 with open bite, 1411
Maxillary retrusion, 1422
 dentoalveolar, anterior, surgical-orthodontic correction of,1433–1439
Maxillary segments, in bilateral cleft lip and palate, 1952, 1953, *1954, 1955*
Maxillary sinus
 epidermoid cancer of, 2767, *2769*
 mucoepidermoid carcinoma of, total maxillary resection for, *2585*
 packing of, in zygomatic fractures, 715, 716, *717*
 relative increase in size of in adult vs. child's skull, *801*
Maxillectomy, total, in malignant maxillary tumors, 2578–2580
 via midfacial degloving incision, *2582, 2583*, 2584, *2584, 2585, 2585, 2586*
Maxillofacial prosthetics, 2917–2949
 ear, 2948
 extraoral, 2937–2942
 history of, 2917, 2918
 indications for, 2918, 2919, *2919*
 limitations of, 2948
 mandibular, 2921–2928
 maxillary, 2929–2937
 nasal, 2946–2948
 orbital restoration in, 2942–2946
 postoperative care in, 2948
 techniques of fixation in, 2919–2921
Maxillomandibular disharmony, correction of, 1466, 1467, *1467, 1468*
Mayer view, of temporomandibular joint, 623, 624, *624*
Meckel's cartilage, 815, *816*, 817, *818*, 2369, 2370
Meckel's diverticulum, 3728
Median cleft, false, 2132, *2133*
Median cleft face syndrome, 2128, 2129

Median nerve, 2961, 2975
 acroparesthesia or compressive neuropathy of at wrist. See *Carpal tunnel syndrome.*
 repair of, 3215–3242
Median nerve paralysis, splinting in, 2997
Median neuritis. See *Carpal tunnel syndrome.*
Mee's lines, 2978
Meibomian glands, 861
Melanocytes, 154
Melanoma(s)
 juvenile, benign, 2802, *2802*
 malignant, 2841–2853
  amelanotic, 2846
  chemotherapy of, 2853
  classification of, 2843–2849
  diagnosis of, 2843
  etiology of, 2842, 2843
  immunotherapy of, 2851–2853
  in nevus, 2842, 2846, *2846*
  incidence of, 2841, 2842
  lentigo, 2844, *2844*
  level of microscopic invasion in, 2846–2849
  nodular, 2845, *2845*
  of eyelids, 880
  of hand and forearm, 3464–3468
  preexisting nevi and, 2842
  primary therapy in, 2849–2853
  radiation therapy of, 2853
  regional node dissection in, 2849, 2850
  regional perfusion in, 2851
  spreading, superficial, 2844, *2845*
  subungual, 2845, *2845*, 2846
  sunlight and, 2842, 2843
  trauma and, 2842
 of cheek, *2630*
 of floor of mouth, 2636, *2637*
 of head and neck, 2636, *2637*
Melanosis of Dubreuilh, precancerous, 2805, *2805*, 2806, *2806*
Melanotic freckle, of eyelids, 878
 of Hutchinson, 2805, *2805*, 2806, *2806*
Meloschisis, 2142, 2145
Mendelian ratios, 117, 118
Meningioma, craniofacial surgical techniques in, 2490
Meningocele, 3750, *3750*
 surgical treatment of, 3753, *3754*
Meningomyelocele, 3750, 3751, *3751*
 surgical treatment of, 3753, *3755, 3760*
Meniscus, 661, 1521, 1522, *1522*
Mentalis muscle, 1781
Menton, 28, *28*, 1289, *1290*
6-Mercaptopurine (6–MP), and immunosuppression, 138
Mesenchymal bone, 313
Mesenchymoma, 2841
 of hand and forearm, 3482
Mesh grafts, 174, 175, *175*
Mesioclusion, 647, *647, 1292*, 1293
Mesonephros, 3828, *3828*, 3829
Mesotenon, 268, *269, 271*
Metacarpal arch, 2961
Metacarpal head, third, as anatomic center of hand, 2959, *2959, 2969*
Metacarpals, 2958, *2958*
 fractures of, 2970, *2970, 2971*, 3050–3053
Metacarpophalangeal joint arthroplasty, in arthritic hand, 3516
Metacarpophalangeal joint flexion, 3015, 3278–3280, *3281, 3282*
Metacarpophalangeal joint hyperextension, splinting in prevention of, *2996*, 2998, *2998*

Metacarpophalangeal joint stiffness, in burns of hand,
  3370, 3371, *3371*, 3377, *3377*, 3378, *3378*
Metacarpophalangeal joints, 2960
  divisions of extensor tendons at, 3064
  mobility of, 2970, *2972*
Metacarpophalangeal prostheses, in arthritic hand, 3516,
  3517, *3517*
Metacarpus, 2967
Metanephros, 3828, *3828*
Methionine, and wound healing, 93
Methohexital sodium, 587
Methotrexate, in treatment of skin cancer, 2839
Methoxyflurane, 587
Methyl α-cyanoacrylate implants, 393
Methylmethacrylate implants, 393
Michigan splint, 3390, *3390*
Microgenia, 1294, 1384–1404
  chin augmentation in, 1384, 1385
  diagnosis and preoperative planning in, 1384
  mandibular prognathism with, 1338
  technique of contour restoration in, 1385–1404
    by horizontal advancement osteotomy, 1387–1399
    by skin graft inlay and dental prosthesis, *1402*, 1403,
      1403, 1404
    using cartilage or bone grafts, 1385–1387
    using inorganic implant, 1399–1403
Micrognathia, *30*, *683*
  in mandibulofacial dysostosis, treatment of, 2422–2424
  mandibular. See *Mandibular micrognathia.*
  maxillary. See *Maxillary micrognathia.*
Micrognathia and glossoptosis with airway obstruction.
  See *Pierre Robin anomalad.*
Microlymphatic surgery, 384–388
Micromastia, unilateral, 3706, *3706*, 3707
Microphthalmos, 962–968
  operative procedure for correction of, 2460, *2461*, 2462
Micropore adhesive tape tube, in facial nerve repair,
  1795, 1796, *1796*
Microsomia, craniofacial. See *Craniofacial microsomia.*
  hemicraniofacial. See *Craniofacial microsomia.*
  hemifacial, 1676, *1677*
Microsutures, 346–348, *349*
Microtia, 1676–1705
  age factor in, 1678, 1679
  alternative methods of reconstruction in, 1696–1702
  avoidance of scarring in, 1679
  bilateral, 1709, 1710
  cartilage allografts in repair of, 1701
  clinical characteristics of, 1676, 1677, *1677*
  complications in, 1702, 1703
  correlation of with correction of associated deformities,
    1679
  hearing problem in, 1677, 1678
  in craniofacial microsomia, 2361–2366, *2393*
  inorganic implants in repair of, 1696, 1699, 1701, *1701*
  preservation of auricular contour in, 1679, *1680*
  preserved cartilage in repair of, 1701, 1702
  psychologic preparation of patient with, 1678
  reconstruction of with autogenous cartilage, 1683–1696
  secondary reconstruction in, 1703–1705
  skin cover in, 1679, 1680, *1681*, *1682*
  use of orientation markings in, 1680, *1683*
Microvascular clamps, 344, *344*, 345, *345*
Microvascular fascicular nerve grafting, 1797
Microvascular free bone grafts, 379–384
Microvascular free flaps. See *Flap, microvascular free.*
Microvascular needle holder, 343, *344*, 345
Microvascular occlusions, pathophysiology of, 348–354
Microvascular repair, 354–365
Microvascular surgery
  and replantation of amputated auricle, 1732

Microvascular surgery *(Continued)*
  anticoagulation in, 365–370
  history of, 340–343
  in contractures of cervical region, 1654, *1658*
  instrumentation for, 343–348
  patency rates in, 343t, 353, 353t, 354
  postoperative care in, 370–372
  principles of, 340–391
  technique of, 356–364
Midface, duplication of, 2135, *2135*, 2136, *2136*, 2137,
  2137, 2156, *2157*
  malunited fractures of, craniofacial surgical techniques
    in, 2488
Midfacial skeleton, deformities of, 1421–1470
  fractures of in children, 805–808
Midpalatal suture, absence of in cleft palate, 1964
Mid-sagittal plane, 28, *28*
Migration inhibitory factor, 134, *135*
Mikulicz's disease, 2530, *2530*, 2541, 2542
Milia, 454, 459, 2786
Millard island flap, 2273, 2277
Millard method of repair of incomplete bilateral clefts,
  2075, *2076*, 2077
Millard neurovascular island technique in cleft palate
  repair, *2101*, 2102
Millard rotation-advancement operation for cleft lip,
  2019, *2022*, 2028, *2028*, 2029, *2029*, *2030*, *2031*, 2032,
  2033, *2042*, 2043, *2044*, 2045
Millard two-stage repair of complete bilateral cleft lips,
  2077, *2077*, 2078, *2078*
Milroy's disease, 2873
Mirault-Brown-McDowell repair of cleft lip, 2017, 2019,
  2026, 2027, 2032, 2035, *2036*, 2037
Mirault operation for cleft lip, 2017, *2017*
Mitogenic factor, 134, *135*
Mitten deformity, 2322, 2325, 2326, *2326*, 2327
Mixed leukocyte culture test (MLC), 130, *130*
Möbius syndrome, *1810*, 2327–2332, *2333–2336*
  associated anomalies in, 2329, *2331*
  clinical course and physical characteristics of, 2327,
    2327, 2328
  diagnosis of in children, 2328, *2328*, 2329, *2329*, *2330*,
    2331
  diagnosis of in infants, 2328
  etiopathogenesis of, 2329–2332
  history of, 2327
  treatment of, 2332, *2333–2336*
Mohs chemosurgery. See *Chemosurgery, Mohs.*
Moles, pigmented, extensive, dermal overgrafting for,
  186
Molluscum contagiosum, 2781, *2781*
Molluscum sebaceum, 2814, 2815, *2815*, 2857, 2858
Monks-Esser island flap, 959, *961*, 962
Morestin, 10
Morris biphase fixation appliance, in maxillofacial
  prosthetics, 2921
Morris external fixation splint, *1476*, 1477, *1477–1480*
Mouth
  angle of, carcinoma of, tongue flap in reconstruction of,
    2674
  behavior of transplanted skin in, 2684
  burn contractures around, prevention of, 1608, *1608*
  deltopectoral flap in reconstruction of, 2739–2743,
    2744, 2745
  distortion of corner of, 1545, 1546, *1547*, 1559
  floor of, cancer of, 2609–2613, 2620, *2620*
    melanoma of, 2636, *2637*
    squamous cell carcinoma of, *2669*, *2678*
    tumors of, forehead flap in, 2668, 2669, *2669*
      nasolabial flaps in reconstruction of, *2683*
  reconstruction of corner of, 1573–1575

Mouth (*Continued*)
  reconstruction of paralyzed elevators of angle of, 1845–1848
  skin grafting in, 2651–2657
Mouth and cheek muscles, reanimation of in facial paralysis, 1852, 1853, *1853*
Mucoepidermoid carcinoma, of maxillary sinus, 2585
  of parotid gland, 2528, *2529*
Mucoperichondrial splint, principle of, *1122*, 1123, *1123*, *1124*
Mucoperiosteal flaps, in cleft palate repair, 2199, *2199*, *2200*
Mucoperiosteum, 1988
Mucopolysaccharide ground substance, 70, 89
Mucosal flap, apron, 1576, *1576*
  bipedicle, 1576, *1577*
Mucosal graft. See *Graft, mucosal.*
Mucotome, Castroviejo, 917, *918*
Mucous cysts. See *Cyst, mucous.*
Mucous membrane, nasal, 1053
Mucous membrane tube flap, 1576, *1576*
Müllerian ducts, 3828
Müller's muscle, *860*, 864, *864*, 865, *865*
Muscle(s)
  abductor digiti minimi, flap of in foot, 3558, *3558*
  abductor hallucis, mobilization of for flap, *3556*, 3557
  anterior digastric, 1782
  arrector pili, 154, 155, *249*
  auricular, 1782
  biceps femoris, muscle flap of, in pressure sore, *3788*
    myocutaneous flap of, 3561, *3561*, 3562
  buccinator, 1781
  caninus, 1781
  corrugator supercilii, 1782
  depressor septi nasi, 1051, *1051*, 1052, 1781
  digastric, 660, *661*, 1782
  dilator, 1781
  extensor carpi radialis, 2961, 2969
  extensor digitorum brevis, 297, *297*, 298
    graft of in eyelid paralysis, 1841, *1841–1844*
  extensor digitorum longus, flap of in leg defect, *3557*, 3558
  extensor pollicis longus, 2969
  external oblique, 3728
  extraocular, 752, *753*
    imbalance of, 708, 1000, 1001
    injury to, 1009
  facial, 1780–1782
  fat graft buried in, *256*
  flexor carpi radialis, 2961, 2969
  flexor digitorum longus, mobilization of for flap, 3556
  flexor digitorum profundus, 2961, 2962
  flexor hallucis longus, mobilization of for flap, 3557
  flexor pollicis longus, 2962
  frontalis, 931, 936–940, 1782, 1818
  gastrocnemius, mobilization of for flap, 3553, 3554, *3554*
    myocutaneous flap of, 3563, *3563*, *3564*
  genioglossus, 660, *661*
  geniohyoid, 660, *661*
  gluteus maximus, *3791*
  gracilis, myocutaneous flap of, 3562, *3562*, 3926–3929
  Horner's 862, *862*
  hypothenar, 2961
  in limb replantation, 3247
  internal oblique, 3728
  latissimus dorsi, flap of in chest wall reconstruction, *3623*
  levator palpebrae superioris. See *Levator palpebrae superioris.*

Muscle(s) (*Continued*)
  levator veli palatini, *1977*, *1978*, 1979–1981, *1982*, 1987, 1988
  lumbrical, 2962, 3128, 3129, *3131*, 3172
  mandibular, 659, *659*, 660, *661*
  masseter. See *Masseter muscle.*
  mentalis, 1781
  Müller's, *860*, 864, *864*, 865, *865*
  mylohyoid, 660, *661*
  nasalis, 1781
  occipitalis, 1782
  occipitofrontalis, 822, *822*, 823
  of abdominal wall, 3728, 3729
  of hand, 2971–2974
    in rheumatoid arthritis, 3513–3515
  of lip, 1542, 1543, 1966–1975
  of mastication, 659, *659*, 660, 1782, *1782*, 1783
    in craniofacial microsomia, 2374
  of mouth and cheek, 1852, 1853, *1853*
  of nose, 1043, 1044, *1046*, *1047*
  of palate, 1975, *1977*, 1978–1988
  of palatopharyngeal region, *1977*, 1978, *1978*
  orbicularis oculi. See *Orbicularis oculi muscle.*
  orbicularis oris. See *Orbicularis oris muscle.*
  palatoglossus, *1977*, 1984, *1986*, 1987, 1988
  palatopharyngeus, *1977*, 1982–1984, *1985*, 1987, 1988
  palmaris longus, 298, 299, 1844, 1845, *1845*
  pectoral, *3624*, *3625*
  pharyngopalatinus, *1977*, 1982–1984, *1985*, 1987, 1988
  pilomotor, 249, *249*
  platysma, 1781
  preseptal, 861, *861*, 862, *862*, 863
  pretarsal, 861, *861*, 862, *862*
  procerus, 1782
  pronator teres, *295*, 296, 297
  pterygoid, in craniofacial microsomia, 2374
    medial and lateral, *659*, 660
  pyramidalis, 3728, 3729
  quadratus labii inferioris, 1780, 1781
  quadratus labii superioris, 1781
  rectus abdominis, 3728, 3729
  rectus femoris, myocutaneous flap of, 3560, 3561, *3561*
  risorius, 1781
  serratus, *3626*
  skeletal, transplantation of, 293–300
  soleus, mobilization of for flap, 3554, *3555*, 3556, *3556*
  superior oblique, *859*, 860
  superior pharyngeal constrictor, *1977*, *1978*, 1984, 1988
  temporalis. See *Temporalis muscle.*
  tensor fascia lata, 332
  tensor tarsi, 862
  tensor veli palatini, *1977*, 1978, *1978*, 1979, *1979*, 1987
  thenar, 2961, 2975
  transversus, 3728
  triangularis, 1780
  uvular, *1977*, 1984
  zygomaticus, 1781
Muscle arrangement, in cleft palate, 1984, 1987, 1988
Muscle atrophies, denervated, 1784
Muscle contracture, intrinsic, in hand, 3126, 3128, *3129*, *3130*
Muscle deformities, in Romberg's disease, 2339
Muscle fiber length, in transplantation, 294
Muscle flaps. See *Flap, muscle.*
Muscle grafts, autogenous, in reconstruction of paralyzed face, 1841–1848
  cross-zygomaticus, in oral paralysis, 1846, 1847, *1847*
  denervation of, 294–299
Muscle necrosis, causes of, 3560
Muscle transplantation, neurotization in, 1807

Muscle transposition, cross-face nerve transplantation in combination with, 1855, 1857, 1858
   fate of, 3560
   functional disability associated with, 3560
   in facial palsy, 1806–1819
Muscle-rib flap, in chest wall reconstruction, *3626*
Muscular deficits, and speech, 2262
Musculature, extrinsic, of hand, 3130–3137
   intrinsic, of hand, 3124–3129
   of cleft lip and palate, 1966–1988
Musculocutaneous arteries, 192, *193*
Musculofascial flaps, in reconstruction of abdominal wall, 3732–3735
Myectomy, in facial palsy, 1827, 1828
Myelocele, 3751, *3751*, 3752
   surgical treatment of, 3753–3760
Myeloma, multiple, of jaws, 2570, *2570*
Myelomeningocele, 3750, 3751, *3751*
   surgical treatment of, 3753, *3755*, *3760*
Mylar implants, 392
Mylohyoid muscle, 660, *661*
Myoblastoma, granular cell, 2796, 2797, *2797*
   of hand and forearm, 3473, 3474
   of tongue, 2622, *2622*
Myocutaneous flap, 219, *220*, *221*, 222
   gracilis, vaginal reconstruction by, 3926–3929
   in reconstruction of lower extremity, 3560–3563
Myofibril, length of, in transplantation, 294
Myofibroblast, 84, 85, *85*, 283
   in Dupuytren's contracture, 3405, 3406
Myonecrosis, clostridial, of abdominal wall, 3739–3741
Myxoid cysts, 2792
   of hand and forearm, 3470, *3470*, 3471, *3471*
Myxoma, of hand and forearm, 3489
   of jaws, 2554, *2554*, *2555*
Myxosarcoma, 2840

Naffziger-Poppen Craig intracranial approach to orbital decompression, *972*, 973, 974
Nail bed, tumors of, 2979, 2980
Nail plate, fungal infections of, 2979
Nail-patella syndrome, 2980
Nails, of hand, anatomy of, 2976, 2977, *2977*
   color of, 2978
   deformity of, 3144, *3144*
   examination of, 2976–2980
   growth of, 2978
   hardness of, 2977, 2978
   injuries of, 3017, 3018
   occupational hazards to, 2979
   shape and surface contour of, 2979
   of toe, ingrown, 3530
Narcotics, 586
Naris (nares)
   anterior, 2307
   burn contractures around, prevention of, 1608, *1609*
   external, 1042, *1042*, 1052, *1052*
   internal, 1052, *1052*
   posterior, primitive, 2306, 2307
Nasal. See also *Nose.*
Nasal ala (alae)
   correction of in cleft lip-nose, 2180, *2180*, 2181, *2181*
   defect of, 1215, *1215*, *1216*, *1217*
   reconstruction of, 1246–1250
   resection of base of, 1091, *1092*, 1093
   retracted, secondary rhinoplasty for, 1157
Nasal alar margin, sculpturing of, 1093, *1093*

Nasal bones and cartilages, 1042, 1043, *1043*, *1044*, 1047, 1048, *1048*
   axial projection of, 616, *616*
   fractures of, *637*, *638*, 720–732
      anesthesia for, 726, *727*
      comminuted, 730, 731, *731*, *732*
      complications of, 731, 732
      compound, 731
      delayed treatment of, 731
      diagnosis of, 725, 726, *726*
      in children, 806, 807
      instrumentation for reduction of, 726–728
      malunited, 1130, 1131, *1131*
      treatment of, 726–731
      types and locations of, 723–725
   lateral views of, 613, 616, *616*
   squamous cell carcinoma of, *2833*
Nasal bridge, rib cartilage supporting, 303, *304*, *305*
Nasal cartilages. See also *Nasal bones and cartilages* and *Nasal septal cartilage.*
   accessory, *1045*, 1049, *1049*, *1050*
   alar, 1043, *1045*, 1048, 1049, *1049*, *1050*
   lateral, 1043, 1044, *1045*, *1046*, 1047, *1047*, 1048, *1048*
   septal, 1044, 1045, 1047, *1047*, 1048, *1048*
   sesamoid, 1049, *1049*
Nasal cavities, role of in speech, 2254, 2255
Nasal contour restoration, costal cartilage grafts for, 1147, 1148, *1148*
   iliac bone graft for, 1141–1147
Nasal deviations, 1117–1135
   classification of, 1117, 1118
   complications following corrective surgery for, 1134, 1135, *1136*, *1137*
   corrective surgery for, 1130, 1131, *1131*
   of bony portion of nose, 1118, *1118*
   of cartilaginous portions of nose, 1118–1120
   septum and, 1120–1122
   types of, 1117, *1117*
Nasal dorsum, 1041, *1042*
   cartilaginous, depression of, 1135, 1138–1140
   contour restoration of, in malunited naso-orbital fractures, 1016, *1018*
   depressed, 1135–1141
      various applications of iliac bone grafts for correction of, *1146*, 1147, *1147*
   excessive reduction of, correction of, 1157, 1158, *1158*
   osteocartilaginous, depression of, 1140
Nasal emission, 2269
Nasal escape, 2269
Nasal glioma, 1169, 1170, *1170*, 1171, *1171*, 1173
   orbital hypertelorism secondary to, *2459*
Nasal mucous membrane, 1053
Nasal placodes, 2304
   in cleft lip and palate, 1948, *1948*
Nasal processes, 2304
Nasal prostheses, 2946–2948
Nasal reconstruction, 1040–1287
   by methods other than forehead flap, 1266–1268
   forehead flaps for, 1226–1234
      island, with subcutaneous tissue pedicle, 1231–1233
      median, 1228–1231, 1233, 1234, *1234*, *1235*
      scalping, 1234–1263
         following extensive radiation, 1254, *1254*, 1255
      timing of reconstruction in, 1227, 1228
   in children, 1184
   subtotal, scalping forehead flap in, 1244–1256
   total, 1263–1268
Nasal sac, 2306

Nasal septal angle, 1042
Nasal septal cartilage
 dislocation of caudal end of, 1127–1129
 excessive resection of caudal end of, correction of,
  1158, 1159, *1159*
 total resection and transplantation of over dorsum of
  nose, *1128*, 1129, *1129*, 1130
 transplantation of, 305, 306
  to dorsum of nose, 1129, *1129*, 1138
Nasal septal flap, for restoration of skeletal framework of
 nose, 1256, *1256*, *1257*
Nasal septal framework, as transplant to increase
 projection of nasal dorsum, 1157, 1158, *1158*
 fractures and dislocation of, treatment of, 728–731
Nasal septal framework resection, and osteotomy, bone
 and cartilage grafting in conjunction with, 1148, 1149
Nasal septal graft, composite, *1246–1249*
 as lining for median forehead flap in nasal
  reconstruction, 1234, *1234*, *1235*
Nasal septal procedures, conservative, 1122–1127
Nasal septal surgery, in rhinoplasty, 1131–1134
Nasal septal-turbinate synechiae, traumatic, 1150
Nasal septum, 1044, 1045, 1047, *1047*
 and deviated nose, 1120–1122
 bony and cartilaginous, 721, *723*
 collapse of, *1121*
 embryonic development of, 2307, 2311
 fracture of, 725, *725*
 hematoma of, 728, 730, *730*
 in bilateral cleft lip and palate, *1951*, 1952
 in unilateral cleft lip and palate, 1957, 1958, 1959,
  1959, *1960*
 membranous, 1053
 perforation of, 1150–1152
 sensory innervation of, *1061*
 submucous resection and other techniques used in
  straightening of, 1121, 1122, 1132–1134
 use of for skeletal support of lower portion of nose,
  1256, *1256*, *1257*
 used for framework and lining in lateral nasal defect,
  1251
Nasal skeletal framework, 778, *778*
 anatomy of, 721, *722*
 primary grafting of, in subtotal and total rhinoplasty,
  1263, 1264, *1265*, *1266*
 restoration of by forehead flaps, 1256–1263
Nasal speech, in cleft palate, 2096, 2103
Nasal spine, protrusive, 1095, *1095*
Nasal splint, 728, *729*
Nasal stenosis, correction of, 1199, 1200, *1200*
Nasal surgery, corrective, 1055–1063
 anesthesia in, 1059–1063
 examination and diagnosis in, 1056
 in Crouzon's disease, 2485
 planning of operation in, 1056–1059
Nasal tip, 1042, *1042*
 bifid, correction of, 1116, *1116*
 broad or bulbous, correction of, *1109*, 1110, 1111, *1111*
 composite graft for repair of defect of, *1222*, 1223
 deformities of in cleft lip-nose, 2177, *2177*
 degloving of, 1108, *1108*
 deviated, correction of, 1116, 1117
 excessively pointed, correction of, 1116, *1116*
 increasing projection of, 1110, 1111, *1111*
 pinched, secondary rhinoplasty for, 1156, *1156*, 1157
 "plunging," correction of, 1113, *1113*, 1114
  secondary rhinoplasty for, 1158, 1159, *1159*
 projecting, correction of, 1114, 1115, *1115*, 1116
 round, correction of, 1111, *1111*, 1112, *1112*
 secondary deformities of, 1156, *1156*, 1157
 "smiling" or mobile, correction of, 1114, *1114*

Nasal tip exposure, complete, through rim incision, 1108,
 1108
 variations in technique of in corrective rhinoplasty,
  1105–1117
Nasal tip remodeling operation, 1110, *1110*
Nasal tissue, full-thickness loss of, 1209–1281
 evolution of forehead flap in, 1210–1214
 historical background of, 1209, 1210
 small to moderate-sized defects of, 1214–1225
Nasal valve, 1052, *1052*, 1053
Nasal ventilation, anatomical factors influencing, 1055
Nasal wall, lateral, scalping and median forehead flaps in
 repair of defects of, 1250, *1250*, 1251, *1251*
Nasalis muscle, 1781
Nasality, 2262
Nasion, 28, *28*, 1042, 1289, *1290*
Nasoalveolar cyst, 2565
Nasociliary nerve, 866
Nasofrontal angle, 1041
 prominent, deepening of, 1098, *1098*, *1099*
 transverse folds and redundant tissue at, correction of,
  1922
Nasolabial angle, 1042, *1042*
Nasolabial flaps. See *Flap, nasolabial.*
Nasolabial fold, *1042*
 basal cell epithelioma of, *2758*
Nasolabial reconstruction, use of wedge composite graft
 in, 1224, *1224*, 1225
Nasolacrimal duct, *980*, 981, 2307
Nasolacrimal furrow, 2307
Nasomaxillary complex, postnatal growth of, 819
Nasomaxillary dysostosis, 2465, *2466*, *2467*
Nasomaxillary hypoplasia, *1276*, 1277, *1459*, *1460*
Nasomaxillary skin graft inlay, 1201–1205
Naso-orbital cleft, and orbital hypertelorism, *2460*
Naso-orbital fractures, 776–785
 clinical examination in, 781, 782
 complications of, 789–792
 conjunctivorhinostomy following, 988, *988*, 989
 dacryocystorhinostomy following, 986
 diagnosis of, 781, 782
 in children, 806, 807
 malunited, 1005–1012
  and orbital fractures, complicated cases of, 1020–1026
 roentgenographic examination in, 782
 structural aspects of, 776–778, *1005*
 surgical pathology of, 778–781
 treatment of, 782–785
Naso-orbito-maxillary osteotomy, 1455–1458
Nasopalatine duct cyst, 2564, *2565*
Nasopharynx, cancer of, 2697, 2698
 reconstructive surgery of, 2697–2756
Neck, 597–2949. See also *Head and neck.*
 congenital cysts and tumors of, 2902–2916
  branchial. See *Branchial cysts and fistulas.*
  branchiogenic carcinoma, 2914–2916
  embryology of, 2902–2905
  of thyroglossal duct, 2905–2908
 congenital webbing of, 1659–1661
 deltopectoral flap in defect of, *2745*, 2747
Neck deformities, in Romberg's disease, 2339
Neck dissection, in parotid tumor surgery, 2536
 radical, 2593–2599
  accompanying deltopectoral flap in oropharyngoesophageal reconstructive surgery, 2734, *2734*,
   2735, *2735*, *2736*
  bilateral, 2598, *2598*, 2599, *2599*
  complications of, 2599
  incisions for, 2593, *2593*, *2594*
  partial and complete, 2593
  technique of, 2595–2598

Neck *(Continued)*
  radical, therapeutic and prophylactic, 2593, 2595
Neck flap, 2679, *2680*, 2682, 2719–2723
Neck skin, anterior, total loss of, 1643, 1644
Necrosis, and failure of skin graft, 180
  failure of flap transfer due to, 225, 226
Needle electrode examination, of hand, 2982, *2982*
Needle holder, microvascular, 343, *344, 345*
Neoplastic disease, lymphedema in, 3583, *3584*, 3585,
  3585. See also *Cancer, Carcinoma,* and *Tumors.*
Nerve(s)
  alveolar, 1470
  auricular, posterior, 1777
  biological processes in healing of, 99–101
  cable graft of, 3231
  cervicofacial, 1777
  cranial, anomalies of in craniofacial microsomia, 2376,
    2376, 2377
  digital, *3011*, 3012, 3237
  facial. See *Facial nerve.*
  frontal, 866, *867*
  in limb replantation, 3250, *3250*, 3251, *3251*
  infraorbital, 750, *750*, 866, *866*, 867
    anesthesia of, 1001, *1001*, 1002
      following orbital fractures, 791
    in zygomatic fractures, 711, *711*
  lacrimal, 866
  maxillary, 866, 867
  median. See *Median nerve.*
  mobilization of, 3230
  nasociliary, 866
  of abdominal wall, 3729
  of hand, 2974, 2975
    injuries to, 3009, 3078–3084
  olfactory, 2433, *2433*
  ophthalmic, 866, *866*
  peripheral, of hand and forearm, 3215–3242
    anatomy of, 3215–3217
    classification of injuries of, 3220
    factors influencing timing and results of repair of,
      3220, 3221
    metabolic changes in, 3217–3220
    results of repair of, 3223–3225
    special problems in repair of, 3225–3227
    technique of repair of, 3222, 3223
    tumors of, 3493–3496
  petrosal, greater superficial, 1775, 1786
  radial, 2975, 2996, 2997, *2997*, 3215–3242, 3269–3275,
    3276–3278
  repaired, when to explore, 3225, 3226
  supratrochlear and supraorbital, *859*, 860
  temporofacial, 1777
  to stapedius, 1775, 1777, 1786
  trigeminal, 1782, *1782*
  ulnar. See *Ulnar nerve.*
  zygomatic, 866, 867
Nerve action potential, evoked (NAP), 1789
Nerve anastomosis, 1860
Nerve branches, choice of in cross-face nerve
  transplantation in facial palsy, 1861, 1862
Nerve conduction test, in facial palsy, 1788, 1789
Nerve defects, management of, 3229–3234
Nerve entrapment syndrome, of hand, 3428–3448
Nerve grafting
  autogenous, vs. end-to-end suture in, 3228, 3229
  facial. See *Facial nerve grafts.*
  fascicular. See *Fascicular nerve grafting.*
  following resection of body of mandible and bone graft
    reconstruction, 1497
  in hand, 3227–3240

Nerve grafting *(Continued)*
  in hand, allografts and xenografts in, 3230, 3231
    procuring donor autografts in, 3231, 3232
    results of, 3234–3240
    tension at suture site in, 3227–3229
  interfascicular, 3231–3234, 3238, 3240
  sural, in facial paralysis, *1850*, 1852, *1852, 1859*
Nerve injuries
  following maxillary tumor surgery, 2587, 2588
  in proximal palm, wrist, and forearm, 3206–3212
  of hands, 3009, 3078–3084
  peripheral, electrodiagnosis of, 2986–2989
    of hand, Dupuytren's contracture after, 3407, *3407*
Nerve loss, following face lift operation, 1925, 1926
Nerve repair
  age and, 3220, 3221
  in hand, 3215–3242
  level of injury and, 3221
  primary vs. secondary, 3221
  special problems in, 3225–3227
  species and, 3221
  technique of, 3221–3223
  type of trauma and, 3221
Nerve severance, in hand, 3206, 3207, *3207*
Nerve sheath tumor, specific, of hand and forearm, 3493,
  3494
Nerve stumps, techniques used to reduce distance between,
  3230–3234
Nerve supply, in tendon, 269
Nerve transplantation, cross-face, in facial paralysis,
  1848–1864
Nerve transplants, choice of, 1861
Nerve-muscle transplantation, free, in combination with
  cross-face nerve grafting, 1855, *1856, 1857, 1858*
Nervous system deformities, in craniofacial microsomia,
  2375–2377
Nesbit procedure for correction of chordee, 3836, *3837*
Neural groove, of embryo face, 2302, *2302*
Neural tissue tumors, 2796, 2797, *2797*
Neurapraxia, 1784, 2966, 2986
Neurectomy, in facial palsy, 1827
Neurilemoma, of hand and forearm, 3493, *3494*
Neuritis, median. See *Carpal tunnel syndrome.*
Neuroblastoma, of mandible, 2624, *2625*
Neurofibroma, 2879, *2879*
  of eyelids, 874–877
  of hand and forearm, 3494, *3494, 3495*
  of nose, *1173*, 1175
  of thorax, 3654, *3655*
Neurofibromatosis, 2879, *2879*, 3494, 3495, 3654,
  3655
Neurogenic fibrosarcoma, of chest wall, 3652, *3652*
Neuroleptanalgesia, 588
Neurologic deficits, and speech, 2262
Neurologic disorders, in Crouzon's disease, 2317, 2318
Neurologic lesion, electrodiagnosis in location of,
  2984–2986
Neurolysis, 3226, 3227
Neuroma, in continuity, when to explore and when to
  resect a nerve with, 3226
  transplant, 1852, *1852, 1853*
  traumatic, amputation and, 3149–3151
Neurotization, *1861*, 1862, *1862*
  muscular and neural, *1856*
Neurotmesis, 1784, 2986
Neurotrophic ulcers, plantar, 3530
Neurovascular island flap, 219, *219*
Neutroclusion, 647, *647*, 1292, *1292*
Nevocellular nevi, 2797–2802
Nevoid basal cell epithelioma syndrome, 2822

Nevus (nevi)
  basal cell, linear, 2822
  blue, 2800, *2800*, 2801, 2861
    malignant, 2846
  darkening of after chemical planing, 460
  hairy, *30*
    coverage of by advancement flap, 203, *203*, *204*
    giant, malignant melanoma in, 2846, *2846*
  halo, 2801, *2801*
  intradermal, *2859*, 2860
  junctional, *2859*, 2861, *2861*
  linear, *2860*, 2861
  malignant melanoma in, 2842
  nevocellular, 2797–2802
  pigmented, 2859–2865
    dermabrasion of, 447, 449
    giant, 2800
    hairy, *2860–2865*
    of hand and forearm, 3464–3468
  sebaceous, senile, 2786, *2786*
  spider, 2795, 2796
  treatment of, 2861–2865
Nevus araneus, 2795–2796
Nevus cell nevus, 2798, 2799
Nevus cells, origin of, 2859
Nevus flammeus, 2792, 2793, *2793*. 2865, 2866, *2871*
Nevus sebaceus, 2787, *2787*
Nevus unius lateris, 2786, 2787
Nevus verrucosus, 2786, 2787
Nipple
  formation of by serial application of split-thickness
    grafts, *3722*, 3723
  Paget's disease of, 2812
  transplantation of as free composite graft, 3684,
    3685–3688
  transposition of on pedicle vs. transplantation as free
    composite graft, 3665, 3666
Nodular fasciitis, pseudosarcomatous, of hand and
    forearm, 3475
Nodulus cutaneus, 2790, *2790*, 2791
Norethandrolone, 284
Nose. See also *Nasal.*
  anatomy of, 1041–1055
    and nasal ventilation, 1055
    bony structures of, 1042, 1043, *1043*, *1044*, 1047,
      1048, *1048*. See also *Nasal bones and cartilages.*
    cartilaginous structures of, 1043–1049. See also
      Nasal bones and cartilages, Nasal cartilage, and
      Nasal septal cartilage.
    central pillar of, 1047
    columella of. See *Columella.*
    covering soft tissues of, 1041
    essential external landmarks of, 1041, 1042, *1042*
    individual and ethnic variations in, 1053, 1054
    membranous septum of, 1053
    muscles of, 1043, 1044, *1046*, *1047*
    nostril border of, 1049–1051
    physiologic considerations in, 1054, 1055
    structural framework of, 1042, 1043, *1043*
    vestibule of, 1052, *1052*, 1053
  bifid, 1178–1184
    in orbital hypertelorism, 2453, *2454*, 2455, *2456*,
      2460
  bone and cartilage grafting to, complications following,
    1149, 1150
  bony, defects of, secondary rhinoplasty for, 1154
  burn deformities of, 1636, *1636*, *1637*
  cartilaginous, defects of, secondary rhinoplasty for,
    1154, 1156
  chemosurgery on, 2883, 2884, *2884*, *2885*, *2892*

Nose *(Continued)*
  cleft. See *Cleft lip and nose.*
  congenital absence of, 1178, 1179, *1180*, 1181–1184
  cutaneous scars of, 1195, *1195*, 1196, *1196*
  deformities of, congenital, 1178–1184
    in mandibulofacial dysostosis, treatment of, 2424,
      2424
    of lining, 1199–1208
    of skin, 1195–1199
  deltopectoral flap in reconstruction of, *2746*, 2747
  early operations on, 4–8
  embryologic formation of, 1948, *1948*, 1949
  flat, 1135–1141
  foreshortened, 1271–1281
    burned, lengthening of, 1278, 1279, *1279*, *1280*
    external incisions in repair of, 1274, *1274*
    lengthening bony framework in repair of, *1276*, 1277,
      1278
    lengthening cartilaginous framework in repair of,
      1274–1277
    lengthening of after loss of nasal tissue, 1278
    postoperative, 1279, 1280, *1281*
  hump, rhinoplasty for. See *Rhinoplasty, for hump nose.*
  lacerations of, 635, *638*
  large full-thickness defects of, reconstructive rhinoplasty
    for, 1225–1268
  muscles of, 1043, 1044, *1046*, *1047*
  postchemosurgery reconstruction of, 2891, *2892*, 2893
  reticulum cell sarcoma of, *2838*
  saddle. See *Saddle nose deformity.*
  sensory innervation of, *1060*
  skin grafting within, 1200, 1201, *1201*
  small to moderate-sized full-thickness defects of lower
    portion of, 1214–1225
  soft triangle of, 1050, 1051, *1051*
  suspensory ligament of, 1051, *1051*
  tip-columella angle of, *1051*, 1052
  tumors of, benign, 1184
    congenital, 1169–1178
      embryology of, 1169, 1170, *1170*
      of mesodermic origin, 1177, 1178
      of neurogenic origin, 1170–1175
    malignant, 1192–1195
      basal cell epithelioma, 1192, 1193, *1262*, 1263,
        2824, *2825*
      choice of methods of repair of, 1194
      timing of reconstruction in, 1194, 1195
  weak triangle of, 1051, *1051*
Nose repair, arm flap technique of, 5, 6
Nose-chin relationships, *1057*
Nostril, embryonic development of, 2306
Nostril border, 1049–1051
Nové-Josserand method of reconstruction of urethra,
  3842, *3843*
Nylon implants, 392

Obturator, cleft palate, 2283–2293
  preparation of, 2284–2287
Obwegeser-Dal Pont sagittal osteotomy of ramus,
  1325–1334
Occipital artery, 1779
Occipitalis muscle, 1782
Occipitofrontalis muscles, 822, *822*, 823
Occlusion, functional, cleft palate repair and, 2094
Ocular complications, following orbital fractures, 790, 791
Ocular deformities, in Apert's syndrome, 2322, *2323*,
  2471, *2471*
  in Crouzon's disease, 2317, *2317*, 2471, *2471*

Ocular globe, 752
    injury to following maxillary tumor surgery, 2587
Ocular muscle imbalance, following orbital fractures,
    790
Ocular prostheses, 2942, 2943, *2945*
Oculoauriculovertebral dysplasia, 2408, *2408, 2409*
Oculomandibulodyscephaly with hypotrichosis, 2408
Odontogenic cysts, of jaws, 2563, 2564, *2564*
Odontomas, of jaws, 2553, *2553, 2554*
Olecranon, bone graft removed from, 1145, *1146*
    ulcer over, 3792, *3793*
Olecranon process grafts, 334
Olfactory nerves, 2433, *2433*
Olfactory pits, 2304
Olfactory placodes, 2304
Ombrédanne's method of reconstruction of urethra, 3839,
    3840
Omental autotransplant, in scalp defect, 837, *840*
Omental flap, in chest wall reconstruction, 3614, 3615,
    3615
    transposition of in lymphedema, 3593
Omentum, greater, closure of chest wall defect with,
    3614, 3615, *3615*
Omphalocele, 3741–3747
    closure of abdominal wall in, 3746, *3746*, 3747
    embryology of, 3741, *3742*, 3743
    preoperative management of, 3743, 3744, *3744*
    surgical correction of, 3744–3746
    with exstrophy of bladder, 3871, *3872*
Open bite, 682, *682*, 1295, 1406–1421
    anterior, 1406, *1407*
        dentoalveolar osteotomy for correction of, *1304*
        mandibular laterognathism with, 1420, *1424*
        mandibular prognathism with, *1309*
    complex mandibular deformity associated with, *1360*
    dentoalveolar, surgical-orthodontic correction of,
        1408–1411
    etiology of, 1406
    mandibular micrognathia with, 1421
    mandibular prognathism with, *1309*, 1338, *1417*,
        1418–1421
    maxillary micrognathia with, 1411
    skeletal, surgical correction of, 1411–1421
    surgical-orthodontic treatment of, 1407, 1408, *1408*
    traumatic, 1406, 1407, *1407*
Open reduction, and interosseous wire fixation, in
        fractures of zygoma, 715, *716*, 719
    in mandibular fractures, 674–676
    in maxillary fractures, 702, *704*
    in multiple facial fractures, 736–741
    of condylar fractures, 684, 685, *686*
    of mandibular fractures, 670, *672*
Open-sky technique, in treatment of naso-orbital fractures,
    783–785, *786, 787*
Ophthalmic nerve, 866, *866*
Ophthalmic prostheses, 2942, 2943, *2945*
Optic canal, 752
Optic cup, 2304
Optic foramen, 752
Optic foramen-oblique orbital position, 612, 613, *614*
Optic placode, 2304
Optic stalk, 2304
Optic sulcus, 2304
Optic system, embryonic development of, 2304, *2305*
Optic vesicle, 2304
Oral fissure, elongation of, *1573, 1574*, 1575, *1575*
Oral paralysis, treatment of, 1844–1848
Oral plate, 2303
Oral sphincter, reconstruction of, 1823–1826, 1844, 1845,
    1845, 1846

Orbicularis oculi muscle, *860*, 861–864, 1781, 1782
    hypertrophy of, *1879*, 1880
    reinnervation of, in eyelid paralysis, 1842–1844
        in facial paralysis, *1850*, 1851, *1851*, 1852, *1852,
            1853*
Orbicularis oris muscle, 1781, 1966, *1966, 1967, 1968*
    advancement flap of, in reconstructed lower lip, 1577,
        1578, *1578*
    dissection of with cleft lip repair, 2024, 2025
    in cleft lip, 2166, *2167*
Orbicularis sphincter, circumorbital Silastic string
    reconstruction of, 1838, 1839, *1839, 1840*
Orbit(s)
    bony, 2433–2435
    deformities of, 962–989
    exenteration of, 903–907
        in malignant maxillary tumors, 2580, 2581, *2581*
    floor of, 750, *750*, 2435
        blowout fractures of, 752–775
            associated with zygomatic fracture, *722*
            clinical examination in, 761–764
            diagnosis of, 761–766
            diplopia in, 757, 757t, 758
            enophthalmos in, 757t, 758–761
            "impure," 756, *757*
            in children, 756, *757*
            indications for surgical intervention in, 762, 763,
                763, 764
            mechanism of production of, 754, 755, 755t
            operative technique in, 767–773
            radiologic examination in, 764, 765, 766, *766, 767*
            sensory nerve conduction loss in, 763, 764
            surgical pathology of, 757–761
            timing of surgery in, 766, 767
            treatment of, 766–773
        extensive loss of, 1002–1005
    fractures of, blowout. See *Orbit, floor of, blowout
        fractures of.*
        in children, 807, 808, 813
        malunited, 990–1005
            surgical treatment of, 995–1005
        without blowout fracture, 775, 776
    osteotomy of in orbital hypertelorism, 2452, *2452*
    reconstruction of, *1510, 1512, 1513*
    fracture-dislocation of, malunited, 1031, *1032*
    fractures of, 748–793, 807, 808
        anatomical considerations in, 749–752
        blowout, 752–775, *991, 996, 997*
        classification of, 755t
        complications of, 789–792
        malunited, 989–1033
            and naso-orbital fractures, complicated cases of,
                1020–1026
    in Crouzon's disease and Apert's syndrome, 2469–2471
    injuries to soft tissues of, 632, 633, 635, *637*
    lateral wall of, 751, *751, 752*, 2434, 2435
        fractures of, 774
            malunited, 1026–1031
        osteotomy of in orbital hypertelorism, 2450, 2452,
            2452
        sagittal split of in orbital hypertelorism, 2447, *2448*,
            2449
        total mobilization of in orbital hypertelorism, 2449,
            2449, 2450
    medial wall of, 750, 751, *751*, 2435
        fractures of, 773, 774, *774*
            displacement of in naso-orbital fractures, 784, 785,
                785
            osteotomy of in orbital hypertelorism, 2450, 2452,
                2452

Orbits *(Continued)*
  roof of, 751, 2433, 2434, *2434*
    fractures of, 774, 775, *775*
      malunited, 990
    tumors of, 874–882
Orbital contents, advanced lesions involving, 903–907
Orbital decompression operations, 972–978
Orbital fat, 752
  protrusion of, *1879*, 1880
Orbital hypertelorism, *30, 32,* 2129, 2132, *2132,* 2138,
  2139, 2150–2153, *2154,* 2436–2459
  classification of based on interorbital distance, 2441,
    2441t
  in Apert's syndrome, 2322, *2323,* 2437, *2439, 2443*
  measurement of interorbital distance in, 2437, *2439*
  operative procedures for correction of, 2441–2459,
    2485, 2486
    bifid nose and bone grafting in, 2453, *2454,* 2455
    bone resection from anterior wall of interorbital space
      and exenteration of intranasal structures in, 2450,
      2451
    combined intra- and extracranial approach in, 2443,
      2444
    development of, 2441, 2442, *2442*
    exposure of skeletal framework in, 2444–2447
    extracranial (subcranial) approach in, 2443
    final procedures in, 2455, *2456*
    in children, 2455
    infraorbital osteotomy in, 2450, *2450*
    interosseous fixation and bone grafting in, 2453, *2453*
    intracranial approach in, 2442, 2443, *2443*
    medial canthoplasties in, 2453, *2454*
    mobilization of functional orbits in, 2452
    neurosurgical stage of, 2444, *2444, 2445*
    osteotomies of anterior cranial fossa and medial and
      lateral orbital walls in, 2450, 2452, *2452*
    osteotomy of orbital floor in, 2452, *2452*
    sagittal split of lateral orbital walls in, 2447, *2448,*
      2449
    subcranial approach in, 2443, 2455, 2457, *2457*
    supraorbital osteotomy in, 2447, *2448*
    total mobilization of lateral orbital wall in, 2449,
      2449, 2450
  pathologic anatomy of, 2437, *2440,* 2441
  postoperative treatment in, 2455
  preoperative radiographic planning in, 2457, *2458,*
    2459, 2460
  traumatic, 1031–1033
    craniofacial surgical techniques in, 2488
Orbital hypotelorism, 2120, 2132, *2133,* 2462–2465
  associated anomalies in, 2462, *2462,* 2463, *2463, 2464*
  correction of, 2476
  definition of, 2462
  differential diagnosis of, 2462t
  embryologic aspects of, 2463, 2464, *2464*
  surgical correction of, 2464, 2465, *2465, 2466, 2467*
Orbital restoration, 2942–2946
Orbital septum, *859,* 860, *860*
Orbitale, 28, *28,* 1289, *1290*
Orbitomaxillary region, anaplastic carcinoma of, *2727*
Orbitomaxillary resection, radical, deltopectoral flap
  following, *2748*
Orentreich punch, 229, *229,* 230, *230*
Oriental eyelid, surgical correction of, 947–956
Orientals, corrective rhinoplasty in, 1163
Oromandibular tumors
  anesthesia in, 2589, 2590, 2590t
  biopsy of, 2592, 2593
  composite operation for, 2624
  flaps in, 2624–2636

Oromandibular tumors *(Continued)*
  radical neck dissection in, 2593–2599
  reconstructive aspects of, 2589–2641
  tracheotomy in, 2590–2592
Oronasal fistulas, in cleft palate, 2198–2201
Oronasal membrane, 2306
Oropharyngoesophageal reconstructive surgery,
  2697–2756. See also *Esophagus* and *Pharynx.*
  carotid artery rupture following, 2754
  chylous fistula following, 2752
  complications of and their management, 2751–2755
  deltopectoral skin flap in, 2731–2747, *2748–2750*
    delay of, 2732, 2734
    design of, 2732, *2732, 2733*
    radical neck dissection accompanying, 2734, *2734,*
      2735, *2735, 2736*
  early hemorrhage following, 2751, 2752
  full-thickness skin grafts in, 2715
  general therapeutic considerations in, 2698, 2699
  infection and necrosis following, 2752–2754
  methods of repair in, 2699–2747, *2748–2750*
    local tissue techniques, 2699–2707
    transplantation of gastrointestinal tract, 2707–2712
    transplantation of skin, 2712–2747, *2748–2750*
  pathologic and anatomical considerations in, 2697,
    2698
  skin flaps in, 2715–2747, *2748–2750*
  skin graft inlay technique in, 2712–2715
  stenoses and fistulas following, 2754, 2755
Oropharynx, cancer of, 2698
  reconstructive surgery of, 2697–2756
Orthodontic appliance, edgewise, 1357, *1357*
  in Le Fort I osteotomy, *1445*
Orthodontics
  effect of on facial growth in cleft lip and palate, 2011
  in cleft lip and palate children, 2213–2234
  in jaw deformities, 1302–1305
  in mandibular prognathism, 1310, 1312
Orthopedics, effect of on facial growth in cleft lip and
  palate, 2011
Orthoplast isoprene splint, 1652, *1652*
Orthostatic lines of face and neck, 1870, *1870*
Orthovoltage, 532
Os magnum, 2969, *2969*
Osseous tumors, of jaws, 2566, *2566, 2567*
Ossicles, deformity of, 1720, *1720*
Ostectomy, of mandibular body, 1318, 1319, *1319*
Osteitis, in mandibular fractures, 693
  radiation, 535, 536
Osteoblasts, 314, 320–323
Osteocartilaginous exostosis, of hand and forearm, 3499
Osteochondroma, of hand and forearm, 3499
Osteoclasts, 314
Osteocytes, 313
Osteogenesis, 314–317
Osteogenic sarcoma. See *Sarcoma, osteogenic.*
Osteoma, of jaws, 2556, *2556, 2557*
  osteoid, of hand and forearm, 3499
Osteomyelitis
  chronic, ulcers associated with, 3553, *3554*
  in frontal bone defects, 848, 849, *851*
  of lower extremity, 3526, 3527, *3527*
  of mandible, 693
Osteon, 313, *313*
Osteoperiosteal flap, in correction of mandibular
  hypoplasia, 2423, *2423*
Osteoperiosteal grafts, in defects of cranium, 838, 839
Osteoradionecrosis, 535, 536
Osteotome, guarded, for internal lateral osteotomy, *1080,*
  1081, 1082

Osteotome *(Continued)*
  3-mm, for lateral osteotomy, *1080*
Osteotome technique, of resecting bony hump of nose,
  1076, 1077, *1077, 1078*
Osteotomy (osteotomies)
  advancement, horizontal, in correction of microgenia,
    1387–1399
    maxillary, choice of technique of, 1458, 1459
    naso-orbito-maxillary, 1455–1458
    premolar, 1433–1436
    segmental, premolar, in cleft palate repair, 2198,
      2198
      retromolar, *1448*
  and reduction of malunited fractures of zygoma, 1027,
    1027, 1028
  and septal framework resection, bone and cartilage
    grafting in conjunction with, 1148, 1149
  anterior segmental alveolar, for closure of mandibular
    dentoalveolar open bite, 1410, 1411
    for closure of maxillary open bite, 1410, *1410*
  C-shaped, for elongation of mandible, 1367, 1368,
    1369, 1370
  combined, 1453, 1454, *1454*
  cortical, in jaw deformities, 1304, 1305, *1305, 1306*
  dentoalveolar, in jaw deformities, 1304, *1304*
    set-back, *1428*
  double-step, in correction of microgenia, 1391, *1392,*
    1393
  elongation, of body of mandible, in mandibular
    micrognathia, 1347–1353
  expansion, 1453, 1454, *1454*
  for malunited naso-orbital fracture, 1013, *1013*
  in condylar region for prognathism, 1319, *1320*
  infraorbital, in orbital hypertelorism, 2450, *2450*
  interdental, in correction of mandibular micrognathia,
    1356, 1357
  L, 1347, *1348*
  lateral, in correction of hump nose, 1077–1083
  Le Fort I. See *Le Fort osteotomy.*
  mandibular, in intraoral carcinoma, 2690
  maxillary, complete horizontal low, 1442–1445
    segmental premolar (set-back), *1355*
    teeth in, 1452, 1453
    to correct skeletal deformities, 1442–1459
  medial, in correction of hump nose, 1081–1083
  midline palatal splitting, 1431, *1431*
  naso-orbito-maxillary, 1455–1458
  O-shaped, in orbital hypertelorism, 2443, 2457
  oblique, in microgenia, 1391, *1391*
    of mandible, 1362, *1363*
  of anterior cranial fossa and medial and lateral orbital
    walls, in orbital hypertelorism, 2450, 2452, *2452*
  of body of mandible in prognathism, 1317–1319
  of jaws, in craniofacial microsomia, 2377–2385,
    2394–2398
  of mandibular ramus for prognathism, 1319–1334
    horizontal, 1319, 1320
    oblique, 1323–1325
    sagittal-split, 1325–1334
    vertical, 1320–1325
  of orbital floor, in orbital hypertelorism, 2452, *2542*
  orbital, rectangular, 1031, *1032*
  perinasal, in repair of foreshortened nose, *1276,* 1277,
    1278
  posterior segmental alveolar, for correction of maxillary
    anterior or lateral dentoalveolar open bite, 1409, *1409,*
    1410
  premolar recession (set-back), 1428–1431
  premolar segmental, 1459
  recession, horizontal, in correction of macrogenia, 1404
  reverse-step, for closure of open bite, 1413, *1413*

Osteotomy (osteotomies) *(Continued)*
  sagittal, of mandibular ramus, 1325–1334
  sagittal-split, of mandibular body, 1347, *1349*
    of mandibular ramus, 1366, *1366,* 1367, *1367–1369*
  segmental, maxillary, complications of, 1436
    subnasal dentoalveolar, 1431–1433
    to correct maxillary dentoalveolar deformities, 1427,
      1428
  step, 1347, *1348*
    combined with horizontal advancement osteotomy,
      1395, *1395*
    retromolar, in correction of mandibular micrognathia,
      1361, *1361,* 1362, *1362*
  subcranial, in orbital hypertelorism, 2457, *2457*
  supraorbital, in orbital hypertelorism, 2447, *2448*
  transverse posterior palatal, for closure of anterior
    open bite, 1413, 1414, *1414, 1415, 1416*
    for closure of posterior open bite, 1414
  tripartite, in Crouzon's disease, 2480, *2480,* 2481, *2481*
  types of, for surgical-orthodontic correction in jaw
    deformities, 1303–1305
  U-shaped, in orbital hypertelorism, 2443, 2457, *2457*
  vertical, of mandibular ramus, 1364, *1364,* 1365, 1366
  vertical spur, of lateral orbital wall, 2475, 2476, *2476*
  Wassmund's reversed L-shaped, *1363,* 1364
  with bone grafting to correct maxillary hypoplasia in
    cleft palate, 2208, 2209
Otic capsule, structures derived from, 2369t
Otic pit, 2304
Otic placode, 2304
Otic vesicles, 2304
Otis urethrotome, 3888, *3889*
Otocyst, 1672, 2304
Otohematoma, 1732, 1735
Otomandibular dysostosis, 2407
Otoplasty, corrective, for prominent ear, 1713–1717
Outfracture, in corrective rhinoplasty, 1081–1083
Overbite, *1298*
  in cleft lip and palate, *2230,* 2231
Overgrafting
  composite, repeated, in repair of alar defects, 1225
  dermal. See *Dermal overgrafting.*
  in cheek defect, 1580
  in rhinophyma, 1191
  of skin flaps, 223
Overhealing, 89, *89. 90,* 91, *91*
Overjet, 1295, *1298*
  in cleft lip and palate, *2230,* 2231
Owens operation, for cleft lip, 2018, *2018*
  in complete loss of lower lip, 1570, 1571, *1571*
  in cheek defect, *1591,* 1592
Oxford technique of cleft palate repair, 2095, 2273, 2274,
  2277
Oxycephaly, 2502, *2505, 2506*
  in Apert's syndrome, *2469*
  in Crouzon's disease, 2468, *2468*
Oxygen, hyperbaric, 202

Pachydermatocele, of thorax, 3654, 3656, *3656*
Padgett, Earl C., 14
Padgett skin graft mesher, 174, 175, *175*
Padgett-Hood dermatome, 14, 167, *167,* 171, 172
Paget's disease, extramammary, 2812, *2812*
  of nipple, 2812
Palatal appliance, for newborn with cleft lip and palate,
  2221, 2222, *2222,* 2223
  lift, 2291–2293
  split-plate, 1305, *1306*
Palatal lengthening procedures, 2092

Palatal process(es), 2309
  in unilateral cleft lip and palate, 1959
  positional change in, growth, and fusion of, 1947, *1947*
Palatal push-back procedures, 2272–2274, 2277
Palate
  cleft. See *Cleft palate, Cleft lip and palate,* and *Cleft lip, bilateral, with bilateral cleft of primary palate.*
  deltopectoral flap in defect of, *2748*
  hard, oblique superoinferior posterior occlusal view of, 617, *618*
    reconstruction of, *1510,* 1511, *1511, 1512,* 1513, *1513*
    superior inferior occlusal views of, 616, 617, *617, 618*
  muscles of, 1975, *1977,* 1978–1988
  primary, bilateral cleft of, with bilateral cleft lip. See *Cleft lip, bilateral, with bilateral cleft of primary palate.*
  formation of, 1934, *1934*
  primitive, 2307, 2312
Palate reconstruction, effect of on maxillary complex, 2000–2002
  with compund cervical flap, 2723–2730
Palate repair, anterior, in bilateral cleft lip with bilateral cleft of primary palate, 2060, *2061,* 2062, *2062*
Palatofacial reconstruction, forehead flap in, *2716*
Palatoglossus muscle, *1977,* 1984, *1986,* 1987, 1988
Palatopharyngeal region, muscles of, *1977,* 1978, *1978*
Palatopharyngeus muscle, *1977,* 1982–1984, *1985,* 1987, 1988
Palatoplasty and primary pharyngeal flap, in cleft palate repair, 2096–2102
Palm, flexor tendon injuries in, 3070
  proximal, nerve and tendon injuries in, 3206–3212
Palmar amputations, transverse and ulnar oblique, *3147,* 3148, *3148,* 3149, *3149*
Palmar fasciotomy, in Dupuytren's contracture, 3413, 3419, *3419*
Palmaris longus muscle, 298, 299
Palmaris longus muscle graft, in oral paralysis, 1844, 1845, *1845*
Palmaris longus tendon, *269,* 272–275
  as free graft, 3198, 3199, *3199*
Palpebral deformities, in facial palsy, correction of, 1832–1834
Palpebral fissure, closure of, 864, 865, *865*
  elongation of, in burn ectropion of eyelids, 1630, *1631*
Palsy, facial. See *Facial palsy.*
Panniculus adiposus, 155
Panniculus carnosus, 155
Papillary cystadenoma lymphomatosum, of parotid gland, 2527, *2527*
Papillary layer, *153,* 154
Papilloma, basal cell, 2781–2783
Paralysis
  facial. See *Facial palsy.*
  median nerve, 2997
  of eyelid. See *Eyelid, paralyzed.*
  of hand. See *Hand, partially paralyzed.*
  oral, treatment of, 1844–1848
  radial nerve, 2996, 2997, *2997,* 3269–3275, *3276–3278*
  ulnar nerve, 2998, *3281, 3300,* 3301, *3301, 3302*
Paralytic ectropion, 909
Paranasal sinuses, advanced cancers of, 2767–2770
  malignant tumors of, 2574
Paraplegia, and pressure sores, 3767–3769
Paratenon, 266, 271, *271*
Parathyroid gland, early development of, 2904, *2904*
Paré, Ambroise, 5, 46, 47, *47*
Parotid duct, lacerations of, 630–632, *635, 636*
  transposition of for correction of excessive drooling, 2543, 2544, *2544*

Parotid gland, anatomy of, 2523, *2523,* 2524
  embryology of, 2524, 2525
  tumors of, 2522–2538
    benign, 2525t, 2527, 2528
    chemotherapy of, 2536
    complications of surgery for, 2537, 2538
    diagnosis of, 2530, *2530,* 2531, 2531t
    differential diagnosis of, 2530, *2530,* 2531, 2531t
    history of, 2522
    malignant, 2526t, 2528–2530
    mixed, 2525, *2526,* 2527, *2527, 2532*
    pathology of, 2525, 2525t, 2526t
    radiation therapy of, 2536
    results of surgery for, 2536, 2537, *2537*
    treatment of, 2531–2537
Parotitis, suppurative, acute, 2540, 2541, *2541*
Passavant's pad, *1986,* 1988
Passavant's ridge, 2271, *2272*
Pectoral muscle flap, in chest wall reconstruction, *3624, 3625*
Pectus carinatum, 3646–3652
  etiology of, 3646
  surgical techniques in, 3647–3652
  symptoms and signs of, 3646
  types of, 3646, *3646*
Pectus excavatum, 3633–3645
  cardiopulmonary function in, 3635, 3636
  etiology of, 3634
  funnel costoplasty in, 3641, *3643*
  indications for surgical correction of, 3636
  internal and external fixation in, 3641–3645
  operative procedure in, 3636–3645
  Ravitch technique of correction of, 3637, *3638–3640,* 3641
  roentgenographic studies in, 3636
  silicone prostheses in, 3644, *3645*
  sternoturnover procedure in, 3641, *3642*
  Strib internal fixation in, 3643, *3644, 3645*
  symptoms of, 3635
Pedicle flap. See *Flap, pedicle.*
Pendulum flap, 2174, *2176*
Penetrance, genetic, 119
Penicillamine, 93, 94
Penile rod, construction of for impotence, *3966*
Penis, *3828, 3829, 3831*
  chordee of. See *Chordee.*
  correction of in hypospadias, 3835, 3836, *3836, 3837*
  degloved, *3903*
  double, 3832
  fibrous plaque of, 3895–3900
  radical excision of for carcinoma, *3914*
  reconstruction of, 3909–3919
    complications in, 3918, 3919
    etiology of, 3909
    history of, 3909, 3910
    in true hermaphroditism, *3947, 3950*
    technique of, 3910–3916
  replantation of, 384, *385,* 3916, 3918, *3918*
  resurfacing shaft of with scrotal skin, 3906, *3907, 3908*
  skin grafting of after avulsion, *3905*
  squamous cell carcinoma of, *3908*
Penoscrotal skin, combined avulsion of, 3906–3908
Penrose drain, as finger tourniquet, 3012, *3013*
Pentadactyly, 3338, *3339*
Pentazocine, 586
Penthrane, 587
Pentothal sodium, 587
Perforators, 192, 193
Perichondrium, joining nasal accessory cartilages, 1049, *1050*
Pericranium, *822,* 823

Periderm, 2312
Perilunate dislocations, 3045, 3046, *3046*
Perineurium, 3216, *3216*
Periodontal disease, and temporomandibular joint
    pain, 1524
Perioral region
    .burn contractures of, 1608, *1608, 1609*
    burn deformities of, 1636–1638
    electrical burns of, 1639, 1640
    postchemosurgery reconstruction of, *2893*, 2894
Periorbita, 752, 2435, *2435*
Periorbital region, chemosurgery in, 2884, 2886
Periosteal elevator, 1068, *1068*
    Joseph, *1102, 1103*
Periosteal flap, in chest wall reconstruction, *3627*
Periosteum, in osseous regeneration, 320
Peripheral nerve blocks, in acute hand injuries, 3010,
    3011, 3012
Peripheral nerves of hand. See *Nerves, peripheral, of
    hand.*
Persantin, in microvascular surgery, 365, 368, 369
Petrosal nerve, greater superficial, 1775, 1786
Peutz-Jeghers syndrome, melanin nail bands in,
    2978
Peyronie's disease, 3895–3900
    diagnosis of, 3895, 3896, *3896*
    etiology of, 3895
    pathologic physiology of, 3896
    results of surgery for, 3900
    signs and symptoms of, 3895
    surgical technique in, 3897–3900
    .treatment of, 3896
Pfeiffer's syndrome, 2466, 2468
Phalangeal ligament, distal, 2977, *2977*
Phalanx (phalanges), 2967
    delta, 3332, *3332*
    fractures of, 3053–3056
    proximal, extensor tendon injuries over, 3064
    ungual, composite injuries of, 3143, *3143*, 3144
Phalloplasty, reconstructive, 3909–3919
Phallus, 3831
Pharyngeal constrictor muscle, superior, *1977, 1978*,
    1984, 1988
Pharyngeal flap. See *Flap, pharyngeal.*
Pharyngeal wall, early development of, 2902, *2903*
    faulty development of, 2909, *2910*
    tumors of, forehead flap in, 2669–2671, *2671, 2680*,
    2681
Pharyngobucco-orbicularis oris sphincter, 1781, *1781*
Pharyngopalatinus muscle, *1977*, 1982–1984, *1985*,
    1987, 1988
Pharyngoplasty, 2092, 2271, 2272, *2272, 2273*, 2777,
    2278
    augmentation, 2274, *2274*, 2277
Pharynx. See also *Oropharyngoesophageal reconstruc-
    tive surgery.*
    malignant lesions of, 2697, 2698
    reconstructive surgery of, 2697–2756
    retrocricoid, laryngotracheal substitution for, 2705–
    2707
Phenol, 454, 455, *455*, 457, 458
Phenoxybenzamine, 198
Phenylalanine mustard, in treatment of malignant
    ·melanoma, 2851
Philtral ridges, formation of, *1945*, 1946
Philtrum, reconstruction of in cleft lip, 2169–2171
Photography, in facial injuries, 625, 626
    medical, 35–38, *40, 41*
Photons, 532
Photoplethysmograph, in evaluation of flap circulation,
    195

Pierre Robin anomalad, 1660, *1663, 1963*, 1964, 2005,
    2005, 2006, 2235–2245
    associated congenital defects in, 2239
    cleft palate prosthetics in, 2286, *2286*, 2287, *2287*
    complications in, 2243, 2244
    diagnosis of, 2238, *2238*, 2239
    etiology of, 2237, 2238
    fascia transplantation in, 262
    feeding problems in, 2238
    growth and development in, 2241, 2243
    historical aspects of, 2236, 2237
    operative technique in, 2241, *2242*
    respiratory obstruction in, 2238
    tongue displacement in, 2238, 2239
    treatment of, 2239–2241
Pigeon breast. See *Pectus carinatum.*
Pigment formation, after dermabrasion, 444
Pilar cysts, 2784–2786
Pilomatrixoma, 2787, 2788
Pilomotor function, in skin grafts and flaps, 228
Pilomotor muscles, in dermis graft, 249, *249*
Pin fixation, external, in mandibular fractures, 692, *692*
    of fractures of zygoma, 719
Pin fixation appliances, external, in mandibular
    fractures, 669, *670*, 676
Pinched tip deformity, 1156, *1156*, 1157
Pinna, primitive, 2313
Pitanguy technique of breast reduction, 3676, *3677–3680*
Plagiocephaly, 2502, *2505, 2506*
    in Crouzon's disease, 2468, *2468*
Planing, chemical. See *Chemical planing.*
    surgical. See *Dermabrasion.*
Plantaris tendon, 275–277
Plasmatic circulation, 157, 158
Plastic, polyvinyl, in maxillofacial prosthetics, *2940*,
    2941, 2942, *2944*
Plastic surgery
    airway management in, 588–591
    anesthesiologist's role in, 585–595
    anesthetic agents used in, 587, 588
    ·bleeding problem in, 591, 592, 592t
    definition of, 3, 4
    general principles of, 1–595
    history of, 4–21
        during nineteenth century, 6–9
        during Renaissance, 5, 6
        during seventeenth and eighteenth centuries, 6
        during twentieth century, 9–21
    induced hypotension in, 592, 593
    introduction to, 3–68
    nasal intubation in, 589, *590*
    oral intubation in, 588, *589, 590*
    premedication in, 586, 587
    psychiatric aspects of, 549–564
        concept of deformity in, 550–552
        in postoperative period, 554, 555
        neurotic or psychotic patient in, 555–557
        problem patient in, 557–562
        psychosocial sequelae to, 562, 563
        surgeon-patient relationship in, 552–554
    scope of, 21–23
    social science approach to, 565–584
    technique of, 46–64
        infections in, 50, 51
        pressure dressings in, 49, 50
        raw area, straight line, and wound tension in, 54–64
        repeated partial excisions in, 64
        suturing in, 46–49
        transplantation in, 52–54
        W-plasty in, 60–64
        Z-plasty in, 54–60

Plastic tape, in wound closure, 641, *646*
Platelets, and microvascular occlusion, 349
Platysma muscle, 1781
Pleural space, closure of in chest wall reconstruction, 3617, 3621, *3622*, 3623, *3623–3625*
Plexiform ameloblastoma, of jaws, 2550, *2551*
Plummer-Vinson syndrome, nails in, 2979
Plunging tip deformity, secondary rhinoplasty for, 1158, 1159, *1159*
Pluronic F-68, in microvascular surgery, 369, 370
  in treatment of cold injury, 524, 526
Pneumothorax, 3610
Pocket ear, 1709, *1709*
Pockmarks, dermabrasion for, 446, 447
Pogonion, 28, *28*
Poland's syndrome, hand deformities in, 3311, *3311*, 3313
Polydactyly, surgical management of, 3319–3325
Polyethylene implants, 392, 393
Polyfluroethylene, 402
Polyglycerylmethacrylate, 410
Polymastia, 3707
Polymorphism, 139
Polymorphonuclear leukocytes, sex differences in, 3932, 3933, *3933*
Polypropylene implants, 392, 393
Polythelia, 3707
Polyvinyl alcohol synthetic material, in treatment of Romberg's disease, *2345*
Polyvinyl plastic, in maxillofacial prosthetics, *2940*, 2941, 2942, *2944*
Popliteal lymph nodes, *3575*
Porcine skin, 190, 191
Pore prominence, after chemical planing, 460
Poroma, eccrine, 2788, *2788*, 2789
Port-wine stain, 2792, 2793, *2793*, 2865, 2866, *2871*
  dermabrasion of, 449
Postauricular flap, 1581, *1582*, *1584*, 1739, *1739*
Pouce floutant, 3338, *3339*
Preauricular flap, 1581, *1582*
Preauricular sinuses, 2910, 2911, *2911*
Premaxilla, in bilateral cleft lip with bilateral cleft of primary palate, 2048, *2049*, 2050–2059, 2087
  surgical setback of, in bilateral cleft lip repair, 2055, *2055, 2056*, 2057
Premaxillary displacement, in complete bilateral cleft lip and palate, 1991, *1991*, 1992, *1992*
Premaxillary malformation, in bilateral cleft lip and palate, 1950, 1951, *1951*, 1952
Premaxillary protrusion, in bilateral cleft lip and palate, cause of, 1956, 1957
Premaxillary segment, in bilateral cleft lip and palate, 1955, *1955, 1956, 1956*
  in unilateral cleft lip and palate, 1957, 1958, *1958*
Prepuce, 3832, *3833*
Preputial skin, as donor site for full-thickness skin grafts, 165
Preseptal muscle, 861, *861*, 862, *862, 863*
Pressure bolus grafting, in intraoral tumor surgery, 2655–2657, *2658*
Pressure dressings, 49, 50
  for split-thickness skin grafts, 177
  using dental appliance, in intraoral reconstructive surgery, 2652–2655
  with full-thickness skin grafts, 165, 166, *166*
Pressure sore, 3763–3799. See also *Ulcers.*
  anemia in, 3774
  bipedicle flaps in, 3781, *3781*
  clinical aspects of, 3766, 3767, 3772, 3773
  closed by rotation flap, scar in, 421, 422, *422*
  complications of, 3796, 3797
  double rotation flaps in, 3781, *3781, 3790*

Pressure sore *(Continued)*
  etiology of, 3764–3770
  excision and closure of, 3780
  experimental studies of, 3765, 3766
  history of, 3763, 3764
  multiple, 3792–3796
  muscle flap in, *3788, 3791*
  neurovascular island flaps and free flaps in, 3781, 3782
  nutritional measures in, 3773, 3774
  paraplegia in relation to, 3767–3769
  pathology of, 3770–3772
  relief of pressure in, 3775–3778
  relief of spasm in, 3774, 3775
  roentgenographic studies of, 3778
  skin grafts in, 3780
  spasticity and, 3769
  treatment of, 3773–3797
    local, 3778–3797
      conservative, 3778, 3779
      surgical, 3779–3797
    systemic, 3773–3778
  tube flaps in, 3780, 3781
  tumbler flaps in, 3781
  V-Y advancement flaps in, 3781
Pretarsal muscle, 861, *861*, 862, *862*
Pretibial ulcers, 3792
Prickle cell epithelioma, 2812–2814
Prickle cell layer, 153
Primordial cysts, of jaws, 2563
Proboscis, bilateral, *1180*, 1181
Procerus muscle, 1782
Procollagen peptidase, 88
Progeria, 1877
Prognathism, 1294, 1295
  mandibular. See *Mandibular prognathism.*
  pseudomandibular, 1295, 1310
Prolabial mucosal advancement flap, in repair of deficient buccal sulcus, 2172, *2172*
Prolabium, in bilateral cleft lip, 1970–1975
  with bilateral cleft of primary palate, 2048, *2049*, 2050
Promethazine, 284
Pronator teres muscle, transplantation of, *295, 296*, 297
Pronephros, 3828, *3828*
Proplast, 402
Propranolol, 586, 587
Prosencephalon, 2128
Prostaglandins, 85
Prostate, metastatic carcinoma to jaws from, *2572*
Prostatic urethra, 3883, *3884*
Prostheses. See also *Implants, inorganic.*
  auricular, 1750
  ·dental, and skin graft inlay, in microgenia, *1402*, 1403, *1403*, 1404
  ear, 2948
  for hand, 3090–3096, *3097–3099*
  in reconstruction of abdominal wall, 3737–3739, *3739*
  mandibular. See *Mandibular prostheses.*
  maxillary. See *Maxillary prostheses.*
  metacarpophalangeal, 3516, 3517, *3517*
  nasal, 2946–2948
  ocular, 2942, 2943, *2945*
  ophthalmic, 2942, 2943, *2945*
  silicone, in pectus excavatum, 3644, *3645*
Prosthetic implants, in augmentation mammaplasty, 3694–3698, *3698–3702*
  in chest wall reconstruction, 3627, 3628
Prosthetic replacement, in arthritic hand, 3508, 3509, *3509*, 3510, *3510*, 3516, 3517, *3517*
Prosthetics, cleft palate. See *Cleft palate prosthetics.*
  maxillofacial. See *Maxillofacial prosthetics.*

Prosthodontic treatment, of maxillary micrognathia, 1440, *1440*, 1441
Prosthodontics, and surgery, in correction of jaw deformities, 1303
Protective position, of hand, temporary immobilization ·in, 3014, 3015
Protein, fibrous, structure and synthesis of, 86–89
Protein depletion, and wound healing, 93
Pseudo-Crouzon's disease, 2465
Pseudohypernasality, 2271
Pseudomandibular prognathism, 1295, 1310
Pseudosarcomatous nodular fasciitis, of hand and forearm, 3475
Pterygium colli, 1659–1661
Pterygoid muscles, *659*, 660, 2374
Ptosis
    congenital, construction of supratarsal fold in, *953*, 954
    following esthetic blepharoplasty, 1894
    levator resection operation for, 922–931
    of breasts, *3812*
    of eyebrows, *1879*, 1880
    of upper eyelid, 918–920, 920t, 1009, *1011*
        in Crouzon's disease and Apert's syndrome, 2472, *2479*, 2485
        traumatic, primary and late primary repair of, 921, 922, *922*
Punch graft technique, 229, *229*
Punctum, cicatricial stenosis of, 982, 983
Purine analogues, and immunosuppression, 138
Pyogenic granuloma. See *Granuloma, pyogenic.*
Pyramidalis muscle, 3728, 3729
Pyrex beads, for correction of enophthalmos in nonseeing eye, 998, *999, 1000*
Pyriform aperture, 1043, *1044*
Pyrimidine analogues, and immunosuppression, 138
Pyrolytic graphite, 402

Q-banding, 111, *112, 114*
Quadratus labii inferioris muscle, 1780, 1781
Quadratus labii superioris muscle, 1781
Quilted grafting, in intraoral tumor surgery, 2657, *2659*

R-banding, 111, *113, 114*
Rad, 532
Radial artery, 2976
Radial longitudinal deficiencies, 3337–3348
Radial nerve, 2975
    repair of, 3215–3242
Radial nerve paralysis, 3269–3275, *3276–3278*
    splinting in, 2996, 2997, *2997*
Radial ray deficiency state, 3333–3335
Radiation. See also *Roentgen rays.*
    and rare craniofacial clefts, 2121, 2122
    biological effects of, 532, 533
    extensive, reconstruction of nose following, 1254, *1254*, 1255
Radiation effects, 531–548
    and malignant transformation, 534, 535, 546, *546*, 547
    diagnosis of, 533
    etiology of, 532
Radiation injury, local effects of, 533, 534
    systemic effects of, 534
    treatment of, 536–547
Radiation osteitis, 535, 536
Radiation therapy
    of keloids, 429
    of malignant melanoma, 2853

Radiation therapy *(Continued)*
    of maxillary tumors, 2585, 2586
    of parotid gland tumors, 2536
    planned surgery after, 541–543
Radiation ulcers, treatment of, 543–545
Radicular cyst, of jaws, 2565, *2565*
Radioactive isotope clearance studies, of flap circulation, 196
Radiocarpal joint, 2961
Radiodermatitis, and chest wall reconstruction, 3611, *3612*
    chronic, and carcinoma, 2856
        dermal overgrafting for, 187, *187*
    dermabrasion of, 453
Radioulnar joint, 2961
Radium, in treatment of skin cancer, 2830
Radix nasi, 1042, *1042*
Ramus. See *Mandibular ramus.*
Randall-Graham lip adhesion, in cleft lip repair, 2021, *2022*, 2032, 2033, *2033*
Random pattern flaps, 202–217
Raphé, 3832, *3833*
Rasp, curved, to deepen nasofrontal angle, *1099*
    for determining degree of lowering of nasal profile, 1100, *1100*
Rasp technique of resecting bony hump of nose, 1077, *1078, 1079*
Ray, first, aplasia or hypoplasia of, 3337–3348
Recombination, 140
Reconstructive surgery, definition of, 4
Rectus abdominis muscles, 3728, 3729
Rectus femoris myocutaneous flap, 3560, 3561, *3561*
Rectus sheath, 3729
    transplantation within, *252, 254, 255*
Reese dermatome, 167–171
Reichert's cartilage, 2369
Reinnervation of skin transplants, 226–229
Remodeling, in tendon, 282, 283
    of bone, 315
Renal failure, in thermal burns, 481, 482
Repair
    choice of method of, 45, 46
    microvascular, 354–365
    planning of, 23–26
    timing of, 44
Repair and regeneration, 78–103
Replant, microvascular. See *Microvascular surgery.*
Replantation
    definition of, 52, 53
    digital. See *Digital replantation.*
    major limb. See *Limb replantation.*
    of amputated auricle. See *Auricle, amputated, replantation of.*
    of amputated parts of hand, 3084, *3085, 3086*
    of auricular cartilage, *1729, 1730*
    of auricular tissue, 1727, *1728*
    of penis, 384, *385*, 3916, 3918, *3918*
Replantation surgery, 3243–3265
    anesthesia in, 3246
    anticoagulants in, 3256
    arterial insufficiency in, 3256, 3257
    casualty treatment in, 3245, 3246
    decompression in, 3262, 3263
    first aid in, 3245
    infection in, 3263
    instrumentation in, 3246, 3247
    magnification and debridement in, 3247
    operative technique in, 3246
    postoperative complications in, 3256, 3257
    postoperative management in, 3256, 3257
    preoperative management in, 3245–3247

Replantation surgery *(Continued)*
  results of, 3257–3259
  revascularization in, 3259, 3262
  secondary reconstruction in, 3263
  sequence of vein or artery repairs in, 3259, 3260
  skin closure in, 3262
  swelling in, 3256
  venous inadequacy in, 3257
Respiratory and laryngeal mechanisms, and speech
    production, 2255
Rete pegs, 154
Rethi exposure, of nasal tip, 1108, *1108,* 1109
Reticular layer, *153,* 154
Reticulum cell sarcoma, of nose, *2838,* 2840
Retina, embryonic development of, 2304
Retinacula cutis, 155
Retractor, angulated, *1070*
Retroauricular area, as donor site for full-thickness skin
    grafts, 164, *164*
Retroauricular skin, advancement of in auricular
    reconstruction, 1736, 1737, *1738,* 1739, 1743, *1743*
Retrobulbar hemorrhage, following esthetic blepharo-
    plasty, 1897
Retrognathia, 2235, 2236
  mandibular, 1294, 1341–1373
  maxillary, 1295, 1411, 1424
Retrograde technique, of nasal tip exposure, 1106, *1106*
Retromaxillism, 1424
Revascularization, of autograft tendon, 279, 280
  of skin transplants, 157–163
Rh factor, 119, 120
Rhabdomyosarcoma, of hand and forearm, 3490
Rheobase, 1787
Rheumatoid arthritis, of hand, 3511–3518
Rhinolalia aperta, 2096, 2103
Rhinophyma, 1185–1192, 2783, 2784, *2784, 2785,*
    2875, *2875*
  complications after correction of, 1191, 1192
  dermabrasion of, 450
  diagnosis of, 1185, *1186,* 1187, *1187, 1188, 1189,*
    1189t
  operative technique in, 1188–1191
  pathology of, 1185
  planning operation for, 1188
  secondary procedures in, 1191
  types of operations for, 1187
Rhinoplasty
  corrective, 1040–1163
    early complications following, 1090, 1091
    historical considerations in, 1040, 1041
    in long face with deficiency of chin, *1057*
    in non-Caucasians, 1162, *1162,* 1163
    secondary, 1152–1161
      basic ground rules in, 1154
      correction of some basic mistakes made in primary
        rhinoplasty in, 1154–1157
      decision to operate in, 1153, 1154
    technique of, 1063–1066
    three most frequent errors in, 1157–1160
    variations in, 1098–1117
      double hump operation, 1099
      postoperative splinting in, 1105, *1105*
      recession of nasal dorsum in, 1104, 1105
      saw technique for lateral osteotomy in, 1102–1104
      Sheen's technique of, 1100, *1100*
      single hump operation, 1099
      submucous approach in, 1101, *1101,* 1102
      supracartilaginous approach in, 1102
      tip exposure in, 1105–1117
      transfixion incision in, 1100, 1101, *1101*
  for hump nose, 1066–1117
Rhinoplasty *(Continued)*
    for hump nose, correction of columella-ala triangle,
        septum, and protrusive nasal spine invading upper
        lip after, 1093, 1094, *1094,* 1095, *1095*
      correction of hanging columella after, 1095, *1095*
      correction of retruded and retracted columella after,
        1095–1098
      correction of wide columellar base after, 1093, *1094*
      deepening of prominent nasofrontal angle after,
        1098, *1098, 1099*
      freeing lateral cartilages from attachment to septum
        in, 1070–1073
      invagination procedure after, 1091, *1092*
      lateral (and medial) osteotomies of lateral walls of
        nose in, 1077–1083
      lowering septal profile, shortening septum, and
        correcting nasal tip in, 1070–1076
      resection of base of alae after, 1091, *1092,* 1093
      resection of bony hump in, 1076, 1077, *1077, 1078,*
        1079
      sculpturing of alar margin after, 1093, *1093*
      splinting of nose in, 1086–1091
      tip operation in, 1073–1076
      trimming dorsal borders of septal cartilage and
        medial borders of lateral cartilages in, 1083–1086
      uncovering nasal framework in, 1067–1070
  history of, 8
  reconstructive, for large full-thickness defects of nose,
    1225–1268
  total, *1262,* 1263, *1263,* 1264, *1265, 1266*
  septal surgery in, 1131–1134
  subtotal, four basic principles of, 1239–1244
    secondary grafting of skeletal framework in, 1259,
      1260, 1261, 1262, 1263
Rhinoscope, *1064*
Rhytidectomy, 1898
Rhytidoplasty, 1898
Rib, as stabilizing factor in chest wall reconstruction,
    3623, *3626,* 3627, *3627*
Rib cage, chondroma of, 3652
Rib cartilage, diced, 305, *306*
  transplantation of, 303, 304, *304,* 305, *305, 306*
Rib grafts. See *Graft, rib.*
Ribonucleic acid (RNA), 116
"Riding breeches" deformity, 3811–3820
Rim resection, of mandible, 2689–2695
Ring avulsion injury, 3019, *3020, 3021, 3021*
Ring constrictions, of hand, congenital, 3328, *3328,*
    3329
Risdon approach, 685, 686, *686, 687*
  to mandibular ramus, 1308
Risorius muscle, 1781
RNA (ribonucleic acid), 116
Robin anomalad. See *Pierre Robin anomalad.*
Rochet's procedure for reconstruction of urethra, 3838,
    3839
Rodent ulcer, 2820, 2831
Roentgen ray therapy, of basal cell epithelioma, 2809,
    2810
  of skin cancer, 2830
Roentgen rays, 532. See also *Radiation.*
  and skin cancer, 2818, 2819
Roentgenographic positions, 611–624
Romberg's disease, 2337–2349, *2350–2353*
  associated pathologic manifestations in, 2339, 2340
  bone and cartilage grafts in, 2342, 2343, *2343,* 2344,
    2344
  bone deformities in, 2338, 2339
  cartilage deformities in, 2338, *2338, 2339*
  clinical course and physical characteristics of, 2337–
    2340

Romberg's disease *(Continued)*
  dermis, fat, and fascia grafts in, 254, *258*, 2344, *2344*, 2345, *2345*
  etiopathogenesis of, 2340, 2341
  free dermis-fat flaps in, 2348
  history of, 2337
  muscle deformities in, 2339
  neck, trunk, and extremity deformities in, 2339
  silicone fluid injections in, 2348, 2349, *2350–2353*
  skin and subcutaneous tissue deformities in, 2337, 2338, *2338*
  treatment of, 2342–2349, *2350–2353*
  tube and local flaps in, 2345–2348
Rongeur, for resecting wedge of bone from root of nose, 1082, *1083*
Rose's procedure for repairing cleft lip, 2017, *2017*, 2018
Rose-Thompson straight line repair of cleft lip, *2025*, 2027, *2028*, *2029*, 2032, 2033, *2034*, 2035, *2035*
Rotation flaps. See *Flap, rotation.*
Rowe's disimpaction forceps, 702, *705*
Rubber band traction, in maxillary fractures, 700, *701*
  with intermaxillary fixation, in mandibular fractures, *653*

S-plasty, 58, *59*
Saccule, 2306
Sacral ulcers, 3789, *3789*, 3790, *3790*, *3791*
Saddle nose deformity, 1135–1141, *1273*
  transplantation of dermis in correction of, 240, *241*, *242*, 244, *245*
  transplants and implants for repair of, 1140, 1141, *1141*
  traumatic, *1273*
Saethre-Chotzen syndrome, 2468
Safian tip operation, 1107, *1107*, 1108
Sagittal synostosis, strip craniectomies for, 2493, *2495*
Sagittal-split osteotomy, 1347, *1349*, 1366, *1366*, 1367, *1367–1369*
Salabrasion, 456
Saline wheal test, of flap circulation, 195
Salivary cysts, following face lift operation, 1926
Salivary duct trauma and fistulas, 2542, 2543
Salivary glands
  calculi of, 2542, *2543*
  minor, tumors of, 2539, 2540, *2540*
  non-neoplastic diseases of surgical importance in, 2540–2544
  surgical treatment of disease of, 2521–2546
  tumors of, 2521, 2522
Salivation, excessive, 2543, 2544, *2544*
Salute position, for transfer of abdominal tube flap to nose, 1267, *1267*
Sandwich flap, 2273, 2277
Sanvenero-Rosselli, 12, *12*, *13*, 17, 18, *20*
Saphenous system, greater, normal lymphangiogram of, *3573*
Sarcoma, 2840, 2841
  Ewing's, of jaws, 2567, *2568*, 2569, *2569*
  hemangioendothelial, of chest wall, 3652, *3653*
  Kaposi's, 2841
    of hand and forearm, 3488, *3488*, 3489
  of face, deltopectoral flap in repair of, *2750*
  of head and neck, 2636–2638
  of posterior pharyngeal wall, *2613*
  of soft tissues of hand and forearm, 3489–3491, *3492*, *3493*
  osteogenic, of hand and forearm, 3499
    of jaws, 2566, *2566*, *2567*
    of mandible, 2637, *2637*

Sarcoma *(Continued)*
  reticulum cell, 2840
    of nose, *2838*
  synovial, of hand and forearm, 3490, 3491, *3491–3493*
Saw, angulated, 1103, *1103*, *1104*
Saw guide, Joseph, 1103, *1103*
Sayoc eyelid fixation forceps, *950*, 951, *951*
Scalp
  advanced cancers of, 2763–2767
    pathology of, 2763, *2764*, *2765*
    reconstruction of defects of, 2767
    technique of resection of, *2766*, 2767
  anatomy of, 822, *822*, 823
  burn deformities of, 1618
  congenital absence of, 828–831
  congenital aplasia of, 827, 828
  congenital defects of, 824–832
  deformities of, 822–857
Scalp autografts, full-thickness, 230, *230*
Scalp avulsion, 832–837, *838–840*
Scalp flaps. See *Flap, scalp.*
Scalp graft, 1618, *1618*, 1619, *1619*
Scalping flap. See *Flap, forehead, scalping.*
Scapha, deformity of, 1708, 1709
Scaphal cartilage tubing, in correction of prominent ear, *1711*, 1712, *1715*
Scaphocephaly, in Crouzon's disease, 2468, *2468*
Scaphoid, *2968*, 2969
Scaphoid fossa, 1978
Scaphoid fractures, 3047
Scapular tube flap, *211*
Scapular ulcer, 3792
Scar contraction, physical basis of, 415–420
Scar contractures, after chemical planing, 460
  of cervical region, 1643, 1644, *1645*
Scar formation, in healed tendon, 282, 283
Scar irregularity, chemical planing for, 461, *461*
Scar revision, 430–438
  complications of, 436–438
  dermal buttressing of, 436, *437*
  edge dermal undermining in, 436, *437*
  sebaceous hypertrophy excision in, 437, *437*
Scarification, 442
Scarpa's fascia, 3728
Scars, 413–441
  burn. See *Burn scars.*
  cancer in, 415, 2819
  contracted, 430, 431, *432*, 434, 1644, *1645*, 2966, *2967*. See also *Contracture* and *Contraction.*
  cutaneous, basic observations on, 413–415
    of nose, 1195, *1195*, 1196, *1196*
  depressed, 430, *431*, 434
    dermabrasion of, 447, *449*, *450*
    of partially avulsed trapdoor flaps, Z-plasty and W-plasty in, 64
    transplantation of dermis in treatment of, 240, *241*
  dermabrasion for, 446, 447, *448–452*
  electric dermatome in shaving of, 172
  elevated, 430, 432, *432*, 436
  extensive, dermal overgrafting for, 186
  fibrosarcoma in, 415
  hypertrophic, 89, *90*, 430, *432*, 434
    after chemical planing, 460
    after dermabrasion, 454
    in burn injury, 1599–1601
      of hand, 3389
      treatment of, 1640, 1641
    wide, excision, Z plasty, and skin grafting in, 63
  linear, of upper lip, 1544, *1545*
  multiple curve excision of, *434*, 435, *435*
  pigmented, 432, *433*

Scars *(Continued)*
  relationship of to sarcomas, 2840
  spread, 430, *431*, 433, *433*
  synthesis of, 79
  trapdoor, 418, 419, *420*, 432, *433*, 434–436
Schwannoma, malignant, of hand and forearm, 3495, 3496, *3496*
  of hand and forearm, 3493, *3494*
Scissors, angulated, for tip surgery, *1074*
    for trimming dorsal border of septum, *1071*
  blunt-tip (Stevens), *1075*
Scleral lens, *938*, 940
"Scleral show," 1001
Scoville clamps, 345, *345*
Scrotal skin, in reconstruction of male urethra, 3916, *3916*, *3917*
  resurfacing shaft of penis with, 3906, *3907*, *3908*
Scrotum, 3832, *3833*
  construction of in true hermaphroditism, *3948–3950*
  partial loss of, *3903*
Sebaceous adenoma, 2875
Sebaceous cysts, 2784–2786, 2877, 2878
  of auricle, 1766
Sebaceous gland carcinoma, 2875
  of hand and forearm, 3464
Sebaceous gland function, in skin grafts and flaps, 229
Sebaceous gland hyperplasia. See *Rhinophyma.*
Sebaceous gland tumors, 2875, *2875*
  of hand and forearm, 3453
Sebaceous glands, *153*, 154, 155
  in transplanted dermis, 247, 248
Sebaceous hyperplasia, 2786, *2786*
Sebaceous hypertrophy, in scar revision, 437, *437*
Sebaceous nevi, senile, 2786, *2786*
Seborrheic keratosis, 2781–2783, 2857, *2858*
  of hand and forearm, 3453, 3455, *3455*
Seborrheic wart, 2781–2783
Segregation of alleles, 140, 140t
Semi-axial (superoinferior) projection, 613, *614*
Semicircular ducts, 2306
Senile ectropion, 908, 909
Senior syndrome, 2980
Sensory nerve loss, following corrective surgery of jaws, 1470
Septal flap technique, for repair of full-thickness defects of lower portion of nose, 1215, 1218, *1218*
Septal graft, 1129, *1129*, 1138, 1234, *1234*, *1235*, *1246–1249*
Septum. See *Nasal septum.*
Septum orbitale, 752, *859*, 860, *860*
Septum-premaxillary relationship, in normal infants and those with bilateral cleft, 2051, *2051*, 2052
Serologically defined (SD) antigen, 130, 131, 142–147
Serotonin creatinine sulfate, 85
Serratus muscle-split rib flap, in chest wall reconstruction, *3626*
Serum imbibition, 157–159
Sewall operation for orbital decompression, *972*, 973–975
Sex, gonadal, 3934–3936, *3937*
  hormonal, 3937, 3938
Sex assignment, problem of, 3938
Sex chromatin mass, 3932–3934
Sex identification, chromosomes in, 3930, 3931
  verification of, 3931–3938
    chromosome karyotype in, 3934, *3935*, *3936*
    gonadal sex in, 3934–3936, *3937*
    hormonal sex in, 3937, 3938
    sex chromatin mass in, 3932–3934
Sheen's technique of corrective rhinoplasty, 1100, *1100*

Shell ear, 1710, 1717, 1718
Shock, prevention and control of, in severe facial injuries, 608
Shoulder-back flap, *1656*
Sialadenitis, chronic, 2541, 2542
Sialolithiasis, 2542, *2543*
Sickle flap, 1226, *1227*, *1547*
Silastic cuff, in repair of nerves of hand, 3223
Silastic implants, *809*, 810, *1025*, 1026
  following mandibular resection, 2692–2694
  in augmentation mammaplasty, 3697
  in breast after radical mastectomy, 3716, 3720
  in joints, 102
  in microgenia, 1395, *1396*
  in microtia, 1699, *1701*
  in naso-orbital fractures, 772, 790
  in orbital fractures, 995–997, *997*
Silicone, in maxillofacial prosthetics, *2940*, 2941
  room temperature vulcanizing (RTV), 394
Silicone balloon prosthesis, for mammary augmentation, 3697, *3698–3702*
Silicone cyst, 396, *396*
Silicone fluid, injectable, 254, 394, 395, *395*
    in mammary augmentation, 3690
    in Romberg's disease, 2348, 2349, *2350–2353*
    technique and complications of, 401
  use of for correction of minor irregularities of nose
    after corrective rhinoplasty, 1160, 1161, *1161*, *1162*
Silicone gel prosthesis of Cronin, for mammary augmentation, 3697, *3698*, *3699*, *3702*, *3706*
Silicone implants, 393–401
  body response to, 394
  effects of on vascular system, 399, 401
  hematologic effects of, 398, 399, *400*
  in mandibulofacial dysostosis, 2416, *2417*, *2418*
  in microgenia, 1395, *1396*, 1399–1403
  reaction of adipose tissue to, 397, 398, *398*
  soft, in rabbits, 402, *403*, *404*, 405
  tissue response to, 395–401
  visceral and systemic distribution of, 398, *399*
Silicone rubber, 394
"Siliconoma," 409, 410
Silk implants, 392
Silver nitrate, in thermal burns, 488, 488t, 489, *489*, 489t, 490, 3372
Silver sulfadiazine, in facial burns, 1603
  in thermal burn, 491, 491t, 492t
Simiansim, surgical-orthodontic treatment of, 1436–1439
Simonart's bar, *1961*, 1962, *1962*, 1963
Sinus (sinuses)
  cervical, 2306, 2903, *2903*
  dermoid of nose, *1174*, 1175, *1175*, 1176, 1177
  ethmoidal, 777, 778
  frontal, 777, *778*. See *Frontal sinus.*
  lip, congenital, 1540–1543
  maxillary. See *Maxillary sinus.*
  paranasal, 2574, 2767–2770
  preauricular, 2910, 2911, *2911*
  skin, 2876–2878
Skeletal deformities, in Apert's syndrome, 2322–2324
Skeletal injuries, of hand, 3004, *3005*
Skeletal muscle, transplantation of, 293–300
Skeletal osteotomy, in jaw deformities, 1303, *1303*, 1304
Skeletal traction, in skin grafting after thermal burns, 500–503, *504*
Skeleton, facial. See *Facial skeleton.*
  jaw, 1509–1513
  of hand, 2957–2961
    injuries to, 3004, *3005*, 3059, 3060

Skin
  aging, histologic and histochemical characteristics of,
      1873–1875
  biological principles in healing of, 94–99
  blanching of, 74, 75
  color and texture match of, 45
  elasticity, extensibility, and resiliency of, 38–44
  elephant, 3654, 3656, *3656*
  grafted, contraction of, 182, 183
  in limb replantation, 3251, 3252
  of hand, examination of, 2966, 2967, *2967*
      injuries to, *3003*, 3004, *3004*
  of nose, deformities of, 1195–1199
  physical properties of, 69–77
  plastic surgeon and, 38–44
  sensitivity of, 2962, 2963
  stress-strain curve for, 68, *72*
  surgical and chemical planing of, 442–463
  tattoos of, 2815, *2816*. See also *Tattoo.*
  tumors of, 2776–2901. See also *Skin cancer.*
    basal cell epithelioma. See *Basal cell epithelioma.*
    Bowen's disease, 2810, 2811, *2811*
    carcinoma, 2817–2839. See also *Carcinoma.*
      basosquamous, 2828
      chemosurgery in, 2830
      chemotherapy of, 2838, 2839, *2839*
      classification of, 2819–2828
      clinical signs of, 2828
      diagnosis of, 2828, 2830
      electrodessication and cautery of, 2830
      incidence and etiology of, 2817–2819
      radium in treatment of, 2830
      roentgen therapy of, 2830
      squamous cell. See *Squamous cell carcinoma.*
      surgical excision of, 2830–2838
      treatment of, 2830–2839
    chemosurgery for. See *Chemosurgery, for Skin
        Cancer.*
    chronic radiodermatitis and carcinoma, 2856
    cysts, fistulas, and sinuses, 2876–2878
    epidermal and pilar cysts, 2784–2786
    epidermal appendage, 2786–2788
    erythroplasia of Queyrat, 2811, 2812, *2812*
    hair follicle, 2874, 2975
    histiocytoma, 2790, *2790*, 2791
    keratoacanthoma, 2814, 2815, *2815*
    keratoses, 2856–2858
    lymphangiomas, 2873, *2873*, 2874, *2874*
    malignant melanoma. See *Melanoma, malignant.*
    melanotic freckle of Hutchinson, 2805, *2805*, 2806,
        2806
    milia, 454, 459, 2786
    mucous cysts, 2791, *2791*, 2792
    myxoid cysts, 2792
    neural tissue, 2796, 2797, *2797*
    nevocellular nevi and selected pigmented lesions,
        2797–2802
    of thorax, 3654–3657
    Paget's disease of nipple and extramammary Paget's
        disease, 2812, *2812*
    pigmented nevi, 2859–2865
    rhinophyma, 2783, 2784, *2784*, *2785*
    sarcoma, 2840, 2841
    sebaceous gland, 2875, *2875*
    seborrheic keratosis, 2781–2783
    skin tags, 2791, *2791*
    squamous cell carcinoma. See *Squamous cell
        carcinoma.*
    superficial, 2853, *2854*, *2855*, 2856
    sweat gland, 2788–2790, 2874

Skin *(Continued)*
    tumors of, tattoos, 2815, *2816*
      vascular, 2792–2796, 2865–2873
        treatment of, 2869–2873
      viral, 2776–2781
      warts, 2876
      xanthomatoses, 2876
    visco-elastic properties of, 70, 71, *75*, *76*
  Skin allograft rejection reactions, 128, 129
  Skin anatomy, 152–156
  Skin appendages, aging of, 1874, 1875
    tumors of, 2874, 2875, *2875*
  Skin cancer. See also *Skin, tumors of.*
    age and sex and, 2818
    chemicals and, 2819
    chemosurgery for. See *Chemosurgery, for skin cancer.*
    chemotherapy of, 2838, 2839, *2839*
    heredity and, 2818
    invasive, treatment of, 2760, 2761
    pigmentation and, 2818
    roentgen ray therapy of, 2830
    roentgen rays and, 2818, 2819
    scars and ulcerations and, 2819
    sunlight and, 2818
    superficial forms of, 2853, *2854*, *2855*, 2856
    ulcerations and, 2819
  Skin cancer surgery, for carcinoma, 2830–2838
  Skin closure, Steri-tape technique of, 47, *48*
  Skin deformities, in Romberg's disease, 2337, 2338, *2338*
  Skin extensibility, 75–77
  Skin flaps. See *Flaps, skin.*
  Skin folds and wrinkles, 1870–1873
  Skin graft inlay, and dental prosthesis, in correction of
      microgenia, *1402*, 1403, *1403*, 1404
    nasomaxillary, 1201–1205
  Skin graft inlay technique, 178, *178*
    in mandibular reconstruction, 1503–1507
    in oropharyngoesophageal reconstructive surgery,
        2712–2715
  Skin graft outlay technique, 178, *178*
  Skin grafts. See *Grafts, skin.*
  Skin injuries, of hand, *3003*, 3004, *3004*
  Skin preservation, cryobiologic, 181, 182
  Skin replacement, in burns of hand, 3373–3376
    timing of, 224, 225
  Skin sinuses, 2876–2878
  Skin slough, following face lift operation, 1925
  Skin suture marks, 420–424
  Skin tags, 2791, *2791*
  Skin tension, 71–75
  Skin transplants, 53, 54. See also *Grafts, skin.*
    behavior of in mouth, 2684
    in oropharyngoesophageal reconstructive surgery,
        2712–2747, 2748–2750
    reinnervation of, 226–229
    revascularization of, 157–163
  Skin varnish, use of in splinting of nose, 1087, 1088,
      1089
  Skin-fat graft, 1269, *1269*
  Skoog method of bilateral cleft lip repair, 2078, *2080*,
      2081, *2081*
  Skull
    adult vs. child, *797–801*
    base of, submentovertex and verticosubmental positions
        for, 617, *619*
    cloverleaf, 2493, *2494*
    embryonic, *816*, *817*
  Skull deformities, in Apert's syndrome, 2322, *2326*,
      2468–2472
    in Crouzon's disease, 2316, 2317, 2468–2472

Sleeve procedure, for correction of columellar retrusion, 1097, *1097*
Sling flap, 1749, *1750*
Smith, Ferris, 12, *12*, 13, *15*
Smith's modification of Fasanella-Servat operation, *926*, *927*, 928
Socket reconstruction, 968–970
Soft tissue crush injuries, of hand, 3021, 3022
Soft tissue deformities, in craniofacial microsomia, 2377
Soft tissue replacement, in acute hand injuries, 3023–3041
Soft tissue tumors, benign, 2878–2880
Soft tissue wounds, facial, debridement of, 627, 628, *628, 629, 630*
    dressings in, 641, 643
    extensive, care of, 637, 639, 640, *643, 644, 645*
    nonsuture technique of closure of, 640, 641, *646*
    treatment of, 625, 627–645
    in infants and children, 795, 796
    of hand, 3017–3022
Soft tissues, nonepithelial, of hand and forearm, tumors of, 3468–3482
Solar keratosis, 2802
Soleus muscle, mobilization of for flap, 3554, *3555*, 3556, *3556*
Spastic ectropion, 908, 909
Spasticity, and pressure sores, 3769
Spatula deformity, 2323, *2323*
Spectrometer, mass, in evaluation of flap circulation, 196
Speech, "normal" and "acceptable," 2248
Speech mechanism, 2253–2257
Speech problems, in cleft lip and palate, 2246–2267
Speech process, 2249–2257
    development of articulation skills in, 2250, 2251, 2251t
Speech sound articulation, testing of, 2263
Speech sounds, classification of, 2251, 2252, 2252t, 2253
Speech therapy, 2264, 2265
Sphenoid bone, 2431, *2432*
Sphenomandibular ligament, and relapse in mandibular micrognathia, 1373
Spider nevus, 2795, 2796
Spider telangiectasis, 2795, 2796, 2866
Spina bifida, 3749–3760
    differential diagnosis of, 3752
    embryology of, 3749
    medical management of, 3752, 3753
    surgical treatment of, 3753–3760
Spina bifida cystica, 3750–3752
Spina bifida occulta, 3749, *3749*, 3750
    surgical treatment of, 3753
Spinal block, 594
Spinal concussion, 3768
Spinal cord injuries, experimental studies dealing with production, prophylaxis, and therapy of, 3769, 3770
Spinal shock, 3767
Spina's method of bilateral cleft lip repair, 2083, *2083*, *2084*
Spine-costal margin, ulcer of, 3792
Splint(s)
    acrylic, 1477, *1478, 1479*, 2920
        in correction of jaw deformities, 1301, *1301, 1302*
    in adduction contracture of thumb, 2998, *2998*
    in burn scar contracture of neck, 1650–1652
    in corrective rhinoplasty, 1086–1091, 1105, *1105*
    in hand, 2991–2993, 2995–2999
    in maintenance of intermaxillary fixation, 652, *657*
    in mandibular fractures, 669
    in maxillofacial prosthetics, 2920, *2920*, 2921
    in radical nerve paralysis, 2996, 2997, *2997*
    internal, in deviated nose, 1126, 1127, *1127*

Splint(s) *(Continued)*
    isoprene, in burn scar contracture of neck, 1644, *1645*, 1647, 1652, *1652*
    Michigan, in burns of hand, 3390, *3390*
    Morris external fixation, *1476*, 1477, *1477–1480*
    mucoperichondrial, *1122*, 1123, *1123, 1124*
    nasal, 728, *729*
    Roger Anderson, extraoral, in mandibular tumor surgery, 2616, 2618
    sectional, in mandibular defects involving soft tissue loss, 1498, *1498*
    "stick-and-carrot," 2396, 2398
    tantalum, in mandibular reconstruction, 1485, *1488*, *1489*
    vitallium, 1357, *1358*
Split hand complexes, 3335–3337
Split-plate appliance, palatal, 1305, *1306*
Split rib grafts. See *Graft, split-rib.*
Sponge implants, 407
Springs, spiral, in retention of maxillary prosthesis, 2934, *2935*
Squamous cell carcinoma
    forehead flap in defect of, *2832*
    involving craniofacial skeleton, 2758, 2759, *2760, 2761*
    metastatic, *2571*
    of alveolus, 2656, 2669
    of buccal mucosa, 2608, 2658, 2659, 2677
    of eyelids, 880
    of faucial region and pharyngeal wall, *2671, 2680, 2681*
    of finger, chemosurgery for, 2885, 2886
    of floor of mouth, 2669, 2678
    of hands and forearms, 3459, *3459*, 3460, *3460–3464*
    of lip, *2600*, 2603, *2834–2836*, *2839*
    of maxilla, *2574, 2575, 2586*, 2653
    of nose, 1193, *2833*
    of penis, *3908*
    of skin, 2812–2814, 2828, *2829*
    of thorax, *3614*
    of thumb, *3459*
    of tongue, 2609, *2610*, 2611, *2669*
    of zygoma, *2832, 2833, 2837*
    radiation-induced, *546*, 547
    repair of by gull-shaped median forehead flap, 1258, *1258*
Stapedius, nerve to, 1775, 1777, 1786
Staphylococcus aureus, 50
Staphylorrhaphy, 2091
Staphyloschisis, 2091
Steatoma, 2784–2786, 2877, 2878
Steel implants, 392, 393
Stein operation, in repair of lower lip defect, 1565, *1566*
Stein-Abbé lip flap, 223
Stein-Kazanjian flap, *1572*, 1573
Stensen's duct, 2542, 2543, *2543*, 2544, *2544*
    lacerations of, *635*
    ligation of, 813
Step osteotomy. See *Osteotomy, step.*
Steri-strips, 47, *48*, 641, *646*
Sternal defects, reconstruction of, 3628–3631
Sternal dehiscence, 3632
Sternal tumors, 3628
Sternocleidomastoid "tumor," *1665*, 1666, 1667
Sternomastoid flap, in intraoral tumor surgery, 2645, *2646*, 2647
Sternotomy, median, 3632
Sternum, keloid of, 3654, *3654*
    total resection of, 3630, 3631, *3631, 3632*
Steroids, adrenal, and immunosuppression, 138
    and rare craniofacial clefts, 2122, 2123
    in keloid therapy, 430

Stick-and-carrot appliance, *1355*, 1357, *1358*, 1395, *1395*
Stitch abscess, 422
Stomodeum, 2303
Stout method of intermaxillary fixation, 651, *654*
Straddling technique, of dermabrasion, 447, *450*
Stratum corneum, 153
Stratum germinativum, 153
Stratum granulosum, 153
Stratum lucidum, 153
Stratum spinosum, 153
Strawberry marks, 2793, *2793*, 2794, 2795
"Stress relaxation," 71, *75*
Striae, 74
Strömbeck operation for breast reduction, 3672–3676, *3676*
Stryker dermabrader, 445, *449*
Stryker right-angle oscillating saw, 1324, *1324*
Stryker turbine dermatome, 173
Sturge-Weber syndrome, 2793, 2867
Stylomastoid artery, 1779
Subcondylar fracture, 687
Subcutaneous flap, *2171*
Subcutaneous tissue, aging of, 1875, *1875*
Subcutaneous tissue deformities, in Romberg's disease, 2337, 2338, *2338*
Subepicranial space, 822, *822*, 823
Submandibular apron flap, 2645, *2646*
Submandibular gland, tumors of, 2538, 2539
Submaxillary duct injuries, 632
Submaxillary gland, tumors of, 2538, 2539
Submental depression, following face lift operation, 1925
Submental lipectomy, and resection of redundant skin, 1915, 1916, *1916*, *1917*, *1919*
Subnasale, 28, *28*, 1042, 1289, *1290*
Succinic dehydrogenase, *247*, 248
Succinylcholine chloride, 587
Sulfadiazine, in burn therapy, 3372
Sulfamylon, in burn therapy, 490, 490t, 491, 1603, 3372
Sunlight, and malignant melanoma, 2842, 2843
and skin cancer, 2818
Superior oblique muscle, *859*, 860
Supervoltage, 532
Supraclavicular area, as donor site for full-thickness skin graft, 164, *165*
Supramid implants, in naso-orbital fractures, 772, 790
Supraorbital fractures, 785, 788, 789
Supraorbital nerve, *859*, 860
Supratarsal fixation, following esthetic blepharoplasty, 1895, *1895*, 1896, *1896*
Supratarsal folds, asymmetry of, following esthetic blepharoplasty, 1894, 1895
construction of, 949–955
Supratip area, of nose, 1042, *1042*
Supratip protrusion, correction of, 1159, *1159*, 1160, *1160*, *1161*
following corrective rhinoplasty, 1085, *1085*, 1091
Supratrochlear nerve, *859*, 860
Sural nerve graft, in facial paralysis, *1850*, 1852, *1852*, *1859*
Surgery
esthetic, 4, 1868–1929
microlymphatic, 384–388
microvascular. See *Microvascular surgery.*
plastic. See *Plastic surgery.*
reconstructive, definition of, 4
replantation. See *Replantation surgery.*
Surgical planing. See *Dermabrasion.*
Suspension method, of reduction of fractures of zygoma, 717, 718, *718*, 719

Suture(s)
buried, subcuticular, 47, *50*
end-to-end, vs. autogenous nerve graft, 3228, 3229
epineural, in nerves of hand, 3222
figure-of-eight, 46, *47*
funicular, in nerves of hand, 3222
in microvascular surgery, 346–348
interrupted, everting, 47, *49*
inverting, 47, *49*
mattress, horizontal, with dermal component, 47, *51*
vertical, 47, *50*
midpalatal, absence of in cleft palate, 1964
nonabsorbable, and scar formation, 423
occlusive lid, 868, *869*
running, continuous, 48, *51*
selection and placement of, 95
subcuticular, continuous, removable, 48, *51*, *52*
Suture marks, skin, 420–424
Suture tension and spacing, 423, *423*
in microvascular surgery, 357–359
Suturing, 46–49
variations in technique of, 49, *52*, *53*
Swan-neck deformity, 3175–3180, 3513, *3513*, 3514
Sweat (eccrine and apocrine) glands, *153*, 155
function of, in skin grafts and flaps, 228
in dermis graft, *246*, 247, *247*, 248
tumors of, 2788–2790, 2874, 2875
of hand and forearm, 3453, 3464
Swinging door operation, 1123–1126
"Switch" flap, of lower eyelid, in repair of upper lid defects, 889, 890, *890*, 891, *892*
Symblepharon, 915–918, *919*
Symbrachydactyly, in Poland's syndrome, 3311, *3311*
Symphalangism, 3331
Symphyseal region, tumors of, forehead flap in, 2673
Syndactyly, first web, 3338, *3338*
surgical management of, 3313–3319
Syndrome arcade of Frohse, 3446
Synechiae, septal-turbinate, traumatic, 1150
Syngeneic, 141
Syngenesiotransplantation, 52
Synovectomy, in arthritic hand, 3512, 3513
Synovial cysts, of hand and forearm, 3470
Synovial membrane, 661
Synovial sarcoma, of hand and forearm, 3490, 3491, *3491–3493*
Synovial sheath, 271, 272
Syringoma, 2788, *2788*
of eyelids, 879
Syringomyelocele, 3751

T bar of Kazanjian, 679, *679*
T cells, 133, 134
Tagliacotian brachial flap, 1199, 1266, 1267, *1267*
Tagliacozzi, Gaspare, 5, 6
Talwin, 586
Tantalum implants, 392
Tantalum plate, in treatment of Romberg's disease, 2343, 2344, *2344*
Tantalum tray, combined with cancellous bone chips, use of in restoration of continuity of mandible, 1473, 1474, *1488*, *1489*
Tarsal glands, 861
Tarsal plates, 860, *861*
average dimensions of, 948t
Tarsoconjunctival flap. See *Flap, tarsoconjunctival.*
Tarsoconjunctival wedge operation, for correction of entropion, 914, *915*

Tarsorrhaphy, 868, 869, *870*
 inadvisability of in lower eyelid burn ectropion, 1629,
  1629, 1630
Tattoo(s)
 accidental, *628, 632*
 dermabrasion of, 447, *453*
 dermal overgrafting for, 187, 188
 of skin, 2815, *2816*
 treatment of, 442, 443
Teeth. See also *Dentition.*
 buccolingual relationships of, *1297*
 congenital absence of in cleft lip and palate,
  2217, *2218*
 damage to in mandibular fractures, 664, 665
 ectopic, in cleft lip and palate, 2217, 2219, *2220*
 fused, in cleft lip and palate, 2217, *2219*
 in maxillary osteotomies, 1452, 1453
 injuries of, in alveolar fractures in children, 805
 loss of following corrective surgery of jaws, 1469, 1470
 permanent, position of in skull, *797, 798, 799, 800*
 role of in speech, 2253, 2254
 rotated, in cleft lip and palate, 2217, *2218, 2219*
 supernumerary, in cleft lip and palate, 2217, *2218*
 transposed, in cleft lip and palate, 2219, *2220*
Teflon implants, 392, 401, 402
 in blowout fractures of orbital floor, 772, *773*, 789, 790
Telangiectases, after chemical planing, 460
 spider, 2795, 2796, 2866
Telecanthus, traumatic, 723, *725*, 780, 781, *782, 785*,
 1008, *1009, 1010*, 1021, 1022, *1022*
Temporal artery, superficial, 217, *217*, 1779
Temporal bone, 1521
 cancers of, 2770–2772
Temporal branches, of facial nerve, 1778
Temporal flap. See *Flap, forehead.*
Temporalis muscle, *659*, 660, 1782, *1782*
 in craniofacial microsomia, 2374
Temporalis muscle reinnervation, in eyelid paralysis,
 1841, *1841*, 1842
Temporalis muscle tendon and coronoid process transfer,
 in facial palsy, 1818, 1819, *1819*
Temporalis muscle transposition, *1858*
 in facial palsy, 1810–1818, *1859*
Temporofacial nerve, 1777
Temporomandibular arthrosis, 1529, *1529*
Temporomandibular joint, 660, 661, *662*
 disturbances of, 1521–1539
 fractures of, in children, 802–805
 functional anatomy of, 1521–1523
 injury to, 1528, 1529, *1529*
 radiographic anatomy of, 1522, *1522*, 1523, *1523, 1524*
 roentgenographic positions for, *622, 623, 623*, 624, *624*
 surgical approach to, 1525, *1525*, 1526
  complications and causes of failures in, 1537
Temporomandibular joint ankylosis, 693, 803, 804, *804*,
 1529–1537
 diagnosis and type of, 1530, *1530*
 treatment of, 1530–1536
Temporomandibular joint pain, 1523–1525
Tendon(s)
 autograft, revascularization of, 279, 280
 biochemistry and physiology of, 269–271
 biological principles in healing of, 99
 canthal, medial and lateral, *859, 863, 864*
 donor, 272–278
 extensor digiti minimi, 278
 extensor digitorum longus to second, third, and fourth
  toes, 277, *277*, 278
 extensor indicis, 278

Tendon(s) *(Continued)*
 flexor, composite allografts of, 287, 288
  injuries to, *2992, 2994*
 flexor digitorum profundus, 3073, 3075, *3076*
 flexor digitorum superficialis, 278
 flexor pollicis longus, 3075, 3077, *3077*
 gliding mechanism of, 271, *271*, 272
 ground substance in, 267, 270
 in limb replantation, 3247
 lymph drainage in, 269
 lyophilization of, 285
 morphology, histology, and ultrastructure of, 266–269
 nerve supply in, 269
 of hand, 2971–2974
  extensor, deformities of, 3325, 3326, *3326*
  flexor, grafting of, 3193–3206
  in rheumatoid arthritis, 3512, 3513
  injuries of, See *Hand injuries, acute, of tendons.*
  repair of in children, 3191, 3192
  severance of, 3206, 3207, *3207*
  transplantation of, 2989
 palmaris longus, *269*, 272–275, 3198, 3199, *3199*
 plantaris, 275–277
 preservation of, 285–287
 remodeling in, 282, 283
 scar formation in, 282, 283
 transplantation of, 266–292, 3193–3206
  allograft, 284–288
  autograft, 278–284
  in burns of hand, 3379, *3379*
  in hand, 2989, 3268, 3269, *3269*
  timing of, 2989
  xenograft, 288
Tendon bundles, 267
Tendon ends, healing of, 280, 281
Tendon entrapment syndrome, of hand, 3428–3448
Tendon fibers, 267
Tendon graft. See *Tendon, transplantation of.*
Tendon injuries, in proximal palm, wrist, and forearm,
 3206–3212
 of hand, 3004–3009
Tendon sheath, of hand, giant cell tumor of, 3472, *3472,*
 3473, 3473, 3474
 in rheumatoid arthritis, 3512, 3513
Tendovaginitis, digital, stenosing, 3440–3443
Tennison operation for cleft lip, 2019, *2028*, 2033, *2069*,
 2070–2073
Tenocytes, 267, 270, 271
Tenodesis, in partially paralyzed hand, 3303, 3304
Tenon's capsule, 752
Tensor fasciae latae muscle, 332
Tensor tarsi muscle, 862
Tensor veli palatini muscle, *1977*, 1978, *1978*, 1979,
 1979, 1987
Teratoma, of eyelids, 877
Tessier classification of craniofacial clefts. See
 Craniofacial clefts, rare, Tessier classification of.
Testes, burial of in thigh pocket, 3906, 3907
Testicle, undescended, 3834
Testicularism, feminizing, 3954–3956, *3957*
Tetanus prophylaxis, in facial injuries, 624, 625
 in thermal burn, 482, 483
Thalidomide, 2123, 3306, 3307
Thalidomide embryopathy, 3334
Thenar flap, *216*, 217, 3027–3033
Thenar muscles, 2961, 2975
Thermal burns. See *Burns, thermal.*
Thermography, infrared, in evaluation of flap circulation,
 196

Thiersch skin graft, 14
Thiersch-Duplay technique of repair of hypospadias, 3848, *3849*
Thiersch's operation for glanular hypospadias, 3837, *3838*
Thigh, as donor site for full-thickness skin grafts, 164, 165
  dermolipectomy of, 3811–3820
  fascia lata from, 263
Thigh flap, total, *3794*
Thiopental sodium, 587
Thompson's procedure for repairing cleft lip, 2018, *2018*
Thoracic duct, *3577*
  obstruction of, 3586–3590
Thoracic duct lymph flow, *3571*
Thoracic wall defects, reconstruction of, 3609–3660
Thoracoabdominal tube flap, in chest wall reconstruction, 3617, *3619*
Thoracobrachial flap, in arm repair, 215, *215*
Thoracoepigastric flap, *1656*
Thorax, benign tumors of skin of, 3654–3657
  injuries of, 3609, 3610, *3610*
  recurrent squamous cell carcinoma of, *3614*
Thrombosis, in microvascular surgery, 349–354
Thumb
  adduction contracture of, 3117–3124
    in burns of hand, 3376, *3376*, 3377
    splinting in, 2998, *2998*
    treatment of, 3119–3124
  fractures of, 3048, *3048*, *3049*
  in arthritic hand, 3517, 3518
  ligamentous injuries of, 3048–3050
  palmar abduction of, 3014, 3015
  relationship of to fixed unit of hand, 3115–3124
  squamous cell carcinoma of, *3459*
  traumatic loss of, reconstruction of, 3350–3367
    by finger transfer, 3355–3363, *3364*, *3365*
    by tubed pedicle flap and bone graft, 3365, *3366*, 3367
    history of, 3350–3352
    neurovascular pedicle method of, 3352, *3353–3355*
  trigger, 3325, *3325*
  triphalangeal, 3320, *3322*, 3324, 3325
Thumb amputation, levels of, 3355
Thumb aplasia, 3338, *3338*
Thumb movement, biomechanics of, 3280–3285
Thumb opposition, restoration of, 3285–3301
Thymus gland, early development of, 2904, *2904*, 2905
Thyroglossal duct, early development of, 2904
Thyroglossal duct cysts and fistulas, 2877, *2877*, 2905–2908
Thyroid gland, early development of, 2904, *2904*
Thyrotoxic exophthalmos, 970–978
Tibia, fracture of, osteomyelitis in, 3527, *3527*
Tibial bone graft struts, in reconstruction of sternal defects, 3629, *3629*
Tibial bone grafts, 326, 327, *327*
Tinel's sign, 2974
Tip, of nose. See *Nasal tip.*
Titanium implants, 392
Titterington position, 613, *614*
Toenail, ingrown, 3530
Toes, amputation of, to resurface defect of plantar surface of metatarsal head, *3536*
  supernumerary, 3527, 3529
Tomography, axial, computerized, in craniofacial surgery, 2428, *2428*
Tongue
  blood supply of, 2701, *2701*
  cancer of, 2609–2613, 2622, *2622*, *2628*, *2629*, *2634*
  embryonic development of, 2312

Tongue *(Continued)*
  role of in speech, 2254
  tumors of, forehead flap in, 2668–2671
Tongue flaps. See *Flap, tongue.*
"Tongue in groove" advancement, for correction of coronal synostosis, 2495, *2497*, *2504*
Tongue stimulation, galvanic, in facial palsy, 1787, 1788
Tongue-tie, 2254
Tonofibrils, 153
Tooth. See *Teeth.*
Torticollis, muscular, congenital, 1664–1668
Tracheoesophageal fistula, 2239
Tracheotomy, 601–607
  complications of, 606, 607
  elective, 602–606
  emergency, 601, 602, *602*
  in head and neck surgery, 2590–2592
  in multiple facial fractures in children, 811, 813
  indications for, 602
  low, 602, 603, *603*
  techniques of, 602–606
Traction appliances, external, 1371, *1371*, 1372, *1372*
Tragion, 28, 1289, *1290*
Tranquilizers, 586
  and rare craniofacial clefts, 2123
Transabdominal flap, *1657*
Transfer factor, 134, *135*
Transfixion incision, in rhinoplasty, 1068–1070
  variations in, 1100, 1101, *1101*
Transplant rejection, mechanism of, 132–135
  modification of process of, 135–138
Transplantation, 52–54
  genetics of, 139–147
  of bone, 313–339
  of cartilage. See *Cartilage, transplantation of.*
  of dermis. See *Dermis, transplantation of.*
  of fascia. See *Fascia, transplantation of.*
  of fat. See *Fat, transplantation of.*
  of hair, 229–232
  of joints, 102
  of nerve, 1861. See also *Nerve grafting.*
  of rib cartilage, 303–305, *305*, *306*
  of skeletal muscle, 293–300
  of tendon. See *Tendon, transplantation of.*
  skin, mediate and immediate, 53, 54
Transplantation antigens, 129
Transplantation biology, 126–151
Transplants
  autogenous, in treatment of orbital fractures, 995–997
  for repair of saddle nose deformities, 1140, 1141, *1141*
  skin. See *Skin transplants.*
  tumor, 127
Transposition flaps. See *Flap, transposition.*
Transscaphoid-perilunate dislocations, 3046, 3047
Transsexualism, 3960–3965, *3966*
Transversalis fascia, 3729
Transversus muscle, 3728
Trapdoor effect, 418, 419, *420*, 432, *433*, 434–436
Trapdoor flap, 64, 1023, *1024*, *1025*, *1501*
Trauner operation for cleft lip, 2019, 2028, 2029
Treacher Collins syndrome, 2121, 2124, 2145, 2149, *2150*, 2158, 2160, 2359, 2401–2426
  abortive form of, 2405
  antimongoloid slant of palpebral fissures in, 2401, 2402
  associated syndromes in, 2407, *2407*, 2408, *2408*, *2409*
  atypical form of, 2406
  auricular deformities in, treatment of, 2419, 2422
  classification of, 2403–2408
  coloboma in, 2401
  etiology of, 2408–2411

Treacher Collins syndrome *(Continued)*
  eyelid deformities in, treatment of, 2416–2419, *2420–2422*
  Franceschetti and Klein classification of, 2404–2406
  hypoplasia of malar bones in, 2402
  incomplete form of, 2405, *2405*
  malar, maxillary, and infraorbital rim deficiencies in, treatment of, 2413–2416
  mandibular hypoplasia in, treatment of, 2422–2424
  nasal deformities in, treatment of, 2424, *2424*
  pathogenesis of, 2411–2413
  treatment of, 2413–2424
  unilateral form of, 2405, 2406, *2406*
Trench foot, 517
Triamcinolone acetonide, in treatment of keloids, 430
Triangular flap, repair of cleft lip, 2019, *2028*, 2038, 2039, *2040*, 2041, *2041*, 2043
Triangularis muscle, 1780
Triazene, 2122, 2123
Trichiasis, epilation for, 914
Trichion, 28, *28*, 1289, *1290*
Trichloroacetic acid, 456
Trichoepithelioma, 2789, 2790, 2874, 2875
  of eyelids, 879
Trigeminal nerve, 1782, *1782*
Trigonocephaly, in Crouzon's disease, 2468, *2468*
  orbital hypotelorism in, 2462
Tripartite osteotomy, in Crouzon's disease, 2480, *2480*, 2481, *2481*
Tripier flap, bipedicle, in eyelid reconstruction, 885, *887*, 888
Trismus, following maxillary tumor surgery, 2588
Trochanter, greater, grafts of, 334
Trochanteric defect, muscle flap in, 3549, 3550, *3550*, *3551*
Trochanteric lipodystrophy, 3811–3820
Trochanteric ulcers, 3790, 3792, *3792*
Trochlea, *859*, 860
Trocinate, 86
Tropocollagen. See *Collagen.*
Trunk, 3607–3823
  as donor site of flaps, 212–215
Trunk deformities, in Romberg's disease, 2339
Tube flaps. See *Flap, tube.*
Tuberculum impar, 2306
d-Tubocurarine, 587
Tumbler flap, 3781
Tumor(s)
  Brooke's, 2874, 2875
  Buschke-Lowenstein, 2778
  carotid body, 2638, 2639
  connective tissue, of jaws, 2567–2569
  desmoid, 2879
  epidermal appendage, 2786–2788
  epithelial, of hand and forearm, 3450–3464
  giant cell, of bone of hand and forearm, 3499, 3500
    of tendon sheath of hand, 3472, *3472*, 3473, *3473*, *3474*
  glomus, 2796, *2796*, 2869, 3485, *3485*, 3486, *3486*, *3487*
  helical, 1768, *1768*
  intraoral. See *Intraoral tumors.*
  involving craniofacial skeleton, 2757–2775
  localized, in rhinophyma, *1187*, *1189*
  metastatic to jaws, *2571, 2572, 2572*
  of auricle, 1766–1768, *1768*
  of buccal mucosa, 2607, *2608, 2609*, 2671–2673
  of cheek, *2672, 2674*
  of chest wall, 3652–3657
  of ethmoid sinus, 2490

Tumor(s) *(Continued)*
  of eyelids, 874–882
  of faucial region, 2669–2671
  of floor of mouth, 2668, 2669, *2669*, 2683
  of fronto-ethmoid area, craniofacial surgical techniques in, 2490
  of hair follicles, 2874, 2875
  of hand and forearm. See *Hand and forearm, tumors of.*
  of head and neck, in children, 2622–2624
  of hypopharynx, 2613, *2613, 2614, 2615*
  of jaws. See *Jaws, tumors of.*
  of lip, 2601, *2601, 2602*, 2603–2607
  of lower extremity, 3526
  of mandible. See *Mandible, tumors of.*
  of maxilla. See *Maxilla, tumors of.*
  of nail bed, 2979, 2980
  of neck, congenital. See *Neck, congenital cysts and tumors of.*
  of neural tissue, 2796, 2797, *2797*
  of nose. See *Nose, tumors of.*
  of orbit, 874–882
  of paranasal sinuses, 2574
  of parotid gland. See *Parotid gland, tumors of.*
  of pharyngeal wall, 2669–2671
  of salivary glands, 2521, 2522, 2539, 2540, *2540*
  of sebaceous glands, 2875, *2875*, 3453
  of skin. See *Skin, tumors of.*
  of skin appendages, 2874, 2875, *2875*
  of submandibular (submaxillary) gland, 2538, 2539
  of sweat glands, 2788–2790, 2874, 2875, 3453, 3464
  of symphyseal region, 2673
  of thorax, 3654–3657
  of vascular system, 2865–2873
  oromandibular. See *Oromandibular tumors.*
  soft tissue, benign, 2878–2880
  sternal, 3628
  sternocleidomastoid, *1665*, 1666, 1667
  turban, 2789, *2789*
  vagal body, 2638, 2639, *2639, 2640*
  Warthin's, 2527, *2527*
Tumor resection, primary bone grafting following, in mandible, *1481, 1482*, 1483, *1483*, 1484, *1484*
Tumor transplants, 127
Tumorectomy, in breast, 3710
Tunnel procedure, in auricular reconstruction, *1757*, 1758–1761
Turban tumor, 2789, *2789*
Turbine dermatomes, 173
Turner's syndrome, 109, 1660, *1661, 1662*, 3931, 3934, 3938, 3956, *3958–3960*
Turribrachycephaly, 2322
Turricephaly, 2502, *2503*
  in Crouzon's disease, 2468, *2468*

Ulcer(s)
  and skin cancer, 2819
  associated with chronic osteomyelitis, 3553, *3554*
  calcaneal, *3559*
  Curling's, 509
  decubitus. See *Pressure sore.*
  elbow, 3792, *3793*
  foot, 3792
  heel, 3792
  ischial, 3784, *3785–3788*, 3789
  knee, 3792, *3792*
  neurotrophic, plantar, 3530
  of scapula, iliac crest, and spine-costal margin, 3792
  over olecranon, 3792, *3793*

Ulcer(s) (*Continued*)
  pretibial, 3792
  radiation, treatment of, 543–545
  rodent, 2820, 2831
  sacral, 3789, *3789*, 3790, *3790, 3791*
  trochanteric, 3790, 3792, *3792*
  varicose, normal intralymphatic pressures associated
    with, *3569*
  venous stasis, dermal overgrafting for, 186, *186*, 187
    of lower extremity, 3523–3525, *3525, 3532*, 3552,
    3553
Ulna, 2961
Ulnar artery, 2976
Ulnar deficiency state, *3335*
Ulnar dimelia, 3323, *3324*
Ulnar drift, in arthritic hand, 3514, 3515, *3515*
Ulnar nerve, 2961, 2975
  repair of, 3215–3242
Ulnar nerve paralysis, *3281, 3300*, 3301, *3301, 3302*
  splinting in, 2998
Ulnar tunnel syndrome, 3437–3440
Ulrich-Noonan syndrome, 1660, *1661, 1662*
Ultrasound, noninvasive, in measurement of velo-
  pharyngeal incompetence, 2270
Umbilicus, 3728
Ungual phalanx, composite injuries of, 3143, *3143*, 3144
Upper extremity. See *Extremity, upper.*
Uranoplasty, 2091, 2092
Uranoschisis, 2091
Urethra
  bulbous, 3883, *3884, 3885*
    strictures of, surgical techniques in, 3891–3893
  glanular, 3837, 3883, *3886*
  male, anatomy of, 3883, *3884–3886*
    construction of in true hermaphroditism, *3948, 3949*
    reconstruction of using scrotal skin, 3916, *3916,
      3917*
    strictures of, 3883–3901
      diagnosis of, 3886, *3887*
      dilatation in, 3888
      excision in, 3888, 3889, *3889, 3890*
      external urethrotomy in, 3889
      incision and graft in, 3889
      internal urethrotomy in, 3888, *3889*
      marsupialization in, 3889
      pathology of, 3886, *3887*
      surgical techniques in, 3890–3895
      treatment of, 3886–3889
  membranous, 3883, *3884*
    strictures of, surgical techniques in, 3893, *3894*, 3895
  pendulous, 3883, *3884, 3885*
    strictures of, surgical techniques in, 3890, 3891,
      3891
  prostatic, 3883, *3884*
  reconstruction of in hypospadias, 3835–3843
Urethral meatus, strictures of, surgical techniques in,
  3890
Urethroplasty
  Badenoch, *3889*
  Leadbetter, *3893*
  patch graft, *3894*
  Waterhouse, *3890*
Urethrotomy, external, in strictures of male urethra,
  3889
  internal, in strictures of male urethra, 3888, *3889*
Urinary tract anomalies, embryology of, 3828–3831
Urogenital membrane, 3831, *3832*
Urogenital ridge, 3828
Uterus, metastatic carcinoma to jaws from, *2573*
Utricle, 2306
Uvular muscle, *1977*, 1984

V–Y advancement flaps. See *Flaps, advancement, V–Y.*
V–Y retroposition ("push-back") procedure, in cleft
  palate repair, 2095, 2096, *2096, 2097*
V–Y technique, in repair of cheek defect, 1581, *1582*
V–Z advancement, in repair of deficient buccal sulcus,
  2171, 2172, *2172*
Vacutome, 172
Vagal body tumor, 2638, 2639, *2639, 2640*
Vagina, congenital absence of, 3922, 3923
Vaginal construction, in transsexualism, 3964, *3964,
  3965, 3965, 3966*
  in true hermaphroditism, 3942–3944, *3945*
Vaginal reconstruction, following vaginectomy, 3926–
  3929
Vaginoplasty, in feminizing testicularism, *3957*
Valium, 586, *2123*
Varicose ulcer, *3569*
Vascular injuries, of hand, 3004, 3084–3090
Vascular system, of hand and forearm, tumors of,
  3482–3489
  tumors of, 2865–2873
Vasculature, cutaneous, *192*, 193, *193*
  segmental, 191, *191*, 192
Vasomotor function, in skin grafts and flaps, 228
Vasopressors, and craniofacial clefts, 2123
Veau, Victor, 17
Veau classification of clefts of lip and palate, 1935, *1935*
Veau II operation for bilateral cleft lip repair, 2084,
  2085, *2085*, 2086
Veau III operation for bilateral cleft lip repair, *2058,
  2059–2067, 2068, 2069*
Veau-Wardill-Kilner operation for cleft of secondary
  palate, 2095, *2096*
Vein grafts, 356, *357*
Veins, microvascular repair patency rates for, 353, 353t,
  354
  of abdominal wall, 3729
Vellus, 154
Velopharyngeal function, influence of on speech, 2261
Velopharyngeal incompetence, 2268–2295
  causes of, 2269
  definition of, 2269
  determination of port size and shape in, 2276, 2277
  evaluation of surgical results in, 2276–2279
  following maxillary advancement, 1451, *1451*, 1452,
    1452, 1453
  measurement of, 2269–2271
  operative technique in, 2279–2283
Velopharyngeal port mechanism, and speech production,
  2255–2257
Velopharyngeal sphincter, reconstruction of, 2274, 2276,
  2278
Velopharyngeal valve, air- and water-tight, construction
  of in cleft palate, 2093
Veloplasty, intravelar, 2271, 2272, *2272, 2273*
  in cleft palate repair, 2095
Venous congestion, in microvascular replants, 371
Venous defect, primary, in chronic edema, 3579
Venous repair, microvascular, 358, 359, *363, 364*
Venous stasis, chronic, increased intralymphatic pres-
  sures associated with, *3570*
Venous stasis ulcers, dermal overgrafting for, 186, *186,*
  187
  of lower extremity, 3523–3535, *3525, 3532*, 3552, 3553
Vermilion advancement, in cleft lip reconstruction, *2171,
  2173*
Vermilion border, defects of, 1575, 1576, *1576, 1577,
  1578*
  notching of, 1576, *1577, 1578*
Verruca pigmentosa, of hand and forearm, 3453, 3455,
  3455

Verruca planae, 2777, *2777*, 2778, 2779
  of hand and forearm, 3450
Verruca vulgaris, 2776–2781, 2876
  of hand and forearm, 3450, *3451*
Verrucous carcinoma, 2778, 2779
Verrucous hemangioma, 2795
Vessel wall, changes in during microsurgery, 351, 352
Vestibule, of nose, 1052, *1052*, 1053
Vincristine, 2122
Vincula, 268
Vision, loss of, following esthetic blepharoplasty, 1897, 1898
Vitallium implants, 392
Vitallium splint, 1357, *1358*
Vitamin A, and craniofacial clefts, 2123
Vitelline duct, 3728
Volar wrist crease, as donor site for full-thickness skin grafts, 165
Volkmann's canals, 313, *314*
Volkmann's contracture, 3130–3137
  treatment of, 3132–3137
Vomer, 1047, *1047*
  in bilateral cleft lip and palate, *1951*, 1952, *1953*
  in unilateral cleft lip and palate, 1959, *1960*
Von Graefe, 3, 8
Von Hippel-Lindau disease, 2867
Von Langenbeck, 8
Von Recklinghausen's disease, 2879, *2879*, 3494, 3495, 3654, *3655*

W-plasty, 60–64
  for cutaneous scars of nose, 1195
  for pigmented spread scar, *433*
  in scar revision, *434*, 435
  indications and contraindications for, 61–63
Walsham forceps, 727, *728*
Walsh-Ogura operation for orbital decompression, 975, *975*, 976,·*976*, 977
Warthin's tumor, 2527, *2527*
Warts, 2876
  acuminate, 2777, 2778, *2778*, 2780, 2781
  common, 2776–2781
  digitate and filiform, 2777
  of hand and forearm, 3450, *3451*
  plane, 2777, *2777*, 2778, 2779
  plantar, 2777, *2778*, *2779*, 2780, 2876, 3529
  seborrheic, 2781–2783
  treatment of, 2876
Waterhouse urethroplasty, *3890*
Waters position, 611, *611*
  reverse, 612, *613*
Waters view, in fractures of zygoma, 712, *713*
  of blowout fracture of orbital floor, 765, *767*
Weber-Ferguson-Longmire incision, 2578, *2579*
Wehrbein-Smith procedure for repair of hypospadias, 3850, 3852, *3852*
Wen, 2784–2786, 2877, 2878
Werner's syndrome, 1877
Whistle deformity, 2087, *2173*, 2174, *2174*, *2175*, 2176, *2176*
"White eye" syndrome, 1001
Wiener technique of breast reduction, 3676, *3683*
Williston's law, 823
Wilson's disease, nail color in, 2978
Wire(s)
  cable arch, in mandibular fractures, 667, *668*
  figure-of-eight, *675*, 676
    Kirschner, 676
  stainless steel, buried, infection and, 693

Wire extension, forked, in mandibular fractures, 673
Wire fixation
  circumferential, 1393, *1394*
    in facial bone fractures in children, 800, *802*
    in mandibular fractures, 680, *680*, 689, *689*, 690, *690*
      use of splint or dentures with, 673, 674, *674*
  dental, in jaw fractures, 648–652
  eyelet, 800, *809*
  interdental, horizontal, in mandibular fractures, 665, *666*
  internal, in maxillary fractures, 701, *702*, *704*
  interosseous, direct, in mandibular fractures, 690, *690*, 691, *691*
    in fractured edentulous maxilla, 706, *707*
    in multiple facial fractures, *809*, 810
    intraoral, in mandibular fractures, 676, *676*, *677*
    open reduction and, in fractures of zygoma, 715, *716*, 719
      in mandibular fractures, 674–676
        with arch bar, *672*
      in maxillary fractures, 702, *704*
      in multiple facial fractures, 736–741
  through-and-through, over plates, in nasal fractures, 731, *731*, *732*
  transalveolar, in mandibular fractures, *680*
  transosseous, for medial canthopexy, 1014–1016
Wire ligatures, for intermaxillary fixation, 651, 652, *655–657*
Wire suspension, internal, in fractured edentulous maxilla, 706, *707*
Wolfe, graft, in Dupuytren's contracture, 3417, *3417*, *3418*, 3419, *3419*, 3422, *3423*
Wolffian ducts, 3828, 3829
Wound, burn, excision of, 493, *494*. See also *Burns*.
  cutaneous, 7 day old, *96*
    10 day old, *97*
Wound closure
  correct and incorrect, *645*
  delayed primary, in facial injuries, 622, 623
  geometric broken line, *434*, 435
  nonsuture technique of, 640, 641, *646*
  timing of skin replacement in, 225
Wound contraction, 79, 83–86. See also *Contraction*.
Wound healing
  ascorbic acid depletion and, 92, 93
  by first and second intention, 415, 416
  dermis and, 95
  following thermal burns, 1596–1601
  protein depletion and, 93
Wound tension, in plastic surgery, 54–64
Wrinkles, 1870–1873
  deep forehead, correction of, 1921
  fine, dermabrasion of, 450
Wrist, 2960, 2961
  indications for repair of severed structures at, 3209, 3210, *3211*
  nerve injuries in, 3206–3212
  reconstructive surgery of, 3112–3115
  technique of implantation of end of tube flap into, *213*
  tendon injuries in, 3063, *3063*, 3064, 3069, *3069*, 3070, 3206–3212
Wrist crease, volar, as donar site for full-thickness skin grafts, 165
Wrist flexion, role of in finger extension, 3169, *3169*
Wrist flexion-extension, 3112, 3113, *3113*
Wrist fusion, 3113–3115
Wynn operation for cleft lip, 2019, 2028, 2029, 2081, 2082, *2082*, 2083

X chromosome, 139, 3932
X-rays, definition of, 532. See also *Radiation.*
Xanthelasma, 2876
Xanthoma
    fibrous, of hand and forearm, 3472, *3472*
    juvenile, 2876
    of eyelids, 879
    of hand and forearm, 3471
Xanthoma diabeticorum, 2876
Xanthoma disseminatum, 2876
Xanthoma palpebrarum, 2876
Xanthomatoses, 2876
Xenograft(s), 126
    after thermal burn, 505
    definition of, 52, 156
    of bone, immune response to, 323, 324
    of cartilage, 307
    of fascia, 263
    of tendon, 288
    skin, 188–191
Xeroderma pigmentosum, reconstruction of nose in
    patient with, *1262*
Xylocaine, 627

Y chromosome, 139, 3932

Z-plasty, 54–60
    amount of elongation in, 56
    compound right angle, 60, *62*
    development of, 55
    double opposing, 58, *60*
        in eyelid burns, *1628*, 1629
        in traumatic epicanthus, 941, 942, *943*
    for congenital constricting bands, *3528*
    four-flap, 58, 60, *60, 61, 62*
    in burn contractures, 1610, 1611
    in cleft lip repair, 2019, 2027, *2027*, 2028, *2028*, 2033,
        2035

Z-plasty *(Continued)*
    in cross-joint scar, 418, *419*
    in cutaneous scars of nose, 1195, *1195, 1196*
    in Dupuytren's contracture, 3417, *3418*
    in eyebrow distortion, 956, *956*
    in hypertrophied scar contracture, *432*
    in linear scar contracture of nose, 1199, 1200, *1200*
    in symblepharon, 915, *916*
    in upper lip defect, 1548, *1548*, 2172, *2173, 2174*
    in vermilion border notching, 1576, *1577*
    indications and contraindications for, 61–63
    multiple, 56, *56, 57*
    technique of, *54, 55, 55, 56, 56*
    to realign scar within lines of minimal tension, 56, 57,
        57, 58
    variations in, 58, *58, 59,* 60, *60, 61, 62*
    with advancement flap, in eyelid reconstruction, 885,
        885
    with unequal triangles, 58, *58, 59*
Zigzag method of repair of bilateral cleft lip, *2069,*
    2070–2073
Zimany flap, 206, *208*
Zimmer skin graft mesher, 174, *175*
Zygoma, fractures of, 708–720
    classification of, 711
    comminuted, 715–719
    complications of, 719, 720, *721, 722*
    compound comminuted, 719, *720*
    delayed treatment of, 719
    in children, 807, 808
    diagnosis of, 711, 712, *712, 713*
    malunited, 713, *713,* 720, *721, 722*
        depressed, 1029–1031
    methods of reduction of, 713–715, *716*
    roentgenographic examination of, 712, *713*
    surgical pathology of, 709–711
    treatment of, 712–719
    reconstruction of, *1510, 1513*
    squamous cell carcinoma of, *2832, 2833, 2837*
Zygomatic branches, of facial nerve, 1778
Zygomatic nerve, 866, 867
Zygomaticus muscle, 1781